ANESTHESIA
for the
CARDIAC
PATIENT

Visit our website at **www.mosby.com**

ANESTHESIA for the CARDIAC PATIENT

CHRISTOPHER A. TROIANOS, M.D.

Vice Chair, Department of Anesthesiology
Chief, Division of Cardiovascular Anesthesia
Director, Intraoperative Echocardiography
The Mercy Hospital of Pittsburgh
Pittsburgh, Pennsylvania

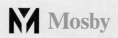 Mosby

An Imprint of Elsevier Science

St. Louis   London   Philadelphia   Sydney   Toronto

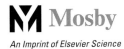
An Imprint of Elsevier Science

Acquisitions Editor: Allan Ross
Developmental Editor: Josh Hawkins
Publishing Services Manager: Patricia Tannian
Book Design Manager: Gail Morey Hudson
Cover Designer: Mark Oberkrom

NOTICE

Anesthesiology is an ever-changing field. Standard safety precautions must be followed, but as new research and clinical experience broaden our knowledge, changes in treatment and drug therapy may become necessary or appropriate. Readers are advised to check the most current product information provided by the manufacturer of each drug to be administered to verify the recommended dose, the method and duration of administration, and contraindications. It is the responsibility of the licensed prescriber, relying on experience and knowledge of the patient, to determine dosages and the best treatment for each individual patient. Neither the publisher nor the editor assumes any liability for any injury and/or damage to persons or property arising from this publication.

Mosby, Inc.
An Imprint of Elsevier Science
11830 Westline Industrial Drive
St. Louis, MO 63146

Printed in United States of America

Library of Congress Cataloging in Publication Data

Anesthesia for the cardiac patient / [edited by] Christopher A. Troianos.—1st ed.
        p. ; cm.
    Includes bibliographical references and index.
    ISBN 0-323-00874-7
    1. Anesthesia in cardiology. 2. Heart—Surgery. I. Troianos, Christopher A.
    [DNLM: 1. Anesthesia. 2. Heart Diseases. 3. Anesthetics—pharmacology. 4.
Perioperative Care. WO 240 A5792 2002]
RD87.3.H43 A53 2002
617.9′67412—dc21
                                                    2001055836

02 03 04 05 06 GW/MV-Y 9 8 7 6 5 4 3 2 1

To
Barb, Rachael, Andrew, and **Rebecca**
and my parents,
Evangeline and **Achilles**

Contributors

JOHN L. ATLEE, M.D.
Professor of Anesthesiology
Medical College of Wisconsin
Milwaukee, Wisconsin

JOHN G. AUGOUSTIDES, M.D.
Assistant Professor of Anesthesiology
University of Pennsylvania School of Medicine
Philadelphia, Pennsylvania

PAUL G. BARASH, M.D.
Professor of Anesthesiology
Yale University School of Medicine
New Haven, Connecticut

REBECCA A. BARNETT, M.B.CH.B.
Assistant Professor of Anesthesia
University of Pennsylvania School of Medicine
Philadelphia, Pennsylvania

VICTOR C. BAUM, M.D.
Professor of Anesthesiology and Pediatrics
University of Virginia
Charlottesville, Virginia

ALBERT T. CHEUNG, M.D.
Associate Professor of Anesthesiology
University of Pennsylvania School of Medicine
Philadelphia, Pennsylvania

THOMAS J. CONAHAN, M.D.
Associate Professor of Anesthesia
University of Pennsylvania School of Medicine
Philadelphia, Pennsylvania

REGINA Y. FRAGNETO, M.D.
Associate Professor
Director, Obstetric Anesthesia
Department of Anesthesiology
University of Kentucky College of Medicine
Lexington, Kentucky

ASHRAF M. GHOBASHY, M.D.
Assistant Professor, Cardiac Anesthesia
Department of Anesthesiology
Yale University School of Medicine
New Haven, Connecticut

LORIN GRAEF, M.D.
Clinical Fellow
Johns Hopkins University School of Medicine
Baltimore, Maryland

C. WILLIAM HANSON III, M.D.
Professor of Anesthesia, Surgery, and Internal Medicine
University of Pennsylvania School of Medicine
Philadelphia, Pennsylvania

ELIZABETH HERRERA, M.D.
Assistant Professor of Anesthesiology
Emory University School of Medicine
Atlanta, Georgia

WILLIAM D. HETRICK, M.D.
Clinical Associate Professor
Department of Anesthesiology/Critical Care Medicine
University of Pittsburgh School of Medicine
Pittsburgh, Pennsylvania

INGRID HOLLINGER, M.D.
Professor of Anesthesiology
Mount Sinai Medical School
New York, New York

W. ANDREW KOFKE, M.D.
Professor of Anesthesia
University of Pennsylvania School of Medicine
Philadelphia, Pennsylvania

JAN KOMTEBEDDE, D.V.M.
Vice President, Marketing and Business Development
Evalve, Inc.
Redwood City, California

GLENN S. MADARA, M.D.
Staff and Cardiac Anesthesiologist
College Anesthesia Associates
Lancaster, Pennsylvania

HEATHER E. MANSPEIZER, M.D.
Private Practice
New York, New York

THOMAS M. MCLOUGHLIN, JR., M.D.
Clinical Associate Professor of Anesthesia
Pennsylvania State University College of Medicine
Hershey, Pennsylvania

DAVID MOSKOWITZ, M.D.
Director, Cardiothoracic Anesthesia
Department of Anesthesiology
Englewood Hospital and Medical Center
Englewood, New Jersey

E. ANDREW OCHROCH, M.D.
Assistant Professor of Anesthesia
University of Pennsylvania School of Medicine
Philadelphia, Pennsylvania

CHRISTOPHER J. O'CONNOR, M.D.
Associate Professor of Anesthesiology
Rush Medical College
Chicago, Illinois

DAVID L. REICH, M.D.
Professor of Anesthesiology
Mount Sinai School of Medicine
New York, New York

ALAN F. ROSS, M.D.
Associate Professor
Department of Anesthesia
University of Iowa
Iowa City, Iowa

IVAN S. SALGO, M.D.
Assistant Professor of Anesthesia
University of Pennsylvania School of Medicine
Philadelphia, Pennsylvania

JACK S. SHANEWISE, M.D.
Associate Professor of Anesthesiology
Emory University School of Medicine
Atlanta, Georgia

LINDA SHORE-LESSERSON, M.D.
Assistant Professor of Anesthesiology
Mount Sinai School of Medicine
New York, New York

LAWRENCE C. SIEGEL, M.D.
Attending Anesthesiologist
Stanford University Medical Center
Stanford, California

PETER S. STAATS, M.D.
Associate Professor
Johns Hopkins University School of Medicine
Baltimore, Maryland

CHRISTOPHER A. TROIANOS, M.D.
Vice Chair, Department of Anesthesiology
Chief, Division of Cardiovascular Anesthesia
Director, Intraoperative Echocardiography
The Mercy Hospital of Pittsburgh
Pittsburgh, Pennsylvania

KENNETH J. TUMAN, M.D.
Professor of Anesthesiology
Rush Medical College
Chicago, Illinois

ROBERT A. VANCE, M.D.
Associate Professor and Vice Chair
Department of Anesthesiology
West Virginia University
Morgantown, West Virginia

Foreword

A classic definition of anesthesia is "to render a patient insensible to the manipulation of the surgeon." Just how inadequate that definition is today can readily be appreciated by perusing the pages of *Anesthesia for the Cardiac Patient*. The concept of perioperative medicine, with all that it encompasses, is repeatedly emphasized. Christopher A. Troianos, M.D., has recruited a group of recognized authorities from 14 institutions across the United States whose chapters reflect their expertise on the topics they present. The overall design of the book, as well as that of each chapter, highlights the importance of a comprehensive approach to each patient—including preoperative evaluation and preparations, intraoperative care with as much emphasis on monitoring as on administration of anesthesia, and postoperative care.

The all-encompassing nature of the contents is perhaps best demonstrated in the fourth section, where patients with cardiac disease, documented or potential (e.g., chest trauma), undergoing noncardiac surgery or care are discussed. Here, as in the other three sections, the consequences of cardiac pathophysiology and the effects of anesthesia on those consequences are detailed in a clear manner. This book helps clinicians to understand with equal clarity the anesthetic management options available to care for a parturient with mitral stenosis requiring anesthesia for mitral valve replacement or delivery of a term infant.

In 50 years of open-heart surgery using cardiopulmonary bypass, cardiac surgery has changed markedly. Concentrating originally on corrections of simple and later of complex congenital defects, cardiac surgery progressed to valve replacements and myocardial revascularization, then heart transplants, and now permanent artifical hearts are on the horizon.

As surgery was evolving, so was cardiac anesthesia, with progress in both anesthetic drugs and monitoring techniques. Although the volatile agents have improved considerably, a greater change was the advent of high-dose narcotic anesthesia, first with morphine and then with the fentanyl family.

Equally important have been the monitoring changes. The inability of the central venous pressure to provide information on function of the left side of the heart was understood early. Although left atrial pressure lines compensated for this inadequacy, they could be used only in cardiac patients and only after the chest was opened. The 1970 description of a balloon-tipped, flow-directed, pulmonary artery catheter was a giant step forward in monitoring. The addition of a thermistor on the tip permitted convenient serial measurements of cardiac output.

The next major improvement in monitoring was the introduction of echocardiography, first transthoracic and then transesophageal (TEE). TEE permits direct visualization of cardiac performance in real time intraoperatively, facilitating definitive diagnosis, correction of inadequate surgical repair before chest closure, and determination of volume status.

All anesthesiologists and their patients have benefited from these developments in cardiac anesthesia. Experience gained in caring for patients with cardiac disease having cardiac surgery has been quickly exported to other areas of the operating room and to intensive care units, medical as well as surgical.

On a personal note, Chris Troianos, a graduate of the University of Pittsburgh School of Medicine, completed a fellowship in cardiac anesthesia at the University of Pennsylvania in 1990 and returned to Mercy Hospital in Pittsburgh, where he had taken his anesthesia residency. He quickly established himself as a leader in the subspecialty of cardiac anesthesia, with special expertise in TEE interpretation. *Anesthesia for the Cardiac Patient* is just the most recent of his accomplishments that demonstrate his position as a leader in cardiac anesthesia.

Norig Ellison, M.D.
Emeritus Professor of Anesthesia
University of Pennsylvania
Philadelphia, Pennsylvania

Preface

Cardiac disease is prevalent in an increasing proportion of candidates for surgery as advances in medicine and technology increase life expectancy and decrease perioperative risk. Newer, minimally invasive techniques allow surgery to be performed on patients whose risk was previously considered prohibitive for surgery and anesthesia. Concerns over rising health care costs, which led to increased surgical volume in outpatient settings and reduced hospital lengths of stay, create the need for new approaches in the anesthetic management of patients with cardiac disease. Patients with cardiac disease, who previously would have been thought to be at a higher risk for perioperative morbidity and mortality, currently undergo surgery in ambulatory, neurosurgical, thoracic, vascular, and obstetrical suites. New technologies within the subspecialty of cardiac anesthesia enhance the care of patients with cardiac disease during both cardiac and noncardiac surgery. Milestones in technological development include extracorporeal support of the circulation, pulmonary artery catheterization and cardiac output determination, transesophageal echocardiography, and minimally invasive surgical techniques. As the name implies, the purpose of *Anesthesia for the Cardiac Patient* is to advance the care and anesthetic management of patients with cardiac disease, regardless of whether they are undergoing cardiac or noncardiac surgery.

The book is divided into four sections that address specific aspects of care. Section I, "Perioperative Care of the Cardiac Patient," includes preoperative evaluation, cardiovascular medications, intraoperative monitoring, perioperative transesophageal echocardiography, postoperative care, and pain management. The relative importance of various preoperative screening tests and implications of test results is covered in Chapter 1, on preoperative evaluation of the cardiac patient. Cardiovascular medications are discussed in Chapter 2 from both the perspective of maintenance (usually oral) cardiac medications and implications during perioperative care, and vasoactive medications used to treat acute cardiovascular problems encountered in the perioperative setting. Chapter 3, on intraoperative monitoring, covers all aspects of cardiovascular monitoring, encompassing both invasive and noninvasive modalities, indications, contraindications, and insertion techniques.

Chapter 4, on perioperative transesophageal echocardiography (TEE), is a comprehensive discussion that includes preoperative, intraoperative, and postoperative indications in both cardiac and noncardiac surgery. The physics of ultrasound is presented in a clinically oriented approach, providing the basis for understanding TEE evaluation. The comprehensive TEE examination is discussed in detail, giving the reader all the necessary information to perform a complete evaluation of cardiac structures and common lesions. The chapter includes the TEE evaluation of both stenotic and regurgitant lesions of all four cardiac valves and the systolic and diastolic function of the left and right ventricles, atrial septum, thoracic aorta, and prosthetic valves. Development of an intraoperative echocardiography service, including training issues, reporting, and billing, completes the discussion of perioperative TEE. The chapter is based on my experience in learning and teaching TEE to a varied audience of anesthesia providers over the past 12 years. A collection of echocardiograms in color is provided to enhance the educational value of this chapter.

Chapter 5, on postoperative care, focuses on the important period immediately after surgery when complications related to cardiac disease are often manifested. Transport of critically ill patients with cardiac disease and management of common cardiovascular problems are included in this discussion. Pain management is presented in Chapter 6 from a unique perspective that follows the same theme as the rest of the book. The importance of and approach to pain management in patients with cardiac disease experiencing surgical pain are emphasized. A unique aspect of this chapter is the treatment of anginal pain using traditional anesthesia pain management modalities.

Section II of the book provides information for the anesthetic management of cardiac disease processes. These include coronary artery disease, valvular heart disease, electrophysiologic problems, congenital heart lesions, and less common cardiac problems such as constrictive pericarditis, hypertrophic obstructive cardiomyopathy, and tamponade. Anesthetic management of each disease process is discussed from the perspective of basic hemodynamic goals and of anesthesia in cardiac and noncardiac surgical settings. For example, the section on electrophysiologic problems discusses the anesthetic management of patients undergoing implantation of a pacemaker and automatic internal cardiac defibrillator (AICD), but also discusses the management of patients with a preexisting pacemaker or AICD undergoing noncardiac surgery. The same theme is used for patients with coronary artery disease undergoing either coronary artery bypass surgery or noncardiac surgery and patients with valvular heart disease undergoing either valvular or noncardiac surgery. Anesthetic management of patients with congenital heart lesions is presented from the perspective of congenital heart disease requiring repair and the concerns regarding previously repaired lesions.

Section III addresses topics specifically applicable to cardiac surgical settings. These include management of cardiopulmonary bypass, minimally invasive cardiac surgery, cardiac transplantation, and the cardiothoracic intensive care unit. Thoracic aortic surgery is included in this section because management for these surgical procedures shares many of the same issues and techniques employed during cardiac surgery.

Section IV addresses the issues and anesthetic management of the patient with cardiac disease specifically undergoing noncardiac surgery. The presence of cardiac disease is common and challenging in vascular and thoracic surgical settings. The chapter on trauma deals with patients suffering cardiac trauma as well as patients with underlying heart disease who sustain noncardiac trauma. The special anesthetic requirements for the neurosurgical patient, such as induced hypotension during aneurysm clipping, are affected by the presence of cardiac disease. Neurologic processes such as intracranial hypertension can produce profound cardiovascular effects, including ECG changes and arterial hypertension. The obstetrical patient with cardiac disease presents unique challenges in terms of anesthetic management for labor, delivery, the fetus, and the mother. Management of the obstetrical patient requiring cardiac surgery and cardiopulmonary resuscitation is discussed, along with management of peripartum cardiomyopathy. The management of the parturient with a cardiac transplant is also addressed.

This text would not have become a reality without the time, dedication, research, thoughtfulness, and expertise of all of the first-class contributors. Their efforts and hard work will benefit many practitioners and countless cardiac patients who require anesthesia. I thank each and every one from the inferior surface (bottom) of my heart. I thank Laurel Craven for her encouragement to move forward with this project and Allan Ross for keeping the project on track and for bringing it to fruition. I also thank my many mentors, colleagues, residents, and fellows that I have worked with throughout my career, whose example and love of anesthesia encouraged me to learn as much as possible. I hope this text is a reflection of their belief and trust in me. Finally, I thank my family for their love, understanding, and support during the countless hours spent on the book at home. So read and enjoy for your benefit and the benefit of your patients with cardiac disease.

Christopher A. Troianos, M.D.

Contents

Perioperative Care
of the Cardiac Patient

CHAPTER 1

Preoperative Evaluation of the Cardiac Patient

Alan F. Ross, M.D.

OUTLINE

Continued

Patients with cardiac disease present for surgery in several preoperative settings. General surgical patients with a history of cardiac disease require preoperative assessment of problems that may affect postoperative outcome and long-term health. Patients scheduled for cardiac surgery have a variety of signs and symptoms that characterize the particular cardiac lesion. Preoperative assessment provides information that allows administration of the optimal anesthetic that matches the cardiovascular needs. The third type of cardiac patient has no documented history of cardiac disease but has vague symptoms suggestive of occult heart disease. The anesthesiologist alert to cardiovascular assessment is in a key position to positively influence perioperative outcome.

RISK INDEX MODELS AND GUIDELINES
Clinical Studies Before 1975

When did the concern for cardiac risk associated with surgery begin? A task force of the American Heart Association, American College of Cardiology,[1] and the American College of Physicians[2] reviewed the available literature since the mid-1970s as a basis for their preoperative guidelines. Yet the significance of cardiac disease on perioperative outcome dates back to 1912, when a Mayo Clinic pathologist noted that an embolism to a coronary artery was the cause of postoperative mortality.[3] Our present understanding of cardiac risk includes significant developments between these dates. The most important was the identification that myocardial infarction (MI) within 6 months of surgery greatly increased the risk of adverse outcome. Anesthesiologists played a major role in defining this factor.

During the 1930s, clinicians recognized that surgery performed on patients with acute MI resulted in exceed-ingly high mortality.[4] In 1938, Master et al evaluated 35 patients with postoperative MI; common features included age greater than 60 years, prior coronary artery disease, cardiac enlargement, and preoperative electrocardiogram (ECG) abnormalities.[5-7] Mortality was 65%, and most adverse events occurred within 3 days of surgery. Etsten and Proger reported that a recent MI increased the risk of postoperative cardiac death by 20 times as compared with an older MI.[8]

In 1951, Ernstene of the Cleveland Clinic predicted that the future would bring an inexpensive oscilloscope (ECG monitor) into "every anesthetist's armamentarium."

This prediction came into fruition, and major advances in cardiac monitoring occurred during the 1960s.[9] Coronary care units provided continuous ECG monitoring and allowed early intervention for patients with acute MI.[10,11] Driscoll et al in 1961 used preoperative and postoperative ECGs in 496 unselected surgical patients to demonstrate that the incidence of postoperative MI was much higher than symptoms alone indicated. Although only six patients had clinical symptoms of chest pain, hypotension, or respiratory distress, the ECG demonstrated 12 definite new infarctions and 30 possible infarctions (persistent postoperative T-wave inversions).[12]

In 1964, Skinner and Pearce determined a list of risk factors that contributed to increased surgical mortality. An assessment of 25 parameters was performed on all patients who had received a preoperative cardiac assessment. Many of the factors noted by Skinner and Pierce are still recognized today[13] (Box 1-1).

In contrast, not all early studies and conclusions were on track. In 1963, the following remarks were published in the *American Journal of Cardiology:* "The present philosophy seems to indicate that all antihypertensive medications should be withdrawn preoperatively when possible."[14]

In the mid 1960s, four studies reported the risks of a recent preoperative MI (less than 3 months or less than 6 months) before noncardiac surgery. Each demon-

strated a worse outcome in patients with recent preoperative MIs.[13,15-17] Anesthesiologists at the Mayo Clinic provided the definitive studies quantifying the risk of a recent preoperative MI.[18] The first report in 1972 reviewed 422 patients who had a history of MI *before* general anesthesia for noncardiac surgery.[19] Twenty-eight patients (6.6%) reinfarcted the week after surgery. The important discovery from this study was that a more recent preoperative MI had a much higher risk of reinfarction. *A person who had experienced an MI within 3 months of noncardiac surgery had a 30% incidence of reinfarction.* Postoperative infarction was most common on the third postoperative day and had a mortality of more than 50%.[19] The second report in 1978 reviewed an additional 587 patients who had a history of MI before noncardiac surgery.[20] Despite optimism over the advances in anesthesia, medicine, and surgery, in 1978 Steen et al reported that the incidence of perioperative reinfarction was unchanged. The rates of reinfarction were remarkably similar to those in the first study.[20] Combining these data of the Mayo Clinic provides a series of more than 1000 patients illustrating that *recent MI* is a major risk to noncardiac surgery[19,20] (Table 1-1).

An interesting finding was the high (10.8%) incidence of reinfarction in patients whose previous MI was described as "old" or of unknown timing. Conceivably, some of the "unknown" infarctions were in fact recent but clinically silent.

Goldman and Detsky Risk Index Methods

The Goldman Cardiac Risk Index. In 1977, Goldman et al reported their landmark study, which established the Cardiac Risk Index (CRI). Nine independent preop-

---

BOX 1-1
Surgical Risk in the Cardiac Patient

- Mortality is high with intraperitoneal and intrathoracic surgery.
- Cases of healed myocardial infarction have 14% mortality. Acute preoperative myocardial infarction (less than 3 months) has a mortality of 40%.
- Higher mortality occurs in patients with systolic pressure <100 mm Hg or diastolic pressure <50 mmHg. This represents patients in shock despite efforts to stabilize blood pressure.
- Mitral valvular disease is relatively safe, but patients with aortic valve disease do not tolerate major procedures well.
- Patients with chronic pulmonary disease having an intrathoracic or intraabdominal procedure have 37% mortality.
- Patients in CHF have increased mortality in proportion to the severity of CHF. Mild CHF versus severe CHF has mortality of 4% versus 67%.
- ECG abnormalities of atrial fibrillation, atrial flutter, heart block, or bundle-branch block increase mortality compared with patients with normal ECGs.
- Emergency surgery is not well tolerated.

From Skinner JF, Pearce ML: *J Chronic Disease* 17:57, 1964.
CHF, Congestive heart failure; *ECG,* electrocardiogram.

TABLE 1-1
Risk of Recent Myocardial Reinfarction (MI)—Mayo Clinic Studies

TIME OF PRIOR MI BEFORE SURGERY (mo)	TARHAN ET AL,[19] 1967-1968* (n = 422)	STEEN ET AL,[20] 1974-1975* (n = 587)	COMBINED MAYO DATA* (n = 1009)	PERCENTAGE OF REINFARCTION†
0-3	3/8	4/15	7/23	30
4-6	3/19	2/18	5/37	13
7-12	2/42	2/31	4/73	5.5
13-18	1/27	1/30	2/57	3.5
19-24	1/21	1/17	2/38	5.3
25+	10/232	15/383	25/615	4.1
Old or unknown	7/73	11/93	18/160	10.8

*Denominator indicates the number of patients who had preoperative myocardial infarction in the indicated time period. Numerator indicates the number of these patients who had a perioperative reinfarction.
†Pertains to the combined Mayo Clinic data. Note the highest risk for reinfarction was prior myocardial infarction within 3 months of noncardiac surgery. This risk levels off after 6 months.

TABLE 1-2
Goldman Variables by "Point" Value

VARIABLE	POINTS	LIFE-THREATENING COMPLICATIONS*	CARDIAC DEATHS*
Third heart sound or jugular venous distention	11	5/35	7/35
Recent myocardial infarction	10	3/22	5/22
Nonsinus rhythm or premature atrial contractions on electrocardiogram	7	11/112	10/112
>5 premature ventricular contractions	7	7/44	6/44
Age >70 yr	5	19/324	16/324
Emergency operation	4	16/197	10/197
Poor general medical condition	3	25/362	13/362
Intraperitoneal, intrathoracic, or aortic operation	3	32/437	11/437
Important valvular aortic stenosis	3	1/23	3/23

*The denominator indicates the number of patients who possessed the risk factor. The numerator indicates the number of patients with that risk factor who experienced a complication.

erative characteristics were identified that predicted *outcome* of surgery for 1001 patients older than 40 years of age who underwent major noncardiac surgery[21-23] (Table 1-2). Adverse cardiac outcomes occurred in 58, or 5.8% of the overall group and included postoperative MI, pulmonary edema, or ventricular tachycardia. Four risk classes were established based on the total number of points accumulated for preoperative characteristics (Table 1-3).

Factors that did not increase the risk of adverse cardiac outcome are also of interest. These were present in many patients and included smoking, diabetes, hypertension, stable angina, peripheral vascular disease, bundle-branch blocks, digitalis use, and congestive heart failure (CHF) *without* a third heart sound or jugular venous distention (JVD). The factor "cardiac dyspnea" also did not increase risk. Some factors, such as angina, were clearly markers for cardiovascular disease and yet did not predict an adverse outcome.[21-23] This later became a major point of contention by Detsky et al in creation of their proposed index.

Success of the CRI. Why did the Goldman index become so widely used when most of the cardiac risk factors had been already identified by prior studies? The CRI greatly simplified and organized the process of preoperative evaluation. First, many variables, such as angina, hypertension, and ST changes on the ECG, were *not* found to be *statistically significant* in a large number of patients. Clinicians could then confidently focus their attention on the nine Goldman variables. Second, the CRI provided a simple, arithmetic method to quantitatively predict outcome. A similar risk analysis method proposed at the same time by Cooperman et al received

TABLE 1-3
Goldman Predictive Classes and Point Ranges

CLASS	POINT RANGE	ADVERSE OUTCOME* (PATIENTS IN CLASS)	CARDIAC COMPLICATION (%)
I	0-5	5/537	1
II	6-12	21/316	7
III	13-25	18/130	14
IV	>26	14/18	78
TOTAL		58/1001	6

*Denominator indicates the total number of patients in the risk class. The numerator indicates the number of patients in that class that experienced an adverse cardiac outcome.

very little attention, probably because of its complicated application.[24]

Limitations of CRI. First, the strongest risk factors were derived from relatively small numbers of patients. For example, "recent MI" was present in only 22 patients for Goldman, compared with 422 patients in the study by the Mayo Clinic group. Goldman's strongest predictor, "third heart sound or jugular venous distention," was present in only 35 patients, which was 3.5% of the population preoperatively.

Second, some important risk factors depended on the clinical skills of the examining physician. Assessment of a third heart sound, severity of JVD, or differentiation of aortic stenosis from a benign systolic ejection murmur could differ among physicians.

Finally, ECGs and cardiac enzymes were not obtained unless symptoms or clinical suspicion warranted assessment.[25] Numerous investigators have demonstrated that chest pain does not necessarily occur with postoperative MI.[12,26,27] About 25% of the postoperative reinfarctions studied by Tarhan et al were not associated with chest pain.[19] Likewise, studies using Holter monitoring have demonstrated that many dysrhythmias are clinically silent. Thus the number of complications detected in the Goldman study was likely underestimated.

Application of the Goldman CRI. Clinicians were eager to test the Goldman CRI in real patient populations. The first prospective application by Waters et al in 1981 compared the American Society of Anesthesiologists (ASA) Physical Status Classification with the Goldman index in a large series of patients undergoing noncardiac surgery at a university hospital.[28] The ASA classification was as effective as the Goldman index in predicting adverse cardiac outcomes. In addition, the Waters study showed a higher incidence of cardiac complications following abdominal aortic aneurysm surgery than the Goldman index predicted.[28]

In 1983, Jeffrey et al prospectively applied the Goldman CRI to 99 patients undergoing abdominal aortic aneurysm surgery at the same hospital as Goldman's original series.[29] Significantly more adverse cardiac events occurred in these patients than predicted by the Goldman risk index. These findings should not be surprising. The CRI was created from the study of consecutive, *nonselected* surgery patients. Jeffrey studied *selected* patients with known vascular disease. A higher-risk population is expected to have a higher incidence of adverse outcomes.[30]

Note that in practice, the CRI is always applied to the individual patient, *selected* because of perceived cardiac risk.

Over the years, many others have applied the CRI with varying degrees of success. These include Zeldin in 1984,[31] Detsky in 1986,[32,33] Beebe in 1992,[34] Cohen in 1992,[35] Takase in 1993,[36] Musser in 1994,[37] and Shackelford in 1995.[38] The largest study that found the Goldman CRI to be predictive of adverse cardiac outcome was that of Zeldin. In 1140 consecutive patients undergoing noncardiac surgery for whom Zeldin was the primary surgeon, Goldman classes I, II, and III were predictive of adverse outcome.[31] However, in the highest-risk class IV patients, adverse cardiac events occurred less often than predicted. Zeldin postulated that awareness of the high risk may have created a bias for enhanced care. An alternative explanation is that patients with postoperative *low* cardiac output were excluded from analysis.[31]

Few studies have addressed cardiac risk in women. However, Shackelford, in 1995, studied 406 female patients undergoing elective vaginal surgery.[38] Here, neither the Goldman index nor the New York Heart Association (NYHA) functional class was predictive of adverse outcome. However, in a subgroup of 168 postmenopausal women, hypertension and ischemic heart disease were predictors of cardiac morbidity.[38]

The Detsky Modified Cardiac Risk Index. The other major risk index for noncardiac surgery is that of Detsky et al,[32,33] who judged the Goldman CRI to be unsatisfactory when they used it during preoperative medical consultation. Based on the consensus opinion of their cardiology consultation team, a "Modified Cardiac Risk Index" that had several significant changes was proposed in 1986. First, several risk factors were added, including clinical angina, history of pulmonary edema, and old MI. These factors had been found "not significant" by the Goldman multivariate analysis. In the Detsky index, angina (Canadian classes[39] III and IV) was assigned high point values. Second, the Goldman factors JVD, third heart sound (S_3), and type of surgery (intraabdominal, intrathoracic, or aortic surgery) were deleted. Notably, JVD and S_3 had been the strongest predictors in the Goldman analysis. Third, "significant" aortic stenosis was changed to "critical" aortic stenosis, requiring a history of syncope, angina, or congestive failure. This newly defined variable was awarded a much higher point value in the Detsky index.

Overall, this new index depended more on historic information than physical findings (Table 1-4). On one hand, this removed some potential variability but also eliminated Goldman's sensitive indicators (JVD or S_3) of ongoing ventricular dysfunction. Were the changes justified? Recall that Goldman's factors were derived from statistical multivariate analysis. In contrast, the Detsky index was based on opinions of experienced clinicians. Finally, appropriate application of the Detsky index requires knowledge of usual cardiac risk for a particular surgical procedure at a particular hospital ("pretest probability"). A "likelihood ratio nomogram" is then applied to calculate the "posttest probability" of adverse outcome. Although this process may contribute to the accuracy of the Detsky index, it removed the key element of *simplicity*, which was a major benefit of the Goldman index.[32,33] Thus, despite superficial resemblance, the Detsky Modified Cardiac Risk Index represents major differences from the Goldman CRI.

Application of the Detsky Index. Wong and Detsky reviewed the various methods of cardiac risk stratification for patients undergoing peripheral vascular surgery.[40] Patients were judged to be at high risk for cardiac death or MI after vascular surgery if they had a Goldman index greater than 12, a Detsky index greater than 15, or

TABLE 1-4
Detsky's Modified Multifactorial Index Arranged According to Point Value

VARIABLES	POINTS
Class IV angina*	20
Suspected critical aortic stenosis	20
Myocardial infarction within 6 mo	10
Alveolar pulmonary edema within 1 wk	10
Unstable angina within 3 mo	10
Class III angina*	10
Emergency operation	10
Myocardial infarction >6 mo ago	5
Alveolar pulmonary edema ever	5
Sinus plus atrial premature beats or rhythm other than sinus on last preoperative electrocardiogram	5
> 5 ventricular premature beats any time before surgery	5
Poor general medical status†	5
Age >70 yr	5

*Canadian Cardiovascular Society classification for angina. From Campeau L: *Circulation* 54:522, 1976.
†Po$_2$, <60 mm Hg; Pco$_2$, >50 mm Hg; serum potassium, <3.0 mEq/L; serum bicarbonate, <20 mEq/L ; serum urea nitrogen, >50 mg/dl; serum creatinine, >3 mg/dl; aspartate aminotransferase abnormality; signs of chronic liver disease; and/or bedridden from noncardiac causes. From Detsky AS, Abrams HB, McLaughlin JR et al: *J Gen Intern Med* 1:211, 1986; Destsky AS, Abrams HB, Forbath N et al: *Arch Intern Med* 146:2131, 1986.

BOX 1-2
The Six Risk Factors of the Revised Cardiac Risk Index

- High-risk type of operation
- History of ischemic heart disease
- History of congestive heart failure
- History of cerebrovascular disease
- Preoperative treatment with insulin
- Preoperative serum creatinine >2 mg/dl

From Lee TH, Marcantonio ER, Mangione CM et al: *Circulation* 100:1043, 1999.

TABLE 1-5
Risk Classifications of the Revised Cardiac Risk Index

NO. OF RISK FACTORS	DERIVATION COHORT COMPLICATION RATE (%)	VALIDATION COHORT COMPLICATION RATE (%)
0	0.5	0.4
1	1.3	0.9
2	4	7
≥3	9	11

From Lee TH, Marcantonio ER, Mangione CM et al: *Circulation* 100: 1043, 1999.

more than three of the Eagle criteria[41] (age greater than 70 years, diabetes, angina, Q waves on electrocardiogram, or ventricular dysrhythmias).

The definition of low risk was more difficult. Patients were considered to *possibly* be at low risk if they had low scores by both the risk index methods and none of Eagle's criteria. The authors cautioned that the "low-risk" definition had not been reproduced by independent studies. The truth was that neither the Detsky nor Goldman indexes were satisfactory to describe patients at "low risk." In other words, for both indexes, adverse cardiac outcomes occurred in the lowest-risk class patients.

The Revised Index and Comparisons

The Revised Cardiac Risk Index by Lee et al, 1999.

The most recent preoperative risk stratification tool is the Revised Cardiac Risk Index published by Lee et al in 1999.[42] In this study, 4315 patients aged 50 years or older undergoing major noncardiac procedures were assessed for major cardiac complications, including MI, pulmonary edema, ventricular fibrillation or primary cardiac arrest, and complete heart block. Six independent predictors of complications were identified (Box 1-2).

Statistical analysis provided a satisfactory model for risk assessment when the six factors were given equal prognostic importance. A particular patient's risk was determined by adding the number of risk factors[42] (Table 1-5).

The new Revised Cardiac Risk Index differs significantly from the original Goldman CRI and the Modified CRI of Detsky. Age, aortic stenosis, and dysrhythmia characteristics are not included. Severity of illness variables such as Goldman's S$_3$ or JVD, Detsky's definition of "critical aortic stenosis," and "recent versus old MI" in both indexes are also not included. New variables of diabetes (requiring insulin), renal insufficiency, and cerebrovascular disease were not in either of the prior indexes.

Perhaps the major benefit of the new index is a lowered threshold for risk identification. Both of the earlier Goldman and Detsky indexes focused on variables that

TABLE 1-6
Comparison of Four Risk Stratification Methods

	PATIENTS* (% TOTAL)	COMPLICATIONS	RATE COMPLICATIONS (%)
Cardiac Risk Index			
(Goldman et al)			
Class I	2200 (76)	31	1.4†
Class II	561 (19)	20	3.6
Class III	127 (4.4)	5	3.9
Class IV	5 (0.2)	0	0
Modified Risk Index			
(Detsky et al)			
Class I	2786 (96)	49	1.8†
Class II	95 (3.3)	6	6.3
Class III	12 (0.4)	1	8.3
American Society of Anesthesiologists (ASA) Classification			
Class I	140 (4.9)	0	0†
Class II	1558 (55)	14	0.9
Class III	1078 (38)	35	3.3
Class IV	81 (2.8)	7	8.6
Revised Risk Index			
(Lee et al)			
Class I	1071 (37)	5	0.5†
Class II	1106 (38)	14	1.3
Class III	506 (17)	18	3.6
Class IV	210 (7)	19	9.1

Modified from Lee TH, Marcantonio ER, Mangione CM et al: *Circulation* 100:1043, 1999.
*For each index model, patients were distributed according to their risk class. Note that for the original Goldman and Detsky models, a large majority (76%-96%) of the patients were grouped into the lowest-risk class.
†Note that cardiac complications occur in the lowest risk class for each index method except the ASA Classification.

identified high-risk patients. As a result, patients with lesser degrees of cardiovascular disease fell into the lowest-risk classification group along with patients who were entirely without cardiac disease. Neither the Goldman nor Detsky index was able to accurately identify the true "low-risk" patient.

Comparison of Risk Index Methods. A recent study[43] compared four methods: (1) ASA physical status,[44] (2) Goldman CRI, (3) the Detsky modified index, and (4) the Canadian Cardiovascular Society[39] index for predicting cardiac adverse events after noncardiac surgery. In this study, 2035 patients referred for preoperative medical consultation in two Canadian[43] teaching hospitals were prospectively assigned scores by each of the risk indexes. Adverse cardiac events included MI, unstable angina, acute pulmonary edema, and death. The authors concluded that each risk index method was better than chance at predicting cardiac complications

but that no index was significantly better than another. The authors stated, "The most striking finding of our study was the generally poor degree of accuracy of existing cardiac risk prediction methods."[43]

In the study by Lee et al,[42] the authors compared their new Revised Cardiac Risk Index to three other risk stratification tools: the original CRI of Goldman et al, the Modified Cardiac Risk Index of Detsky et al, and the ASA Physical Status Classification (Table 1-6). Analysis by the receiver operator curve (ROC) method suggested superiority of the new Revised Cardiac Risk Index. However, this analysis method also found the ASA classification to be superior to the original Goldman index and the Detsky modified index. Simple observation of the data is revealing. The original Goldman and the Detsky indexes stratified a large majority of patients into the lowest (class I) risk category. Despite being the lowest risk category, cardiac complications were still noted. The new index of Lee et al provided more even distribution of patients into risk classes. However, only the ASA Physical Status Classification method identified a low-risk class in which no cardiac complications occurred.[42]

Guidelines for Noncardiac Surgery

Clinical preoperative evaluation for noncardiac surgery used risk index methods in the late 1970s. By the mid-1980s, noninvasive tests such as dipyridamole thallium and later dobutamine stress echocardiography (DSE) were popularized. In 1993, an editorial in *Circulation* titled "Risk Stratification for Noncardiac Surgery" estimated that performing one noninvasive test in vascular surgery patients would cost $200 to $400 million annually in the United States.[45] Recognizing the need for guidance, the American College of Cardiology (ACC) and the American Heart Association (AHA) published guidelines in 1996.[1,46] In 1997, the American College of Physicians (ACP) published its own set of preoperative guidelines.[2] Although the themes are similar, the two versions differ significantly.

1996 ACC/AHA Guidelines for Perioperative Cardiovascular Evaluation for Noncardiac Surgery[1]

The ACC/AHA guidelines represented a review of Medline information from 1975 through 1994. This document provided the clinician with an organized approach to the preoperative assessment that was economically responsible. From the Executive Summary[1]:

> The overriding theme of these guidelines is that intervention is rarely necessary to lower the risk of surgery. The goal of the task force is the rational use of testing in an era of cost containment.

A stepwise approach is described for preoperative cardiac assessment. Key considerations include clinical predictors of risk, functional activity of the patient, and degree of surgical stress. These guide the decision process to various pathways in the algorithm shown in Fig. 1-1. The steps listed in Box 1-3 correspond to the algorithm process.

The algorithm can be separated into several compartments. The first three steps pertain to circumstances (emergency operation, prior coronary revascularization, recent cardiac evaluation) that allow the patient to proceed directly to surgery without further evaluation. "Clinical Predictors of Risk" (Box 1-4) are used in the rest of the algorithm. Step 4 seeks the presence of Major Clinical Predictors such as unstable angina, recent MI, or decompensated CHF. These are rather severe conditions that may warrant hospitalization regardless of surgery. Major clinical predictors must be evaluated before elective noncardiac surgery is performed.

Patients with intermediate predictors of risk are the subject of steps 5 and 6. Intermediate predictors are characteristics that clearly establish the presence of coronary artery disease. Consideration of the type of surgery is key (Box 1-5). Low-risk surgery does not require workup, but high-risk operations warrant further noninvasive testing (Fig. 1-1). Intermediate risk surgery is a broad category accounting for a large share of operations performed in a typical hospital. Consideration of functional capacity (Box 1-6) is used to assess intermediate-risk surgery. Poor exercise capacity requires noninvasive testing; good exercise capacity does not.

Step 7 pertains to minor clinical predictors. These characteristics are associated with coronary disease, and type of operation is key. The patient with only minor predictors can proceed with low- or intermediate-risk surgery regardless of functional capacity, but high-risk surgery is acceptable only if exercise tolerance is good. Noninvasive testing is indicated for the patient facing high-risk surgery *and* who has poor functional capacity.

Probably the most difficult aspect of the ACC/AHA guidelines is the treatment of preoperative MI. The definition of *recent MI* is "greater than 7 days but less than or equal to 1 month (30 days)." Recent MI is appropriately considered a major clinical predictor. A "prior MI" is the only other category and is considered an intermediate predictor. This implies that an MI 6 *weeks* before noncardiac surgery carries the same risk as an MI 6 *months* prior, despite the fact that prior large clinical studies established an increased risk for MI less than 6 months before noncardiac surgery.[15-20]

1997 American College of Physicians Guidelines for Assessing Perioperative Risk Associated with Major Noncardiac Surgery

The second major set of guidelines is that of the ACP published in 1997.[2] These guidelines represent a Medline review of clinical studies between 1977 and 1996. The Modified Cardiac Risk Index by Detsky et al[32,33] is the main clinical risk stratification tool used for these guidelines. An important issue when considering the ACP guidelines is that the three risk classes of the Detsky index do not correspond to low-, intermediate-, and high-risk stratification for adverse perioperative events in the algorithm of the ACP guidelines (Fig. 1-2).

Class II (20-30 points) and class III (>30 points) patients by the Detsky index are both considered to represent high-risk patients with a greater than 15% chance of adverse perioperative cardiac events, such as MI and death. Such high-risk patients are treated according by an algorithm based on the nature of their risk variables (Fig. 1-3).

Patients who have low point scores by the Detsky modified risk index (class I, 0-15 points) are not necessarily at low risk for adverse perioperative cardiac events.

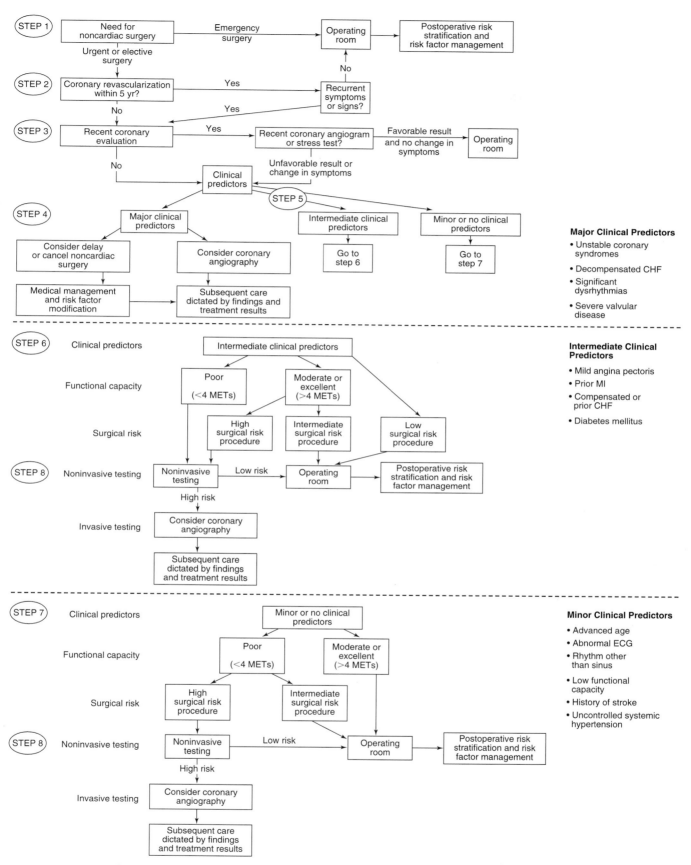

FIG. 1-1 Stepwise approach to preoperative cardiac assessment. *CHF,* Congestive heart failure; *ECG,* electrocardiogram; *METs,* metabolic equivalents; *MI,* myocardial infarction. (From *Circulation* 93:1284, 1996.)

BOX 1-3
Stepwise Approach to Preoperative Cardiac Assessment

Step 1. What is the urgency of noncardiac surgery? Certain emergencies do not allow time for preoperative cardiac evaluation. Postoperative risk stratification may be appropriate for some patients who have not had such an assessment before.

Step 2. Has the patient undergone coronary revascularization in the past 5 years? If so, and if clinical status has remained stable without recurrent symptoms/signs of ischemia, further cardiac testing is generally not necessary.

Step 3. Has the patient had a coronary evaluation in the past 2 years? If coronary risk was adequately assessed and the findings were favorable, it is usually not necessary to repeat testing unless the patient has experienced a change or new symptoms of coronary ischemia since the previous evaluation.

Step 4. Does the patient have an unstable coronary syndrome or a major clinical predictor of risk? When elective noncardiac surgery is being considered, the presence of unstable coronary disease, decompensated CHF, symptomatic arrhythmias, and/or severe valvular heart disease usually leads to cancellation or delay of surgery until the problem has been identified and treated.

Step 5. Does the patient have *intermediate clinical predictors of risk*? The presence or absence of prior MI by history or ECG, angina pectoris, compensated or prior CHF, and/or diabetes mellitus helps further stratify clinical risk for perioperative coronary events. Consideration of *functional*

capacity and level of *surgery-specific risk* allows a rational approach to identifying patients most likely to benefit from further noninvasive testing.

Step 6. Patients without major but with intermediate predictors of clinical risk and moderate or excellent functional capacity can generally undergo intermediate-risk surgery with little likelihood of perioperative death or MI. Conversely, further noninvasive testing is often considered for patients with poor functional capacity or moderate functional capacity but higher-risk surgery, and especially for patients with two or more intermediate predictors.

Step 7. Noncardiac surgery is generally safe for patients with neither major nor intermediate predictors of clinical risk and moderate or excellent functional capacity (≥ 4 METs). Further testing may be considered on an individual basis for patients without clinical markers but poor functional capacity who are facing higher-risk operations, particularly those with several minor clinical predictors of risk who are to undergo vascular surgery.

Step 8. The results of noninvasive testing can be used to determine further preoperative management. Alternatively, the results may lead to a recommendation to proceed with surgery. In some patients, the risk of coronary intervention or corrective cardiac surgery may approach or even exceed the risk of the proposed noncardiac surgery. This approach may be appropriate, however, if it also significantly improves the patient's long-term prognosis.

From Eagle KA, Brundage BH, Chaitman RB et al: *J Am Coll Cardiol* 27:910-948, 1996.
CHF, Congestive heart failure; *ECG,* electrocardiogram; *METs,* metabolic equivalents; *MI,* myocardial infarction.
Note: This material represents the steps used in the guidelines algorithm. Bold type has been added for emphasis. If the patient is identified as high risk, "subsequent care" is recommended. This may include cancellation or delay of surgery, coronary revascularization followed by noncardiac surgery, or intensive care.

BOX 1-4
Clinical Predictors of Increased Perioperative Cardiovascular Risk

Major
Unstable coronary syndromes
    Recent myocardial infarction* with evidence of
        important ischemic risk by clinical symptoms or
        noninvasive study
    Unstable or severe† angina (Canadian class III
        or IV)‡
Decompensated congestive heart failure
Significant dysrhythmias
    High-grade atrioventricular block
    Symptomatic ventricular dysrhythmias in the presence
        of underlying heart disease
    Supraventricular dysrhythmias with uncontrolled
        ventricular rate
Severe valvular disease

Intermediate
Mild angina pectoris (Canadian class I or II)
Prior myocardial infarction by history or pathologic Q waves
Compensated or prior congestive heart failure
Diabetes mellitus

Minor
Advanced age
Abnormal ECG (left ventricular hypertrophy, left bundle-
    branch block, ST-T abnormalities)
Rhythm other than sinus (e.g., atrial fibrillation)
Low functional capacity (e.g., inability to climb one flight of
    stairs with a bag of groceries)
History of stroke
Uncontrolled systemic hypertension

Adapted from Eagle KA, Brundage BH, Chaitman RB et al: *J Am Coll Cardiol* 27:910-948, 1996; *Circulation* 93:1278-1317, 1996.
ECG, Electrocardiogram.
*The American College of Cardiology National Database Library defines *recent myocardial infarction* as greater than 7 days but less than or equal to 1 month (30 days).
†May include "stable" angina in patients who are unusually sedentary.
‡Campeau L: *Circulation* 54:522-523, 1976.

BOX 1-5
Cardiac Risk* Stratification for Noncardiac Surgical Procedures

High Risk (Reported Cardiac Risk Often >5%)

- Emergent major operations, particularly in the elderly
- Aortic and other major vascular procedures
- Peripheral vascular surgery
- Anticipated prolonged surgical procedures associated with large fluid shifts and/or blood loss

Intermediate (Reported Cardiac Risk Generally <5%)

- Carotid endarterectomy
- Head and neck surgery
- Intraperitoneal and intrathoracic procedures
- Orthopedic surgery
- Prostate surgery

Low Risk[†] (Reported Cardiac Risk Generally <1%)

- Endoscopic procedures
- Superficial procedures
- Cataract removal
- Breast surgery

Adapted from Eagle KA, Brundage BH, Chaitman RB et al: *J am Coll Cardiol* 27:910-948, 1996.
*Combined incidence of cardiac death and nonfatal myocardial infarction.
†Do not generally require further preoperative cardiac testing.

BOX 1-6
Estimated Energy Requirements for Various Activities

1 MET   Can you take care of yourself?
         Eat, dress, or use the toilet?
         Walk indoors around the house?
         Walk a block or two on level ground at 2-3 mph
              or 3.2-4.8 km/hr?
         Do light work around the house, such as dust-
4 METs   ing or washing dishes?

4 METs   Climb a flight of stairs or walk up a hill?
         Walk on level ground at 4 mph or 6.4 km/hr?
         Run a short distance?
         Do heavy work around the house, such as
              scrubbing floors or lifting or moving heavy
              furniture?
         Participate in moderate recreational activities
              such as playing golf, bowling, dancing, play-
              ing doubles tennis, or throwing a baseball or
              football?
         Participate in strenuous sports such as swim-
              ming, singles tennis, football, basketball, or
>10 METs   skiing?

Adapted from Eagle KA, Brundage BH, Chaitman RB et al: *J Am Coll Cardiol* 27:910-948, 1996; *Circulation* 93:1278-1317, 1996; Hlatky MA, Boineau RE, Higginbotham MB et al: *Am J Cardiol* 64:651-654, 1989; Fletcher GH, Balady G, Froelicher VF et al: *Circuation* 91:580-615, 1995.
MET, Metabolic equivalents.

For this reason, the ACP guidelines recommends that such patients be further assessed for "Low-risk variables" (Table 1-7). If patients have no or one low-risk variable, they are considered **low risk** (<3%) for perioperative cardiac events and can proceed to surgery without further testing.

If patients have two or more low-risk variables, they are considered **intermediate risk** (3%-15%) for perioperative events. If such patients are undergoing nonvascular surgery, no further testing is recommended before surgery. If such patients are undergoing vascular surgery, noninvasive testing by dipyridamole thallium or DSE is

recommended. If these tests are "negative," the patient can proceed to surgery. If positive, the patient is considered high risk and evaluated according to the high-risk algorithm.

Which guideline system is better for preoperative risk assessment? A major difference between the ACC/AHA guidelines and the ACP guidelines is the management of intermediate-risk patients scheduled for vascular versus nonvascular surgery. In the ACC/AHA guidelines, noninvasive testing is done for all intermediate-risk patients scheduled for high-risk surgery. In the ACP guidelines, intermediate-risk patients receive noninvasive testing

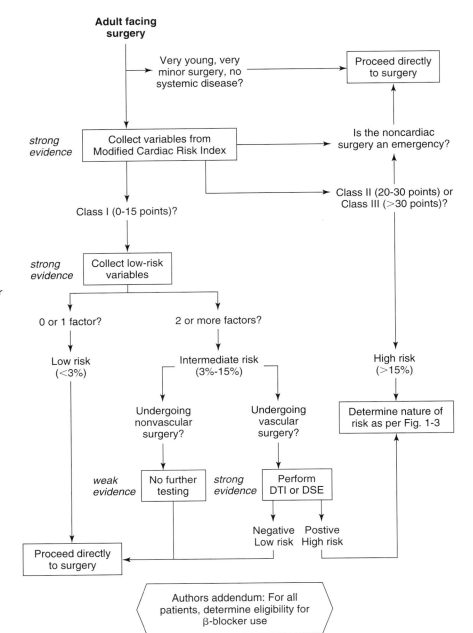

FIG. 1-2   Algorithm for the risk assessment and management of patients at low or intermediate risk for perioperative cardiac events. *DSE,* Dobutamine stress echocardiography; *DTI,* dipyridamole thallium imaging.

(From American College of Physicians: *Ann Intern Med* 127:311, 1997.)

only if scheduled for vascular surgery. Another difference is that ACP guidelines do not use "functional capacity" in the algorithm. Finally, the surgery-specific risks differ. Both guidelines recognize vascular surgery as high risk. However, the ACP guidelines regard orthopedic procedures as high risk (>13%), whereas the ACC/AHA guidelines rate orthopedic surgery as an intermediate risk.

Cardiac Surgery Risk Index Models

Coronary artery bypass graft (CABG) surgery has been the focus of increasing health care attention because of its frequency and expense. In 1987, the Health Care Financing Administration published a list of hospitals with higher-than-expected CABG mortality rates in Medicare patients. The report was criticized by the Society of Thoracic Surgeons because the data did not adequately address severity of illness:

> Use of such data without consideration of risk factors that are predictors of hospital mortality and of other indices of quality of care is inappropriate and misleading and may adversely affect the care of the high-risk cardiac surgical patient.[48]

A number of models were subsequently developed to identify patient risk characteristics[49] that contribute to outcome of CABG operation.

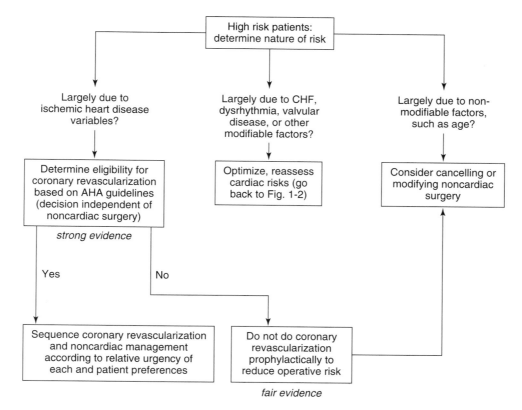

FIG. 1-3   Algorithm for the management of patients at high risk for perioperative cardiac events. *AHA,* American Heart Association; *CHF,* congestive heart failure.

(From American College of Physicians: *Ann Intern Med* 127:311, 1997.)

Risk Stratification Models for Cardiac Surgery. The Parsonnet model was an early system of risk stratification that emphasized objective and easily obtainable criteria.[50] From a group of 3500 consecutive patients, 14 risk factors were determined. Each factor was assigned a "point value," and five risk groups were created (Table 1-8). Mortality (within 30 days of operation), complication rate, and hospital length of stay were assessed.

Parsonnet et al[50] emphasized that factors in the model must be simple, objective, and broadly applicable. Chronic obstructive lung disease was excluded because it lacked a single clinical feature to quantitate severity and many patients did not receive preoperative pulmonary evaluation. Cerebrovascular disease, left ventricular end-diastolic pressure (LVEDP), and degree of left main coronary stenosis were excluded for similar reasons.

The highest risk was "catastrophic states," which included cardiogenic shock and a range of 10 to 50 points. Age greater than 80 years was the next highest risk category, with 20 points. In contrast, an ejection fraction of less than 30% was assigned a score of 4 points. A total score of more than 20 points was associated with a predicted mortality of greater than 20%.

TABLE 1-7
Low-Risk Variables

EAGLE CRITERIA[41]	VANZETTO CRITERIA[47]
Age >70 yr	Age >70 yr
History of angina	History of angina
Diabetes mellitus	Diabetes mellitus
Q waves on the electrocardiogram	Q waves on the electrocardiogram
History of ventricular ectopy	History of myocardial infarction
	ST-segment ischemia on resting electrocardiogram
	Hypertension with severe left ventricular hypertrophy
	History of congestive heart failure

Modified from American College of Physicians: *Ann Intern Med* 127: 311, 1997.

Note that four of the variables are shared by both the Eagle and Vanzetto studies.

TABLE 1-8
The Parsonnet Model for Cardiac Surgery

RISK FACTOR	ASSIGNED WEIGHT
Female gender	1
Morbid obesity (>1.5 × ideal body weight)	3
Diabetes (type not specified)	3
Hypertension (systolic blood pressure >140 mm Hg)	3
Ejection fraction:	
Good (>0.50)	0
Fair (0.30-0.49)	2
Poor (<0.30)	4
Age (yr):	
70-74	7
75-79	12
>80	20
Reoperation:	
First	5
Second	10
Balloon pump preoperatively	2
Left ventricular aneurysm (if resection planned)	5
Emergency surgery	10
Dialysis (hemodialysis or peritoneal)	10
Catastrophic states	10-50
Other rare conditions (e.g., paraplegia, pacemaker, congenital heart disease, asthma)	2-10
Valve surgery	
Mitral	5
Pulmonary artery pressure >60 mm Hg	8
Aortic valve gradient >120 mm Hg	7
Coronary artery bypass graft at the time of valve surgery	2

From Parsonnet V, Dean D, Bernstein AD: *Circulation* 79(suppl I): I-3, 1989.

TABLE 1-9
The Cleveland Clinic Model

RISK FACTOR	POINT SCORE
Emergency surgery	6
Serum creatinine	
≥1.6 and ≤1.8 mg/dl	1
≥1.9 mg/dl	4
Severe left ventricular dysfunction	3
Reoperation	3
Operative mitral insufficiency	3
Age ≥65 and ≤74 yr	1
Age ≥75 yr	2
Prior vascular surgery	2
Chronic obstructive pulmonary disease	2
Anemia (hematocrit ≤0.34)	2
Operative aortic stenosis	1
Weight ≤65 kg	1
Diabetes (oral or insulin therapy)	1
Cerebrovascular disease	1

From Higgins TL, Estafanous FG, Loop FD et al: *JAMA* 276:2344, 1992.

Parsonnet et al prospectively tested the model at their hospital and two other hospitals. The potential utilities of this model included (1) a means to provide an objective informed consent to patients, (2) the ability to identify patients whose operative risk is unacceptably high, and (3) the ability to quantify severity of disease for billing purposes.

From New York State's Cardiac Surgery Reporting System, Hannan et al[51] used preoperative risk factors and postoperative outcome to compare 28 hospitals performing heart surgery. The clinical variables were similar to those used by Parsonnet. Increased risk of death was associated with increased age, female gender, MI in the previous week, diabetes, dialysis, unstable angina, CHF, and greater than 90% stenosis of the left main coronary artery. The highest risk factor was "disasters," which included cardiogenic shock and gunshot wounds. The im-

portant finding of this study was that several hospitals had higher-than-expected mortality.[52,53]

O'Conner derived a model from the Northern New England Cardiovascular Disease Study Group, which included data from five regional medical centers and represented all cardiothoracic surgery performed in Maine, New Hampshire, and Vermont.[54] Predictors of in-hospital mortality included increased age, female gender, small body surface area, greater comorbidity, poor cardiac function as evidenced by low ejection fraction and increased LVEDP, and emergent or urgent surgery. In this model, noncardiac variables such as diabetes and renal disease were combined into a "comorbidity index" and were less represented than cardiac variables. The major finding of this study was that differences in case mix, defined by the aforementioned variables, could not account for differences of in-hospital mortality rates among institutions and surgeons of northern New England.[54-56]

Higgins et al[57] provided an index from data of adult patients undergoing CABG surgery at the Cleveland Clinic between 1986 and 1990. Morbidity and mortality were assessed. Morbidity included (1) cardiac complications such as MI and low cardiac output requiring mechanical assistance, (2) prolonged ventilatory support for 3 days or longer, (3) central nervous system (CNS) complications, (4) renal failure, and (5) serious infection. The study identified 13 preoperative variables that contributed significantly to adverse outcome and assigned a weight (point score) to each[57] (Table 1-9).

TABLE 1-10
Comparison of Variables Used in Four CABG Models

VARIABLE	CLEVELAND	NEW YORK	NEW ENGLAND	PARSONETTE
Age	+	+	+	+
LV function	+	+	+	+
Body habitus	+	+	+	+
Reoperation	+	+	+	+
Gender	−	+	+	+
Renal function	+	+	−	+
Diabetes	+	+	−	+
Priority	+	−	+	−
Preoperative IABP	−	+	−	+
COPD	+	−	+	−
Coronary anatomy	−	+	+	−

From Orr RK, Maini BS, Sottile FD et al: *Arch Surg* 130: 301-306, 1995. A plus sign (+) indicates that the model utilized the variable to calculate CABG risks.
CABG, Coronary artery bypass graft; *COPD,* chronic obstructive pulmonary disease; *IABP,* intraaortic balloon pump; *LV,* left ventricular.

The Edwards risk factor index[58-60] was derived from data of the Society of Thoracic Surgeons (STS) National Cardiac Surgery Database. This represented data from more than 300,000 patients undergoing isolated CABG surgery from 1990 to 1994.

Assessment of Cardiac Surgery Risk Prediction Models. The previously discussed models differ in several characteristics (Table 1-10). The Parsonette and Cleveland Clinic data were collected from single institutions and used a simple "point score" method for risk calculation. The New York, Northern New England, and STS models used data from multiple institutions. In 1995, Orr et al compared these models by applying them to a population of 865 consecutive CABG patients at institutions different from those that developed the models.[61]

The Parsonette model consistently predicted a higher mortality rate than was observed. The authors speculated that improvements in CABG surgery may have occurred after the data collection of this early model. The best fitting models were the New York and New England models. However, when individual patients were classified, risk could be minimal (<1%) or relatively high risk (14%) depending on the model used (Table 1-11).

Problems with these various models included the following: different variables were judged to be important; definitions were not standard; and some variables, such as angina severity and acuteness of illness, were subjective and might overestimate or underestimate risk. In 1993, representatives from seven large cardiovascular database models joined the Cooperative CABG Database Project to form a consensus opinion. Their

TABLE 1-11
Comparison of Four CABG Risk Prediction Models

MODEL	PREDICTED MORTALITY (%)	OBSERVED MORTALITY (%)
Cleveland Clinic	2.9	4.0
New York State	2.8	3.7
Northern New England	5.9	3.7
Parsonette	9.2	3.0

From Orr RK, Maini BS, Sottile FD et al: *Arch Surg* 130:301-306, 1995.

findings were reported by Jones et al in 1996.[62] Three types of preoperative variables were described:

Core variables were those "unequivocally related to operative mortality. These variables *should* be in the data base record of every patient undergoing CABG." These seven variables are age, gender, previous heart operation, left ventricular ejection fraction, percentage of stenosis of left main coronary, number of major coronary arteries with stenosis greater than 70%, and acuity of operation (e.g., elective, urgent, emergent).

Level 1 variables were those shown to "have a likely relation to short-term CABG mortality. These variables are *suggested* for inclusion in the data base record of every patient undergoing CABG." These

13 variables are height, weight, percutaneous transluminal coronary angioplasty (PTCA) during same admission, date of most recent MI, angina history, serious ventricular dysrhythmias, CHF, mitral regurgitation (MR), diabetes, cerebrovascular disease, peripheral vascular disease, chronic obstructive pulmonary disease (COPD), and creatinine levels.

Level 2 variables were those "not clearly shown to relate directly to short-term CABG mortality but with potential research or administrative interest. These variables are *optional* for inclusion in the data base record of patients undergoing CABG." Some of these 24 variables are race, institution where CABG is performed, surgeon responsible for CABG, payment source, LVEDP, smoking history, hypertension, pacemaker, liver disease, and malignancy.

Several of the core variables accounted for the majority of the risk prediction. These variables were acuity of operation, history of previous cardiac surgery, and patient age. The more important Level 1 variables were cerebrovascular disease, number of previous MIs, and CHF.

MEDICAL HISTORY AND SYMPTOM REVIEW

The history constitutes a major component of any medical evaluation,[63] and often contributes more than the physical examination or laboratory tests.[64] The history involves review of *known medical and surgical conditions* and *assessment of symptoms*. Cardinal symptoms of cardiovascular disease include dyspnea, fatigue, cough and hemoptysis, cyanosis, chest pain, palpitations, syncope, edema, and claudication.[65] Obtaining an accurate medical history is a skill. Variability can be improved by using plain words rather than medical or suggestive terminology.[66] The patient's own description of chest discomfort may be more revealing than a direct question about the occurrence of "angina." Despite clear and well-understood questions, patients occasionally provide different answers.[67] The key to a valuable history thus involves careful listening to and interpretation of the patient's story.

Cerebrovascular Disease

Cerebrovascular disease has been implicated as a risk factor for adverse CNS outcomes for both noncardiac[68] and cardiac surgery.[69] For noncardiac surgery, it is a marker for atherosclerosis and thus potential adverse cardiac outcome. For cardiac surgery, it is associated with an increased risk of stroke. Cerebrovascular disease includes prior stroke, asymptomatic carotid bruit, and transient ischemic attack.

Asymptomatic Bruit. Stroke is the third leading cause of mortality in the United States.[70] However, an asymptomatic bruit is problematic because it may not indicate a carotid stenosis.[71,72] In a study of 1000 normal patients, a bruit was heard in 87% of patients younger than 5 years of age and 22% of patients aged 30 to 34.[73] Another study determined the presence of a cervical venous hum in 27% of young adults.[74] Hemodialysis patients often have a bruit in their neck, presumably because of the high-output circulatory state.[75] A carotid Doppler study of asymptomatic bruits demonstrated that the strongest predictor of a stenotic lesion was bilateral upper neck bruits (stenotic lesion in 76% of cases). A unilateral neck bruit correlated with an ipsilateral stenotic lesion in 61% of cases. However, a stenotic lesion was found on the *opposite*, clinically silent side in 28% of cases.[76]

Large epidemiologic studies demonstrated the presence of an asymptomatic cervical bruit in about 5% of patients, which was associated with increased risk of stroke.[77,78] However, most often the stroke was from cardiac embolism, from ruptured aneurysm, or in a vascular territory *not* related to the bruit.

Chambers and Norris followed 500 patients with asymptomatic bruits for up to 4 years.[79] Patients were grouped according to the initial severity of stenosis. Neurologic events were more common in patients with severe stenoses. However, even in patients with the most severe stenoses, the initial neurologic event was usually a TIA rather than stroke. MIs were significantly more common than strokes[79] (Table 1-12).

Transient Ischemic Attack. A first-time transient ischemic attack (TIA) is more worrisome than an asymp-

TABLE 1-12
Asymptomatic Carotid Bruit—One-Year Sequelae According to Degree of Stenosis

OUTCOME	SEVERITY OF INITIAL CAROTID STENOSIS		
	0%-29%	30%-74%	75%-100%
TIA only	2	6	16
Stroke after TIA	1	1	2 (1)*
Stroke without TIA	2 (1)*	2	4 (1)*
Nonfatal MI	4	8	4
Fatal MI	7	8	12

From Chambers BR, Norris JW: *N Engl J Med* 315:960, 1986.
MI, Myocardial infarction; *TIA*, transient ischemic attack. Numbers indicate the number of events per each category of stenosis.
*A total of three strokes were fatal.

tomatic bruit.[80,81] The incidence of TIA is about 3 per 10,000 annually, but older persons are more often affected.[82] The risk of stroke is highest in the early months after a first-time TIA.[83] Whisnant reported that 36% of patients with TIA developed a stroke over 5 years. The first month was the period of greatest risk, and half of the strokes occurred during the first year.[82]

In summary, a new TIA clearly represents an increased risk for a neurologic event in the near future. An asymptomatic bruit represents lesser risk. Both are important markers of atherosclerosis.[84] Carotid endarterectomy has been a matter of considerable controversy, particularly in patients with an asymptomatic bruit.[85-88]

Cerebrovascular Disease and Cardiac Surgery. In cardiac surgery, perioperative stroke is a major adverse outcome. The incidence varies between 0.4% and 5.4%.[89]

Gardner et al reported a 10-year study of 3279 consecutive patients who underwent isolated CABG surgery from 1974 to 1983.[90] Operative mortality decreased from 3.9% to 2.6%, but the risk of perioperative stroke *increased* from less than 1% to 2.4%. Risk factors for stroke were increased age, preexisting cerebrovascular disease, severe atherosclerosis of the ascending aorta, prolonged cardiopulmonary bypass time, and severe perioperative hypotension. The increased stroke rate was thought to be related to the increasing age of the surgical population.[90]

In 1996, Roach et al reported a multiinstitutional (24 centers) study of stroke after elective CABG surgery.[89] The incidence was 6.1% in the 2108 patients prospectively studied. Two types of neurologic outcome were defined: type I outcomes included fatal cerebral injury and nonfatal strokes, and type II outcomes were new deterioration in intellectual function or new onset of seizures. Both outcome types increased mortality and length of stay.

Type I adverse outcomes were associated with severe proximal aortic atherosclerosis, suggesting embolic events occurring during surgery. A history of diabetes, preoperative stroke, or TIA was also associated with type I adverse cerebral outcomes. Here the mechanism was postulated to be inadequate cerebral or collateral blood flow or impaired autoregulation. Advanced age, especially age greater than 70 years, was associated with both type I and II adverse outcomes, perhaps because of increased atherosclerosis, increased embolic events, or altered autoregulation. Hypertension and pulmonary disease were also associated with both type I and II adverse outcomes[89] (Table 1-13).

Congestive Heart Failure

Congestive heart failure has been a major predictor of adverse outcome for both cardiac[91-94] and noncardiac surgery.[13,21,33] The Agency for Health Care Policy and Research defines heart failure[95] as a clinical syndrome or condition characterized by one of the following:

1. Signs and symptoms of intravascular and interstitial volume overload, including shortness of breath, rales, and edema
2. Manifestations of inadequate tissue perfusion, such as fatigue or poor exercise tolerance (These signs and symptoms result when the heart is unable to generate a cardiac output sufficient to meet the body's demands.[95])

The Framingham Heart Study determined that coronary artery disease and long-standing hypertension were

---

TABLE 1-13
Adjusted Odds Ratio for Adverse Cerebral Outcomes

SIGNIFICANT FACTOR	TYPE I OUTCOME (FATAL + NONFATAL STROKE)	TYPE II OUTCOME (INTELLECT OR SEIZURE)
Proximal aortic atherosclerosis	4.52	
History of neurologic disease	3.19	
Use of intraaortic balloon pump	2.60	
Diabetes	2.59	
History of hypertension	2.31	
History of pulmonary disease	2.09	2.37
History of unstable angina	1.83	
Age (per additional decade)	1.75	2.20
Admission systolic blood pressure >180 mm Hg		3.47
History of excessive alcohol intake		2.64
History of coronary artery bypass graft		2.18
Dysrhythmia on day of surgery		1.97
Antihypertensive therapy		1.78

TABLE 1-14
Framingham Criteria for Congestive Heart Failure

MAJOR CRITERIA	MINOR CRITERIA
Orthopnea	Ankle edema
Paroxysmal nocturnal dyspnea	Night cough
Neck vein distention	Dyspnea on exertion
Rales	Hepatomegaly
Cardiomegaly on CXR	Pleural effusion
Acute pulmonary edema	Decreased vital capacity
S_3 gallop	Tachycardia (>120 beats/min)
Increased venous pressure (>16 cm H_2O)	
Circulation time >25 sec	
Hepatojugular reflux	
Weight loss of ≥ 4.5 kg in 5 days in response to treatment of congestive heart failure.	

From Ho KKL, Pinsky JL, Kannel WB et al: *J Am Coll Cardiol* 22(suppl A):6A-13A, 1993.
The diagnosis of congestive heart failure required two major criteria or one major and two minor criteria concurrently. Minor criteria were acceptable only if not the result of another medical condition.

common causes of CHF.[96] Significant CHF had a 6-year mortality rate of 82% in men and 67% in women. The risk of stroke and MI was four to five times higher than that of the general population. Characteristics associated with developing cardiac failure include an enlarged heart, ECG abnormalities such as left ventricular hypertrophy (LVH), decreased vital capacity reflecting engorgement of pulmonary vasculature, and a rapid resting heart rate. Modifiable risk factors for CHF include hypertension, impaired glucose tolerance, smoking, obesity, elevated serum cholesterol, elevated low-density lipoprotein cholesterol, and both low and high hematocrit levels.[97]

The Framingham Study also established major and minor criteria for CHF [98] (Table 1-14). The Agency for Health Care Policy and Research adds symptoms suggestive of heart failure: decreased exercise tolerance; unexplained confusion, altered mental status, or fatigue in an elderly person; and abdominal symptoms such as nausea or pain associated with ascites and/or hepatic engorgement.[95] Left ventricular failure is expected to produce pulmonary congestion and signs of reduced forward flow, such as fatigue.[99] Pallor, oliguria, and postprandial abdominal discomfort may occur because of vasoconstriction.[100] Right ventricular failure causes JVD, liver enlargement, peripheral edema, and abnormal neck vein distention when pressure is applied to the periumbilical region.[101]

Many patients with significantly impaired cardiac function may be asymptomatic. In one study, 20% of patients with an ejection fraction of less than 40% did not have clinical criteria of heart failure.[102] In another study, less than half of the patients with an ejection fraction of less than 30% had dyspnea on exertion.[103] The explanation is that patients gradually reduce activity or perform daily activities more slowly to prevent symptom occurrence. This gives a false impression of adequate compensation.

Similarly, physical signs of heart failure are not reliable to estimate the hemodynamics of chronic heart failure. A study of 50 known CHF patients with ventricular dilation and an ejection fraction of less than 30% is illustrative.[104] Of the 43 patients with a pulmonary capillary wedge pressure (PCWP) greater than 22 mm Hg, 18 patients (40%) lacked rales, edema, or elevated jugular venous pressure.[104] A third heart sound was present in 48 patients but failed to distinguish patients with low versus high PCWP. Elevated jugular venous pressure was present in half of the patients. Peripheral edema or rales was absent in 80% of patients. The most reliable indicator of increased PCWP was recent orthopnea. This was present in 43 patients (91%) with a PCWP of 22 mm Hg or greater and was absent in 7 patients with lower PCWPs. The authors found that the patient's pulse pressure correlated with the cardiac index.[104]

An explanation for these findings is that compensatory mechanisms modify the chronic state of CHF. For example, increased lymphatic drainage accommodates chronic fluid exudation in the lung. Therefore estimation of ejection fraction is based on symptoms rather than physical findings. One study found that cardiologists were more likely than internists or family physicians to use echocardiography, radionuclide ejection fraction, or exercise testing to follow patients with heart failure.[105]

Practice guidelines for CHF have recommended treatment with angiotensin converting enzyme (ACE) inhibitor.[106] However, recent reports indicate underutilization of this therapy.[107] Cardiologists prescribe ACE inhibitors for CHF more frequently than do primary care physicians.[108,109] More recently, β-blocker drugs have been demonstrated to improve survival of CHF patients.[110,111]

Congestive Heart Failure After Noncardiac Surgery.
The original Goldman analysis determined that the presence of a third heart sound or JVD was the best predictor of adverse cardiac outcome after noncardiac surgery.[21] In a subsequent analysis Goldman et al correlated other preoperative CHF indicators to postoperative pulmonary edema.[22,23] NYHA functional classification[112] was a good predictor (Box 1-7). Patients with NYHA classes II and III had a 6% to 7% incidence of pulmonary edema, whereas patients with class IV had a

BOX 1-7
New York Heart Association Functional Classification

Class I

Patients with cardiac disease but without resulting limitations of physical activity. Ordinary physical activity does not cause undue fatigue, palpitation, dyspnea, or anginal pain.

Class II

Patients with cardiac disease resulting in slight limitation of physical activity. They are comfortable at rest. Ordinary physical activity results in fatigue, palpitation, dyspnea, or anginal pain.

Class III

Patients with cardiac disease resulting in marked limitation of physical activity. They are comfortable at rest. Less than ordinary physical activity causes fatigue, palpitation, dyspnea, or anginal pain.

Class IV

Patients with cardiac disease resulting in inability to carry on any physical activity without discomfort. Symptoms of cardiac insufficiency or of anginal syndrome may be present even at rest. If any physical activity is undertaken, discomfort is increased.

From The criteria of the New York Heart Association: *Nomenclature and criterial for diagnosis*, ed 9, Boston, 1994, Little Brown.

TABLE 1-15
Preoperative Signs of Congestive Failure and Postoperative Cardiogenic Pulmonary Edema

PREOPERATIVE VARIABLE	PATIENTS WITH VARIABLE	PERCENTAGE DEVELOPING PULMONARY EDEMA
S_3 gallop	17	35
Jugular venous distention and signs of left-sided heart failure	23	30
NYHA functional class IV for congestive heart failure	17	25
History of pulmonary edema	22	25
Left-sided heart failure by preoperative physical examination or chest X-ray	66	16
History of left-sided heart failure but not evident on preoperative examination or chest X-ray	87	6
NYHA functional class for congestive heart failure		
III	34	6
II	15	7
I	935	3
No history of congestive heart failure	853	2

From Goldman L: *Ann Intern Med* 98:504-513, 1983.
NYHA, New York Heart Association.

25% incidence (Table 1-15). This study also noted that 20% to 25% of patients who had mitral stenosis or regurgitation, or aortic stenosis or regurgitation, developed new or worsened postoperative CHF.[22,23]

Risk Factors for Ischemic Heart Disease

Framingham Heart Study. Occasionally, a patient without a history of cardiac disease has vague chest discomfort or nonspecific ECG abnormalities that might be consistent with ischemic heart disease. An assessment for "risk factors" is helpful to guide interpretation. Since 1948, the Framingham Heart Study[113] has followed a group of 5209 men and women with biennial cardiovascular examinations that included blood tests,

ECG, and chest X-ray studies. These persons were considered free of heart disease at the start of the study. A report after the first 18 years found that in 259 patients, the initial manifestation of coronary disease was MI.[114] The infarction was unrecognized in 25% and diagnosed by routine ECG. Half of these unrecognized infarctions were clinically silent. Patients with diabetes or high blood pressure seemed more likely to have an unrecognized infarction.[114] A similar proportion of unrecognized infarctions occurred after 30 years. The incidence was higher in women than in men.[115] Clearly, lack of symptoms does not eliminate the possibility of coronary artery disease. However, Framingham and other studies[116] clearly establish the risk factors for coronary artery disease[117] (Box 1-8).

BOX 1-8
Established Risk Factors for Coronary Artery Disease

Fixed
Age (risk increases with age)
Gender (male > female)
Family history of coronary disease

Modifiable
Elevated cholesterol, hyperlipidemia, elevated triglycerides
Hypertension
Smoking
Glucose intolerance and diabetes
Obesity
Sedentary lifestyle
Personality/behavior type
Gout
Estrogen status (postmenopausal)
Left ventricular hypertrophy

BOX 1-9
Novel Risk Factors for Coronary Artery Disease

Elevated homocysteine[123]
Elevated fibrinogen[125,126]
Elevated lipoprotein(a)
Markers of fibrinolytic function (e.g., D-dimer)[120]
Markers of inflammation (e.g., C-reactive protein)

Major Independent and Predisposing Risk Factors. The previously described risk factors were recently studied for their independence and strength of prediction. "Major independent risk factors" include cigarette smoking, elevated blood pressure, elevated serum cholesterol, elevated low-density lipoprotein cholesterol, reduced high-density lipoprotein cholesterol, diabetes, and advanced age. These major factors are quantitative (higher cholesterol imparts greater risk) and additive in their ability to predict coronary disease. A recent Framingham report described point values for each of the major independent factors. A person's probability of developing coronary disease in the next 10 years can be determined by adding these point scores.[118,119]

Gender differences are important for the major risk factors. Factors that affect greater risk in women than in men include diabetes, age greater than 45 years, and low levels of high-density lipoprotein cholesterol.

Other risk factors that are not independent or quantitative predictors are regarded as "predisposing risk factors." These include obesity, physical inactivity,[120] family history of premature coronary disease,[121] ethnic characteristics, and psychosocial factors. Predisposing risk factors worsen the risk defined by major independent factors. Obesity, for example, affects other risk factors by increasing blood pressure and elevating cholesterol levels, and is associated with type 2 diabetes. Although not an independent predictor, the AHA lists obesity as a major target for intervention.[122]

Novel Risk Factors. A group of novel risk factors have also been associated with coronary disease (Box 1-9). These are described as "conditional risk factors" because their characteristics have not been evaluated thoroughly.

Homocysteine is an amino acid that is produced with metabolism of the essential amino acid methionine. Total plasma homocysteine levels are elevated in patients with occlusive vascular disease, men versus women, and cigarette smokers. In a review of 35 human studies, total homocysteine levels were consistently higher in patients with atherosclerotic diseases.[123] One study found that intraoperative nitrous oxide transiently increased plasma homocysteine.[124]

Fibrinogen has a number of key roles in blood viscosity and the coagulation process.[125] Fibrinogen levels are increased with smoking, diabetes, obesity, and increased age and serum low-density lipoprotein cholesterol. Levels are decreased with alcohol use, exercise, weight loss, and smoking cessation. The Framingham population demonstrated a correlation between fibrinogen level and the risk of cardiovascular events.[126]

Fibrinolysis activity is another new risk factor. Appropriate reorganization of blood clots depends on a balance between fibrinolytic enzymes such as tissue-type plasminogen activator (t-PA) and its inhibitor PAI-1. Levels of PAI-1 are increased in patients with obesity and insulin resistance.[127]

Recent contributions from the Framingham studies include evidence for impaired fibrinolysis in hypertensive patients,[128] association of pulse pressure,[129] and attenuated exercise heart rate response[130] with coronary heart disease.

Diabetes

Diabetes is a relentless, progressive disorder contributing to coronary artery disease, stroke, renal disease, and blindness. Diabetes is included in cardiac surgery risk index models but with a relatively low weight.[50,51,57] In contrast, Eagle et al listed diabetes as one of their key clinical variables to determine cardiac risk with noncardiac surgery.[41] Diabetes requiring insulin is also included in the recent Modified Cardiac Risk Index of Lee et al.[42] A key aspect of diabetes is that significant coronary artery ischemia can occur without obvious symptoms.[131,132]

TABLE 1-16
Diabetic Patients and Angioplasty, Six-Month Follow-Up

	GROUP 1 (n = 162)	GROUP 2 (n = 257)	GROUP 3 (n = 94)
Angiogram at 6 mo	No restenosis	Nonocclusive restenosis	Coronary occlusion
Baseline Characteristics			
Retinopathy	15%	21%	21%
Nephropathy	17%	23%	26%
Neuropathy	7%	11%	9%
Symptoms at 6 mo			
No angina	106 (65%)	84 (33%)	29 (31%)
Stable angina	46 (29%)	108 (42%)	28 (30%)
Unstable angina or acute myocardial infarction	10 (6%)	65 (25%)	37 (39%)
Mortality after 6.5 yr	17%	26%	45%

From Van Belle E, Ketelers R, Bauters C et al: *Circulation* 103:1218-1224, 2001.

Diabetes is associated with increased morbidity and mortality after CABG surgery[133,134] and an increased incidence of restenosis after PTCA[135-137] or stent placement.[138] Diabetic patients also have a higher incidence of mortality after MI than do nondiabetic patients.[139,140] Aggressive therapy to control diabetes with insulin and risk factor reduction is associated with reduced coronary mortality from diabetes.

Diabetes and CABG versus PTCA. In the Bypass Angioplasty Revascularization Investigation (BARI), patients with coronary disease were randomized to either CABG or PTCA.[141] A subgroup of 353 patients had diabetes that required treatment with oral hypoglycemic agents or insulin.[142] Follow-up after 5.4 years demonstrated that patients with diabetes who received CABG had significantly better outcome (5.8% mortality) than those who received PTCA (20.6% mortality).[142] Both of these groups had higher mortality than patients without a history of treated diabetes (CABG mortality, 4.7%; PTCA mortality, 4.8%). However, the most important finding of this study was that the benefit of CABG in diabetic patients was significantly related to whether the patient had received an internal mammary artery (IMA) graft with CABG. Patients with treated diabetes undergoing CABG with at least one IMA graft had a mortality of 2.9%, whereas patients undergoing CABG with only vein grafts had a mortality of 18.2%.[142]

Diabetes and Angioplasty. Another follow-up study of 513 diabetic patients treated by standard angioplasty without coronary stents illustrates the problems associated with a lack of symptoms.[143] Six months after coronary angioplasty, an angiogram study demonstrated complete occlusion in 18%, nonocclusive restenosis in 50%, and no restenosis in 32% of patients. Clinical symptoms did not distinguish the groups. However, patients with evidence of end-organ damage at baseline were more likely to develop restenosis (Table 1-16). The 6-month angiogram was more likely to predict long-term (6.5 years) mortality than clinical symptoms.[143]

Hypertension

The 1996 AHA/ACC guidelines for perioperative cardiovascular evaluation addresses hypertension before noncardiac surgery.[1] Numerous clinical studies do not indicate that moderate hypertension is an independent risk factor for cardiovascular complications.[22,144] However, hypertension is a marker for potential coronary artery disease. Thus the AHA/ACC guidelines indicate that mild or moderate hypertension is not a significant perioperative problem, but further assessment is recommended for higher pressures:

If more severe hypertension (e.g., diastolic blood pressure greater than or equal to 110 mm Hg) exists before elective noncardiac surgery, it is prudent to control it before surgery.[1]

Hypertension is the most prevalent cardiovascular disease in the United States, affecting nearly 50 million people. It is an important risk factor for coronary artery disease, stroke, CHF, and renal failure.[145] Over the last 30 years, significant decreases in the incidence of stroke and (to a lesser degree) coronary artery disease have occurred because of hypertension awareness and therapy. The Sixth Joint National Committee on Prevention, Detection, Evaluation and Treatment of High Blood Pressure (JNC VI) warns that these favorable trends have leveled off.[146] Less than one third of hypertensive persons have satisfactory blood pressure control (systolic pressure less than 140 mm Hg and diastolic pressure less than 90 mm Hg).[147] Coincidently, the incidence of end-stage renal disease and heart failure has increased.[148] In 1999 the ACC published a "Call to Action" for cardiologists to address these challenges.[147] Because hypertension is asymptomatic, its discovery during preoperative assessment is an important opportunity for clinicians to favorably affect a patient's health.

Definitions. In adults, *hypertension* is systolic pressure greater than 140 mm Hg, diastolic pressure greater than or equal to 90 mm Hg, or use of medication for treatment of high blood pressure[146] (Table 1-17). Hypertension is common in older persons in the United States. More than 60% of persons older than 60 years of age have hypertension. The incidence is greater than 70% for older African Americans.[146] An elevated pulse pressure is a better predictor of risk than either systolic or diastolic pressure in older persons. The incidence of hypertension in children is low but represents an opportunity for significant risk reduction with early treatment[149-151] (Table 1-18).

Therapy. Physiologic changes with hypertension include altered baroreflex function,[152] changes in autoregulation of the cerebral[153] and coronary[154] circulations, altered renal function,[155] and LVH. The older "stepped therapy" for hypertension has been replaced by individualized therapy that considers coexisting conditions that influence the choice of the antihypertensive agent(s).[156-158] For example, patients with MI benefit from β-blocker therapy, whereas those with systolic dysfunction also benefit from an ACE inhibitor. For patients without special considerations, initial therapy recommended for hypertension is a diuretic and a β-blocker.[159]

Approach to Hypertension. Several important steps are in order when hypertension is identified.[160] The JNC recommends (1) identification of known causes of hypertension, (2) assessment for target-organ damage and cardiovascular disease, and (3) identification of other risk factors and disorders to guide therapy and prognosis.

Medications that predispose and contribute to hypertension include immunosuppressive drugs (e.g., cyclosporine, tacrolimus, steroids), oral contraceptives, erythropoietin, mineralocorticoids, nonsteroidal antiinflammatory drugs, dermatologic or anabolic steroids, and some herbal remedies. Habits such as excessive alcohol intake, cigarette smoking, and stimulant drug use are also implicated.[146]

TABLE 1-17
Blood Pressure in Adults Aged 18 Years and Older*

CATEGORY	SYSTOLIC (mm Hg)		DIASTOLIC (mm Hg)
Optimal	<120	and	<80
Normal	<130	and	<85
High-normal	130-139	or	85-89
Stage 1 hypertension	140-159	or	90-99
Stage 2 hypertension	160-179	or	100-109
Stage 3 hypertension	≥180	or	≥110

From the Sixth Report of the Joint National Committee on Detection, Evaluation, and Treatment of High Blood Pressure: *Arch Intern Med* 157:2417, 1997.

*Pertains to persons not taking antihypertensive drugs and not acutely ill. If systolic and diastolic pressures fall into different categories, the higher category should be selected for classification. In addition to classification, the presence or absence of target-organ disease and additional risk factors should be specified. Classification based on the average of two or more readings taken at each of two or more visits after an initial screening.

TABLE 1-18
Pediatric Hypertension Classification

	SIGNIFICANT HYPERTENSION		SEVERE HYPERTENSION	
	DIASTOLIC (mm Hg)	SYSTOLIC (mm Hg)	DIASTOLIC (mm Hg)	SYSTOLIC (mm Hg)
Newborn				
7 days	—	≥96	—	≥106
8-40 days	—	>104	—	≥110
Infants	≥74	≥112	≥82	≥118
Children				
3-5 yr	≥76	≥116	≥84	≥124
6-9 yr	≥78	≥122	≥86	≥130
10-12 yr	≥82	≥126	≥90	≥134
13-15 yr	≥86	≥136	≥92	≥144
16-18 yr	≥92	≥142	≥98	≥150

From Task Force on Blood Pressure Control in Children: *Pediatrics* 79:1-25,1987.

Secondary causes of hypertension account for 5% of hypertensive patients. Such causes are potentially curable and may be indicated by physical examination. Medical conditions that cause hypertension include renal artery stenosis,[161] primary aldosteronism,[162] Cushing's syndrome,[163] pheochromocytoma,[164] coarctation of the aorta,[165] acromegaly, and hyperparathyroidism.

Evidence for target-organ damage may be found with a fundoscopic examination indicating hypertensive retinopathy,[166] with a cardiac examination indicating cardiomegaly or LVH,[167] or with basic laboratory tests such as urinalysis, blood chemistry (serum creatinine), and ECG (LVH).[146] Target-organ involvement indicates that an elevated blood pressure reading is likely because of long-standing hypertension.

Renal Disease

Renal disease is often associated with the cardiac patient.[168] Hypertension and diabetes are common to both cardiac and renal disease. Aspects of chronic renal failure such as hypertension, hyperlipidemia, secondary hyperparathyroidism, and dialysis accelerate atherosclerosis.[169] Renal failure requiring dialysis after cardiac surgery greatly increases mortality.[170] Cardiac surgery risk models also list preoperative dialysis as a significant risk factor.[50,51,57] The recent noncardiac surgery Revised Cardiac Risk Index lists elevated serum creatinine as a significant risk factor for adverse events.[42] Renal insufficiency and chronic renal failure are therefore significant preoperative risk factors. Surgery can contribute to worsened renal function because of blood or fluid loss[171] or increased intraabdominal pressure,[172,173] or major renal stresses such as aortic cross-clamping for aortic aneurysm repair and cardiopulmonary bypass. Yet even in carotid endarterectomy renal insufficiency increases risk.[174]

Renal Failure After Cardiac Surgery. A large study of 43,642 patients who underwent coronary bypass or valve surgery at 43 Veterans Affairs medical centers identified preoperative risk factors that were predictive of postoperative acute renal failure (ARF) requiring dialysis.[175] Overall, the risk of ARF was 0.9% for coronary patients and 2.0% for valve patients. Patients who developed ARF requiring dialysis had an overall operative mortality of 63.7% versus a 4.3% mortality in patients without this complication. The risks of postoperative MI, reoperation for bleeding, and mediastinitis were higher in patients who developed ARF. Independent predictors of postoperative ARF were determined[175,176] (Table 1-19).

Another study of 24 U.S. medical centers identified five preoperative risk factors for renal insufficiency after CABG: advanced age, CHF, prior CABG, elevated serum glucose, and elevated serum creatinine. Patients

who developed renal insufficiency (not dialysis) after CABG had intensive care unit and hospital stays twice as long as patients who did not develop renal insufficiency.[177] Preoperative blood urea nitrogen (BUN) has also been described as a risk factor for mortality after CABG surgery.[178]

Cardiac Surgery in Dialysis Patients. A large study examined dialysis-dependent renal failure patients undergoing CABG surgery.[179] Preoperatively, the 279 patients with renal failure had more severe cardiac disease (MI, CHF, unstable angina) and medical problems (diabetes, COPD, vascular disease) than the other 15,271 patients. Postoperatively, renal failure patients had higher mortality and increased incidence of stroke and mediastinitis. This relationship was maintained even after adjustment for preoperative risk characteristics. The incidence of reexploration for bleeding was not statistically different[179] (Table 1-20). It should be noted that troponin levels are known to be higher in dialysis patients than in patients with renal insufficiency not on

TABLE 1-19
Independent Risk Factors for Acute Renal Failure Requiring Dialysis after Cardiac Surgery

PARAMETER	OR
Valvular surgery	1.98
Creatinine clearance (ml/min)	
>100	1.00
80-100	1.31
60-80	1.81
40-60	3.38
<40	5.80
Intraaortic balloon pump	3.19
Reoperation	1.93
NYHA class IV	1.55
Peripheral vascular disease	1.51
Ejection fraction <35%	1.45
Pulmonary rales	1.37
COPD	1.26
Systolic BP (mm Hg)	
120-139	1.00
140-159	1.27
<120 valve surgery	1.42
<120 CABG surgery	0.72
≥160 valve surgery	1.03
≥160 CABG surgery	1.98

From Chertow GM, Lazarus JM, Christiansen CL, et al: *Circulation* 95:878-884, 1997.
BP, Blood pressure; *CABG,* coronary artery bypass graft; *COPD,* chronic obstructive pulmonary disease; *NYHA,* New York Heart Association; *OR,* odds ratio.

	NONRENAL FAILURE	RENAL FAILURE
Number of patients	15,271	279
Age (yr)	64.8	66.7
Male gender (%)	72.0	66.3
Preoperative Characteristics		
COPD	11.8%	27.2%
Diabetes	28.2%	48.0%
Peripheral vascular disease	12.5%	40.9%
Liver disease	0.4%	1.1%
Preoperative Cardiac Profile		
Ejection fraction	53.5%	47.6%
LVEDP	16.9 mm Hg	20.0 mm Hg
CHF	12.4%	37.3%
Prior myocardial infarction	50.8%	65.5%
Unstable angina	48.1%	57.7%
Intravenous nitroglycerin	20.1%	28.7%
Postoperative Outcomes		
In-hospital mortality	3.0%	12.2%
Mediastinitis	1.2%	3.6%
Stroke	1.7%	4.3%
Bleeding	2.9%	3.6%

From Liu JY, Birkmeyer NJO, Sanders JH et al: *Circulation* 102:2973, 2000.
CABG, Coronary artery bypass graft; *CHF,* congestive heart failure; *COPD,* chronic obstructive pulmonary disease; *LVEDP,* left ventricular end-diastolic pressure.

dialysis. Still, troponin levels are considered a useful predictor of cardiac events in dialysis patients.[180]

Valvular Heart Disease

The presence of valvular heart disease has implications for management, monitoring, and endocarditis antibiotic prophylaxis.[181-184] Symptoms and signs of valvular heart disease include history of heart murmur, exertional dyspnea, palpitations, fatigue, chest pain, family history of heart disease or early death, and history of rheumatic fever.[185,186] Syncope may occur from aortic stenosis.[187,188] The patient's awareness of an exaggerated, bounding pulse suggests aortic insufficiency.[189] Hemoptysis or evidence of systemic emboli is suggestive of mitral stenosis.[190] Chronic mitral or aortic re-

gurgitation can be moderate to severe without significant symptoms. In contrast, similar degrees of *acute* insufficiency cause severe symptoms (e.g., papillary muscle dysfunction or endocarditis). Cardiac surgery for mitral valve replacement (MVR) is considered higher risk than aortic valve replacement (AVR).[191,192] When cardiac surgery is valve replacement *with* CABG, operative mortality of MVR plus CABG is substantially higher than that for AVR plus CABG. However, for noncardiac surgery, only valvular aortic stenosis increases the incidence of postoperative adverse cardiac outcome.[21,22,32,33]

Aortic Stenosis. Aortic stenosis can be congenital or acquired. A congenital bicuspid aortic valve is commonly not obstructive in childhood but becomes stenotic as fibrosis and calcification occur later in life. Acquired aortic stenosis from rheumatic heart disease is characterized by fusion of the valve commissures leaving a small triangular opening that is often insufficient as well as stenotic. In acquired degenerative calcific aortic stenosis, calcium deposition on the leaflets restricts opening but the commissures are not fused.[193]

Adults with an aortic stenosis murmur may be asymptomatic for years because progressive concentric LVH compensates for the outflow obstruction.[187,194] In the sixth decade of life, symptoms of angina, syncope, and CHF occur. Without operative treatment, survival is limited to 5 years or less[194,195] (Fig. 1-4). This progression of severity explains the difference between the Goldman and Detsky cardiac risk indexes concerning aortic stenosis. Goldman used only a characteristic grade 2 of 6 systolic murmur to define aortic stenosis, whereas Detsky required evidence for suspected critical aortic stenosis (e.g., syncope). Thus aortic stenosis was a minor risk factor for Goldman but a major factor for Detsky.[21,22,32,33]

The reduced left ventricular compliance of LVH requires increased filling pressure and sinus rhythm to maintain adequate preload. Maximal coronary vasodilation may be required to maintain adequate resting blood flow to the hypertrophied myocardium.[196] Patients with long-standing aortic stenosis may experience angina despite normal coronary arteries.[197] Hypovolemia, anemia, and dysrhythmias are poorly tolerated. Chest compressions for cardiopulmonary resusitation (CPR) in patients with aortic stenosis are less effective than in patients without aortic stenosis.

Echocardiographic and exercise predictors have been found to be useful prognostic indicators in asymptomatic aortic stenosis patients. Patients with an aortic valve jet velocity <3.0 m/sec were unlikely to develop symptoms from aortic stenosis over a subsequent 5 year period. Patients with a jet velocity >4.0 m/sec had greater than a 50% incidence of developing symptoms or death in 2 years.[198]

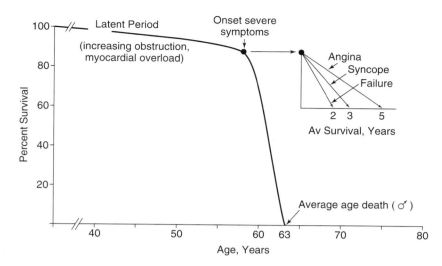

FIG. 1-4   Average course of valvular aortic stenosis in adults. Data assembled from post-mortem studies.

(From Ross J, Braunwald E: *Circulation* 38[suppl V]:61, 1968.)

Aortic Insufficiency. Left ventricular filling occurs from the left atrium and from the aorta in patients with aortic insufficiency. Chronic volume overload causes left ventricular dilation. Net forward cardiac flow is the difference between the forward stroke volume and the backward regurgitant volume. Determination of cardiac output by thermodilution is valid in aortic insufficiency because right ventricular output equals net left ventricular forward flow. The regurgitant volume depends on the size of the regurgitant orifice, the diastolic time, and the pressure difference between the aorta and left ventricle during diastole.[200] Regurgitation causes the aortic diastolic pressure to decline and the left ventricular pressure to rise, thus decreasing coronary perfusion pressure. Aortic insufficiency reduces the effectiveness of antegrade cardioplegia[201] during cardiac surgery and causes left ventricular distention if a left ventricular vent is not used.

Echocardiographic measures have improved follow-up prognosis in asymptomatic patients with aortic insufficiency. A left ventricular end systolic dimension of greater than or equal to 55 mm or an LVEF less than 55% predicts poor prognosis.[199,202]

Mitral Stenosis. A narrowed mitral orifice creates a pressure gradient between the left atrium and the left ventricle. Left atrial dilation and reduced left ventricular filling lead to decreased cardiac output and pulmonary vascular congestion. Tachycardia shortens the diastolic time for flow through the mitral valve, and worsens pulmonary vascular congestion and systemic hypotension. Atrial fibrillation is poorly tolerated because of tachycardia *and* loss of atrial contraction.[203,204] Although elevated left atrial pressure can cause dyspnea, a key point is that the left atrial pressure must be sufficient to force blood across the stenotic mitral orifice for left ventricular filling. Preoperative diuretics are poorly tolerated during anesthesia because they increase the risk

of inadequate left ventricular filling. Peripheral vasodilation is also poorly tolerated in mitral stenosis because the cardiac output cannot promptly increase to compensate. Thus afterload reduction is not likely to improve cardiac output in patients with mitral stenosis, in contrast to its demonstrated effectiveness in patients with MR.[205] Some improvement in cardiac output may occur with gentle vasodilation, suggesting the presence of vasoconstriction in mitral stenosis.[206]

Patients with long-standing mitral stenosis may develop pulmonary hypertension, right ventricular hypertrophy or failure, and tricuspid insufficiency. Rheumatic fever also affects the myocardium. The rigid "mitral valve complex" including chordae tendineae and papillary muscles immoblizes the posterobasal myocardial region.[207] Thus MVR for long-standing mitral stenosis provides a significant anesthetic challenge.

Mitral Insufficiency. Appropriate mitral valve function requires coordination of all six components of the mitral value complex: the left atrial wall, annulus, leaflets, chordae tendineae, papillary muscles, and left ventricular wall.[208] The left atrium is markedly enlarged and compliant in patients with chronic mitral insufficiency.[209] A significant mitral insufficiency jet can be accommodated by the compliant left atrium without a significant increase in left atrial pressure. Patients with chronic mitral insufficiency may be relatively asymptomatic, although limited in their ability to exercise. In contrast, acute MR into a small and noncompliant atrium causes large increases in left atrial pressure (V waves) and pulmonary vascular congestion.[210] The differences in left atrial compliance explain the lack of correlation between the presence and height of V waves and the degree of mitral insufficiency.[211-213]

The left ventricle has two outlets for ejection in patients with mitral insufficiency: the aorta and the incompetent mitral valve. Thus a "normal" ejection fraction does not necessarily indicate normal left ventricular function.[214,215] MVR eliminates the "low-resistance" outlet and may unmask ventricular dysfunction. Afterload reduction with vasodilator therapy is important for patients with mitral insufficiency.[216] An intraaortic balloon pump is ideal therapy because it provides afterload reduction *and* augments coronary perfusion pressure.

Vascular Disease

Patients undergoing vascular surgery have long been recognized as having increased risk for adverse cardiac outcome.[28,29,217] In 1982, Hertzer reported a 6- to 11-year follow-up on 273 consecutive patients who had undergone lower extremity vascular surgery. Coronary disease and MI accounted for half of the early postoperative deaths and half of the late mortalities.[218] Waters and Jeffrey et al demonstrated that the Goldman CRI underestimated the risk of adverse cardiac outcome when applied to populations of patients undergoing abdominal aortic vascular surgery[28,29] (Table 1-21).

Some investigators routinely performed coronary angiography in vascular surgery patients to better define coronary risk.[219-221] The largest study was that of Hertzer et al in 1984, which included 1000 patients before elective vascular surgery.[220] A 70% stenosis of at least one coronary artery was found in more than half of the patients. Operable coronary disease was mostly found in patients with suspected cardiac disease but was also found in some patients who had no evidence of prior MI, angina, or ECG abnormality. Coronary disease was found in patients with abdominal aortic aneurysm, lower extremity ischemia, and cerebrovascular disease.[220]

TABLE 1-21
Prospective Evaluation of Goldman Index in Abdominal Aortic Surgery Patients

GOLDMAN CLASS	NO. OF PATIENTS	GOLDMAN PREDICTION NUMBER EVENTS	ACTUAL EVENTS FOUND
1	56	0-1 (1%)*	4 (7%)
2	35	2-3 (7%)	4 (11%)
3	8	1 (14%)	3 (38%)

From Jeffrey CC, Kunsman J, Cullen DJ et al: *Anesthesiology* 55:A343, 1981.
*The number in parentheses is the percentage of patients in the class that the Cardiac Risk Index predicted would have an adverse event. For the 56 patients in Goldman Class I, the CRI predicted 1% incidence of adverse events (0-1 events). Note that the actual number of events was higher for each Goldman class.

Similar coronary angiography findings were demonstrated in a series of 506 patients with extracranial cerebrovascular disease.[221] In a follow-up of carotid endarterectomy surgery, cardiac problems accounted for 72% of late deaths.[222] Similar findings occurred in a follow-up of 500 patients with asymptomatic carotid bruits. Stroke caused three deaths, but MI accounted for 27.[79] Sirna et al warned that MI is the leading cause of death in patients with asymptomatic bruits, TIA, and ischemic cerebrovascular accidents, and they recommended assessment for coronary artery disease in all patients with ischemic cerebrovascular disease.[84]

Two large studies of patients with vascular and coronary artery disease have been reported by Rihal et al.[223,224] A 1995 analysis focused on a subgroup of Coronary Artery Surgery Study (CASS) patients who had both coronary and vascular disease.[223] *Vascular disease* was defined as "peripheral" by a history of intermittent claudication or absent peripheral pulses, or "cerebrovascular" by a history of TIAs or stroke. These 1834 patients underwent either CABG surgery or medical management of their coronary artery disease. For the CABG patients with vascular disease, perioperative mortality was 4.2%. This was higher than the 2.9% mortality noted for other CASS patients without vascular disease who underwent CABG. However, the most important observation of the study was that patients with vascular disease who received CABG had better long-term outcomes (follow-up of 10.4 years) than those managed medically. The respective estimated probabilities of 4-, 8-, 12-, and 16-year survival rates were 88%, 72%, 55%, and 41% after CABG and 73%, 57%, 44%, and 34% for medical management. An analysis of subgroups showed that these survival benefits of surgery were limited to patients with three-vessel coronary disease and were inversely related to ejection fraction.[223]

The second series assessed a subgroup of 550 patients with coronary and vascular disease from the BARI who underwent either CABG surgery or PTCA for their coronary artery disease.[224] Vascular patients included 268 patients with lower extremity disease and 349 patients with cerebrovascular disease who were treated with either CABG surgery or PTCA. For patients treated with PTCA, the risk of a major complication (e.g., death, MI, stroke, coma, emergency CABG) was 11.7% for patients with vascular disease, compared with 7.8% for patients without vascular disease. This included an increased incidence of abrupt closure of the dilated vessel. For patients treated with CABG surgery, the risk of major complications in patients with vascular disease was 12%, markedly higher than the 6.1% risk for patients without vascular disease. Within the group of CABG patients with vascular disease, those with carotid disease had a higher incidence of neurologic complications than those with lower extremity disease (6.2% vs. 1.3%). Neurologic complications occurred both in patients with prior neurologic symptoms (2.1% incidence) and in those without prior symptoms (1.7% incidence).[224]

For noncardiac surgery, preoperative exercise testing and assessment of functional status may be limited in vascular patients because of claudication.[225,226] Effective risk stratification for such patients by the thallium dipyridamole scan was a major advancement. Such noninvasive tests have had major applications for preoperative cardiac risk assessment of vascular patients. The 1996 AHA/ACC guidelines for preoperative assessment categorize major and peripheral vascular surgery as high-risk operations.[1] Thus all patients with intermediate predictors (mild angina, prior MI, compensated CHF, diabetes) are recommended for noninvasive testing before vascular surgery. Patients with minor predictors (advanced age, abnormal ECG, nonsinus rhythm, low functional capacity, stroke history, uncontrolled hypertension) are also recommended for noninvasive testing before vascular surgery if their exercise tolerance is poor.[1] One study determined that the long-term (50-month) cardiac event-free survival after vascular surgery was similar for men and women.[227]

Chest Discomfort

In noncardiac surgery patients, chest discomfort symptoms should be stable. In patients scheduled for coronary bypass surgery, a history of increasing symptoms is expected. However, a significant change in symptoms could occur in either setting and represent an unstable condition that requires attention. Recognizing and differentiating angina pectoris from noncardiac causes is of major importance.

Distinction of Angina. The causes of chest discomfort range from benign conditions such as gastric hyperacidity to critical conditions such as acute MI. Identification of angina is challenging, and some myocardial ischemia is clinically silent.[228] Differentiating angina pectoris from noncardiac causes of chest discomfort can be made by assessing quality, location, timing, duration, provoking and relieving factors, and associated symptoms.[229,230]

The *quality* of the discomfort is a key characteristic. The term *angina* means "choking" or "tightening" rather than pain.[229] *Levine's sign* is described as a patient holding a clenched fist in front of the sternum. This is a strong indicator of angina. In diabetic patients with neuropathy or cardiac transplant patients, these symptoms may be absent. Another symptom such as dyspnea may be their "angina equivalent." Sharp, jabbing, or knifelike pain is not usually indicative of angina.

The *location* of angina is generally midchest or substernal.[229] Sensory transmission occurs via sympathetic afferent nerves rather than somatic nerves. Anginal discomfort is therefore diffuse rather than specifically localized. Pain localized to a particular site, such as the left breast, may be attributable to noncardiac causes. Radiation of anginal pain usually extends to the left side of the chest and ulnar aspect of the left arm, although radiation to the jaw, epigastrium, back, and right side of the chest can occur. A recent study attempted to correlate the location of chest pain to the site of coronary occlusion. The occluded artery could not reliably be identified.[231]

The *duration* of angina is brief, approximately 2 to 10 minutes.[229] Pain that is very brief (seconds) is not suggestive of angina. Prolonged pain (hours) may indicate infarction. Recent guidelines from the ACC/AHA report that chest pain of 20 minutes' duration may represent an acute coronary syndrome such as MI or unstable angina. Such patients should be evaluated immediately by a physician and a 12-lead ECG performed.[232]

Factors that *provoke* angina are exertion and other stresses such as cold exposure, walking against the wind, meals, or emotional stress. Activities such as shoveling snow, mowing the lawn, walking briskly, and climbing stairs are provocative. Relief usually occurs with cessation of the activity. Severe coronary artery disease is suggested when angina occurs with progressively less exertion. Angina that occurs at rest is considered unstable and demands prompt evaluation.[229,230] Printzmetal's angina (variant angina) representing coronary vasospasm differs from classic angina in that it can occur at rest or during the early morning hours of sleep.[232,233]

Pain occuring after exercise or in certain body positions is not suggestive of angina. Pain that occurs with a deep inspiration or with coughing may represent a pleural or diaphragmatic cause or pulmonary embolism. Pain elicited by applying pressure over a rib, sternum, or cartilage is consistent with a musculoskeletal etiology.[229,230]

Anginal pain is typically relieved with rest and sublingual nitroglycerin. However, nitroglycerin is also effective for relief of pain associated with esophageal spasm. Pain relief with food, antacids, H_2 antagonists, or belching suggests a gastrointestinal etiology. Pericardial pain improves with leaning the patient forward. Pain relief with antiinflammatory analgesics suggests a musculoskeletal etiology or pericarditis.[229,230]

Associated symptoms such as diaphoresis, syncope, nausea, dyspnea, or pallor may be indicative of an MI. Other possibilities, such as pulmonary embolism or pneumothorax, are considered when the onset of chest discomfort is abrupt and occurs with dyspnea. The presence of a fever suggests other diagnoses such as pneumonia or pericarditis.[229,230]

Mimics of Angina. A number of conditions resemble the chest discomfort of angina pectoris[234] because of

TABLE 1-22
Chest Pain Conditions Resembling Angina Pectoris

ETIOLOGY	DURATION	QUALITY	PROVOCATION	RELIEF	LOCATION
Mitral prolapse	Minutes to hours	Superficial variable	Spontaneous	Time	Left anterior
Esophageal reflux	10 min-1 hr	Visceral, rarely radiates	Recumbency, lack of food	Food, antacid	Substernal epigastric
Esophageal spasm	5-60 min	Visceral, mimics angina	Spontaneous, cold liquids, exercise	Nitroglycerin	Substernal radiates
Peptic ulcer	Hours	Visceral burning	Lack of food, "acid" foods	Food, antacids	Epigastric substernal
Biliary disease	1 hr	Visceral (wax and wane) colic	Spontaneous food	Time, analgesia	Epigastric ? radiates
Cervical disc	Variable (gradually subsides)	Superficial, not relieved by rest	Head and neck movement, palpation	Time, analgesics	Arm, neck
Hyperventilation	2-3 min	Visceral with facial paresthesia	Emotion tachypnea	Stimulus removal	Substernal
Musculoskeletal	Variable	Superficial, tenderness	Movement palpation	Time, analgesia	Multiple sites
Pulmonary disease	>30 min	Visceral (pressure) with dyspnea	Often spontaneous	Rest, time, bronchodilator	Substernal

From Christie LG, Conti CR: *Am Heart J* 102:897, 1981.

common sympathetic pathways, interconnecting in cervical and thoracic ganglia. Pain of cardiac origin is perceived within a T1 to T6 dermatomal band. Shared ascending pathways means that left arm pain is *not* pathognomonic of angina but may occur from other visceral organs.[235] Nitroglycerin relieves pain caused by either angina or esophageal spasm, another T1 to T6 dermatomal condition known to mimic angina pectoris. The various conditions that mimic angina can be organized according to quality, location, duration, provocation, and relief of symptoms[234-237] (Table 1-22).

Unstable Angina. An acute coronary syndrome should be considered when anginal symptoms are greater than 20 minutes' duration. These symptoms may represent either unstable angina or acute MI.[232] Unstable angina and non–ST-segment elevation myocardial infarction (NSTEMI) represent an imbalance of myocardial oxygen demand and supply. The most common cause is a nonocclusive thrombus originating from a disrupted atherosclerotic coronary artery plaque.[238,239] The distinction between unstable angina and NSTEMI is determined by the release of myocardial enzymes (troponin I, troponin T, creatine kinase-MB isoenzyme), indicating myocardial damage. NSTEMI is associated with enzyme release, whereas unstable angina is not. A patient with symptoms of an acute coronary syndrome should be immediately referred to an emergency

department for ECG assessment. Findings consistent with acute MI make the patient eligible for reperfusion therapy.[232]

Unstable angina has five possible causes.[240] An important concept is that unstable angina may represent a combination of these five factors. The most common cause is reduced myocardial perfusion resulting from a nonocclusive thrombus originating from a recently fissured or eroded plaque that previously had been only mildly or moderately occlusive. Therapy focuses on antithrombotic treatment, such as unfractionated heparin and low-molecular-weight heparin, and antiplatelet medications, such as aspirin, ticlopidine, or glycoprotein IIb/IIIa inhibitors. The second cause of unstable angina is a dynamic obstruction caused by coronary vasoconstriction. Treatment includes nitrates and calcium antagonists. The third form of unstable angina represents severe progressive luminal narrowing as may occur during restenosis after PTCA. Treatment focuses on mechanical therapy such as transluminal or surgical revascularization. The fourth form of unstable angina involves an inflammatory or infectious etiology. Potential pathogens include *Chlamydia pneumoniae*, virulent strains of *Helicobacter pylori*, herpes simplex virus, and cytomegalovirus. Elevation of inflammation markers such as C-reactive protein is associated with a poor prognosis in patients with unstable angina. The fifth cause of unstable angina represents extrinsic conditions

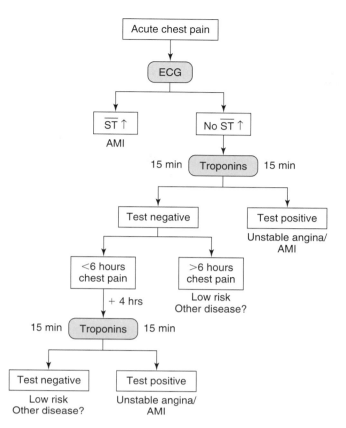

FIG. 1-5   Algorithm to risk stratify patients with unstable angina based on electrocardiogram (ECG) and repeated troponin measurements. If ST-segment elevation is excluded, serial testing for troponin allows identification of subgroups with different risk. *AMI,* Acute myocardial infarction.

(From Hamm CW, Braunwald E: *Circulation* 102:118, 2000.)

TABLE 1-23
Pulmonary versus Cardiovascular Causes of Dyspnea

PULMONARY	CARDIOVASCULAR
Upper Airway	**Valvular**
Sleep apnea	Mitral stenosis or regurgitation
Vascular ring	Aortic stenosis or regurgitation
Lower Airway	**Congenital**
Asthma	Patent ductus arteriosus
Bronchitis	Atrioventricular canal, ventricular
Emphysema	septal defect
	Cyanotic lesions
Alveolar	
Pneumonia	**Myocardial**
	Myocardial ischemia
Interstitial	Cardiomyopathy, hypertrophy
Pulmonary fibrosis	Congestive failure, diastolic
Sarcoidosis	dysfunction
Pulmonary edema	
	Vascular
Other	Fluid overload
Myasthenia gravis	Pulmonary hypertension
Scoliosis	Anemia
Obesity	Pulmonary embolism

that cause an imbalance of myocardial oxygen supply and demand. Increased demand occurs with fever, tachycardia, sympathetic stimulation, and hypertension. Decreased supply occurs with tachycardia, hypotension, anemia, and hypoxemia. This fifth etiology of unstable angina is a major factor during the perioperative period. β-Adrenergic blockade is therefore an important component of perioperative therapy.[240]

A clinical risk stratification scheme for patients with unstable angina was proposed by Braunwald in 1989.[241] This was based on the clinical history, presence or absence of ECG changes, and the intensity of antiischemia treatment. Several studies validated this classification method.[242,243] More recently, an updated classification scheme has been proposed (Fig. 1-5) based on ECG and troponin information.

Dyspnea

Etiology. Dyspnea is "an uncomfortable sensation of breathing"[245] and may be an indicator of significant cardiac or pulmonary disease.[246,247] A history

of dyspnea is associated with increased mortality from cardiovascular,[248-250] pulmonary,[251] and other causes.[252] The patient with dyspnea warrants further evaluation to elucidate a cardiac or pulmonary etiology (Table 1-23). Because the cardiac and pulmonary systems are interdependent, signs and symptoms often overlap.[253] The infant with respiratory signs of tachypnea and nasal flaring may have primary congenital cardiac disease such as atrioventricular (AV) canal or ventricular septal defect (VSD) causing pulmonary congestion.[254] Although wheezing is typical of asthma, airway edema from CHF can cause "cardiac asthma." Exertional dyspnea may occur from myocardial ischemia but is also characteristic of the asthmatic patient with bronchospasm.

A pulmonary cause of dyspnea is suggested by the presence of a chronic productive cough, smoking history, bronchodilator use, or known history of restrictive or obstructive lung disease. Chronic coughing in a smoker suggests chronic bronchitis, whereas in a young nonsmoker, recurrent cough may be the sole presenting symptom of asthma.[255] Cough is also associated with ACE inhibitor medications.[256]

The chest X-ray film and ECG provide important information to differentiate the cause of dyspnea. Cardiomegaly and pulmonary vascular congestion are suggestive of a cardiac cause, whereas hyperinflation of the lung fields and a normal-sized heart are suggestive of a pulmonary cause. Pulmonary function tests and echocardiography provide even more specific information. Doppler echocardiographic assessment is useful to identify diastolic dysfunction when systolic function is normal.

A trial of bronchodilator,[257] diuretic, or antibiotic therapy may help clarify the cause of dyspnea. If the cause of dyspnea is still uncertain, exercise testing may be useful.[246,253,258,259] The cardiac patient will discontinue exercise because of muscular fatigue and lactic acidosis before he or she reaches maximum ventilatory capacity. The pulmonary patient will stop because maximum ventilatory capacity is reached and gas exchange is insufficient to sustain exercise demands.[253]

Cardiac Dyspnea. Cardiac dyspnea usually occurs because of pulmonary vascular congestion resulting from elevated left atrial and pulmonary venous pressure.[260] The increased hydrostatic pressure forces fluid into the interstitial space of the lung, reducing pulmonary compliance and increasing the effort of breathing. Elevated left atrial pressure can occur in a variety of circumstances, including myocardial ischemia, LVH, diastolic dysfunction, mitral stenosis and cor triatriatum, mitral or aortic insufficiency, and fluid overload. Congenital heart lesions with excessive pulmonary blood flow and congenital obstructed pulmonary venous drainage can also cause pulmonary congestion.

Dyspnea without pulmonary congestion can also be present in patients with cyanotic congenital heart disease.[261-263] During a cyanotic "spell" in a patient with tetrology of Fallot, dyspnea occurs when pulmonary blood flow is reduced (right-to-left shunt through a VSD). Squatting reestablishes pulmonary flow and the spell resolves. Dyspnea without pulmonary congestion can also occur in patients with a fixed low cardiac output such as right ventricular failure.

The circumstances associated with dyspnea are useful for making a diagnosis.[264] The presence of lower extremity edema indicates an etiology of CHF. Patients with valvular heart disease often have a murmur, palpitations, and exertional fatigue. Sudden onset of dyspnea may indicate pulmonary embolism, pneumothorax, dysrhythmia such as atrial fibrillation, or acute pulmonary edema from severe myocardial ischemia. Abrupt onset of dyspnea when assuming a particular position may be consistent with a left atrial myxoma. In contrast, dyspnea from CHF is chronic and slowly progressive. *Orthopnea* is the onset of dyspnea with a recumbent position. In patients with CHF, redistribution of blood from the extremities to central circulation precipitates pulmonary congestion. Worsening heart failure is indicated by a progressive increase in the number of pillows

used to sleep. *Paroxysmal nocturnal dyspnea* (PND) is a common symptom in patients with CHF. Several hours after going to bed, the patient is awakened by dyspnea and anxiety. Sitting upright at the side of the bed or at an open window causes gradual resolution over 20 to 30 minutes. Proposed mechanisms of PND include reabsorption of lower body edema fluid causing pulmonary congestion.

Noncardiac disorders can also cause orthopnea such as obesity, pleural effusion, and COPD. Patients with COPD may awaken at night to cough to clear bronchial secretions. *Nocturia* may also indicate the presence of heart failure. During daytime activity, renal vasoconstriction reduces urine output, whereas during the night, renal excretion resumes, leading to nocturia. Prostate hypertrophy may also cause nocturia, but this can usually be elucidated by careful history-taking.

A key aspect of the preoperative evaluation is to ascertain whether dyspnea occurs when the patient experiences angina. Ischemia decreases ventricular compliance as a result of impaired ventricular relaxation. If a sufficient amount of myocardium is affected, LVEDP rises and leads to pulmonary congestion. Dyspnea associated with myocardial ischemia suggests that a large portion of the myocardium is involved. Other confirming signs include increased PCWP and increased LVEDP during cardiac catheterization. The finding of dyspnea during angina indicates ventricular dysfunction and may warrant intraoperative monitoring with a pulmonary artery catheter.

Obstructive Sleep Apnea. Finally, an important syndrome of disordered respiration is that of obstructive sleep apnea (OSA), which is estimated to affect 2% to 4% of the U.S. adult population.[265-267] Dyspnea may not be recognized because obstructed breathing occurs during sleep. Daytime somnolence occurs because of interrupted sleep. Observation by a family member of prominent snoring, and particularly, apneic episodes during sleep, is significant. Clinical features may not reliably distinguish patients with OSA from those without OSA.[268] Obstructive sleep apnea is associated with pulmonary hypertension[269] and coronary artery disease.[270] A history of snoring has been implicated as a risk factor in ischemic heart disease.[271]

Edema

Edema is a swelling of the skin caused by an excess accumulation of interstitial fluid.[272] Causes of peripheral edema include water and salt retention as in CHF, a reduction in albumin as in renal disease or poor nutrition, and obstruction of venous or lymphatic drainage. Because the location of the edema is influenced by gravity, ambulatory patients may describe difficulty in putting on shoes. Associated symptoms are helpful for differentiating cardiac causes from noncardiac causes. Edema with dyspnea indicates CHF with pulmonary congestion. Cardiac causes of edema without dyspnea include tricuspid valve disease, pericardial effusion, and constrictive pericarditis. Edema with jaundice indicates hepatic involvement. Passive hepatic congestion can occur from right-sided heart dysfunction, but edema and jaundice may also occur in patients with primary liver disease such as cirrhosis. Renal disease such as nephrotic syndrome or glomerulonephritis can produce edema of the face and eyes. Facial edema can also occur with obstruction of the superior vena cava (SVC syndrome) caused by aneurysm of the ascending aorta or lung cancer. Angioneurotic edema is associated with medications such as ACE inhibitors, stress, or certain food allergies. A Glenn shunt for congenital heart disease or severe hypothyroidism, known as *myxedema*, can also cause facial edema. When localized to one extremity, the cause of edema is usually obstruction of lymphatic drainage or venous thrombosis. Edema of the legs associated with chronic skin ulcers occurs with chronic venous insufficiency.[273] The menstrual cycle causes mild cyclical edema.

Gastrointestinal Problems

Some cardiac patients are prone to gastrointestinal problems. Adult patients with congenital heart disease and polycythemia develop gallstones, which are a common cause for surgery.[274] Heart transplant recipients with chronic steroid immunosuppression are at risk for ulcer disease and bowel perforation.[275] A variety of gastrointestinal conditions may also coexist with cardiac disease, such as hiatal hernia and esophageal reflux. An unusual circumstance is the liver transplant recipient who requires cardiac surgery.[276]

Gastroesophageal Reflux. Aspiration of gastric contents remains a significant risk for general anesthesia. Mortality estimates for aspiration in general surgical patients[277] underestimate the risk for patients with cardiac disease. Preoperative identification of risk factors is important. Insulin-dependent diabetic patients and patients who experience stress have delayed gastric emptying. The patient presenting for cardiac transplantation may not have satisfactory NPO (nothing-by-mouth) status. The patient emergently arriving to the operating room after a prolonged catheterization laboratory procedure may also be a risk for aspiration. Nausea may accompany ischemia of the right coronary artery.

Jaundice. Jaundice occurs in the cardiac patient as a result of: liver congestion, as in CHF, pericarditis, or

tricuspid valve disease; hemolysis caused by malfunctioning prosthetic heart valve or paravalvular leak; or bile stones; it may also occur after cardiopulmonary bypass.[278-282] A history of jaundice raises concern for primary liver disease, viral hepatitis, or a drug or toxin etiology. Although distinctly unusual, jaundice following general anesthesia may represent hepatic sensitivity to halogenated anesthetic agents. Perioperative blood transfusion is another consideration. The presence of significant ascites suggests liver disease, but lesser amounts of ascites can occur with CHF, constrictive pericarditis, and renal disease.

Dysphagia. The frequent intraoperative use of transesophageal echocardiography (TEE) makes preoperative identification of swallowing problems essential. In cases such as mitral valve repair, in which intraoperative TEE is essential, a history suggestive of esophageal stricture requires a preoperative barium swallow radiograph and possible esophageal dilation. The pediatric cardiac patient with a history of tracheoesophageal fistula has increased risk associated with use of intraoperative TEE. Intraoperative TEE use is associated with postoperative dysphagia and pulmonary aspiration.[283] Preoperative identification of problems will benefit postoperative assessment.

Syncope

Syncope is a transient loss of consciousness associated with the inability to maintain an upright posture. Determination of the cause can be challenging and expensive.[284] Although many patients may describe "feeling faint" during illness, an actual loss of consciousness is not common. In the Framingham Study, 3% of men and women experienced syncope.[285] Another study of 3000 healthy Air Force personnel found that 7% had experienced at least one episode of syncope.[286] Most episodes are benign. However, because syncope may be the presenting symptom of serious cardiovascular disease, evaluation is important. A review of six population-based studies found that, overall, the history and physical examination can identify the cause of syncope in 45% of patients[284] (Box 1-10).

Postural symptoms usually indicate etiologies that include medications, orthostatic, or vasovagal syncope. One study implicated antihypertensive and antidepressant drugs as the most common medication causes of syncope.[287] β-Blockade may also be a causative factor. Postictal symptoms usually indicate a neurologic cause. Observation of a seizure establishes the diagnosis. A noncardiac cause is suspected when syncope occurs during hyperventilation, anxiety, coughing, urination, swallowing, or abrupt or prolonged standing.[288,289]

A cardiac cause is suspected when syncope occurs

Cardiovascular Etiology
Heart Disease (associated with exertion, dyspnea, chest
   pain, family history, murmur)
Aortic stenosis
Hypertrophic obstructive cardiomyopathy
Pulmonary hypertension
Myxoma
Anomalous coronary anatomy
Myocardial infarction
Pulmonary embolism

Dysrhythmia (associated with palpitations or
   slow pulse)
Heart block (congenital or acquired)
Sick sinus syndrome
Long QT interval
Accessory pathway (e.g., Wolff-Parkinson-White
   syndrome)
Ventricular tachycardia
Supraventricular tachycardia
Pacemaker malfunction

Noncardiovascular Etiology
Reflex-Causes (associated with pain, fear, provocative
activity [e.g., neck pressure])
Vasovagal
Cough, micturition, defecation, swallowing
Carotid sinus hypersensitivity

Neurologic (associated with seizure, headache, diplopia)
Migraines
Transient ischemic attack
Seizure
Subclavian steal

Orthostatic (symptoms occur with standing)

Psychiatric (frequent symptoms without injury)

Adapted from Linzer M, Young EH, Estes NA III et al: *Ann Intern
Med* 126:989-996, 1997.

3%.[295] Hypertrophic cardiomyopathy was the most common cause of sudden death in a group of 29 competitive athletes reviewed by Maron et al.[296]

Palpitations and awareness of a slow pulse usually indicate a dysrhythmia, which is a major category among cardiac etiologies.[297] Elderly persons are more likely to acquire sick sinus syndrome. Younger patients are susceptible to tachydysrhythmias in cases of obstructive cardiomyopathy, mitral valve prolapse, prolonged QT interval, and WPW syndrome.[285,298,299] Heart block can be congenital or acquired and occurs in young and elderly patients. Some antidysrhythmic medications may predispose patients to dysrhythmias.[300]

The physical examination in patients with syncope should assess orthostatic changes in blood pressure, abnormalities of the pulse, the presence of a cardiac murmur, presence of a bruit, and abnormalities of carotid upstroke. In one study of patients with syncope, 31% were found to have orthostatic hypotension, defined as a 20-mm Hg decrease in systolic blood pressure with standing.[301] Although carotid sinus massage is a diagnostic tool in elderly patients, the ACP does not recommend this maneuver if carotid bruits are present, if the patient has a history of ventricular tachycardia, or after a recent stroke or MI.[284]

Electrocardiography is recommended by the ACP for almost all patients with syncope.[284] This test provides valuable information for the diagnosis of dysrhythmias, repolarization or conduction abnormalities (WPW and bundle-branch block), MI, and ventricular hypertrophy.[302,303] In 134 patients with hypertrophic cardiomyopathy, normal ECGs were extremely uncommon.[304] In contrast, tests such as electroencephalography, carotid ultrasound, computed tomography (CT) and magnetic resonance imaging (MRI) scans are not recommended except to investigate a history of seizures, carotid bruit, or focal neurologic deficits.[284] A history suggestive of a cardiac cause of syncope warrants further cardiac evaluation. Echocardiography is performed in patients with exertional syncope before exercise stress testing. Syncope can occur in the supine position during pregnancy as a result of aortocaval compression by the uterus in the supine position. Testing for pregnancy is recommended in "obese" women of childbearing age.[284]

Four studies analyzed the outcome of patients evaluated for syncope.[305-308] In up to one third of cases, the etiology was cardiac and included ventricular dysrhythmias; bradycardias, including sick sinus syndrome and heart block; aortic stenosis; supraventricular tachycardia; and MI. The cause of syncope remained unexplained in about half the cases. Mortality after 1 year was increased if syncope resulted from a cardiac cause rather than an unexplained or noncardiac cause. Further workup is therefore indicated for cardiac causes of syn-

during exercise or is associated with a positive family history of cardiac disease or premature sudden death. Examples of cardiac syncope include aortic stenosis,[290] hypertrophic cardiomyopathy,[291] coronary artery disease, pulmonary hypertension,[292] congenital heart disease,[293] prolonged QT syndromes, accessory conduction pathway such as Wolf-Parkinson-White (WPW) syndrome, or anomalous coronary anatomy.[294] Syncope in a younger person is a concern. In patients known to have hypertrophic cardiomyopathy, the annual incidence of premature sudden death is 2% to

cope. Difficult cases may benefit from electrophysiologic and tilt-table studies.

Medications

Patient medications must be reviewed before anesthesia (Box 1-11). Medications such as β-blockers, nitrates, calcium channel blockers, and certain antihypertensive medications are usually continued throughout the perioperative period because abrupt withdrawal may have adverse consequences. Discontinuing β-blocker medications during the perioperative period may precipitate angina and even MI. Abrupt withdrawal of clonidine can cause rebound hypertension.

In some cases, the anesthesiologist may desire to hold or modify medication administration during the perioperative period. Diuretics are commonly withheld because hypovolemia is undesirable during anesthesia and surgery. Intraoperative hypotension may occur with use of ACE inhibitors. The decision to continue or withhold a particular medication must be individualized. Continuation of diuretics or ACE inhibitors may be appropriate under certain circumstances when prescribed for control of CHF.

Anticoagulant medications require special consideration because these agents are usually prescribed to prevent serious cardiovascular consequences.[309-311] Examples include embolic stroke from atrial fibrillation, pulmonary embolism, vascular graft occlusion, and thrombosis of mechanical heart valves. Aspirin, an antiplatelet drug, is also usually prescribed for similar purposes or for prophylactic prevention of stroke. A study of patients with newly implanted coronary stents suggested that the practice of discontinuing antiplatelet medications predisposes patients to serious thrombosis. Patients receiving warfarin are usually prescribed intravenous heparin before planned surgery as warfarin is discontinued. A policy regarding anticoagulant medications requires careful discussion between the anesthesiologist, the prescribing physician, and the surgeon.

Physical Examination

The anesthesiologist performs a *directed physical examination* to focus on specific areas while maintaining a vigilance for subtle clues of other diseases. Specific goals are to identify the presence of cardiac and pulmonary disorders, degree of cardiopulmonary compensation, and indications for cost-effective utilization of further cardiac tests.[312] Information obtained from the physical examination is also necessary for risk assessment by the indexes of Goldman and Detsky and the ACC/AHA guidelines for noncardiac surgery.[313,314] A thorough assessment can identify new diagnoses such as carotid

---

BOX 1-11
Various Preoperative Medications and Their Adverse Perioperative Consequences

Antihypertensive Agents

Clonidine	Rebound hypertension upon withdrawal
MAO inhibitors	Severe interactions with indirect sympathomimetics (e.g., ephedrine)
Diuretic	Hypovolemia, hypokalemia
Reserpine	Catecholamine depletion

Antiischemic Agents

β-Blockers, nitrates, and calcium channel blockers	Potential myocardial ischemia upon withdrawal

Hypoglycemic Agents

Metformin	Serious lactic acidosis, discontinue preoperatively
Insulin	Need provisions to prevent hypoglycemia

Chemotherapy Agents

Adriamycin (doxorubicin)	Cardiac toxicity
Bleomycin	Pulmonary toxicity

Antidysrhythmic Agents

Amiodarone	Pulmonary toxicity, bradycardia
Disopyramide	Myocardial depression
Procainamide	Lupus syndrome

Anticoagulants

Aspirin	Assess risk of thrombosis if discontinued
Antiplatelet medications	Potential major issues for thrombosis of coronary stents if discontinued; possible bleeding if continued.
Warfarin	Requires time, vitamin K, or fresh frozen plasma to reverse; often requires heparin as substitute
Enoxaparin	Poses risk for epidural analgesia

Antiinflammatory Agents

Corticosteroids	Soft tissue enlargement, airway risk; requires perioperative supplementation
Nonsteroidal agents	Ulcer, renal toxicity, platelet dysfunction

Other

Digoxin	Potential toxicity with renal insufficiency
Theophylline	Tachycardia, diuresis

artery disease and valvular heart disease that have significant implications for a patient's long-term health.

Vital Signs

The traditional vital signs, blood pressure, heart rate, respiratory rate, and temperature, are objective measurements that provide quantitative physiologic information. Pulse oximetry is regarded as a vital sign for this discussion.

Blood Pressure. Accurate blood pressure measurement requires an appropriate-sized cuff (see Chapter 3), a comfortable and relaxed patient, and an appreciation of the auscultatory gap. Neither an invasive arterial catheter nor a blood pressure cuff is recognized as more accurate than the other. It is important not to ignore hypotension by either method. Another issue to consider is what is "normal" blood pressure for an individual patient.[157] A blood pressure of 110/60 mm Hg may be *abnormal* for the chronic hypertensive patient whose usual blood pressure is 170/90 mm Hg.

Environmental circumstances (e.g., presence of a physician) may influence blood pressure measurement (white coat hypertension). The finding of significant hypertension directs the physical examination to identify conditions that cause secondary hypertension, such as palpable kidney, abdominal bruit, lability in blood pressure, weight loss, pallor, truncal obesity, pigmented abdominal striae, acromegalic features, absent lower extremity pulses, and differences in blood pressure between the arms and legs.[161-165]

Blood pressure should routinely be measured in both arms. A significant difference can occur because of subclavian stenosis or aortic dissection.[315] Discovery of a potential subclavian stenosis may preclude use of the internal mammary artery on the affected side and warrants Doppler assessment.[316] If blood pressure is low in both arms, an assessment of the femoral pulse is necessary to rule out the unusual case of bilateral subclavian stenosis. In pediatric patients, upper and lower extremity blood pressure are often measured to identify aortic coarctation.

Orthostatic blood pressure measurements are used to identify hypovolemia. Blood pressure is measured with the patient in a supine position and then in a sitting position. A significant drop in blood pressure with the sitting position may indicate reduced venous return because of hypovolemia. Alternatively, elevation of the legs in adults may increase blood pressure in patients with hypovolemia.

Pulsus paradox is a marked change in systolic blood pressure during the cycle of respiration.[273] As the blood pressure cuff is slowly deflated only systolic beats occurring during exhalation are heard initially. As the cuff is further deflated, systolic beats are heard throughout the respiratory cycle. A pulse paradox exists when the difference in cuff inflation pressure between these patterns is significant. The classic description of a paradoxical pulse is associated with cardiac tamponade.[317] However, significant hypovolemia, mediastinal mass, or acute asthma can also produce this finding.

Heart Rate. Heart rate determination is obtained from the ECG, the peripheral pulse, and the pulse oximeter. Because premature atrial or ventricular contractions and certain dysrhythmias may not generate an adequate pulse with every heartbeat, the peripheral pulse rate and pulse oximeter rate may underestimate the true heart rate. Most elective surgical patients have a relatively normal heart rate. The urgent cardiac patient from the cardiac catheterization lab may have had various therapies affecting heart rate, such as medications, electrical pacing, or cardioversion. There are numerous causes for tachycardia and bradycardia. Two points deserve emphasis for the anesthesiologist. First, if bradycardia is present, *hypoxemia must be ruled out.*[318] Second, resting tachycardia should not be dismissed as preoperative anxiety without consideration of other causes (Table 1-24).

TABLE 1-24
Various Causes of Heart Rate Alterations

TACHYCARDIAS	BRADYCARDIAS
Anemia	Aortic stenosis
Anxiety	Bezold-Jarish reflex
Atrial fibrillation	Electrolyte imbalance
Bypass tracts (e.g.,	(hyperkalemia)
Wolff-Parkinson-White	Heart block
syndrome)	Hypertension
Congestive heart failure	Hypothermia
Electrolyte imbalance (hypo-	Hypoxemia
kalemia, premature beats)	Medications (amiodarone,
Fever, malignant	β-blocker, calcium
hyperthermia	channel blocker, digoxin
Hypovolemia	toxicity, cholinesterase
Medications (anticholinergic	inhibitor)
and sympathomimetic)	Sick sinus syndrome
Other drugs (alcohol with-	Intracranial hypertension
drawal, amphetamine,	Vagal reflex
cocaine)	
Pain	
Respiratory insufficiency	
Tamponade	
Thyroid hormone excess	
Vasodilation	
Ventricular tachycardia	

Respiratory Rate. The respiratory rate reflects the status of the cardiac and pulmonary systems. Elevation of left atrial pressure (left ventricular ischemia, left ventricular failure, or atrial fibrillation) is transmitted to the pulmonary veins, shifting the hydrostatic balance toward the interstitial space of the lung. Increased interstitial fluid reduces lung compliance, which may be perceived by the patient as mild dyspnea. Even if dyspnea is not reported, subtle increases in respiratory rate alone may be a sign of elevated left atrial pressure. Other stimuli of respiratory drive include hypoxemia, hypercarbia, metabolic acidosis, sympathetic stimulation, anemia, fever, pregnancy, head injury, sepsis, and drugs such as theophylline, caffeine, amphetamine, and cocaine.

Tachypnea in a pediatric patient with reduced pulmonary blood flow (e.g., patient scheduled for Blalock-Taussig shunt) may represent compensation for pulmonary dead space. Although both lungs are being ventilated, a significant amount of the ventilation may be ineffective because reduced pulmonary blood flow limits the amount of gas exchange possible.

Oxygen Saturation. Similar to other vital signs, pulse oximetry provides valuable information about pulmonary and cardiovascular status. In the adult patient, decreases in saturation are often related to pulmonary processes. Cardiac causes of pulmonary congestion also reduce oxygen saturation. Deep breathing or coughing may improve saturation if the etiology is airway secretions or simple atelectasis. Patients with pneumonia, CHF, or pleural effusion will not improve oxygen saturation with these maneuvers.

Patients with congenital heart disease require a knowledge of the specific cardiac lesion for appropriate management of oxygen saturation. For example, patients with transposition have separation of their pulmonary and systemic circulations except for mixing interfaces. The measured systemic saturation will be low despite the highest possible inspired oxygen concentration. In other congenital heart lesions, high oxygen saturation is undesirable. Patients with hypoplastic left heart syndrome (HLHS), for example, have a circulatory system that allows blood to go either to the lungs or the body.[319] If inspired oxygen is increased, pulmonary resistance is reduced and blood flows preferentially to the lungs rather than the body; severe metabolic acidosis ensues. To prevent this "overperfusion" of the lungs, the F_IO_2 is kept at a minimum. Finally, alterations of oximetry saturation indicate a dynamic physiology. When not provoked, the patient with tetrology of Fallot may have a normal oximetry saturation. However, during a "spell," resistance to pulmonary blood flow is severely increased and venous blood is shunted across the VSD to the left ventricle. Mixing of the venous and oxygenated blood in the left ventricle results in reduced oxygen saturation. Treatment of the spell will restore normal saturation.

Temperature. Temperature varies depending on the site of measurement. Oral temperature is typically a degree lower than rectal temperature. Oral temperature may be even lower with mouth breathing. Both oral and rectal sites are preferable over axillary temperature measurement. Devices that measure tympanic temperature avoid common problems.

Fever in the preoperative cardiac patient may indicate occult infection. If the planned surgery includes implantation of prosthetic material such as a heart valve, pacemaker, or aortic graft, treatment of the infection before surgery is indicated.

Another cause of fever in the pediatric patient is dehydration. Reduced cutaneous perfusion reduces normal dissipation of body heat. Other signs of dehydration, such as a sunken fontanelle and decreased skin moisture, will aid the diagnosis. Anticholinergic drugs such as atropine may contribute to temperature elevation by reducing heat dissipation.

Skin and Extremities

Skin. Skin inspection is another useful evaluation in patients with cardiac disease.[320] Radiation therapy to the chest (breast or skin cancer or Hodgkin's disease) is of particular interest because of the association between radiation and ostial stenoses of the coronary arteries, even in younger patients. Atherosclerosis is suggested by subcutaneous or tendinous xanthomas of hypercholesteremia. Trophic changes of the skin of lower extremities may be caused by impaired arterial perfusion. Mild jaundice may occur with hepatic congestion caused by right ventricular failure or hemolysis from a prosthetic heart valve or paravalvular regurgitation. Pigmentation described as "slate" or "bronze" may occur with hemochromatosis (associated with constrictive cardiomyopathy). Chronic amiodarone therapy can also produce a skin discoloration. This should be distinguished from true cyanosis because amiodarone also can cause pulmonary disease.

Cyanosis is a bluish skin color resulting from the presence of desaturated hemoglobin (>3 g/dl).[321] Patients with *peripheral* cyanosis have normal arterial oxygen saturation, but peripheral vasoconstriction and oxygen extraction produce a cyanotic appearance. Warming the extremity may relieve peripheral cyanosis. Patients with *central* cyanosis have reduced arterial oxygen saturation. Right-to-left shunting of venous blood to the systemic arterial system occurs because of an intracardiac lesion or pulmonary shunt. Patients with *differential* cyanosis have one region of the body that is blue while a different region is pink. In an infant, this could occur with coarctation and patent ductus arteriosis (PDA). A right-to-left shunt through the PDA causes the lower extremities to be cyanotic while the arms are pink. Differential cyanosis can occur in the adult with a long-standing PDA and Eisenmenger syndrome. The right arm is pink, while the legs are blue.

Cool and damp skin is a concern because it may indicate increased sympathetic nervous system activity. A normal hemodynamic profile may become unstable when anesthesia blunts the sympathetic support. Alternatively, skin that is hot and dry indicates use of an anticholinergic medication such as atropine. This is a useful finding in pediatric patients because dissipation of body heat may be impaired.

Pulse. Palpation of the pulse should be assessed before administration of anesthesia because it provides a rapid assessment of the hemodynamic circulation during anesthesia and surgery. A variety of pulse characteristics have been correlated to various cardiac disorders.[322]

A wide pulse pressure (high systolic and low diastolic) is characteristic of aortic insufficiency. Regurgitation of the aortic valve decreases diastolic pressure and contributes to left ventricular filling, thus augmenting stroke volume. This type of pulse is easily palpated and is described as a "water-hammer" pulse. Other circumstances also produce a bounding pulse: anemia, fever, sepsis, exercise, PDA, AV dialysis fistula, and Paget's disease. Mitral insufficiency can also produce a bounding pulse, but it is of short duration and is described as "small water-hammer" pulse.

In contrast, the pulse of a patient with aortic stenosis is late peaking, with a narrow pulse pressure. This pulse is less palpable and is described as "parvus et tardis," meaning "small and late." The diminished pulse pressure indicates that the left ventricle may be unable to compensate for any degree of hypotension. The patient with aortic stenosis and a relatively normal pulse pressure may also have aortic insufficiency.

A pulse characterized by two peaks is known as a *bisferiens* pulse and has been associated with aortic insufficiency and hypertrophic obstructive cardiomyopathy (HOCM). Intraaortic balloon pump counterpulsation can also produce this type of pulse. Lack of the bisferiens pulse does not eliminate the possibility of HOCM. Another characteristic of HOCM is the Brockenbraugh pulse.[323] Normally, the pulse that follows a premature ventricular contraction (PVC) is more prominent because of enhanced cardiac contractility. In HOCM, increased contractility worsens left ventricular outflow obstruction, so the pulse after a PVC is diminished.

Perfusion Indicators. Skin temperature is an important indicator of perfusion. An obvious example is the cool leg on the side of a femoral intraaortic balloon pump. The presence of occlusive peripheral vascular disease is another. However, in the absence of mechanical obstruction, comparison of skin temperature between the proximal and distal extremity is a good method for estimating adequacy of cardiac output. The skin temperature of the foot, calf, and lower thigh are assessed. Ideally, all should be the same temperature. A cool foot *and* calf indicates *worse* perfusion than a cool foot alone. Reduced perfusion may be related to low cardiac output or excessive vasoconstrictor drug levels. The key point is to repeat the skin temperature comparisons over time. With appropriate therapy, the distal extremity should warm over time. If, instead, the area of warmth is retreating, further intervention is necessary.

Capillary refill is another method of assessing perfusion. The skin is compressed briefly and then observed for a return of pink color over 1 or 2 seconds. A caveat is that venous obstruction can lead to misinterpretation. For example, when a venous tourniquet is wrapped securely around the arm, compression and release of the skin of a finger is accompanied by an immediate capillary refill. Rather than representing arterial perfusion, this refill is caused by elevated venous pressure and does not represent tissue well-being.

Edema. Edema of the lower extremities may indicate fluid retention associated with CHF, reduced serum albumin concentration, or obstruction of venous or lymphatic drainage. The patient with an ascending or aortic arch aneurysm may present with upper extremity edema resulting from obstruction of upper body venous drainage (SVC syndrome).[324]

Head and Neck

Head appearance may also indicate cardiac disease. A bobbing head coincident with the pulse can occur with severe aortic insufficiency. A facial rash with a butterfly shape may indicate systemic lupus. The fontanelle of the pediatric patient provides an assessment of fluid status.

Eye Examination. Unequal pupil size attributable to anisocoria or after cataract surgery should be noted preoperatively. A ring around the iris, a circumferential arcus senilis, in persons younger than 50 years of age is associated with atherosclerosis. Bilaterally dilated pupils can occur with anticholinergic medication, especially intravenous scopolamine. This is an important finding because dilated pupils may also indicate sympathetic stimulation (e.g., light anesthesia) or cerebral injury (e.g., hypoxemia).

Funduscopic examination is usually performed by the internist. An abnormal light reflex as well as an abnormal vessel caliber and tortuosity are associated with coronary artery disease.[325] Retinal changes representing the end-organ effects of significant hypertension may also be evident.[167] "Roth spots" are hemorrhagic areas with white centers that can occur from emboli of bacterial endocarditis as well as leukemia.[320]

Nose. The nose represents an important alternative pathway for intubation. The old adage "a difficult oral intubation is likely an easy nasal intubation" should not be forgotten. The nasal pathway of pediatric patients with choanal atresia may not provide this option. If a nasal intubation is anticipated, direct fiberoptic nasal inspection may be useful.

Ears. Pediatric patients with congenital heart disease may have characteristics of the ears that are associated with the congenital heart lesions. Movement of the ear-lobes laterally coincident with the heartbeat may indicate severe tricuspid insufficiency.[320] In adult patients, a diagonal crease in the earlobe has been associated with the presence of atherosclerosis, although this is a controversial association.[326-328]

Neck Inspection. The neck provides important sites for central venous access. Prior neck procedures such as carotid endarterectomy, neck dissection, thyroidectomy, and especially prior catheterization (Hickman line, temporary dialysis catheter, temporary pacemaker) may contribute to difficult access. A caveat is that although a distended neck vein may appear an appealing puncture site, it may also represent distal obstruction.

Airway. A high-arched palate may be associated with congenital heart disease. Hoarseness may be indicative of recurrent laryngeal nerve involvement with an aneurysm of the descending aorta or a significantly enlarged left atrium.

Airway management is a primary responsibility of the anesthesiologist, and preoperative airway assessment is essential.[329] Mobility of the neck to achieve the "sniffing position" is important for laryngoscopy and intubation. Fullness in the anterior neck may indicate an enlarged thyroid gland. Tracheal deviation warns of possible airway compression. A tracheostomy scar is a key finding. It may represent emergency airway access in the past, and prior tracheostomy may be associated with subglottic stenosis of the airway.

Atlantoaxial subluxation of the cervical spine can occur in rheumatoid arthritis,[330] infections of the posterior pharynx, neck trauma, and some congenital syndromes (e.g. Down's syndrome).[331] Although symptoms of pain, stiffness, or paresthesia may occur, these situations may also be asymptomatic. Cervical spine flexion and extension films are useful for evaluating these circumstances.

Carotid Artery. Auscultation over the carotid arteries can identify a carotid bruit, possibly indicating narrowing of the carotid artery. Bilateral upper neck bruits are the strongest predictor of a stenotic lesion.[76]

Neck Veins. Examination of the neck veins gives important information about filling of the right side of the heart.[332] Internal jugular vein observation is preferable when the patient is seated at about 45 degrees. A double undulation is seen at the top of the venous column when a sinus rhythm is present. Central venous (right atrial) pressure is estimated by the height of column (centimeters of water) above the right atrium (assumed 5 cm below the sternal angle).[320] In practice, the exact number is less important than assessment of satisfactory volume status. If the patient must be positioned horizontally or with legs elevated to observe venous pulsations, hypovolemia is present. Neck vein distention while sitting upright may indicate hypervolemia. Other causes of elevated venous pressure include CHF, cor pulmonale, tricuspid stenosis or insufficiency, constrictive pericarditis, pericardial effusion, pulmonary hypertension, tamponade, and SVC syndrome from thoracic aortic aneurysm.

Hepatojugular reflux or the abdominojugular maneuver involves observing the neck veins while applying firm pressure over the liver.[333] In normal circumstances, a transient rise in jugular venous pressure returns rapidly (<10 seconds) to baseline pressure. A sustained increase in JVD is most commonly caused by CHF or dilated cardiomyopathy but can also occur with tricuspid stenosis and right ventricular dysfunction from pulmonary hypertension or infarction.

Venous pulsations in the neck consist of three positive (outward bulge) waves: "a wave," atrial contraction; "c wave," corresponding to ventricular contraction (likely representing transmission of the carotid pulse); and "v wave," representing atrial filling prior to opening of the tricuspid valve. Two negative waves (inward movement) are the "x descent," representing atrial relaxation, and the "y descent," representing opening of the tricuspid valve (see Chapter 3). Abnormal pulsations such as a prominent v wave in tricuspid insufficiency are more easily appreciated by transducing the pressure within a central venous catheter, rather than simple bedside observation. In contrast, a "cannon a wave" may be easily visible by bedside observation. A cannon a wave occurs when the right atrium contracts against a closed tricuspid valve (e.g., junctional rhythm), causing transmission of the pressure wave into the neck veins.[320,322]

The Heart and Lungs

Heart Examination. Assessment of the cardiovascular system includes cardiac rhythm and rate, volume status, contractility, blood pressure, and peripheral perfusion. Auscultation of the heart provides information regarding valvular function and aspects of CHF, and can indi-

	Origin of Murmur				
	Right-sided	Aortic stenosis	Hypertrophic cardiomyopathy	Mitral regurgitation	Ventricular septal defect
Inspiration	↑	↓	↓	↓	↓
Expiration	↓	↑	↑	↑	↑
Muller maneuver	—	↓	↓	—	↓
Valsalva maneuver	↓	↓	—	↓	↓
Squatting to standing	—	↓	↑	—	—
Standing to squatting	—	↑	↓	—	—
Leg elevation	—	—	↓	—	—
Handgrip	—	—	↓	↑	↑
Transient arterial occlusion	—	—	—	↑	↑
Amyl nitrate inhalation	↑	—	↑	↓	↓

FIG. 1-6   Provocative maneuvers to distinguish systolic murmurs. Arrows indicate the predominant change in murmur intensity for maneuver. A dash (—) indicates a mixed response or no change in intensity.
(Modified from Lembo NJ, Dell'Italia LJ, Crawford MH et al: *N Engl J Med* 318:1512, 1988.)

cate pericarditis if a friction rub is heard. Auscultation of a murmur identifies the location, intensity or loudness, timing, radiation pattern, pitch, and auditory shape. Heart murmurs are classified as systolic, diastolic, and continuous.[181,193]

Systolic Murmurs. The murmur of aortic stenosis causes a midsystolic, crescendo-decrescendo murmur that radiates to the carotid arteries. The murmur may have a harsh sound at the right second intercostal space because of turbulence. At the same time, a musical quality is heard at the lower left side of the sternum at the ventricular apex. The loudness of the murmur is increased after longer diastolic periods (e.g., after a premature contraction). The benign murmur of "aortic sclerosis" is also midsystolic.[320,193]

The murmur of mitral regurgitation (MR) is holosystolic. Radiation of the murmur depends on the direction of the regurgitant jet as observed with echocardiography. A posterolateral jet radiates to the axilla, whereas an anteromedial jet toward the aorta radiates to the left sternal edge.[193,320] The MR murmur of a patient with ischemic papillary muscle dysfunction is heard only during chest pain.[334] Mitral valve prolapse is a late systolic murmur accompanied by a midsystolic click.

Tricuspid insufficiency produces a systolic murmur that increases during inspiration because of the increased right ventricular volume. The increased loudness during inspiration is *Carvallo sign*. The murmur of a restrictive VSD is also holosystolic.[193,320]

Distinction between the systolic murmurs of hypertrophic cardiomyopathy, VSD, MR, and aortic stenosis can be facilitated by provocative maneuvers. These maneuvers include inspiration and exhalation, Valsalva and Mueller maneuvers, squatting and standing, leg elevation, handgrip, transient arterial occlusion, and amyl nitrate inhalation[335] (Fig. 1-6).

Diastolic Murmurs. Diastolic murmurs require more subtle auscultation skills. The murmur of aortic insufficiency is early, soft, diastolic, and decrescendo in shape. It is best heard with the patient seated, leaning forward, at end exhalation. The murmur of mitral stenosis is a low-frequency murmur described as a middiastolic rumble that follows an opening snap.[193]

Continuous Murmurs. The most common type of normal continuous murmur is a cervical venous hum, which is typical in healthy children and young adults. An abnormal continuous murmur is that of a PDA murmur representing a connection between the aorta and pulmonary artery. The development of pulmonary hypertension with long-standing PDA initially causes a reduction in the loudness of the murmur, followed by a resumption as Eisenmenger syndrome of right-to-left shunting develops.[193]

Auscultation is a skill that improves with experience. A study of five experienced physicians demonstrated significant disagreement in auscultation findings when 32 patients were examined. Mitral stenosis was diagnosed in two normal patients in whom a phono-

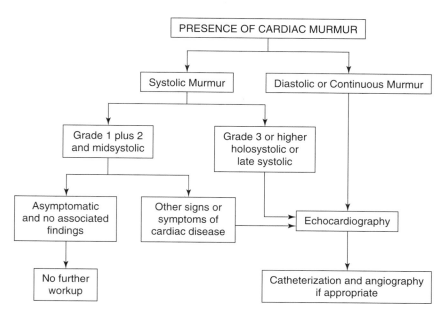

FIG. 1-7   Indications for echocardiographic assessment of heart murmur.

(From Bonow RO, Carabello B, DeLeon AC et al: *JACC* 32:1493, 1998.)

cardiogram did not detect the murmur.[336] These findings suggest that cardiac murmurs may often deserve further diagnostic evaluation. Perhaps the current emphasis on technology has deemphasized the importance of cardiac auscultation skills.[337-340] One approach is to use echocardiography for diastolic or continuous murmurs. Soft (grade I or II) midsystolic murmurs do not require further workup unless the patient is symptomatic or the ECG and chest radiograph were abnormal. Louder (grade III or higher), holosystolic, or late systolic murmurs require echocardiographic evaluation[180] (Fig. 1-7).

Indications of Congestive Heart Failure. Palpation of the chest wall for location of the ventricular impulse and percussion can identify cardiomegaly. An S_3 gallop is heard with auscultation. These findings, as well as pulmonary rales, JVD, and peripheral edema, have been correlated to reduced ejection fraction.[341-343] A study of patients with CHF found that the presence of a third heart sound was common despite a lack of other signs such as rales, edema, or elevated jugular pressure.[102] Another study advocated precordial percussion over palpation to determine cardiomegaly.[344] The Valsalva maneuver can also be used to distinguish CHF. In normal patients, this maneuver produces a characteristic decrease and then overshoot of the blood pressure and heart rate. In CHF, a square wave change in pressure occurs.[345]

CHF can occur because of systolic or diastolic dysfunction.[346] A reduced ejection fraction (EF) indicates systolic dysfunction. A normal EF but elevated filling pressures indicate diastolic dysfunction in the absence of other causes such as valve disease. A review of the best clinical methods to diagnose CHF reported that increased filling pressures were indicated by chest X-ray redistribution[347] and jugular venous distension.[348] Re-

duced EF was indicated by cardiomegaly, abnormal apical impulse (especially sustained duration), chest X-ray redistribution, and anterior Q waves or left bundle-branch block on ECG.[342,349] Diastolic failure was also identified by the presence of elevated blood pressure during heart failure.[346]

Respiratory Examination

Inspection. The patient's general appearance often may reveal important aspects of pulmonary function. Prior chest tube or thoracotomy scars indicate a significant pulmonary history.[350] Kyphoscoliosis, obesity, and pectus excavatum, suggest restrictive physiology. Accessory muscles are used in patients with restrictive disorders such as pulmonary congestion, pneumothorax, and diaphragmatic dysfunction. A barrel-shaped thorax and pursed-lip expiratory breathing indicate chronic obstructive lung disease (COPD). The physical signs of patients with COPD (tracheal descent, scalene muscle contraction, costal margin movement, and location of most prominent cardiac contraction) can be correlated to the degree of airflow obstruction and spirometric lung volumes.[351] Tachypnea is indicated when the patient must pause midsentence to inspire. Orthopnea occurs when the patient uses extra pillows or inclines the head of the bed. The patient who "must sit up" may have pulmonary edema or cardiac tamponade. The ability to breathe deeply and vigorously cough indicates the ability to clear secretions and atelectasis and is predictive of postoperative pulmonary complications.[352]

Palpation. Palpation identifies asymmetric chest excursion, accessory muscle use, and diaphragmatic function. Abnormal tactile fremitus is present in lung disease.

Percussion. Percussion is particularly useful to detect a pleural effusion, which may be a prominent cause of dyspnea. Lung consolidation and diaphragmatic excursion can also be assessed.

Auscultation. Auscultation of normal breathing reveals "vesicular" breath sounds, which are described as a "whishing" sound. Inspiration is longer and louder than exhalation with normal, quiet breathing. The exhalation phase of patients with "asthmatic breathing" is much longer than inspiration, and exhalation is accompanied by wheezing.[272] Forced exhalation may provoke wheezing that is otherwise silent. The loudness of wheezing does not necessarily correlate with the severity of obstruction. Very severe obstruction reduces airflow, diminishing the amount of sound produced.[353] In a study of asthmatic patients during acute bronchospasm, the only sign that correlated with severe impairment was retraction of the sternocleidomastoid muscle. Wheezing was still present even when patients believed the attack had resolved.[354] The absence of preoperative wheezing does not guarantee that an episode will not occur intraoperatively. The asymptomatic patient with reactive airways may develop significant bronchospasm with tracheal intubation.

"Crackles" occur when an abnormally closed airway opens during inspiration or closes at the end of expiration. These abnormal breath sounds occur with atelectasis, pneumonia, pulmonary edema, or CHF. The timing and pitch of breath sounds distinguish various pulmonary abnormalities.[355,356] When auscultation abnormalities are heard, evaluation with a chest X-ray film is appropriate.

Variability in auscultation among clinicians is characteristic of the respiratory examination.[350] One study of 9 physicians examining 13 patients with emphysema demonstrated significant disagreement as to whether a particular sign was present.[357] More than 40% of the physicians disagreed on the presence of rales, hyperresonance, barrel chest, and use of accessory muscles in a patient with known severe emphysema. Nearly half of the physicians disagreed on the presence of hyperresonance, diminished breath sounds, and rales in a patient who was known to be without disease.

Abdominal Examination

Inspection for surgical scars should accompany the patient interview regarding prior abdominal operations and anesthetics. Upper abdominal scars indicate procedures such as partial gastectomy, Nissen fundoplication, Heller myotomy, or gastric stapling, which may pose a risk to the use of intraoperative TEE. Lower abdominal scars may indicate prior vascular operations such as repair of an abdominal aortic aneurysm, which may increase the risk of femoral arterial cannulation or placement of an intraaortic balloon pump. Physical examination should also seek indicators of liver disease, such as

jaundice, spider angiomas, or superficial veins on the abdomen. Portal hypertension from liver disease or vena caval obstruction may cause prominent superficial abdominal veins. Abdominal striae caused by previous pregnancy are white. Striae that are red or purple indicate excess cortisol levels that would suggest a diagnosis of Cushing's syndrome in a hypertensive patient.

A distended abdomen increases the risk for gastroesophageal reflux.[358] Possible etiologies include delayed gastric emptying (anxiety, pain, or narcotics), bowel obstruction, ascites, swallowed air, obesity or pregnancy.[359] Auscultation of bowel sounds facilitates this diagnosis. Obesity may predispose the patient to increased surgical risk with noncardiac surgery.[360] However, a recent large study found that obese (body mass index [BMI] 75th to 94th percentile) and severely obese (BMI 95th to 100th percentile) patients undergoing CABG surgery were not at increased risk for mortality or stroke. The incidence of sternal wound infection was increased but the incidence of postoperative bleeding was significantly less than in nonobese patients.[361]

Abdominal palpation should assess the liver for increased size or tenderness. Palpation of liver size of the pediatric patient in particular is a good indication of the degree of right-sided heart failure. In contrast, estimation of liver size by percussion in the adult patient is more accurate than palpation of the liver below the rib margin.[362] Painful palpation may be caused by liver congestion from ventricular failure,[280] inflammation from infectious hepatitis, or gallbladder disease. The presence of preoperative jaundice deserves explanation.[363] A history of excessive alcohol ingestion, recent blood transfusion, or recent anesthetic exposure is important. Hemolysis from a prosthetic heart valve can also produce jaundice.[364] Evaluation of liver function tests is appropriate with positive findings.[359] Infectious hepatitis represents a risk to both the patient and the health care team.[365]

Urinary tract infection (UTI) should be suspected with the finding of tenderness over the suprapubic region or the abdominal flank. A history of dysuria or prior UTI is notable. Bladder distention may be attributable to prostatic disease, neurogenic dysfunction, or polyuria of diabetes. These diagnoses may predispose patients to bladder distention during the perioperative period, a potent stimulus for hypertension.[336] Auscultation for abdominal bruits may reveal an abdominal aortic aneurysm or renal artery stenosis.

Ascites is free fluid in the abdominal cavity and may occur with heart failure, liver disease, nephrotic syndrome, or malignancy. Accumulation of fluid occurs because of increased hydrostatic pressures, reduced osmotic pressure, or processes that produce fluid in excess of reabsorption capacity.[367]

Gastrointestinal complications are known to occur

after cardiac surgery and may be related to reduced perfusion during cardiopulmonary bypass.[368,369] One study found that patients with preoperative elevated right atrial pressure and multiple valve replacements were at increased risk for postoperative hyperbilirubinemia.[370] Another study related postoperative pancreatitis to increased administration of calcium.[371]

Neurologic and Musculoskeletal Systems

Directed Neurologic Examination. A baseline assessment of preoperative neurologic function is important before carotid artery surgery, thoracic aortic cross-clamping, and cardiopulmonary bypass, where complications such as perioperative stroke or spinal cord ischemia with paraplegia can occur. Documentation of preoperative deficits greatly assist postoperative assessment.[89,90,372]

Abnormalities in mental alertness and orientation, speech quality, eye movements, facial appearance, and coordination are often immediately obvious. Pupil size (anisocoria) and reactivity are useful indicators of anesthetic depth and deserve specific observation. Pressure applied to the anesthetic face mask may cause facial nerve dysfunction. Diabetic neuropathy affects lower extremity sensory discrimination. Preoperative lower extremity sensory or motor deficits may make regional techniques less desirable for medicolegal reasons, unless the deficits are well documented.

Directed Musculoskeletal Examination. The musculoskeletal system may indicate the presence of systemic diseases[373] and neuromuscular processes that increase the risk of anesthesia.[374,375] Patients with acromegaly and Marfan syndrome have characteristic features. Joint deformities indicating rheumatoid arthritis raise concerns for atlantooccipital instability.[330] The distinctive kyphosis of ankylosing spondylitis may be associated with difficulties in airway management and aortic insufficiency.[376] Pectus excavatum is associated with congenital cardiac abnormalities as well as respiratory changes. Patients with muscular dystrophy may have significant cardiac disease.[377]

Duchenne's muscular dystrophy is early onset and progressive muscle weakness disorder despite "pseudohypertrophy" of certain muscle groups (e.g., calf muscles).[377] Cardiac involvement includes cardiomyopathy[378,379] and dysrhythmias including accelerated AV conduction.[380] Cardiac arrest has been reported during anesthesia induction in patients with Duchenne's muscular dystrophy.[381,382] Myotonic muscular dystrophy is a relatively common neuromuscular disease (5 per 100,000) and characterized by delayed muscle relaxation after contraction.[377] Conduction abnormalities causing AV block are characteristic and evidenced by

ECG PR interval prolongation, left anterior fascicular block, and QRS widening.[377,383,384] Patients with neuromuscular disease are considered at risk for malignant hyperthermia.[385]

Simple maneuvers by physical examination may localize symptoms of muscle weakness. Proximal muscle strength is tested by the ability to abduct arms and perform supine leg raising. Distal muscle strength is tested by spreading the fingers and dorsiflexing the foot. Muscle reflexes are delayed in patients with hypothyroidism and may be diminished in patients with muscular disease. Reflexes are increased with hyperthyroidism and upper motor neuron diseases.

TECHNOLOGY AND CARDIAC RISK

Clinical assessment is a very useful but limited diagnostic tool. Warner et al reviewed the morbidity and mortality of 38,598 ambulatory surgery patients at the Mayo Clinic.[386] Fourteen MIs accounted for 45% of major morbidity and all of the medical causes of mortality. Although the incidence was low, this study reiterates the fact that adverse cardiac complications occur, even among patients who are presumed to be healthy. Half of the infarctions, including both fatal infarctions, occurred in ASA class 2 patients. Preoperative risk factors were few and no risk factors were present in five of the patients.[386]

Technology greatly extends the physician's ability to diagnose and quantify cardiac disease. For noncardiac surgery, patients with intermediate clinical risk factors derive the most benefit from noninvasive testing[387] such as dipyridamole thallium or DSE. Noninvasive tests identify which patients should have definitive assessment with cardiac catheterization. There are also different levels of assessment for patients undergoing cardiac surgery.[388] For example, aortic valve replacement in an otherwise young, healthy patient may proceed without preoperative coronary angiography. In contrast, the high-risk cardiac patient with advanced coronary artery disease may require myocardial viability testing to determine whether CABG surgery would be of benefit.[389] Technologic advancements provide a continuum of cardiac testing. It is worth noting that the ECG and the chest radiograph were regarded in past years as "laboratory tests." Current literature includes both of these tests as integral parts of the clinical assessment.

Resting ECG, Exercise Stress Test, Ambulatory Monitoring

ECG. The resting ECG provides valuable information: evidence of MI and LVH, rhythm disturbances, and conduction abnormalities.[390,391] The ECG defines an ACC/AHA intermediate-risk predictor (Q waves indicating prior MI) and several minor-risk predictors (LVH, left bundle-branch block, ST-T abnormalities, rhythm other than sinus).[1] The ECG is also used to identify low-risk variables (Q waves and ST-segment ischemia) for the ACP guidelines.[2] Although the discovery of an acute MI with the preoperative ECG would be rare, such a finding would be extremely important and a major risk indicator. In one study, patients with an abnormal preoperative ECG were 3.2 times more likely to have a perioperative cardiac event.[392,393]

The significance of a preexisting bundle-branch block is controversial. Several authors suggest that bundle-branch block (including right bundle-branch block with left axis) does not increase the risk of complete heart block during anesthesia and surgery.[394-396] One study reported a single episode of "complete heart block" that occurred during intubation.

The presence of a left bundle-branch block, especially one of new onset, is associated with ischemic heart disease. A recent study evaluated the outcomes of medical patients with right bundle-branch block or left bundle-branch block on the admission ECG. Both types were associated with higher risk.[397,398]

Exercise ECG. The treadmill stress test adds the provocative stress of exercise to ECG assessment.[225,399-402] Specific ECG changes distinguish an ischemic response from nonspecific changes.[403,404] Horizontal or downsloping ST depression greater than 0.1 mV, particularly with low levels of exercise, indicates a risk for ischemia. ECG changes during other provocative noninvasive tests, such as dipyridamole thallium, may also indicate a risk for ischemia. The major problem with the exercise ECG is that the highest-risk vascular patients are often unable to exercise at peak stress because of lower extremity claudication.[405]

Ambulatory Holter ECG. Another approach to evaluating the ambulatory cardiac patient is the use of Holter ECG recording.[406-408] Raby et al demonstrated that preoperative ambulatory ECG monitoring correlated with outcome after elective vascular surgery.[409] Patients were monitored for 24 to 48 hours within 9 days before surgery. ECG ischemia was often asymptomatic and occurred in 18% of patients. Ischemia was more common in patients 70 years of age or older, or those with a history of hypertension, prior carotid artery surgery, CHF, angina, MI, prior coronary bypass surgery, or any coronary disease. Postoperative cardiac events (MI, unstable angina, or ischemic pulmonary edema) occurred in 38% of patients who had preoperative ischemia (Table 1-25). The most significant variable that correlated with postoperative adverse events was preoperative Holter ischemia. Importantly, the absence of preoperative ischemia predicted a good outcome. Ambulatory ECG is one fifth as costly as other noninvasive tests

TABLE 1-25
Correlation of Preoperative Ambulatory Ischemia to Postoperative Cardiac Events

	PREOPERATIVE ISCHEMIA ON AMBULATORY ECG?*	
	YES (*n* = 32)	NO (*n* = 144)
Postoperative cardiac event	12 (38%)	1 (1%)
No event	20 (63%)	143 (99%)†

From Raby KE, Goldman L, Craeger MA et al: *N Engl J Med* 321:1296, 1989.
ECG, Electrocardiogram.
*Ambulatory ECG monitoring in 176 consecutive patients for elective vascular surgery.
†The absence of preoperative ambulatory ischemia was associated with no cardiac event in 99% of cases.

such as thallium dipyridamole.[409] Other authors have also demonstrated a good correlation between ambulatory ECG and outcome. A key finding from these studies is that a significant amount of ischemia occurs without symptoms.[410-412]

Radionucleotide Ejection Fraction

The resting left ventricular ejection fraction (EF) is a useful predictor of outcome for patients undergoing cardiac surgery.[413] The preoperative EF might also be a prognostic guide for patients undergoing noncardiac surgery.[414] Although early studies suggested a strong correlation between EF and good outcome for patients undergoing repair of abdominal aortic aneurysm, other authors have not found a similar relationship.

A normal EF clearly does not exclude the presence of severe coronary artery disease.[415] A patient with significant coronary disease may have a normal EF at rest but a severely reduced EF during ischemia provoked by exercise.[416] Franco et al studied resting gated blood pool EFs in 85 patients having vascular surgery.[417] The patients were classified into three groups according to their EF. The incidence of postoperative MIs was similar for each group, but cardiac deaths occurred only in the low EF group (Table 1-26). Thus a low preoperative EF predicts poor outcome, but a normal EF does not guarantee good outcome.

Dipyridamole Thallium Scan

Before 1985, preoperative risk assessment of the vascular surgery patient was unsatisfactory. Clinical assessment by the Goldman CRI underestimated risk.[28,29] Cardiac catheterization for all patients represented con-

GROUP	NO. OF PATIENTS	MYOCARDIAL INFARCTIONS	DEATHS
I EF = 0.56-0.92	50	9 (18%)	0
II EF = 0.37-0.55	20	3 (15%)	0
III EF = 0.20-0.35	15	3 (20%)	2

From Franco CD, Goldsmith J, Veith FJ et al: *J Vasc Surg* 10:656, 1989.

Note that postoperative myocardial infarctions occurred at a rate of 15-20% in each ejection fraction group. Thus preoperative ejection fraction did not correlate to this outcome. In contrast, mortality occurred only in the lowest ejection fraction group.

siderable expense and risk.[220,221] Because of this, the 1985 risk stratification study by Boucher et al using noninvasive dipyridamole thallium cardiac imaging, was a landmark contribution.[418] Myocardial uptake of thallium-201 is *linearly* related to regional myocardial blood flow and is detected by a nuclear medicine gamma camera.[419] Regions of reduced blood flow appear as "defects" during scanning. Dipyridamole is a potent coronary vasodilator that exaggerates regional differences in coronary blood flow. Consequently, myocardium supplied by a stenotic coronary artery becomes ischemic and appears as a defect compared with normal myocardium because the stenotic artery cannot dilate. As dipyridamole dissipates (redistribution), blood flow to this ischemic region improves and the "defect" appears normal. These "reversible defects" indicate viable myocardium at risk for ischemia. "Fixed" defects are areas that do not normalize with redistribution of dipyridamole and represent previously infarcted, nonviable myocardium.[420,421]

Boucher's study of 54 vascular surgery patients demonstrated that "reversible defects" were strong predictors of perioperative cardiac events.[418] Persistent or fixed defects were characteristic of a prior MI, but did not correlate with perioperative ischemic events. In 6 of the 22 patients with reversible defects, the scan results were so significant that the managing physician removed the patients from the study to undergo cardiac catheterization. Severe multivessel coronary artery disease was discovered in all of these patients.[418]

Eagle et al reported that a reversible defect on a dipyridamole thallium scan was the most significant predic-

tor of postoperative ischemic events in 61 patients having major aortic surgery.[422] Several historic variables also correlated with outcome and included Q wave on ECG, CHF, diabetes, angina, and prior MI. The absence of historic variables identified a low-risk population that would not benefit further from the dipyridamole thallium scan. Eagle et al tested this hypothesis on 50 other patients.[422]

A follow-up study on 200 vascular surgery patients identified seven factors as independent predictors of postoperative cardiac events.[41] Five clinical risk factors were advanced age, Q wave on ECG, diabetes, angina, and history of ventricular dysrhythmias. Two dipyridamole thallium scan factors were redistribution defects and ischemic ECG changes during dipyridamole infusion. Absence of any clinical factor identified a low-risk patient. A high-risk patient was identified by three or more clinical risk factors. Dipyridamole thallium scanning was deemed unnecessary in the low- and high-risk groups because the incidence of ischemic events was adequately predicted by clinical characteristics. The major utility of the dipyridamole thallium scan was in the intermediate-risk group, characterized by one or two clinical risk factors[41] (Table 1-27).

The algorithm in Table 1-27 improved the predictive accuracy of the dipyridamole thallium scan by eliminating some of the false-positive and false-negative results. Leppo et al also recommended testing in intermediate risk patients.[423]

The issue of false-negative results was raised by Fleisher and Mangano.[424,425] Both authors reported patients with either normal scans or "fixed defects" (no reperfusion defects) who sustained MIs after noncardiac surgery.[424,425] The report by Fleisher described three patients with various clinical risk factors, such as age greater than 70, diabetes, hypertension, prior MI, and ventricular ectopy.[424]

The study by Mangano et al was prospective in 60 vascular surgery patients, and managing clinicians were blinded to the results of the scan. Half of the adverse outcomes of MI, severe ischemia or unstable angina, or CHF occurred in patients without redistribution defects (Table 1-28).[425] Editorial remarks[426] criticized the study by Mangano because it excluded patients with unstable heart disease and included "soft" outcome events such as unstable angina and CHF. Nonetheless the Mangano study demonstrated that the dipyridamole-thallium scan is not infallible.[427]

Few complications have been reported in patients undergoing dipyridamole thallium scanning, thus indicating the procedure's overall safety.[428] Symptoms of angina occur in 16% to 41% of patients but are relieved with intravenous aminophylline.[429] Ventricular ectopy,[430] ventricular fibrillation, and acute cardiac arrest have been reported.[431] The two mechanisms by which dipyridamole exacerbates myocardial ischemia

TABLE 1-27
Combination of Clinical Factors and Thallium Scan Results for Prediction of Cardiac Risk for Noncardiac Surgery

	CLINICAL RISK			
	LOW* (*n* = 64)	INTERMEDIATE† (*n* = 116)		HIGH‡ (*n* = 20)
Thallium scan redistribution	—	No	Yes	—
Number of ischemic events	2/64 (3.1%)	2/62 (3.2%)	16/54 (29.6%)	10/20 (50%)

From Eagle KA, Coley CM, Newell JB et al: *Ann Intern Med* 110:859, 1989.
Note: In this algorithm, three clinical risk categories are established by the presence of clinical factors. The dipyridamole thallium scan was not recommended for either the high or the low clinical risk groups. Dipyridamole thallium scanning was recommended for the intermediate clinical risk group, and divided this group according to whether a redistribution defect was demonstrated.
*No factors.
†One or two clinical factors.
‡Three or more clinical factors.

TABLE 1-28
Adverse Cardiac Outcomes after Preoperative Dipyridamole Thallium Scans

	REDISTRIBUTION DEFECT (*n* = 22)	FIXED DEFECT (*n* = 18)	NO DEFECT (*n* = 20)
Myocardial infarction	1	1	1*
Severe ischemia/ unstable angina	3	1	1
Congestive heart failure	2	2	1

Data from Mangano DT, London MJ, Tubau JF et al: *Circulation* 84: 493, 1991.
*Indicates fatal myocardial infarction. When multiple events occurred, only the most serious is listed.

are "coronary steal" and peripheral vasodilation causing hypotension.

Many studies have used the dipyridamole thallium scan to stratify cardiac risk before noncardiac surgery. Shaw et al reported a meta-analysis of 10 studies using dipyridamole thallium imaging before vascular surgery, published between 1985 and 1994 (Table 1-29).[432] Editorial remarks by Goldman emphasized patient selection issues.[433] In patients referred for testing (selected patients), a redistribution defect on the dipyridamole thallium scan was associated with approximately a ninefold increase in relative risk for major adverse cardiac events. When used for unselected, consecutive vascular surgery patients, the value of the test is less significant.[433,434]

Early and late outcomes after vascular surgery were assessed by L'Italien et al in 1995.[435] From two medical centers, 547 patients underwent aortic (321 patients), infrainguinal (177 patients), or carotid (49 patients) vascular surgery. Perioperative MI occurred in 6% of aortic and carotid cases and 13% of infrainguinal cases. MI was predicted by a history of angina, reversible *and* fixed defects on dipyridamole thallium scanning, and ischemic ST-segment depression during the scan. Four-year follow-up found predictors of late MI to be a history of angina, CHF, diabetes, fixed defect on dipyridamole thallium scanning, and perioperative MI. Infrainguinal procedures had a greater risk for late adverse events. The authors determined that comorbid factors contributed to the increased risk for infrainguinal procedures.[435]

Dobutamine Stress Echocardiography

Preoperative Cardiac Risk Stratification. Echocardiography combined with various provocative measures such as exercise, pacing, dobutamine infusion, or dipyridamole infusion facilitates the diagnosis of coronary artery disease.[427,436] The provocative stress creates an imbalance between myocardial oxygen supply and demand, and the resulting regional wall-motion abnormalities are detected by ultrasound imaging. Although clinical experience with stress echocardiography for preoperative risk assessment is less than that with nuclear perfusion imaging methods, the technique offers advantages by its assessment of valvular and ventricular function.

TABLE 1-29
Meta-Analysis of Dipyridamole Thallium-201 Imaging (1985 to 1994)

AUTHOR, YEAR	NUMBER PATIENTS	FIXED DEFECT				REVERSIBLE DEFECT		
		NO. OF PATIENTS	ALL EVENTS (%)*	DEATH OR MI (%)†		NO. OF PATIENTS	ALL EVENTS (%)*	DEATH OR MI (%)†
Boucher, 1985	54	12	0.0	0.0		16	50.0	18.8
Eagle, 1989	254	67	20.9	11.9		82	30.5	12.4
Lane, 1989	101	10	0.0	0.0		71	14.1	12.7
Younis, 1990	130	20	10	10		40	15.0	15.0
McEnroe, 1990	95	15	46.7	26.7		34	26.5	8.8
Mangano, 1991	60	18	22.2	5.6		22	27.3	4.5
Hendel, 1992	360	167	11.7	11.7		171	14.4	14.4
Kresowik, 1993	190	38	2.6	2.6		87	3.4	3.4
Baron, 1994	513	94	24.5	12.8		160	19.4	8.8
Bry, 1994	237	30	16.7	16.7		110	10.9	10.9
TOTAL	1994	471				793		
% EVENTS			11	7			18	9

Adapted from Shaw LJ, Eagle KA, Gersh BJ et al: *J Am Coll Cardiol* 27:787, 1996.
*Includes all cardiac complications measured by the individual study, such as congestive heart failure, myocardial ischemia, nonfatal myocardial infarction, and cardiac death.
†Cardiac death or myocardial infarction.

Lane et al reported the initial application of DSE to cardiac risk stratification of patients undergoing noncardiac surgery.[437] This study involved 57 patients undergoing vascular, intraabdominal, or major orthopedic surgery who could not perform traditional exercise testing. Most patients had some cardiac risk factor (prior MI in 40%), but none had unstable angina or severe heart failure. Dobutamine was administered up to a maximum of 40 µg/kg/min. Three groups were distinguished:

Group 1: normal wall motion at rest and normal during dobutamine infusion

Group 2: abnormality at rest but no new abnormality with dobutamine

Group 3: new abnormal wall motion during dobutamine infusion in regions that had been normal at baseline

Adverse postoperative cardiac events occurred in 21% of group 3 patients but not in groups 1 or 2.[437]

A larger series was reported by Poldermans et al in 1993 in which 136 patients presented for major vascular surgery.[438] Patients were assessed by the Detsky Modified Cardiac Risk Index and DSE. DSE was more useful for risk assessment than clinical information. All adverse cardiac events (15 patients) occurred in patients who had a positive test. By multivariate analysis, only two variables were independent predictors of a cardiac event: (1) new wall-motion abnormalities with DSE and (2) age greater than 70 years.[438]

Poldermans et al later reported that the addition of atropine improved cardiac risk stratification by DSE for vascular surgery patients.[439] Atropine facilitated heart rate increases for the test. Clinical risk assessment was attempted by the Detsky method as well as by that proposed by Eagle for the dipyridamole thallium scan. The Eagle variables were helpful, but the Detsky system was insensitive. Absence of clinical variables identified a low-risk group. A negative DSE also predicted a low risk of adverse events (Table 1-30). Poldermans noted that the heart rate threshold at which ischemic changes occurred was important. A positive test at a low ischemic threshold (defined as <70% of age-corrected maximal heart rate) indicated extremely high risk.[439]

Shaw et al reviewed five studies of preoperative DSE for vascular surgery that were published between 1991 and 1994 (Table 1-31).[432] Editorial remarks by Goldman emphasized that a positive result with stress echocardiography suggests a higher risk than a positive result with dipyridamole thallium scanning. Patients in the clinical intermediate-risk category benefited most from the DSE.[433]

DSE has been shown to predict long-term outcome after vascular surgery.[440] Poldermans studied 316 patients and identified three groups based on clinical risk factors and DSE:

Low risk: no history of prior MI and normal DSE, *or* either history of prior MI or limited ischemia on DSE

Moderate risk: history of prior MI and limited ischemia on DSE, *or* more extensive ischemia on DSE without prior MI

High risk: history of prior MI plus extensive ischemia on DSE

Follow-up for 19 months demonstrated 32 adverse events, including 11 cardiac deaths, 11 nonfatal MIs, and 10 episodes of unstable angina. The incidence of adverse events was 4.9% in low-risk patients, 20% in moderate-risk patients, and 52% in high-risk patients. The heart rate threshold for ischemia was not an independent predictor in this study.[440,441]

DSE and Outcome from Known or Suspected Coronary Disease. Decision making for the patient with known or suspected coronary disease is challenging. In a large series of 860 patients, DSE using a 16-segment model for wall-motion assessment predicted an increased incidence of MI and cardiac death during a mean follow-up of 24 months. By multivariate analysis, independent predictors of cardiac events were a history of CHF, the percentage of abnormal wall segments at peak stress, and an abnormal left ventricular end-systolic volume response to stress.[442]

Cardiac Catheterization

Right-Sided Heart Catheterization. Cardiac catheterization is the gold standard for assessment of patients with cardiac disease. Catheterization of the right side of the heart with a flow-directed, balloon-tipped catheter provides cardiac filling pressures, pulmonary artery

TABLE 1-30
Perioperative Cardiac Outcomes and Dobutamine-Atropine Stress Echocardiography

	CLINICAL RISK VARIABLES CLASSIFICATION (TOTAL PATIENTS = 300)					
	0 (100 PATIENTS)		1 OR 2 (179 PATIENTS)		3 OR MORE (21 PATIENTS)	
	(−)	(+)	(−)	(+)	(−)	(+)
Results of dobutamine stress echocardiography	88	12	130	49	10	11
All adverse cardiac events*	0	1	0	20	0	6
Cardiac death or myocardial infarction	0	0	0	11	0	6

From Poldermans D, Arnese M, Fioretti PM et al: *Am Coll Cardiol* 26:648, 1995.
*Adverse cardiac events of cardiac death, myocardial infarction, or unstable angina occurred in 27 patients. Clinical risk variables are those of Eagle and include age greater than 70 years, angina, diabetes requiring therapy, Q wave on electrocardiogram, and history of ventricular ectopy.

TABLE 1-31
Cardiac Complications and Dobutamine Stress Echocardiography

AUTHOR, YEAR	NO. OF PATIENTS	NO DYSSYNERGY			NEW DYSSYNERGY		
		NO. OF PATIENTS	ALL EVENTS (%)*	DEATH OR MI (%)†	NO. OF PATIENTS	ALL EVENTS (%)*	DEATH OR MI (%)†
Lalka, 1992	60	22	4.6	4.6	38	29.0	23.7
Eichelberger, 1993	75	48	0	0	27	19.0	7.0
Langan, 1993	81	31	0	0	50	6.0	6.0
Poldermans, 1993	136	99	0	0	35	42.9	14.3
Davila-Roman, 1993	93	70	0	0	23	20.0	4.0
TOTAL	445	270			173		
% EVENT			<1	<1		23.4	11.0

Adapted from Shaw LJ, Eagle KA, Gersh BJ et al: *J Am Coll Cardiol* 27:787, 1996.
MI, Myocardial infarction.
*Includes all cardiac complications measured by the individual study, such as congestive heart failure, myocardial ischemia, nonfatal myocardial infarction, and cardiac death.
†Cardiac death or myocardial infarction.

pressure, thermodilution cardiac output; oxygen saturations, Fick determination of cardiac output, calculation of systemic and pulmonary vascular resistances, and the degree of intracardiac shunts. The left atrial pressure is estimated by the PCWP.[443]

Comparison of the values obtained at catheterization to normal values (Box 1-12) helps characterize baseline cardiac function. The concept of the Starling curve is useful for understanding hemodynamic status. A normal cardiac output and low filling pressures indicate normal cardiac function. A low cardiac output with high filling pressures characterize some degree of heart failure. Elevated wedge or pulmonary artery diastolic pressure may indicate left ventricular dysfunction from CHF, myocardial ischemia, or valvular disease. In circumstances of ventricular hypertrophy, such as aortic stenosis, elevated left ventricular filling pressures that represent reduced compliance may be normal for that particular patient. Elevated right atrial pressure indicates right ventricular dysfunction or tricuspid or pulmonic valve disease. The etiology of right ventricular dysfunction includes myocardial ischemia and pulmonary hypertension. Elevated pulmonary artery pressures with elevated wedge pressure suggests left ventricular dysfunction from ischemia or valvular (mitral, aortic) heart disease. Elevated pulmonary artery pressures with a low wedge pressure indicates increased pulmonary vascular resistance.

Patients with a known abnormality such as the classic hemodynamic subsets of patients with acute MI provide a useful source for comparison (Table 1-32).

Left-Sided Heart Catheterization. Catheterization of the left ventricle is accomplished by fluoroscopic guidance of a catheter advanced from the femoral or brachial artery.[443] Left-sided heart catheterization provides pressure measurements, angiography of the coronary arteries, and contrast injection of the left ventricle. Pressure measurements include left ventricular systolic and diastolic pressures and aortic systolic and diastolic pressures. Aortic valve stenosis creates a gradient between the left ventricular systolic and aortic systolic pressure that is measured by pull-back of the catheter from the left ventricular to the proximal aorta (peak-to-peak gradient; see Chapter 4).

Coronary anatomy is defined by contrast dye injection into the right or left coronary ostia. A cineangiogram of the dye injection is reviewed for exact location and degree of coronary stenoses. Because coronary atherosclerotic lesions are eccentric, several views are obtained. Interpretation of the angiogram by different observers may yield variable interpretations.[445]

"Triple-vessel disease" indicates significant coronary stenoses of the three major coronary vessels: the left anterior descending (LAD) artery, the left circumflex artery, and the right coronary artery (RCA). Severe "left main coronary" disease is of great importance because the left main coronary divides to form the LAD and the circumflex arteries. Reduced left main coronary perfusion causes ischemia of the majority of the left ventricle

---

BOX 1-12
Normal Cardiac Catheterization Measurements*

Pressures (mm Hg)

Right atrium (mean)	2-8
Right ventricle (systolic/diastolic)	15/2-30/8
Pulmonary artery (systolic/ diastolic)	15/4-30/12
Left atrium or wedge (mean)	2-10
Left ventricle (systolic/diastolic)	100/3-140/12
Systolic arterial (systolic/diastolic)	100/60-140/90

Blood Flows

Cardiac index	2.6-4.2 L/min/m^2
Stroke index	30-65 ml/beat/m^2

From Grossman W: *Cardiac catheterization and angiography*, ed 3, Philadelphia, 1986, Lippincott Williams & Wilkins.
*Normal values should be determined in each individual laboratory.

TABLE 1-32
Hemodynamic Subsets of Acute Myocardial Infarction

CLASS	CLINICAL DEFINITION	CARDIAC INDEX (L/min/m^2)	PCWP (mm Hg)	MORTALITY (%)
I	No pulmonary congestion or systemic hypoperfusion	>2.2	<18	3
II	Pulmonary congestion only, good perfusion	>2.2	>18	9
III	Reduced perfusion only, no pulmonary congestion	<2.2	<18	23
IV	Both pulmonary edema and hypoperfusion (shock)	<2.2	>18	51

From Forrester JS, Diamond G, Chatterjee K et al: *N Engl J Med* 295:1404, 1976.
PCWP, Pulmonary capillary wedge pressure.

TABLE 1-33
Abnormalities of Wall Motion on the Left Ventriculogram

TERM	DEFINITION
Hypokinesis	Region of the myocardium contracts during systole, but the contraction is less than that of neighboring regions.
Akinesis	Region of myocardium does not contract during systole.
Dyskinesis	Region of myocardium bulges outward during systole and thus moves in the opposite direction compared with adjacent regions of myocardium.

From Franch RH, Douglas JS, King SB: Cardiac catheterization and coronary arteriography. In Alexander WR, Schlant RC, Fuster V, editors: *Hurst's the heart*, New York, 1998, McGraw-Hill.
Note: Typically, hypokinetic regions are interpreted as ischemic areas, akinetic regions as infarcted myocardium, and dyskinetic areas as either very severely ischemic or a ventricular aneurysm.

TABLE 1-34
Grades of Mitral Insufficiency

GRADE	DESCRIPTION
Mild (1+)	A trace of contrast dye is visible in the atrium but clears during each beat and never opacifies the entire left atrium.
Moderate (2+)	Contrast dye does not clear with each beat and generally opacifies the left atrium after several beats, although opacification is not equal to that of the left ventricle.
Moderately severe (3+)	Left atrium is completely opacified, and opacification becomes more dense with each cardiac cycle.
Severe (4+)	Contrast agent completely opacifies the atrium during the first cardiac cycle.

From Grossman W: *Cardiac catheterization and angiography*, ed 3, Philadelphia, 1986, Lippincott Williams & Wilkins.

with resulting hypotension and further decreased perfusion. Myocardium supplied by a completely stenosed artery may receive perfusion from collateral vessels from another coronary artery. The circumstance of "left main equivalent" stenosis occurs when both the LAD and circumflex arteries are severely stenosed and receive collateral flow from the RCA, which itself is significantly narrowed.[446]

Injection of contrast dye into the cavity of the left ventricle generates the "left ventriculogram" from which the left ventricular EF and regional wall motion are determined. Reversible ischemia usually causes hypokinesis, whereas akinesis (no movement) represents previous MI; dyskinesis (outward bulging) may indicate a ventricular aneurysm (Table 1-33). A key issue in interpretation is that myocardial ischemia alone can cause any of these wall-motion abnormalities. The presence of a completely occluded coronary artery by angiography supports but does not guarantee that an akinetic or dyskinetic region represents myocardial scar. Viability testing may be necessary to make the distinction.[389] The LVEDP is often measured before and after injection of contrast dye for the ventriculogram. Radiographic contrast dye may acutely worsen left ventricular function because of a lack of oxygen carriage, chelation of calcium, or direct effect on the myocardium. An increase in LVEDP after contrast injection indicates more severe cardiac disease.

Injection of contrast dye is also used to characterize valvular heart lesions. The time taken for dye injected into the left ventricle to opacify the left atrium is a measure of mitral insufficiency (Table 1-34).[447] To

assess aortic valve insufficiency, dye is injected into the root of the aorta and observed to opacify the left ventricle.

It is important that cardiac catheterization data be correlated to the clinical assessment. For example, it is possible to have a low EF with regional areas of dyskinesis and yet a normal cardiac output. This might occur if a left ventricular aneurysm bulges during systole but has enough normal surrounding myocardium so that forward stroke volume is satisfactory. Absence of fatigue or exercise intolerance suggests that the cardiac output measurement is appropriate. In contrast, a patient could have a normal EF and normal cardiac output yet have elevated filling pressures and clinical symptoms of ventricular failure. Here a postinfarction VSD contributes to a false elevation of the cardiac output measurement. When clinical information and catheterization are not consistent, additional diagnoses should be considered.

Myocardial Viability Assessment

Hibernating Myocardium. An important issue for the patient with coronary artery disease is whether CABG surgery will be beneficial. Ideally, cardiac catheterization localizes discrete coronary stenoses supplying contracting myocardium that benefit from bypass grafts. In contrast, areas of myocardium that are nonfunctional and represent scar from MI do not benefit. Patients with "hibernating" or "stunned" myocardium have viable myocardial muscle that does not contract because of severe ischemia. The distinction between viable myocardium from nonviable scar is key. In some cases, viability assessment may convert a "nonoperable" patient into a CABG candidate.

Positron emission tomography (PET) scanning uses nuclear scanning techniques to identify myocardium in which metabolism is ongoing. Another method uses DSE. Here "contractile reserve" indicates viability and represents improved systolic thickening in regions of depressed left ventricular function during dobutamine infusion. Contractile reserve demonstrated with preoperative DSE is associated with improved systolic wall thickening after coronary revascularization.[448]

Dobutamine MRI. The most recent method of myocardial assessment uses cine MRI to provide tomographic assessments of regional myocardial function. The addition of dobutamine as a provocative stress makes dobutamine MRI the latest method of noninvasively assessing coronary artery disease. The first report of dobutamine MRI was that of Pennell et al in 1992, who studied 25 patients with exertional chest discomfort and abnormal exercise ECGs. The dobutamine dosage was 20 μg/kg/min. Areas of abnormal wall motion on the dobutamine MRI corresponded with good agreement to areas of decreased perfusion by dobutamine thallium scanning and coronary angiography.[449]

The first report of high-dose dobutamine (up to 40 μg/kg/min plus atropine) with MRI was that of Nagel et al in 1999.[450] Dobutamine MRI was compared with DSE in 208 patients with suspected coronary disease. Patients subsequently underwent cardiac catheterization to define coronary anatomy. Dobutamine MRI was better than DSE for diagnosing coronary artery disease. In this study, 18 patients could not undergo dobutamine MRI scanning because of claustrophobia or body habitus. Also, 18 patients could not be assessed by DSE because of poor image quality.[450]

An accompanying editorial summarized the strengths and weaknesses of dobutamine MRI. The major strengths included good image quality that did not depend on a satisfactory window, as does transthoracic echocardiography, and more diagnostic accuracy. Weaknesses included the necessity of repeated breath-holding (16 seconds) to acquire MRI images, current MRI technology prevents analysis of ST-segment monitoring during the procedure, and real-time wall motion cannot be displayed. However, the future of MRI holds promise of real-time imaging.[451,452]

NONCARDIAC SURGERY IN SPECIAL GROUPS
Aortic Stenosis and Noncardiac Surgery

The presence of aortic stenosis in patients undergoing noncardiac surgery deserves special consideration. O'Keefe et al studied 48 consecutive patients with significant aortic stenosis undergoing elective noncardiac surgeries at the Mayo Clinic.[453] *Significant aortic stenosis* was defined as either moderate (peak Doppler-derived gradient velocity of 3.5 to 4.4 m/s or calculated aortic valve area of 0.76-0.99 cm^2) or severe (peak Doppler-derived gradient velocity of 4.5 m/s or a calculated aortic valve area of ≤0.75 cm^2). More than half of the procedures were minor, using local anesthesia with sedation. General anesthesia was used in 22 patients, and 1 patient received spinal anesthesia. No deaths occurred, but five patients (four general anesthesia, one spinal) experienced intraoperative hypotension. Four of the patients with hypotensive episodes responded to fluids and vasopressor drugs, but one patient (general anesthesia for abdominal aortic aneurysm repair) remained hypotensive, required dopamine for 24 hours, and had borderline elevation of CK-MB enzyme. The authors concluded that selected patients with severe aortic stenosis can undergo noncardiac procedures with a reasonably low risk of complications with careful monitoring.[453]

A more recent investigation by Torsher et al (also from the Mayo Clinic) studied 19 patients with severe aortic stenosis (aortic valve area index <0.5 cm^2/m^2 or mean gradient >50 mm Hg determined by Doppler echocardiography or cardiac catheterization).[454] Most patients had normal ventricular function (EF >0.55 in 15 patients, EF <0.3 in 1 patient, and not reported in three cases). General anesthesia was used in 26 patients and continuous spinal in 2. Operations were elective in 22 cases and emergent in 6. Intraoperative hypotension requiring vasoconstrictor therapy occurred in 14 patients (two thirds of the cases). Bradycardia occurred in two cases, one of which required temporary pacing. Postoperative cardiac complications occurred in two patients. An 81-year-old man developed an MI after bilateral total knee arthroplasties and died 17 days later. Another 90-year-old man developed multiple-organ failure and died after emergent laparotomy and superior mesenteric artery embolectomy. Overall mortality was 11%.[454]

In the same report, Torsher et al also described three additional aortic stenosis patients who underwent emergent aortic balloon valvuloplasty *after* undergoing an elective noncardiac surgical procedure. In two cases the surgery was characterized as "uneventful," and in the third, a 20-minute period of hypotension occurred and was treated with phenylephrine. The diagnosis of aortic stenosis was not apparent preoperatively in any of these patients, although a systolic murmur was documented. All three patients developed pulmonary edema either immediately postoperatively or shortly after hospital discharge. One of these patients sustained an MI and died, despite aortic balloon valvuloplasty; the other two patients recovered.[454]

These scenarios are thought provoking for several reasons. Clearly, aortic stenosis can be a minor or major risk factor depending on its severity. Yet how can the severity be accurately judged? The three additional patients described by Tosher et al indicate that the preoperative history and physical were either incomplete or insensitive. If Tosher et al had included all the patients in their report, the mortality would have been 13.5% (3 deaths in 22 patients).[454] Is this significant? Consider that, in 1988, Craver et al reported surgical replacement of the aortic valve in 188 patients older than 70 years of age had a 30-day mortality of 10.1%.[455]

Another recent study by Raymer and Yang was a retrospective review of 55 patients with the diagnosis of aortic stenosis who underwent noncardiac surgery.[456] The severity was established by the most recent echocardiogram and was described as mild in 18 patients (aortic valve area 1.0-1.6 cm^2), moderate in 13 patients (0.8-0.99 cm^2), and severe in 24 patients (<0.8 cm^2). The authors used matching control patients and found that cardiac complications occurred in five aortic stenosis patients and six controls. Unfortunately, they did not note what type of anesthetic (general, regional, or conscious sedation) was performed in patients with varying degrees of aortic stenosis (mild, moderate, or severe). Nonetheless, the complications for aortic stenosis patients were significant: CHF, four patients; MI, two patients; ventricular fibrillation, one patient; and death, one patient. Although the authors concluded that there was no difference in complications between patients with aortic stenosis and matched controls, both groups had undesirable morbidity.[456]

Valvuloplasty Before Noncardiac Surgery. For patients with severe valvular aortic stenosis, the approach of percutaneous valvuloplasty before noncardiac surgery has been explored. Levine et al,[457] and Roth et al,[458] reported mostly successful outcomes, but Hayes et al[459] reported a relatively high incidence of cardiac tamponade with perforation of the left ventricle. The Mansfield Valvuloplasty Registry[460,461] indicates that the results of valvuloplasty are best in patients with better ventricular function, larger valve areas, and a lower incidence of MI *before valvuloplasty*. In one assessment, long-term results were best in patients with a PCWP of less than 18 mm Hg and a baseline aortic systolic pressure of 140 mm Hg or greater.[462] These patients had event-free survival rates of 65% at 1 year and 41% at 2 years. In patients with PCWP of 25 mm Hg or greater and baseline aortic systolic blood pressure of less than 110 mm Hg, predicted event-free survival rates were 23% at 1 year and 4% at 2 years. These patients should undergo surgical aortic valve replacement for better long-term survival.[462]

Noncardiac Surgery After Prior Coronary Bypass

A number of studies have indicated that noncardiac surgery in patients with prior CABG has a lower risk of cardiac complications.[463,464] Hertzer et al demonstrated improved outcome when patients with severe coronary

disease underwent coronary bypass before vascular surgery.[218,221] Mahar et al, compared outcomes after noncardiac surgery in patients who had prior CABG versus patients with medically treated coronary disease.[465] Patients with prior CABG did not sustain an MI, whereas patients with medically treated coronary disease had a 5% infarction rate. Schoeppel et al also reported no postoperative MIs after noncardiac surgery in patients with prior CABG.[466]

The CASS database has followed a large number of patients with suspected coronary disease who were treated medically or with CABG. Foster et al reviewed the outcomes of 1600 CASS patients who had undergone major noncardiac surgery.[467] Group I had no angiographic evidence of coronary disease. Group II included patients with prior CABG. Group III included patients with angiographically confirmed coronary disease who received only medical therapy. There was no statistical difference in the incidence of MI, heart failure, or rhythm disturbances among the groups. However, cardiac deaths and overall mortality were similar for CABG patients and patients without coronary disease (Table 1-35). Cardiac deaths and overall mortality were higher in group III patients who had coronary disease but not CABG. These data suggest that successful CABG reduces the risk of subsequent noncardiac surgery.

Eagle et al reported a 10-year follow-up of 3368 CASS patients who had undergone noncardiac surgery.[468] Abdominal (36%), urologic (21%), orthopedic (15%), and vascular procedures were most common. This study had several important findings. First, "high-risk" noncardiac operations were distinguished from "low-risk" operations on the basis of a combined MI and death rate of 4% or greater in medically treated patients with known coronary disease. High-risk noncardiac operations included abdominal, vascular, thoracic, head, and

TABLE 1-35
Noncardiac Surgery in 1600 Patients from CASS Registry

VARIABLE	GROUP 1* ($n = 399$)	GROUP 2† ($n = 743$)	GROUP 3‡ ($n = 458$)
Operative mortality	2 (0.5)	7 (0.9)	11 (2.4)
Cardiac deaths	1 (0.25)	4 (0.54)	9 (1.9)

From Foster ED, Davis KB, Carpenter JA et al: *Ann Thorac Surg* 41: 42, 1986.
Number in parentheses indicates the percent of the group that had an event.
*No coronary disease.
†Prior coronary artery bypass graft.
‡Angiographic coronary disease.

neck operations. Low-risk surgeries included urologic, orthopedic, breast, and skin operations.[468]

The second finding (Fig. 1-8) was that for high-risk surgery; patients with coronary disease and prior CABG surgery had better outcomes (death, 1.7%; MI rate, 0.8%) than patients with medically managed coronary disease (death, 3.3%; MI rate, 2.7%). For lower-risk surgery, there was no significant difference in outcome. Multivariate analysis identified several predictors of 30-day death or MI after high-risk surgery: medical versus CABG treatment of coronary disease, CHF score, hypertension, and smoking history. The elapsed time between the original CABG revascularization and noncardiac surgery was assessed. After 6 years, there was a trend toward increased incidence of perioperative MI. The risk of perioperative death (<2%) was unchanged over these periods.[468]

The authors qualify the study findings in several ways. First, patients were enrolled in the CASS registry 15 years before the retrospective review. Significant advances in medical and surgical therapy occurred during those years. Second, their study did not examine the risk of CABG surgery.[468] The CASS registry demonstrated an average operative mortality of 2.3% for patients undergoing CABG surgery.[469] The authors concluded that if coronary revascularization is warranted on the basis of symptoms or coronary anatomy, coronary artery revascularization should be performed before noncardiac surgery.[468,470]

Prior PTCA Revascularization Before Noncardiac Surgery

A retrospective review of hospital discharge data by Posner et al compared 30-day outcomes after noncardiac surgery among PTCA patients, patients with unrevascularized coronary disease, and normal controls.[471] Patients were matched on the basis of age, gender, and year

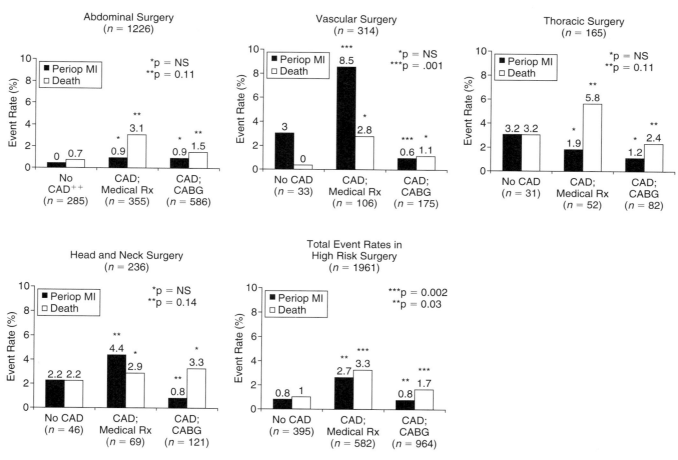

FIG. 1-8 Adverse outcomes for high-risk operations in CASS patients. Shows rates of myocardial infarction (MI) or death among patients undergoing abdominal, vascular, thoracic, and head and neck surgeries. Groups are No CAD, indicating no coronary artery disease; CAD Medical Rx, indicating medical treatment of coronary artery disease; and CAD CABG, indicating that coronary artery bypass graft surgery had been performed. Note the marked incidence of MI in medically treated coronary patients who underwent vascular surgery.

(From Eagle KA, Rihal CS, Mickel MC et al: Circulation 96:1884, 1997.)

and type of noncardiac surgery. Adverse cardiac outcomes included MI, angina, CHF, malignant dysrhythmia, cardiogenic shock, or "unspecified cardiac complication." Overall, patients who had angioplasty were less likely to have angina, CHF, or MI after noncardiac surgery than matched patients with unrevascularized coronary disease. However, patients with "recent PTCA" (<90 days) had adverse cardiac outcomes similar to those of patients with unrevascularized coronary disease. Normal controls had fewer adverse cardiac outcomes than PTCA patients.[471] It is worth questioning the validity of their "matching" process. Patients were presumably treated with PTCA as an appropriate therapy of significant coronary disease. Patients who did not have PTCA presumably did not have the same degree of coronary disease to warrant the procedure.

The authors concluded that PTCA did not render the patients "good as new" in terms of risk of cardiac complications after noncardiac surgery. Posner et al also emphasized that the risk of prophylatic PTCA before noncardiac surgery should include both the risk of the PTCA procedure and the risk of the noncardiac surgery. This combined risk may be greater than the risk of proceeding directly to noncardiac surgery without PTCA.[471] A recent study by Van Norman supports these findings.[472]

Huber et al studied 55 patients with high cardiac risk by clinical assessment or noninvasive testing who underwent PTCA before noncardiac surgery.[473] Multivessel disease was identified by cardiac catheterization in 76% of patients. Angioplasty was successful in 50 patients who subsequently underwent noncardiac surgery. Of these, one patient had a fatal MI nearly 3 weeks after abdominal aortic aneurysm repair. Two others had nonfatal, non–Q-wave infarctions 1 to 2 days after noncardiac surgery. This yielded a perioperative cardiac mortality of 1.9% and a nonfatal infarction rate of 5.6%. In the five cases in which angioplasty was unsuccessful, the patients underwent emergency coronary artery bypass surgery, and all survived.[473]

The BARI trial was designed to compare CABG versus PTCA as treatment of symptomatic two- or three-vessel coronary disease. All angioplasties were performed without the use of coronary stents. A subset of 501 patients, originally randomized to either CABG or angioplasty, subsequently underwent 1049 noncardiac operations.[474] After the first noncardiac surgery, the rate of adverse cardiac events (death and nonfatal MI) was 1.6% in both groups (Table 1-36). When all noncardiac procedures were considered, the incidence of adverse outcomes was also similar.[474]

There was a tendency for more cardiac events to occur after surgical procedures regarded as "high risk," such as thoracic and vascular procedures (Table 1-37). The low incidence of adverse events after abdominal procedures may be related to the fact that more than one third were

TABLE 1-36
Noncardiac Surgery after CABG or PTCA

ADVERSE EVENTS AFTER FIRST NONCARDIAC SURGERY	CABG GROUP ($n = 250$)	PTCA GROUP ($n = 251$)
Death	2 (0.8)	2 (0.8)
Nonfatal MI	2 (0.8)	2 (0.8)
Total events	4 (1.6)	4 (1.6)

From Hassan SA, Hlatky MA, Boothroyd DB et al: *Am J Med* 110: 260, 2001.
CABG, Coronary artery bypass graft; MI, myocardial infarction; PTCA, percutaneous transluminal coronary angioplasty.

TABLE 1-37
Type of Noncardiac Operation after CABG or PTCA

SURGERY TYPE	NO. OF PROCEDURES	NO. OF EVENTS (%)
Thoracic	22	1 (5)
Vascular	120	5 (4)
Urologic	131	3 (2)
Abdominal	162	2 (1)
Orthopedic	173	1 (1)
Eye	228	2 (1)
Head and neck	48	0
Breast	14	0

From Hassan SA, Hlatky MA, Boothroyd DB et al: *Am J Med* 110: 260, 2001.
CABG, Coronary artery bypass graft; PTCA, percutaneous transluminal coronary angioplasty.

simple hernia repairs. Longer periods of time between revascularization and noncardiac surgery were associated with an increased incidence of cardiac events. Noncardiac surgery performed within 4 years of revascularization was associated with a complication rate of less than 1%, whereas surgery performed after 4 years had a cardiac event rate of 3.6%. In addition, the vast majority (90%) of patients had noncardiac surgical procedures performed more than 6 months after their coronary revascularization, beyond the period of early angioplasty restenosis.[474]

PTCA with Coronary Stenting. The use of coronary stents has become a widespread practice during coro-

TABLE 1-38
Adverse Surgery Outcomes Early after Coronary Stent

AGE (yr)	STENT TO SURGERY (days)	OPERATION	COMPLICATIONS
82	1	Femoral artery	MI, death
62	1	Carotid artery	MI, bleeding, death
72	1	Mitral valve	Bleeding, death
68	1	Carotid artery	MI, bleeding, death
67	2	TAA	MI
67	3	TAA	MI, bleeding, death
72	5	Colectomy	MI, death
62	6	Lung transplant	MI, bleeding, death
74	11	TAA	Bleeding, death

From Kaluza GL, Jane J, Lee JR et al: *J Am Coll Cardiol* 35:1288, 2000.

MI, Myocardial infarction; *TAA,* thoracoabdominal aneurysm.

nary angioplasty. Improved techniques and antiplatelet drugs have resolved initial problems with thrombosis.[311] However, Kaluza et al reported that noncardiac surgery immediately after a coronary stent procedure was associated with a high incidence of major adverse outcomes.[475] The study evaluated 40 patients who had received a coronary stent less than 6 weeks before their noncardiac surgery. All patients received aspirin at the time of the stent procedure and at least one dose of ticlodipine after stenting. Postoperative MIs occurred in seven patients, six of which were fatal. All of the fatal MIs occurred in patients who underwent surgery within 1 week of the coronary stent procedure (Table 1-38).[475]

Although antiplatelet therapy is recommended for at least 14 days after coronary stent placement and for 30 days in high-risk patients,[476] a number of patients in this study had one or both antiplatelet drugs discontinued immediately before surgery and restarted afterward.[475] The authors presumed that stent thrombosis was the cause of all the MIs, but this was confirmed by angiography in only two cases.[475] Excessive bleeding was reported in 11 cases, 2 of which attributed bleeding to the cause of death.

It is important to note that the cases in this series were not all "noncardiac" surgery. The patient undergoing MVR had systemic heparin and cardiopulmonary bypass. The three thoracoabdominal aneurysm repairs and one lung transplantation may have had other bleeding causes in addition to the antiplatelet drugs. The important "take home message" is that discontinuation of antiplatelet medicines risks thrombosis, whereas continuation of antiplatelet therapy risks bleeding. Kaluza et al recommend that elective surgery be delayed for 2 to 4 weeks after the placement of a coronary stent. Because PTCA without stenting is not associated with the same potential for thrombosis, stent placement should be avoided if noncardiac surgery is anticipated soon afterward.[475]

Hypertrophic Obstructive Cardiomyopathy (HOCM)

Description. HOCM, also described as idiopathic hypertrophic subaortic stenosis (IHSS), is a special entity in the group of cardiac disorders known as *cardiomyopathies*.[477,478] Cardiomyopathy refers to diseases of the heart muscle, rather than secondary responses to conditions such as hypertension, ischemia, or valvular heart disease. There are three types of cardiomyopathy. Dilated cardiomyopathy is most common (60%) and is characterized by decreased contractility and ventricular dilation. Restrictive cardiomyopathy is least common and is characterized by reduced ventricular compliance and diastolic dysfunction. Hypertrophic cardiomyopathy is characterized by significant hypertrophy of the left ventricle, including the interventricular septum. Systolic function is preserved or hyperdynamic, and diastolic filling is impaired. There is a significant genetic component to the occurrence of hypertrophic cardiomyopathy, which suggests that other family members may be affected.[477,478]

Within the category of hypertrophic cardiomyopathy is a subgroup in which hypertrophy of the intraventricular septum creates a dynamic left ventricular outflow tract (LVOT) obstruction. Patients with HOCM represent only about 25% of those with hypertrophic cardiomyopathy but are extremely important to identify because of the risk of sudden death even in a young individual.[477,478]

Physiology. The LVOT obstruction in patients with HOCM is variable and depends on ventricular contractility, ventricular filling, and systemic vascular resistance. Braunwald et al demonstrated that circumstances that increase contractility, such as digoxin, exercise, and isoproterenol, worsen the obstruction.[479] Arterial hypotension occurs despite markedly increased intraventricular pressure. β-Blockade decreases contractility and therefore reduces outflow tract obstruction. Nitroglycerin and the Valsalva maneuver reduce ventricular filling, and worsen the obstruction. α-Vasoconstrictors (methoxamine, phenylephrine) also reduce the obstruction. Significant LVOT obstruction in an awake patient was relieved by general anesthesia because of the decreased contractility caused by the inhalation agent.[479]

Anesthesia for Noncardiac Surgery. A number of reports address the issue of anesthetic technique for patients with HOCM undergoing noncardiac surgery. Thompson et al reviewed 35 patients with a discharge diagnosis of HOCM who had undergone noncardiac surgery.[480] The diagnosis of HOCM was based on a dynamic LVOT gradient (baseline gradient 30 mm Hg, 80 mm Hg when provoked) in 22 patients and the ratio of septal wall thickness to the posterior wall in the other 13 patients. General anesthesia was used in 32 patients and spinal anesthesia in 3. One case of angina and several cases of dysrhythmias occurred in the general anesthesia group. Perioperative MI occurred in the one patient who received spinal anesthesia. The authors concluded that general anesthesia was relatively safe but cautioned the use of spinal anesthesia.[480]

A different conclusion was reached by Haering et al.[481] They reviewed 77 patients with echocardiographic evidence of asymmetric septal hypertrophy (septum-to-posterior wall thickness ratio >1.5) who had undergone noncardiac surgery. Adverse events were relatively frequent (ischemia, 12%; hypotension, 14%; CHF, 16%; stable dysrhythmia, 25%), but only one patient sustained an MI. The authors concluded that severe outcomes were uncommon. Thus surgery should not be discouraged, but a high incidence of postoperative CHF should be anticipated. They also reasoned that regional anesthesia was acceptable provided that hemodynamics were controlled.[481] Several other annecdotal reports describe the use of general or regional anesthesia in patients with varying degrees of success and adverse outcome.

The key issue in the all of these reports is whether truly significant LVOT obstruction was present. Only 25% of patients with hypertrophic cardiomyopathy have characteristics of obstruction. Thus in Thompson's population, 63% of cases had known LVOT gradients that were approximately 30 mm Hg at rest and 80 mm Hg when provoked.[480] In Haering's population, 39% of cases had an LVOT gradient of 10 mm Hg or greater.[481] This suggests that the patients in Thompson's series were at higher risk than those of Haering's. It is probably inappropriate to plan an anesthetic for a patient with severe dynamic LVOT obstruction based on the experiences of patients with significantly lesser degrees of obstruction.

When planning an anesthetic for the patient with true HOCM, the potential for dynamic LVOT obstruction should be assessed. Each anesthetic has expected physiologic responses. General inhalational anesthesia causes decreased myocardial contractility, a characteristic expected to reduce dynamic obstruction. Spinal or epidural techniques are characterized by venous and arterial vasodilation, characteristics expected to provoke obstruction. Further considerations for anesthetic management are discussed in Chapter 11.

Noncardiac Surgery in Congenital Heart Disease

Preoperative Assessment. Patients with repaired or unrepaired congential heart disease occasionally present for noncardiac operation.[482] Review of the specific heart disorder is helpful before evaluating the patient[483] (see Chapter 10). For example, conventional auscultation of the left side of the chest may not detect a significant heart murmur in a patient with dextrocardia. In "situs inversus," both the thoracic and abdominal organs are in a mirror-image position from normal. Thus palpation for liver distention would be performed in the upper *left* abdominal quadrant. If lung surgery is planned, the reversed right and left bronchi will influence the choice of double-lumen tube. Patients who have received a Blalock-Taussig systemic-to-pulmonary shunt may have a diminished pulse in the arm on the side of the operation.

Residua. The term *residua* refers to conditions that remain or are left over after successful corrective surgery for congential heart disease.[484] An example would be a congenital bicuspid aortic valve in a patient who has undergone coarctation repair in childhood. Although the aortic valve was not an issue during coarctation repair, it may have become hemodynamically significant over time. Patients who have had successful coarctation repair may also have systemic hypertension. Rupture of a circle of Willis aneurysm has been reported after distant repair of coarctation.[485] Mild aortic insufficiency may remain after surgery for tetralogy of Fallot, truncus arteriosus, or perimembranous VSD.[484]

Sequelae. The term *sequelae* is a consequence that has occurred because of the congenital heart repair. Atrial dysrhythmias may be common in patients who have undergone a Mustard or Senning atrial baffle procedure for transposition of the great arteries.[484] In patients who have undergone a Fontan procedure, pulmonary blood flow depends on systemic venous pressure. Such patients will be vulnerable to dehydration, blood loss, and circumstances that increase pulmonary vascular resistance, such as hypercarbia, acidosis, and hypoxemia. A respiratory illness in such patients poses potentially serious problems and should preclude elective surgery.

Eisenmenger Syndrome. The term *Eisenmenger complex* originated from a 1897 description of a 32-year-old man who died suddenly after a long history of dyspnea and cyanosis. A large VSD was found at autopsy. Wood described "pulmonary hypertension at the systemic level due to a high pulmonary vascular resistance, with reversed or bi-directional shunting through a large ventricular septal defect." The term *Eisenmenger syndrome* describes the circumstance of increased pulmonary vascular resistance that has caused reversal of shunt flow across any systemic-pulmonary connection (e.g., PDA).

Cyanosis with erythrocytosis is a characteristic finding in patients with Eisenmenger syndrome. Hyperviscosity may cause thromboembolism and symptoms of headache, dizziness, and fatigue. Treatment includes careful phlebotomy and fluid replacement with an equal volume of saline. Phlebotomy without volume replacement may worsen cardiac output,[274] and over-aggressive phlebotomy can cause cardiovascular collapse.[486] Patients are at risk for bleeding because of defects involving platelets, the coagulation system, and fibrinolysis. Other issues include hemoptysis, hyperuricemia, cholelithiasis, arthralgias, renal dysfunction, and risk of paradoxical embolism with stroke. Medicines such as calcium channel blockers, lower systemic vascular resistance and may worsen right-to-left shunting.

Causes of death include complications associated with pregnancy. Maternal mortality is high: 33% for vaginal delivery and 47% for cesarean section. Noncardiac surgery is avoided when possible because of high perioperative mortality (19%). Anesthetic considerations are summarized in Box 1-13.

Noncardiac Surgery and Eisenmenger Syndrome.
Ammash et al reviewed their experience with 24 adult patients with Eisenmenger syndrome undergoing noncardiac surgery.[487] The patients were 17 to 55 years of age and underwent surgery for tubal ligation (nine cases), craniotomy (three cases), cholecystectomy (three cases), vasectomy (three cases), hysterectomy (three cases), spinal fusion, appendectomy, eye enucleation, hernia, hand, tonsillectomy, and therapeutic abortion. The most common primary congenital heart defects were VSD (seven cases), atrial septal defect (six cases), and PDA (three cases).[487]

Preoperative characteristics included hematocrit, 42% to 73%; arterial saturation, 63% to 92%; platelet count, 81 to 314 K; and left ventricle EF, 40% to 64%. Right ventricular dysfunction was moderate in five patients and severe in three. Arterial pressure was monitored continuously in more than half the patients and central venous pressure monitored in fewer than half. Five patients developed transient intraoperative hypotension to 90 mm Hg. One death occurred postoperatively in a patient who underwent spinal fusion. This procedure lasted more than 8 hours, with significant blood and fluid transfusion and persistent intraoperative hypotension requiring dopamine. These more complicated procedures were performed at the Mayo Clinic; other, less complicated procedures were performed outside the Mayo Clinic. One death occurred outside of the clinic following appendectomy. The authors emphasize that patients with Eisenmenger syndrome who require surgery should be referred to centers familiar with caring for such patients.[487]

Surgery in Heart Transplant Recipients
Noncardiac and Cardiac Surgery. Cardiac transplantation began in 1967 and has become the major therapy for end-stage heart disease. Cardiac transplant patients may require a variety of noncardiac surgery procedures. One report described that general surgical problems occurred in cardiac transplant recipients 10 times more often than nontransplant cardiac surgery. Corticosteroid use is associated with gastrointestinal bleeding, peptic ulcer, bowel perforation, and pancreatitis. Osteoporosis and aseptic necrosis can lead to total hip and total knee replacement.

Heart transplant recipients may also require cardiac surgery. Accelerated coronary atherosclerosis is characteristic of the heart transplant recipient. Although focal lesions may be amenable to angioplasty or CABG surgery,[488,489] the characteristic lesion is a concentric intimal proliferation throughout the entire coronary artery and smaller branches. Repeat cardiac transplantation may be the only option in such cases.[490]

Anesthetic Considerations. The transplanted heart is denervated and is not influenced by sympathetic or parasympathetic nerves. Indirect-acting drugs such as atropine will be ineffective, but the transplanted heart will respond to direct-acting drugs such as epinephrine. Autonomic influence persists in what remains of the recipient's native heart such as a portion of the atrium, visible on the ECG as a second p wave. Denervation of afferent fibers implies that these patients will not experience the typical symptoms of angina. Instead, ischemia may present with the symptoms of CHF.

Hypertension develops frequently in transplant recipients. The normal decrease in blood pressure that occurs during sleep is absent. The process of atherosclerosis is increased, and endothelial dysfunction is characteristic. A normal coronary artery will dilate in response to acetylcholine, but after transplantation, a vasoconstrictor response occurs. Coronary arteries of the transplanted heart dilate in response to nitroglycerin.[491]

The transplanted heart differs from the normal heart in response to exercise. An increase in cardiac output occurs in both, but by different mechanisms. In normal patients, exercise initiates an immediate increase in heart rate with a stable stroke volume. In cardiac transplant patients, heart rate is unchanged but stroke volume increases because of increased venous return. The transplanted heart depends on the Starling mechanism. The heart rate of the transplanted patient increases over time because of catecholamines released from the adrenal glands.[492] Dependence on circulating catecholamines means that β-blocking agents are poorly tolerated. Immunosuppression in these patients mandates strict adherence to appropriate sterile technique for line placement.

KEY POINTS

1. The consensus guidelines of the AHA/ACC and ACP for preoperative assessment of the cardiac patient undergoing noncardiac surgery differ in their handling of functional capacity, assessment of the intermediate-risk patient, and whether the procedure involves vascular surgery. Preoperative assessment must be individualized for the patient and surgical procedure.

2. A recent MI significantly increases the risk of a perioperative cardiac event. Elective surgery should *ideally* be postponed for 6 months after an MI. This applies only to noncardiac surgery—not cardiac surgery.

3. The best-known clinical methods for assessing risk of the cardiac patient undergoing noncardiac surgery are the Goldman CRI and the Detsky Modified Risk Index. The more recently proposed Revised Cardiac Index by Lee et al uses the type of surgery, history of ischemic heart disease, CHF, cerebrovascular disease, preoperative insulin therapy, and serum creatinine greater than 2 mg/dl to calculate operative risk.

4. Core variables related to outcome with cardiac surgery include age, gender, previous cardiac surgery, left ventricular EF, percentage of stenosis of the left main coronary artery, the number of major coronary arteries with greater than 70% stenosis, and the acuity of the operation.

5. The history and physical examination provide the foundation upon which the rest of the preoperative evaluation is based. Although cardiac and pulmonic disease processes are often interrelated, specific signs and symptoms of heart failure and ischemic heart disease must be identified.

6. A variety of tests are available to assess risk and cardiac function. Dipyridamole thallium scanning and DSE are useful for identifying myocardium at risk for ischemia and assessing ventricular function. These tests are most beneficial for patients with intermediate risk (one or two clinical risk factors).

7. Cardiac catheterization is the definitive test for evaluating coronary artery disease and left ventricular function. This diagnostic tool can also be used to determine intracardiac pressures and shunts, valvular gradients, and vascular resistances.

8. Newer technology includes dobutamine MRI and PET, which is used to distinguish viable from scarred myocardium.

9. The risk of noncardiac surgery in patients with prior CABG is similar to that for patients who lack coronary artery disease. Outcome is also similar for patients who had multivessel PTCA at least 6 months before noncardiac surgery. Patients with medically managed coronary artery disease have worse outcomes after high-risk noncardiac surgery than patients with prior CABG.

10. There is a high incidence of adverse cardiac outcomes in patients undergoing noncardiac surgery shortly (1-6 weeks) after coronary artery stenting. The decision to discontinue antiplatelet medication for noncardiac surgery shortly after coronary stenting is a dilemma between the risks of increased surgical bleeding and stent thrombosis.

11. Noncardiac surgery can be performed safely in patients with aortic stenosis or HOCM, but with increased risk of adverse outcome. Careful preoperative assessment of the severity of the disease and strong consideration of the necessity of the surgery are warranted to optimize risk versus benefit.

KEY REFERENCES

Abraham SA, Coles NA, Coley CM et al: Coronary risk of noncardiac surgery, *Prog Cardiovasc Dis* 34:205-234, 1991.

American College of Physicians: Guidelines for assessing and managing the perioperative risk from coronary artery disease associated with major noncardiac surgery, *Ann Intern Med* 127:309-312, 1997.

Badgett RG, Lucey, CR, Mulrow CD: Can the clinical examination diagnose left-sided heart failure in adults? *JAMA* 277: 1712-1719, 1997.

Brown KA: Prognostic value of thallium-201 myocardial perfusion imaging, *Circulation* 83:363, 1991.

Carabello BA, Crawford FA: Medical progress: valvular heart disease, *N Engl J Med* 337:32-41, 1997.

Chertow GM, Levy EM, Hammermeister KE et al: Independent association between acute renal failure and mortality following cardiac surgery, *Am J Med* 104:343-348, 1998.

Dajani AS, Taubert KA, Wilson W et al: Prevention of bacterial endocarditis, *JAMA* 227:1794-1801, 1997.

Detsky AS, Abrams HB, Forbath N et al: Cardiac assessment for patients undergoing noncardiac surgery, a multifactorial clinical risk index, *Arch Intern Med* 146:2131, 1986.

Eagle K, Brundage BH, Chaitman BR et al: Guidelines for perioperative cardiovascular evaluation for noncardiac surgery: report of the American College of Cardiology/American Heart Association Task Force on Practice Guidelines, *J Am Coll Cardiol* 27:910-948, 1996.

Eagle KA, Coley CM, Newell JB et al: Combining clinical and thallium data optimizes preoperative assessment of cardiac risk before major vascular surgery, *Ann Intern Med* 110:859, 1989.

Goldman L, Caldera DL, Nussbaum SR et al: Multifactorial index of cardiac risk in noncardiac surgical procedures, *N Engl J Med* 297:845, 1977.

Hamm CW, Braunwald E: A classification of unstable angina revisited, *Circulation* 102:118-122, 2000.

Jones RH, Hannan EL, Hammermeister KE et al: Identification of preoperative variables needed for risk adjustment of short-term mortality after coronary artery bypass graft surgery, *J Am Coll Cardiol* 28:1478-1487, 1996.

Kaluza GL, Jane J, Lee JR et al: Catastrophic outcomes of noncardiac surgery soon after coronary stenting, *J Am Coll Cardiol* 35:1288, 2000.

Lee TH, Marcantonio ER, Mangione CM et al: Derivation and prospective validation of a simple index for prediction of cardiac risk of major noncardiac surgery, *Circulation* 100: 1043, 1999.

Lembo NJ, Dell'Italia LJ, Crawford MH et al: Bedside diagnosis of systolic murmurs, *N Engl J Med* 318:1572, 1988.

Marcus ML, Doty D, Hiratzka LF et al: Decreased coronary reserve—a mechanism for angina pectoris in patients with aortic stenosis and normal coronary arteries, *N Engl J Med* 307:1362, 1982.

Parsonnet V, Dean D, Bernstein AD: A method of uniform stratification of risk for evaluating the results of surgery in acquired adult heart disease, *Circulation* 79(suppl I):I-3, 1989.

Rihal CS, Sutton-Tyrrell K, Guo P et al: Increased incidence of periprocedural complications among patients with peripheral vascular disease undergoing myocardial revascularization in the bypass angioplasty revascularization investigation, *Circulation* 100:171-177, 1999.

Roach GW, Kanchuger M, Mora Mangano C et al: Adverse cerebral outcomes after coronary bypass surgery, *N Engl J Med* 335:1857, 1996.

Roberts WC, Perloff JK: Mitral valvular disease, *Ann Intern Med* 77:939, 1972.

Steen PA, Tinker JH, Tarhan S: Myocardial reinfarction after anesthesia and surgery, *JAMA* 239:2566, 1978.

Van Norman GA, Posner K: Coronary stenting or percutaneous transluminal coronary angioplasty prior to noncardiac surgery increases adverse perioperative cardiac events: the evidence is mounting, *J Am Coll Cardiol* 35:1288-1294, 2000.

References

1. Eagle KA, Brundage BH, Chaitman RB et al: Guidelines for perioperative cardiovascular evaluation for noncardiac surgery: report of the American College of Cardiology/American Heart Association Task Force on Practice Guidelines, *J Am Coll Cardiol* 27:910-948, 1996.

2. American College of Physicians: Guidelines for assessing and managing the perioperative risk from coronary artery disease associated with major noncardiac surgery, *Ann Intern Med* 127: 309-312, 1997.

3. Wilson, LB: Fatal post-operative embolism, *Ann Surg* 56:809-817, 1912.

4. Butler S, Feeney N, Levine SA: The patient with heart disease as a surgical risk, *JAMA* 95:85, 1930.

5. Wenger NK: A 50 year old useful report on coronary risk for noncardiac surgery, *Am J Cardiol* 66:1375, 1990.

6. Master AM, Dack S, Jaffe HL: Factors and events associated with onset of coronary artery thrombosis, *JAMA* 109:546, 1937.

7. Master AM, Dack S, Jaffe HL: Postoperative coronary artery occlusion, *JAMA* 110:1415, 1938.

8. Etsten B, Proger S: Operative risk in patients with coronary heart disease, *JAMA* 159:845, 1955.

9. Ernstene AC: The management of cardiac patients in relation to surgery, *Circulation* 4:430, 1951.

10. Brown K, MacMillan RL, Forbath N: Coronary unit, an intensive care centre for acute myocardial infarction, *Lancet* 2:349, 1963.

11. Day HW: An intensive coronary care area, *Dis Chest* 44:423, 1963.

12. Driscoll AC, Hobika JH, Etsten BE et al: Clinically unrecognized myocardial infarction following surgery, *N Engl J Med* 264:633, 1961.

13. Skinner JF, Pearce ML: Surgical risk in the cardiac patient, *J Chron Dis* 17:57, 1964.

14. Oaks WW, Mills LC: Symposium on cardiovascular-pulmonary problems before and after surgery, *Am J Cardiol* 12:277, 1963.

15. Knapp RB, Topkins RJ, Artusio JF: The cerebrovascular accident and coronary occlusion in anesthesia, *JAMA* 182:332, 1962.

16. Arkins R, Smessaert AA, Hicks RG: Mortality and morbidity in surgical patients with coronary artery disease, *JAMA* 190:485, 1964.

17. Topkins RJ, Artusio JF: Myocardial infarction and surgery: a five year study, *Anesth Analg* 43:716, 1964.
18. Tinker JH: Perioperative myocardial infarction, *Semin Anesth* 1:253, 1982.
19. Tarhan S, Moffitt EA, Taylor WF et al: Myocardial infarction after general anesthesia, *JAMA* 220:1451, 1972.
20. Steen PA, Tinker JH, Tarhan S: Myocardial reinfarction after anesthesia and surgery, *JAMA* 239:2566, 1978.
21. Goldman L, Caldera DL, Nussbaum SR et al: Multifactorial index of cardiac risk in noncardiac surgical procedures, *N Engl J Med* 297:845, 1977.
22. Goldman L, Caldera DL, Southwick FS et al: Cardiac risk factors and complications in non-cardiac surgery, *Medicine* 57:357, 1978.
23. Goldman L: Cardiac risks and complications of noncardiac surgery, *Ann Intern Med* 98:504, 1983.
24. Cooperman M, Pflug B, Martin EW et al: Cardiovascular risk factors in patients with peripheral vascular disease, *Surgery* 84:505, 1978.
25. Charlson ME, MacKenzie CR, Ales K et al: Surveillance for postoperative myocardial infarction after noncardiac operations, *Surgery, Gynecology, and Obstetrics* 167:407, 1988.
26. Wasserman F, Bellet S, Saichek RP: Postoperative myocardial infarction: report of 25 cases, *N Engl J Med* 252:967, 1955.
27. Wroblewski F, LaDue JS: Myocardial infarction as a postoperative complication of major surgery, *JAMA* 150:1212, 1952.
28. Waters J, Wilkinson C, Golmon M et al: Evaluation of cardiac risk in noncardiac surgical patients, *Anesthesiology* 55:A343, 1981.
29. Jeffrey CC, Kunsman J, Cullen DJ et al: A prospective evaluation of cardiac risk index, *Anesthesiology* 58:462, 1983.
30. Charlson ME, Ales KA, Simon R et al: Why predictive indexes perform less well in validation studies, *Arch Intern Med* 147:2155, 1987.
31. Zeldin RA: Assessing cardiac risk in patients who undergo noncardiac surgical procedures, *Can J Surg* 27:402, 1984.
32. Detsky AS, Abrams HB, McLaughlin JR et al: Predicting cardiac complications in patients undergoing noncardiac surgery, *J Gen Intern Med* 1:211, 1986.
33. Detsky AS, Abrams HB, Forbath N et al: Cardiac assessment for patients undergoing noncardiac surgery, a multifactorial clinical risk index, *Arch Intern Med* 146:2131, 1986.
34. Beebe DS, Belani KG, Lao JC et al: Complications and mortality of the in-situ saphenous vein bypass for lower extremity ischemia, *Minn Med* 75:27-30, 1992.
35. Cohen JR, Cooper B, Sardari F: Risk factors for myocardial infarction after distal arterial reconstructive procedures, *Am Surg* 58:478-483, 1992.
36. Takase B, Younis LT, Byers SL et al: Comparative prognostic value of clinical risk indexes, resting two-dimensional echocardiography, and dipyridamole stress thallium-201 myocardial imaging for perioperative cardiac events in major nonvascular surgery patients, *Am Heart J* 126:1099-1106, 1993.
37. Musser DJ, Nicholas GG, Reed III JF: Death and adverse cardiac events after carotid endarterectomy, *J Vasc Surg* 19:615-622, 1994.
38. Shackelford DP, Hoffman MK, Kramer Jr PR et al: Evaluation of preoperative cardiac index values in patients undergoing vaginal surgery, *Am J Obstet Gynecol* 173:80-84, 1995.
39. Campeau L: Grading of angina pectoris, *Circulation* 54:522, 1976 (letter).
40. Wong T, Detsky AS: Preoperative cardiac risk assessment for patients having peripheral vascular surgery, *Ann Int Med* 116:743-753, 1992 (review).
41. Eagle KA, Coley CM, Newell JB et al: Combining clinical and thallium data optimizes preoperative assessment of cardiac risk before major vascular surgery, *Ann Intern Med* 110:859, 1989.
42. Lee TH, Marcantonio ER, Mangione CM et al: Derivation and prospective validation of a simple index for prediction of cardiac risk of major noncardiac surgery, *Circulation* 100:1043, 1999.
43. Gilbert K, Larocque BJ, Patrick LT: Prospective evaluation of cardiac risk indices for patients undergoing noncardiac surgery, *Ann Intern Med* 133:356, 2000.
44. Saklad M: Grading of patients for surgical procedures, *Anesthesia* 2:281, 1941.
45. Massie BM, Mangano DT: Risk stratification for noncardiac surgery: how (and why)? *Circulation* 87:1752, 1993 (editorial).
46. Guidelines for perioperative cardiovascular evaluation for noncardiac surgery: report of the American College of Cardiology/American Heart Association Task Force on Practice Guidelines, *Circulation* 93:1278-1317, 1996.
47. Vanzetto G, Machecourt J, Blendea D et al: Additive value of thallium single-photon emission computed tomography myocardial imaging for prediction of perioperative events in clinically selected high cardiac risk patients having abdominal aortic surgery, *Am J Cardio* 77:143, 1996.
48. Kouchoukos NT, Ebert PA, Grover FL et al: Report of the Ad Hoc committee on risk factors for coronary artery bypass surgery, *Ann Thorac Surg* 45:348, 1988.
49. Kennedy JW, Kaiser GC, Fischer LD et al: Multivariate discriminant analysis of the clinical and angiographic predictors of operative mortality from the Collaborative Study in Coronary Artery Surgery (CASS), *J Thorac Cardiovasc Surg* 80:876, 1980.
50. Parsonnet V, Dean D, Bernstein AD: A method of uniform stratification of risk for evaluating the results of surgery in acquired adult heart disease, *Circulation* 79(suppl I):I-3, 1989.
51. Hannan EL, Kiburn Jr. H, O'Donnell JF et al: Adult open heart surgery in New York state: an analysis of risk factors and hospital mortality rates, *JAMA* 264:2768, 1990.
52. Hannan EL, Kiburn Jr. H, Racz M et al: Improving the outcomes of coronary artery bypass surgery in New York State, *JAMA* 271:761, 1994.
53. Hannan EL, Kumar D, Racz M et al: New York state's cardiac surgery reporting system: four years later, *Ann Thorac Surg* 58:1852, 1994.
54. O'Conner GT, Plume SK, Olmstead EM et al: A regional prospective study on in-hospital mortality associated with coronary artery bypass grafting, *JAMA* 266:803, 1991.
55. O'Conner GT, Plume SK, Olmstead EM et al: Multivariate prediction of in-hospital mortality associated with coronary artery bypass graft surgery, *Circulation* 85:2110, 1992.
56. O'Conner GT, Plume SK, Olmstead EM et al: A regional intervention to improve the hospital mortality associated with coronary artery bypass graft surgery, *JAMA* 275:841, 1996.
57. Higgins TL, Estafanous FG, Loop FD et al: Stratification of morbidity and mortality outcome by preoperative risk factors in coronary artery bypass patients: a clinical severity score, *JAMA* 267:2344, 1992.
58. Edwards FH, Clark RE, Schwartz M: Coronary artery bypass grafting: The Society of Thoracic Surgeons national database experience, *Ann Thorac Surg* 57:12, 1994.
59. Edwards FH, Grover FL, Shroyer LW et al: The Society of Thoracic Surgeons national cardiac surgery database: current risk assessment, *Ann Thorac Surg* 63:903, 1997.
60. Clark, RE: The Society of Thoracic Surgeons national database status report, *Ann Thorac Surg* 57:20, 1994.
61. Orr RK, Maini BS, Sottile FD et al: A comparison of four severity-adjusted models to predict mortality after coronary artery bypass graft surgery, *Arch Surg* 130:301, 1995.
62. Jones RH, Hannan EL, Hammermeister KE et al: Identification of preoperative variables needed for risk adjustment of short-term mortality after coronary artery bypass graft surgery, *J Am Coll Cardiol* 28:1478-1487, 1996.

63. Sandler G: The importance of the history in the medical clinic and the cost of unnecessary tests, *Am Heart J* 100:828, 1980.

64. Hampton JR, Harrison MJG, Mitchell JRA et al: Relative contributions of history-taking, physical examination, and laboratory investigation to diagnosis and management of medical outpatients, *Br Med J* 2:486, 1975.

65. Smith, TW: Approach to the patient with cardiovascular disease. In Wyngaarden JB, Smith LH, editors: *Cecil textbook of medicine,* ed 18, Philadelphia, 1988, WB Saunders.

66. Koudstaal PJ, Van Gijn J, Staal A et al: Diagnosis of transient ischemic attacks: improvement of interobserver agreement by a check-list in ordinary language, *Stroke* 17:723, 1986.

67. Fairbairn AS, Wood CH, Fletcher CM: Variability in answers to a questionnaire on respiratory symptoms, *Br J Prev Soc Med* 13:175, 1959.

68. Larsen SF, Zaric D, Boysen G: Postoperative cerebrovascular accidents in general surgery, *Acta Anaesthesiol Scand* 32:698, 1988.

69. Newman DC, Hicks RG: Combined carotid and coronary artery surgery: a review of the literature, *Ann Thorac Surg* 45:574, 1988.

70. Nadeau SE: Stroke, *Med Clin North Am* 73:1351, 1989.

71. Sandok BA, Whisnant JP, Furlan AJ et al: Carotid artery bruits, *Mayo Clin Proc* 57:227, 1982.

72. Fisher M, editor: Screening for cerebrovascular diseases. In *Guide to clinical prevention services: an assessment of the effectiveness of 169 interventions, report of the U.S. Prevention Services Task Force,* Baltimore, 1989, Williams and Wilkins.

73. Hammond JH, Eisinger RP: Carotid bruits in 1000 normal subjects, *Arch Intern Med* 109:109, 1962.

74. Jones FL: Frequency characteristics and importance of the cervical venous hum in adults, *N Engl J Med* 267:658, 1962.

75. Mavra MB, Zerofsky RA: Supraclavicular and carotid bruits in hemodialysis patients, *Ann Neurol* 2:535, 1977.

76. Chambers BR, Norris JW: Clinical significance of asymptomatic neck bruits, *Neurology* 35:742, 1985.

77. Heyman A, Wilkenson WE, Heyden S et al: Risk of stroke in asymptomatic persons with cervical arterial bruits, *N Engl J Med* 302:838, 1980.

78. Wolf PA, Kannel WB, Sorlie P et al: Asymptomatic carotid bruit and risk of stroke, *JAMA* 245:1442, 1981.

79. Chambers RB, Norris JW: Outcome in patients with asymptomatic neck bruits, *N Engl J Med* 315:860, 1986.

80. Canadian Cooperative Study Group: A randomized trial of aspirin and sulfinpyrazone in threatened stroke, *N Engl J Med* 299:53, 1978.

81. Fields WS, Lemak NA, Frankowski RF et al: Controlled trial of aspirin in cerebral ischemia, *Stroke* 8:301, 1977.

82. Whisnant JP: Epidemiology of stroke: emphasis on transient cerebral ischemic attacks and hypertension, *Stroke* 5:68, 1974.

83. Cebul RD, Whisnant JP: Carotid endarterectomy, *Ann Intern Med* 111:660, 1989.

84. Sirna S, Biller J, Skorton DJ et al: Cardiac evaluation of the patient with stroke, *Stroke* 21:14, 1990.

85. Beebe HG, Clagett P, DeWeese JA et al: Assessing risk associated with carotid endarterectomy, *Circulation* 79:472, 1989.

86. Barnett HJM, Plum F, Walton JV: Carotid endarterectomy: an expression of concern, *Stroke* 15:941, 1984.

87. Moore WS, Barnett HJ, Beebe HG et al: Guidelines for carotid endarterectomy: a multidisciplinary consensus statement from the ad hoc committee, American Heart Association, *Stroke* 26:188-201, 1995.

88. Executive Committee for the Asymptomatic Carotid Atherosclerosis Study: Endarterectomy for asymptomatic carotid artery stenosis, *JAMA* 273:1421-1428, 1995.

89. Roach GW, Kanchuger M, Mora Mangano C et al: Adverse cerebral outcomes after coronary bypass surgery, *N Engl J Med* 335:1857, 1996.

90. Gardner, TJ, Horneffer PJ, Manolio TA et al: Stroke following coronary artery bypass grafting: a ten year study, *Ann Thorac Surg* 40:574, 1985.

91. Kennedy JW, Kaiser GC, Fisher LD et al: Clinical and angiographic predictors of operative mortality from the collaborative study in coronary artery surgery (CASS), *Circulation* 63:793-802, 1981.

92. Alderman EL, Fisher LD, Litwin P et al: Results of coronary artery surgery in patients with poor left ventricular function (CASS), *Circulation* 68:785-795, 1983.

93. Johnson WD, Brenowitz JB, Kayser KL: Factors influencing long-term (10-year to 15-year) survival after a successful coronary artery bypass operation, *Ann Thorac Surg* 48:19-25, 1989.

94. Wechsler AS, Junod FL: Coronary bypass grafting in patients with chronic congestive heart failure, *Circulation* 79(suppl I):I-92-I-96, 1989.

95. Kasper EK, editor: *Heart failure: evaluation and care of patients with left ventricular systolic dysfunction: commentary on the Agency for Health Care Policy and Research clinical practice guidelines,* New York, 1997, Chapman and Hall.

96. McGee PA, Castelli WP, McNamara PM et al: The natural history of congestive heart failure: the Framingham study, *N Engl J Med* 26:1441, 1971.

97. Kannel WB: Epidemiological aspects of heart failure, *Cardiol Clin* 7:1, 1989.

98. Ho KKL, Pinsky JL, Kannel WB et al: The epidemiology of heart failure: the Framingham Study, *J Am Coll Cardiol* 22(suppl A):6A-13A, 1993.

99. Shub C: Heart failure and abnormal ventricular function, *Chest* 96:636, 1989.

100. Zelis R, Sinoway L, Musch T et al: Vasoconstrictor mechanism in congestive heart failure, *Modern Concepts of Cardiovascular Disease* 58:7, 1989.

101. Kaplati MM: Liver dysfunction secondary to congestive heart failure, *Prac Cardiol* 6:39, 1980.

102. Marantz PR, Tobin JN, Wassertheil S et al: The relationship between left ventricular systolic function and congestive heart failure diagnosed by clinical criteria, *Circulation* 77:607, 1988.

103. Mattleman SJ, Hakki AH, Iskandrian AS et al: Reliability of bedside evaluation in determining left ventricular function: correlation with left ventricular ejection fraction determined by radionuclide ventriculography, *J Am Coll Cardiol* 1:417-420, 1983.

104. Stevenson LW, Perloff JK: The limited reliability of physical signs for estimating hemodynamics in chronic heart failure, *JAMA* 261:884, 1989.

105. Fleg JL, Hinton PC, Lakatta EG et al: Physician utilization of laboratory procedures to monitor outpatients with congestive heart failure, *Arch Intern Med* 149:393-396, 1989.

106. Baker DW, Konstam MA, Bottorff M et al: Management of heart failure, I: pharmacologic treatment, *JAMA* 272:1361-1366, 1994.

107. Deedwania PC: Underutilization of evidence-based therapy in heart failure: an opportunity to deal a winning hand with ace up your sleeve, *Arch Intern Med* 157:2409-2412, 1997.

108. Stafford RS, Saglam D, Blumenthal D: National patterns of angiotensin-converting enzyme inhibitor use in congestive heart failure, *Arch Intern Med* 157:2460-2464, 1997.

109. Edep ME, Shah ND, Tateoi IM et al: Differences between primary care physicians and cardiologists in the management of CHF: relationship to practice guidelines, *J Am Coll Cardiol* 30:518-526, 1997.

110. Hjalmarson A et al for the MERIT-HF Study Group: Effects of controlled-release metoprolol on total mortality, hospitalizations, and well-being in patients with heart failure: the metoprolol CR/XL randomized intervention trial in congestive heart failure (MERIT-HF), *JAMA* 283:1295-1302, 2000.

111. Bristow MR: β-Adrenergic receptor blockade in chronic heart failure, *Circulation* 101:558-569, 2000.

112. The Criteria Committee of the New York Heart Association: Nonmenclature and criterial for diagnosis, ed 9, Boston, 1994, Little, Brown.

113. Inter-Society Commission for Heart Disease Resources: Primary prevention of atherosclerotic disease, *Circulation* 42:1-42, 1970.

114. Margolis JR, Kannel WB, Feinleib M et al: Clinical features of unrecognized myocardial infarction—silent and symptomatic, *Am J Cardiol* 32:1, 1973.

115. Kannel WB, Abbott RD: Incidence and prognosis of unrecognized myocardial infarction, *N Engl J Med* 311:1144, 1984.

116. Stamler J, Wentworth D, Neaton JD: Is relationship between serum cholesterol and risk of premature death from coronary heart disease continuous and graded? Findings in 356,222 primary screenees of the Multiple Risk Factor Intervention Trial (MRFIT), *JAMA* 256: 2823-2828, 1986.

117. Fuster V, Pearson TA: 27th Bethesda Conference: matching the intensity of risk factor management with the hazard for coronary disease events, *J Am Coll Cardiol* 27:957-1047, 1996.

118. Wilson PW, D'Agostino RB, Levy D et al: Prediction of coronary heart disease using risk factor categories, *Circulation* 97:1837-1847, 1998.

119. Grundy SM, Pasternak R, Greenland P et al: Assessment of cardiovascular risk by use of multiple-risk-factor assessment equations: a statement for healthcare professionals from the American Heart Association and the American College of Cardiology, *J Am Coll Cardiol* 34:1348-1359, 1999.

120. Fletcher GF, Balady G, Blair SN et al: Statement on exercise: benefits and recommendations for physical activity programs for all Americans: a statement for health professionals by the Committee on Exercise and Cardiac Rehabilitation of the Council on Clinical Cardiology, American Heart Association, *Circulation* 94:857-862, 1996.

121. Myers RH, Kiely DK, Cupples LA et al: Parental history is an independent risk factor for coronary artery disease: the Framingham Study, *Am Heart J* 120:963-969, 1990.

122. Eckel RH: Obesity and heart disease: a statement for healthcare professionals from the Nutrition Committee, American Heart Association, *Circulation* 96:3248-3250, 1997.

123. Moghadasian MH, McManus BM, Frohlich JJ: Homocysteine and coronary artery disease, *Arch Intern Med* 157: 2299, 1997.

124. Badner NH, Drader K, Freeman D et al: The use of intraoperative nitrous oxide leads to postoperative increases in plasma homocysteine, *Anesth Analg* 87:711-713, 1998.

125. Ernst E, Resch KL: Fibrinogen as a cardiovascular risk factor: a metaanalysis and review of the literature, *Ann intern Med* 118: 956, 1993.   .

126. Kannel WB, Wolf PA, Castelli WP et al: Fibrinogen and risk of cardiovascular disease: the Framingham Study, *JAMA* 258:1183, 1987.

127. Ridker PM, Genest J, Libby Peter: Risk factors for atheroscerotic disease. In Bruanwald, Zipes, Libby, editors: *Heart disease*, ed 6, Philadelphia, 2001, WB Saunders.

128. Poli KA, Tofler GH, Larson MG et al: Association of blood pressure with fibrinolytic potential in the Framingham offspring population, *Circulation* 101:264-269, 2000.

129. Franklin SS, Khan SA, Wong ND et al: Is pulse pressure useful in predicting risk for coronary heart disease? The Framingham heart study. *Circulation* 100:354-360, 1999.

130. Lauer MS, Okin PM, Larson MG et al: Impaired heart rate response to graded exercise. Prognostic implications of chronotropic incompetence in the Framingham Heart Study, *Circulation* 93:1520-1526, 1996.

131. Bradley RF, Schonfeld A: Diminished pain in diabetic patients with acute myocardial infarction, *Geriatrics* 17:322-326, 1962.

132. Faerman I, Faccio E, Milei J et al: Autonomic neuropathy and painless myocardial infarction in diabetic patients, *Diabetes* 26: 1147-1158, 1977.

133. Chychota MN, Gan GT, Pluth JR et al: Myocardial revascularization: comparison of operability and surgical results in diabetic and nondiabetic patients, *J Thorac Cardiovasc Surg* 65:856-862, 1973.

134. Verska JJ, Walker WJ: Aortocoronary bypass in the diabetic patient, *Am J Cardiol* 35:774-777, 1975.

135. Kip K, Faxon D, Detre K et al: Coronary angioplasty in diabetic patients (PTCA): the NHLBI PTCA Registry, *Circulation* 94:1818-1825, 1996.

136. Stein B, Weintraub WS, Gebhart SP et al: Influence of diabetes on early and late outcome after percutaneous transluminal coronary angioplasty, *Circulation* 91:979-989, 1995.

137. Califf RM, Fortin DF, Frid DJ et al: Restenosis after coronary angioplasty: an overview, *J Am Coll Cardiol* 17:2B-13B, 1991.

138. Carrozza JP, Kuntz KE, Fishman RF et al: Restenosis after arterial injury caused by coronary stenting in patients with diabetes mellitus, *Ann Intern Med* 118:344-349, 1993.

139. Abbott RD, Donahue RP, Kannel WB et al: The impact of diabetes on survival following myocardial infarction in men vs. women: the Framingham Study, *JAMA* 260:3456-3460, 1988.

140. Butler WJ, Osrander Jr LD, Carman WJ et al: Mortality from coronary heart disease in the Tecumseh Study: long-term effect of diabetes mellitus, glucose intolerance and other risk factors, *Am J Epidemiol* 121:541-547, 1985.

141. The BARI Investigators: Comparison of coronary bypass surgery with angioplasty in patients with multivessel disease, *N Engl J Med* 335:217-225, 1996.

142. The BARI Investigators: Influence of diabetes on 5-year mortality and morbidity in a randomized trial comparing CABG and PTCA in patients with multivessel disease, *Circulation* 96:1761-1769, 1997.

143. Van Belle E, Ketelers R, Bauters C et al: Patency of percutaneous tranluminal coronary angioplasty sites at 6-month angiographic follow-up: a key determinant of survival in diabetics after coronary balloon angioplasty, *Circulation* 103:1218-1224, 2001.

144. Goldman L, Caldera DL: Risk of general anesthesia and elective operation in the hypertensive patient, *Anesthesiology* 50:285, 1979.

145. National High Blood Pressure Education Program Working Group: National high blood pressure education program working group report on primary prevention of hypertension, *Arch Intern Med* 153:186-208, 1993.

146. The Sixth Report of the Joint National Committee on Prevention, Detection, Evaluation and Treatment of High Blood Pressure, *Arch Intern Med* 157:2413, 1977.

147. Levy D, Merz C, Cody R et al: Hypertension detection, treatment and control: a call to action for cardiovascular specialists, *J Am Coll Cardiol* 34:1360, 1999.

148. Levy D, Larson MG, Vasan RS et al: The progression from hypertension to congestive heart failure, *JAMA* 275:1557, 1996.

149. Task Force on Blood Pressure Control in Children (from the National Heart, Lung, and Blood Institute, Bethesda, Md): Report of the Second Task Force on Blood Pressure Control in Children—1987, *Pediatrics* 79:1, 1987.

150. National High Blood Pressure Education Program Working Group on Hypertension Control in Children: Update on the 1987 task force report on high blood pressure in children and adolescents, *Pediatrics* 98:649-658, 1996.

151. Sorof JM, Portman RJ: Ambulatory blood pressure monitoring in the pediatric patient, *J Pediatr* 136:578-586, 2000.

152. Eckberg DW: Carotid baroreflex function in young men with borderline blood pressure elevation, *Circulation* 59:632, 1979.

153. Strandgaard S: Autoregulation of cerebral blood flow in hypertensive patients, *Circulation* 53:720, 1976.
154. Harrison DG, Florentine MS, Brooks LA et al: The effect of hypertension and left ventricular hypertrophy on the lower range of coronary autoregulation, *Circulation* 77:1108, 1988.
155. Guyton A: Renal function curve—a key to understanding the pathogenesis of hypertension, *Hypertension* 10:1, 1987.
156. Hollenberg NK: Evolution of the treatment of hypertension: what really matters in the 1990s? *Am J Med* 93:4S-10S, 1992 (review).
157. Weber MA: Antihypertensive treatment, *Circulation* 80(suppl IV):120, 127, 1989.
158. Weber MA: Hypertension: steps forward and steps backward: the Joint National Committee Fifth Report, *Arch Intern Med* 153:149, 1993.
159. Fagan, TC: Evolution of the Joint National Committee Reports, 1988-1997: evolution of the science of treating hypertension, *Arch Intern Med* 157:2401, 1997.
160. Joint National Committee of the National High Blood Pressure Education Program: The 1988 Report of the Joint National Committee on Detection, Evaluation, and Treatment of High Blood Pressure, *Arch Intern Med* 148:1023, 1988.
161. Working Group on Renovascular Hypertension: Detection, evaluation and treatment of renovascular hypertension, *Arch Intern Med* 147:820, 1987.
162. Weinberg MH, Grim CE, Hollified JW et al: Primary aldosteronism: diagnosis, localization and treatment, *Ann Intern Med* 90:386, 1979.
163. Krakoff LR, Elijovich F: Cushing's syndrome and exogenous glucocorticoid hypertension, *Clin Endocrinol Metab* 10:479, 1981.
164. Bravo EL, Gifford RW: Pheochromocytoma: diagnosis, localization, and management, *N Engl J Med* 311:1298, 1984.
165. Liberthson RR, Pennington DG, Jacobs ML et al: Coarctation of the aorta: review of 234 patients and clarification of management problems, *Am J Cardiol* 43:835, 1979.
166. Kirkendall WM, Armstrong ML: Vascular changes in the eye of treated and untreated patients with essential hypertension, *Am J Cardiol* 9:663, 1962.
167. Larson AW, Strong CG: Initial assessment of the patient with hypertension, *Mayo Clin Proc* 64:1533, 1989.
168. Kennedy R, Case C, Fathi R et al: Does renal failure cause an atherosclerotic milieu in patients with end-stage renal disease? *Am J Med* 110:198-204, 2001.
169. Huysmans K, Lins R, Daelemans R et al: Hypertension and accelerated atherogenesis in endstage renal disease, *J Nephrol* 11:185-195, 1998.
170. Lindner A, Charra B, Sherrar DJ et al: Accelerated atherosclerosis in prolonged maintenance hemodialysis, *N Engl J Med* 290:697, 1974.
171. Charlson ME, MacKenzie CR, Gold JP et al: Postoperative renal dysfunction can be predicted, *Surgery, Gynecology and Obstetrics* 169:303,1989.
172. Richards WO, Scovill W, Shin B et al: Acute renal failure associated with increased intra-abdominal pressure, *Ann Surg* 197:183, 1983.
173. Harman PK, Kron IL, McLachlan HD et al: Elevated intra-abdominal pressure and renal function, *Ann Surg* 196:594, 1982.
174. Hamdan AD, Pomposelli FB, Gibbons GW et al: Renal insufficiency and altered postoperative risk in carotid endarterectomy, *J Vasc Surg* 29:1006-1011, 1999.
175. Chertow GM, Lazarus JM, Christiansen CL et al: Preoperative renal risk stratification, *Circulation* 95:878-884, 1997.
176. Chertow GM, Levy EM, Hammermeister KE et al: Independent association between acute renal failure and mortality following cardiac surgery, *Am J Med* 104:343-348, 1998.
177. Magano CM, Diamondstone LS, Ramsay JG et al: Renal dysfunction after myocardial revascularization: risk factors, adverse outcomes, and hospital resource utilization, *Ann Intern Med* 128:194-203, 1998.
178. Hartz AJ, Kuhn EM, Kayser KL et al: BUN as a risk factor for mortality after coronary artery bypass grafting, *Ann Thorac Surg* 60:398-404, 1995.
179. Liu JY, Birkmeyer, NJO, Sanders JH et al: Risks of morbidity and mortality in dialysis patients undergoing coronary artery bypass surgery: *Circulation* 102:2973, 2000.
180. Roppolo LP, Fitzgerald R, Dillow J et al: A comparison of troponin T and troponin I as predictors of cardiac events in patients undergoing chronic dialysis at a veteran's hospital: a pilot study, *J Am Coll Cardiol* 34:448-454, 1999.
181. A Report of the American College of Cardiology/American Heart Association Task Force on Practice Guidelines (Committee on Management of Patients with Valvular Heart Disease): ACC/AHA guidelines for the management of patients with valvular heart disease, *J Am Coll Cardiol* 32:1486-1588, 1998.
182. Carabello BA, Crawford FA: Medical progress: valvular heart disease, *N Engl J Med* 337:32 41, 1997.
183. Dajani AS, Taubert KA, Wilson W et al: Prevention of bacterial endocarditis, *Circulation* 96:358-366, 1997.
184. Dajani AS, Taubert KA, Wilson W et al: Prevention of bacterial endocarditis, *JAMA* 227:1794-1801, 1997.
185. Bisno AL, Shulman ST, Dajani AS: The rise and fall (and rise?) of rheumatic fever, *JAMA* 259:728, 1988.
186. Wallace MR, Garst PD, Papadimos TJ et al: The return of acute rheumatic fever in young adults, *JAMA* 262:2557, 1989.
187. Lombard JT, Selzer A: Valvular aortic stenosis: a clinical and hemodynamic profile of patients, *Ann Intern Med* 106:292, 1987.
188. Selzer A: Changing aspect of the natural history of valvular aortic stenosis, *N Engl J Med* 317:91, 1987.
189. Spagnuolo M, Kloth H, Taranta A et al: Natural history of rheumatic aortic regurgitation, *Circulation* 44:368, 1971.
190. Selzer A, Cohn KE: Natural history of mitral stenosis: a review, *Circulation* 45:878, 1972.
191. Kirklin JW, Pacifico AD: Surgery for acquired valvular heart disease (second of two parts), *N Engl J Med* 288:194, 1973.
192. Junod FL, Harlan BJ, Payne et al: Preoperative risk assessment in cardiac surgery: comparison of predicted and observed results, *Ann Thorac Surg* 43:59, 1987.
193. Braunwald E: Valvular heart disease. In Braunwald E, Zipes DP, Libby P, editors: *Heart disease*, ed 6, Philadelphia, 2001, WB Saunders.
194. Pellikka PA, Nishimura RA, Bailey KR et al: The natural history of adults with asymptomatic, hemodynamically significant aortic stenosis, *J Am Coll Cardiol* 15:1012-1017, 1990.
195. Ross Jr J, Braunwald E: The influence of corrective operations on the natural history of aortic stenosis, *Circulation* 38(suppl V):61, 1968.
196. Marcus ML, Doty D, Hirazka LF et al: Decreased coronary reserve—a mechanism for angina pectoris in patients with aortic stenosis and normal coronary arteries, *N Engl J Med* 307:1362, 1982.
197. Julius BK, Spillmann M, Vassalli G et al: Angina pectoris in patients with aortic stenosis and normal coronary arteries, *Circulation* 95:892, 1997.
198. Otto CM, Burwash IG, Legget ME et al: Prospective study of asymptomatic valvular aortic stenosis: clinical, echocardiographic, and exercise predictors of outcome, *Circulation* 95:2262-2270, 1997.
199. Carbello BA: Timing of valve replacement in aortic stenosis: moving closer to perfection *Circulation* 95:2241-2243, 1997.
200. Laniado S, Yellin EL, Yoran C et al: Physiologic mechanism in aortic insufficiency, *Circulation* 66:226, 1982.

201. Moisa RB, Zeldis SM, Alper SA et al: Aortic regurgitation in coronary artery bypass grafting: implications for cardioplegia administration, *Ann Thorac Surg* 60:665-668, 1995.

202. Bonow RO, Lakatos E, Maron BJ et al: Serial long-term assessment of the natural history of asymptomatic patients with chronic aortic regurgitation and normal left ventricular systolic function, *Circulation* 84:1625-1635, 1991.

203. Paris TM, McAllister M, Ross JJ et al: Doppler-echocardiographic evaluation of left atrial contribution to left ventricular filling in mitral stenosis at rest and during exercise, *Am J Cardiol* 64:1058, 1989.

204. Stott DK, Marpole DGF, Bristow JD et al: The roles of left atrial transport in aortic and mitral stenosis, *Circulation* 61:1031, 1970.

205. Bolen JL, Lopes MG, Harrison DC et al: Analysis of left ventricular function in response to afterload changes in patients with mitral stenosis, *Circulation* 52:894, 1975.

206. Stone GJ, Hoar PF, Faltas AN et al: Nitroprusside and mitral stenosis, *Anesth Analg* 59:662, 1980.

207. Heller SJ, Carleton RA: Abnormal left ventricular contraction in patients with mitral stenosis, *Circulation* 42:1099, 1970.

208. Perloff JK, Roberts WC: The mitral apparatus: functional anatomy of mitral regurgitation, *Circulation* 46:227, 1972.

209. Braunwald E: The syndrome of severe mitral regurgitation with normal left atrial pressure, *Circulation* 27:29, 1963.

210. Roberts WC, Perloff JK: Mitral valvular disease, *Ann Intern Med* 77:939, 1972.

211. Fuchs RM, Heuser RR, Yin FCP et al: Limitations of pulmonary wedge v waves in diagnosing mitral regurgitation, *Am J Cardiol* 49:849, 1982.

212. Pichard AD, Kay R, Smith H et al: Large v waves in the pulmonary wedge pressure tracing in the absence of mitral regurgitation, *Am J Cardiol* 50:1044, 1982.

213. Grose R, Strain J, Cohen MV: Pulmonary arterial v waves in mitral regurgitation: clinical and experimental observations, *Circulation* 69:214, 1984.

214. Ross Jr J: Left ventricular function and the timing of surgical treatment in valvular heart disease, *Ann Intern Med* 94:498, 1981.

215. Vokonas PS, Gorlin R, Cohn PF et al: Dynamic geometry of the left ventricle in mitral regurgitation, *Circulation* 48:786, 1973.

216. Chatterjee K, Parmley WW, Swan HJC et al: Beneficial effects of vasodilator agents in severe mitral regurgitation due to dysfunction of subvalvular apparatus, *Circulation* 48:684, 1973.

217. Domaingue CM, Davies MJ, Cronin KD: Cardiovascular risk factors in patients for vascular surgery, *Anaesth Intensive Care* 10:324, 1982.

218. Hertzer NR: Fatal myocardial infarction following peripheral vascular operations—a study of 951 patients followed 6-11 years postoperatively, *Cleve Clin Q* 49:1, 1982.

219. Tomatis LA, Fierens EE, Verbrugge GP: Evaluation of surgical risk in peripheral vascular disease by coronary angiography: a series of 100 cases, *Surgery* 71:429, 1972.

220. Hertzer NR, Beven EG, Young JR et al: Coronary artery disease in peripheral vascular patients—a classification of 1,000 coronary angiograms and results of surgical management, *Ann Surg* 199:233, 1984.

221. Hertzer NR, Young JR, Beven EG et al: Coronary angiography in 506 patients with extracranial cerebrovascular disease, *Arch Intern Med* 145:849, 1985.

222. Thompson JE, Patman RD, Talkington CM: Asymptomatic carotid bruit: long-term outcome of patients having endarterectomy compared with unoperated controls, *Ann Surg* 188:308, 1978.

223. Rihal CS, Eagle KA, Mickel MC et al: Surgical therapy for coronary artery disease among patients with combined coronary artery and peripheral vascular disease, *Circulation* 91:46-53, 1995.

224. Rihal CS, Sutton-Tyrrell K, Guo P et al: Increased incidence of periprocedural complications among patients with peripheral vascular disease undergoing myocardial revascularization in the bypass angioplasty revascularization investigation, *Circulation* 100:171-177, 1999.

225. McPhail N, Calvin JE, Scheriatmadar A et al: The use of preoperative exercise testing to predict cardiac complications after arterial reconstruction, *J Vasc Surg* 7:60, 1988.

226. McPhail NV, Ruddy TD, Calvin JE et al: A comparison of dipyridamole-thallium imaging exercise testing in the prediction of postoperative cardiac complications in patients requiring arterial reconstruction, *J Vasc Surg* 10:51, 1989.

227. Hendel RC, Chen MH, L'Italien GJ et al: Sex differences in perioperative and long-term cardiac event-free survival in vascular surgery patients: an analysis of clinical and scintigraphic variables, *Circulation* 91:1044-1051, 1995.

228. Cohn PF: Severe asymptomatic coronary artery disease: a diagnostic, prognostic and therapeutic puzzle, *Am J Med* 62:565, 1977.

229. Braunwald E: This history. In Braunwald E, Zipes DD, Libby P, editors: *Heart disease,* ed 6, Philadelphia, 2001, WB Saunders.

230. Shub C: Stable angina pectoris: clinical patterns, *Mayo Clin Proc* 64:233, 1990.

231. Lichstein E, Breibart S, Shani J et al: Relationship between location of chest pain and site of coronary artery occlusion, *Am Heart J* 115:564-568, 1988.

232. A Report of the American College of Cardiology/American Heart Association Task Force on Practice Guidelines (Committee on the Management of Patients with Unstable Angina): ACC/AHA guidelines for the management of patients with unstable angina and non-ST-segment elevation myocardial infarction: executive summary and recommendations, *Circulation* 102:1193-1209, 2000.

233. Yasue H, Omote S, Takizaw A et al: Cardiac variations of exercise capacity in patients with Prinzmetal's variant angina: role of exercise-induced coronary arterial spasm, *Circulation* 59:938, 1979.

234. Christie LG, Conti CR: Systemic approach to evaluation of angina-like chest pain: pathophysiology and clinical testing with emphasis on objective documentation of myocardial ischemia, *Am Heart J* 102:897, 1981.

235. Sampson JJ, Cheitlin MD: Pathophysiology and differential diagnosis of cardiac pain, *Prog Cardiovasc Dis* 13:507, 1971.

236. Frøbert O, Funch-Jensen P, Bagger JP: Diagnostic value of esophageal studies in patients with angina-like chest pain and normal coronary angiograms, *Ann Intern Med* 124:959-969, 1996.

237. Singh S, Richter JE, Hewson EG et al: The contribution of gastroesophageal reflux to chest pain in patients with coronary artery disease, *Ann Intern Med* 117:824-830, 1992.

238. Yeghiazarians Y, Braunstein JB, Askari A et al: Unstable angina pectoris, *N Engl J Med* 342:101-114, 2001.

239. Rentrop KP: Thrombi in acute coronary syndromes, *Circulation* 101:1619-1626, 2000.

240. Braunwald E: Unstable angina: an etiologic approach to management, *Circulation* 98:2219-2222, 1998.

241. Braunwald E: Unstable angina: a classification, *Circulation* 80:410-414, 1989.

242. Calvin JE, Klein LW, Vandenberg BJ et al: Risk stratification in unstable angina: prospective validation of the Braunwald classification, *JAMA* 273:136-141, 1995.

243. Miltenburg-van Zijl AJ, Simoons ML, Veerhoek RJ et al: Incidence and follow-up of Braunwald subgroups in unstable angina pectoris, *J Am Coll Cardiol* 25:1286-1292, 1995.

244. Hamm CW, Braunwald E: A classification of unstable angina revisited, *Circulation* 102:118-122, 2000.

245. Manning HL, Schwartzstein RM: Pathophysiology of dyspnea, *N Engl J Med* 333:1547-1553, 1995.

246. Mahler DA, Horowitz MB: Clinical evaluation of exertional dyspnea, *Clin Chest Med* 15:259-269, 1994 (review).

247. Wasserman K: Dyspnea on exertion: is it the heart or the lung? *JAMA* 248:2039-2043, 1982.

248. Cook DG, Shaper AG: Breathlessness, lung function, and the risk of a heart attack, *Eur Heart J* 9:1215, 1988.

249. Ebi-Kryston KL, Hawthorne VM, Rose G et al: Breathlessness, chronic bronchitis, and reduced pulmonary function as predictors of cardiovascular disease mortality among men in England, Scotland and United States, *Int J Epidemiol* 18:84, 1989.

250. Higgins MW, Keller JB: Predictors of mortality in the adult population of Tecumseh, *Arch Environ Health* 21:418, 1970.

251. Carpenter L, Beral V, Stracham D et al: Respiratory symptoms as predictors of 27 year mortality in a representative sample of British adults, *Br Med J* 299:357, 1989.

252. Ferris BG, Speizer FE, Worcester J et al: Adult mortality in Berlin, NH, from 1961 to 1967, *Arch Environ Health* 23:434, 1967.

253. Staats BA: Dyspnea—heart or lungs? *Int J Cardiol* 19:13, 1988.

254. Artman M, Graham T: Congestive heart failure in infancy: recognition and management, *Am Heart J* 103:1040, 1982.

255. Corrao WM, Braman SS, Irwin RS: Chronic cough as the sole presenting manifestation of bronchial asthma, *N Engl J Med* 300:633, 1979.

256. Israili ZH, Hall WD: Cough and angioneurotic edema associated with angiotensin-converting enzyme inhibitor therapy, *Ann Intern Med* 117:234-242, 1992.

257. Parks DP, Ahrens RC, Humphries CT et al: Chronic cough in childhood: approaches to diagnosis and treatment, *J Pediatrics* 115:856, 1989.

258. Gallagher CG: Exercise limitation and clinical exercise testing in chronic obstructive pulmonary disease, *Clin Chest Med* 15:305-326, 1994 (review).

259. Epstein SK, Celli BR: Cardiopulmonary exercise testing in patients with chronic obstructive pulmonary disease, *Cleve Clin J Med* 60:119-128, 1993 (review).

260. Lauer MB, Hallowell P, Goldblatt A: Pulmonary dysfunction secondary to heart disease, *Anesthesiology* 33:161, 1970.

261. Davies HH, Gazetopoulos N: Dyspnoea in cyanotic congenital heart disease, *Br Heart J* 27:28, 1964.

262. Gold WM, Mattioli LF, Price AC: Response to exercise in patients with tetralogy of Fallot with systemic-pulmonary anastomoses, *Pediatrics* 43:781-793, 1969.

263. Perloff JK, Child JS: *Congenital heart disease in adults*, Philadelphia, 1991, WB Saunders.

264. Topol EJ: The history. In Topol EJ, editor: *Comprehensive cardiovascular medicine*, Philadelphia, 1998, Lippincott-Raven.

265. Kaplan J, Staats BA: Obstructive sleep apnea syndrome, *Mayo Clin Proc* 65:1087-1094, 1990.

266. Piccirillo JF, Duntley S, Schotland H: Obstructive sleep apnea, *JAMA* 284:1492-1494, 2000.

267. Young T, Palta M, Dempsey J et al: The occurrence of sleep-disordered breathing among middle-aged adults, *N Engl J Med* 328:1230-1235, 1993.

268. Viner S, Szalai JP, Hoffstein V: Are history and physical examination a good screening test for sleep apnea? *Ann Intern Med* 115:356-359, 1991.

269. Sanner BM, Doberauer C, Konermann M et al: Pulmonary hypertension in patients with obstructive sleep apnea syndrome, *Arch Intern Med* 157:2483-2487, 1997.

270. Hung J, Whitford EG, Parsons RW et al: Association of sleep apnoea with myocardial infarction in men, *Lancet* 336:261-264, 1990.

271. Hu FB et al: Snoring and risk of cardiovascular disease in women, *J Am Coll Cardiol* 35:308-313, 2000.

272. DeGowin EL, DeGowin RL: *Bedside diagnostic examination*, New York, 1976, MacMillan.

273. O'Rourke RA, Shaver JA, Salerni R et al: The history, physical examination, and cardiac auscultation. In Alexander WR, Schlant RC, Fuster V et al, editors: *Hurst's the heart*, ed 9, New York, 1998, McGraw-Hill.

274. Vongpatanasin W, Brickner ME, Hillis LD et al: The Eisenmenger syndrome in adults, *Ann Intern Med* 128:745-755, 1998.

275. Merrell SW, Ames SA, Nelson EW et al: Major abdominal complications following cardiac transplantation, *Arch Surg* 124:889-894, 1989.

276. Prabhakar G, Testa G, Abbasoglu O et al: The safety of cardiac operations in the liver transplant recipient, *Ann Thorac Surg* 65:1060-1064, 1998.

277. Warner MA, Warner ME, Weber JG: Clinical significance of pulmonary aspiration during the perioperative period, *Anesthesiology* 78:56-62, 1993.

278. Ross RM: Hepatic dysfunction secondary to heart failure, *Am J Gastroenterol* 76:511-518, 1981.

279. Kubo SH, Walter BA, John DH et al: Liver function abnormalities in chronic heart failure: influence of systemic hemodynamics, *Arch Intern Med* 147:1227-1230, 1987.

280. Cohen JA, Kaplan MM: Left-sided heart failure presenting as hepatitis, *Gastroenterology* 74:583-587, 1978.

281. Chu CM, Chang CH, Liaw YF et al: Jaundice after open heart surgery: a prospective study, *Thorax* 39:52-56, 1984.

282. Michalopoulos A, Alivizatos P, Geroulanos S: Hepatic dysfunction following cardiac surgery: determinants and consequences, *Hepatogastroenterology* 44:779-783, 1997.

283. Hogue CW, Lappas GD, Creswell LL et al: Swallowing dysfunction after cardiac operations *J Thorac Cardiovasc Surg* 110:517-522, 1997.

284. Linzer M, Yang EH, Estes M et al: Diagnosing syncope, part 1: value of history, physical examination, and electrocardiography, *Ann Intern Med* 126:989-996, 1997.

285. Savage DD, Corwin L, McGee DL et al: Epidemiologic features of isolated syncope: the Framingham study, *Stroke* 16:626, 1985.

286. Dermksian G, Lamb LE: Syncope in a population of healthy young adults: incidence, mechanisms, and significance, *JAMA* 168:1200, 1958.

287. Hanlon JT, Linzer M, MacMillan JP et al: Syncope and presyncope associated with probable adverse drug reactions, *Arch Intern Med* 150:2309-2312, 1990.

288. Ibrahim MM, Tarazi RC, Dustan HP: Orthostatic hypotension: mechanisms and management, *Am Heart J* 90:513, 1975.

289. Wright KE, McIntosh HD: Syncope: a review of pathophysiological mechanisms, *Prog Cardiovasc Dis* 13:580, 1971.

290. Mark AL, Kioschos M, Abboud FM et al: Abnormal vascular responses to exercise in patients with aortic stenosis, *J Clin Invest* 52:1138, 1973.

291. Epstein SE, Maron BJ: Sudden death and the competitive athlete: perspectives on preparticipation screening studies, *J Am Coll Cardiol* 7:220, 1986.

292. Sleeper JC, Orgain ES, McIntosh HD: Primary pulmonary hypertension, *Circulation* 26:1358, 1962.

293. Lambert EC, Menon VA, Wagner HR: Sudden unexpected death from cardiovascular disease in children: a cooperative international study, *Am J Cardiol* 34:89, 1974.

294. Cheitlin MD, Castro CM, McAllister HA: Sudden death as a complication of anomalous left coronary origin from the anterior sinus of valsalva, *Circulation* 50:780, 1974.

295. Maron BJ, Bonow RO, Cannon RO et al: Hypertrophic cardiomyopathy (second of two parts), *N Engl J Med* 316:844, 1987.

296. Maron BJ, Roberts WC, McAllister HA et al: Sudden death in young athletes, *Circulation* 62:218, 1980.

297. DiCarlo LA, Morady F: Evaluation of the patient with syncope, *Cardiol Clin* 3:499, 1985.

298. Kowey PR, Eisenberg R, Engel TR: Sustained arrhythmias in hypertrophic obstructive cardiomyopathy, *N Engl J Med* 310:1566, 1984.

299. Schwartz PJ, Periti M, Malliani A: The long Q-T syndrome, *Am Heart J* 89:378, 1975.

300. Josephson ME: Antiarrhythmic agents and the danger of proarrhythmic events, *Ann Intern Med* 111:101, 1989.

301. Atkins D, Hanusa B, Sefcik T et al: Syncope and orthostatic hypotension, *Am J Med* 91:179-85, 1991.

302. Kapoor WN: Evaluation and outcome of patients with syncope, *Medicine (Baltimore)* 69:160-175, 1990.

303. Strasberg B, Sagie A, Rechavia E et al: The noninvasive evaluation of syncope of suspected cardiovascular origin, *Am Heart J* 117:160, 1989.

304. Savage DD, Seides SF, Clark CE et al: Electrocardiographic findings in patients with obstructive and nonobstructive hypertrophic cardiomyopathy, *Circulation* 58:402, 1978.

305. Day SC, Cook EF, Funkenstein H et al: Evaluation and outcome of emergency room patients with transient loss of consciousness, *Am J Med* 73:15, 1982.

306. Eagle KA, Black HR, Cook EF et al: Evaluation of prognostic classifications for patients with syncope, *Am J Med* 79:455, 1985.

307. Kapoor WN, Karpf M, Weiand S et al: A prospective evaluation and follow-up of patients with syncope, *N Engl J Med* 309:197, 1983.

308. Silverstein MD, Singer DE, Mulley AG et al: Patients with syncope admitted to medical intensive care units, *JAMA* 248:1185, 1982.

309. Kearon C, Hirsh J: Management of antiocoagulation before and after elective surgery, *N Engl J Med* 336:1506-1511, 1997.

310. Quinn MJ, Fitzgerald DJ: Ticlopidine and clopidogrel, *Circulation* 100:1667-1672, 1997.

311. Schror K: Antiplatelet drugs: a comparative review, *Drugs* 50:1-28, 1995.

312. Belzberg H, Rivkind AI: Preoperative cardiac preparation, *Chest* 115:82S-95S, 1999.

313. Eagle KA: Surgical patients with heart disease: summary of the ACC/AHA guidelines, *Am Fam Physician* 56:811-818, 1997.

314. Potyk D, Raudaskoski P: Preoperative cardiac evaluation for elective noncardiac surgery, *Arch Fam Med* 7:164-173, 1998.

315. Roberts WC: Aortic dissection: anatomy, consequences, and causes, *Am Heart J* 101:195, 1981.

316. Amar D, Attai LA, Gupta SK et al: Perioperative diagnosis of subclavian artery stenosis: a contraindication for internal mammary artery-coronary artery bypass graft, *Anesthesiology* 73:783, 1990.

317. Fowler NO: Physiology of cardiac tamponade and pulsus paradoxus. *Modern Concepts of Cardiovascular Disease* 47:109-113, 1978.

318. Keenan RL, Boyan CP: Cardiac arrest due to anesthesia, *JAMA* 253:2373, 1985.

319. Norwood WI: Hypoplastic left heart syndrome, *Ann Thorac Surg* 52:688-695, 1991.

320. Chatterjee K: Physical examination. In Topol EJ, editor: *Comprehensive cardiovascular medicine*, Philadelphia, 1998, Lippincott-Raven.

321. Freed MD, Plauth Jr WH: The pathology, pathophysiology, recognition and treatment of congenital heart disease. In Alexander WR, Schlant RC, Fuster V et al, editors: *Hurst's the heart*, ed 9, New York, 1998, McGraw-Hill.

322. O'Rourke RA, Braunwald E: Physical examination of the heart. In Isselabacher KJ, Adams RD, Braunwald E et al, editors: *Harrison's principles of internal medicine*, New York, 1980, McGraw-Hill.

323. Brockenbrough EC, Braunwald E, Morrow AG: Hemodynamic technic for the detection of hypertrophic subaortic stenosis, *Circulation* 23:189-194, 1961.

324. Parish JM, Marschke Jr RF, Dines DE et al: Etiologic considerations in superior vena cava syndrome, *Mayo Clin Proc* 56:407-413, 1981.

325. Michelson EL, Morganroth J, Nichols CW et al: Retinal arteriolar changes as an indicator of coronary artery disease, *Arch Intern Med* 139:1139, 1979.

326. Lichstein E, Chapman I, Gupta PK et al: Diagonal ear lobe crease and coronary artery sclerosis, *Ann Intern Med* 85:337, 1976.

327. Brady PM, Zive MA, Goldberg RJ et al: A new wrinkle to the earlobe crease, *Arch Intern Med* 147:65-66, 1987.

328. Elliott WJ, Karrison T: Increased all-cause and cardiac morbidity and mortality associated with the diagonal earlobe crease: a prospective cohort study, *Am J Med* 91:247-254, 1991.

329. Salem MR, Mathrubhuthum M, Bennett EJ: Difficult intubation, *N Engl J Med* 295:879, 1976.

330. Jenkins LC, McGraw RW: Anaesthetic management of the patient with rheumatoid arthritis, *Can Anaesth Soc J* 16:407, 1969.

331. Hill SA, Miller CA, Kosnik EJ et al: Pediatric neck injuries: a clinical study, *J Neurosurg* 60:700, 1984.

332. Cook DJ, Simel DL: Does this patient have abnormal central venous pressure? *JAMA* 275:630-634, 1996.

333. Sochowski RA, Dubbin JD, Naqvi SZ: Clinical and hemodynamic assessment of the hepatojugular reflux, *Am J Cardiol* 66:1002-1006, 1990.

334. Martin CE, Shaver JA, Leonard JJ: Physical signs, apex cardiography, phonocardiography and systolic time intervals in angina pectoris, *Circulation* 46:1098, 1972.

335. Lembo NJ, Dell'Italia LJ, Crawford MH et al: Bedside diagnosis of systolic murmurs, *N Engl J Med* 318:1572, 1988.

336. Raftery EB, Holland WW: Examination of the heart: an investigation into variation, *Am J Epidemiol* 85:438, 1967.

337. Craig E: Should auscultation be rehabilitated? *N Eng J Med* 318:1611-1613, 1988.

338. Mangione S, Nieman Z, Gracely E et al: The teaching and practice of cardiac auscultation during internal medicine and cardiology training, *Ann Intern Med* 119:47-54, 1993.

339. Mangione S: Cardiac ausculatory skills of physicians-in-training: a comparison of three English-speaking countries, *Am J Med* 110:210-216, 2001.

340. Schneiderman H: Cardiac auscultation and teaching rounds: how can cardiac auscultation be resuscitated? *Am J Med* 110:233-235, 2001.

341. Cease KB, Nicklas JM: Prediction of left ventricular ejection fraction using simple quantitative clinical information, *Am J Med* 81:429, 1986.

342. Eagle KA, Quertermous T, Singer DE et al: Left ventricular ejection fraction: physician estimates compared with gated blood pool scar measurements, *Arch Intern Med* 148:882, 1988.

343. Perloff JF: The physiologic mechanisms of cardiac and vascular physical signs, *J Am Coll Cardiol* 1:184, 1983.

344. Heckerling PS, Wiener SL, Moses VK et al: Accuracy of precordial percussion in detecting cardiomegaly, *Am J Med* 91:328-334, 1991.

345. Nishimura RA, Tajik AJ: The valsalva maneuver and response revisited, *Mayo Clin Proc* 61:211-217, 1986.

346. Badgett RG, Lucey, CR, Mulrow CD: Can the clinical examination diagnose left-sided heart failure in adults? *JAMA* 277:1712-1719, 1997.

347. Chakko S, Woska D, Martinez H et al: Clinical, radiographic, and hemodynamic correlations in chronic congestive heart failure, *Am J Med* 90:353-359, 1991.

348. Butman SM, Ewy GA, Standen JR et al: Bedside cardiovascular examination in patients with severe chronic heart failure, *J Am Coll Cardiol* 22:968-974, 1993.

349. Rihal CS, Davis KB, Kennedy JW et al: The utility of clinical, electrocardiographic, and roentrgenographic variables in the prediction of left ventricular function, *Am J Cardiol* 75:220-223, 1995.

350. Maitre B, Similowski T, Derenne JP: Physical examination of the adult patient with respiratory diseases: inspection and palpation, *Eur Respir J* 8:1584-1593, 1995 (review).

351. Stubbing DG, Mathur PN, Roberts RS et al: Some physical signs in patients with chronic airflow obstruction, *Am Rev Respir Dis* 125:549, 1982.

352. Greene BA, Berkowitz S: The preanesthetic induced cough as a method of diagnosis of preoperative bronchitis, *Ann Intern Med* 37:723, 1952.

353. McFadden Jr ER, Gilbert IA: Asthma, *N Engl J Med* 327:1928-1937, 1992 (review).

354. McFadden ER, Kiser R, DeGroot WJ: Acute bronchial asthma, *N Engl J Med* 288:221, 1973.

355. Piirila P, Sovijarvi AR: Crackles: recording, analysis and clinical significance, *Eur Respir J* 8:2139-2148, 1995 (review).

356. Bettencort PE, Del Bono EA, Spiegelman D et al: Clinical utility of chest auscultation in common pulmonary diseases, *Am J Respir Crit Care Med* 150:1291-1297, 1994.

357. Schneider IC, Anderson AE: Correlation of clinical signs with ventilatory function in obstructive lung disease, *Ann Intern Med* 62:477, 1965.

358. Richter JE, Castell DO: Gastroesophageal reflux—pathogenesis, diagnosis and therapy, *Ann Intern Med* 97:93, 1982.

359. Landa SE: Preanesthetic assessment of the patient with gastrointestinal disease, *Anesthesiology Clinics of North America* 8:713, 1990.

360. Pasulka PS, Bistrian BR, Benotti PN et al: The risks of surgery in obese patients, *Ann Intern Med* 106:540, 1986.

361. Birkmeyer NJO, Charlesworth DC, Hernandez F et al: Obesity and risk of adverse outcomes associated with coronary artery bypass surgery, *Circulation* 97:1689-1694, 1998.

362. Castell DO, O'Brien KD, Muench H et al: Estimation of liver size by percussion in normal individuals, *Ann Intern Med* 70:1183, 1969.

363. Frank BB: Clinical evaluation of jaundice, *JAMA* 262:3031, 1989.

364. Jacobs MR, Kotler IA: Evaluation of hemolysis in patients with prosthetic heart valves, *Clin Cardiol* 21:387-392, 1998.

365. Friedman LS, Maddrey WC: Surgery in the patient with liver disease, *Med Clin N Am* 71:453, 1987.

366. Fagius J, Karhuvaara S: Sympathetic activity and blood pressure increases with bladder distension in humans, *Hypertension* 14:511, 1989.

367. Williams JW, Simel DL: Dies this patient have ascites? *JAMA* 267:2645, 1992.

368. Gaer, JAR, Shaw ADS, Wild R et al: Effect of cardiopulmonary bypass on gastrointestinal perfusion and function, *Ann Thorac Surg* 57:371-375, 1994.

369. Christenson JT, Schmuziger M, Maurice J et al: Gastrointestinal complications after coronary artery bypass grafting, *J Thorac Cardiovasc Surg* 108:899-906, 1994.

370. Wang MJ, Chao A, Huang CH et al: Hyperbilirubinemia after cardiac operation: incidence, risk factor, and clinical significance, *J Thorac Cardiovasc Surg* 108:429-436, 1994.

371. Fernandez-del Castillo C, Harringer W, Warshaw AL et al: Risk factors for pancreatic cellular injury after cardiopulmonary bypass, *N Engl J Med* 325:382, 1991.

372. Gold JP, Charlson ME, Williams-Russo P et al: Improvement of outcomes after coronary artery bypass: a randomized trial comparing intraoperative high versus low mean arterial pressure, *J Thorac Cardiovasc Surg* 110:1302-1314, 1995.

373. Merli GJ, Bell RD: Preoperative management of the surgical patient with neurologic disease, *Med Clin N Am* 71:511, 1987.

374. Cooperman LH: Succinylcholine-induced hyperkalemia in neuromuscular disease, *JAMA* 213:1867, 1970.

375. Ellis FR: Neuromuscular disease and anaesthesia, *Br J Anaesth* 46:603, 1974.

376. Tucker CR, Towles RE, Cahn A et al: Aortitis in ankylosing spondylitis: early detection of aortic root abnormalities with two dimensional echocardiography, *Am J Cardiol* 49:680, 1982.

377. Perloff JK: Neurological disorders and heart disease. In Braunwald E, editor: *Heart disease*, ed 4, Philadelphia, 1992, WB Saunders.

378. Perloff JD, deLeon AC, O'Doherty D: The cardiomyopathy of progressive muscular dystrophy, *Circulation* 33:625, 1966.

379. Riggs T: Cardiomyopahty and pulmonary emboli in terminal Duchenne's muscular dystrohy, *Am Heart J* 119:690, 1990.

380. Perloff JK: Cardiac rhythm and conduction in Duchennes' muscular dystrophy, *J Am Coll Cardiol* 3:1263, 1984.

381. Chalkiadis GA, Branch KG: Cardiac arrest after isoflurane anaesthesia in a patient with Duchenne's muscular dystrophy, *Anaesthesia* 45:22, 1990.

382. Sethna NF, Rockoff MA: Cardiac arrest following inhalation induction of anaesthesia in a child with Duchenne's Muscular dystrophy, *Cn Anaesth Soc J* 33:799, 1986.

383. Moorman JF, Coleman RE, Packer DL et al: Cardiac involvement in myotonic muscular dystrophy, *Medicine* 64:371, 1985.

384. Nguyen HH, Wolfe III JT, Holmes Jr DR et al: Pathology of the cardiac conduction system in myotonic dystrophy: a study of 12 cases, *J Am Coll Cardiol* 11:662, 1998.

385. Gronert GA: Malignant hyperthermia, *Anesthesiology* 53:395, 1980.

386. Warner MA, Shields SE, Chute CG: Major morbidity and mortality within 1 month of ambulatory surgery and anesthesia, *JAMA* 270:1437-1441, 1993.

387. Abraham SA, Coles NA, Coley CM et al: Coronary risk of noncardiac surgery, *Prog Cardiovasc Dis* 34:205-234, 1991.

388. Dupuis JY, Wang F, Nathan H: The cardiac anesthesia risk evaluation score, *Anesthesiology* 94:194-204, 2001.

389. Lee KS, Marwick TH, Cook SA et al: Prognosis of patients with left ventricular dysfunction with and without viable myocardium after myocardial infarction: relative efficacy of medical therapy and revascularization, *Circulation* 90:2687-2694, 1994.

390. Hurst JW: Electrocardiographic crotchets or common errors made in the interpretation of the electrocardiogram, *Clin Cardiol* 21:211-216, 1998.

391. Goldberger AL, O'Konski M: Utility of the routine electrocardiogram before surgery and on general hospital admission, *Ann Intern Med* 105:552, 1986.

392. Carliner NH, Fisher ML, Plotnick GD et al: Routine preoperative exercise testing in patients undergoing major noncardiac surgery, *Am J Cardiol* 56:51, 1985.

393. Carliner NH, Fisher ML, Plotnick GD et al: The preoperative electrocardiogram as an indicator of risk in major noncardiac surgery, *Can J Cardiol* 2:134, 1986.

394. Berg GR, Kotler MN: The significance of bilateral bundle branch block in perioperative patients, *Chest* 59:62, 1971.

395. Rooney SM: Relationship of right bundle branch block and marked left axis deviation to complete heart block during general anesthesia, *Anesthesiology* 44:64, 1976.

396. Pastore JO, Yurchak PM, Janis KM et al: The risk of advanced heart block in surgical patients with right bundle branch block and left axis deviation, *Circulation* 57:677, 1978.

397. Hesse B, Diaz LA, Snader CE et al: Complete bundle branch block as an independent predictor of all-cause mortality: report of 7,073 patients referred for nuclear exercise testing, *Am J Med* 110:253-259, 2001.

398. Behar S: Are right and left bundle branch block similarly associated with increased risk of mortality? *Am J Med* 110:318-319, 2001.

399. Gerson MC, Hurst JM, Hertzberg VS et al: Cardiac prognosis in noncardiac geriatric surgery, *Ann Intern Med* 103:832, 1985.

400. Gerson MC, Hurst JM, Hertzberg VS et al: Prediction of cardiac and pulmonary complications related to elective abdominal and noncardiac thoracic surgery in geriatric patients, *Am J Med* 88:101, 1990.

401. Cutler BS, Wheeler HB, Paraskos JA et al: Applicability and interpretation of electrocardiographic stress testing in patients with peripheral vascular disease, *Am J Surg* 141:501, 1981.

402. Gauss A, Röhm H, Schäuffelen A: Electrocardiographic exercise stress testing for cardiac risk assessment in patients undergoing noncardiac surgery, *Anesthesiology* 94:38-46, 2001.

403. Goldschlager N, Selzer A, Cohn K: Treadmill stress tests as indicators of presence and severity of coronary artery disease, *Ann Intern Med* 85:277-286, 1976.

404. Goldschlager N: Use of the treatmill test in the diagnosis of coronary artery disease in patients with chest pains, *Ann Intern Med* 97:383-388, 1982.

405. Leppo J, Plaja J, Gionet M et al: Noninvasive evaluation of cardiac risk before elective vascular surgery, *J Am Coll Cardiol* 9:269, 1987.

406. Kennedy HL, Wiens RD: Ambulatory (Holter) electrocardiography and myocardial ischemia, *Am Heart J* 117:164, 1989.

407. Fleisher LA, Rosenbaum SH, Nelson AH et al: Preoperative dipyridamole thallium imaging and ambulatory electrocardiographic monitoring as a predictor of perioperative cardiac events and long-term outcome, *Anesthesiology* 83:906-917, 1995.

408. Mangano DT, Hollenberg M, Fegert G et al: Perioperative myocardial ischemia in patients undergoing noncardiac surgery: incidence and severity during the 4 day perioperative period: *J Am Coll Cardiol* 17:843-850, 1991.

409. Raby KE, Goldman L, Creager MA et al: Correlation between preoperative ischemia and major cardiac events after peripheral vascular surgery, *N Engl J Med* 321:1296, 1989.

410. Raby KE, Barry J, Creager MA et al: Detection and significance of intraoperative and postoperative myocardial ischemia in peripheral vascular surgery, *JAMA* 268:222, 1992.

411. Ouyang P, Gerstenblith G, Furman WR et al: Frequency and significance of early postoperative silent myocardial ischemia in patients having peripheral vascular surgery, *Am J Cardiol* 64:1113, 1989.

412. Muir AD, Reeder MK, Foex P et al: Preoperative silent myocardial ischae mia: incidence and predictors in a general surgical population, *Br J Anaesth* 67:373, 1991.

413. Cohn PF, Gorlin R, Cohn LH et al: Left ventricular ejection fraction as a prognostic guide in surgical treatment of coronary and valvular heart disease, *Am J Cardiol* 34:136, 1974.

414. Lazor L, Russell JC, DaSilva J et al: Use of the multiple uptake gated acquisition scan for the preoperative assessment of cardiac risk, *Surg Gynecol Obstet* 167:234, 1988.

415. Moraski RE, Russell RO, Smith M et al: Left ventricular function in patients with and without myocardial infarction and one, two, or three vessel coronary artery disease, *Am J Cardiol* 35:1, 1975.

416. Upton M, Rerych S, Newman G et al: Detecting abnormalities in left ventricular function during exercise before angina and ST-depression, *Circulation* 62:341, 1980.

417. Franco CD, Goldsmith J, Veith FJ et al: Resting gated pool ejection fraction: a poor predictor of perioperative myocardial infarction in patients undergoing vascular surgery for infrainguinal bypass grafting, *J Vasc Surg* 10:656, 1989.

418. Boucher CA, Brewster DC, Darling RC et al: Determination of cardiac risk by dipyridamole-thallium imaging before peripheral vascular surgery, *N Engl J Med* 312:389, 1985.

419. Brown KA: Prognostic value of thallium-201 myocardial perfusion imaging, *Circulation* 83:363, 1991.

420. Brown KA, Rowen M: Extent of jeopardized viable myocardium determined by myocardial perfusion imaging best predicts perioperative cardiac events in patients undergoing noncardiac surgery, *J Am Coll Cardiol* 21:325-330, 1993.

421. Levinson JR, Guiney TE, Boucher CA: Functional tests for myocardial Ischemia, *Annu Rev Med* 42:119-126, 1991.

422. Eagle KA, Singer DE, Brewster DC et al: Dipyridamole-thallium scanning in patients undergoing vascular surgery, *JAMA* 257:2185, 1987.

423. Leppo JA, Dahlberg ST: The questions: to test or not to test in preoperative cardiac risk evaluation, *J Nucl Cardiol* 5:332, 1998.

424. Fleisher LA, Nelson AH, Rosenbaum SH: Failure of negative dipyridamole thallium scans to predict perioperative myocardial ischaemia and infarction, *Can J Anaesth* 39:179, 1992.

425. Mangano DT, London MJ, Taubau JF et al: Dipyridamole thallium-201 scintigraphy as a preoperative screening test, a reexamination of its predictive potential, *Circulation* 84:493, 1991.

426. Pohost GM: Dipyridamole thallium test: is it useful for predicting coronary events after vascular surgery? *Circulation* 84:931, 1991 (editorial comment).

427. Bolognese L, Sarasso G, Bongo AS: Dipyridamole echocardiography test, *Circulation* 84:1100, 1991.

428. Homma S, Gilliland Y, Guiney TE et al: Safety of intravenous dipyridamole for stress testing with thallium imaging, *Am J Cardiol* 59:152, 1987.

429. Keltz TN, Innerfield M, Gitler B et al: Dipyridamole-induced myocardial ischemia, *JAMA* 257:1515, 1987.

430. Bayliss J, Pearson M, Sutton GC: Ventricular dysrhythmias following intravenous dipyridamole during "stress" myocardial imaging, *Br J Radiol* 56:686, 1983.

431. Blumenthal MS, McCauley CS: Cardiac arrest during dipyridamole imaging, *Chest* 93:1103, 1988.

432. Shaw JL, Eagle KA, Gersh BJ et al: Meta-analysis of intravenous dipyridamole-thallium 201 imaging (1985 to 1994) and dobutamine echocardiography (1991 to 1994) for risk stratification before vascular surgery, *J Am Coll Card* 27:787-798, 1996.

433. Goldman L: Cardiac risk for vascular surgery, *J Am Coll Cardiol* 27:799-802, 1996.

434. L'Ilalien GJ, Paul SD, Hendel RC et al: Development and validation of a Bayesian model for perioperative cardiac risk assessment in a cohort of 1,081 vascular surgical candidates, *J Am Coll Cardiol* 27:779-786, 1996.

435. L'Italien GJ, Cambria RP, Cutler BS et al: Comparative early and late cardiac morbidity among patients requiring different vascular surgery procedures, *J Vasc Surg* 21:935-944, 1995.

436. Sawada SG, Segar DS, Ryan T et al: Echocardiographic detection of coronary artery disease during dobutamine infusion, *Circulation* 83:1605, 1991.

437. Lane RT, Sawada SG, Segar DS et al: Dobutamine stress echocardiography for assessment of cardiac risk before noncardiac surgery, *Am J Cardiol* 68:976, 1991.

438. Poldermans D, Fioretti PM, Forster T et al: Dobutamine stress echocardiography for assessment of perioperative cardiac risk in patients undergoing major vascular surgery, *Circulation* 87:1506-1512, 1993.

439. Poldermans D, Arnese M, Fioretti PM et al: Improved cardiac risk stratification in major vascular surgery with dobutamine-atropine stress echocardiography, *J Am Coll Cardiol* 26:648-653, 1995.

440. Poldermans D, Karnese M, Pioretti PM et al: Sustained prognostic value of dobutamine stress echocardiography for late cardiac events after major noncardiac vascular surgery, *Circulation* 95:53-58, 1997.

441. Bach DS, Eagle KA: Dobutamine stress echocardiography, *Circulation* 95:8-10, 1997.

442. Chuah SC, Pillikka PA, Roger VL et al: Role of dobutamine stress echocardiography in predicting outcome in 860 patients with known or suspected coronary artery disease, *Circulation* 97:1474, 1998.
443. Grossman W: *Cardiac catheterization and angiography,* ed 3, Philadelphia, 1986, Lea and Febiger.
444. Forrester JS, Diamond G, Chatterjee K et al: Medical therapy of acute myocardial infarction by application of hemodynamic subsets, *N Engl J Med* 295:1404, 1976.
445. Wright C, White C, Furda J et al: Can the coronary angiogram predict the functional significance of a coronary stenosis? *Circulation* 62:214, 1980.
446. Hutter Jr AM: Is there a left main equivalent? *Circulation* 62:207, 1980.
447. Franch RH, Douglas JS, King SB: Cardiac catheterization and coronary arteriography. In Alexander, WR, Schlant RC, Fuster V, editors: *Hurst's the heart,* New York, 1998, McGraw-Hill.
448. Cigarroa CG, deFilippi CR, Brickner ME et al: Dobutamine stress echocardiography identifies hibernating myocardium and predicts recovery of left ventricular function after coronary revascularization, *Circulation* 88:430-436, 1993.
449. Pennell DJ, Underwood SR, Manzara CC et al: Magnetic resonance imaging during dobutamine stress in coronary artery disease, *Am J Cardiol* 70:34-40, 1992.
450. Nagel E, Lehmkuhl HB, Bocksch W et al: Noninvasive diagnosis of ischemia-induced wall motion abnormalities with the use of high-dose dobutamine stress MRI, comparison with dobutamine stress echocardiography, *Circulation* 99:763-770, 1999.
451. Zoghbi WA, Barasch E: Dobutamine MRI: a serious contender in pharmacological stress imaging? *Circulation* 99:730-732, 1999.
452. Pohost GM, Biederman WW: The role of cardiac MRI stress testing "Make a better mouse trap," *Circulation* 100:1676-1679, 1999.
453. O'Keefe JH, Shub C, Rettke SR: Risk of noncardiac surgical procedures in patients with aortic stenosis, *Mayo Clin Proc* 64: 400, 1989.
454. Torsher LC, Shub C, Rettke SR et al: Risk of patients with severe aortic stenosis undergoing noncardiac surgery, *Am J Cardiol* 81:448-452, 1998.
455. Craver JM, Weintraub WS, Jones EL et al: Predictors of mortality, complications and length of stay in aortic valve replacement for aortic sterosis, *Circulation* 78(suppl I):85, 1988.
456. Raymer K, Yang H: Patients with aortic stenosis: cardiac complications in non-cardiac surgery, *Can J Anaesth* 45:855-859, 1998.
457. Levine MJ, Berman AD, Safian RD et al: Palliation of valvular aortic stenosis by balloon valvuloplasty as preoperative preparation for noncardiac surgery, *Am J Cardiol* 62:1309, 1988.
458. Roth RB, Palacios IF, Block PC: Percutaneous aortic balloon valvulo plasty: its role in the management of patients with aortic stenosis requiring major noncardiac surgery, *J Am Coll Cardiol* 13:1039, 1989.
459. Hayes SN, Holmes DR, Nishimura RA et al: Palliative percutaneous aortic balloon valvuloplasty before noncardiac operations and intensive diagnostic procedures, *Mayo Clin Proc* 64: 753, 1989.
460. McKay RG: The Mansfield scientific aortic valvuloplasty registry: overview of acute hemodynamic results and procedural complications, *J Am Coll Cardiol* 17:485, 1991.
461. O'Neill WW: Predictors of long-term survival after percutaneous aortic valvuloplasty: report of the Mansfield scientific balloon aortic valvuloplasty registry, *J Am Coll Cardiol* 17:193, 1991.
462. Kuntz RE, Tosteson AN, Berman AD et al: Predictors of event-free survival after balloon aortic valvuloplasty, *N Engl J Med* 325:17, 1991.
463. McCollum CH, Garcia-Rinaldi R, Graham JM et al: Myocardial revascularization prior to subsequent major surgery in patients with coronary artery disease, *Surgery* 81:302, 1977.
464. Scher KS, Tice DA: Operative risk in patients with previous coronary artery bypass, *Arch Surg* 3:807, 1976.
465. Mahar LJ, Steen PA, Tinker JH et al: Perioperative myocardial infarction in patients with coronary artery disease with and without aorta-coronary artery bypass grafts, *J Thorac Cardiovasc Surg* 76:533, 1978.
466. Schoeppel SL, Wilkinson C, Waters J et al: Effects of myocardial infarction on perioperative cardiac complications, *Anesth Analg* 62:493, 1983.
467. Foster ED, Davis KB, Carpenter JA et al: Risk of noncardiac operation in patients with defined coronary disease: the Coronary Artery Surgery Study (CASS) registry experience, *Ann Thorac Surg* 41:42, 1986.
468. Eagle KA, Rihal CS, Mickel MC et al: Cardiac risk of noncardiac surgery. Influence of coronary disease and type of surgery in 3368 operations, *Circulation* 96:1882-1887, 1997.
469. CASS Principle Investigators and Their Associates: Myocardial infarction and mortality in the Coronary Artery Surgery Study (CASS) randomized trial, *N Engl J Med* 310:750, 1984.
470. Mangano DT, Goldman L: Preoperative assessment of patients with known or suspected coronary disease, *N Eng J Med* 333: 1750-1756, 1995.
471. Posner KL, Van Norman GA, Chan V: Adverse cardiac outcomes after noncardiac surgery in patients with prior percutaneous tranluminal coronary angioplasty, *Anesth Analg* 89:553-560, 1999.
472. Van Norman GA, Posner K: Coronary stenting or percutaneous transluminal coronary angioplasty prior to noncardiac surgery increases adverse perioperative cardiac events: the evidence is mounting, *J Am Coll Cardiol* 35:1288-1294, 2000.
473. Huber KC, Evans MA, Bresnahan JF et al: Outcome of noncardiac operations in patients with severe coronary artery disease successfully treated preoperatively with coronary angioplasty, *Mayo Clin Proc* 67:15-21, 1992.
474. Hassan SA, Hlatky MA, Boothroyd DB et al: Outcome of noncardiac surgery after coronary bypass surgery or coronary angioplasy in the bypass angioplasty revascularization investigation (BARI), *Am J Med* 110:260, 2001.
475. Kaluza GL, Jane J, Lee JR et al: Catastrophic outcomes of noncardiac surgery soon after coronary stenting, *J Am Coll Cardiol* 35:1288, 2000.
476. Popma JJ, Weitz J, Bittl JA et al: Antithrombotic therapy in patients undergoing coronary angioplasty, *Chest* 114: 728S-741S, 1998.
477. Spirito P, Seidman CE, McKenna WJ et al: The management of hypertrophic cardiomyopathy, *N Eng J Med* 336:775-785, 1997 (review).
478. Maron B: Hypertrophic cardiomyopathy, *Curr Probl Cardiol* 18: 641-704, 1993.
479. Braunwald E, Lambrew CT, Rockoff SD et al: Idiopathic hypertrophic subaortic stenosis: a description of the disease based upon an analysis of 64 patients, *Circulation* 29-30(suppl IV):3-207, 1964.
480. Thompson RC, Liberthson RR, Lowenstein E: Perioperative anesthetic risk of noncardiac surgery in hypertrophic obstructive cardiomyopathy, *JAMA* 254:2419, 1985.
481. Haering JM, Comunale ME, Parker RA et al: Cardiac risk of noncardiac surgery in patients with asymmetric septal hypertrophy, *Anesthesiology* 85:254-259, 1996.
482. Baum VC, Barton DM, Gutgesell HP: Influence of congenital heart disease on mortality after noncardiac surgery in hospitalized children, *Pediatrics* 105:332-335, 2000.
483. Brickner ME, Hillis LD, Lange RA: Congenital heart disease in adults, *N Engl J Med* 342:256-263, 2000.
484. Perloff JK: Residua and sequelae. In Perloff JK, Child JS, editors:*Congenital heart disease in adults,* Philadelphia, 1991, WB Saunders.

485. Simon AB, Zloto AE: Coarctation of the aorta: longitudinal assessment of operated patients, *Circulation* 50:456, 1974.

486. Deanfield JE, Gersh BJ, Warnes CA et al: Congenital heart disease in adults. In Alexander WR, Schlant RC, Fuster V et al, editors: *Hurst's the heart,* ed 9, New York, 1998, McGraw-Hill.

487. Ammash NM, Connolly HM, Abel MD et al: Noncardiac surgery in Eisenmenger syndrome, *J Am Coll Cardiol* 33:222-227, 1999.

488. Copeland JG, Butman SM, Sethi G: Successful coronary artery bypass grafting for high risk left main coronary artery atherosclerosis after cardiac transplantation, *Ann Thorac Surg* 49:106-110, 1990.

489. Vetrovec GH, Cowley MJ, Newton CM et al: Applications of percutaneous transluminal coronary angioplasty in cardiac transplantation, *Circulation* 78(suppl 3):83-86, 1988.

490. Billingham ME: Cardiac transplant atherosclerosis, *Transplant Proc* XIX:19-25, 1987.

491. Fish RD, Nabel EG, Selwyn AP et al: Responses of coronary arteries of cardiac transplant patients to acetylcholine, *J Clin Invest* 81:21-31,1988.

492. Schroeder JC: Hemodynamic performance of the human transplanted heart, *Transplant Proc* XI:304-308, 1979.

CHAPTER 2

Cardiovascular Medications

Thomas M. McLoughlin, Jr., M.D.

OUTLINE

Patients with cardiac disease present the anesthesiologist with the greatest opportunity, and often the greatest need, to administer drugs that specifically alter cardiac rhythm, myocardial contractility, and vascular tone. For many years, cardiovascular pharmacology was essentially described as autonomic pharmacology. An understanding of the autonomic nervous system, its receptor subclasses, and the effects of drugs on them was in many ways sufficient to have a grasp on the perioperative vasoactive drug management of the patient with cardiac disease. More recently, our enhanced appreciation for the role of the endothelium, as well as the development and clinical introduction of nonadrenergic inotropic agents, has broadened the foundation of physiology necessary to understand the actions of cardiovascular drugs and has expanded our ability to achieve desired effects.

For organizational purposes, this chapter is broadly divided into preoperative medications (i.e., maintenance oral medications) and perioperative medications, although this distinction is somewhat artificial and many preoperative maintenance medications may be administered parentally in the perioperative period. Also, the broad topic of cardiac antiarrhythmic medications is not covered in this chapter but is addressed in depth elsewhere (see Chapter 9).

PREOPERATIVE MEDICATIONS
Nitrates

Nitroglycerin and longer-acting oral nitrates (e.g., isosorbide dinitrate) belong to a larger group of compounds referred to as *nitrovasodilators*. All agents within this group act to release nitric oxide (NO), which diffuses to vascular smooth muscle and other target tissues, yielding increased production of cyclic guanosine 3'5'-monophosphate (cGMP) and, consequently, vasodilation.[1] Preoperative nitrates are administered by many routes, including sublingual tablets and sprays, transdermal patch delivery systems, and longer-acting swallowed preparations. Sublingual tablets and sprays result in peak plasma levels within 5 minutes and are thus useful in the treatment of acute, recurrent angina pectoris. Isosorbide dinitrate is the most commonly prescribed long-acting prophylactic nitrate, and it acts in concert with its active hepatic metabolite (isosorbide-5-mononitrate) to provide clinical effects lasting 4 to 6 hours after an oral dose.

Nitrates alleviate myocardial ischemia in three principal ways: (1) by producing venodilation that results in decreased left ventricular end-diastolic pressure and thus decreased left ventricular wall stress; (2) by inducing selective epicardial and collateral coronary vasodilation that results in redistribution of coronary blood flow to ischemic regions; and (3) at higher dosages by causing arterial vasodilation that results in decreased cardiac afterload, and again, decreased wall stress. Tolerance to nitroglycerin administered by any route is a common problem that decreases the vascular effects of a chronically administered dose, and many prescription regimens include a "nitrate-free period" to combat this problem.[2,3]

An important consideration with any preoperative medication is whether it is advisable to have patients continue taking their medication through the morning of surgery. It is most commonly recommended that chronically administered nitrates be continued. However, an important study by Weightman et al.[4] found that preoperative nitrate treatment was an independent predictor of perioperative death in patients who have coronary artery bypass surgery. In their review of 1593 consecutive patients undergoing coronary artery bypass surgery, the relative risk of in-hospital mortality was 3.8-fold higher (95% confidence interval = 1.5-9.6) in patients receiving regular, daily nitrate treatment before surgery. Although it is possible that preoperative chronic nitrate administration served as a marker for more severe coronary artery disease not amenable to surgical repair, this explanation fails to explain why other preop-

erative antianginal therapies (e.g., calcium entry blockers, β-adrenergic antagonists) failed to similarly serve as markers for patients likely to have an adverse outcome in the study. The results more likely suggest that cessation of oral or transdermal nitrates may result in rebound vascular and coronary vasoconstriction, or that tolerance to the effects of nitrates occurring during chronic administration may lead to reduced effectiveness of perioperatively administered nitrovasodilators.[4]

Digoxin

Digoxin is the prototypical example and most commonly prescribed member of a group of drugs called *cardiac glycosides.* These drugs are found naturally as an extract of foxglove, milkweed, lily of the valley, oleander, and many other plants. Digoxin is most often used in the treatment of congestive heart failure (Fig. 2-1) and for control of the ventricular response rate to supraventricular arrhythmias, especially atrial fibrillation. It is useful for improving both right and left ventricular function, and can be used safely in the setting of pulmonary hypertension.[5] It is well absorbed orally, with peak plasma levels occurring 1 to 2 hours after administration. However, approximately 10% of patients show reduced bioavailability of an ingested dose, secondary to inactivation of the drug by enteric bacteria.[6] Bioavailability may increase following antibiotic administration, complicating the management of dosing this drug, which is notorious for its low therapeutic index and risk of toxic side effects. Digoxin is principally excreted un-

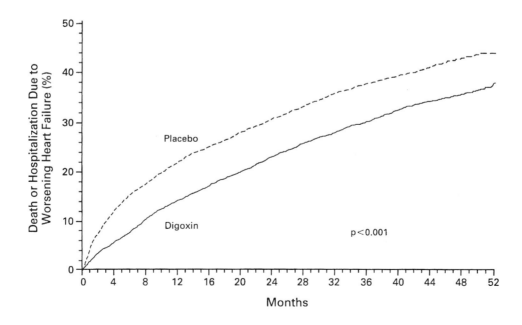

FIG. 2-1 Incidence of death or hospitalization resulting from worsening heart failure in 3397 patients treated with digoxin versus 3403 patients treated with placebo.
(From The Digitalis Investigation Group: *N Engl J Med* 336:525-533, 1997.)

changed by the kidney, and maintenance dosing must be decreased with declining creatinine clearance.

The cardiovascular actions of digoxin are complex but can be classified primarily into direct effects on cardiac tissue, resulting in increased inotropy and indirect cardiac electrophysiologic effects mediated through increased parasympathetic tone. Cardiac glycosides principally exert their inotropic effect through inhibition of membrane-bound sodium-potassium-adenosine triphosphatase, resulting in accumulation of intracellular sodium and calcium, and thus intensifying the reaction between actin and myosin in cardiac sarcomeres. Their electrophysiologic effects are mediated through central vagal nuclei stimulation, sensitization of peripheral baroreceptors, and facilitation of muscarinic transmission in cardiac tissue.

Complications of digoxin therapy can be life threatening and difficult to diagnose and treat. This is particularly concerning given the narrow window of safety between therapeutic and toxic blood levels. Therapeutic digoxin levels are approximately one third of toxic levels, and cardiac arrhythmias begin to manifest at approximately two thirds of the toxic level.[7] Aggravating conditions that predispose to digoxin toxicity include hypomagnesemia, hypercalcemia, and especially hypokalemia. Treatment of digoxin toxicity, which manifests as almost any arrhythmia, consists of correcting any accompanying electrolyte disturbances, administration of cardiac antiarrhythmic drugs such as phenytoin, and, in severe cases, administration of commercially prepared antibodies (Fab fragments) to digoxin.

Because of the narrow therapeutic index of cardiac glycosides, digoxin is no longer considered a first-line agent for treatment of congestive heart failure by many clinicians and is instead reserved for patients whose failure persists despite treatment with alternative agents such as β-adrenergic antagonists and angiotensin-converting enzyme inhibitors.[8,9] Recommending discontinuation of digoxin therapy preoperatively remains controversial. Although discontinuation is advised by many clinicians, there is no evidence that continuing therapy in patients without toxic manifestations is deleterious, and maintaining digitization may be particularly important in those patients receiving the drug for heart rate control.[7]

β-Adrenergic Antagonist Drugs (β-Blockers)

β-Blockers are a group of drugs chemically resembling the β-adrenoceptor agonist isoproterenol but which act to competitively antagonize the action of catecholamines at β_1 and β_2 receptors. β_1 Receptors are more commonly located in cardiac tissue, and their blockade leads to decreased heart rate and inotropy, and thus to decreased myocardial oxygen consumption. β_2 Receptors are mostly located in bronchial and vascular smooth muscle, where their blockade leads to increased airway resistance and mild vasoconstriction, respectively. Predominance of the β_1 effect, as well as antagonism of renin release, reliably leads to decreased blood pressure when nonselective β-blockers are administered. Some β-blockers have an increased affinity for the β_1 receptor, and are thus termed *cardioselective*. These drugs have a reduced tendency to induce bronchospastic complications in patients with reactive airways disease, although no β-blocker is devoid of antagonism at the β_2 receptor. Also, some β-blockers retain partial agonist activity at β receptors and are referred to as having intrinsic sympathomimetic activity, which can lessen the decrease in cardiac output seen with pure antagonists. Finally, many β-blockers possess local anesthetic (or "membrane-stabilizing") properties secondary to sodium channel blockade, but this effect is not evident with the low tissue levels achieved during systemic administration. The pharmacologic properties of commonly prescribed β-blockers are summarized in Table 2-1.

The most significant risks of β-blocker administration are bronchoconstriction and excessive myocardial depression or bradycardia. Therefore, the most significant contraindications to β-blockers are asthma or coadministration of calcium entry-blocking drugs such as verapamil or diltiazem. Traditional contraindications to β-blockade, such as diabetes and peripheral vascular disease, have been relaxed as the value of β-blockers in these patients has been increasingly proven and because these drugs are better tolerated than once suspected. β-Blockers are also well tolerated in most patients with chronic obstructive pulmonary disease. Unfortunately, β-blockers remain underused both chronically and perioperatively, especially in women and the elderly.[10]

β-Blockers are among the most useful agents in the chronic and perioperative management of patients with cardiovascular disease. For patients in acute and postmyocardial infarction conditions, β-blockers have been shown to decrease total mortality, cardiovascular mortality, sudden arrhythmic death, and recurrent myocardial infarction.[11] They decrease the incidence and severity of myocardial ischemia during daily activities in patients with coronary artery disease.[12] A recent meta-analysis concluded that patients with stable angina maintained on β-blockers have similar rates of cardiac death and myocardial infarction as do patients on calcium entry blockers, but they discontinue their drug because of adverse events less often.[13] Although β-blockers must be avoided or used with caution in patients with acute heart failure, they improve both ejection fraction and survival in chronic congestive heart failure.[14] Suggested mechanisms for their beneficial effects in heart failure include (1) antagonism of high, possibly cardiotoxic, circulating levels of catechola-

TABLE 2-1
Properties of Commonly Prescribed β-Adrenergic Antagonist Drugs

DRUG	β₁ SELECTIVE	PARTIAL AGONIST	CLEARANCE	HALF-LIFE	ORAL BIOAVAILABILITY	IV USE
Propranolol	No	No	Hepatic	3-6 hr	30%	Yes
Atenolol	Yes	No	Renal	6-9 hr	40%	Yes
Metoprolol	Yes	No	Hepatic	3-4 hr	50%	Yes
Nadolol	No	No	Renal	16-24 hr	33%	No
Sotalol	No	No	Renal	8-12 hr	90%	No
Pindolol	No	Yes	Hepatic, renal	3-4 hr	90%	No
Timolol	No	Mild	Hepatic	3-5 hr	50%	No
Esmolol	Yes	No	Plasma	10 min	0%*	Yes
Labetalol†	No	No	Hepatic	4-6 hr	30%	Yes

IV, Intravenous.
*IV administration only.
†Combined nonselective β-adrenergic blocking drug and selective α₁-adrenergic blocking drug.

mines; (2) improved diastolic filling; (3) antagonism of catecholamine-induced vasoconstriction and activation of the renin-angiotensin system; and (4) upregulation of β-receptor populations.[15,16] Established β-blockade helps preserve myocardial function following an acute ischemic insult.[17] β-Blockade is being increasingly used in coronary artery bypass surgery to optimize surgical conditions for beating heart surgery, and when intense β-blockade is used instead of cardioplegic arrest, there may be reduced risk of post–cardiopulmonary bypass (CPB) ischemia and myocardial edema formation.[18]

Patients taking β-blockers should have their therapy continued through the morning of both cardiac and noncardiac surgery. Preoperative administration of chronically administered β-blockers does not compromise myocardial performance after CPB. Acute discontinuation of these agents is often accompanied by hypertension and tachycardia. Perioperative cardiac ischemia most commonly derives from conditions of tachycardia and increased myocardial oxygen demand, rather than from abrupt loss of oxygen supply.[19] In fact, physicians should consider perioperative β-blockade in almost all patients with cardiovascular disease, even those not taking these drugs chronically. The incidence of perioperative myocardial ischemia in untreated hypertensive patients can be reduced with preoperative β-blocker administration.[20] Recently, investigators with the Multi-Center Study of Perioperative Ischemia research group conducted a prospective, randomized, double-blind, and placebo-controlled trial of 200 men undergoing major noncardiac surgery. The men either had known coronary artery disease or risk factors such as hypertension and diabetes without known coronary artery disease. They were randomized to receive either placebo or atenolol preoperatively and every 12 hours until hospital discharge or up to 7 days postoperatively. In two important reports of the findings in this study population, the investigators found a reduced incidence of postoperative myocardial ischemia in the atenolol group, and a survival benefit that extended at least 2 years postoperatively (Fig. 2-2).[21,22]

Angiotensin-Converting Enzyme Inhibitors

Angiotensin-converting enzyme (ACE) inhibitor drugs inhibit the enzyme peptidyl dipeptidase, which hydrolyzes angiotensin I to angiotensin II, preventing angiotensin II-induced vasoconstriction. These drugs reduce peripheral vascular resistance but, unlike direct vasodilators, do not induce reflex sympathetic activation and tachycardia. The most significant difference between drugs within this class lies in their duration of effect (Table 2-2). They have become standard treatment in the chronic management of essential hypertension, congestive heart failure, and mitral regurgitant lesions. The intravenous form of enalapril (enalaprilat) has become a common acute antihypertensive agent in the operating room and postanesthesia care unit. ACE inhibitors are especially useful because of their favorable side effect profile. Adverse effects such as bronchospasm, bradycardia, insomnia, depression, and sexual dysfunction, which may complicate other antihypertensive regimens, are rarely seen with ACE inhibitors. The most significant contraindications to their use are pregnancy and renal artery stenosis (in which renal failure may be induced). Severe hypotension can complicate initial dosing of ACE inhibitors, especially in patients who are hypovolemic or who have high renin activity. A persistent cough

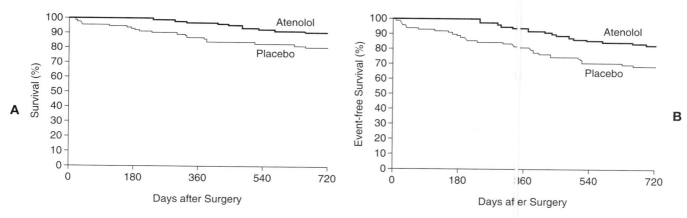

FIG. 2-2 **A,** Overall survival and **B,** cardiac event–free survival after hospital discharge among 192 patients receiving perioperative atenolol versus placebo.

(From Mangano DT, Layug EL, Wallace A et al: *N Engl J Med* 335:1713-1720, 1996.)

TABLE 2-2
Pharmacologic Profile of Common Angiotensin-Converting Enzyme Inhibitors

DRUG	USUAL ORAL DOSE	TIME TO PEAK	DURATION OF EFFECT
Captopril	100 mg	1-2 hr	6-10 hr
Enalapril	20 mg	4-8 hr	18-30 hr
Lisinopril	10 mg	2-4 hr	18-30 hr
Ramipril	20 mg	3-8 hr	24-60 hr

Adapted from Stoelting RK: *Pharmacology and physiology in anesthetic practice,* ed 3, Philadelphia, 1999, Lippincott-Raven, p 308.

and wheezing are seen in some patients, and rarely angioedema may develop.[23]

Whether to continue ACE inhibitor therapy through the morning of surgery is debatable. Anecdotal experience, as well as several published reports, indicates that severe hypotension, particularly at the time of anesthetic induction, can complicate the care of patients taking these drugs.[24,25] In a more recent study of anesthetic induction in patients with ischemic heart failure, a larger average drop in blood pressure and cardiac index was seen in ACE inhibitor–treated versus untreated patients, but the incidence of "severe" hypotension was not different.[26] Some authors continue to advise withholding ACE inhibitors on the day of surgery.[27] Although this recommendation remains controversial, there exist no studies demonstrating a benefit to ACE inhibitor continuation.

Calcium Entry Blockers

Calcium entry blockers are a diverse group of compounds (Fig. 2-3) that act to block calcium flux across L-type calcium channels, predominantly located in cardiac and vascular smooth muscle. To greater or lesser degrees, their administration leads to coronary and systemic vasodilation, and decreased chronotropy, inotropy, and dromotropy. The dihydropyridine calcium entry blockers (e.g., nifedipine, nicardipine, amlodipine, nimodipine) are most commonly used as antihypertensive and antianginal medications. Nimodipine is highly lipid soluble and is thus useful in conditions requiring a central nervous system effect, such as cerebral vasospasm. The dihydropyridines share potent vasodilating properties, and little or no effect on sinoatrial and atrioventricular nodal conduction. Their potent vasodilation can lead to reflex sympathetic activation and tachycardia. Verapamil, a phenylalkylamine, was the first clinically introduced calcium entry blocker. Unlike the dihydropyridines, verapamil displays modest vasodilating effects, but depresses inotropy, chronotropy, and atrioventricular conduction. It is prescribed as an antihypertensive and antianginal agent, but its properties also favor its use as an antiarrhythmic. Diltiazem, a benzothiazepine, yields effects that are intermediate between verapamil and the dihyropyridines, both with regard to its vasodilation and to its effects on cardiac conduction and contractility.

Perioperatively, calcium entry blockers can be useful for the acute treatment of hypertension, tachycardia, supraventricular arrhythmias, and myocardial ischemia. They are also used by practitioners to attenuate the hemodynamic responses to surgical stimulation and tracheal intubation or extubation.[28,29] Diltiazem administration results in more rapid control of atrial fibril-

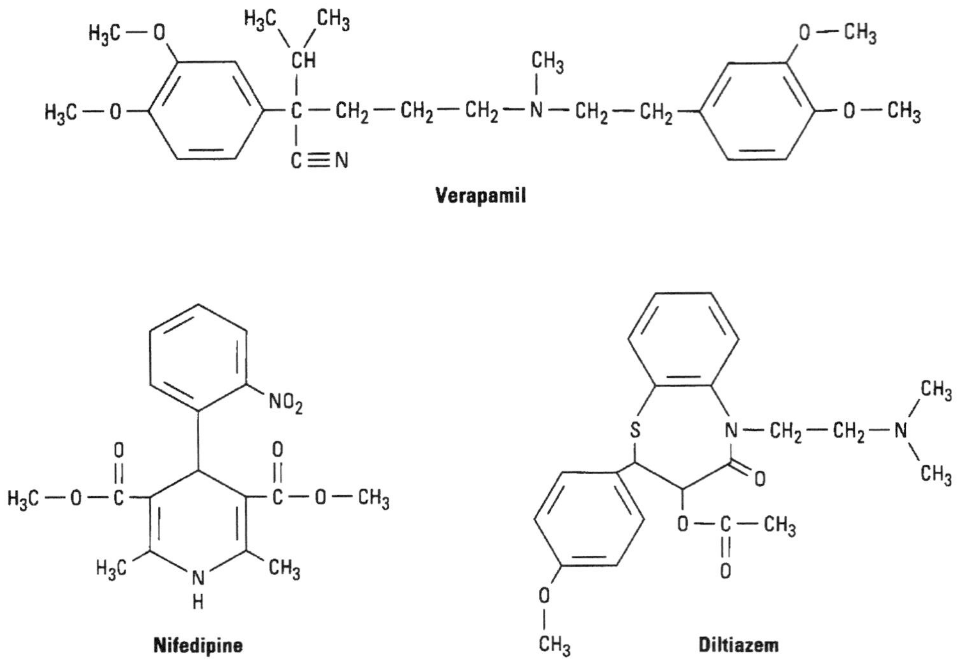

FIG. 2-3 Structural formulas of prototypical calcium entry blocking drugs. *Verapamil*, Benzothiazepine; *nifedipine*, dihydropyridine; *diltiazem*, phenylalkylamine.

lation that complicates coronary bypass surgery than does digoxin administration.[30]

Adverse effects of the calcium entry blockers are usually direct extensions of their therapeutic actions. Diltiazem and verapamil may cause excessive myocardial depression and bradycardia or atrioventricular block. Their myocardial depression can be more pronounced in conjunction with inhaled anesthetics. Diltiazem and verapamil inhibit the cytochrome P450 3A enzymes, which metabolize midazolam and alfentanil among other drugs, and may prolong the clinical effect of these anesthetic agents, resulting in delayed emergence.[31] Prophylactic intravenous diltiazem during cardiac surgery may increase the risk of postoperative renal dysfunction.[32] As the indications for perioperative infusion of calcium entry blockers grow, such as to prevent spasm of radial artery–free grafts, these considerations become increasingly important. Nifedipine and the other dihydropyridines may cause excessive hypotension or complications related to excessive reflex sympathetic stimulation. In fact, administration of nifedipine actually increases mortality in patients recovering from myocardial infarction and increases the risk of cardiovascular complications in hypertensive patients receiving chronic therapy.[33-35] Despite these cautions, it is most commonly recommended that patients taking calcium entry blockers preoperatively have their maintenance dosing continued through the morning of surgery.

Diuretics

Diuretics are a heterogenous group of compounds that act on various parts of the renal tubular transport system to increase urine flow (Fig. 2-4). Thiazide diuretics remain commonly prescribed agents in patients with cardiovascular disease, although they are rarely used as first-line antihypertensive therapy, as they once were. Thiazide diuretics (e.g., hydrochlorothiazide) inhibit reabsorption of sodium and chloride, principally in the renal cortical ascending loop. Their antihypertensive effect is initially due to loss of extravascular and intravascular fluid; however, this short-lived effect is replaced by a chronic, mild attenuation of sympathetic nervous system activity. Important side effects include metabolic alkalosis, hypokalemia (especially important in patients also receiving digoxin), increased serum cholesterol, hyponatremia, muscular weakness, and potentiation of nondepolarizing neuromuscular blocking drugs. Combination drugs often include a thiazide diuretic with a potassium-sparing diuretic (aldosterone antagonist) to produce diuresis with less significant side effects. Loop diuretics (e.g., furosemide) are prescribed almost exclusively for treatment of chronic extracellular fluid accumulation, or they may be administered intravenously acutely for the treatment of pulmonary edema or to rapidly induce urine flow. They are no longer prescribed as antihypertensives. They act by inhibiting sodium and chloride reabsorption in the ascending loop of Henle. Important side effects can include severe hypokalemia, metabolic alkalosis, hypomagnesemia,

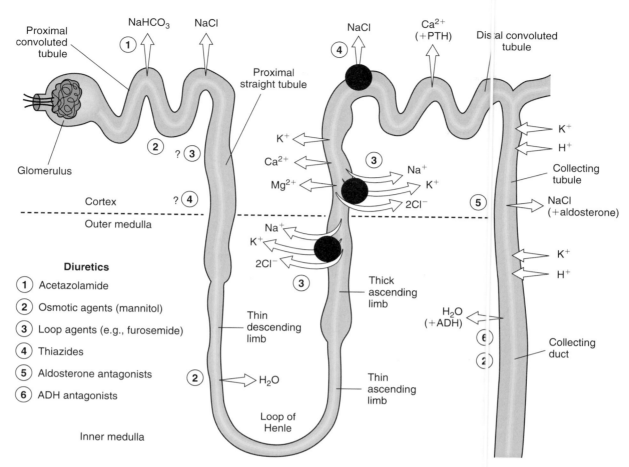

FIG. 2-4   Renal tubular transport systems and the sites of action of diuretics. *ADH*, Antidiuretic hormone; *PTH*, parathyroid hormone.

(From Ives HE: Diuretic agents. In Katzung BG, editor: *Basic and clinical pharmacology*, ed 7, Stamford, Conn, 1998, Appleton and Lange, p 243.)

and rarely, ototoxicity leading to deafness. Mannitol, a six-carbon sugar, is the most commonly used osmotic diuretic. It is not metabolized but eliminated only by glomerular filtration. Because it is not reabsorbed from the renal tubules, it increases the osmolarity of the fluid within the tubules and promotes diuresis. Its effect to increase plasma osmolarity also promotes fluid movement from extracellular collections and the central nervous system. Although mannitol is often administered perioperatively as a renal protective agent, there is little evidence that mannitol provides additional protection from ischemic renal injury over volume expansion alone.[36]

PERIOPERATIVE MEDICATIONS
Sympathomimetics

A narrative of the anatomy and physiology of the autonomic nervous system is beyond the scope of this chapter, but the reader is referred to such a discussion.[37] In brief, the anatomic distribution and effects of adrenoceptor stimulation are shown in Table 2-3.

Adrenergics
A summary table of the comparative pharmacology of direct- and indirect-acting adrenergic sympathomimetics is presented in Table 2-4. Fig. 2-5 graphically depicts the effects on heart rate and blood pressure typically seen with bolus administration of a mixed α and β agonist versus a selective α- or selective β-agonist drug.

α Agonists. Phenylephrine is the most commonly used α agonist. It is a synthetic, direct-acting agonist at α_1 receptors with much less significant activity at the α_2 receptor. It produces rapid and significant venoconstriction and less pronounced arteriolar constriction. It increases preload and mean arterial pressure, but can decrease cardiac output, especially in patients with ischemic cardiac disease.[38] Still, it is useful in rapidly restoring coronary perfusion pressure in acute perioperative

TABLE 2-3
Anatomic Distribution and Actions of Adrenoceptors

RECEPTOR	TISSUE LOCATIONS	RESULTS OF STIMULATION
α_1	Vascular smooth muscle	Vasoconstriction
	Heart	Mild inotropy
	Pupillary muscle	Pupillary dilation
	Hair follicles	Piloerection
α_2	Central nervous system	Complex
		Inhibition of norepinephrine release
		Sedation
	Fat	Inhibition of lipolysis
	Platelets	Aggregation
β_1	Heart	Chronotropy
		Inotropy
β_2	Heart ($\beta_1 > \beta_2$)	Chronotropy
		Inotropy
	Vascular smooth muscle	Vasodilation
	Bronchial smooth muscle	Bronchodilation
	Liver	Glycogenolysis
β_3	White and brown fat	Lipolysis
	Intestines	Intestinal relaxation
Dopaminergic$_1$	Vascular smooth muscle	Vasodilation
Dopaminergic$_2$	Sympathetic nerve endings	Inhibition of norepinephrine release

hypotension, and in supporting cerebral perfusion pressure during CPB.

β Agonists. Isoproterenol is a synthetic catecholamine with potent nonselective agonist properties at β receptors and essentially no activity at α receptors. At infused dosages of 1 to 5 μg/kg/min, isoproterenol causes increased heart rate and myocardial contractility, resulting in increased cardiac output. The effect on cardiac output can result in higher blood pressure, although the β_2 stimulation decreases vascular resistance. Its use in adults with coronary vascular disease is limited because its effects reliably increase myocardial oxygen consumption (and may decrease oxygen supply if the β_2 stimulation decreases diastolic blood pressure). However, the drug is useful for treating bradycardia that is poorly responsive to atropine and for increasing idioventricular escape rate in complete heart block. It is also often used in pediatric cardiac surgery because of its ability to increase heart rate and cardiac output while decreasing vascular resistance (particularly pulmonary vascular resistance).[39] β_2 Agonism also results in bronchodilation; specific β_2 agonists, such as terbutaline, may help improve oxygenation in postoperative cardiac surgical patients.[40]

Mixed Agonists. Adrenergic sympathomimetic agents with mixed effects at α and β receptors include naturally occurring compounds such as epinephrine, norepinephrine, and dopamine, as well as synthetic agents such as dobutamine and ephedrine. Their relative potencies at α and β receptors are displayed in Table 2-4. Although multiple adrenergic agonist drugs are often infused simultaneously in critically ill and cardiac surgical patients, recent evidence suggests that these drugs may antagonize each other, resulting in subadditive clinical effects during coadministration.[41]

Epinephrine is often considered the prototypical adrenergic agonist, yielding potent nonselective β stimulation and less pronounced α agonism. It is a potent inotrope and chronotrope. Effects on vascular resistance are dose dependent, with β_2 effects yielding decreased systemic vascular resistance at low dosages (<2 μg/min in adults) and vasoconstriction at higher dosages. Caution must be exercised in patients receiving β-blockers. β-Blockade may attenuate the β_2 effects seen with low-dose epinephrine, and "unmask" predominantly α effects leading to vasoconstriction, thus attenuating or eliminating expected increases in cardiac output.[42] Also, α effects predominate in the renal vasculature even at low dosages, and renal blood flow is substantially reduced by epinephrine, even in the absence of changes in systemic blood pressure.[43] Nevertheless, epinephrine increases cardiac index more reliably than does dopamine or dobutamine after separation from CPB,[44] and it is the agent of choice in many practices for this purpose.[45]

Norepinephrine and epinephrine have similar properties at β_1 receptors; however, norepinephrine shows

TABLE 2-4
Comparative Pharmacology of Adrenergic Sympathomimetic Agents

	RECEPTORS STIMULATED			MECHANISM OF ACTION	CARDIAC EFFECTS			PERIPHERAL VASCULAR RESISTANCE	RENAL BLOOD FLOW	MEAN ARTERIAL PRESSURE	AIRWAY RESISTANCE	CENTRAL NERVOUS SYSTEM STIMULATION	SINGLE INTRAVENOUS DOSE (70-KG ADULT)	CONTINUOUS INFUSION DOSE (70-KG ADULT)
	α	β_1	β_2		CARDIAC OUTPUT	HEART RATE	DYSRHYTHMIAS							
Natural Catecholamines														
Epinephrine	+	++	++	Direct	++	++	+++	±	---	+	---	Yes	2-8 µg	1-20 µg/min
Norepinephrine	+++	++	+	Direct	-	-	+	+++	---	+++	NC	No	2-8 µg	1-16 µg/min
Dopamine	++	++	+	Direct	+++	+	+	+	+++	+	NC	No	Not used	2-20 µg/kg/min
Synthetic Catecholamines														
Isoproterenol	0	+++	+++	Direct	+++	+++	+++	---	-	±	----	Yes	1-4 µg	1-5 µg/min
Dobutamine	+	+++	+	Direct	+++	+	±	NC	++	+	NC	No	Not used	2-10 µg/kg/min
Synthetic Noncatecholamines														
Indirect Acting														
Ephedrine	++	+	+	Indirect some direct	++	++	++	+	--	++	--	Yes	10-25 mg	Not used
Mephentermine	++	++	+	Indirect	++	++	++	+	--	++	-	Yes	10-25 mg	Not used
Metaraminol	++	++	+	Indirect, direct	-	-	+	+++	---	++	NC	No	1.5-5.0 mg	40-500 µg/kg/min
Direct Acting														
Phenylephrine	+++	0	0	Direct	-	-	NC	+++	---	++	NC	No	50-100 µg	20-50 µg/min
Methoxamine	+++	0	0	Direct	-	-	NC	+++	---	+++	NC	No	5-10 mg	

Adapted from Stoelting RK: *Pharmacology and physiology in anesthetic practice*, ed 3, Philadelphia, 1999, Lippincott-Raven, p 260.
0, None; +, minimal increase; ++, moderate increase; +++, marked increase; −, minimal decrease; −−, moderate decrease; −−−, marked decrease; NC, no change.

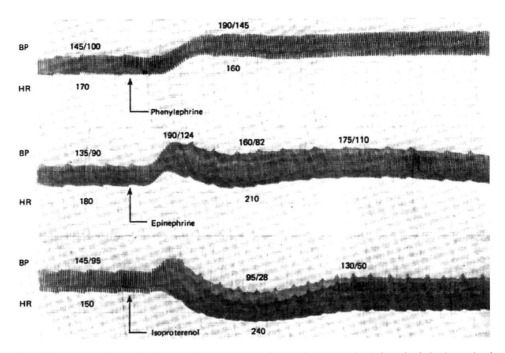

FIG. 2-5   Hemodynamic effects of a selective α-adrenergic antagonist (phenylephrine), a mixed agonist (epinephrine), and a β agonist (isoproterenol), given as a bolus intravenous injection. *BP,* Blood pressure; *HR,* heart rate.

(From Hoffman BB: Adrenoceptor-activating and other sympathomimetic drugs. In Katzung BG, editor: *Basic and clinical pharmacology,* ed 7, Stamford, Conn, 1998, Appleton and Lange, p 126.)

reduced activity at β_2 receptors and much greater agonism at α receptors. Thus, norepinephrine increases peripheral resistance and blood pressure more than does epinephrine, whereas compensatory vagal responses tend to limit increases in heart rate.

Dopamine is the immediate metabolic precursor of norepinephrine. Although possessing activity at α, β, and dopaminergic receptors, at dosages less than 3 μg/kg/min, the dopaminergic effects predominate, leading to decreased vascular resistance and increased renal blood flow. This effect is not antagonized by α stimulation, and thus renal blood flow can be augmented with low-dose dopamine infusions even as other adrenergic medications are given.[46] However, the prophylactic use of dopamine as a protective agent against development of perioperative renal failure remains largely unsupported in the literature.[47,48] Mesenteric and coronary vasodilation are also seen with low-dose dopamine. At higher dosages, α effects begin to predominate, which may attenuate β-induced increases in cardiac output secondary to vasoconstriction.

Dobutamine is a synthetic agent with mixed-agonist properties, yielding increased inotropy and chronotropy through its major effect on β_1 receptors, typically accompanied by mild vasodilation secondary to its β_2 stimulation. Thus, dobutamine is effective in raising cardiac output without the accompanying increases in pulmo-

nary vascular resistance often seen with epinephrine and norepinephrine use.[49] However, associated tachycardia may be more severe than that seen with epinephrine.[50]

Nonadrenergics

Phosphodiesterase Inhibitors.   Phosphodiesterase is the enzyme that hydrolyzes cyclic adenosine monophosphate (cAMP), whose intracellular concentration is increased as a result of β-adrenergic stimulation. At least five isoenzymes exist, with phosphodiesterase isoenzyme III (PDE III) being found principally in cardiac and vascular smooth muscle. Amrinone and milrinone are specific inhibitors of PDE III, resulting in increased intracellular cAMP and increased inward calcium flux, and thus increased inotropy. Their effect on cAMP accumulation in vascular smooth muscle also results in vasodilation, both effects combining to improve cardiac output[51,52] (Fig. 2-6). PDE III inhibitors produce increases in heart rate comparable to dobutamine, but may result in greater increases in cardiac index, especially in patients with pulmonary hypertension.[53] Because the PDE III inhibitors act through mechanisms complementary to β-adrenergic agonists, the addition of a PDE III inhibitor to the treatment of a patient receiving an adrenergic drug such as epinephrine may increase cardiac performance to a greater degree than would the addition of another adrenergic sympathomimetic.[54]

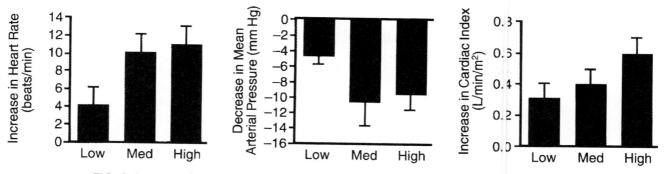

FIG. 2-6 Hemodynamic effect of amrinone in 39 patients recovering from coronary artery bypass surgery (low dose = 0.75 mg/kg loading dose, 10 µg/kg/min infusion; medium dose = 1.5 mg/kg loading dose, 10 µg/kg/min infusion; high dose = 2.25 mg/kg loading dose, 20 µg/kg/min infusion). Measurements made at baseline and at steady state during drug infusion; all hemodynamic changes significantly different from baseline at all doses.

(From Butterworth JF: *J Cardiothorac Vasc Anesth* 7[suppl 1]:1-7, 1993.)

Tachycardia induced by PDE III inhibitors can be problematic, especially in patients with ischemic coronary disease. Cardioselective β-blockers can be administered in cases of excessive tachycardia without ablating improvements in cardiac index.[55] In a randomized, blind comparison of milrinone and amrinone, the hemodynamic effects of administration were not sufficiently different to recommend one drug over the other[56] (Fig. 2-7), although thrombocytopenia and elevation of liver enzymes seem to occur more frequently with administration of amrinone.[57] The hemodynamic effects of various amrinone dosing regimens are indicated in Fig. 2-6. Milrinone is administered as a loading dose of 50 µg/kg over 10 minutes followed by a maintenance infusion of 0.5 µg/kg/min. The range for the milrinone infusion dose is 0.375 to 0.75 µg/kg/min. Dosing is adjusted downward in patients with reduced creatinine clearance.

Calcium. Calcium salts are frequently administered to cardiac surgical patients, especially on separation from CPB, or to antagonize the hypotensive effects of drugs such as protamine or propofol.[58] However, little data support the routine, or even frequent, use of calcium to improve cardiac performance. Calcium administration increases arterial pressure after CPB but does not increase cardiac index.[59] Modest doses of ephedrine actually improve right ventricular ejection fraction after CPB more than does 600 mg of calcium chloride.[60] In fact, calcium administration antagonizes the improvements in cardiac index seen with β-adrenergic agonists such as epinephrine and dobutamine.[61,62]

Calcium administration after CPB also confers risks. Intravenous calcium may induce postoperative vasospasm of native and graft coronary vessels.[63,64] The role of calcium in ischemic reperfusion injury is being extensively studied. Finally, post-CPB calcium administration may be an important causal factor in the development

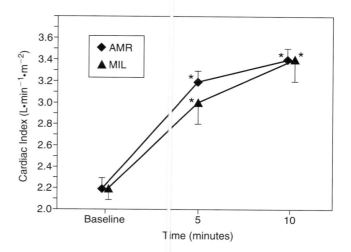

FIG. 2-7 Cardiac index after administration of two sequential doses of either amrinone (*AMR*, 0.75 mg/kg, n = 22 patients) or milrinone (*MIL*, 25 µg/kg, n = 22 patients), following separation from cardiopulmonary bypass. The first AMR or MIL dose was given immediately after baseline hemodynamic measurements were taken; the second dose was given immediately after the 5-minute measurements. *$p < 0.05$.

(From Rathmell JP, Prielipp RC, Butterworth JF et al: *Anesth Analg* 86:683-690, 1998.)

of pancreatitis, which complicates recovery from cardiac surgery[65,66] (Fig. 2-8).

Glucagon. Glucagon is a natural pancreatic peptide hormone that increases adenyl cyclase activity and production of intracellular cAMP. Its effect is independent of β-adrenoceptor stimulation and is not related to inhibition of PDE III. It does not have a role in the clinical management of heart failure, but is used in cases of severe bradycardia, especially that caused by β-blocker or calcium entry–blocker toxicity due to overdose.[67,68]

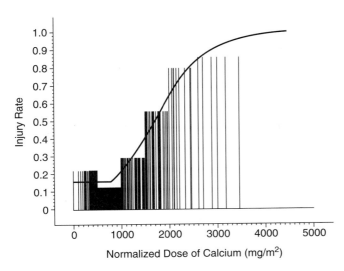

FIG. 2-8   Logistic regression of the rate of pancreatic cellular injury on the total normalized calcium dose (during surgery and in the first 24 postoperative hours) in 300 prospectively studied patients.

(From Castillo CF, Harringer W, Warshaw AL et al: *N Engl J Med* 325:382-387, 1991.)

Triiodothyronine. Triiodothyronine (T_3) is the biologically active form of thyroid hormone, 85% of which is derived outside the thyroid by conversion from T_4, with the remaining 15% secreted directly by the thyroid. Through complex effects on cellular protein synthesis, T_3 regulates cellular oxygen use. Many clinical situations, including acute illness, fasting, heart failure, and CPB, produce acute hypothyroidism (or "euthyroid sick syndrome") characterized by low T_3, normal or low T_4, and normal thyroid-stimulating hormone levels.[69] Early clinical reports[70] and animal studies[71] suggested that T_3 had useful clinical inotropic properties. T_3 has been studied as a treatment for congestive heart failure[72] and as an adjunct to the resuscitation of donor hearts in cardiac transplantation.[73,74] Perioperative T_3 may decrease the incidence of post-CPB atrial fibrillation.[75] However, a recent randomized, double-blind, placebo-controlled trial of T_3 in 211 high-risk patients undergoing coronary bypass surgery failed to reveal any significant effects on post-CPB hemodynamic variables[76] (Table 2-5). These results, and the high cost of T_3 administration,[77] argue against common use of this agent. Some authors continue to advocate its use as a "rescue" agent, in patients who are having difficulty or failing to wean from CPB.[78]

Vasodilators

Nitric Oxide Donors

Intravenously administered nitroglycerin (NTG) and sodium nitroprusside (SNP) both act to produce vasodilation through release of NO, formerly known as *endothelium-derived relaxing factor*.[79] NTG is an indirect

NO donor, requiring breakdown of the drug in the presence of thiol compounds to produce NO, whereas SNP is a direct NO donor on exposure to oxyhemoglobin.[80] The tolerance to chronic oral or transdermal nitrate administration described earlier is also seen with intravenous NTG administration, and may be explained by gradual depletion of intracellular thiol groups necessary to allow release of active NO.[80] Tolerance is not seen with prolonged SNP infusion. Perioperative infusion of L-arginine, the biologic precursor for NO, is also being investigated and shows promise as a coronary vasodilator in patients undergoing coronary bypass grafting.[81]

NTG or SNP may be administered intraoperatively or postoperatively to control hypertension and reduce myocardial oxygen consumption. Clinically, SNP is a more potent dilator of arterioles than NTG, whereas NTG acts principally as a dilator of venous capacitance vessels until higher dosages are given. The potent arteriolar relaxation properties of SNP may result in coronary steal secondary to dilation of epicardial resistance vessels and diversion of flow from ischemic subendocardium. NTG has not been shown to produce coronary steal. Consequently, NTG is often considered the vasodilator of choice in the treatment of myocardial ischemia or mild hypertension in patients after revascularization procedures, whereas SNP is often chosen for reliable, potent afterload reduction in patients recovering from extensive aortotomy or valvular replacement procedures.

SNP is composed of five cyanide moieties and a nitrosyl group surrounding a ferrous iron center, and a well-known potential complication of SNP infusion is cyanide toxicity. Cyanide can be metabolized by the liver at a rate of up to 2 µg/kg/min; accumulation may occur when infusion rates exceed this level, leading to poisoning of oxidative phosphorylation.[82] Cyanide toxicity is identified by increasing tolerance, metabolic acidosis, and increased tissue oxygen consumption as evidenced by decreasing mixed venous oxygen saturation. Inhaled amyl nitrate or slow intravenous infusions of sodium nitrite (5 mg/kg) or sodium thiosulfate (150 mg/kg) are treatments for cyanide toxicity.

Inhaled Nitric Oxide

NO is now appreciated as a vital endogenous regulator of vascular tone and as a potentially useful pharmacologic agent.[83] Its ultra-short half-life (seconds) and its nature as a gas lend it to be administered as an inhaled agent for the production of selective pulmonary vasodilation. Inhaled NO reliably reduces pulmonary vascular resistance with essentially no effect on the systemic circulation[84] (Fig. 2-9). Its administration has been studied in the treatment of numerous disease states characterized by high pulmonary vascular resistance, including primary pulmonary hypertension,[85] lung and heart transplantation,[86] acute

TABLE 2-5

Hemodynamic Measurements (+/− SEM) in Patients Randomized after Coronary Bypass Surgery to an Infusion of Triiodothyronine or Placebo

HEMODYNAMIC PARAMETER	TIME OF MEASUREMENT	T_3 (n = 66)	PLACEBO (n = 71)	P
Heart rate	Baseline	68 +/− 1.9	65 +/− 1.7	NS
	Off CPB	91 +/− 1.4	89 +/− 1.4	NS
	ICU	92 +/− 1.2	90 +/− 1.9	NS
	Hour 4	98 +/− 1.2	94 +/− 1.8	NS
	Hour 6	100 +/− 1.5	96 +/− 1.8	NS
Cardiac index (L/min/m²)	Baseline	2.4 +/− 0.08	2.4 +/− 0.07	NS
	Off CPB	2.7 +/− 0.08	2.8 +/− 0.08	NS
	ICU	2.6 +/− 0.07	2.5 +/− 0.07	NS
	Hour 4	2.6 +/− 0.08	2.6 +/− 0.08	NS
	Hour 6	2.8 +/− 0.08	2.6 +/− 0.07	NS
Mean arterial pressure (mm Hg)	Baseline	98 +/− 2.5	93 +/− 2.1	NS
	Off CPB	73 +/− 1.5	73 +/− 1.3	NS
	ICU	80 +/− 1.7	81 +/− 1.3	NS
	Hour 4	80 +/− 1.7	82 +/− 1.2	NS
	Hour 6	77 +/− 1.3	78 +/− 1.1	NS
Pulmonary artery diastolic pressure (mm Hg)	Baseline	18 +/− 1.0	15 +/− 0.8	NS
	Off CPB	15 +/− 0.5	15 +/− 0.5	NS
	ICU	17 +/− 0.6	15 +/− 0.5	NS
	Hour 4	15 +/− 0.5	14 +/− 0.5	NS
	Hour 6	16 +/− 0.5	14 +/− 0.5	NS
Systemic vascular resistance (dyne × sec × cm⁻⁵)	Baseline	1710 +/− 77	1600 +/− 56	NS
	Off CPB	1040 +/− 40	1060 +/− 43	NS
	ICU	1230 +/− 57	1280 +/− 52	NS
	Hour 4	1200 +/− 51	1330 +/− 53	NS
	Hour 6	1090 +/− 40	1170 +/− 43	NS

Adapted from Bennett-Guerrero E, Jimenez JL, White WD et al: *JAMA* 275:687-692, 1996.

T_3, Triiodothyronine (0.8 µg/kg followed by 0.12 µg/kg/hr for 6 hr); *p*, probability; *CPB*, cardiopulmonary bypass; *ICU*, intensive care unit; *NS*, no statistically significant difference between groups.

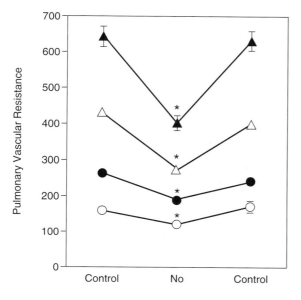

FIG. 2-9   Pulmonary vascular resistance (PVR, dyne × cm × sec⁻⁵) in 25 patients before, during, and after inhalation of nitric oxide (NO, 20 ppm), when precardiopulmonary and postcardiopulmonary bypass data are combined and grouped by baseline PVR. All groups are significantly different from baseline after inhalation of NO ($p < 0.05$). The magnitude of effect of NO inhalation in decreasing PVR is proportional to baseline PVR.

(From Rich GF, Murphy GD, Roos CM et al: *Anesthesiology* 78:1028-1035, 1993.)

respiratory distress syndromes,[87] and pulmonary hypertension complicating adult and pediatric cardiac surgery.[88,89] Inhaled NO may also be useful in improving ventilation-perfusion matching in patients after CPB but has not been shown to have an impact on outcome in this setting.[90,91] Inhaled NO delivery systems typically allow for delivery of 1 to 100 ppm, although NO is most commonly delivered in doses of 10 to 40 ppm. Concerns surrounding widespread clinical use of in-

haled NO center around potential toxicity. NO is known to be directly toxic to pulmonary tissues in high concentrations, to produce methemoglobinemia, and to spontaneously form nitrogen dioxide on reaction with oxygen, another agent with known pulmonary toxic effects.[92] The total dose of NO may be reduced by "spiking" each breath with a short burst of NO in concentrations of 100 ppm. This technique was as effective in dilating the pulmonary vasculature as 40 ppm of

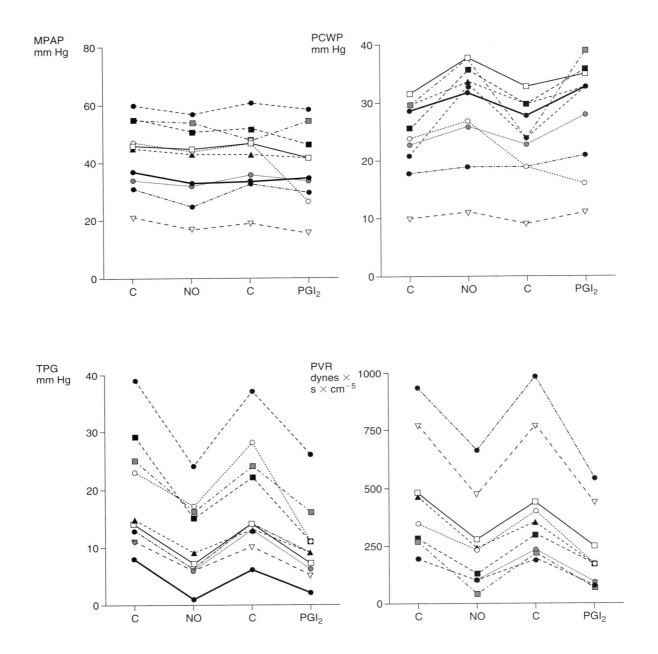

FIG. 2-10 Individual data from 10 heart transplant candidates showing the effect of inhaled nitric oxide (*NO*, 40 ppm) and inhaled prostacyclin (*PGI₂*, 10 μg/ml) on mean pulmonary artery pressure *(MPAP)*, pulmonary capillary wedge pressure *(PCWP)*, total transpulmonary gradient *(TPG)*, and pulmonary vascular resistance *(PVR)*. *C*, Control.

(From Haraldsson A, Kieler-Jensen N, Nathorst-Westfelt U et al: *Chest* 114:780-786, 1998.)

NO delivered throughout inhalation, but it reduced the total dose of NO fortyfold.[93]

Prostaglandin E₁ and Prostacyclin

Prostaglandin E_1 (PGE_1, alprostadil) acts on specific prostaglandin receptors to produce potent vasodilation of both the pulmonary and systemic vasculatures. It is principally used at dosages of 0.1 to 0.4 μg/kg/min to maintain patency of the ductus arteriosus in patients with ductal-dependent congenital heart lesions such as pulmonary atresia and hypoplastic left heart syndrome.

Inhaled PGE_1 and prostacycline are being investigated as alternatives to inhaled NO as selective pulmonary vasodilating drugs, in large measure stimulated by the toxicity concerns of NO, as discussed earlier[94-96] (Fig. 2-10).

α-Adrenergic Antagonists

Phentolamine is a nonselective α-adrenergic antagonist that produces rapid vasodilation when given intravenously. It may be used in doses of 10 to 40 μg/kg to treat severe hypertension, but its usefulness is limited by occasionally severe accompanying tachycardia induced both as a baroreceptor reflex and through central α_2-receptor blockade. This disadvantage is unimportant in patients on CPB, in whom phentolamine given in doses of 50 to 100 μg/kg reliably reduces blood pressure for approximately 20 minutes. In this setting, phentolamine is sometimes used to reduce excessive systemic vascular resistance and facilitate extracorporeal perfusion, or to promote more uniform cooling and rewarming. Chlorpromazine has been similarly used for its α-adrenergic blocking properties, but is now rarely used.

Dopamine Agonists

Fenoldopam is a new, selective dopamine₁-receptor agonist that rapidly produces vasodilation on intravenous administration (see Table 2-3). It is typically infused at dosages of 0.1 to 0.4 μg/kg/min (no bolus dose is recommended) and is useful in the treatment of most hypertensive emergencies, and for continuous control of hypertension that complicates cardiac surgery for up to 48 hours.[97] Its principal advantage over alternative vasodilators seems to be that it effectively reduces blood pressure without concomitant decreases in renal blood flow. Caution should be exercised in patients with glaucoma because fenoldopam administration reliably increases intraocular pressure. Its role in the future of perioperative cardiac surgical care remains to be defined by clinical investigation.

KEY POINTS

1. Preoperative maintenance nitrate therapy correlates with increased mortality in patients having coronary bypass surgery, perhaps because nitrate tolerance renders perioperative nitrovasodilators less effective or because abrupt cessation causes vasoconstriction.

2. Digoxin is effective in reducing mortality in patients with chronic congestive heart failure, but is no longer a first-line agent because of its narrow therapeutic index.

3. β-Adrenergic antagonists should not be discontinued before surgery, and in fact should be considered for prophylaxis against perioperative myocardial ischemia in all patients with known or suspected coronary artery disease.

4. No drug has been demonstrated to be superior to epinephrine in facilitating separation from CPB.

5. Amrinone and milrinone yield clinical effects that are not distinguishable in a blinded comparison.

6. Calcium raises arterial blood pressure but not cardiac index after CPB; its administration is poorly supported in the literature unless serum ionized calcium is low.

7. Despite initial enthusiasm, T_3 does not improve cardiac performance sufficiently to justify common use, particularly given its high cost.

8. NO release accounts for the vasodilating properties of NTG and SNP; the biologic precursor of NO, L-arginine, may become a useful intravenous vasodilator.

9. Inhaled NO is being extensively studied in the laboratory and in clinical trials as a selective pulmonary vasodilator.

KEY REFERENCES

Bennett-Guerrero E, Jimenez J, White W et al: Cardiovascular effects of intravenous triiodothyronine in patients undergoing coronary artery bypass graft surgery, *JAMA* 275:687-692, 1996.

The Digitalis Investigation Group: The effect of digoxin on mortality and morbidity in patients with heart failure, *N Engl J Med* 336:525-533, 1997.

Fullerton D, McIntyre R: Inhaled nitric oxide: therapeutic applications in cardiothoracic surgery, *Ann Thorac Surg* 61: 1856-1864, 1996.

Gibson R: Current status of calcium channel-blocking drugs after q wave and non-q wave myocardial infarction, *Circulation* 80:IV107-IV119, 1989.

Heidenreich P, McDonald K, Hastie T et al: Meta-analysis of

trials comparing β-blockers, calcium antagonists, and nitrates for stable angina, *JAMA* 281:1927-1936, 1999.

Mangano D, Layug E, Wallace A et al: Effect of atenolol on mortality and cardiovascular morbidity after noncardiac surgery, *N Engl J Med* 335:1713-1720, 1996.

Palmer R, Ferrige A, Moncada S: Nitric oxide release accounts for the biological activity of endothelium-derived relaxing factor, *Nature* 327:524-526, 1987.

Rathmell J, Prielipp R, Butterworth J et al: A multicenter, randomized blind comparison of amrinone with milrinone after elective cardiac surgery, *Anesth Analg* 86:683-690, 1998.

Steen P, Tinker J, Pluth J: Efficacy of dopamine, dobutamine, and epinephrine during emergence from cardiopulmonary bypass in man, *Circulation* 57:378-384, 1978.

Wallace A, Layug B, Tateo I et al: Prophylactic atenolol reduces postoperative myocardial ischemia, *Anesthesiology* 88:7-17, 1998.

Weightman W, Gibbs N, Sheminant M et al: Drug therapy before coronary artery surgery: nitrates are independent predictors of mortality and β-adrenergic blockers predict survival, *Anesth Analg* 88:286-291, 1999.

References

1. Harrison D, Bates J: The nitrovasodilators: new ideas about old drugs, *Circulation* 87:1461-1467, 1993.
2. Mehra A, Shotan A, Ostrzega E et al: Escalating nitrate dose overcomes early attenuation of hemodynamic effect caused by nitrate tolerance in patients with heart failure, *Am Heart J* 130:798-805, 1995.
3. Nordlander R, Walter M: Once versus twice daily administration of controlled release isosorbide-5-mononitrate in the treatment of stable angina pectoris: a randomized, double-blind, crossover study, *Eur Heart J* 15:108-113, 1994.
4. Weightman W, Gibbs N, Sheminant M et al: Drug therapy before coronary artery surgery: nitrates are independent predictors of mortality and β-adrenergic blockers predict survival, *Anesth Analg* 88:286-291, 1999.
5. Rich S, Seidlitz M, Dodin E et al: The short term effects of digoxin in patients with right ventricular dysfunction from pulmonary hypertension, *Chest* 114:787-792, 1998.
6. Lindenbaum J, Rund D, Butler V et al: Inactivation of digoxin by the gut flora: reversal by antibiotic therapy, *N Engl J Med* 305:789-794, 1981.
7. Stoelting R: *Pharmacology and physiology in anesthetic practice*, Philadelphia, 1999, Lippincott-Raven, p 282.
8. The Digitalis Investigation Group: The effect of digoxin on mortality and morbidity in patients with heart failure, *N Engl J Med* 336:525-533, 1997.
9. Packer M: End of the oldest controversy in medicine: are we ready to conclude the debate on digitalis? *N Engl J Med* 336:575-576, 1997.
10. Warltier D: β-adrenergic-blocking drugs: incredibly useful, incredibly underutilized, *Anesthesiology* 88:2-5, 1998.
11. Kennedy H: β-blocker prevention of proarrhythmia and pro-ischemia: clues from CAST, CAMIAT, and EMIAT, *Am J Cardiol* 80:1208-1211, 1997.
12. Deedwania P, Carbajal E: Role of beta blockade in the treatment of myocardial ischemia, *Am J Cardiol* 80(9B):23J-28J, 1997.
13. Heidenreich P, McDonald K, Hastie T et al: Meta-analysis of trials comparing β-blockers, calcium antagonists, and nitrates for stable angina, *JAMA* 281:1927-1936, 1999.
14. Cleland J, McGowan J, Cowburn P: β-Blockers for chronic heart failure: from prejudice to enlightenment, *J Cardiovasc Pharmacol* 32:S52-S60, 1998.
15. vanCampen L, Visser F, Visser C: Ejection fraction improvement by β-blocker treatment in patients with heart failure: an analysis of studies published in the literature, *J Cardiovasc Pharmacol* 32:S31-S35, 1998.
16. Emilien G, Maloteaux J: Current therapeutic uses and potential of β-adrenergic agonists and antagonists, *Eur J Pharmacol* 53:389-404, 1998.
17. Toleikis P, Tomlinson C: Myocardial functional preservation during ischemia: influence of beta blocking agents, *Mol Cell Biochem* 176:205-210, 1997.
18. Warters R, Allen S, Davis K et al: β-Blockade as an alternative to cardioplegic arrest during cardiopulmonary bypass, *Ann Thorac Surg* 65:961-966, 1998.
19. Cohen A: Prevention of perioperative myocardial ischaemia and its complications, *Lancet* 351:385-386, 1998.
20. Stone J, Foex P, Sear J et al: Myocardial ischemia in untreated hypertensive patients: effect of a single small oral dose of a β-adrenergic blocking agent, *Anesthesiology* 68:495-500, 1988.
21. Mangano D, Layug E, Wallace A et al: Effect of atenolol on mortality and cardiovascular morbidity after noncardiac surgery, *N Engl J Med* 335:1713-1720, 1996.
22. Wallace A, Layug B, Tateo I et al: Prophylactic atenolol reduces postoperative myocardial ischemia, *Anesthesiology* 88:7-17, 1998.
23. Brown N, Snowden M, Griffin M: Recurrent angiotensin-converting enzyme inhibitor-associated angioedema, *JAMA* 278:232-233, 1997.
24. Colson P, Saussine M, Seguin J et al: Hemodynamic effects of anesthesia in patients chronically treated with angiotensin-converting enzyme inhibitors, *Anesth Analg* 74:805-808, 1992.
25. Coriat P, Richer C, Douraki T et al: Influence of chronic angiotensin-converting enzyme inhibition on anesthetic induction, *Anesthesiology* 81:299-307, 1994.
26. Ryckwaert F, Colson P: Hemodynamic effects of anesthesia in patients with ischemic heart failure chronically treated with angiotensin-converting enzyme inhibitors, *Anesth Analg* 84:945-949, 1997.
27. Whalley D, Maurer W: Hemodynamic effects of anesthesia in patients receiving angiotensin-converting enzyme inhibitors, *Anesth Analg* 86:215-216, 1998.
28. Mikawa K, Nishina K, Maekawa N et al: Attenuation of cardiovascular responses to tracheal extubation: verapamil versus diltiazem, *Anesth Analg* 82:1205-1210, 1996.
29. Song D, Singh H, White P et al: Optimal dose of nicardipine for maintenance of hemodynamic stability after tracheal intubation and skin incision, *Anesth Analg* 85:1247-1251, 1997.
30. Tisdale J, Padhi D, Goldberg A et al: A randomized, double-blind comparison of intravenous diltiazem and digoxin for atrial fibrillation after coronary artery bypass surgery, *Am Heart J* 135:739-747, 1998.
31. Ahonen J, Olkkola K, Salmenpera M et al: Effect of diltiazem on midazolam and alfentanil disposition in patients undergoing coronary artery bypass grafting, *Anesthesiology* 85:1246-1252, 1996.
32. Young E, Diab A, Kirsh M: Intravenous diltiazem and acute renal failure after cardiac operations, *Ann Thorac Surg* 65:1316-1319, 1998.

33. Gibson R: Current status of calcium channel-blocking drugs after q wave and non-q wave myocardial infarction, *Circulation* 80: IV107-IV119, 1989.

34. Furberg C, Posaty B, Meyer J: Nifedipine: dose-related increase in mortality in patients with coronary artery disease, *Circulation* 92: 1326-1331, 1995.

35. Psaty B, Heckbert S, Koepsell T et al: The risk of myocardial infarction associated with antihypertensive drug therapies, *JAMA* 274:620-625, 1995.

36. Paul M, Mazer D, Byrick R et al: Influence of mannitol and dopamine on renal function during elective infrarenal aortic clamping in man, *Am J Nephrol* 6:427-434, 1986.

37. Lawson N, Meyer D: Autonomic nervous system: physiology and pharmacology. In Barash P, Cullen B, Stoelting R, editors: *Clinical anesthesia*, Philadelphia, 1997, Lippincott-Raven, pp 243-310.

38. Schwinn D, Reves J: Time course and hemodynamic effects of α-1 adrenergic bolus administration in anesthetized patients with myocardial disease, *Anesth Analg* 68:571-578, 1989.

39. Daoud F, Reeves J, Kelly D: Isoproterenol as a potential vasodilator in primary pulmonary hypertension, *Am J Cardiol* 42:817-822, 1978.

40. Waller D, Saunders N: Terbutaline improves efficiency of oxygenation after coronary artery bypass surgery, *J Cardiovasc Surg* 37: 59-62, 1996.

41. Prielipp R, MacGregor D, Royster R et al: Dobutamine antagonizes epinephrine's biochemical and cardiotonic effects, *Anesthesiology* 89:49-57, 1998.

42. Tarnow J, Muller R: Cardiovascular effects of low-dose epinephrine infusions in relation to the extent of preoperative β-adrenoceptor blockade, *Anesthesiology* 74:1035-1043, 1991.

43. Stoelting R: *Pharmacology and physiology in anesthetic practice*, Philadelphia, 1999, Lippincott-Raven, p 265.

44. Steen P, Tinker J, Pluth J: Efficacy of dopamine, dobutamine, and epinephrine during emergence from cardiopulmonary bypass in man, *Circulation* 57:378-384, 1978.

45. Tinker J: Strong inotropes (i.e., epinephrine) should be drugs of first choice during emergence from cardiopulmonary bypass, *J Cardiothorac Anesth* 1:256-258, 1987.

46. Schaer G, Fink M, Parillo J: Norepinephrine alone versus norepinephrine plus low-dose dopamine: enhanced renal blood flow with combination pressor therapy, *Crit Care Med* 13:492-496, 1985.

47. Baldwin L, Henderson A, Hickman P: Effect of postoperative low-dose dopamine on renal function after elective major vascular surgery, *Ann Intern Med* 120:744-747, 1994.

48. Byrick R, Rose D: Pathophysiology and prevention of acute renal failure: the role of the anaesthetist, *Can J Anaesth* 37:457-467, 1990.

49. Schwenzer K, Miller E: Hemodynamic effects of dobutamine in patients following mitral valve replacement, *Anesth Analg* 68: 467-472, 1989.

50. Butterworth J, Prielipp R, Royster R et al: Dobutamine increases heart rate more than epinephrine in patients recovering from aortocoronary bypass surgery, *J Cardiothorac Vasc Anesth* 6:535-541, 1992.

51. Butterworth J: Use of amrinone in cardiac surgery patients, *J Cardiothorac Vasc Anesth* 7(suppl 1):1-7, 1993.

52. Butterworth J, Royster R, Prielipp R et al: Amrinone in cardiac surgical patients with left-ventricular dysfunction: a prospective, randomized placebo-controlled trial, *Chest* 104:1660-1667, 1993.

53. Jenkins I, Dolman J, O'Connor J et al: Amrinone versus dobutamine in cardiac surgical patients with severe pulmonary hypertension after cardiopulmonary bypass: a prospective, randomized double-blinded trial, *Anaesth Intensive Care* 25:245-249, 1997.

54. Royster R, Butterworth J, Prielipp R et al: Combined inotropic effects of amrinone and epinephrine after cardiopulmonary bypass in humans, *Anesth Analg* 77:662-672, 1993.

55. Alhashemi J, Hooper J: Treatment of milrinone-associated tachycardia with β-blockers, *Can J Anaesth* 45:67-70, 1998.

56. Rathmell J, Prielipp R, Butterworth J et al: A multicenter, randomized blind comparison of amrinone with milrinone after elective cardiac surgery, *Anesth Analg* 86:683-690, 1998.

57. Katzung B, Parmley W: Cardiac glycosides and other drugs used in congestive heart failure. In Katzung B, editor: *Basic and clinical pharmacology*, ed 7, Stamford, Conn, 1998, Appleton and Lange, pp 197-215.

58. Tritapepe L, Voci P, Marino P et al: Calcium chloride minimizes the hemodynamic effects of propofol in patients undergoing coronary artery bypass grafting, *J Cardiothorac Vasc Anesth* 13: 150-153, 1999.

59. Royster R, Butterworth J, Prielipp R et al: A randomized, blinded, placebo-controlled evaluation of calcium chloride and epinephrine for inotropic support after emergence from cardiopulmonary bypass, *Anesth Analg* 74:3-13, 1992.

60. Johnston W, Robertie P, Butterworth J et al: Is calcium or ephedrine superior to placebo for emergence from cardiopulmonary bypass? *J Cardiothorac Vasc Anesth* 6:528-534, 1992.

61. Zaloga G, Strickland R, Butterworth J et al: Calcium attenuates epinephrine's β-adrenergic effects in postoperative heart surgery patients, *Circulation* 81:196-200, 1990.

62. Butterworth J, Zaloga G, Prielipp R et al: Calcium inhibits the cardiac stimulating properties of dobutamine but not amrinone, *Chest* 101:174-180, 1992.

63. Buxton A, Goldberg S, Marken A et al: Coronary vasospasm immediately after myocardial revascularization, *N Engl J Med* 304: 1249-1253, 1981.

64. Boulanger M, Maille J, Pelletier G et al: Vasospastic angina after calcium injection, *Anesth Analg* 63:1124-1126, 1984.

65. Reber H: Acute pancreatitis: another piece of the puzzle? *N Engl J Med* 325:423-424, 1991.

66. Castillo C, Harringer W, Warshaw W et al: Risk factors for pancreatic cellular injury after cardiopulmonary bypass, *N Engl J Med* 325:382-387, 1991.

67. Love J, Sachdeva D, Bessman E et al: A potential role for glucagon in the treatment of drug-induced symptomatic bradycardia, *Chest* 114:323-326, 1998.

68. Mahr N, Valdes A, Lamas G: Use of glucagon for acute intravenous diltiazem toxicity, *Am J Cardiol* 79:1570-1571, 1997.

69. Burman K: Is triiodothyronine administration beneficial in patients undergoing coronary artery bypass surgery? *JAMA* 275: 723-724, 1996.

70. Novitzky D, Cooper D, Barton C et al: Triiodothyronine as an inotropic agent after open heart surgery, *J Thorac Cardiovasc Surg* 98:972-978, 1989.

71. Morkin E, Pennock G, Raya T et al: Development of a thyroid hormone analog for the treatment of congestive heart failure, *Thyroid* 6:521-526, 1996.

72. Klein I, Ojamaa K: Thyroid hormone treatment of congestive heart failure, *Am J Cardiol* 81:490-491, 1998.

73. Novitzky D: Novel actions of thyroid hormone: the role of triiodothyronine in cardiac transplantation, *Thyroid* 6:531-536, 1996.

74. Jeevanandam H: Triiodothyronine: spectrum of use in heart transplantation, *Thyroid* 7:139-145, 1997.

75. Klemperer J, Klein I, Ojamaa K et al: Triiodothyronine therapy lowers the incidence of atrial fibrillation after cardiac operations, *Ann Thorac Surg* 61:1323-2329, 1996.

76. Bennett-Guerrero E, Jimenez J, White W et al: Cardiovascular effects of intravenous triiodothyronine in patients undergoing coronary artery bypass graft surgery, *JAMA* 275:687-692, 1996.

77. Boylston B: Triiodothyronine and cardiac surgery (letter), *JAMA* 276:100, 1996.

78. Broderick T, Wechsler A: Triiodothyronine in cardiac surgery, *Thyroid* 7:133-137, 1997.

79. Palmer R, Ferrige A, Moncada S: Nitric oxide release accounts for the biological activity of endothelium-derived relaxing factor, *Nature* 327:524-526, 1987.

80. Young J: Nitric oxide and related vasodilators, *Can J Anaesth* 44:R23-R28, 1997.

81. Wallace A, Ratcliffe M, Galindez D et al: L-Arginine infusion dilates coronary vasculature in patients undergoing coronary bypass surgery, *Anesthesiology* 90:1577-1586, 1999.

82. Stoelting R: *Pharmacology and physiology in anesthetic practice*, ed 3, Philadelphia, 1999, Lippincott-Raven, p 317.

83. McHugh J, Cheek D: Nitric oxide and regulation of vascular tone: pharmacologic and physiologic considerations, *Am J Crit Care* 7:131-140, 1998.

84. Rich G, Murphy G, Roos C et al: Inhaled nitric oxide: selective pulmonary vasodilation in cardiac surgical patients, *Anesthesiology* 78:1028-1035, 1993.

85. Cockrill B: The use of nitric oxide in primary pulmonary hypertension, *Respir Care Clin N Amer* 3:505-519, 1997.

86. Bacha E, Head C: Use of inhaled nitric oxide for lung transplantation and cardiac surgery, *Respir Care Clin N Amer* 3:521-536, 1997.

87. Troncy E, Francoeur M, Blaise G: Inhaled nitric oxide: clinical applications, indications, and toxicology, *Can J Anaesth* 44: 973-988, 1997.

88. Fullerton D, McIntyre R: Inhaled nitric oxide: therapeutic applications in cardiothoracic surgery, *Ann Thorac Surg* 61:1856-1864, 1996.

89. Carmona M, Auler J: Effects of inhaled nitric oxide on respiratory system mechanics, hemodynamics, and gas exchange after cardiac surgery, *J Cardiothorac Vasc Anesth* 12:157-161, 1998.

90. Westphal K, Martens S, Strouhal U et al: Nitric oxide inhalation in acute pulmonary hypertension after cardiac surgery reduces oxygen concentration and improves mechanical ventilation but not mortality, *Thorac Cardiovasc Surg* 46:70-73, 1998.

91. Bender K, Alexander J, Enos J et al: Effects of inhaled nitric oxide in patients with hypoxemia and pulmonary hypertension after cardiac surgery, *Am J Crit Care* 6:127-131, 1997.

92. Hess D, Bigatello L, Hurford W: Toxicity and complications of inhaled nitric oxide, *Respir Care Clin N Amer* 3:487-502, 1997.

93. Katayama Y, Higgenbottam T, Cremona G et al: Minimizing the inhaled dose of NO with breath-by-breath delivery of spikes of concentrated gas, *Circulation* 98:2429-2432, 1998.

94. Haraldsson A, Kieler-Jensen N, Ricksten S: Inhaled prostacyclin for treatment of pulmonary hypertension after cardiac surgery or heart transplantation: a pharmacologic study, *J Cardiothorac Vasc Anesth* 10:864-868, 1996.

95. Haraldsson A, Kieler-Jensen N, Nathorst-Westfelt U et al: Comparison of inhaled nitric oxide and inhaled aerosolized prostacyclin in the evaluation of heart transplant candidates with elevated pulmonary resistance, *Chest* 114:780-786, 1998.

96. Krieg P, Wahlers T, Giess W et al: Inhaled nitric oxide and inhaled prostaglandin E_1: effect on left ventricular contractility when used for treatment of experimental pulmonary hypertension, *Eur J Cardiothorac Surg* 14:494-502, 1998.

97. Post J, Frishman W: Fenoldopam: a new dopamine agonist for the treatment of hypertensive urgencies and emergencies, *J Clin Pharmacol* 38:2-13, 1998.

CHAPTER 3

Intraoperative Monitoring

Christopher A. Troianos, M.D.

OUTLINE

Intraoperative hemodynamic monitoring is an important aspect of the anesthetic management of the cardiac patient. The degree of cardiovascular monitoring is generally predicated upon both the medical condition of the patient and the nature of surgery. Severe medical debilitation alone is insufficient reason for full cardiovascular monitoring. Patients with severe cardiac disease undergoing relatively minor or outpatient procedures often require only the standard American Society of Anesthesiologists (ASA) monitors, electrocardiography (ECG), noninvasive blood pressure monitoring, and pulse oximetry. Conversely, patients with only mild systemic disease require full invasive monitoring when undergoing relatively complicated surgical procedures, including cardiac surgery, aortic cross-clamping, induced hypotension, trauma, or transplant surgery.

The advent of more sophisticated and automated monitoring devices has created less reliance on the more basic and reliable monitors of palpation, auscultation, and visual inspection. Yet the "finger on the pulse" remains a valuable tool for assessing blood pressure and pulse, particularly in the absence of more invasive monitoring. The palpated pulse provides continuous indication of blood pressure during the induction of anesthesia similar to invasive arterial monitoring. The palpated pulse yields blood pressure information faster than an automated blood pressure device. Capillary refill is a reflection of cardiac output by assessment of peripheral perfusion. Adequate cardiac output provides good peripheral perfusion, whereas decreased cardiac output compromises peripheral perfusion. Visual inspection of the patient, particularly the mucous membranes, nail beds, and jugular veins, provides valuable information regarding oxygenation, dehydration, hemoglobin level, and volume overload. Auscultation of the heart may reveal murmurs associated with stenotic or regurgitant valvular lesions, volume overload with the presence of an S_3 gallop, or a pericardial friction rub. All of these diagnoses have important implications in terms of anesthetic management. Intraoperative monitoring of the patient under general anesthesia with an esophageal stethoscope generally reveals louder heart tones with rising blood pressure in a hyperdynamic state. Blood pressure is also dependent on systemic vascular resistance. Both noninvasive and invasive techniques are employed to measure blood pressure.

Cardiac output is determined by ventricular contractility, preload, afterload, and heart rate. Each of these parameters can be measured or estimated in the cardiac patient by using echocardiography, electrocardiography, and arterial, central venous, pulmonary artery occlusion, and left atrial pressure monitoring. Mixed venous oxygen saturation is a reflection of cardiac output, oxygen delivery, and oxygen extraction by the tissues. A lower cardiac output results in lower mixed venous oxygen saturation because tissue extraction is greater. This chapter reviews these aspects of hemodynamic monitoring in the patient with cardiac disease undergoing cardiac and noncardiac surgery.

NONINVASIVE BLOOD PRESSURE MONITORING

All patients undergoing anesthesia and surgery, regardless of their cardiac disease status, require noninvasive blood pressure (NIBP) measurement. NIBP is a broad indicator of cardiovascular function that encompasses cardiac output and systemic vascular resistance. NIBP cannot be used when patient anatomy precludes occlusion of blood flow in an extremity (e.g., presence of arteriovenous fistula, surgically excised lymphatic system, or morbid obesity). NIBP is often not used when invasive blood pressure monitoring is available, and cannot be used in the absence of pulsatile flow during cardiopulmonary bypass. Air is pumped into an inflatable bladder within a cuff that encircles an extremity until blood flow ceases in the major artery passing through the extremity. Correct blood pressure cuff sizing is important for accurate determination of blood pressure. The American Heart Association recommends that the cuff width equal 40% of the arm circumference at the midpoint of the limb and the bladder length be twice the recommended width or 80% of the circumference.[1] Korotkoff described the sounds heard with a stethoscope over an artery distal to the occlusion as the cuff was slowly released.[2] The pressure at which the sounds are first heard is the systolic pressure (SBP), whereas the pressure at which the sounds disappear is the diastolic pressure (DBP).[1] In the past, the pressure at which the sounds become muffled was considered the diastolic pressure.[3] Despite the controversy over when the diastolic sound is heard, most authorities currently agree that the cuff pressure when the sounds become inaudible is the best index of DBP in adults. The pressure at the onset of muffling is considered the diastolic pressure only if the sounds do not completely disappear as the cuff is deflated to zero pressure. For children, the onset of muffling is still considered the best index of DBP.[1] In addition to auscultation, various other methods can be used to detect flow in the artery distal to the occlusive cuff. These include palpation, oscillometry (including automated oscillometry), ultrasound, and plethysmography.

Variation exists as to when the systolic and diastolic blood pressures occur using automated NIBP devices. This determination is dependent on the technique and the proprietary algorithm of each automated system. The systolic pressure using the palpation method is the pressure at which the first pulse is palpable. The oscillometric technique uses pressure fluctuation within the inflated bladder to detect flow through the extremity as the cuff is slowly deflated. Three separate variables are used to determine systolic, diastolic, and mean arterial pressures.[4] Systolic pressure is the pressure at which there is a rapid increase in the oscillation amplitude, mean arterial pressure is the lowest pressure at which maximum oscillations occur, and diastolic pressure is the pressure at which there is a rapid decrease in oscillation amplitude[4] (Fig. 3-1). Doppler techniques use an ultrasound beam to measure velocity in the artery, as described in Chapter 4, as the cuff is deflated. Blood pressure determinations using Doppler techniques are higher than those measured by palpation, but lower than those measured by invasive techniques.[5]

Auscultation and ultrasound methods must calculate mean arterial pressure (MAP) from the equation $MAP = [SBP + (2 \times DBP)]/3$. For this reason, oscillometry is the noninvasive technique of choice for comparing MAP to invasive measurement of MAP[6-9] (see Fig. 3-1). Noninvasive measurements often do not equal invasive measurements of blood pressure (Table 3-1). Noninvasive measurement of SBP equals or slightly underestimates SBP in normotensive patients when compared with invasive measurement. Noninvasive measurement underestimates systolic pressure in hypertensive patients and overestimates systolic pressure in hypotensive patients when compared with invasive measurement.[6-8] Noninvasive determination of MAP generally equals or slightly overestimates invasive determination of MAP.[10]

Plethysmography is another noninvasive technique for determining blood pressure. The Finapres system consists of a circumferential cuff applied to a finger that contains an infrared light source opposite a light detector (photoplethysmography).[11] Pressure in the cuff varies, but is maintained throughout the cardiac cycle by a computer chip that provides sufficient pressure to maintain the artery in a constant state of minimal compression. The cuff pressure thus reflects the pressure within the artery. The system provides an arterial waveform in addition to the display of the various pressures.

Pulse pressure is the difference between the systolic and diastolic pressure. Pulse pressure is increased in

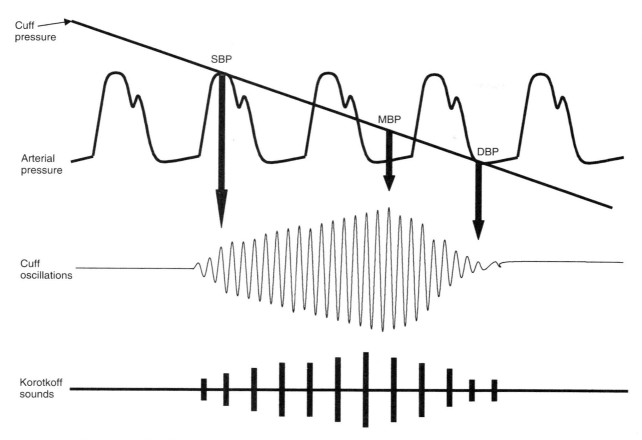

FIG. 3-1   The relation between arterial pressure, cuff pressure, cuff oscillations, and Korotkoff sounds. *DBP*, Diastolic blood pressure; *MBP*, mean blood pressure; *SBP*, systolic blood pressure.

TABLE 3-1
Relation between NIBP and Invasive Systolic Blood Pressure

HEMODYNAMIC STATE	NIBP VS. INVASIVE
Normotensive	NIBP ≤ Invasive
Hypertensive	NIBP << Invasive
Hypotensive	NIBP >> Invasive

NIBP, Noninvasive blood pressure.

patients with aortic insufficiency and decreased in patients with low systemic vascular resistance. DBP monitoring is important because it determines coronary perfusion (coronary perfusion pressure = aortic diastolic blood pressure minus left ventricular diastolic pressure). Noninvasive measurement of DBP slightly overestimates measurement by invasive techniques.[10]

INVASIVE BLOOD PRESSURE MONITORING
Indications

Direct intraarterial blood pressure monitoring is indicated for reasons related to the medical condition of the patient, the nature of surgery, or both (Box 3-1). Invasive monitoring is also indicated when NIBP measurement is impossible, difficult, or unreliable. Extensive adipose tissue surrounding the artery of morbidly obese patients makes blood pressure measurement with a cuff difficult or unreliable. Patients with limb amputation and unavailability of multiple limbs because of the site of surgery, trauma, burns, or excised lymph nodes are additional examples of inability to measure blood pressure with noninvasive techniques.

Patients undergoing surgery with unstable angina, recent myocardial infarction, active congestive heart failure, severe valvular heart disease, and shock require invasive blood pressure monitoring, except for minor surgical procedures. This type of patient often requires urgent or emergent surgery that precludes optimization of the medical condition. Patients who require frequent blood sampling, particularly arterial blood gases intraoperatively or postoperatively, should have an intraarterial catheter placed for surgery. These patients may include diabetic patients receiving intravenous insulin; patients with chronic obstructive pulmonary disease, particularly patients who retain carbon dioxide; and patients with acid-base disorders or electrolyte abnormalities.

Surgical procedures that involve aortic cross-clamping, cardiac surgery, large fluid shifts, massive blood loss, or induced hypotension require intraarterial monitoring of blood pressure during the surgical procedure. It is paramount to manage arterial blood pressure accurately and aggressively in patients undergoing cross-clamping of their aorta. The acute increased afterload imposed by the cross-clamp can lead to myocardial ischemia or heart failure. Aggressive management to lower the blood pressure to appropriate levels, but not lower the pressure too far, requires continuous and direct blood pressure measurement. Continuous monitoring is also important when the cross-clamp is removed to allow rapid treatment of hypotension and thus avoid myocardial ischemia, particularly in the patient with coronary artery disease or aortic insufficiency. Procedures that require induced hypotension require invasive monitoring to avoid overzealous lowering of the pressure, which is deleterious to the patient with coronary artery disease. Invasive monitoring is required during cardiac surgery for the patient indications related to cardiac disease (see Box 3-1), but also because of cardiopulmonary bypass. Blood pressure is nonpulsatile during cardiopulmonary bypass and is therefore not obtainable by noninvasive techniques that require pulsatile flow.

Cannulation Site

Invasive access for intraarterial cannulation varies according to the surgical procedure and preference of the clinician. The radial artery is most often used during anesthesia because of its accessibility and ease of localization during many surgical procedures, collateral flow to the hand by the ulnar artery, and because anesthesia personnel are most familiar with this cannulation site. The axillary and femoral arteries are considered "end-arteries" because another artery does not provide collateral flow to the same tissue distribution. These arteries are of sufficient diameter in adults that thrombosis is relatively rare. The brachial artery is also an end-artery, but its smaller diameter increases the concern for vascular insufficiency. Brachial artery systolic and mean pressures are higher than radial artery measurements 2 minutes after cardiopulmonary bypass, but the pressure difference normalizes after 60 minutes.[12] Although mean and diastolic blood pressures may be about the same throughout the arterial vasculature,[13] systolic pressure is higher in the periphery of young patients as compared with ascending aortic pressure because of arterial resonance.[14] The systolic pressure in the ascending aorta of elderly patients and patients with chronic hypertension is more similar to the pressure in peripheral arteries, because the energy from the efferent pulse is reflected back to the ascending aorta during systole.[15] The difference between radial and aortic systolic pressures in elderly, hypertensive patients is increased by nitroglycerin because of decreased stroke volume index, not by a decrease in wave reflection.[16] A large discrepancy between femoral and radial arterial pressures may also be observed in patients with massive ascites, presumably from a compartment-like syndrome impeding arterial blood flow to the lower extremities.[17]

Either the radial or ulnar arteries can be cannulated because of their similar diameters and collateral flow, although the ulnar artery provides more blood flow to the hand in most patients.[18] Cannulation attempts should not be made for both arteries in the same hand because the collateral flow may be compromised after a failed cannulation attempt in the other artery. The Allen's test was routinely recommended in the past to determine collateral flow to the hand.[19,20] The test is performed by asking the patient to make a tight fist to exsanguinate the hand as the radial and ulnar arteries are occluded by digital pressure. The patient is then asked to relax the hand. The pressure is released either on the ulnar artery to evaluate flow through the ulnar artery, or the radial artery to evaluate flow through the radial artery. The hand is observed for reperfusion within 5 to 10 seconds. Lack of reperfusion after 15 to 20 seconds suggests a lack of collateral flow. The problem with using this test to determine the safety of radial artery cannulation is that the results of the Allen's test do not correlate with complications.[21,22] No complications occurred in a small series of patients with a poor Allen's test.[21] Conversely, severe vascular insufficiency may occur despite a normal Allen's test.[22] Radial artery cannulation is contraindicated in patients with Raynaud's disease because of the potential for digital amputation secondary to ischemia.[23] Thrombocytosis may also predispose patients to radial artery thrombosis.[24] The radial artery of the nondominant hand is not used for catheter placement when a radial artery harvest is planned for coronary artery bypass grafting.

Other arteries may or may not be used depending on the surgical procedure. For example, the femoral artery is not used during abdominal aortic surgery or vascular procedures on the ipsilateral lower extremity because vascular clamping interferes with pressure monitoring. The brachial or axillary artery is used when the radial and femoral arteries cannot be cannulated. The left axillary artery is preferable over the right axillary artery because flushing the line may unintentionally embolize particles into the vascular circulation. Embolization to the cerebral vasculature is more common with a right axillary artery catheter than with a left axillary line. Vigorous flushing of even a radial artery catheter can cause reversal of flow retrograde to the aortic arch with the potential for carotid artery embolization.[25] Many clinicians prefer to use the left radial artery to avoid embolization to the cerebral vessels and because the left hand is most commonly the nondominant hand. A "pulsatile" or low-pressure, gentle flushing technique should be used to clear radial, brachial, and axillary artery lines. Cannulation of the dorsalis pedis artery is most often considered for craniotomy procedures. Umbilical artery cannulation is limited to the newborn.

Catheter Placement

Various techniques have been described to insert intraarterial catheters. Aseptic technique and local anesthesia are used for all techniques performed in awake patients. Advancing a "catheter-over-needle" assembly through the skin toward the palpable pulse is termed *direct cannulation.* This is the most common technique used to cannulate the radial and brachial arteries. The unit is advanced until bright red pulsatile blood is observed in the needle. The 45-degree insertion angle is decreased and the unit is slightly advanced within the artery as blood flow through the needle is maintained. The catheter is advanced into the artery with a rolling motion while the needle is held in a fixed position. The catheter should advance to the hub without resistance. The needle is removed and placement is confirmed by observing pulsatile blood flowing out of the needle hub. The catheter is connected to pressure tubing and aspirated for air.

The Seldinger technique is commonly used to cannulate the axillary and femoral arteries. A hollow needle is directed toward a palpable pulse until bright red pulsatile flow is encountered. A wire is inserted into the hollow needle without resistance, and the needle is removed. A catheter is then passed over the wire into the artery and the wire is removed. Correct placement is confirmed by observing pulsatile blood flowing out of the needle hub and an arterial waveform on the monitor when the catheter is connected to a pressure transducer. The system is aspirated for air and flushed with saline. The success rate of arterial cannulation is increased with the Seldinger technique over the direct technique.[26] Commercially available systems include a wire within the assembly that is advanced through the hollow needle as a single unit, before the catheter is advanced (Fig. 3-2).

Doppler and two-dimensional ultrasound can also be used to help locate arterial and venous vessels. Doppler ultrasound produces an audible signal characteristic of arterial or venous flow. The artery is localized when the maximal audible arterial signal is obtained by scanning the skin surface with the Doppler probe. The catheter is inserted through the skin, distal to the Doppler probe, and advanced in the direction of the probe at a 30- to 40-degree angle with the skin. Two-dimensional ultrasound is commonly used to locate the internal and subclavian veins, as will be discussed in a later section of this chapter. Commercial systems exist that provide needle guides that direct the angulation of the needle according to the depth of the vessel under the skin (SiteRite, Dymax Corp, Pittsburgh, Pa.). Two-dimensional ultrasound is used to locate the vessel and depth markers on the screen indicate the depth of the vessel. A higher-frequency 9-MHz probe used to cannulate pediatric jugular veins is used to locate the radial, brachial, axillary, or femoral arteries. The appropriate needle guide is used to direct the catheter toward the vessel. The Doppler and two-dimensional ultrasound techniques are useful in patients with low cardiac output or peripheral vasoconstriction and obese patients in whom palpation is not helpful in locating the artery.

Surgical incision and exposure is a last resort when direct arterial cannulation is required and all other techniques have failed. The tissue over the vessel is dissected until the artery is exposed. A direct cannulation technique is employed to insert the catheter into the artery.

Complications

Complications related to invasive direct arterial cannulation include thrombosis or ischemia distal to the cannulation site, hematoma, nerve injury, infection, bleeding, and inaccurate pressure monitoring. Opening a stopcock to air near the transducer allows the transducer system to be electronically zeroed. The transducer must be placed at the same level above the ground as the pressure to be measured. For example, the transducer is

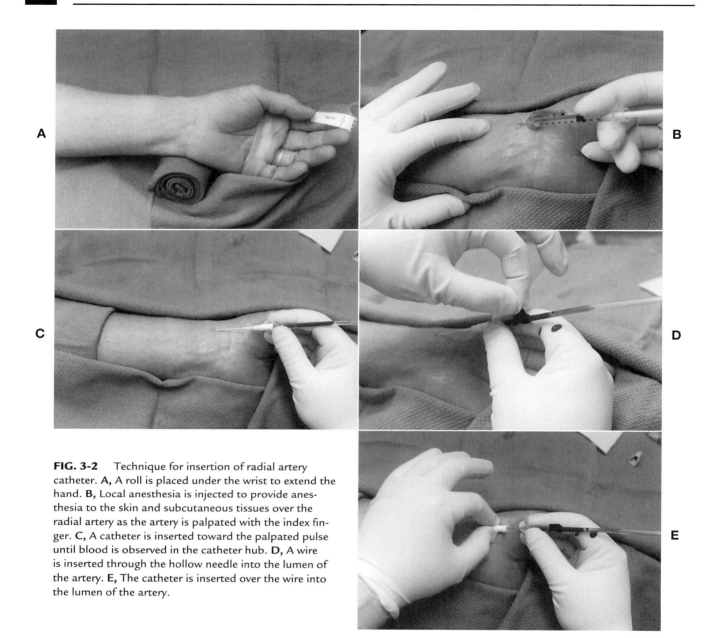

FIG. 3-2   Technique for insertion of radial artery catheter. **A,** A roll is placed under the wrist to extend the hand. **B,** Local anesthesia is injected to provide anesthesia to the skin and subcutaneous tissues over the radial artery as the artery is palpated with the index finger. **C,** A catheter is inserted toward the palpated pulse until blood is observed in the catheter hub. **D,** A wire is inserted through the hollow needle into the lumen of the artery. **E,** The catheter is inserted over the wire into the lumen of the artery.

placed at the level of the head for a patient undergoing a sitting craniotomy if the clinician desires accurate measurement of intracerebral pressures, but placed at the level of the heart or pulmonary artery if intracardiac pressures are most important. Radial artery dampening may occur with severe chest wall retraction during internal mammary artery harvesting if the ipsilateral radial artery is cannulated. This phenomenon is recognized by the temporal relation of decreased blood pressure measurement and chest wall retraction. Thrombosis and vascular insufficiency are of greatest concern when an end-artery is used for cannulation. The median nerve may be injured because it is near the brachial artery. The patient, who is awake, will usually complain of a pares-

thesia during attempted cannulation in the distribution of the median nerve.

CENTRAL VENOUS CATHETERIZATION
Central Venous Pressure Monitoring

Central venous pressure (CVP) catheters are inserted to measure right-sided filling pressures as an estimate of intravascular volume and to provide direct access to the central circulation for administration of vasoactive medications. CVP catheters are particularly useful in patients with cardiac disease when an immediate drug effect is desirable. The catheter tip located in the distal superior vena cava or proximal right atrium reflects in-

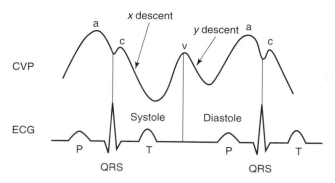

FIG. 3-3 A normal central venous pressure (*CVP*) waveform consists of three systolic components (c wave, x descent, and v wave) and two diastolic components (y descent, a wave). *ECG*, Electrocardiogram.

(Modified from Mark JB: *J Cardiothorac Vasc Anesth* 5:163-173, 1991.)

trathoracic pressure, right atrial pressure, right ventricular end-diastolic pressure, pericardial pressure, and left heart pressures. A pressure change in any one of these chambers is reflected by a pressure change in the CVP. Therefore an increase in CVP does not necessarily indicate an increase in intravascular volume because other factors also influence the CVP. Conversely, an increase in intravascular volume is not always indicated by an increase in CVP because of the compliance of the right atrium and right ventricle.

The information derived from CVP catheters exceeds that of merely monitoring an absolute number, but is enhanced by observing the waveform, which provides valuable information regarding right heart function. There are five components to a normal CVP tracing during each cardiac cycle: three waves or peaks and two descents or downward deflections[27] (Fig. 3-3). Each wave reflects a cardiac event that causes that particular peak or descent. The *a wave* is caused by right atrial contraction and is observed after the *P* wave on the ECG. The right atrium relaxes after the a-wave peak, causing the right atrial pressure to decrease. The *c wave* occurs during isovolumic contraction of the right ventricle and is observed after the R wave on the ECG. The onset of ventricular systole causes the tricuspid valve to close and billow toward the right atrium, causing a slight increase in right atrial pressure. Right ventricular contraction causes radial shortening of the ventricular chamber and displacement of the tricuspid valve away from the right atrium, leading to a decrease in right atrial pressure (*x descent*). Venous inflow into the right atrium produces the *v wave* during late systole, while the tricuspid valve remains closed, and is observed after the T wave on the ECG. The *y descent* occurs when the tricuspid valve opens and blood flows passively from the right atrium to the right ventricle.

Changes in the components of the CVP waveform provide valuable insight and information regarding right heart function.[27] For example, a large v wave indicates severe tricuspid regurgitation that may be caused by right heart failure, pulmonary hypertension, or right ventricular ischemia. The absence of an a wave indicates lack of atrial contraction because of a nodal rhythm, atrial fibrillation, or atrial flutter, whereas a large a wave occurs with atrial-ventricular (A-V) dissociation and tricuspid stenosis, when the atrium contracts against a closed or stenotic tricuspid valve, respectively. A large a wave may also occur in patients with decreased right ventricular compliance from pulmonary hypertension or pericardial constriction or restriction.

Central Venous Cannulation

Multiple insertion sites are possible for central venous access. The chosen site depends on the surgical procedure and preference of the clinician. The right internal jugular (RIJ) vein is commonly used during anesthesia because of its accessibility during many surgical procedures, direct route into the right atrium, and predictable location. The left internal jugular vein is a commonly used alternative when the surgical site precludes cannulation of the RIJ vein or when cannulation of the RIJ is unsuccessful. External jugular veins are also an option and may be preferable because of a lower complication rate for cannulation[28] and because they are often visible without special equipment. Subclavian veins are often preferred for cannulation by surgeons, but this carries the risk of pneumothorax. The left subclavian vein is preferred over the right when placement of a pulmonary artery catheter is planned because the curved catheter follows a similarly curved path into the right heart from the left subclavian vein. The subclavian vein is also chosen according to the site of a previously existing chest tube. The ipsilateral side is chosen because treatment for the pneumothorax complication is already in place. The disadvantage of the subclavian route for placement of a pulmonary artery catheter during cardiac surgery is kinking of the catheter during sternal retraction. Cardiac output determination may not be possible because the cold injectate cannot be forced through the kinked catheter. Femoral or antecubital sites are chosen for surgical procedures on the head and neck. These vessels will also accommodate large-bore catheters. Long CVP catheters are used to access thoracic vessels from these insertion sites. The median antecubital vein is selected over the lateral antecubital vein, because the median antecubital vein leads to the deep axillary vein, whereas the lateral antecubital vein leads to the cephalic vein. The acute angle formed by the insertion of the cephalic vein into the subclavian vein makes it difficult to pass long CVP catheters beyond this point[29] (Fig. 3-4).

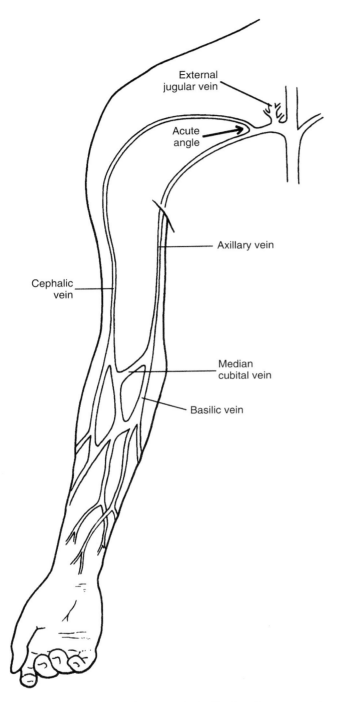

FIG. 3-4 Anatomy of the arm veins indicating the acute angle formed by the insertion of the cephalic vein into the subclavian vein.

(Modified from Rosen M, Latto P, Ng S: *Handbook of percutaneous central venous catheterisation*, London, 1992, WB Saunders.)

Internal Jugular Vein

The RIJ vein is commonly used during anesthesia because of its accessibility during many surgical procedures, direct route into the right atrium, and predictable location. The left internal jugular vein is a

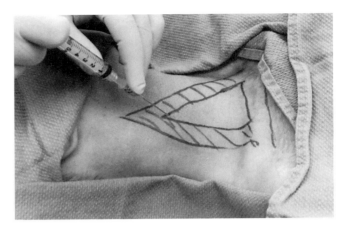

FIG. 3-5 Cannulation of the internal jugular vein is performed by inserting a needle at the apex of a triangle formed by the two divisions of the sternocleidomastoid muscle and the clavicle. The needle is inserted at a 45-degree angle toward the ipsilateral nipple with the head turned to the contralateral side.

commonly used alternative when the surgical site precludes cannulation of the RIJ vein or when cannulation of the RIJ is unsuccessful. The standard approach to the RIJ vein uses visual and palpable landmarks to guide needle placement and is associated with a 95% success rate.[28] Unintentional puncture of surrounding structures accounts for the most serious complications of this technique.[28,30,31]

English and colleagues first described cannulation of the internal jugular vein in 1969. They described both an elective method and an alternative method.[32] The elective method was used during general anesthesia with muscle relaxation and involved palpation of the carotid artery and internal jugular vein via a *high central approach*. The alternative method was a *low central approach* performed with local anesthesia in awake patients, when the elective method was unsuccessful, or when the vein could not be palpated. A needle is inserted just inferior to the apex of the angle formed by the division of the sternocleidomastoid muscle with the patient in a 25° Trendelenburg position. A needle is inserted through a local anesthetic wheal at a 30° to 40° angle directed toward the inner border of the anterior end of the first rib behind the clavicle. A *high, central, or anterior approach* described by Prince and colleagues[33] is the technique most commonly used by many clinicians. An 18-gauge needle is inserted at the apex of the angle formed by the division of the sternocleidomastoid muscle and directed toward the ipsilateral nipple at a 45° angle with the skin (Fig. 3-5). Blood is aspirated from the catheter and the pressure within the lumen is transduced with a fluid column to confirm venous placement. The Seldinger technique with a J-wire is used to insert a larger-bore catheter after the smaller catheter is removed (Fig. 3-6).

Other anatomic landmark–guided approaches to access the internal jugular vein have been described and

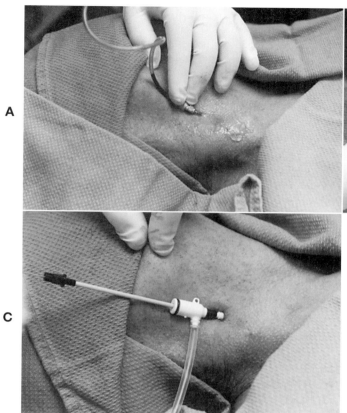

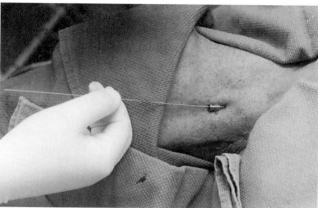

FIG. 3-6   Cannulation of an internal jugular vein with a large-bore catheter using the Seldinger technique. **A,** Tubing is attached to the hub of the catheter and the pressure within the vessel lumen is estimated using a column of blood to confirm venous placement. **B,** A wire is inserted through the catheter, after which the catheter is removed. **C,** A large-bore catheter with an introducer are inserted into the vein over the wire and the introducer is removed with the wire.

are nicely summarized in Rosen, Latto, and Ng's *Handbook of Percutaneous Central Venous Cannulation* (see key references). This paragraph discusses the high, medial, low, central, and lateral approaches to the internal jugular vein described in their book and depicted in Fig. 3-7.[29] A superiority of one landmark-guided technique over the others has not been demonstrated.[34] Boulanger and colleagues described a *high, medial approach* with the advantage of minimizing the risk of pneumothorax and carotid puncture by the higher entry site and lateral insertion angle, respectively.[35] The needle is inserted at the superior border of the thyroid cartilage, along the medial border of the sternocleidomastoid muscle and directed laterally at a 45° angle to the muscle and 10° above the skin. Brinkman and Costley described a *high, lateral approach* with the advantage of minimizing the risk of pneumothorax by a higher entry site cephalad to the junction of the external jugular vein and the sternocleidomastoid muscle.[36] The needle is inserted along the lateral border of the sternocleidomastoid muscle and directed toward the sternal notch and 10° above the skin. Mostert and others described a *high, medial approach* with the advantage of not requiring identification of the sternocleidomastoid muscle.[37] The needle is inserted along the medial border of the sternocleidomastoid muscle at its midpoint, above the level of the cricoid cartilage, and just lateral to the palpable carotid artery pulse. The needle is directed toward the middle portion of the ipsilateral clavicle and 45° above the skin. Civetta and Gabel described a *high, central approach* with the advantage of minimizing excessive trauma with use of a smaller-gauge spinal needle and minimizing the risk of pneumothorax by a higher entry site.[38] The needle is inserted 5 cm above the clavicle and 1 cm medial to the lateral border of the sternocleidomastoid muscle. The needle is directed medially, parallel to the medial border of the sternocleidomastoid muscle 30° above the skin. Jernigan and colleagues described a *low, lateral approach* to the internal jugular vein by inserting a needle two fingerbreadths above the clavicle on the lateral border of the clavicular head of the sternocleidomastoid muscle.[39] The needle is directed toward the suprasternal notch and 45° above the skin. A lower approach to the internal jugular vein has the disadvantages of an acute angle of entry into the vein and a greater risk of pneumothorax and carotid puncture. Although cannulation of the internal jugular vein at any level of the neck may cause persistent incompetence of the internal jugular vein valve, the incidence of valve incompetence appears to be higher with a lower approach (75% vs. 41%).[40]

Hayashi and others observed the respiratory jugular venodilation in mechanically ventilated patients and used the most prominent location of venodilation during respiration as their sole landmark for locating the internal jugular vein.[41] Respiratory jugular venodilation was observed in 79% of patients and resulted in cannulation with the first attempt in 83.5% of patients and one carotid puncture (0.6%). For patients in whom respiratory jugular venodilation was not visible, the carotid pulse at the cricoid level was used as the landmark and resulted in a first attempt success of 42.9% with a 9.5% incidence of carotid puncture. Visibility correlates with the extent of the vein's dynamic change during a respiratory cycle, but not with vein size.[42] This study emphasizes the importance of visualizing the structure, but unfortunately is applicable only to mechanically ventilated patients.

Ultrasound allows imaging of the internal jugular vein and carotid artery. Ultrasound-guided placement of central venous catheters improves success rates and decreases the complications associated with internal jugular and subclavian cannulation.[43-53] Commercial equipment specifically designed for this purpose is available and requires a sterile sheath to maintain sterility during real-time use (Fig. 3-8). Clinicians lacking dedicated

equipment for ultrasound-guided cannulation can use echocardiographic equipment used for intraoperative transesophageal echocardiography (TEE).[54] Pediatric transthoracic probes usually work best for this purpose because of the smaller probe size and higher frequency. TEE probes may also be used if transthoracic probes are not available. The use of ultrasound for vessel location alone has no effect on the complication or success rate of subclavian vein cannulation,[55] but must be used in real time during catheter placement to be effective.[56-58] Ultrasonography identifies anatomy conducive for carotid artery puncture, in which the internal jugular vein overlies the carotid artery.[59] The ultrasound probe is adjusted to locate an insertion site with a more favorable anatomic relation between the carotid artery and internal jugular vein (vein lateral to the artery instead of overlying the artery), thereby decreasing the likelihood of carotid puncture by a needle that punctures the posterior wall of the vein. Two-dimensional imaging allows

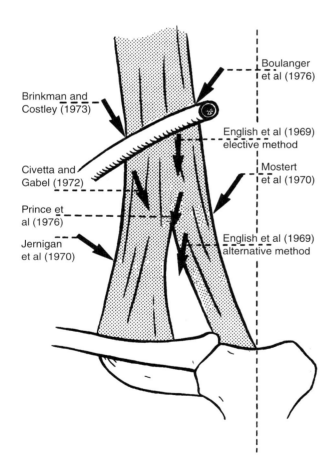

FIG. 3-7 Various approaches to cannulation of the internal jugular vein. See text for details.

(Modified from Rosen M, Latto P, Ng S: *Handbook of percutaneous central venous catheterisation*, London, 1992, WB Saunders.)

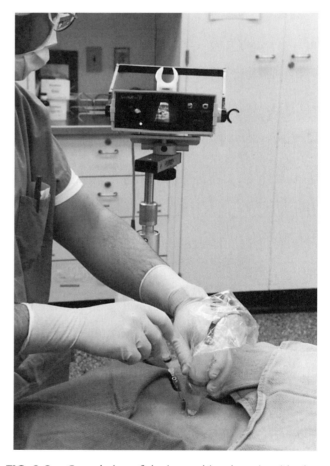

FIG. 3-8 Cannulation of the internal jugular vein with ultrasound guidance. A probe with a needle guide is applied to the skin, and the internal jugular vein and carotid artery are identified by the two-dimensional ultrasound image displayed on the monitor. The ultrasound image is observed in real time as the needle is advanced into the vein.

identification of the carotid artery and internal jugular vein by their relative position, compressibility of the vein, expansion of the vein during Valsalva maneuver, and pulsation of the artery (Fig. 3-9). Ultrasound guidance improves success on the first needle pass[43,50,51,53] and decreases the time to successful cannulation.[43,51,57] The results of a large randomized study comparing ultrasound-guided to landmark-guided RIJ vein cannulation are listed in Table 3-2.

Attempted cannulation of the internal jugular vein carries the risk of venous air embolism and the unintentional puncture of surrounding structures, including the carotid artery, cervical plexus, lung, and thoracic duct (left side only). The incidence of pneumothorax is low with needle insertion sites higher in the neck, but increases with lower insertion sites.[29] Patients usually complain of ipsilateral arm pain when a needle is directed too laterally at the cervical plexus. The most serious and potentially life-threatening complication of internal jugular vein cannulation is arterial puncture. Puncture of the aorta is rare, but may occur with a low (supraclavicular posterior) approach and lead to cardiac tamponade.[60] Arterial puncture of the carotid artery is more common, with an incidence of 2% to 16%.[28,61]

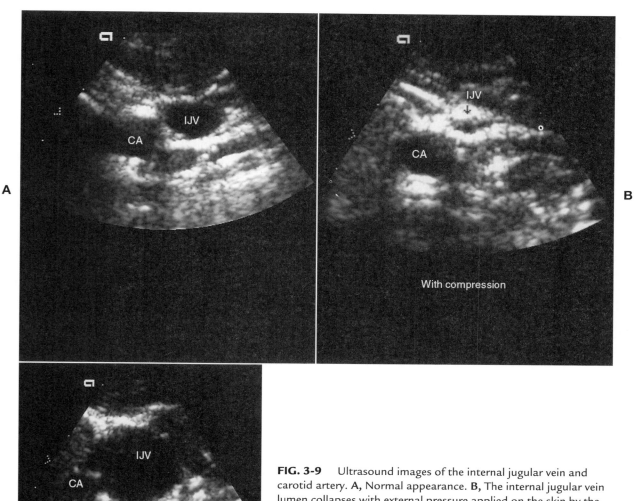

FIG. 3-9   Ultrasound images of the internal jugular vein and carotid artery. **A,** Normal appearance. **B,** The internal jugular vein lumen collapses with external pressure applied on the skin by the ultrasound probe. **C,** The internal jugular vein lumen enlarges with the Valsalva maneuver. *CA,* Carotid artery; *IJV,* internal jugular vein.

TABLE 3-2
Ultrasound-Guided versus Landmark-Guided Cannulation of the Right Internal Jugular Vein

	LANDMARK-GUIDED ($n = 83$)	ULTRASOUND-GUIDED ($n = 77$)
Successful cannulations	80 (96%)	77 (100%)
Success on first attempt ($p < 0.05$)	45 (54%)	56 (73%)
Attempts per cannulation		
Mean ± SD ($p < 0.05$)	2.8 ± 3.0	1.4 ± 0.7
Range	1-15	1-4
Time per cannulation (seconds)		
Mean ± SD ($p < 0.05$)	117 ± 136	61 ± 46
Range	8-400	15-180
Arterial punctures	7 (8%)	1 (1%)

From Troianos CA, Jobes DR, Ellison N: *Anesth Analg* 72:823-826, 1991.
SD, Standard deviation.

Carotid artery puncture is potentially lethal when a large-bore catheter is inserted into the carotid artery.[62] Strategies for reducing the incidence and severity of this complication include the use of ultrasound to guide needle placement, use of a small 25-gauge "finder needle,"[63] transducing the cannulating needle, and using the external jugular vein when possible.[28] Arterial puncture is of greater concern in anticoagulated patients and those with carotid artery disease, and when a large-bore catheter is inserted into the artery. Carotid artery puncture can occur primarily (directly into the carotid artery) or secondarily (after the needle traverses the internal jugular vein [IJV]).[43]

The best management approach to carotid artery puncture is avoidance. Ultrasound-guided techniques decrease the incidence of carotid artery puncture, but the incidence is not zero.[43,50,57] It is therefore important to identify carotid artery puncture with the smaller cannulating needle to avoid insertion of large-bore catheters, which may produce lethal consequences.[28,30,31] The pressure within the cannulating needle should always be transduced with either a fluid column or electrical transducer to verify venous placement.[28,64,65] Observation of the color of the aspirated blood is not a reliable method to confirm venous access, particularly when blood is aspirated into a saline-filled syringe.[66] Syringes that allow insertion of a guide wire into the needle through the barrel without disconnecting the syringe from the needle may also play a role in arterial puncture. The simple act of disconnecting the syringe from the cannulating needle may in itself reveal an arterial puncture. Ultrasound can also be used to confirm correct placement after initially transducing the catheter. Imaging the wire in the vein with the absence of the wire in the artery confirms correct placement.

Carotid artery puncture may occur after the cannulating needle has traversed the internal jugular vein. The ease by which the internal jugular vein is compressed accounts for the initial undetected entry into the vein. Slow needle withdrawal after the initial advance is an important step before advancing the needle too far and into the carotid artery. The mean distance to the internal jugular vein via a high anterior approach is between 15.0 and 21.5 mm, and the initial aspiration of blood is more likely during withdrawal rather than insertion, particularly with larger (16-gauge) needles.[67] It is important not to advance the needle beyond this distance and to withdrawal the needle slowly, allowing the vein to reexpand with the needle tip in the lumen.[68] The close proximity of the two vessels allows for the development of a carotid artery–internal jugular vein fistula as a result of puncture of the posterior wall of the internal jugular vein and the anterior wall of the carotid artery.[69-71] The anatomic position of the IJV is classically described as lateral to the carotid artery.[72] This anatomic relation describes the relation of these structures in the coronal plane and not in the direction of the cannulating needle with the head turned to the contralateral side.[59] Turning the head produces overlap between the two vessels,[59,73] possibly increasing the likelihood of carotid puncture after the needle traverses the IJV (Fig. 3-10). Older patients have a higher incidence of having an internal jugular vein that overlies the carotid artery,[59] presumably because the common carotid artery becomes elongated and tortuous in older patients with arteriosclerosis.[74] Head rotation does not appear to affect the likelihood of cannulating the internal jugular vein.[34] Real-time ultrasound-guided cannulation provides imaging of the IJV and carotid artery, directs placement of the cannulating needle at a

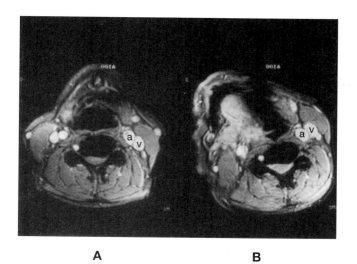

A   **B**

FIG. 3-10   Nuclear magnetic resonance image of the neck at the apex of the division of the sternocleidomastoid muscle, demonstrating the anatomic relation of the carotid artery *(a)* and internal jugular vein *(v)*. **A,** Head facing anteriorly. **B,** Head turned toward left.

(From Troianos CA, Kuwik RJ, Pasqual JR et al: *Anesthesiology* 85:43-48, 1996.)

level in the neck with minimal vessel overlap, monitors compression of the vein during needle advancement, and determines depth of insertion to minimize puncture of an underlying carotid artery. Ultrasound-guided systems that employ needle guides that direct the needle depth by controlling the insertion angle are the most useful for avoiding carotid artery puncture. The depth of the IJV is determined by two-dimensional ultrasound, and the corresponding needle guide (SiteRite, Dymax Corp, Pittsburgh, Pa.) is chosen to direct needle insertion to that particular depth (Fig. 3-11). Use of a needle guide directs the needle to the axis of the ultrasound beam, thus reducing the possibility of operator error.[58] The ultrasound image must be observed continuously during needle advancement until it is imaged within the lumen of the internal jugular vein. The ultrasound probe is removed from the needle and the catheter is advanced into the vein. Blood is aspirated from the catheter and the pressure within the catheter is transduced to confirm venous placement. Ultrasound is also used to confirm correct placement by observing the wire within the lumen of the vein *and* by the absence of the wire in the lumen of the artery. This latter step is important for ensuring that the wire has not traversed the vein and entered the artery. A large-bore introducer and catheter may then be inserted into the vein over the guide wire. Techniques that employ ultrasound to merely localize the entry site on the skin, do not demonstrate a benefit of ultrasound-guided cannulation.[55,58]

Unintentional placement of a large-bore catheter into the carotid artery is best managed by leaving the catheter in place and allowing surgical exploration for removal and repair of the artery to avoid the potentially lethal hemorrhagic consequence of this complication. Although prompt removal of the catheter without surgical exploration may be considered, this noninvasive management is not appropriate for the anticoagulated patient or the patient who is about to receive anticoagulant therapy, such as a large bolus of heparin for cardiopulmonary bypass. Noninvasive management with prolonged external pressure carries the risk of carotid artery compression and bradycardia via the carotid body reflex. Upper airway obstruction is another concern after removing a large-bore catheter from the carotid artery. The external surface anatomy and the patient's breathing must be carefully monitored for signs and symptoms of an expanding hematoma that may require surgical evacuation. Subsequent cannulation of the ipsilateral IJV may be near impossible because of external compression of the relatively low-pressure venous vessel. Ultrasound imaging provides valuable information in this scenario regarding the position and compression of the IJV. Failure to image the vein should preclude further cannulation attempts.

Subclavian Vein

The subclavian vein is commonly used by surgeons and intensivists and may be preferable for long-term use because of the larger diameter of this vessel compared with the IJV. The main disadvantage to cannulating the subclavian vein is the higher incidence of pneumothorax. A chest X-ray is mandatory after placement. Preoperative placement requires review of the chest X-ray to ensure the absence of a pneumothorax before initiating positive pressure ventilation, which may cause a tension pneumothorax.

Although both supraclavicular and infraclavicular techniques have been described, the most common approach is infraclavicular. A roll or blanket is placed behind the supine patient at the center of the back. This allows the shoulders to fall back away from the clavicular area. The sternal notch and clavicle are palpated and a hollow needle is inserted midway to two thirds of the distance between the sternal notch and the end of the clavicle (Fig. 3-12). The needle is directed toward the sternal notch and advanced until the inferior surface of the clavicle is encountered. The needle is then redirected with slight angulation, allowing the needle to pass underneath the clavicle. The syringe is advanced until blood is aspirated. Venous placement is confirmed as previously described for the IJV. The Seldinger technique with a J-wire is used to insert larger-bore catheters into the subclavian vein, also previously described.

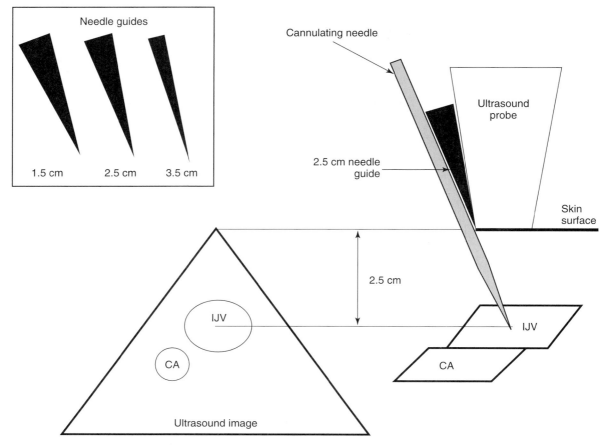

FIG. 3-11 Determination and use of the proper needle guide to perform ultrasound-guided cannulation. The depth from the skin to the lumen of the internal jugular vein *(IJV)* is determined from the ultrasound image (2.5 cm). The appropriate needle guide (2.5 cm) is attached to the ultrasound probe to guide the needle under the skin surface into the IJV within the same plane as the ultrasound image. *CA,* Carotid artery.

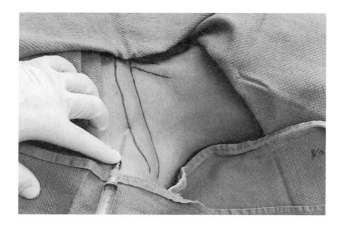

FIG. 3-12 Cannulation of the subclavian vein is performed by inserting a needle one half to two thirds of the distance between the sternal attachment and the distal end of the clavicle. The needle is directed toward the sternal notch as the needle is "walked off" the inferior surface of the clavicle.

Malposition of the catheter tip is more common with the subclavian approach, particularly with the longer (16-20 cm), pliable, smaller-diameter (7.5 Fr) catheters. A cephalad misplacement into the ipsilateral IJV may be recognized by observing the central venous pressure and waveform before and during application of firm external pressure over the supraclavicular area for 5 to 10 seconds. A rise in pressure above baseline within the catheter lumen suggests misplacement into the ipsilateral IJV.[75] This occurs because IJV compression by external pressure impedes venous return and causes pressure within the lumen of the vessel to rise.

Peripheral Venous Pressure

Peripheral venous pressure (PVP) is an alternative to central venous cannulation for estimating CVP. PVP tends to be 2 to 3 mm Hg greater than CVP in mechanically ventilated surgical patients.[76,77] The pressure trends correlate best in cases of significant blood loss ($r = 0.885$) or hemodynamic stability ($r = 0.923$).[76] Correlation is also reliable during intraoperative fluid challenges and in the postanesthesia care unit in spontaneously ventilating patients.[77]

INDICATIONS FOR CENTRAL VENOUS PRESSURE VS. PULMONARY ARTERY PRESSURE MONITORING

Central venous and pulmonary artery pressure monitoring are used to determine volume status, monitor changes in filling pressures, and direct therapy for patients with cardiac disease undergoing cardiac and noncardiac surgery. CVP monitoring reflects intrathoracic, right atrial, right ventricular end-diastolic, pericardial, and left heart pressures. Pulmonary artery pressure monitoring is also affected by intrathoracic and pericardial pressures, but is more reflective of left heart pressures, particularly when the catheter is wedged (pulmonary capillary wedge pressure, or PCWP). This distinction is particularly important in patients with right heart failure, pulmonary hypertension, or pulmonary embolism. A change in ventricular compliance or intrathoracic or pericardial pressure that is reflected by pressure changes in the CVP and PCWP may be unrelated to a change in left ventricular volume. Therefore an increase in filling pressures does not necessarily indicate an increase in intravascular volume because factors other than intravascular volume determine these pressures. Conversely, an increase in intravascular volume is not always indicated by an increase in filling pressure because of left and right ventricular compliance. The PCWP is more accurate than CVP in estimating left ventricular volume status because PCWP is less affected by changes in pulmonary and right ventricular compliance.

The ASA Task Force on Pulmonary Artery Catheterization provided practice guidelines for pulmonary artery catheter insertion (Box 3-2).[78] Use of these guidelines was recommended in surgical settings associated with an increased risk because of complications from hemodynamic changes, and by clinicians competent in safe insertion and accurate interpretation of the data provided. Pulmonary artery pressure monitoring is indicated for reasons related to the medical condition of the patient or the nature of surgery (Box 3-3), but is not recommended when the patient, procedure, and practice setting each pose a low risk for hemodynamic complications.[78] Patients undergoing surgery with unstable angina, recent myocardial infarction, active congestive heart failure, severe coronary or valvular heart disease, massive trauma, severe lung or renal disease, and shock require pulmonary artery blood pressure monitoring, except for minor surgical procedures. This type of patient often requires urgent or emergent surgery that precludes optimization of the medical condition. Surgical

---

BOX 3-2

The American Society of Anesthesiologists Task Force on Pulmonary Artery Catheterization Practice Guidelines for Pulmonary Artery Catheter Insertion[78]

Indications Related to the Patient
Clinical evidence of significant cardiovascular disease
Pulmonary dysfunction
Hypoxia
Renal insufficiency
Other conditions associated with hemodynamic instability (e.g., advanced age, endocrine disorders, sepsis, trauma, burns)

Indications Related to Surgery
Surgical procedures associated with an increased risk of hemodynamic changes, including damage to the heart, kidneys, lungs, or brain

Indications Related to Practice Setting
Physician skills
Duration of procedure
Technical support
Training and experience of nursing staff
Ability to manage potential complications

BOX 3-3

Indications for Pulmonary Arterial Pressure Monitoring

Indications Related to the Patient
Right heart failure
Pulmonary hypertension
Pulmonary embolism
Unstable angina
Recent myocardial infarction
Acute congestive heart failure
Severe coronary artery disease
Severe valvular heart disease
Shock (cardiogenic, septic, or hemorrhagic)
Massive trauma
Severe lung disease
Severe renal disease

Indications Related to Surgery
Major organ transplantation
Aortic cross-clamping procedures
Large fluid shifts
Massive blood loss
Implantation/explantation of ventricular assist device

---

settings that are likely to cause large fluid shifts or blood loss, cross-clamping of the aorta, and major organ transplantation are typical examples. Routine pulmonary artery (PA) catheterization in all patients undergoing coronary artery surgery is not necessary. Outcome after coronary artery surgery is not influenced by routine use of a PA catheter, suggesting its use can be delayed until a clinical need develops.[79]

The ASA Task Force also recommended that PA catheterization not be performed by clinicians who lack competence in safe insertion or accurate interpretation of the results. A 31-question multiple-choice examination administered to 496 physicians in 13 medical facilities revealed marked variation in physicians' understanding of all aspects of pulmonary artery catheterization.[80] Forty-seven percent of clinicians were unable to obtain even the most basic information provided by the PA catheter. Patients who receive a PA catheter tend to incur a longer hospital stay and greater cost. Institutions that place more PA catheters appear to obtain better outcomes related to its use.[81]

PULMONARY ARTERY CATHETERIZATION
Catheter Insertion

Pulmonary artery pressure monitoring requires placement of a large-bore introducer sheath in a large vein as previously described for central venous cannulation. Cardiovascular and catecholamine responses to central venous and pulmonary artery catheterization are the same whether catheterization is performed under local versus general anesthesia.[82] After central venous cannulation, the patient should be taken out of the Trendelenburg position because this position is associated with a significantly higher incidence of malignant dysrhythmias as compared with patients in a right lateral tilt position.[83] A flexible multilumen, balloon-tipped catheter is inserted through a one-way valve in the introducer sheath and advanced 20 cm before the balloon is inflated. The curve in the catheter is used to direct the tip in the direction of the right atrium and tricuspid valve. The convexity of the curve is to the patient's right and slightly anterior when inserting the catheter via the RIJ vein, but cephalad and slightly anterior when inserting the catheter via the left subclavian vein. The catheter may need to be rotated from its initial direction if its course deviates from a direct path. For example, insertion of the catheter via the left internal jugular vein may require that the tip be initially directed toward the patient's right, but then rotated inferiorly and to the patient's left, to direct the catheter toward the right atrium and tricuspid valve.

Insertion of the catheter must always be performed with continuous monitoring of the ECG and the pressure and waveform of the lumen at the catheter tip. The inflated balloon at the catheter tip will generally follow blood flow into the right atrium and through the tricuspid valve. The continuous observation of the pressure waveform identifies the position of the catheter tip by the characteristic waveform patterns of the various car-

diovascular chambers leading to the pulmonary artery (Fig. 3-13). It is important to note premature wedging of the catheter before it enters the right atrium, which indicates misdirection of the catheter away from the right atrium and into a vein or against a vessel wall. The pressure tracing becomes less attenuated and resembles a CVP tracing as the catheter is advanced toward the right atrium. A marked change in the tracing occurs when the catheter enters the right ventricle (25-35 mm insertion from the RIJ approach) and the systolic pressure measurement increases to 25 to 35 mm Hg in normal patients. The right ventricular systolic pressure may be as high as 70 to 90 mm Hg or higher in patients with severe pulmonary hypertension. Advancement of the catheter is hastened through the right ventricle because of the propensity for dysrhythmias. The diastolic pressure increases and a dicrotic notch becomes apparent as the catheter tip passes through the pulmonic valve. The "diastolic step-up" occurs in the pulmonary artery tracing because the pulmonic valve is closed during diastole. Systolic pressures are generally the same between the right ventricle and pulmonary artery because the pulmonic valve is open during systole. Exceptions include patients with pulmonic or infundibular stenosis.

The catheter is advanced into the pulmonary artery until a waveform resembling the CVP tracing is obtained. This indicates the PCWP. It is important to note the catheter insertion depth when the various waveforms are observed. The catheter should enter the pulmonary artery within 10 cm after entering the right ventricle and attain a PCWP within 10 cm thereafter. A greater insertion requirement for obtaining the pulmonary artery or PCWP beyond the "rule of 10 cm" usually indicates catheter coiling and is commonly associated with dysrhythmias. Typical intracardiac pressures obtained during insertion of a pulmonary artery catheter are listed in Table 3-3.

The curve in the PA catheter usually directs the catheter tip into the right main pulmonary artery, and the blood flow directs the balloon tip catheter to the area

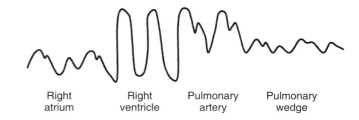

| Right atrium | Right ventricle | Pulmonary artery | Pulmonary wedge |

FIG. 3-13 Pressure waveforms obtained from the distal lumen of a pulmonary artery catheter as it is passes through the right heart. There is a marked change in the systolic pressure as the catheter enters the right ventricle and a marked increase in the diastolic pressure as the catheter enters the pulmonary artery.

with the most blood flow, which is usually posterior in the supine patient and to the right middle or lower lobe.[84] The PCWP reflects left atrial pressure when the catheter tip is located in Zone III, where pulmonary venous pressure exceeds alveolar pressure (Fig. 3-14). For the PCWP to reflect left atrial pressure, vascular patency must exist between the catheter tip wedged in a pulmonary arteriole, the pulmonary venules, the pulmonary veins, and the left atrium. The pulmonary venules are collapsed in areas of the lung where the alveolar pressure exceeds the pulmonary venous pressure (Zones I and II), thereby eliminating the patency between the catheter tip and the left atrium (Fig. 3-14).

TABLE 3-3
Normal Range of Intracardiac Pressures during Pulmonary Artery Catheterization

CHAMBER	PRESSURE (MM HG)
Right atrium	0-10
Right ventricle (systolic/diastolic)	15-30/5-10
Pulmonary artery (systolic/diastolic)	15-30/5-15
Pulmonary capillary wedge pressure	5-15

A chest radiograph is obtained after surgery to determine the position of the catheter tip and to exclude complications such as pneumothorax, hemothorax, vascular perforation, and pulmonary embolism. The pulmonary artery pressure and waveform are continuously monitored for catheter migration until the PA catheter is removed.

Contraindications

Right bundle-branch block (RBBB) occurs in 3% of patients undergoing PA catheterization.[85] Although the incidence of complete heart block during PA catheterization of patients with previous left bundle-branch block (LBBB) is not higher than the incidence of RBBB in patients without underlying conduction defects, placement of a PA catheter in patients with a preexisting LBBB is not recommended unless precautions are taken for the development of complete heart block.[85,86] These include application of transcutaneous pacing pads before the catheter is advanced into the right ventricular outflow tract and use of a PA catheter with pacing electrodes. The presence of a PA catheter or even just the guide wire used for CVP insertion in the right ventricular outflow tract may interfere with right bundle-branch conduction and lead to complete heart block in patients with LBBB.[85-87] An algorithm for PA catheter insertion

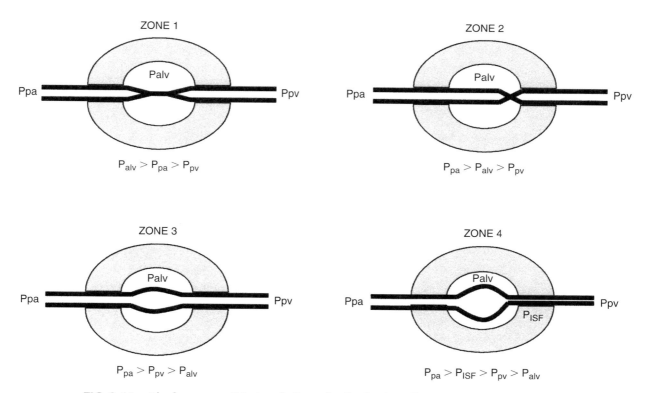

FIG. 3-14   The four zones of the lung indicate the distribution of blood flow to various areas of the lung. The zones are defined by the relation between the pulmonary artery pressure (P_{pa}), alveolar pressure (P_{alv}), pulmonary venous pressure (P_{pv}), and interstitial pressure (P_{ISF}).

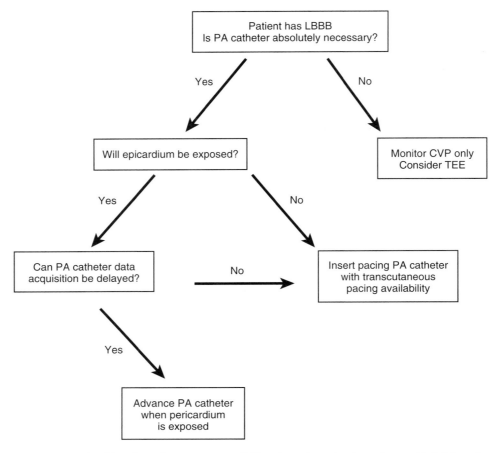

FIG. 3-15 Algorithm for pulmonary artery *(PA)* catheter insertion in patients with left bundle-branch block *(LBBB)*. *TEE,* Transesophageal echocardiography.

in patients with preexisting LBBB is presented in Fig. 3-15. The first decision is whether PA catheter insertion is absolutely necessary. Use of TEE may reduce or eliminate the need for a PA catheter. The next decisions are dependent on whether the PA catheter information is required before the epicardium is exposed and whether the surgical exposure will permit application of epicardial pacing wires by the surgeon. In this situation, a standard PA catheter is inserted to the 20-cm marking before surgery and advanced into the PA after the epicardium is exposed, but delays acquisition of the PA catheter data. Pericardial adhesions from pericarditis or prior cardiac surgery and minimally invasive or thoracotomy approaches may preclude use of this strategy because of the inability to gain rapid access for epicardial pacing. These situations require placement of transcutaneous pacing pads before the catheter is advanced into the right ventricular outflow tract and use of a PA catheter with pacing capability.

Another indication for a PA catheter with pacing electrodes is the surgical patient with a permanent pacemaker who is pacemaker dependent. Electrocautery, commonly used during surgical procedures, will interfere pacemaker function, rendering the patient asystolic during use of the electrocautery. Insertion of a pacing PA catheter allows the clinician to control the heart rate and pacing mode, despite the use of electrocautery. Other options for pacemaker management perioperatively are presented in Chapter 9. PA catheter insertion is generally avoided in patients with newly implanted transvenous pacing wires who are pacemaker dependent because of the risk of lead displacement.

PA catheter insertion is contraindicated in patients with right atrial or right ventricular masses and tetralogy of Fallot. Intracardiac masses such as tumors, particularly atrial myxomas, are easily dislodged, leading to pulmonary embolism. Irritability of the right ventricular outflow tract in patients with tetralogy of Fallot may cause infundibular spasm and lead to cyanosis.

Types of Pulmonary Artery Catheters

A standard PA catheter consists of three lumens (CVP, PA, and balloon) and a thermistor for temperature measurement. A volume infusion port catheter is used by most clinicians because of the additional lumen for infusion of vasoactive medications. The pacing PA catheter is available in two types. In the first type, electrodes are embedded onto the surface of the catheter at locations that typically contact the right atrial and right ventricular walls, permitting atrial and ventricular pacing respectively. Another type of pacing PA catheter (Pace Port) has an additional lumen that allows insertion of a pacing wire into the right ventricle once the PA catheter is appropriately positioned. The author prefers the former type because it is easier to use, pacing can be initiated more rapidly, and the catheter is capable of both atrial and ventricular pacing. Some clinicians fear that the wire inserted via the Pace Port catheter may damage cardiac structures.

Oximetric catheters provide a continuous display of mixed venous oxygen saturation. These catheters are particularly useful for patients affected by simultaneous changes in ventricular function, pulmonary function, hemoglobin content, and preload. The continuous nature of the measurement is a useful monitoring tool in a busy intensive care unit, where frequent determinations of cardiac output are not practical. Continuous monitoring of mixed venous oxygen saturation may indicate an ensuing problem of cardiac, pulmonary, hemoglobin, or volume status before it would otherwise be apparent. Continuous cardiac output catheters provide a measurement of cardiac output at predefined intervals. Heating elements are incorporated onto the catheter surface proximal to the thermistor. A heating period is followed by passive cooling to mimic the temperature changes that occur with a bolus cold injectate technique. Right ventricular ejection catheters provide a rapidly responsive thermistor that can detect temperature changes within a cardiac cycle. Temperature measurements made at the beginning and end of a cardiac cycle allow for determination of right ventricular ejection.

Cardiac Output Determination

PA catheters allow for the determination of several hemodynamic parameters (Table 3-4), but the basis for all of these calculations is measuring cardiac output. Cardiac output (CO) is the amount of blood delivered to the tissues over time and is usually expressed as liters per minute (L/min). Cardiac index is used to determine whether a CO value determined for an individual patient is adequate and is expressed as $L \cdot min^{-1} \cdot m^{-2}$. The cardiac output of larger patients is normally greater than that of smaller patients; however, cardiac index is normalized for body size and allows for individual patient assessment independent of body size. Once an adequate value for CO is determined for an individual patient, cardiac output or index can be used to follow patient trends or response to therapy.

CO determination uses a thermistor located at the tip of the PA catheter to measure blood temperature as a known volume of cold solution is rapidly injected upstream in the blood flowing through the right

TABLE 3-4
Hemodynamic Parameters Provided by a Pulmonary Artery Catheter

HEMODYNAMIC PARAMETER	CALCULATION
Cardiac output (CO)	Computed by integrating temperature change over time
Cardiac index (CI)	$\dfrac{CO}{BSA}$
Stroke volume (SV)	$\dfrac{CO}{HR} \times 100$
Stroke volume index (SVI)	$\dfrac{CI}{HR} \times 100$
Systemic vascular resistance (SVR)	$\dfrac{MAP - CVP}{CO} \times 80$
Systemic vascular resistance index (SVRI)	$SVR \times BSA$
Pulmonary vascular resistance (PVR)	$\dfrac{MPAP - PCWP}{CO}$
Pulmonary vascular resistance index (PVRI)	$PVR \times BSA$
Left ventricular stroke work index (LVSWI)	$\dfrac{(MAP - PCWP) \times SVI}{100} \times 1.36$
Right ventricular stroke work index (RVSWI)	$\dfrac{(MPAP - CVP) \times SVI}{100} \times 1.36$

BSA, Body surface area (m^2); *CO*, cardiac output (L/min); *CVP*, central venous or mean right atrial pressure; *HR*, heart rate (beats/min); *MAP*, mean arterial pressure; *MPAP*, mean pulmonary artery pressure; *PCWP*, pulmonary capillary wedge pressure.

heart.[88,89] The Stewart-Hamilton equation is used to calculate CO[89,90]:

$$CO = \frac{V \times (T_B - T_I) \times S_I \times C_I \times 60}{S_B \times C_B \times \int_0^\infty \Delta T_B(t) dt}$$

where V is the cold injectate volume, T_B is blood temperature, T_I is injectate temperature, S_I is the specific gravity and C_I is the specific heat of the injectate, S_B is the specific gravity and C_B is the specific heat of blood, and the integral from zero to infinity of $\Delta T_B(t)dt$ is the area under the temperature curve plotted over time. Because $T_B(t)dt$ is in the denominator of the Stewart-Hamilton equation, larger areas yield smaller CO determinations. Intuitively, a larger area under the curve suggests that blood flow past the thermistor is reduced, allowing for a greater change in temperature and a slower return to baseline (Fig. 3-16). Conversely, a smaller area under the curve suggests greater blood flow past the thermistor, thus attenuating the temperature change with a more rapid return to baseline temperature. This is an important concept to understand when considering the accuracy of the CO measurement.

Errors in measurement may become apparent with inspection of the temperature versus time curve. A larger area under the curve accurately represents a lower CO, because the colder temperature and a prolonged return to baseline indicate greater injectate influence on thermistor temperature as a result of lower blood flow. An inaccurately low CO is obtained by conditions that produce a similar influence (larger area) on the temperature versus time curve. Examples include a larger injectate volume, colder injectate, tricuspid regurgitation, or intracardiac shunt. A smaller area under the curve accurately represents a higher CO, because the reduce temperature drop and the more rapid return to baseline indicate less injectate influence on blood temperature as a result of higher blood flow. An inaccurately high CO is obtained by conditions that produce a similar influence (smaller area) on the temperature versus time curve. Examples include a smaller injectate volume, warmer injectate, or a partially wedged catheter.

CO measurements are more precise when a 10-ml volume is injected at room temperature or 0° C.[91] Iced injectates, however, tend to lower the heart rate,[92] which has the effect of decreasing CO (CO = HR × SV). This effect may be more pronounced in patients with low cardiac index, low mean pulmonary artery pressure, and high systemic vascular resistance.[93] Smaller injectate

volumes (3 and 5 ml) result in less reproducibility even when the correct computation constant is used for the smaller injectate volume.[91] Using a constant rate and duration of injection[94] and injecting the solution at a specific time in the respiratory cycle[95] improve the precision of thermodilution CO determination. Accuracy, however, is decreased when the injectate is injected at specific times in the respiratory cycle,[95] and when simultaneously administered intravenous fluids cause fluctuations in the baseline temperature.[96] This further emphasizes the importance of observing the temperature versus time curve. CO determination is particularly inaccurate immediately following hypothermic cardiopulmonary bypass. Thermodilution CO is underestimated within the first 10 minutes[97] and the effects of the ventilatory cycle are more pronounced during the first 30 minutes following bypass.[98] Despite an excellent correlation, accuracy, and precision between continuous and intermittent thermodilution CO measurements before and 45 minutes after hypothermic cardiopulmonary bypass, there is a lack of correlation during the early period following cardiopulmonary bypass.[99]

Accurate CO determination allows calculation of other hemodynamic parameters that are used to manage patients with cardiac disease. More important than isolated calculations are repeat measurements in response to perioperative events and therapeutic intervention. This emphasizes the importance of administering the injectate volume in a consistent manner at a specific time in the respiratory cycle and with the same rate and duration of injection. CO determination directly affects all other hemodynamic parameters listed in Table 3-4. CO and wall stress can be determined using echocardiographic data without the use of a PA catheter, as discussed in Chapter 4.

CO data are also obtained with "continuous cardiac output" catheters. These catheters determine CO using the same principle of thermodilution, but instead of injecting a bolus of cold injectate, a heating element warms the blood at predetermined intervals (usually 30 seconds). The change in thermistor temperature at the end of the catheter is plotted over time. A binary heating and cooling curve is used to compute the CO by integrating the area under the curve over time.[100] Because measurements are averaged over a few minutes, rapid changes in CO such as those associated with aortic cross-clamping, may not be apparent for several minutes. Bolus CO determination is probably better suited for rapidly changing hemodynamic conditions, whereas continuous cardiac output determination is better suited for the postoperative intensive care unit setting where hemodynamic changes usually occur gradually. Continuous measurement does not require medical personnel to interrupt other tasks to determine CO. The ongoing generation of CO data may provide an earlier

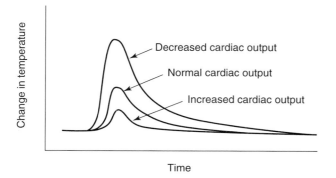

FIG. 3-16 Thermodilution cardiac output curves indicating change in temperature with a bolus injection of a cold solution over time. Decreased cardiac output produces a larger area under the curve, whereas increased cardiac output produces a smaller area under the curve.

warning to an underlying but developing problem that may otherwise not become apparent until arterial blood pressure is compromised.

Mixed Venous Oxygen Saturation

PA catheters allow for the determination of mixed venous oxygen saturation (SV_{O_2}) either by intermittent sampling by blood gas analysis or by a continuous fiber optic measurement. Continuous mixed venous oxygen saturation requires a PA catheter with fiber optic channels that transmit and measure the frequency of reflected light. Oxygenated hemoglobin absorbs nearly all infrared light and reflects nearly all red light, whereas deoxygenated hemoglobin reflects infrared light and absorbs more infrared light. The relative concentration of oxygenated and deoxygenated hemoglobin determines oxygen saturation. Different manufacturers employ either a two- or three-wavelength system to measure oxygen saturation. Both systems function with reasonable accuracy and reproducibility over a wide range of oxygen saturation,[101] although some investigators have found the three-wavelength system to be more accurate and precise than the two-wavelength system.[101-103]

Although CO is one determinant of mixed venous saturation,[104] SV_{O_2} is also affected by oxygen-carrying capacity and metabolic demand of the tissues. SV_{O_2} is therefore a better indicator of tissue oxygenation than CO measurement alone. A decrease in either CO or hemoglobin level or an increase in tissue extraction each signal a problem with tissue oxygenation. Continuous measurement becomes useful in the same manner as described earlier for continuous CO determination, by providing continuous data without interrupting other personnel tasks or having to wait for blood gas results to be reported by the laboratory. A continuous mixed venous oxygen saturation catheter may thus provide earlier warning of an impending problem. Complete reliance on SV_{O_2} data alone to indicate CO may be erroneous because of the influence of oxygen supply and demand. Therefore these catheters often provide continuous CO data along with the mixed venous oxygen saturation.

Clinical situations in which oxygen demand changes rapidly are particularly prone to errors in interpreting changes in SV_{O_2} as changes in CO. The classic example is during liver transplantation. Oxygen demand decreases when the liver is removed and increases after reperfusion. Liver transplantation, resection of an abdominal aortic aneurysm, cardiac surgery, and the intraoperative environment in general are prone to rapid changes in CO. Continuous mixed venous and CO catheters are less useful in these situations because data are collected and averaged over a few minutes. The display of data

indicating a change in CO is delayed. The benefit of these catheters in providing an early warning of CO changes in the more stable postoperative period is a detriment in the rapidly changing intraoperative environment. Intraoperative CO determination with a standard PA catheter using an intermittent bolus technique is more useful and less costly than a continuous mixed venous and CO catheter.

Complications of Pulmonary Artery Catheters

PA catheterization is generally a safe and beneficial monitoring technique commonly employed in anesthesia practice.[105] Complications arise with proper use, improper techniques, or patient conditions that predispose patients to complications. Complications of PA catheterization include those associated with central venous cannulation; dysrhythmias; pulmonary artery rupture; valvular damage; coiling, knotting, or entrapment of the catheter; and misinterpretation of the data. Long-term complications include thrombocytopenia, thrombus formation, and infection. A nonrandom, uncontrolled, observational study suggested that PA catheterization is associated with increased mortality and increased utilization of resources.[106] However, PA catheter use was not dissuaded because of the uncontrolled nature of this observational study.

Central Venous Cannulation Complications. The complications of central venous cannulation were discussed in detail in a previous section. Briefly, these complications include arterial puncture, pneumothorax, nerve injury, bleeding, infection, and dysrhythmias. Dysrhythmias are commonly extraatrial or ventricular contractions that occur because the J-wire used with the Seldinger technique is inserted too far. Contact between the wire and the wall of the right atrium can cause premature atrial contractions, atrial flutter, or atrial fibrillation, whereas contact with the right ventricle can cause premature ventricular contractions, ventricular tachycardia, or ventricular fibrillation. ECG monitoring must be employed during every central venous cannulation, and wire insertion should be minimized to avoid this complication.

Dysrhythmias. Dysrhythmias are also common during insertion of the PA catheter.[107] Premature atrial and ventricular contractions occur as the catheter balloon tip passes through the right atrium and ventricle, respectively. Patients with right ventricular ischemia or recent infarction have increased ventricular ectopy. Although ventricular tachycardia or fibrillation may occur, the use of prophylactic lidocaine is controversial.[108] The Trendelenburg position is associated with a significantly higher incidence of malignant dysrhythmias as compared with a 5-degree head-up and right lateral tilt position.[83] PA catheter insertion in patients with preexisting LBBB was previously discussed as a contraindication to PA catheter insertion, unless provisions are made for the dreaded complication of complete heart block.

Pulmonary Artery Rupture. Pulmonary artery rupture is a potentially lethal complication of PA catheterization that may present with only minor endobronchial bleeding or major hemorrhage. Mortality was reported as 46% in a review of 28 cases, but the rate was 75% in anticoagulated patients.[109] Patient risk factors include pulmonary hypertension, mitral stenosis, advanced age, female gender, and coagulopathy. Some clinicians do not recommend wedging the catheter in these situations. Iatrogenic risk factors involve advancing the catheter too far into the pulmonary arterial vasculature, overinflation of the balloon, and inflating the balloon against resistance. Continuous monitoring of the PA waveform after insertion is important for identifying unintentional catheter wedging as a result of migration. The waveform must always be examined before balloon inflation. Inflating the balloon of a wedged catheter will undoubtedly exert pressure on the vessel wall and may cause vessel rupture. Catheter wedging that requires less than 1.5 ml of air suggests that the catheter is too distal in the vasculature and must be pulled back. The position of the catheter tip is particularly important if cardiopulmonary bypass is anticipated. Concurrent use of TEE permits imaging of the distal tip of the PA catheter, which is easily identified with balloon inflation. The author withdraws the PA catheter, using TEE guidance, to the right pulmonary artery just distal to the bifurcation of the main pulmonary artery to prevent catheter wedging during cardiopulmonary bypass. The potential for PA perforation appears to increase with hypothermia.

Management of endobronchial hemorrhage includes correction of coagulation disorders, placement of a double-lumen endobronchial tube to isolate the lung,[110] positive end-expiratory pressure, pulmonary embolization,[111] and ultimately pulmonary resection.[112] Although most clinicians advocate positive pressure ventilation via a double-lumen endobronchial tube, there is controversy over management involving the PA catheter. Pulling the catheter back would theoretically prevent the catheter from abutting against a susceptible area of the vasculature, which may cause further damage. Leaving the catheter in place permits localization of the bleeding site by X-ray or contrast injection, should a pulmonary resection be required.[110] Others advocate reinflating the balloon to reduce blood flow to the bleeding site. Whatever PA catheter management option is chosen must be accompanied by recognition of the potential morbidity and mortality. Insertion of large-bore intravenous catheters, retrieval of blood from the blood bank, and double-lumen endobronchial intubation with positive pressure ventilation are appropriate steps for this complication.

Valve Damage, Coiling, Knotting, and Entrapment. Valvular damage to the tricuspid[113] or pulmonic[114] valves most easily occurs by withdrawing a PA catheter with the balloon inflated. Another mechanism of valve damage may occur by coiling the catheter around chordae tendineae during insertion and with subsequent knotting of the catheter around the chordae during withdrawal. It is important to maintain the balloon inflated during insertion to minimize the chance of passing the catheter between chordae.[115] Fortunately, knotting of the PA catheter is rare.[116] Knotting is easily diagnosed by X-ray film, but the catheter should not be withdrawn in an attempt to remove the knot.[117] Coiling of the catheter is more likely in patients with dilated right heart chambers. PA catheters can also be entrapped by suturing them within the heart. A common site is the right atrial purse string suture used to secure the venous return cannula for cardiopulmonary bypass. Patients with previous atriotomy are at risk because the sutures are placed within the free wall of the atrium instead of in the atrial appendage. TEE is very useful for diagnosing PA catheter coiling and entrapment by imaging the tip of the PA catheter and the cardiac chambers during catheter withdrawal.[118] The PA catheter tip is imaged as the catheter is withdrawn. The catheter is not likely to be coiled or entrapped if the catheter tip moves proximally as the catheter is withdrawn. A catheter sutured into the right atrial purse string suture will reveal invagination of the atrial free wall by TEE during catheter withdrawal.[118] If TEE is used in patients at risk for PA catheter entrapment and coiling, imaging the catheter tip and right atrium may identify these potential complications before surgical closure of the mediastinum.

Data Misinterpretation. Probably the most common complication of PA catheter use is misinterpretation of the data generated. Errors in measurement can occur from improper calibration of the transducer, improper positioning of the catheter tip (i.e., against a vessel wall or not in Zone III), failing to consider the effects of mechanical ventilation, artifacts, and unrecognized catheter migration. A multicenter study revealed that physicians' understanding of the PA catheter was quite variable and dependent on training, frequency of use, and whether the physician's hospital was a primary medical school affiliate.[80] Misinterpretation of PCWP may lead to patient management decisions that increase morbidity. For example, hyperresonance in the pulmonary artery pressure recording causes the digital display of values that overestimate the systolic pressure or underestimate the diastolic pressure. A PA catheter tip located in the right ventricle instead of the pulmonary artery will also yield pulmonary artery diastolic pressures that underestimate the actual pulmonary artery diastolic filling pressure. These data will direct the clinician to administer more volume, whereas the therapy for accurate data may be opposite. Failure to recognize a V wave in the PCWP causes an overestimation of filling pressure. These examples emphasize the importance of monitoring the graphic display of the PA waveform in addition to the numerical pressure display. Hyperresonance is easily corrected with damping the pressure line, V waves prompt treatment of mitral regurgitation, and a catheter tip in the right ventricle is advanced into the pulmonary artery.

A very important aspect of interpreting PA catheter data is to consider the information in the context of the patient and other hemodynamic data. TEE is particularly useful for supplementing and allowing accurate interpretation of PA catheter data. For example, high PCWP pressure in the context of a normal ejection fraction and a small end-diastolic left ventricular cross-sectional area indicates decreased left ventricular compliance. A hypotensive patient with these echocardiographic findings would require volume loading or an α agonist, therapy that appears contrary to the usual therapy for high PCWP. Even without TEE, one would suspect such a scenario based on patient characteristics that include left ventricular hypertrophy. Patients with chronic hypertension or patients undergoing aortic valve replacement for aortic stenosis classically have decreased left ventricular compliance and should therefore be expected to require higher PCWP for adequate volume loading after valve replacement.

Preload is the myocardial fiber stretch imposed on the ventricle at end-diastole. TEE allows for the closest estimation of the degree of stretch by displaying end-diastolic area. PCWP is a reflection of left atrial pressure, which is a reflection of left ventricular end-diastolic pressure, which is a reflection of left ventricular end-diastolic volume. Multiple assumptions are thus made when one considers the PCWP as preload. Any physiologic conditions that interfere with these pressure and volume correlations invalidate the assumption that PCWP estimates preload.

ELECTROCARDIOGRAPHY

ECG is a safe, noninvasive method of monitoring patients for dysrhythmias and myocardial ischemia perioperatively. Depolarization and repolarization of myocardial cells produce electrical potentials that are recorded on the surface of the body. Two body-surface electrodes detect the depolarization of the heart by measuring the flow of current between the electrodes. The flow of electrical current is depicted as a positive deflec-

tion when the current propagates toward the positive electrode and a negative deflection when the current propagates away from the positive electrode. One cardiac cycle produces a characteristic set of positive and negative deflections, as shown in Fig. 3-17.

Electrodes are placed on the arms and legs to create several monitoring leads based on various combinations of electrodes. Lead I is obtained by placing the positive electrode on the left arm and the negative electrode on the right arm. Lead II is obtained from a positive electrode on the left leg and a negative electrode on the right arm. Lead II is most commonly used for rhythm monitoring because the normal depolarization of the heart follows the same axis as Lead II. Positive deflections occur with depolarization extending from the superior aspect of the heart to the inferior aspect because the positive lead is inferior to the heart (left leg). Lead III is obtained from a positive electrode on the left leg and a negative electrode on the left arm. These three bipolar limb leads constitute Einthoven's triangle (Fig. 3-18). Einthoven's Law defines the center of the heart as the zero reference point, so that the sum of Leads I and III is equivalent to Lead II.[119] The three augmented limb leads (aVR, aVL, and aVF) are unipolar leads that represent an axis from the center of the heart to the positive electrode. The positive electrode is the right arm electrode for the aVR lead, left arm electrode for aVL lead, and the leg electrode for the aVF lead (Fig. 3-19). The flow of electrical current is depicted as a positive deflection when the current propagates toward the positive electrode and a negative deflection when the current propagates away from the positive electrode. The precordial leads are also unipolar leads. These leads are placed across the precordium and measure

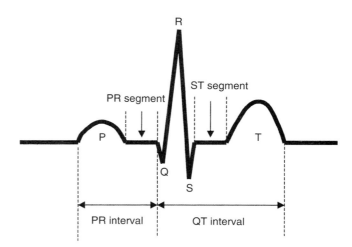

FIG. 3-17 The components of a normal electrocardiogram. The P wave indicates atrial depolarization, the QRS wave indicates ventricular depolarization, and the T wave indicates ventricular repolarization.

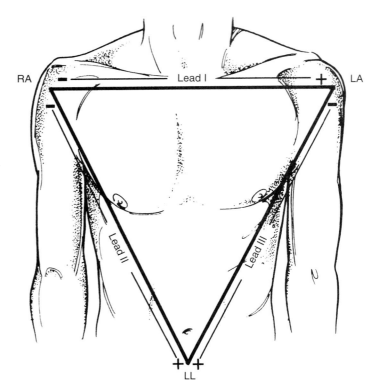

FIG. 3-18 Einthoven's triangle indicating the electrical axes of the bipolar electrocardiogram leads (I, II, and III). *LA*, Left arm lead; *LL*, left leg lead; *RA*, right arm lead.

(From Dasher LA, Slye DA: *ECG, arrhythmia, and ST segment analysis*, Redmond, Wash, 1994, SpaceLabs Medical, Inc.)

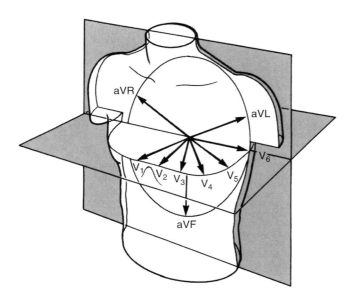

FIG. 3-19 Electrical axes of the unipolar leads. The axes of the augmented leads (aVR, aVL, and aVF) are in the vertical plane and the axes of the precordial leads (V1 through V6) are in the horizontal plane.

(From Anderson ST, Downs WG, Lander P et al: *Advanced electrocardiography*, Redmond, Wash, 1994, SpaceLabs Medical, Inc.)

electrical forces propagating along six different axes in one horizontal plane[120] (Fig. 3-19). One precordial and the four limb electrodes constitute the five-electrode system commonly used for intraoperative monitoring. The V_5 lead is the single preferred precordial lead for monitoring ischemia because this lead is most sensitive for detecting ECG changes indicative of ischemia.[121]

Normal electrical conduction within the heart begins at the sinoatrial (SA) node, propagates to the right atrium, and extends to the left atrium. This atrial depolarization is indicated by a P wave on the ECG (Fig. 3-20). The interval between the P and R waves (PR interval) represents a delay in propagation of the electrical impulse allowing the atria to contract. The atrioventricular node transmits the electrical impulse to the ventricles via the bundle of His and to the left and right bundle branches (Fig. 3-20). The left bundle branch divides into the anterior and posterior fascicles, which carry the electrical impulse to the anterior-superior and posterior-inferior endocardial surfaces of the heart respectively. The impulse terminates in the Purkinje fibers of the ventricles, which propagate the impulse from the endocardial surface, through the myocardium to the epicardial surface. This entire depolarization of the ventricular myocardium is represented by the QRS complex on the ECG (Fig. 3-20). A second delay is observed on the ECG as indicated by the isoelectric ST segment. Ventricular repolarization occurs during the T wave on the ECG, which is occasionally followed by a U wave. The significance of the U wave is unclear. A U wave that occurs in the same direction as the T wave may simply represent terminal ventricular repolarization.[119] However, an inverted U wave may indicate the presence of certain metabolic or cardiovascular disorders such as hypertension, coronary artery disease, or valvular heart disease.[122]

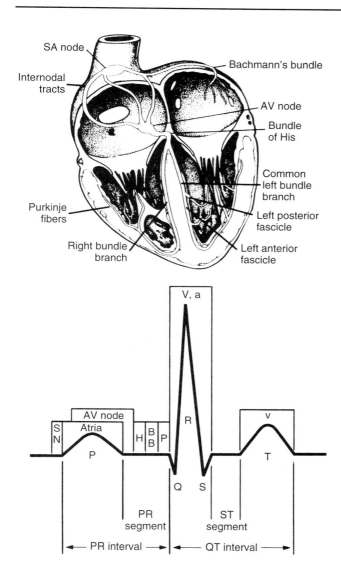

FIG. 3-20   Cardiac conduction system anatomy with associated electrocardiographic waveforms. *AV*, Atrioventricular; *SA*, sinoatrial. Depolarization is indicated by *Atria*, right and left atria; *AV node*, atrioventricular node; *BB*, bundle branches; *H*, bundle of His; *P*, Purkinje network; and *SN*, sinoatrial node; *V*, right and left ventricles. Repolarization is indicated by *a*, right and left atria; *v*, right and left ventricles.

(Modified from Dasher LA, Slye DA: *ECG, arrhythmia, and ST segment analysis*, Redmond, Wash, 1994, SpaceLabs Medical, Inc.)

Ischemia Detection

Detection of myocardial ischemia is an important aspect of intraoperative ECG monitoring. Changes in the ST segment and the T wave provide an early indication of myocardial ischemia, second only to wall motion abnormalities in time of onset (see Chapter 4). As previously mentioned, the electrical impulse normally travels through the myocardium from the endocardium to the epicardium. A subendocardial injury to the myocardium causes a redirection of the electrical impulse such that the current in the area of injury trav-

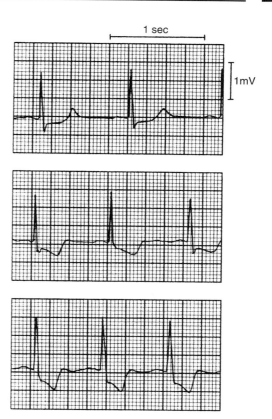

FIG. 3-21   An electrocardiogram of a patient with subendocardial ischemia producing ST-segment depression. The ST segment becomes more depressed and more down-sloping in this patient with left main coronary artery disease as the heart rate increases from 63 beats per minute *(top panel)* to 75 beats per minute *(middle panel)* and finally to 86 beats per minute *(lower panel)* because of increased myocardial oxygen demand.

(From Mark JB: *Atlas of cardiovascular monitoring*, New York, 1998, Churchill Livingston.)

els from the normal epicardium toward the injured subendocardium. This is depicted as ST depression on the ECG[10] (Fig. 3-21), because the direction is opposite from the QRS depolarization. Conversely, a transmural injury originates in the epicardium, causing an injury current in the same direction as the QRS depolarization or ST elevation[10] (Fig. 3-22). Coronary thrombosis and vasospasm cause ST elevation in patients with coronary artery disease undergoing cardiac or noncardiac surgery. Mechanical problems affecting blood flow in coronary bypass grafts are additional causes of ST elevation in patients undergoing cardiac surgery. An ST-segment deviation of at least 1 mm or T-wave inversion is indicative of myocardial ischemia. However, ST- and T-wave changes may also occur in the absence of myocardial ischemia with conditions such as left ventricular hypertrophy, digoxin use, electrolyte abnormalities, bundle-branch blocks, and Wolff-Parkinson-White syndrome.

Ischemia detection with ECG is relatively common in patients with coronary artery disease undergoing surgery.[121,123] Visual detection of ST-segment changes is an unreliable method of monitoring patients for ischemia by ECG. Between 0% and 46% of ischemic episodes are detected by visual inspection alone.[123,124] Computerized analysis of the ST segment is a more reliable method of detecting ECG ischemia, but is dependent on the accuracy of the reproduction of the ECG and the algorithms and filters used.[125] The identification of three points within the ECG complex is required for calculation of the ST-segment deviation: the isoelectric reference line, the J point, and the ST segment (Fig. 3-23). The isoelectric reference is obtained from a horizontal line drawn from the PR segment that occurs before the QRS complex. Various algorithms define the PR point using the QRS complex, R wave, or J point as references. The J point occurs at the junction between the QRS complex and the ST segment. The computer algorithm sets the ST point at which the ST segment is measured, 60 to 80 msec after the J point.[119] Placing the ST point at 60 msec after the J point may yield better sensitivity, whereas placing it at 80 msec may achieve greater specificity.[126] The ST-segment value is calculated by measuring the vertical distance between the PR point (isoelectric line) and the ST point. Accuracy of ST-segment analysis depends on proper placement of these three points within the ECG complex. It is important to review the template selected by the monitor and

to verify any ECG changes by reviewing printed strips of the lead in question.[125]

Lead selection is another important aspect of monitoring patients for myocardial ischemia. London and colleagues used a continuous 12-lead ECG to monitor 105 patients with known or suspected coronary artery disease undergoing major noncardiac surgery.[121] Lead sensitivity for detecting myocardial ischemia was calculated by dividing the number of ischemic episodes in each lead by the total number of ischemic episodes (Fig. 3-24). Lead V_5 had the greatest sensitivity (75%), followed by lead V_4 (61%). Monitoring two leads simultaneously yielded a sensitivity of 80% if leads II and V_5 were monitored, 82% if leads II and V_4 were monitored, and 90% if leads V_4 and V_5 were monitored. A three-lead system that combined leads II, V_4, and V_5 increased the sensitivity to 96%.

The significance of ST-segment changes depends on the patient population. ST-segment changes in a population with a high prevalence of coronary artery disease usually represent myocardial ischemia, whereas ST-segment changes in patients with a low probability of disease may not represent ischemia.[125,127,128] Ischemia monitoring is equally important during local anesthesia with intravenous sedation and in general anesthesia. In an elderly population undergoing cataract surgery and randomly assigned to either local or general anes-

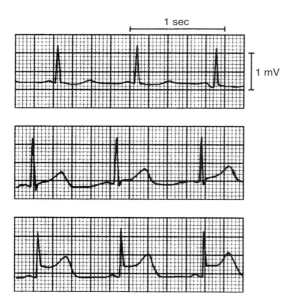

FIG. 3-22 An electrocardiogram of a patient with transmural ischemia producing ST-segment elevation. This patient developed progressive ST-segment elevation *(middle and lower panels)* with occlusion of a patent saphenous vein graft during repeat coronary artery bypass surgery as a result of an interruption in coronary blood supply.

(From Mark JB: *Atlas of cardiovascular monitoring,* New York, 1998, Churchill Livingston.)

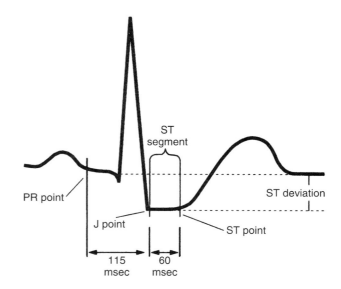

FIG. 3-23 ST-segment measurement points.

(From Dasher LA, Slye DA: *ECG, arrhythmia, and ST segment analysis,* Redmond, Wash, 1994, SpaceLabs Medical, Inc.)

thesia, the incidence or perioperative myocardial ischemia detected by ECG was 31%.[129] Eighty-one percent of these patients had at least two risk factors for ischemic heart disease. Although the incidence of ischemia was similar between groups, the general anesthesia group had significantly more intraoperative events, all of which were associated with tachycardia. Acute reduction in hemoglobin concentration to 5 g/dl may cause ECG ST-segment changes suggestive of ischemia, but may also be related to the associated tachycardia creating an imbalance between oxygen supply and demand.[130] Routine use of TEE during noncardiac surgery provides only minimal additive value over ST-segment monitoring for detecting myocardial ischemia.[131]

Dysrhythmia Detection

A *dysrhythmia* is defined as any cardiac rhythm that is not a normal sinus rhythm. Monitoring cardiac rhythm is important for the cardiac patient because intraoperative dysrhythmias occur more frequently in patients with cardiac disease.[132] Dysrhythmias are most prevalent during tracheal intubation and extubation, but several other intraoperative factors also predispose patients to dysrhythmias. Insertion of central venous catheters commonly involves use of the Seldinger technique, which employs a J-wire that can cause dysrhythmias,

particularly when it is inserted too far. PA catheter insertion uses a balloon-tipped catheter that may cause atrial dysrhythmias, ventricular dysrhythmias, or complete heart block in patients with preexisting left bundle branch. Ventricular dysrhythmias are common with the use of potent inhalational agents, particularly halothane and enflurane.[133] The propensity for dysrhythmias may be increased if the PA catheter is inserted under general anesthesia with these agents. A junctional rhythm is not uncommon during isoflurane anesthesia, whereas bigeminy may occur if the anesthesia is too light. Electrolyte abnormalities and alterations caused by altered respiration, such as hyperventilation, also contribute to intraoperative dysrhythmias. Certain surgical procedures activate cardiac reflexes that produce dysrhythmias. These include abdominal surgery with manipulation of the bowel or retraction of the peritoneum, ophthalmologic surgery, and neck surgery that causes pressure on the carotid body or vagus nerve.

Dysrhythmias may be classified according to their site of origin or involvement. Atrial dysrhythmias include sinus bradycardia, sinus tachycardia, premature atrial contraction, paroxysmal atrial tachycardia, atrial flutter, and atrial fibrillation. Loss of atrial contraction produces a junctional rhythm that usually causes a 15% decrease in CO in patients with normal left ventricular compliance. Ventricular dysrhythmias include

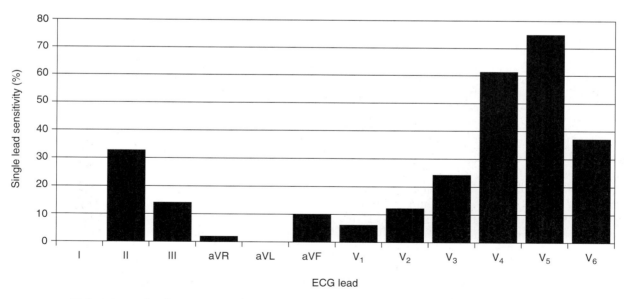

FIG. 3-24   The distribution of ischemic ST-segment changes in each of the 12 ECG leads of 105 patients with known or suspected coronary artery disease undergoing noncardiac surgery with general anesthesia. Sensitivity was calculated from the number of changes in a single lead as a percentage of the total number of episodes obtained with continuous intraoperative recording. (From London MJ, Hollenberg M, Wong MG et al: *Anesthesiology* 69:232-241, 1988.)

premature ventricular contractions, ventricular tachycardia, and ventricular fibrillation. Because monitoring patients with cardiac disease often includes more than ECG monitoring, it is important to observe the waveform and pressure measurement of other hemodynamic monitors such as direct arterial, central venous, and PA catheters. This additional information is valuable for determining whether the dysrhythmia requires prompt or aggressive treatment with either pharmacologic or electrical cardioversion therapy.

Delays or interruptions in transmission of the electrical impulse through the conduction system of the heart produce conduction defects that are classified according to the site of the block. A conduction defect that involves the pathway between the sinus node and ventricles is an AV block. First-degree AV block is a delayed transmission of the sinus impulse that results in a PR interval longer than 0.2 second. Second-degree AV block is an interruption of some, but not all, of the atrial impulses to the ventricles. Progressive lengthening of the PR interval until an impulse is not conducted characterizes a Mobitz Type I AV block. A Mobitz Type II AV block is also manifested by intermittent interruption of atrial impulses to the ventricles, but lacks the progressive lengthening of the PR interval. This block is a more ominous type of AV block because of its propensity to progress to complete heart block. Third-degree heart block (complete heart block) is an interruption of all atrial impulses to the ventricles. Atrial and ventricular depolarizations are observed on the ECG, but they are not related to each other. Intraventricular conduction defects comprise the conduction defects within the bundle branches or fascicles, including left and right bundle-branch blocks and left anterior and posterior fascicular blocks.

ECG artifacts are relatively common in the operative environment because of interference caused by medical equipment and surgical procedures. Application of surgical sterilization solutions can mimic ventricular tachycardia or fibrillation with vigorous application. Prep solution or blood spilled onto the ECG electrodes, causing a loss of skin contact by the electrodes, may give the appearance of asystole on the ECG monitor. Automated fluid pumps used during arthroscopic surgery can create ECG artifacts that mimic atrial flutter or fibrillation.[134] The possibility of ECG rhythm artifacts in the operating room emphasize the importance of integrating information from all available monitors and the patient before initiating unnecessary therapy.

PULSE OXIMETRY

Pulse oximetry is a very valuable monitor for all patients undergoing anesthesia and surgery. High-quality pulse oximeter readings, obtained from the cardiac patient in particular, suggest good distal perfusion, adequate CO, and sufficient oxygen delivery. Oxygen delivery is the product of arterial oxygen content and CO, as shown by the following equation:

$$O_2 \text{ delivery} = [(0.0134 \times Hgb \times Sa_{O_2}) + (0.0031 \times Pa_{O_2})] \times \text{Cardiac Output}$$

where *Hgb* is hemoglobin concentration, Sa_{O_2} is arterial oxygen saturation, and Pa_{O_2} is the partial pressure of oxygen in arterial blood. Ninety-eight percent of the oxygen in arterial blood is bound to hemoglobin, whereas the remaining two percent is dissolved in plasma. Hemoglobin concentration and Sa_{O_2} are therefore the two most important factors for determining arterial oxygen content. Decreased arterial oxygen saturation is compensated by increased CO to maintain oxygen delivery to the tissues. Patients with limited cardiac reserve may not be able to increase their CO and are therefore at risk of inadequate tissue oxygenation, leading to acidosis and further myocardial dysfunction. The main problem with pulse oximeter monitoring is that decreased oxygenation is not detected until the Sa_{O_2} falls below 100%, which corresponds to a Pa_{O_2} of 100 mm Hg. A decrease in Pa_{O_2} from 300 to 100 mm Hg will not be detected by pulse oximeter monitoring because both values yield a Sa_{O_2} of 100%. The Sa_{O_2} declines rapidly with changes in Pa_{O_2} below 60 mm Hg (Fig. 3-25).

A sensor containing two light-emitting diodes and a photodetector are used to determine oxygen saturation. Two wavelengths of light (red and infrared) are used in this method of transmission spectrophotometry, based on the principle that oxygenated hemoglobin absorbs more infrared light than reduced (deoxygenated) hemoglobin, whereas reduced hemoglobin absorbs 10 times as much red light as oxyhemoglobin[135] (Fig. 3-26). Signal processing of the optically transmitted data accounts for the absorption of light by tissue and venous and capillary blood to determine the concentration of oxyhemoglobin in arterial blood. Two wavelengths of light are useful for differentiating all four species of hemoglobin (oxyhemoglobin, reduced hemoglobin, methemoglobin, and carboxyhemoglobin), because methemoglobin absorbs red light to a similar degree as reduced hemoglobin, whereas carboxyhemoglobin absorbs red light to a similar degree as oxyhemoglobin. However, all four species of hemoglobin are differentiated by their differing absorption of infrared light[135] (Fig. 3-26). Hemoglobin saturation provided via blood gas analysis uses a cooximeter with multiple wavelengths to identify each hemoglobin species and provide a value for *fractional oxygen saturation* (Sa_{O_2}) of hemoglobin[135] based on the following equation:

$$Sa_{O_2} = \frac{O_2 Hgb}{O_2 Hgb + RHgb + COHgb + MetHgb + SHgb} \times 100$$

where O_2Hgb is oxyhemoglobin, *RHgb* is reduced hemoglobin, *COHgb* is carboxyhemoglobin, *MetHgb* is methemoglobin, and *SHgb* is sulfhemoglobin.

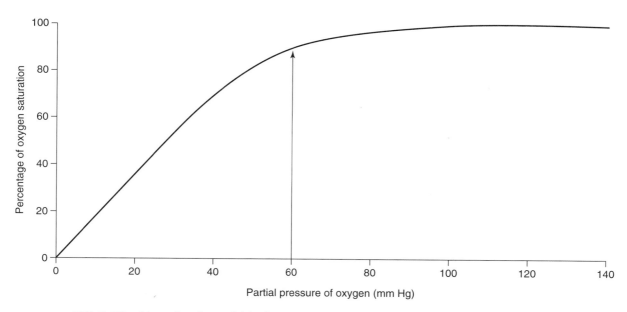

FIG. 3-25 Normal oxyhemoglobin dissociation curve indicating 100% oxygen saturation with partial pressures of oxygen exceeding 100 mm Hg. Saturation declines abruptly as the partial pressure of oxygen decreases below 60 mm Hg.

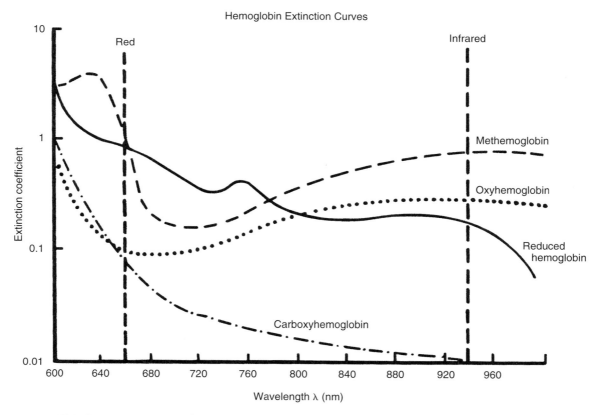

FIG. 3-26 Transmitted light absorbance spectra of four hemoglobin species: oxyhemoglobin, reduced hemoglobin, carboxyhemoglobin, and methemoglobin.

(From Tremper KK, Barker SJ: *Anesthesiology* 70:98-108, 1989. Adapted originally from Barker SJ, Tremper KK: *Int Anesthesiol Clin* 25:155-175, 1987.)

A pulse oximeter that does not differentiate oxyhemoglobin from carboxyhemoglobin and reduced hemoglobin from methemoglobin provides a value termed *functional oxygen saturation* (Spo_2) as follows:

$$Spo_2 = \frac{O_2Hgb}{O_2Hgb + RHgb} \times 100$$

As indicated by the equations, Spo_2 is a greater value than the Sao_2 in the presence of other hemoglobin species. A pulse oximeter that does not recognize other hemoglobin species assumes that the other hemoglobin species are oxyhemoglobin, thereby overestimating the actual oxygen saturation of hemoglobin. This difference is small in the absence of other hemoglobin species and can be ignored for clinical management. This difference may be significant, however, in the presence of methemoglobin, carboxyhemoglobin, or sulfhemoglobin. Arterial blood gas analysis should be performed in such clinical situations to establish the relation between Spo_2 and Sao_2.

Pulse oximetry has a high (31%) incidence of failure among cardiac surgical patients. Hypothermia, hypotension, and hypertension are independent *intraoperative* risk factors of failure,[136] whereas cardiac surgery and patients with an ASA physical status of 3, 4, or 5 are independent *preoperative* predictors of failure. Some systems provide the ability to observe a plethysmograph tracing in addition to the digital display of the oxygen saturation. This tracing is useful for determining the accuracy of the digital display. A good tracing with poor oxygen saturation is more worrisome than the same saturation with a poor tracing. A poor tracing may be more indicative of inaccurate data collection rather than poor saturation. Significant oxygen desaturation is often apparent by visual inspection of the patient. This reliable human monitor of oxygenation must not be forgotten.

Another source of pulse oximeter error is the use of certain vital dyes. Isosulfan blue, a patent blue dye used in identification of the sentinel lymph node, alters the light absorbency of blood and causes pulse oximeter desaturation, which may be interpreted as arterial desaturation.[137,138] Long-term ingestion of metoclopramide is a cause of sulfhemoglobinemia. The presence of this abnormal species of hemoglobin and methemoglobinemia interferes with pulse oximeter readings by affecting the ratio of light absorbencies at the two wavelengths used by the oximeter[139] (Fig. 3-26).

Two novel approaches to pulse oximeter monitoring were recently described. Both employed the use of a disposable pediatric pulse oximeter probe. One technique attached the probe to the left lateral surface of a tracheal tube cuff,[140] whereas the other attached the probe to the back plate of a size 5 LMA.[141] Both approaches were feasible and reported more accurate readings than finger oximetry when compared with arterial blood samples. The recently introduced Masimo Signal Extraction Technology (Masimo SET; Masimo Corporation, Irvine, Calif.) was designed to minimize the effects of artifacts on pulse oximeter readings and provide continuous Spo_2 data, thus reducing the incidence of false alarms. Noise artifacts associated with movement and low perfusion are mathematically manipulated in their proprietary algorithm. A recent comparison between this new technology and conventional pulse oximetry demonstrated a similar incidence and duration of data dropouts, but a reduction in the incidence and duration of false alarms with Masimo SET. The incidence of true alarms was more common with Masimo SET as compared with conventional pulse oximetry.[142]

TEMPERATURE MONITORING

Temperature monitoring is an important aspect of the anesthetic management of the patient with cardiac disease. Hypothermia causes shivering, which increases oxygen demand in the tissues, and vasoconstriction, which increases myocardial wall tension by increasing systemic vascular resistance. These responses to hypothermia are particularly deleterious postoperatively when hypertension and tachycardia resulting from pain are also common. Hyperthermia is less common than hypothermia, but can be associated with equally deleterious consequences in patients with cardiac disease. The best approach to the perioperative management of both hypothermia and hyperthermia is prevention. This requires accurate and reliable intraoperative temperature monitoring.

Core temperature is monitored during general anesthesia to detect hypothermia, prevent hyperthermia resulting from overzealous heating, and detect malignant hyperthermia. The "gold standard" of core temperature monitoring has become the thermistor at the distal end of a PA catheter that measures the temperature of blood in the pulmonary artery. Other monitoring sites for core temperature include the distal esophagus, nasopharynx, and tympanic membrane. These sites are considered core temperature because they have a rich blood supply and temperature is generally higher and more uniform than other monitoring sites within the body.[143] Core temperature monitoring is estimated with reasonable accuracy using bladder, rectal, axillary, and oral temperature probes.[143] These sites are not as reliable when temperature changes are rapid. Bladder temperature in particular is not reliable for detecting rapid changes when the urine output is low, but is similar to the pulmonary artery when urine output is high.[144] Skin temperatures are lower than core temperatures. The difference between skin and core temperature is unpredictable and affected by general anesthesia. Patients are at equal risk of developing hypothermia during spinal anesthesia as during general anesthesia, but patients under spinal anesthesia may remain hypothermic for longer periods.[145] Unfortunately, clinicians often do not monitor patients during regional anesthesia because they underestimate the incidence of hypothermia in these patients.[146] When clinicians do monitor temperature during regional anesthesia, they often monitor skin or axillary temperature.[147] Skin temperature monitoring during spinal anesthesia underestimates core temperature, whereas rectal temperature monitoring is a more accurate and precise method of estimating core temperature during spinal anesthesia.[145]

Although mild hypothermia has beneficial effects in terms of neuronal protection during ischemic events, hypothermia may increase myocardial ischemia[148] and mortality.[149] Ventricular irritability increases at temperatures below 32° C, and cardiac arrest is likely at temperatures below 28° C. The perioperative maintenance of normothermia in patients with cardiac risk factors undergoing noncardiac surgery is associated with a reduced incidence of morbid cardiac events and ventricular tachycardia.[150]

KEY POINTS

1. The degree of cardiovascular monitoring is generally predicated on both the medical condition of the patient and the nature of surgery.
2. The pressure at which Korotkoff sounds are first heard is the systolic blood pressure, whereas the pressure at which the sounds disappear is the diastolic blood pressure.
3. Variation exists as to when the systolic and diastolic blood pressures occur using automated NIBP devices. This determination is dependent on the technique and the proprietary algorithm of each automated system.
4. Patients undergoing surgery with unstable angina, recent myocardial infarction, active congestive heart failure, severe valvular heart disease, and shock require invasive blood pressure monitoring, except for minor surgical procedures. Surgical procedures that involve aortic cross-clamping, cardiac surgery, large fluid shifts, massive blood loss, or induced hypotension also require intraarterial monitoring.
5. There are five components to a normal CVP tracing that occur during each cardiac cycle: three waves or peaks and two descents or downward deflections. Each component reflects a cardiac event that causes a particular peak or descent.
6. The RIJ vein is commonly used during anesthesia because of its accessibility during many surgical procedures, direct route into the right atrium, and predictable location. Unintentional puncture of surrounding structures accounts for the most serious complications of this technique.
7. Ultrasound-guided placement of central venous catheters improves success and decreases the complications associated with internal jugular and subclavian vein cannulation.
8. The most serious and potentially life-threatening complication of internal jugular vein cannulation is arterial puncture. Real-time ultrasound-guided cannulation provides imaging of the internal jugular vein and carotid artery, directs placement of the cannulating needle at a level in the neck with mini-

mal vessel overlap, monitors compression of the vein during needle advancement, and determines depth of insertion to minimize puncture of an underlying carotid artery.
9. The ASA Task Force on Pulmonary Artery Catheterization recommended use of PA catheters in surgeries associated with an increased risk because of complications from hemodynamic changes, and by clinicians competent in safe insertion and accurate interpretation of the data provided.[78]
10. Although the incidence of complete heart block during PA catheterization of patients with previous LBBB is not higher than the incidence of RBBB in patients without underlying conduction defects, placement of a pulmonary artery catheter in patients with a preexisting LBBB is not recommended unless precautions are taken in anticipation of complete heart block.[85,86]
11. Cardiac output measurements are more precise when a 10-ml volume is injected at room temperature or 0° C. Thermodilution cardiac output is underestimated within the first 10 minutes[97] and the effects of the ventilatory cycle are more pronounced during the first 30 minutes following cardiopulmonary bypass.[98]
12. Although cardiac output is one determinant of mixed venous saturation, SV_{O_2} is also affected by oxygen carrying capacity and metabolic demand of the tissues. SV_{O_2} is therefore a better indicator of tissue oxygenation than cardiac output measurement alone.
13. Probably the most common complication of PA catheter use is misinterpretation of the data generated. Errors in measurement can occur from improper calibration of the transducer, improper positioning of the catheter tip, failure to consider the effects of mechanical ventilation, artifacts, and unrecognized catheter migration.
14. Changes in the ST segment and the T wave provide an early indication of myocardial ischemia, second only to wall motion abnormalities in time of onset. Computerized analysis of the ST segment is a more

reliable method of detecting ECG ischemia than visual inspection, but is dependent on the accuracy of the ECG tracing and the algorithms and filters used.[125]

15. Lead V_5 has the greatest sensitivity (75%) for detecting ischemia, followed by lead V_4 (61%). Monitoring two leads simultaneously yields a sensitivity of 80% if leads II and V_5 are monitored, 82% if leads II and V_4 are monitored, and 90% if leads V_4 and V_5 are monitored. A three-lead system that combines leads II, V_4, and V_5 increases the sensitivity to 96%.[121]

16. Pulse oximetry has a high (31%) incidence of failure among cardiac surgical patients. Hypothermia, hypotension, and hypertension are independent *intraoperative* risk factors of failure,[136] whereas cardiac surgery and patients with an ASA physical status of 3, 4, or 5 are independent *preoperative* predictors of failure.

17. The perioperative maintenance of normothermia in patients with cardiac risk factors undergoing noncardiac surgery is associated with a reduced incidence of morbid cardiac events and ventricular tachycardia.[150]

KEY REFERENCES

Amar D, Melendez JA, Zhang H et al: Correlation of peripheral venous pressure and central venous pressure in surgical patients, *J Cardiothorac Vasc Anesth* 15:40-43, 2001.

Eisenberg MJ, London MJ, Leung JM et al: Monitoring for myocardial ischemia during noncardiac surgery. A technology assessment of transesophageal echocardiography and 12-lead electrocardiography. The Study of Perioperative Ischemia Research Group, *JAMA* 268:210-216, 1992.

English IC, Frew RM, Pigott JF et al: Percutaneous catheterisation of the internal jugular vein, *Anaesthesia* 24:521-531, 1969.

Fleisher LA: Real-time intraoperative monitoring of myocardial ischemia in noncardiac surgery, *Anesthesiology* 92:1183-1188, 2000.

Gravlee GP, Wong AB, Adkins TG et al: A comparison of radial, brachial, and aortic pressures after cardiopulmonary bypass, *J Cardiothorac Anesth* 3:20-26, 1989.

Kirkendall WM, Feinleib M, Freis ED et al: Recommendations for human blood pressure determination by sphygmomaneters, *Stroke* 12:555A-564A, 1981.

Iberti TJ, Fischer EP, Leibowitz AB et al: A multicenter study of physicians' knowledge of the pulmonary artery catheter. Pulmonary Artery Catheter Study Group, *JAMA* 264:2928-2932, 1990.

Jobes DR, Ellison N, Troianos CA: Complications and failures of subclavian-vein catheterization, *N Engl J Med* 332:1579-1580, 1995.

Jobes DR, Schwartz AJ, Greenhow DE et al: Safer jugular vein cannulation: recognition of arterial puncture and preferential use of the external jugular route, *Anesthesiology* 59:353-355, 1983.

London MJ, Hollenberg M, Wong MG et al: Intraoperative myocardial ischemia: localization by continuous 12-lead electrocardiography, *Anesthesiology* 69:232-241, 1988.

Mark JB: *Atlas of cardiovascular monitoring*, New York, 1998, Churchill Livingston.

Mark JB: Central venous pressure monitoring: clinical insights beyond the numbers, *J Cardiothorac Vasc Anesth* 5:163-173, 1991.

Pearl RG, Rosenthal MH, Nielson L et al: Effect of injectate volume and temperature on thermodilution cardiac output determination, *Anesthesiology* 64:798-801, 1986.

American Society of Anesthesiologists Task Force on Pulmonary Artery Catheterization: Practice guidelines for pulmonary artery catheterization, *Anesthesiology* 78:380-394, 1993.

Randolph AG, Cook DJ, Gonzales CA et al: Ultrasound guidance for placement of central venous catheters: a meta-analysis of the literature, *Crit Care Med* 24:2053-2058, 1996.

Reich DL, Timcenko A, Bodian CA et al: Predictors of pulse oximetry data failure, *Anesthesiology* 84:859-864, 1996.

Rosen M, Latto P, Ng S: *Handbook of percutaneous central venous catheterisation*, London, 1992, WB Saunders.

Swan HJ, Ganz W, Forrester J et al: Catheterization of the heart in man with use of a flow-directed balloon-tipped catheter, *N Engl J Med* 283:447-451, 1970.

Thomson IR, Dalton BC, Lappas DG et al: Right bundle-branch block and complete heart block caused by the Swan-Ganz catheter, *Anesthesiology* 51:359-362, 1979.

Tremper KK, Barker SJ: Pulse oximetry, *Anesthesiology* 70:98-108, 1989.

Troianos CA, Jobes DR, Ellison N: Ultrasound-guided cannulation of the internal jugular vein. A prospective, randomized study, *Anesth Analg* 72:823-826, 1991.

Troianos CA, Kuwik RJ, Pasqual JR et al: Internal jugular vein and carotid artery anatomic relation as determined by ultrasonography, *Anesthesiology* 85:43-48, 1996.

Troianos CA, Stypula RW Jr: Transesophageal echocardiographic diagnosis of pulmonary artery catheter entrapment and coiling, *Anesthesiology* 79:602-604, 1993.

Tuman KJ, McCarthy RJ, Spiess BD et al: Effect of pulmonary artery catheterization on outcome in patients undergoing coronary artery surgery, *Anesthesiology* 70:199-206, 1989.

References*

1. Kirkendall WM, Feinleib M, Freis ED, et al: Recommendations for human blood pressure determination by sphygmomaneters, *Stroke* 12:555A-564A, 1981.
2. Korotkoff NS: On the subject of methods of determining blood pressure, *Bull Imperial Med Acad* 11:365, 1905.
3. Kirkendall WM, Burton AC, Epstein FH et al: Recommendations for human blood pressure determination by sphygmomaneters, *Circulation* 36:980, 1967.
4. Ramsey M: Blood pressure monitoring: automated oscillometric devices, *J Clin Monit* 7:56-67,1991.
5. Hernandez A, Goldring D, Hartman AF: Measurement of blood pressure in infants and children by the Doppler ultrasound technique, *Pediatrics* 48:788, 1971.
6. Borow KM, Newburger JW: Noninvasive estimation of central aortic pressure using the oscillometric method for analyzing systemic artery pulsatile blood flow: comparative study of indirect systolic, diastolic, and mean brachial artery pressure with simultaneous direct ascending aortic pressure measurements, *Am Heart J* 103:879-86, 1982.
7. Bruner JM, Krenis LJ, Kunsman JM et al: Comparison of direct and indirect measuring arterial blood pressure, *Med Instrum* 15: 11-21, 97-101, 182-188, 1981.
8. Gravlee GP, Brockschmidt JK: Accuracy of four indirect methods of blood pressure measurement, with hemodynamic correlations, *J Clin Monit* 6:284-298, 1990.
9. Yelderman M, Ream AK: Indirect measurement of mean blood pressure in the anesthetized patient, *Anesthesiology* 50:253-256, 1979.
10. Mark JB: *Atlas of cardiovascular monitoring*, New York, 1998, Churchill Livingston.
11. Boehmer RD: Continuous, real-time, noninvasive monitor of blood pressure: Penaz methodology applied to the finger, *J Clin Monit* 3:282-287, 1987.
12. Gravlee GP, Wong AB, Adkins TG et al: A comparison of radial, brachial, and aortic pressures after cardiopulmonary bypass, *J Cardiothorac Anesth* 3:20-26, 1989.
13. Pauca AL, Wallenhaupt SL, Kon ND et al: Does radial artery pressure accurately reflect aortic pressure? *Chest* 102:1193-1198, 1992.
14. O'Rourke MF: What is blood pressure? *Am J Hypertens* 3:803-810, 1990.
15. O'Rourke MF, Kelly RP: Wave reflection in the systemic circulation and its implications in ventricular function, *J Hypertens* 11:327-337, 1993.
16. Soderstrom S, Sellgren J, Ponten J: Aortic and radial pulse contour: different effects of nitroglycerin and prostacyclin, *Anesth Analg* 89:566-572, 1999.
17. Kreisler NS, Stone DJ, Spiekermann BF: Radial to femoral arterial pressure gradient from massive ascites, *Anesthesiology* 92:1508, 2000.
18. Mozersky DJ, Buckley CJ, Hagood CO Jr et al: Ultrasonic evaluation of the palmar circulation. A useful adjunct to radial artery cannulation, *Am J Surg* 126:810-812, 1973.
19. Cable DG, Mullany CJ, Schaff HV: The Allen test, *Ann Thorac Surg* 67:876-877, 1999.
20. Fuhrman TM, Pippin WD, Talmage LA et al: Evaluation of collateral circulation of the hand, *J Clin Monit* 8:28-32, 1992.
21. Slogoff S, Keats AS, Arlund C: On the safety of radial artery cannulation, *Anesthesiology* 59:42-47, 1983.
22. Mangano DT, Hickey RF: Ischemic injury following uncomplicated radial artery catheterization, *Anesth Analg* 58:55-57, 1979.
23. Rose SH: Ischemic complications of radial artery cannulation: an association with a calcinosis, Raynaud's phenomenon, esophageal dysmotility, sclerodactyly, and telangiectasia variant of scleroderma, *Anesthesiology* 78:587-589, 1993.
24. Rehfeldt KH, Sanders MS: Digital gangrene after radial artery catheterization in a patient with thrombocytosis, *Anesth Analg* 90:45-46, 2000.
25. Lowenstein E, Little JW 3rd, Lo HH: Prevention of cerebral embolization from flushing radial-artery cannulas, *N Engl J Med* 285:1414-1415, 1971.
26. Mangar D, Thrush DN, Connell GR et al: Direct or modified Seldinger guide wire-directed technique for arterial catheter insertion, *Anesth Analg* 76:714-717, 1993.
27. Mark JB: Central venous pressure monitoring: clinical insights beyond the numbers, *J Cardiothorac Vasc Anesth* 5:163-173, 1991.
28. Jobes DR, Schwartz AJ, Greenhow DE et al: Safer jugular vein cannulation: recognition of arterial puncture and preferential use of the external jugular route, *Anesthesiology* 59:353-355, 1983.
29. Rosen M, Latto P, Ng S: *Handbook of percutaneous central venous catheterisation*, London, 1992, WB Saunders.
30. McEnany MT, Austen WG: Life-threatening hemorrhage from inadvertent cervical arteriotomy, *Ann Thorac Surg* 24:233-236, 1977.
31. Wisheart JD, Hassan MA, Jackson JW: A complication of percutaneous cannulation of the internal jugular vein, *Thorax* 27:496-499, 1972.
32. English IC, Frew RM, Pigott JF et al: Percutaneous catheterisation of the internal jugular vein, *Anaesthesia* 24:521-531, 1969.
33. Prince SR, Sullivan RL, Hackel A: Percutaneous catheterization of the internal jugular vein in infants and children, *Anesthesiology* 44:170-174, 1976.
34. Metz S, Horrow JC, Balcar I: A controlled comparison of techniques for locating the internal jugular vein using ultrasonography, *Anesth Analg* 63:673-679, 1984.
35. Boulanger M, Delva E, Mailleet et al: A new way of access into the internal jugular vein, *Can Anaesth Soc J* 23:609-615, 1976.
36. Brinkman AJ, Costley DO. Internal jugular venipuncture, *JAMA* 223:182-183, 1973.
37. Mostert JW, Kenny GM, Murphy GP: Safe placement of central venous catheter into internal jugular veins, *Arch Surg* 101: 431-432, 1970.
38. Civetta JM, Gabel JC: Flow directed-pulmonary artery catheterization in surgical patients: indications and modifications of technic, *Ann Surg* 176:753-756, 1972.
39. Jernigan WR, Gardner WC, Mahr MM et al: The internal jugular vein for access to the central venous system, *JAMA* 218:97-98, 1971.
40. Wu X, Studer W, Erb T et al: Competence of the internal jugular vein valve is damaged by cannulation and catheterization of the internal jugular vein, *Anesthesiology* 93:319-324, 2000.
41. Hayashi H, Ootaki C, Tsuzuku M et al: Respiratory jugular venodilation: a new landmark for right internal jugular vein puncture in ventilated patients, *J Cardiothorac Vasc Anesth* 14:40-44, 2000.
42. Hayashi H, Ootaki C, Tsuzuku M et al: Respiratory jugular venodilation: its anatomic rationale as a landmark for right internal jugular vein puncture as determined by ultrasonography, *J Cardiothorac Vasc Anesth* 14:425-427, 2000.
43. Troianos CA, Jobes DR, Ellison N: Ultrasound-guided cannulation of the internal jugular vein. A prospective, randomized study, *Anesth Analg* 72:823-826, 1991.
44. Randolph AG, Cook DJ, Gonzales CA et al: Ultrasound guidance for placement of central venous catheters: a meta-analysis of the literature, *Crit Care Med* 24:2053-2058, 1996.

*The author thanks Peggy Flynn and Barbara Shawhan for their help with the references.

45. Verghese ST, McGill WA, Patel RI et al: Ultrasound-guided internal jugular venous cannulation in infants: a prospective comparison with the traditional palpation method, *Anesthesiology* 91:71-77, 1999.
46. Lin BS, Huang TP, Tang GJ et al: Ultrasound-guided cannulation of the internal jugular vein for dialysis vascular access in uremic patients, *Nephron* 78:423-428, 1998.
47. Gordon AC, Saliken JC, Johns D et al: US-guided puncture of the internal jugular vein: complications and anatomic considerations, *J Vasc Interv Radiol* 9:333-338, 1998.
48. Slama M, Novara A, Safavian A et al: Improvement of internal jugular vein cannulation using an ultrasound-guided technique, *Intensive Care Med* 23:916-919, 1997.
49. Farrell J, Gellens M: Ultrasound-guided cannulation versus the landmark-guided technique for acute haemodialysis access, *Nephrol Dial Transplant* 12:1234-1237, 1997.
50. Gilbert TB, Seneff MG, Becker RB: Facilitation of internal jugular venous cannulation using an audio-guided Doppler ultrasound vascular access device: results from a prospective, dual-center, randomized, crossover clinical study, *Crit Care Med* 23:60-65, 1995.
51. Gratz I, Afshar M, Kidwell P et al: Doppler-guided cannulation of the internal jugular vein: a prospective, randomized trial, *J Clin Monit* 10:185-188, 1994.
52. Denys BG, Uretsky BF, Reddy PS: Ultrasound-assisted cannulation of the internal jugular vein. A prospective comparison to the external landmark-guided technique, *Circulation* 87:1557-1562, 1993.
53. Mallory DL, McGee WT, Shawker TH et al: Ultrasound guidance improves the success rate of internal jugular vein cannulation. A prospective, randomized trial, *Chest* 98:157-160, 1990.
54. Troianos CA, Savino JS: Internal jugular vein cannulation guided by echocardiography, *Anesthesiology* 74:787-789, 1991.
55. Mansfield PF, Hohn DC, Fornage BD et al: Complications and failures of subclavian-vein catheterization, *N Engl J Med* 331:1735-1738, 1994.
56. Gualtieri E, Deppe SA, Sipperly ME et al: Subclavian venous catheterization: greater success rate for less experienced operators using ultrasound guidance, *Crit Care Med* 23:692-697, 1995.
57. Vucevic M, Tehan B, Gamlin F et al: The SMART needle. A new Doppler ultrasound-guided vascular access needle, *Anaesthesia* 49:889-891, 1994.
58. Jobes DR, Ellison N, Troianos CA: Complications and failures of subclavian-vein catheterization, *N Engl J Med* 332:1579-1580, 1995.
59. Troianos CA, Kuwik RJ, Pasqual JR et al: Internal jugular vein and carotid artery anatomic relation as determined by ultrasonography, *Anesthesiology* 85:43-48, 1996.
60. Castelli P: Cardiac tamponade resulting from attempted internal jugular vein catheterization, *J Cardiothorac Vasc Anesth* 11:195-196, 1997.
61. Johnson FE: Internal jugular vein catheterization, *N Y State J Med* 78:2168-2171, 1978.
62. Morgan RN, Morrell DF: Internal jugular catheterization. A review of a potentially lethal hazard, *Anaesthesia* 36:512-517, 1981.
63. Petty C: An alternate method for internal jugular venipuncture for monitoring central venous pressure, *Anesth Analg* 54:157, 1975.
64. Eckhardt WF, Iaconetti J, Kwon JS et al: Inadvertent carotid artery cannulation during pulmonary artery catheter insertion, *J Cardiothorac Vasc Anesth* 10:283-290, 1996.
65. Oliver WC Jr, Nuttall GA, Beynen FM et al: The incidence of artery puncture with central venous cannulation using a modified technique for detection and prevention of arterial cannulation, *J Cardiothorac Vasc Anesth* 11:851-855, 1997.
66. Ho AM, Chung DC, Tay BA et al: Diluted venous blood appears arterial: implications for central venous cannulation, *Anesth Analg* 91:1356-1357, 2000.
67. Maruyama K, Nakajima Y, Hayashi Y et al: A guide to preventing deep insertion of the cannulation needle during catheterization of the internal jugular vein, *J Cardiothorac Vasc Anesth* 11:192-194, 1997.
68. Ellison N, Jobes DR, Troianos CA: Internal jugular vein cannulation, *Anesth Analg* 78:198, 1994.
69. Ezri T, Szmuk P, Cohen Y et al: Carotid artery-internal jugular vein fistula: A complication of internal jugular vein catheterization, *J Cardiothorac Vasc Anesth* 15:231-232, 2001.
70. Oesterle JR, Reddy KS: Double arteriovenous fistula after internal jugular catheterization, *Am J Anesthesiol* 23:135-136, 1996.
71. Gobeil F, Couture P, Girard D et al: Carotid artery-internal jugular fistula: another complication following pulmonary artery catheterization via the internal jugular venous route, *Anesthesiology* 80:230-232, 1994.
72. Goss CM: The veins. In *Gray's anatomy*, Philadelphia, 1973, Lea & Febiger.
73. Sulek CA, Gravenstein N, Blackshear RH et al: Head rotation during internal jugular vein cannulation and the risk of carotid artery puncture, *Anesth Analg* 82:125-128, 1996.
74. Teal JS, Rumbaugh CL, Bergeron RT et al: Lateral position of the external carotid artery: a rare anomaly? *Radiology* 108:77-81, 1973.
75. Pandey JC, Dubey PK: A method for rapid clinical diagnosis of misplaced subclavian vein catheters, *Anesth Analg* 90:229, 2000.
76. Munis JR, Bhatia S, Lozada LJ: Peripheral venous pressure as a hemodynamic variable in neurosurgical patients, *Anesth Analg* 92:172-179, 2001.
77. Amar D, Melendez JA, Zhang H et al: Correlation of peripheral venous pressure and central venous pressure in surgical patients, *J Cardiothorac Vasc Anesth* 15:40-43, 2001.
78. American Society of Anesthesiologists Task Force on Pulmonary Artery Catheterization: Practice guidelines for pulmonary artery catheterization, *Anesthesiology* 78:380-394, 1993.
79. Tuman KJ, McCarthy RJ, Spiess BD et al: Effect of pulmonary artery catheterization on outcome in patients undergoing coronary artery surgery, *Anesthesiology* 70:199-206, 1989.
80. Iberti TJ, Fischer EP, Leibowitz AB et al: A multicenter study of physicians' knowledge of the pulmonary artery catheter. Pulmonary Artery Catheter Study Group, *JAMA* 264:2928-2932, 1990.
81. Ramsey SD, Saint S, Sullivan SD et al: Clinical and economic effects of pulmonary artery catheterization in nonemergent coronary artery bypass graft surgery, *J Cardiothorac Vasc Anesth* 14:113-118, 2000.
82. O'Connor PJ, Welsh KR, Cross MH et al: Cardiovascular responses to pulmonary artery catheterization, *Eur J Anaesthesiol* 17:168-172, 2000.
83. Keusch DJ, Winters S, Thys DM: The patient's position influences the incidence of dysrhythmias during pulmonary artery catheterization, *Anesthesiology* 70:582-584, 1989.
84. Benumof JL, Saidman LJ, Arkin DB et al: Where pulmonary arterial catheters go: intrathoracic distribution, *Anesthesiology* 46:336-338, 1977.
85. Sprung CL, Elser B, Schein RM et al: Risk of right bundle-branch block and complete heart block during pulmonary artery catheterization, *Crit Care Med* 17:1-3, 1989.
86. Thomson IR, Dalton BC, Lappas DG et al: Right bundle-branch block and complete heart block caused by the Swan-Ganz catheter, *Anesthesiology* 51:359-362, 1979.
87. Eissa NT, Kvetan V: Guide wire as a cause of complete heart block in patients with preexisting left bundle branch block, *Anesthesiology* 73:772-774, 1990.

88. Swan HJ, Ganz W, Forrester J et al: Catheterization of the heart in man with use of a flow-directed balloon-tipped catheter, *N Engl J Med* 283:447-451, 1970.

89. Forrester JS, Ganz W, Diamond G et al: Thermodilution cardiac output determination with a single flow-directed catheter, *Am Heart J* 83:306-311, 1972.

90. Ganz W, Donoso R, Marcus HS et al: A new technique for measurement of cardiac output by the thermodilution in man, *Am J Cardiol* 27:392-396, 1971.

91. Pearl RG, Rosenthal MH, Nielson L et al: Effect of injectate volume and temperature on thermodilution cardiac output determination, *Anesthesiology* 64:798-801, 1986.

92. Harris AP, Miller CF, Beattie C et al: The slowing of sinus rhythm during thermodilution cardiac output determination and the effect of altering injectate temperature, *Anesthesiology* 63:540-541, 1985.

93. Nishikawa T, Dohi S: Hemodynamic status susceptible to slowing of heart rate during thermodilution cardiac output determination in anesthetized patients, *Crit Care Med* 18:841-844, 1990.

94. Nelson LD, Houtchens BA: Automatic vs manual injections for thermodilution cardiac output determinations, *Crit Care Med* 10:190-192, 1982.

95. Stevens JH, Raffin TA, Mihm FG et al: Thermodilution cardiac output measurement. Effects of the respiratory cycle on its reproducibility, *JAMA* 253:2240-2242, 1985.

96. Wetzel RC, Latson TW: Major errors in thermodilution cardiac output measurement during rapid volume infusion, *Anesthesiology* 62:684-687, 1985.

97. Bazaral MG, Petre J, Novoa R: Errors in thermodilution cardiac output measurements caused by rapid pulmonary artery temperature decreases after cardiopulmonary bypass, *Anesthesiology* 77:31-37, 1992.

98. Latson TW, Whitten CW, O'Flaherty D: Ventilation, thermal noise, and errors in cardiac output measurements after cardiopulmonary bypass, *Anesthesiology* 79:1233-1243, 1993.

99. Bottiger BW, Rauch H, Bohrer H et al: Continuous versus intermittent cardiac output measurement in cardiac surgical patients undergoing hypothermic cardiopulmo bypass, *J Cardiothorac Vasc Anesth* 9:405-411, 1995.

100. Yelderman ML, Ramsay MA, Quinn MD et al: Continuous thermodilution cardiac output measurement in intensive care unit patients, *J Cardiothorac Vasc Anesth* 6:270-274, 1992.

101. Bongard F, Lee TS, Leighton T et al: Simultaneous in vivo comparison of two- versus three-wavelength mixed venous (SVO_2) oximetry catheters, *J Clin Monit* 11:329-334, 1995.

102. Hecker BR, Brown DL, Wilson D: A comparison of two pulmonary artery mixed venous oxygen saturation catheters during the changing conditions of cardiac surgery, *J Cardiothorac Anesth* 3:269-275, 1989.

103. Gettinger A, DeTraglia MC, Glass DD: In vivo comparison of two mixed venous saturation catheters, *Anesthesiology* 66:373-375, 1987.

104. Krouskop RW, Cabatu EE, Chelliah BP et al: Accuracy and clinical utility of an oxygen saturation catheter, *Crit Care Med* 11:744-749, 1983.

105. Katz JD, Cronau LH, Barash PG et al: Pulmonary artery flow-guided catheters in the perioperative period. Indications and complications, *JAMA* 237:2832-2834, 1977.

106. Connors AF Jr, Speroff T, Dawson NV et al: The effectiveness of right heart catheterization in the initial care of critically ill patients. SUPPORT Investigators, *JAMA* 276:889-897, 1996.

107. Iberti TJ, Benjamin E, Gruppi L et al: Ventricular arrhythmias during pulmonary artery catheterization in the intensive care unit. Prospective study, *Am J Med* 78:451-454, 1985.

108. Salmenpera M, Peltola K, Rosenberg P: Does prophylactic lidocaine control cardiac arrhythmias associated with pulmonary artery catheterization? *Anesthesiology* 56:210-212, 1982.

109. Hannan AT, Brown M, Bigman O: Pulmonary artery catheter-induced hemorrhage, *Chest* 85:128-131, 1984.

110. Stein JM, Lisbon A: Pulmonary hemorrhage from pulmonary artery catheterization treated with endobronchial intubation, *Anesthesiology* 55:698-699, 1981.

111. Carlson TA, Goldenberg IF, Murray PD et al: Catheter-induced delayed recurrent pulmonary artery hemorrhage. Intervention with therapeutic embolism of the pulmonary artery, *JAMA* 261:1943-1945, 1989.

112. Gourin A, Garzon AA: Operative treatment of massive hemoptysis, *Ann Thorac Surg* 18:52-60, 1974.

113. Boscoe MJ, de Lange S: Damage to the tricuspid valve with a Swann-Ganz catheter, *Br Med J* 283:346-347, 1981.

114. O'Toole JD, Wurtzbacher JJ, Wearner NE et al: Pulmonary-valve injury and insufficiency during pulmonary-artery catheterization, *N Engl J Med* 301:1167-1168, 1979.

115. Kainuma M, Yamada M, Miyake T: Pulmonary artery catheter passing between the chordae tendineae of the tricuspid valve, *Anesthesiology* 83:1130-1131, 1995.

116. Lipp H, O'Donoghue K, Resnekov L: Intracardiac knotting of a flow-directed balloon catheter, *N Engl J Med* 284:220, 1971.

117. Lindgren KM, McShane K, Roberts WC: Acute rupture of the pulmonic valve by a balloon-tipped catheter producing a musical diastolic murmur, *Chest* 81:251-253, 1982.

118. Troianos CA, Stypula RW Jr: Transesophageal echocardiographic diagnosis of pulmonary artery catheter entrapment and coiling, *Anesthesiology* 79:602-604, 1993.

119. Dasher LA, Slye DA: *ECG, arrhythmia, and ST segment analysis*, Redmond, Wash, 1994, SpaceLabs Medical, Inc.

120. Anderson ST, Downs WG, Lander P et al: *Advanced electrocardiography*, Redmond, Wash, 1994, SpaceLabs Medical, Inc.

121. London MJ, Hollenberg M, Wong MG et al: Intraoperative myocardial ischemia: localization by continuous 12-lead electrocardiography, *Anesthesiology* 69:232-241, 1988.

122. Surawicz B: U wave: facts, hypotheses, misconceptions, and misnomers, *J Cardiovasc Electrophysiol* 9:1117-1128, 1998.

123. Mangano DT, Hollenberg M, Fegert G et al: Perioperative myocardial ischemia in patients undergoing noncardiac surgery—I: Incidence and severity during the 4 day perioperative period. The Study of Perioperative Ischemia (SPI) Research Group, *J Am Coll Cardiol* 17:843-850, 1991.

124. Mangano DT, Wong MG, London MJ et al: Perioperative myocardial ischemia in patients undergoing noncardiac surgery—II: Incidence and severity during the 1st week after surgery. The Study of Perioperative Ischemia (SPI) Research Group, *J Am Coll Cardiol* 17:851-857, 1991.

125. Fleisher LA: Real-time intraoperative monitoring of myocardial ischemia in noncardiac surgery, *Anesthesiology* 92:1183-1188, 2000.

126. Tisdale LA, Drew BJ: ST segment monitoring for myocardial ischemia, *AACN Clin Issues Crit Care Nurs* 4:34-43, 1993.

127. Mathew JP, Fleisher LA, Rinehouse JA et al: ST segment depression during labor and delivery, *Anesthesiology* 77:635-641, 1992.

128. Fleisher LA, Zielski MM, Schulman SP: Perioperative ST-segment depression is rare and may not indicate myocardial ischemia in moderate-risk patients undergoing noncardiac surgery, *J Cardiothorac Vasc Anesth* 11:155-159, 1997.

129. Glantz L, Drenger B, Gozal Y: Perioperative myocardial ischemia in cataract surgery patients: general versus local anesthesia, *Anesth Analg* 91:1415-1419, 2000.

130. Leung JM, Weiskopf RB, Feiner J et al: Electrocardiographic ST-segment changes during acute, severe isovolemic hemodilution in humans, *Anesthesiology* 93:1004-1010, 2000.

131. Eisenberg MJ, London MJ, Leung JM et al: Monitoring for myocardial ischemia during noncardiac surgery. A technology assessment of transesophageal echocardiography and 12-lead electrocardiography. The Study of Perioperative Ischemia Research Group, *JAMA* 268:210-216, 1992.

132. Bertrand CA, Steiner NV, Jameson AG et al: Disturbances of cardiac rhythm during anesthesia and surgery, *JAMA* 216:1615-1617, 1971.

133. Sigurdsson GH, Carlsson C, Lindahl S et al: Cardiac arrhythmias in non-intubated children during adenoidectomy. A comparison between enflurane and halothane anaesthesia, *Acta Anaesthesiol Scand* 27:75-80, 1983.

134. Toyoyama H, Kariya N, Toyoda Y: Electrocardiographic artifacts during shoulder arthroscopy using a pressure-controlled irrigation pump, *Anesth Analg* 90:856-857, 2000.

135. Tremper KK, Barker SJ: Pulse oximetry, *Anesthesiology* 70:98-108, 1989.

136. Reich DL, Timcenko A, Bodian CA et al: Predictors of pulse oximetry data failure, *Anesthesiology* 84:859-864, 1996.

137. Vokach-Brodsky L, Jeffrey SS, Lemmens HJ et al: Isosulfan blue affects pulse oximetry, *Anesthesiology* 93:1002-1003, 2000.

138. Rizzi RR, Thomas K, Pilnik S: Factious desaturation due to isosulfan dye injection, *Anesthesiology* 93:1146-1147, 2000.

139. Aravindhan N, Chisholm DG: Sulfhemoglobinemia presenting as pulse oximetry desaturation, *Anesthesiology* 93:883-884, 2000.

140. Brimacombe J, Keller C, Margreiter J: A pilot study of left tracheal pulse oximetry, *Anesth Analg* 91:1003-1006, 2000.

141. Keller C, Brimacombe J, Agro F et al: A pilot study of pharyngeal pulse oximetry with the laryngeal mask airway: a comparison with finger oximetry and arterial saturation measurements in healthy anesthetized patients, *Anesth Analg* 90:440-444, 2000.

142. Malviya S, Reynolds PI, Voepel-Lewis T et al: False alarms and sensitivity of conventional pulse oximetry versus the Masimo SET technology in the pediatric postanesthesia care unit, *Anesth Analg* 90:13336-13340, 2000.

143. Cork RC, Vaughan RW, Humphrey LS: Precision and accuracy of intraoperative temperature monitoring, *Anesth Analg* 62:211-214, 1983.

144. Horrow JC, Rosenberg H: Does urinary catheter temperature reflect core temperature during cardiac surgery? *Anesthesiology* 69:986-989, 1988.

145. Cattaneo CG, Frank SM, Hesel TW et al: The accuracy and precision of body temperature monitoring methods during regional and general anesthesia, *Anesth Analg* 90:938-945, 2000.

146. Arkilic CF, Akca O, Taguchi A et al: Temperature monitoring and management during neuraxial anesthesia: an observational study, *Anesth Analg* 91:662-666, 2000.

147. Frank SM, Nguyen JM, Garcia CM et al: Temperature monitoring practices during regional anesthesia, *Anesth Analg* 88:373-377, 1999.

148. Frank SM, Beattie C, Christopherson R et al: Unintentional hypothermia is associated with postoperative myocardial ischemia. The Perioperative Ischemia Randomized Anesthesia Trial Study Group, *Anesthesiology* 78:468-476, 1993.

149. Slotman GJ, Jed EH, Burchard KW: Adverse effects of hypothermia in postoperative patients, *Am J Surg* 149:495-501, 1985.

150. Frank SM, Fleisher LA, Breslow MJ et al: Perioperative maintenance of normothermia reduces the incidence of morbid cardiac events. A randomized clinical trial, *JAMA* 277:1127-1134, 1997.

CHAPTER 4

Perioperative Transesophageal Echocardiography

Christopher A. Troianos, M.D.

OUTLINE

Transesophageal echocardiography (TEE) is a valuable clinical tool for the evaluation of cardiovascular anatomy, myocardial and valvular function, and hemodynamic abnormalities. Perioperative TEE provides definitive diagnoses that prompt surgical intervention, correction of inadequate surgical repair, and reoperation for complications. TEE is a reliable clinical monitor that provides valuable information for appropriate hemodynamic management before, during, and after general anesthesia. This chapter reviews the indications, contraindications, and technique of perioperative TEE in providing a comprehensive examination of cardiac and major vascular structures. Understanding the principles of ultrasound provides the basis for optimal image generation, recognition of artifacts, and interpretation of data. A cogent written report of echocardio-graphic findings, an essential component of the comprehensive TEE examination, communicates the findings to the patient and other health care professionals. The fundamental elements for providing a perioperative service are comprehensive training, ongoing education, maintenance of technical skills, quality review, and quality improvement.

INDICATIONS
Preoperative

The indication for preoperative TEE is to evaluate thoracic structures that are not adequately imaged with transthoracic echocardiography (TTE) to determine the need for surgical intervention, the surgical approach, and myocardial and valvular function. TEE provides superior image quality compared to TTE, particularly for posterior cardiac structures such as the left atrium, mitral valve, and thoracic aorta. Shadows and reverberations from a prosthetic mitral valve that obscure left atrial regurgitant jets, paravalvular leaks, and densities with the transthoracic approach are cast toward the left ventricular aspect of the mitral valve with the transesophageal approach. TEE is more sensitive than TTE for detecting paravalvular abscess in patients with endocarditis.[1] TEE is highly sensitive and specific for the diagnosis of aortic dissection, and provides a rapid and portable means of evaluating the type of aortic dissection, site of intimal tear, extent of dissection, and presence of associated complications. The echocardiographic findings for both of these examples determine the need for surgery.

Detailed evaluation of mitral valve anatomy and severity of regurgitation determine the feasibility of valve repair versus replacement. The etiology of the regurgitation dictates the surgical approach. For example, regurgitation from systolic anterior motion caused by hypertrophic obstructive cardiomyopathy is corrected by myomectomy via a transaortic approach, whereas regurgitation caused by a flail mitral leaflet is repaired via a transatrial approach. The etiology of regurgitation also dictates hemodynamic management during induction of anesthesia. The hemodynamic goals of mitral regurgitation resulting from systolic anterior motion (SAM) are to increase afterload and decrease contractility, whereas regurgitation resulting from a flail leaflet is managed by decreasing afterload and increasing contractility. Preoperative echocardiographic assessment permits appropriate surgical and anesthetic management and allows for rational use of intraoperative monitoring, including intravascular catheters and intraoperative TEE.

Penetrating chest trauma is another indication for preoperative TEE because of associated intracardiac or extracardiac shunts. Early and aggressive use of TEE to evaluate penetrating cardiac injuries can identify otherwise occult lesions that may lead to cardiac tamponade or death. Small defects not identified by TTE or angiography may be identified by TEE.[2,3]

Intraoperative

Cardiac Surgery

Advances in cardiac surgery for correction of mitral regurgitation during the 1980s led to an increase in mitral valve repair over replacement. This prompted the simultaneous need for a rapid, accurate, noninvasive method to evaluate the adequacy of the surgical repair intraoperatively. TEE replaced epicardial echocardiography when advances in ultrasound technology led to the development of TEE probes that no longer required interference with the surgical field. Another advantage to TEE over epicardial echocardiography was

the posterior approach to the mitral valve that permitted unobstructed Doppler analysis of regurgitant jets. This approach was particularly advantageous for the postimplantation evaluation of prosthetic valves for regurgitant lesions and paravalvular leaks.

TEE is used intraoperatively to confirm the presumptive preoperative surgical diagnosis, evaluate the success of the surgical intervention, and detect complications. The practice parameters for perioperative TEE published in 1996 comprised a comprehensive review of the literature and expert opinion.[4] Indications were divided into three categories based on expected usefulness of TEE.

TEE is invaluable during mitral valve repair. Before the surgeon makes an incision, the etiology of the mitral regurgitation is determined, the feasibility of repair is considered, and a surgical plan is formulated. Repair is preferred over replacement because of improved long-term outcome and decreased complications. Retention of the mitral valve apparatus supports left ventricular geometry and contributes to better myocardial contractility. Long-term anticoagulation is not required, thus eliminating the complications associated with anticoagulation and the need for lifelong coagulation monitoring. Myxoid degeneration is the most common cause of mitral regurgitation and is the most amenable to repair. It is important to recognize the etiology of regurgitation to determine the appropriate surgical correction and avoid potential complications. For example, a flail posterior leaflet segment isolated to the middle scallop is the easiest to repair and is associated with the highest success rate.[5] Valves with long redundant anterior and posterior leaflets and chordal elongation affecting both leaflets are at risk for developing SAM after repair. Mitral regurgitation resulting from rheumatic valvulitis is probably the most challenging to repair even in the most experienced hands.[5] After repair, TEE is used to assess the adequacy of repair by evaluating leaflet mobility and quantifying the degree of any residual mitral regurgitation. Transvalvular gradient and effective orifice size are used to evaluate the possibility of stenosis created by the repair.

TEE is used during cardiac surgery to direct cannulation of the coronary sinus for retrograde cardioplegia administration and cannulation of the aorta for cardiopulmonary bypass. TEE directs appropriate positioning of the intraaortic balloon distal to the origin of the left subclavian artery, femoral venous cannula in the right atrium, and special aortic perfusion cannula away from atheromatous plaques. TEE is essential during "port access" cardiac surgery that necessitates the placement of various catheters and cannulae via a percutaneous approach. Removal of intracardiac air before separation from cardiopulmonary bypass is assessed with TEE. Particular attention is given to removing "pockets" of air entrapped in the anterior aspect of cardiac chambers. Common sites for air to collect are the left ventricular apex along the septum, the anterior aspect of the left atrium posterior and to the right of the aortic valve, the left atrial appendage, pulmonary veins, and right coronary sinus of Valsalva.

Decreased ventricular and pulmonary compliance are common after cardiopulmonary bypass, making pulmonary arterial and central venous pressures unreliable indicators of volume status. It is not uncommon for filling pressures to be elevated despite hypovolemia when comparing post-bypass values to pre-bypass values. Patients with left ventricular hypertrophy are particularly vulnerable to discrepancies between post-bypass filling pressures, and volume. TEE is instrumental in guiding fluid therapy based on decreased end-diastolic volume at a time when an elevated pulmonary capillary wedge pressure (PCWP) would suggest hypervolemia. Contractility as determined by TEE is a more reliable indicator of cardiac function than cardiac output measurements. This is particularly true in the immediate post-bypass period when rewarming and reinstitution of pulsatile flow vary the temperature of the venous return, making thermodilution cardiac output measurements unreliable. TEE data are unaffected by these temperature changes because contractility is determined by wall thickening and myocardial excursion.

Noncardiac Surgery

Many elderly patients who undergo noncardiac surgery have coronary, valvular, or multiple cardiac risk factors that increase the incidence of cardiac morbidity and mortality. Physiologic monitors such as electrocardiography, pulmonary artery and central venous pressure monitoring, and arterial pressure monitoring provide useful information in managing the hemodynamic perturbations that occur perioperatively. These monitors have limitations for monitoring certain aspects of cardiac function, such as myocardial wall motion and valvular function. TEE is being used with increasing frequency in noncardiac surgical settings to monitor patients with known cardiac disease or multiple cardiac risk factors, or patients who are undergoing surgical procedures associated with increased cardiac complications (e.g., aortic cross clamping).

The settings in which TEE is used during noncardiac surgery are: (1) anticipated use as a monitor of known cardiac pathology, and (2) unanticipated use in patients suffering cardiac decompensation in which traditional monitors fail to elucidate the diagnosis. TEE has greater impact on the intraoperative management of older patients (>66 years) and patients classified as American Society of Anesthesiologists (ASA) Class 3 or 4 undergoing noncardiac surgery.[6] Table 4-1 summarizes new intraoperative TEE findings in a recent study that examined the use and impact of TEE in 123 patients undergoing noncardiac surgery. Intraoperative TEE had a major impact in 15% of patients, half of whom received treat-

TABLE 4-1 New Intraoperative Findings from TEE: 123 Exams during Noncardiac Surgery	
NEW FINDING	NO.
Patent foramen ovale	3
Global left ventricular dysfunction present on initial exam	12
Global left ventricular dysfunction developed during surgery	3
New regional wall-motion abnormality	2
Intraoperative venous air embolism	1
Right ventricular dysfunction	7
Pleural effusion	1
Absence of ventricular thrombus	1
Valve vegetation	1
Absence of valve vegetation	1
Pulmonary artery thrombus	3
Absence of severe aortic stenosis documented preoperatively	1
Moderate/severe aortic insufficiency	2
Ascending aortic enlargement	3
Mobile aortic plaque	1
Mild/moderate mitral regurgitation	20
Moderate tricuspid regurgitation	3

From Suriani RJ, Neustein S, Shore-Lesserson L et al: Intraoperative transesophageal echocardiography during noncardiac surgery, *J Cardiothorac Vasc Anesth* 12:274-280, 1998. Reproduced by permission.

ment for a potentially life-threatening event.[6] TEE provided information that altered the surgical procedure in two patients. An atrial septal defect was discovered by intraoperative TEE in an elderly patient undergoing total hip arthroplasty after presenting with acute oxygen desaturation.[7]

TEE is particularly useful in monitoring patients with dynamic valvular heart lesions. Functional mitral regurgitation (MR) and MR caused by hypertrophic obstructive cardiomyopathy vary considerably with changes in preload, afterload, and contractility. Precise monitoring of MR and the effects of hemodynamic management are directly assessed with TEE. Elevation of PCWP and decreasing cardiac output are indirect monitors of MR, volume, and contractility, whereas TEE provides a more direct assessment of SAM, septal-leaflet contact, mitral regurgitation, volume, and contractility.

The strong association between perioperative myocardial ischemia and cardiac morbidity, mortality, and long-term prognosis emphasizes the importance of detecting intraoperative episodes of myocardial ischemia.[8,9] Electrocardiography is the most commonly used and simplest intraoperative monitor of myocardial ischemia. Although visual inspection of ST-segment changes is a poor method for detecting ischemia,[10,11] the advent of intraoperative computerized analysis of the electrocardiogram (ECG) has greatly enhanced the ability to accurately and continuously monitor the ECG for ischemia.[12] False-positive ST-segment changes occur because of drug effects, conduction abnormalities, left ventricular hypertrophy, and prior myocardial infarction. An acute increase in PCWP is another indicator of intraoperative myocardial ischemia. This PCWP increase is dependent on a change in left ventricular compliance. Small areas of ischemia may not produce global changes in ventricular compliance, thus reducing sensitivity. Conversely, acute increases in afterload or MR increase PCWP in the absence of myocardial ischemia, thus reducing specificity.

A new regional wall-motion abnormality (RWMA) detected by TEE is considered the earliest sign of myocardial ischemia, making it a more sensitive monitor than the ECG or PCWP. In a study of patients with known coronary artery disease, TEE detected myocardial ischemia more reliably than ECG, even in the absence of hemodynamic perturbations. Persistent wall-motion abnormalities were associated with an adverse outcome in 33% of patients.[13] Limitations to routine use of TEE as an ischemia monitor are false-positives, and the requirements of general anesthesia, expensive equipment, and continuously available specially trained personnel. TEE has minimal additive value over two-lead ECG for detecting ischemia during noncardiac surgery, as demonstrated by a study of 285 high-risk patients, monitored with TEE, 2-lead ECG, and 12-lead ECG.[14] Ten cardiac events occurred in this study, but only one additional cardiac event would have been detected by TEE compared with ECG alone.

Venous air embolism is a risk during any procedure in which the operative field is above the level of the heart. One example is the patient undergoing posterior fossa craniotomy in the sitting position. TEE can be used intraoperatively as a sensitive monitor of venous air embolism and for positioning a right atrial aspiration catheter.[15] The more important role for TEE is for identifying intracardiac defects in patients at risk for venous air embolism and potential paradoxical air embolism to the left heart. Detection of a patent foramen ovale by TEE before incision allows for alterations in the patient's position to minimize the risk of venous air embolism. The likelihood of significant paradoxical air embolism not detected by intraoperative TEE monitoring is remote.[16] Intraoperative TEE during laparoscopic nephrectomy is used to monitor gas embolism, but is more likely to detect changes in tricuspid valve regurgitation.[17]

The incidence of venous embolism during lower extremity surgery performed with a pneumatic tourniquet is relatively common (26%).[18] TEE is useful for detecting venous emboli after tourniquet deflation, but the clinical significance of these events is unclear. Echogenic material resembling fat globules is embolized during placement of intramedullary nails after orthopedic fractures, but not all patients with large emboli detected by TEE develop fat embolism syndrome.[19] Again, the significance is unclear. TEE during surgery for removal of renal cell carcinoma with intracaval extension is indicated to determine the extent of tumor involvement, hemodynamic management, and monitoring for unintentional embolization. TEE detects potentially life-threatening obstruction of the tricuspid valve by tumor extension and prompts alterations in surgical technique.[20]

Endovascular procedures are becoming increasingly common for transaortic stent–grafting for the treatment of aortic aneurysm and dissection. TEE is used during thoracic aortic procedures to determine graft size, guide catheter placement, guide graft tailoring, and evaluate the operative results.[21]

TEE is useful during liver transplantation to detect embolization with allograft reperfusion, transpulmonary air passage, ventricular dysfunction, valvular regurgitation, and intracardiac defects.[22] TEE was used safely in 100 patients undergoing liver transplantation, despite the presence of esophageal varices in 23 patients, 7 of whom had not had variceal sclerotherapy. Coagulation defects were present in the majority of patients. No patient experienced documented variceal hemorrhage, esophageal or gastric perforation, or oropharyngeal trauma in a retrospective chart review.[22]

Pulmonary venous obstruction after lung transplantation is a rare but fatal cause of graft failure, particularly in single-lung transplant recipients.[23] Postoperative chest roentgenogram, perfusion scintigraphic scan, and pulmonary angiography lead clinicians to this diagnosis, but TEE provides real-time information intraoperatively, allowing prompt surgical correction before clinical decompensation.[23] TEE is particularly useful for imaging the right pulmonary artery and right pulmonary venous anastomoses. A pulmonary vein anastomosis diameter less than 0.25 cm can compromise perfusion of the grafted lung.[23] Cardiac transplantation imparts a "snowman" configuration on the left atrium, related to a prominent bulging suture line, but is usually not associated with hemodynamic impairment because of the large size of the atrial anastomosis.[24]

Postoperative

Pericardial effusions after cardiac surgery are "silent" in most (56%) patients. A small percentage subsequently develop cardiac tamponade (1% to 2.5%).[25] Transthoracic echocardiography is used to make the diagnosis of tamponade and guide percutaneous needle drainage in other settings. Conditions after cardiac surgery—such as mechanical ventilation, mediastinal air and drainage tubes, and surgical dressings—make TTE challenging and suboptimal. The transesophageal approach is unaffected by these obstructions and is easily performed in the intubated patient who has not emerged from general anesthesia.[26] TEE of the hypotensive patient quickly identifies the etiology of the hypotension (volume versus contractility) and determines the need for surgical intervention for tamponade, valvular dysfunction, or wall-motion abnormalities. Hypotension in the setting of normal or hypercontractility and adequate volume implies decreased systemic vascular resistance. Continuity in providing perioperative TEE services is encouraged. Postoperative TEE data are considered in the context of acute changes versus persistent intraoperative abnormalities when the postoperative TEE is performed by the intraoperative echocardiographer.

TEE is used after noncardiac surgery in the hemodynamically unstable patient who remains intubated. Mechanical ventilation may interfere with a TTE by hyperinflating the lungs. Extubated patients benefit from an initial assessment by TTE because of the less invasive nature of this procedure and the absence of mechanical ventilation.

CONTRAINDICATIONS AND TECHNIQUE
Contraindications

Contraindications to TEE are esophageal and gastric disorders manifested by impaired swallowing, hematemesis, melena, or recent gastric or esophageal surgery. Esophageal rupture is a risk for patients with stricture, diverticulum, or recent surgery, whereas bleeding is a risk for patients with esophageal tumors, unsclerosed varices, and ulcers. TEE is generally safe when performed properly.[27] The most common complications are sore throat, minor tissue and dental trauma, and damage to the probe. A padded bite block is useful in protecting the gums of edentulous patients under general anesthesia and protecting the probe from dentulous patients having a TEE performed with only intravenous sedation. TEE appears to be an independent risk factor for dysphagia after cardiac surgery.[28] Recurrent laryngeal nerve palsy is more likely to be related to the duration of surgery, cardiopulmonary bypass, and tracheal intubation than to placement of the TEE probe.[29] The probe should never be forced during insertion, manipulation, or withdrawal. Symptoms of esophageal perforation are masked in the anesthetized patient and delays in treatment increase morbidity and mortality.[30] More serious and fatal complications are rare, but have been reported.[31-35]

The complication rate of TEE performed in the emergency department (12.6%) is greater than TEE performed in other clinical settings.[36] An anesthesiologist should not attempt to simultaneously administer anesthesia and perform a TEE in the emergency department without the assistance of another anesthesia or medical provider who can administer and monitor sedation. Complications associated with TEE in this setting include respiratory insufficiency, emesis, agitation, hypotension, cardiac arrhythmias, and even death.[36] The patient with a full stomach and hypotension from a suspected aortic dissection may require invasive monitoring, rapid-sequence induction of anesthesia, and intubation before TEE.

Technique

The TEE probe is inspected for cracks, defects, cleanliness, and unlocked control wheels. Some manufacturers also recommend performing a test for electrical current leakage before each use. The probe is lubricated with ultrasonic gel or other nontoxic lubricating jelly and inserted into the oropharynx. The mandible of the anesthetized intubated patient is displaced anteriorly as the probe is advanced into the esophagus. The anterior neck is observed during insertion and the probe is redirected toward the midline if the lateral aspect of the neck bulges with advancement of the probe. Gentle but firm pressure is applied, but the probe is never advanced against resistance. Unsuccessful attempts may require laryngoscopy for atraumatic insertion of the probe into the esophagus under direct vision.

PRINCIPLES OF ULTRASOUND
Physics

Ultrasound is energy in the form of mechanical vibrations that induce cyclical or alternating compression and expansion (rarefaction) of a medium through which they propagate. As with all types of waves, ultrasound waves are described by frequency, wavelength, and amplitude (Fig. 4-1). *Frequency* refers to the number of cycles per second, measured in hertz. *Wavelength* is the length of one cycle, measured in millimeters. *Amplitude* is the height of the wave perpendicular to the wavelength. Velocity of the wave is dependent on the me-

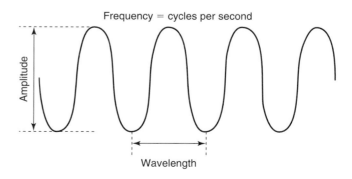

FIG. 4-1   Properties that describe an ultrasound wave.

dium through which the wave travels and is equal to the wavelength times the frequency.

$$\text{Velocity} = \text{Wavelength} \times \text{Frequency}$$

The velocity of propagation of ultrasound through blood is 1540 meters per second. Typical TEE probes have transducers with frequencies from 3.5 to 7.5 megahertz. Because wavelength is calculated as: Wavelength = Velocity/Frequency, transducers with a higher frequency produce ultrasound waves with a shorter wavelength and images with better resolution but less tissue penetration. Lower-frequency transducers produce ultrasound waves with longer wavelength and images with less resolution, but better tissue penetration.

Ultrasound waves encounter various media within the body, such as blood, tissue, air, and bone. Ultrasound energy is reflected back to the transducer at tissue boundaries, allowing the production of ultrasound images. The amount of energy reflected depends on the difference between the acoustic properties of the two tissues. Structures with greater tissue density reflect more ultrasound energy back to the transducer. Refracted ultrasound energy implies that the wave enters the second medium but its path is deflected from a straight line (Fig. 4-2). Absorption of ultrasound energy is referred to as *attenuation* and results in the conversion of ultrasound energy to heat. Greater attenuation occurs with higher-frequency ultrasound, leading to greater heat production and less tissue penetration by the ultrasound wave. Attenuation is the basis for greater tissue penetration by lower-frequency ultrasound waves.

Instrumentation

Ultrasound transducers consist of a piezoelectric crystal that converts electric energy to ultrasound energy by expanding and compressing in response to an alternating electrical current. *Transmission power* is increased by oscillating the piezoelectric crystals at greater amplitude, permitting more tissue penetration by the ultrasound wave. The piezoelectric crystal also functions as a "receiver," converting ultrasound energy reflected from tissues to electrical energy. Manipulation of the *gain setting* affects the amplitude of the received signal; this is similar to raising the volume of a radio. *Time gain compensation* (TGC) is a form of gain control that allows selective amplification of received signals based on their distance from the transducer. Far-field images generally require greater TGC than near-field images.

Computer analysis of the transmitted and reflected ultrasound energy creates an ultrasound image that is continuously updated. The frequency of updating the image is referred to as the *frame rate*. Two-dimensional imaging typically displays 40 to 60 frames per second, whereas M-mode imaging displays 1000 frames per second. *M-mode* is an echocardiographic display of one

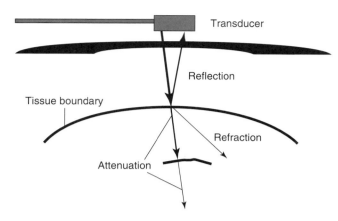

FIG. 4-2 The effects of tissue and tissue boundaries on an ultrasound wave.

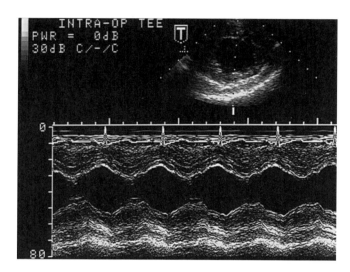

FIG. 4-3 M-mode echocardiogram of normal left ventricular wall motion.

dimension plotted over time (Fig. 4-3). Rapidly moving cardiac structures are more accurately assessed with a faster frame rate, emphasizing the utility of M-mode imaging of cardiac valves. The frame rate for two-dimensional imaging is increased by decreasing the imaging depth, decreasing the sector width and area, decreasing transducer frequency, and turning off Doppler ultrasound analysis. Potential two-dimensional artifacts are listed in Table 4-2.

Doppler Ultrasound

The Doppler effect occurs when a moving object intercepts an ultrasound beam, creating a backscatter to the transducer of a different frequency than the original frequency emitted by the transducer. If the object (blood cell) is moving toward the transducer, the reflected signal has a higher frequency than the signal emitted by the

TABLE 4-2
Two-Dimensional Ultrasound Imaging Artifacts

ARTIFACT	MECHANISM	EXAMPLES
Suboptimal image quality	Poor ultrasound penetration	Gastric air, patient anatomy (hiatal hernia)
Acoustic shadowing	Reflection of all the ultrasound signal by a strong specular reflector	Prosthetic valve Calcification
Reverberations	Reverberation between two strong parallel reflectors	Prosthetic valve
Beam width	Superimposition of structures within the beam profile (including side lobes) into a single tomographic image	Pulmonary artery catheter appears to be in aorta Atheroma appears to be in aortic lumen
Lateral resolution	Displayed width of a point target varies with depth	Excessive width of calcified mass or prosthetic valve
Refraction	Deviation of ultrasound signal from a straight path along the scan line	Double aortic valve or left ventricular image in short-axis view
Range ambiguity	Echo from previous pulse reaches transducer on next cycle	Second, deeper, heart image
Electronic processing	Instrument specific	Variable

Adapted from Otto CM: Principles of echocardiographic image acquisition and Doppler analysis. In Otto CM, editor: *Textbook of clinical echocardiography*, ed 2, Philadelphia, 2000, WB Saunders, pp 1-28.

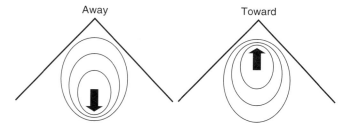

FIG. 4-4 Doppler effect: The reflected signal of an object moving away from the transducer has a lower frequency than the transmitted frequency, whereas the reflected signal of an object moving toward the transducer has a higher frequency than the transmitted signal.

transducer *(positive Doppler shift)*. Conversely, if the object is moving away from the transducer, the Doppler shift is negative because the reflected frequency is less than the original frequency (Fig. 4-4). The relationship between the Doppler shift and the velocity of the moving object is expressed by the Doppler equation:

$$V = \frac{V_{BLOOD}(f_T - f_R)}{2f_T \cos\theta}$$

where V_{BLOOD} is the speed of sound through the medium (1540 meters per second for blood), f_T is the transmitted frequency, f_R is the received frequency, and θ is the angular relation between the ultrasound beam and the direction of blood flow. If the beam is parallel to the direction of blood flow, θ is zero, $\cos\theta$ is 1, and the calculated velocity is an accurate estimate of the blood velocity. An angle θ greater than zero means that $\cos\theta$ is less than one. An underestimation of the blood velocity occurs when $\cos\theta$ is assumed to be 1.0 when the actual angle is greater than zero degrees. An angle up to 20 degrees is acceptable because the calculated velocity is underestimated by 6% or less. Velocity is not measured with TEE if the angle θ is greater than 20 degrees because of the large error in calculation (Fig. 4-5).

Pulsed Doppler echocardiography refers to the alternating aspect of transmitting and receiving "pulses" of ultrasound energy by a single crystal. The Doppler shift is plotted over time in a display termed *spectral analysis* (Fig. 4-6). Markings above the horizontal axis signify positive Doppler shifts indicating blood cells moving toward the transducer, whereas markings below the horizontal axis signify negative Doppler shifts for blood cells moving away from the transducer. The vertical axis indicates the blood flow velocity and the direction of blood flow. Another way of displaying pulsed Doppler analysis is by *color flow mapping* superimposed on a two-dimensional image. By convention, blue is assigned to blood flowing away from the transducer (Fig. 4-7, *A*) and red is assigned to blood flow directed toward the transducer (Fig. 4-7, *B*). Velocity is indicated by the shade bxof red or blue as indicated by a color scale displayed with the image. It is important to follow the manufacturer's recommendation for setting the proper

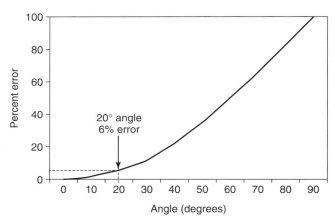

FIG. 4-5   The error from assuming the angular relation between the ultrasound beam and the direction of blood flow to be zero degrees. An angle of up to 20° results in a calculated velocity that is within 6% of the velocity that incorporates the actual angle in the Doppler equation.

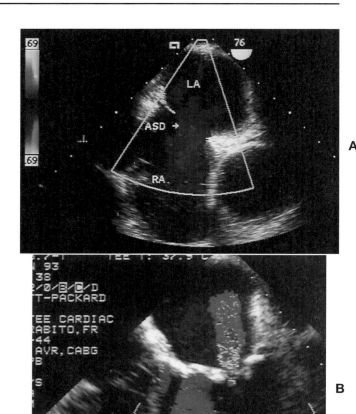

FIG. 4-7   Color Doppler echocardiogram indicating the direction of blood flow. **A**, Blue indicates flow away from the transducer. **B**, Red indicates flow toward the transducer.

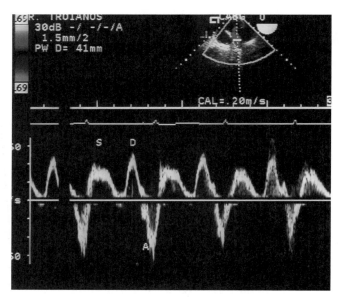

FIG. 4-6   Pulsed-wave Doppler echocardiogram of pulmonary vein flow. Markings above the horizontal axis indicate blood flow toward the transducer, while markings below the horizontal axis indicate blood flow away from the transducer. *A*, Atrial wave; *D*, diastolic wave; *S*, systolic wave.

color Doppler gain; setting the gain too low will underestimate the flow disturbance (Fig. 4-8). A *variance map* includes an additional color (usually yellow or green, as indicated by the color scale) that is added to show excessive variability in velocity. Variance in velocity is observed with turbulent blood flow or high-velocity flow exceeding the limit of measurement. The upper limit of velocity measurement is termed the *Nyquist limit* and is equal to one half the *pulse repetition frequency*

(PRF). The PRF is a single time cycle of ultrasound transmission, an inactive period, and an ultrasound receiving period, because a single crystal functions as the transmitter and receiver. The inactive period is determined by the distance between the site of velocity measurement *(sample volume)* and the transducer. Greater distances require more time between ultrasound transmission and reception, creating a lower PRF and hence a lower Nyquist limit. Velocity sampling closer to the transducer (in the near field), allows for a higher Nyquist limit, enabling higher-velocity measurements. *Aliasing* refers to the phenomenon of velocity exceeding the Nyquist limit and the display of velocity data in the opposite direction from actual blood flow (Fig. 4-9). Aliasing is reduced by increasing PRF, decreasing transducer frequency, and moving the baseline in the direction opposite to that of blood flow.

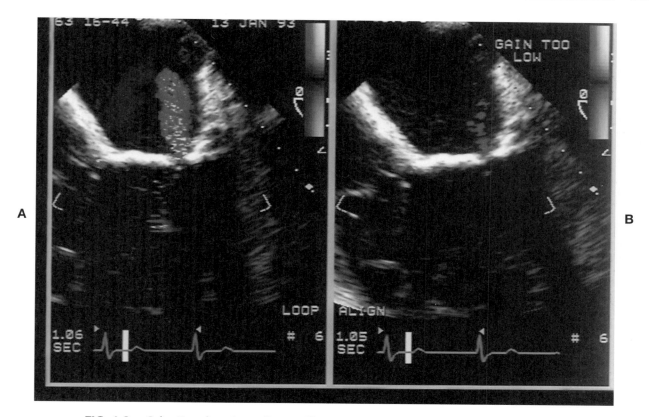

FIG. 4-8   Color Doppler echocardiogram illustrating the effect of color Doppler gain control on the size and character of the regurgitant jet. **A,** Proper gain control. **B,** Gain too low.

Continuous-wave Doppler uses two crystals, one continuously transmitting and another continuously receiving ultrasound signals. Higher-velocity measurements are possible because the upper limit of velocity measurement is not dependent on a PRF that uses one crystal alternating between transmission and reception. The disadvantage of continuous-wave Doppler is the lack of depth discrimination. Velocity measurements are not made at a specific "sample volume" location, but along the entire ultrasound beam. Despite this "overlapping" of velocity data obtained from the entire ultrasound beam, it is possible to differentiate velocities from different locations based on the magnitude, density, and shape of data within the spectral velocity display. One example is velocity analysis of blood flow through the left ventricular outflow tract and a stenotic aortic valve (Fig. 4-10). The lower laminar velocities arise from flow through the wider left ventricular outflow tract, whereas the higher turbulent velocities arise from flow through the small stenotic aortic valve orifice.

The many artifacts that can occur with Doppler ultrasonography relate to the technology's physics, patient anatomy, and the sampling techniques employed. Potential error in measurement and artifacts must be recognized to avoid misinterpretation and inaccurate diagnoses that may lead to unnecessary surgery. Potential spectral Doppler artifacts are listed in Table 4-3.

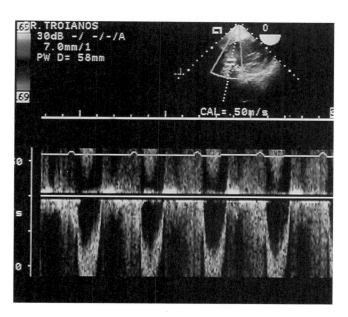

FIG. 4-9   Pulsed-wave Doppler echocardiogram indicating aliasing. The peak of the wave is cut off at the bottom of the figure, but appears at the top of the spectral display on the opposite side of the horizontal axis. Markings on opposite sides of the horizontal axis generally indicate blood flow in opposite directions. In this case, the markings appear on the opposite side of the horizontal axis because the peak velocities exceed the upper limit of the Doppler measurement.

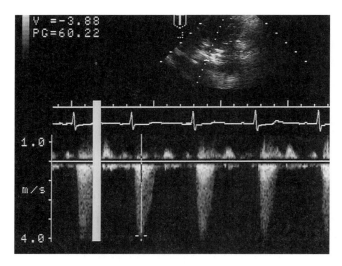

FIG. 4-10 Continuous-wave Doppler echocardiogram, indicating the lack of depth discrimination, of blood flow through the left ventricular outflow tract and aortic valve of a patient with aortic stenosis. The spectral Doppler displays both the aortic valve velocities (higher, fine, feathery appearance) and the left ventricular outflow tract velocities (lower, near the horizontal axis and denser) because velocities along the entire Doppler beam are recorded.

COMPREHENSIVE TEE EXAMINATION

The comprehensive TEE examination is a balance between a fastidious, complete comprehensive examination and expedience.[37] Imaging sites are grouped into four anatomic locations: upper esophageal, midesophageal, transgastric, and deep transgastric (Fig. 4-11). The setting and indication for the examination will determine whether the emphasis should be completeness versus expedience, and the order in which various structures are imaged and evaluated. For example, the thoracic aorta is the first anatomic structure imaged in the conscious, sedated patient undergoing TEE for a suspected aortic dissection, because this information will prompt surgical versus medical treatment. Patient intolerance of the TEE probe may not allow for a complete comprehensive examination. In contrast, the left ventricle and four chambers are the initial views during the evaluation of a hypotensive patient following cardiac surgery, to determine the etiology of hypotension as volume, contractility, or tamponade.

A complete, comprehensive examination that uses 20 standard views (Fig. 4-12) is performed in all patients when feasible. It is helpful for the beginner to develop a regular, consistent examination sequence to include all structures. This provides the beginner with experience imaging normal and abnormal structures

TABLE 4-3	
Spectral Doppler Artifacts	
ARTIFACT	**RESULT**
Nonparallel intercept angle	Underestimation of velocity
Aliasing	Inability to measure maximum velocity
Range ambiguity	Doppler signals from more than one depth along the ultrasound beam are recorded
Beam width	Overlap of Doppler signals from adjacent flows
Mirror image	Spectral display shows unidirectional flow both above and below the baseline
Electronic interference	Bandlike interference signal obscures Doppler flow
Transit-time effect	Change in the velocity of the ultrasound wave as it passes through a moving media results in slight overestimation of Doppler shifts

From Otto CM: Principles of echocardiographic image acquisition and Doppler analysis. In Otto CM, editor: *Textbook of clinical echocardiography*, ed 2, Philadelphia, 2000, WB Saunders, pp 1-28.

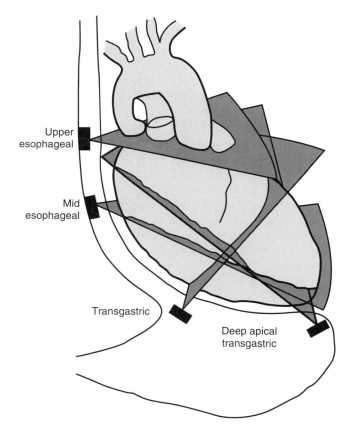

FIG. 4-11 Illustration of the four sites for TEE imaging.

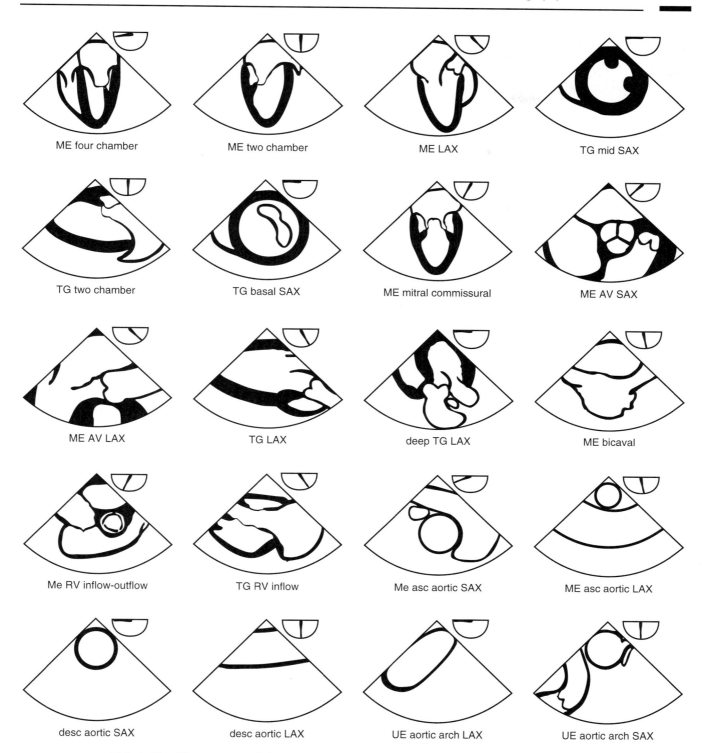

FIG. 4-12 The recommended 20 cross-sectional views that make up the comprehensive TEE examination. The icon adjacent to each view indicates approximate multiplane angle. *asc,* Ascending; *AV,* aortic valve; *desc,* descending; *LAX,* long axis; *ME,* midesophageal; *RV,* right ventricle; *SAX,* short axis; *TG,* transgastric; *UE,* upper esophageal.

(From Shanewise JS, Cheung AT, Aronson S et al: *Anesth Analg* 89:870-884, 1999.)

TABLE 4-4
Comprehensive TEE Examination Sequence

STRUCTURE(S)	EXAMINATION
1. Aortic valve; ascending aorta	Short-axis view (30° to 60°) of aortic valve with planimetry, if indicated; withdraw probe to view ascending aorta; rotate multiplane angle forward to long-axis view (120° to 160°) of aortic valve and ascending aorta; apply color Doppler to aortic valve long-axis and short-axis views
2. Mitral valve	Four-chamber view (0° to 20°) to commissural view (60° to 70°) to two-chamber view (80° to 100°) to long-axis view (120° to 160°) and use spectral Doppler for transmitral flow velocity; apply color Doppler to long-axis, two-chamber, commissural, and four-chamber views
3. Left atrium	Measure size in anterior-posterior and medial-lateral dimensions; examine for thrombi, especially for atrial fibrillation and left atrial appendage; apply spectral pulsed-wave Doppler to pulmonary veins
4. Pulmonary artery	Tip of pulmonary artery catheter in distal main or proximal right pulmonary artery
5. Superior vena cava; intraatrial septum	Follow superior vena cava into right atrium; apply color Doppler to fossa ovalis/septum to identify patent foramen ovale or atrial septal defect; use saline contrast with 20 cm CPAP if indicated
6. Tricuspid valve; right ventricle; pulmonic valve	Four-chamber (0° to 20°) to inflow-outflow (60° to 80°) to bicaval view (90° to 110°); apply color and spectral Doppler to tricuspid and pulmonic valves, as indicated
7. Left ventricle	Four-chamber (0° to 20°) for septal/lateral walls; two-chamber (80° to 100°) for inferior/anterior walls; long-axis (130° to 150°) for posterior/anteroseptal walls; advance probe into stomach for transgastric views: mid, basal, and apical short-axis views; rotate angle forward (80° to 100°) for LV long-axis view to view papillary muscle function; advance deep into stomach and anteflex for deep apical long-axis view for transaortic valve flow velocity
8. Thoracic aorta	Examine ascending aorta in transgastric deep apical long-axis view; undo anteflexion, withdraw probe into esophagus, and turn probe to the left to view descending thoracic aorta in short axis; withdraw probe as descending aorta is examined proximally to aortic arch; turn probe to view aortic arch in long axis; rotate angle forward to 90° to view aortic arch in short axis; turn and advance probe to follow descending aorta to diaphragm, noting origin of left subclavian and intraaortic balloon pump position

CPAP, Continuous positive airway pressure; *LV,* left ventricle.

and ensures a complete TEE examination for the patient. The complete examination is stored in a videotape or digital format for later review or comparison. The ideal sequence for evaluation is developed individually by each echocardiographer, but should possess the characteristics of completeness and consistency. One such nontargeted examination sequence, outlined in Table 4-4, ensures thorough evaluation of most thoracic structures. This examination sequence is based on the close proximity of sequential imaging sites and anatomic structures, minimizing movement of the TEE probe from one imaging site to another. Terminology for probe manipulation is summarized in Fig. 4-13. Normal adult transesophageal measurements[38] are listed in Table 4-5.

Left Ventricle

Evaluation of the left ventricle is one of the most important aspects of the TEE examination. Global assessment of left ventricular function includes contractility,

ejection fraction, circumferential fiber shortening, and cardiac output. Left ventricular function is affected by preload, afterload, ischemia, aortic and mitral valvular dysfunction, pericardial constriction, and cardiac tamponade.[39] Imaging the left ventricle to determine end-diastolic area and contractility provides a prompt diagnosis to guide therapy in the hypotensive patient[39] (Table 4-6).

Preload

Left ventricular preload is estimated with two-dimensional TEE by determining left ventricular cross-sectional area at end-diastole.[40,41] This end-diastolic area (EDA) is most commonly obtained from the transgastric view at the level of the midpapillary muscles. This view uses the papillary muscles as a reference point so subsequent comparisons occur at the same left ventricular cross-sectional area. This view is identified by imaging the papillary muscles in cross section as distinct structures in continuity with the subendocardium (Fig. 4-14). Moving the imaging plane toward the apex de-

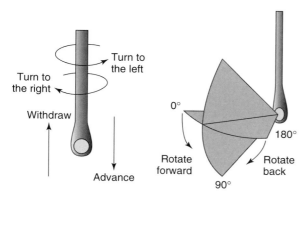

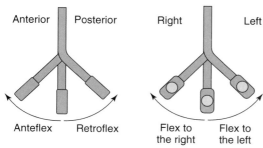

FIG. 4-13 Recommended terminology to describe TEE probe manipulation during image acquisition.

(From Shanewise JS, Cheung AT, Aronson S et al: *Anesth Analg* 89:870-884, 1999.)

TABLE 4-5
Normal Values for Adult TEE

PARAMETER	MEAN ± SD (mm)	RANGE (mm)
Right pulmonary artery	17 ± 3	12-22
Pulmonary vein	11 ± 2	7-16
Length of left atrial appendage	28 ± 5	15-43
Diameter of left atrial appendage	16 ± 5	10-28
Superior vena cava	15 ± 3	8-20
Aortic root	28 ± 3	21-34
Right ventricular outflow tract	27 ± 4	16-36
Left atrium (anteroposterior)	38 ± 6	20-52
Left atrium (medial-lateral)	39 ± 7	24-52
Right atrium (anteroposterior)	38 ± 5	28-52
Right atrium (medial-lateral)	38 ± 6	29-53
Tricuspid annulus (four-chamber view)	28 ± 5	20-40
Mitral annulus (four-chamber view)	29 ± 4	20-38
Coronary sinus	6.6 ± 1.5	4-10
Left ventricle (anteroposterior)-diastole	43 ± 7	33-55
Left ventricle (medial-lateral)-diastole	42 ± 7	23-54
Left ventricle (anteroposterior)-systole	28 ± 6	18-40
Left ventricle (medial-lateral)-systole	27 ± 6	18-42
Proximal descending aorta	21 ± 4	14-30
Distal descending thoracic aorta	20 ± 4	13-28

From Cohen GI, White M, Sochowski RA et al: *J Am Soc Echocardiogr* 8:221-230, 1995.

TABLE 4-6
TEE Evaluation of the Left Ventricle for Hypotension

CONTRACTILITY	END-DIASTOLIC AREA	DIAGNOSIS
Normal to hyperkinetic	Small with systolic obliteration	Hypovolemia or sepsis
Normal	Small with early diastolic collapse of RV	Tamponade
Regional wall-motion abnormality	Normal to dilated	Myocardial ischemia
Global hypokinesis	Dilated	Left ventricular failure

RV, Right ventricle.

---

creases the intraventricular area and the papillary muscles are no longer imaged. Moving the imaging plane toward the base of the heart increases the intraventricular area and the papillary muscles are imaged distinctly separate from the subendocardium. The papillary muscles give rise to the chordae tendineae and mitral valve leaflets as the imaging plane is moved further toward the base of the heart. Consistent measurement of left ventricle (LV) cross-sectional area at the same reference point (midpapillary level) provides credibility to the assumption that changes in EDA occur because of changes in left ventricular volume and not because a different cross section is examined. Changes in left ventricular volume affect the left ventricular short axis to a much greater degree than the long axis.

The echocardiographic end-diastolic area correlates with left ventricular volume determined by radionuclide studies[42] and is a more sensitive estimate of end-diastolic volume than PCWP during abdominal aortic aneurysm repair.[43,44] Adequate left ventricular EDA is dependent on LV function. Patients with severe LV dysfunction require a greater EDA for adequate preload, which is analogous to requiring higher PCWP. Left ventricular EDA of less than 5.5 cm^2/m^2 body surface area indicates hypovolemia.[45] Systolic obliteration of left ventricular cross-sectional area accompanies decreased EDA and is a sign of severe hypovolemia.[45]

Left ventricular short-axis diameter and endocardial circumference also correlate with acute changes in left ventricular volume.[46] It is important to remember that all of these methods of volume assessment infer three-dimensional volume determination from two-dimensional imaging. More accurate measurements require more detailed measurements in multiple axes and imaging planes,[40] but are cumbersome and time consuming to perform. Three-dimensional echocardiography circumvents the geometric assumptions made by two-dimensional echocardiography in determining left ventricular volume.

Diastolic Function

The most important aspect of preload assessment is the integration of pressure and volume data.[47] Decreased diastolic compliance is defined as a decrease in the ratio between changes in volume and changes in pressure (decreased dV/dP). Diastolic dysfunction occurring before systolic dysfunction is a manifestation of certain cardiac diseases and is an important aspect of echocardiographic evaluation. Integration of pulmonary venous and transmitral flow data provides the diagnosis of abnormal diastolic compliance. Left atrial pressure is estimated by pulsed Doppler interrogation of pulmonary venous blood flow.[48-51] Pulmonary venous blood flow is sampled from one pulmonary vein, usually the left upper pulmonary vein, and is characterized by four phases (Fig. 4-15). Diastolic inflow to the left ventricle begins with mitral valve opening and appears on the pulmonary venous Doppler tracing as a positive Doppler shift as blood moves from the lungs to the left atrium. Left atrial contraction causes retrograde flow in the pulmonary vein because of the lack of valves within the pulmonary veins. This retrograde flow appears as a negative Doppler shift on the pulmonary venous Doppler tracing. Systolic inflow into the atrium from the lungs begins with atrial relaxation and is followed by ventricular contraction creating the two positive Doppler peaks during systole.

The spectral velocity display of pulmonary venous blood flow over time is used to estimate left atrial pressure by determining the area under each positive Doppler peak. Area under the systolic phase is the *systolic velocity time integral* (VTI), whereas the area under the diastolic phase is the *diastolic VTI*. The *systolic fraction* of pulmonary vein flow is as follows:

$$\frac{Systolic\ VTI}{Systolic\ VTI + Diastolic\ VTI}$$

A systolic fraction less than 0.55 is a sensitive and specific indicator of left atrial pressure greater than 15 mm Hg.[52] A qualitative assessment of which phase predominates is also used to estimate left atrial pressure. If the systolic phase predominates, left atrial pressures are low (Fig. 4-16, *A*). If the diastolic phase predominates with systolic blunting, left atrial pressures are high (Fig. 4-16, *B*). Age, arterial blood pressure, heart rate, and whether the mediastinum is closed or open do not appear to affect the Doppler variables of pulmonary ve-

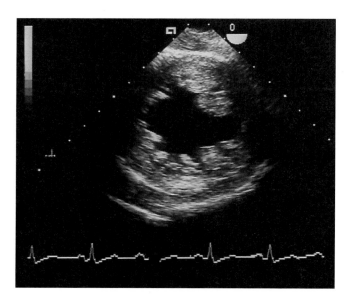

FIG. 4-14 Transesophageal echocardiogram, transgastric short-axis view of the left ventricle at the midpapillary muscle level.

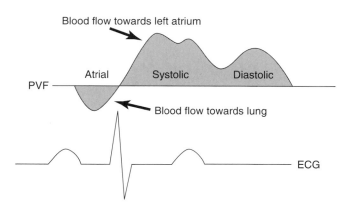

FIG. 4-15 Illustration of pulmonary vein flow *(PVF)* during one cardiac cycle. Blood in the pulmonary veins normally moves towards the left atrium during systole and early diastole and towards the lungs during atrial contraction. Early diastolic flow coincides with mitral valve opening. Atrial contraction causes retrograde flow in the pulmonary veins because of the absence of valves within the pulmonary veins. Systolic flow toward the atrium occurs in two phases: the first with atrial relaxation and the second with ventricular contraction. *ECG,* Electrocardiogram.

nous flow.[52] Acute lung injury and systemic inflammation influence the pulmonary venous flow pattern and its relation to left atrial pressure.[53,54]

Another aspect of diastolic function evaluation is the transmitral Doppler interrogation of ventricular filling. The spectral display pattern consists of two negative Doppler shifts for patients in sinus rhythm (Fig. 4-17). Early ventricular filling is identified by the "E" wave, which occurs in *early* diastole with opening of the mitral valve. Late ventricular filling is identified by the "A" wave, which occurs in late diastole with *atrial* contraction. The A wave is absent in patients with atrial fibrillation or absent atrial contraction. Inflow velocities are sampled with pulsed or continuous-wave Doppler echocardiography. It is important to align the Doppler beam parallel to the mitral valve inflow by using a midesophageal imaging location with retroflexion of the transducer tip. This directs the imaging plane from the posterior aspect of the atrium, through the mitral valve, and toward the left ventricular apex. Both pulsed- and continuous-wave Doppler can be used to measure inflow velocities. The sample volume of pulsed-wave Doppler is placed at the depth of the mitral leaflet tips during diastole, which is usually the site of maximal velocity. Continuous-wave Doppler can also be used to measure inflow velocities. Without depth discrimina-

tion, continuous-wave Doppler displays the maximal velocities along the entire Doppler beam. This may lead to errors in volumetric flow determination, which requires velocity measurement at the site of area determination (mitral annulus).

Normal early diastolic/atrial (E/A) mitral inflow velocity ratio is greater than 1.0, but respiration, heart rate, P-R interval, and age affect this ratio. Young patients with normal left ventricular compliance have a smaller (15%) contribution of atrial contraction to ventricular filling. Older patients and patients with decreased left ventricular compliance require a greater atrial contribution, which decreases the E/A ratio to less than 1.0. Other factors besides left ventricular compliance affect diastolic filling. These include left atrial pressure, and the pressure gradient and blood flow between the left atrium and left ventricle. Increased preload increases early diastolic filling (E-wave velocity) and shortens the time between aortic valve closure and the onset of ventricular filling *(isovolumic relaxation time)*. The deceleration slope of early diastolic filling is steeper and the A-wave velocity is reduced with increased preload because the pressure gradient between the left atrium and

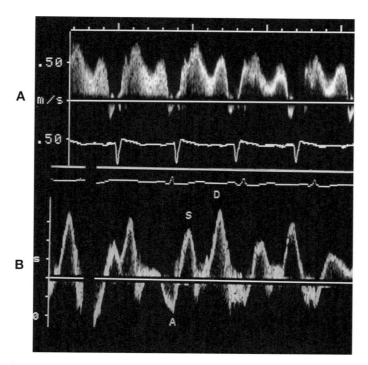

FIG. 4-16 Pulsed-wave Doppler echocardiogram of pulmonary vein flow. **A,** Patient with normal left atrial pressure—S wave is larger than D wave. **B,** Patient with high left atrial pressure—S wave is smaller than D wave. *A,* Atrial wave; *D,* diastolic wave; *S,* systolic wave.

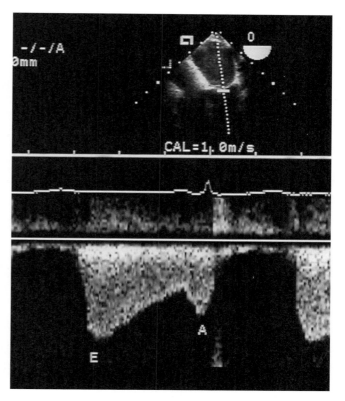

FIG. 4-17 Continuous-wave echocardiogram indicating the velocity of blood flow through a mitral valve. *A,* Atrial wave; *E,* early diastolic wave.

TABLE 4-7
Diastolic Filling Patterns

	NORMAL	IMPAIRED RELAXATION	PSEUDONORMAL PATTERN	RESTRICTIVE FILLING
Deceleration time	160-240 msec*	>240 msec	160-200 msec	<160 msec
Isovolumic relaxation time	70-90 msec	>90 msec	<90 msec	<70 msec
E/A ratio	1-2	<1.0	1-1.5	>1.5
Mitral A duration	≥PVa duration	≥ or <PVa duration†	<PVa duration	<PVa duration
Pulmonary vein flow	PVs2 ≥ PVd‡	PVs2 >> PVd	PVa velocity >35 cm/sec	PVa velocity ≥35 cm/sec§
Effects of preload reduction	normal	decreases E/A ratio	E/A reverses to <1.0	Decreased E/A ratio
Two-dimensional echo findings	normal	decreased EF	LVH, decreased EF	LVH, decreased EF

From Oh JK, Seward JB, Tajik AJ: *The echo manual,* ed 2, Philadelphia, 1999, Lippincott Williams & Wilkins, p 54.
A, Mitral inflow velocity resulting from atrial contraction; *E,* early mitral inflow velocity; *E/A,* early diastolic/atrial; *EF,* ejection fraction; *LVH,* left ventricular hypertrophy; *PVa,* atrial wave of pulmonary vein flow; *PVd,* diastolic wave of pulmonary vein flow; *PVs2,* systolic wave of pulmonary vein flow.
*Can be lower, especially in young persons.
†Depending on LVEDP.
‡PVs2 can be smaller than PVd in young persons.
§Usually, but not always.

left ventricle is decreased and approaches zero more rapidly. Decreased preload results in a lower E-wave velocity and an unaffected or increased A-wave velocity. MR causes increased left atrial pressure and transmitral flow volume, resulting in an increased E-wave velocity, reduced A-wave velocity, and an increased E/A ratio. Other conditions also affect these diastolic parameters and are broadly classified as normal, impaired relaxation, pseudonormal, or restrictive. The associated diastolic characteristics for each classification are listed in Table 4-7.

Global Left Ventricular Function

Global left ventricular function is assessed qualitatively by visual inspection and quantitatively with TEE by fractional shortening (FS) of one dimension, fractional area change, or ejection fraction. FS uses one dimension (ventricular diameter) to describe global contractility in terms of the end-systolic dimension (ESD) and the end-diastolic dimension (EDD):

$$FS = \frac{EDD - ESD}{EDD}$$

The fractional area change (FAC) is a two-dimensional calculation based on the left ventricular cross-sectional end-systolic and end-diastolic areas (ESA and EDA respectively).

$$FAC = \frac{EDA - ESA}{EDA}$$

Ejection fraction (EF) is a three-dimensional assessment that uses end-systole volume (ESV) and end-diastole volume (EDV) measurements:

$$EF = \frac{EDV - ESV}{EDV}$$

Several methods have been described for calculating ventricular volume with two-dimensional echocardiography by measuring multiple dimensions in various imaging planes. These techniques can be cumbersome, time consuming, and require sophisticated computation. Clinically important assessment of left ventricular ejection and filling are detected by visual inspection alone.[55] The left ventricular short-axis view at the mid-papillary muscle cross section is a popular, easily obtained, and reproducible image for making this visual assessment.

Certain ultrasound manufactures provide automated detection of the endocardial border, allowing real-time displays of FAC, EDA, and ESA. Inaccurate data occur when portions of the endocardial border "drops out" or are not imaged because of an inadequate signal or shadowing. Cardiac translation or movement of the heart resulting from respiration, premature contractions, and surgical interference contribute to inconsistencies of measurement. Time-gain compensation settings and adjustments in lateral gain control help to improve endocardial border tracking. Automated detection of the endocardial border permits continuous real-time analysis of left ventricular cross-sectional area changes by displaying values for EDA and FAC.[56,57] Changes in these parameters are monitored over time and provide the clinician with data for patient management by detecting subtle changes before they are apparent by visual observation. Clinically important changes in left ventricular ejection and filling, however, are detected by visual inspection alone.[55] Accuracy of the data depends on quality imaging of a distinct blood-myocardial border obtained from appropriate adjustment of gain settings and probe contact with the gastric mucosa. Poor image quality or inability to maintain consistent border detection makes automated border detection inaccurate or misleading in assessing left ventricular volume and contractility.

Cardiac Output

Cardiac output is determined with echocardiography by estimating stroke volume from two-dimensional images[58] or calculating blood flow through various structures.[39] The *modified Simpson's rule*, a commonly used method for determining ventricular volume, uses three parallel cross-sectional areas for volume calculation:

$$Volume = \frac{L}{3}(MVA + PMA) + \frac{AA}{2} + \frac{\pi \times L^3}{162}$$

where L is the LV long-axis length, MVA is the LV short-axis area at the mitral valve, PMA is the LV short-axis area at the papillary muscles, and AA is the LV short-axis area at the apex.[59] Stroke volume is equal to the difference between the EDV and ESV. Cardiac output is calculated by multiplying the stroke volume by the heart rate. This calculation is most reliable with a regular cardiac rhythm in which the stroke volume is relatively uniform from beat to beat. Three-dimensional echocardiographic techniques compute left ventricular volumes using spatially registered two-dimensional views.[60]

Cardiac output is also determined by calculating blood flow through a cardiac structure such as the pulmonary artery,[61,62] mitral valve,[63,64] left ventricular outflow tract, or aortic valve.[65] The basic method involves determining cross-sectional area (CSA) and blood flow velocity at the same point. The spectral Doppler display of the velocity measurement is used to integrate velocity over time to provide the VTI, which represents the distance blood travels per beat. Cardiac output is calculated as follows:

$$Cardiac\ Output = VTI \times CSA \times heart\ rate$$

Because the pulmonary artery and left ventricular outflow tract are cylindrical structures, the CSA can be determined from the diameter (d): $CSA = \pi \left(\frac{d}{2}\right)^2$. Accurate measurement is important because any error in measurement is squared in the area calculation, which is then multiplied in the cardiac output calculation. Velocity measurements must be obtained at the same location as the area measurement for the equation to be valid. Determining cardiac output through the mitral and aortic valves requires accurate estimates of valvular orifice

TABLE 4-8
Grading Regional Wall Motion

WALL MOTION	RADIAL SHORTENING	MYOCARDIAL THICKENING
Normal	>30%	30%-50%
Mild hypokinesis	10%-30%	30%-50%
Severe hypokinesis	0%-10%	<30%
Akinesis	0	0
Dyskinesis	Outward bulging	Systolic thinning

Data from Smith JS, Cahalan MK, Benefiel DJ et al: Intraoperative detection of myocardial ischemia in high-risk patients: electrocardiography versus two-dimensional echocardiography, *Circulation* 72:1015-1021,1985.

size, most easily obtained from normal valves. A triangular aortic valve orifice is the area that provides the most accurate estimate of cardiac output.[65]

Stroke volume, EF, fractional area change, and cardiac output are global assessments of left ventricular function that are dependent on preload, afterload, and contractility. Left ventricular performance, independent of loading conditions and contractility, is determined by analysis of pressure-volume relations. Because left ventricular volume is difficult to determine on-line, Gorcsan and associates investigated the feasibility and reliability of pressure-area relations and compared them to pressure-volume relations. Pressure-area loops were constructed using TEE automated border detection of left ventricular cross-sectional area and left ventricular pressure. Aortic flow was determined by an electromagnetic probe and comparisons were made to simultaneously derived pressure-volume loops. Stroke work changes calculated by the two methods demonstrated close correlation ($r = 0.99$) and the feasibility of using pressure-area loops to assess left ventricular performance independent of loading conditions.[66]

Regional Left Ventricular Function

Left ventricular regional wall motion is described in terms of *radial shortening* (movement toward the center) and *wall thickening* (during systole). Normal wall motion has greater than 30% radial shortening and a 30% to 50% increase in wall thickness (Table 4-8). An RWMA is a decrement in wall-motion of at least two grades and is considered the earliest sign of myocardial ischemia.[67] RWMAs occur simultaneously with lactate production, several minutes before and sometimes in the absence of electrocardiographic changes.[13,68] For this reason, two-dimensional echocardiography is considered superior to electrocardiography for detecting myocardial ischemia.[13,69,70] Smith and associates used five-lead electrocardiography and intraoperative TEE during predefined intervals and demonstrated a fourfold greater incidence of ischemia with TEE. All patients with electrocardiographic evidence of ischemia had RWMAs. Of 50 patients, 3 had a myocardial infarction, all of which had RWMAs, but only one had electrocardiographic changes.[69] RWMAs may occur in the absence of hemodynamic changes and appear to be predictive of adverse outcome after cardiac surgery.[13]

The midpapillary short-axis view is a popular image for detecting ischemia because myocardium supplied by all three major coronary arteries is represented in this cross section (Fig. 4-18). Approximately one third of all RWMAs are not detected if the midpapillary short-axis view is the only myocardial cross section examined.[71] Multiple planes must be examined by manipulating the

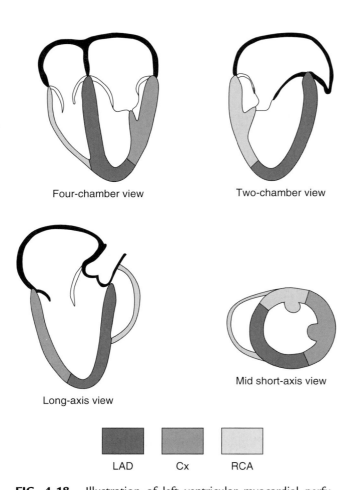

Four-chamber view

Two-chamber view

Long-axis view

Mid short-axis view

LAD   Cx   RCA

FIG. 4-18   Illustration of left ventricular myocardial perfusion by the three major coronary arteries. *Cx,* Left circumflex; *LAD,* left anterior descending; *RCA,* right coronary artery.

(From Shanewise JS, Cheung AT, Aronson S et al: *Anesth Analg* 89:870-84, 1999.)

probe and rotating the transducer. From the position providing a midpapillary image, the probe is withdrawn and/or further anteflexed to obtain images of the basal ventricular segments, and advanced and/or less anteflexed to obtain images of the apical segments. The four-chamber view from the midesophagus provides imaging of the basal, mid, and apical segments of the septum and lateral walls. The multiplane transducer is rotated forward to the two-chamber view (80° to 100°) to provide imaging of the basal, mid, and apical segments of the inferior and anterior walls. Forward rotation to the LV long-axis view (120° to 140°) provides imaging of the basal, and midsegments of the posterior and anteroseptal walls (see Fig. 4-18). Multiplane TEE is superior to biplane TEE in providing a more detailed assessment of left ventricular wall motion, enhancing the evaluation of apical, posterobasal, inferoposterior, and inferolateral wall segments.[72] A 16-segment model is recommended for describing regional wall motion for the entire left ventricle (Fig. 4-19).

Regional wall motion assessed intraoperatively by the qualitative inspection of radial shortening and wall thickening (see Table 4-8) is subjective and dependent on observer experience. M-mode imaging provides a sensitive evaluation of wall motion, but is limited by analysis of wall segments moving parallel to the ultrasound beam. Computerized digitation systems allow for more sensitive analysis of wall motion, such as tardokinesis, not obvious with real-time two-dimensional imaging. *Tardokinesis* represents *delay* in wall motion and usually indicates abnormal function.[73] Color kinesis is an extension of automated border detection technology and provides another qualitative method of assessing regional ventricular function. Temporal color-coding of wall motion is provided during the sequential movement of the endocardial border (Fig. 4-20). Thicker color bands indicate greater excursion, indicative of normal wall motion. Thinner or fewer color bands indicate hypokinesis, absence of color bands indicates akinesis, and the progression of tissue signals to "blood" signals during systole indicates dyskinesis.

Another method used to quantify wall motion is *tissue Doppler imaging,* which permits analysis of wall-motion velocity with color Doppler by filtering out high-velocity blood flow. Low-velocity myocardial motion is preferentially displayed by the filtering. Color is based on the velocity of wall motion and is displayed with varying shades according to the color velocity map. Color is not displayed in akinetic areas resulting from zero velocity. The problems inherent to Doppler echocardiography apply to tissue Doppler imaging. Wall-motion analysis is affected by the angle between the Doppler beam and the direction of wall motion, limiting the evaluation of segments moving orthogonal to the Doppler beam.

Wall-motion abnormalities may be caused by factors

unrelated to ischemia. Bundle-branch blocks, ventricular pacing, tethering, and altered loading conditions cause wall-motion abnormalities in the absence of ischemia. *Tethering* refers to a motion abnormality of a nonischemic wall segment that is adjacent to ischemic or infarcted myocardium. The echocardiographic evaluation of a wall-motion abnormality cannot distinguish between "stunned" or "hibernating" myocardium from ischemic myocardium. Persistence of a wall-motion abnormality after cardiopulmonary bypass and into the intensive care unit in patients undergoing coronary artery bypass grafting provides a clinically important prognostic sign because postbypass TEE ischemia is associated with adverse outcome.[13]

Three-dimensional TEE, which is possible with a number of techniques, provides enhanced imaging but longer and more complicated image generation. Dynamic three-dimensional imaging, sometimes referred to as *four-dimensional imaging,* includes the added dimension of time to provide the perception of motion.[74] Surface rendering techniques allow for quantitative assessment of wall motion and endocardial volume, whereas volume rendering techniques allow for only qualitative assessment and valvular imaging.

Afterload

Systemic vascular resistance (SVR) is often used as an estimate of afterload, but considers blood flow as nonpulsatile in calculation. SVR is calculated from cardiac output, mean arterial pressure (MAP) and central venous pressure (CVP):

$$SVR = \frac{(MAP - CVP) \times 80}{Cardiac\ Output}$$

True afterload is wall stress or force per area that must be overcome to produce ventricular ejection, and considers intracavitary dimensions, wall thickness, and arterial blood pressure. Left ventricular *meridional wall stress*

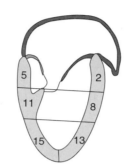

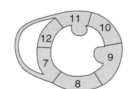

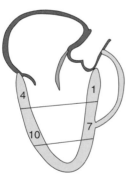

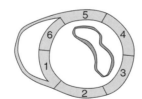

A. Four-chamber view

B. Two-chamber view

C. Long-axis view

D. Mid short-axis view

E. Basal short-axis view

Basal segments	Mid segments	Apical segments
1 basal anteroseptal	7 mid anteroseptal	13 apical anterior
2 basal anterior	8 mid anterior	14 apical lateral
3 basal lateral	9 mid lateral	15 apical inferior
4 basal posterior	10 mid posterior	16 apical septal
5 basal inferior	11 mid inferior	
6 basal septal	12 mid septal	

FIG. 4-19 Nomenclature for left ventricular 16-segment model. **A,** Four-chamber view contains the three septal and three lateral segments. **B,** Two-chamber view contains the three anterior and three inferior segments. **C,** Long-axis view contains the two anteroseptal and two posterior segments. **D,** Mid short-axis view contains six segments at the midpapillary level. **E,** Basal short-axis view contains six segments at the basal level.

(From Shanewise JS, Cheung AT, Aronson S et al: *Anesth Analg* 89:870-84, 1999.)

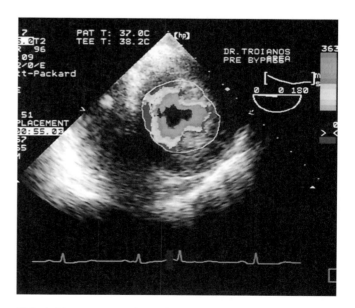

FIG. 4-20 Transesophageal echocardiogram with Color Kinesis (Hewlett-Packard Company, Andover, Mass.) of the transgastric left ventricular mid short axis. Color bands indicate myocardial excursion during one cardiac cycle.

is determined by both echocardiographic (LVd = LV diameter, LVth = LV wall thickness) and systolic arterial pressure (SAP) measurements:

$$Systolic\ Wall\ Stress = \frac{0.334 \times SAP \times LVd}{LVth \left\{ 1 + \frac{LVth}{LVd} \right\}}$$

This determination of systolic wall stress correlates with left ventricular pressure[75] and is expressed as force per unit area (g/cm^2). Expression of wall tension permits comparison between ventricles of varying size and thickness and for the same ventricle with different loading conditions, thus providing the best estimate of left ventricular afterload.[52] In contrast with circumferential wall stress, meridional wall stress is independent of the left ventricular long axis. *Circumferential wall stress* is expressed in g per cm^2 from the long-axis length of the left ventricle (*L*) measured in the four- or two-chamber views as:

$$Systolic\ Wall\ Stress = \frac{1.35 \times SAP \times r \times [1 - (2r^2/L^2)]}{LVth}$$

where *r* is the internal radius calculated as the square root of (endocardial short-axis area/π).[52]

Right Ventricle

The right ventricle (RV) is imaged using the four-chamber, RV inflow-outflow (Fig. 4-21) and transgastric views. The right ventricle appears as an asymmetric crescent-shaped structure that shares the septum with the LV and possesses an anterior free wall, inflow from the tricuspid valve, and an outflow tract to the pulmonic valve. Quantitative evaluation of systolic function is limited because of the nongeometric, asymmetric shape of the RV.

Differences between the RV and LV are the asymmetric shape, thinner free wall, and reduced muscle mass of the RV. The thinner free wall makes diagnosis of subtle regional wall-motion abnormalities difficult to detect. Normal right ventricular wall thickness is ≤5.0 cm and intraventricular cross-sectional area is less than the left ventricular area, determined qualitatively using multiple imaging views. Right ventricular area equal to left ventricular area indicates mild RV dilation, whereas right ventricular area greater than left ventricular area indicates severe right ventricular dilation. The shape of the RV changes as it enlarges. A normal RV appears triangular in the midesophageal four-chamber view, whereas an enlarged RV has a rounded appearance and extends to the cardiac apex. It is important to examine the shape and motion of the septum, which is normally convex toward the RV and moves posterior toward the center of the LV during systole. Septal flattening, curvature reversal, and "paradoxical" anterior motion during systole indicate right ventricular volume overload.

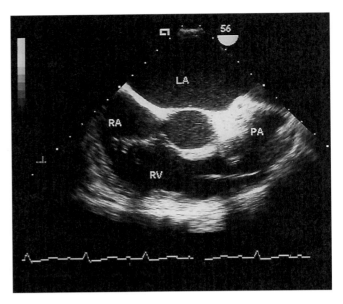

FIG. 4-21 Transesophageal echocardiogram, midesophageal right ventricular inflow-outflow view. *LA,* Left atrium; *PA,* pulmonary artery; *RA,* right atrium; *RV,* right ventricle.

Diastolic filling of the RV is similar to the LV, except for lower inflow velocities, shorter filling time, and reciprocal variation during respiration. Spontaneous inspiration increases venous return, right ventricular filling volume, and velocity over expiratory values. The expiratory phase of positive pressure mechanical ventilation has similar increases in right heart inflow over positive pressure inspiratory values. Right ventricular inflow velocities are lower than left ventricular inflow velocities because the tricuspid valve has a larger orifice area than the mitral valve.

Mitral Valve

TEE provides high-resolution images of the mitral valve apparatus, permitting detailed evaluation of its structure and function. Mitral valve evaluation is invaluable during mitral valve repair surgery, providing insight into the mechanism of valve dysfunction and facilitating the formulation of a repair plan.[77] TEE provides immediate detection of inadequate repair after bypass and allows correction during the same operative setting. Intraoperative TEE is a valuable tool for improving patient outcome and offers the cardiovascular anesthesiologist a role in perioperative surgical decisions.[5]

The mitral valve apparatus consists of two leaflets, chordae tendineae, papillary muscles, and the annulus. Pathology involving any one of these structures leads to valvular dysfunction. The posterior leaflet is composed of three scallops: lateral, middle, and medial, designated P1, P2, and P3, respectively, by the Carpentier nomenclature (Fig. 4-22). The regions of the anterior leaflet corresponding to the three posterior leaflet scallops are

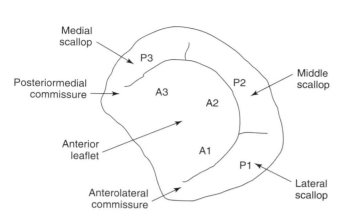

FIG. 4-22   Illustration of mitral valve anatomy as it appears in the transgastric basal short-axis view. Leaflets are labeled according to the Carpentier nomenclature. P1, P2, and P3 are the lateral, middle, and medial scallops of the posterior leaflet, respectively. A1, A2, and A3 are the corresponding regions of the anterior leaflet.

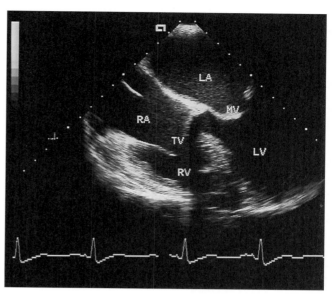

FIG. 4-24   Transesophageal echocardiogram of the midesophageal four-chamber view. *LA,* Left atrium; *LV,* left ventricle; *MV,* mitral valve; *RA,* right atrium; *RV,* right ventricle; *TV,* tricuspid valve.

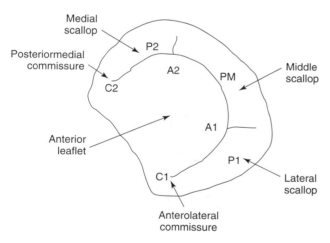

FIG. 4-23   Illustration of mitral valve anatomy as it appears in the transgastric basal short-axis view. Leaflets are labeled according to the Kumar/Duran nomenclature. P1, PM, and P2 are the lateral, middle, and medial scallops of the posterior leaflet, respectively. C1 and C2 refer to the leaflet areas near the anterior and posterior commissures, respectively. A1 refers to the anterior aspect of the anterior leaflet and A2 refers to the posterior aspect of the anterior leaflet.

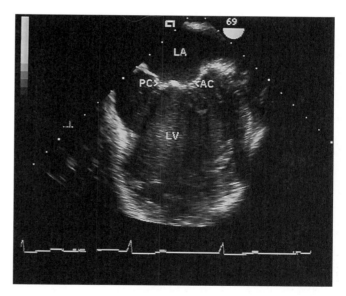

FIG. 4-25   Transesophageal echocardiogram of the midesophageal mitral commissural view. The P1, A2, and P3 regions of the mitral valve are imaged in this view. *AC,* Anterior commissure of the mitral valve; *LA,* left atrium; *LV,* left ventricle; *PC,* posterior commissure of the mitral valve.

similarly designated lateral, medial, and middle or A1, A2, and A3, respectively. Kumar and Duran proposed different terminology,[78] as indicated in Fig. 4-23. For the purpose of this discussion, the Carpentier nomenclature will be used.

The mitral valve apparatus is examined by using the four midesophageal and two transgastric views.[37] The

midesophageal views are obtained at the mid left atrial level by directing the ultrasound plane parallel to the transmitral blood flow and rotating the multiplane imaging angle axially through the mitral valve to acquire the four-chamber view (0° to 20°, Fig. 4-24), the commissural view (60° to 70°, Fig. 4-25), two-chamber view (80° to 100°), and the long-axis view (120° to 160°, Fig.

4-26). Specific posterior leaflet scallops and anterior leaflet regions are examined according to the particular imaging plane that is developed. For example, the commissural view provides imaging of P3, A2, and P1 mitral leaflet segments. The specific valvular lesion that requires repair is thus identified and communicated to the surgeon before the incision is made. The information is important for the surgeon to develop a plan for repair or replacement. Flail or prolapsing posterior leaflet segments (Fig. 4-27) are technically easier to repair and have higher success rates.[5] Bileaflet abnormalities, chordal fusion and shortening, and leaflet calcification are more challenging to repair. Left atrial size indicates the acute versus chronic nature of mitral valve disease and the ease of surgical visualization. Mean left atrial size range is 39 ± 7 cm in the medial to lateral dimension and 38 ± 6 cm in the anteroposterior dimension.[38] A transgastric short-axis view of the mitral valve is shown in Fig. 4-28. This view is used to measure mitral valve area by planimetry and to identify the origin of regurgitant jets.

Examination of the LV for size and regional wall-motion abnormalities provides valuable information in the assessment of mitral valve function. Annular dilation occurs with left ventricular dilation. The posterormedial papillary muscle is more susceptible to ischemia than the anterolateral papillary muscle because the anterior papillary muscle receives blood supply from two coronary arteries (left anterior descending and left circumflex), whereas the posterior papillary muscle receives blood supply from only the posterior descending coronary artery. The diagnosis of papillary

muscle dysfunction is usually associated with a regional wall-motion abnormality in the region of the papillary muscle attachment to the ventricular wall. An imaging plane that transects the muscle in its long axis is most useful to detect dysfunction, which appears as reduced muscle shortening and reduced thickening. The transgastric long-axis view at an 80° to 100° multiplane angle and the midesophageal commissural view are useful for this purpose. Particular papillary muscle dysfunction most commonly affects a region of the mitral valve rather than a particular leaflet. Both leaflets share pri-

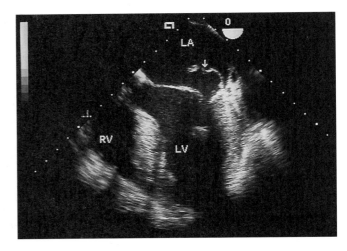

FIG. 4-27 Transesophageal echocardiogram of the midesophageal four-chamber view. Arrow indicates flail posterior leaflet secondary to ruptured chordae tendineae. *LA*, Left atrium; *LV*, left ventricle; *RV*, right ventricle.

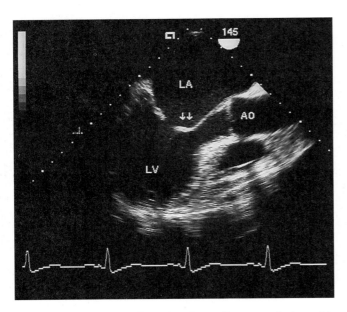

FIG. 4-26 Transesophageal echocardiogram of the midesophageal long-axis view. The P2 (middle) scallop of the posterior leaflet is also imaged in this view. Arrows indicate A2 region of the anterior leaflet of the mitral valve. *AO*, Ascending aorta; *LA*, left atrium; *LV*, left ventricle.

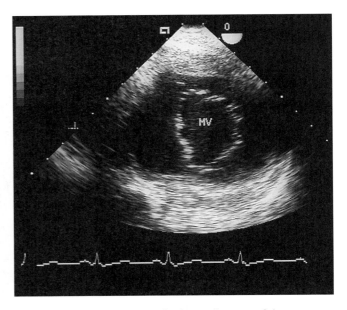

FIG. 4-28 Transesophageal echocardiogram of the transgastric basal short-axis view. The mitral valve *(MV)* is imaged in its short axis during diastole.

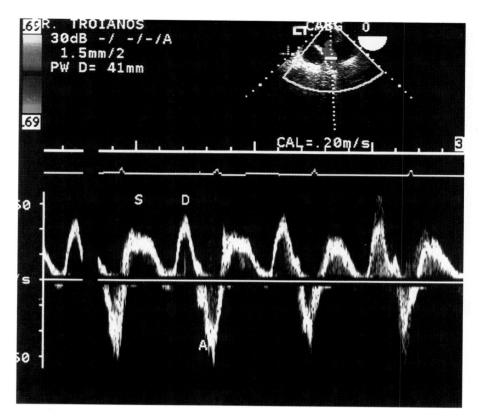

FIG. 4-6 Pulsed-wave Doppler echocardiogram of pulmonary vein flow. Markings above the horizontal axis indicate blood flow toward the transducer, while markings below the horizontal axis indicate blood flow away from the transducer. *A*, Atrial wave; *D*, diastolic wave; *S*, systolic wave.

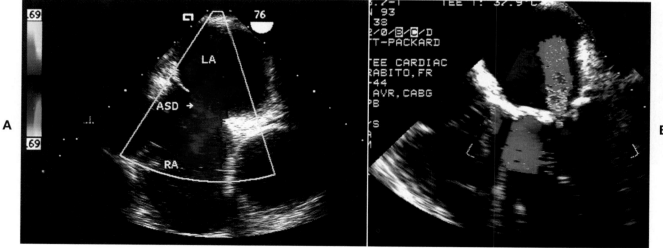

FIG. 4-7 Color Doppler echocardiogram indicating the direction of blood flow. **A**, Blue indicates flow away from the transducer. **B**, Red indicates flow toward the transducer.

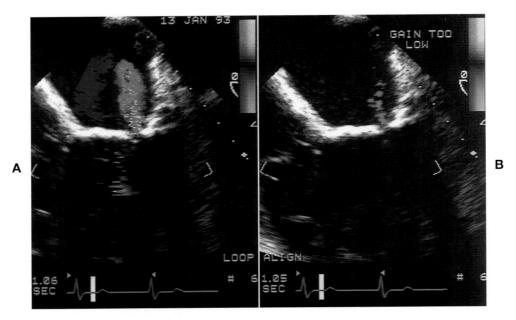

FIG. 4-8 Color Doppler echocardiogram illustrating the effect of color Doppler gain control on the size and character of the regurgitant jet. **A,** Proper gain control. **B,** Gain too low.

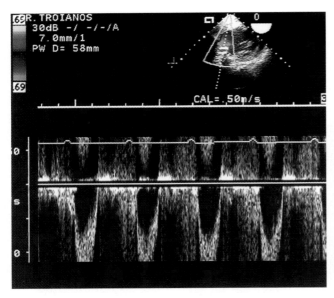

FIG. 4-9 Pulsed-wave Doppler echocardiogram indicating aliasing. The peak of the wave is cut off at the bottom of the figure, but appears at the top of the spectral display on the opposite side of the horizontal axis. Markings on opposite sides of the horizontal axis generally indicate blood flow in opposite directions. In this case, the markings appear on the opposite side of the horizontal axis because the peak velocities exceed the upper limit of the Doppler measurement.

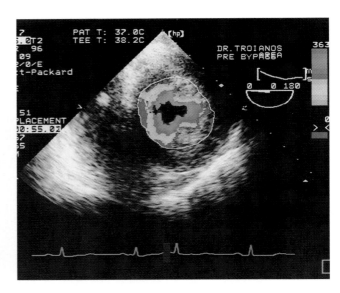

FIG. 4-20 Transesophageal echocardiogram with Color Kinesis (Hewlett-Packard Company, Andover, Mass.) of the transgastric left ventricular mid short axis. Color bands indicate myocardial excursion during one cardiac cycle.

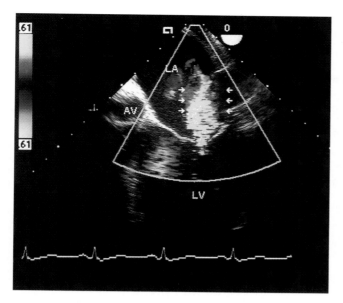

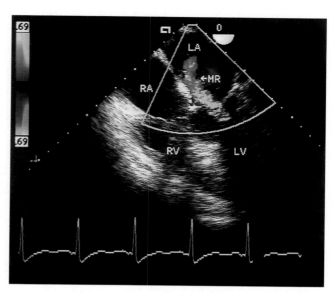

FIG. 4-29 Transesophageal echocardiogram with color flow Doppler. The arrows point to a flow disturbance in the left atrium (LA) that indicates a central mitral regurgitant jet. *LV*, Left ventricle; *AV*, aortic valve.

FIG. 4-30 Transesophageal echocardiogram with color flow Doppler. The arrow points to a flow disturbance in the left atrium *(LA)* that indicates an eccentric mitral regurgitant *(MR)* jet directed toward the atrial septum. *LV*, Left ventricle; *RA*, right atrium; *RV*, right ventricle.

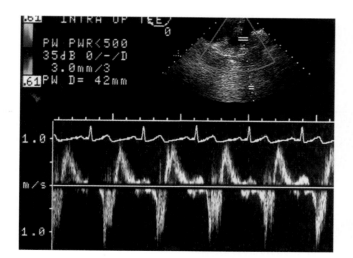

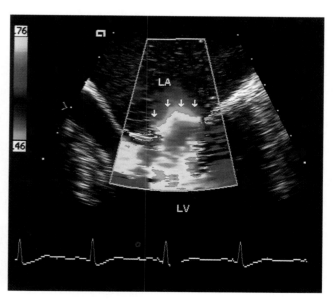

FIG. 4-33 Pulsed-wave spectral Doppler of pulmonary vein flow in a patient with severe mitral regurgitation. The systolic wave occurring after the QRS on the electrocardiogram is directed below the horizontal axis.

FIG. 4-39 Transesophageal echocardiogram in a patient with mitral stenosis. Color flow Doppler identifies flow convergence on the left atrial *(LA)* side of the mitral valve. The *arrows* indicate the isovelocity hemisphere with an aliasing velocity of 0.46 m/sec (see Nyquist limit on color velocity map).

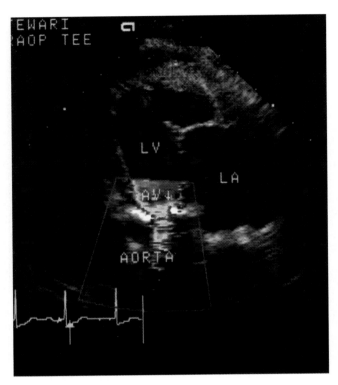

FIG. 4-50 Transesophageal echocardiogram of the deep apical transgastric view with color flow Doppler applied over the stenotic aortic valve. The flow disturbance within the aortic valve *(AV)* identifies the stenotic orifice. *LA,* Left atrium; *LV,* left ventricle.

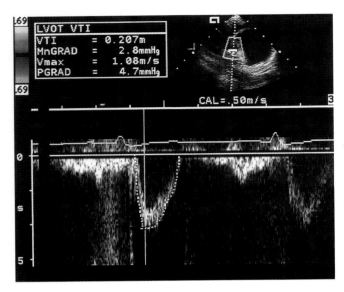

FIG. 4-54 Planimetry of the pulsed-wave spectral Doppler velocities in the left ventricular outflow tract *(LVOT)* provides the velocity time integral *(VTI)* of LVOT flow.

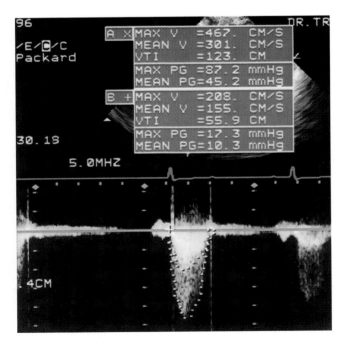

FIG. 4-55 Planimetry of both the aortic valve and left ventricular outflow tract velocities is performed on the same cardiac beat using continuous-wave spectral Doppler.

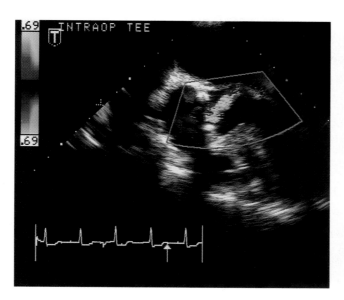

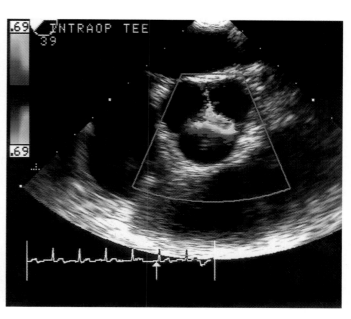

FIG. 4-56 Transesophageal echocardiogram with a color flow Doppler in a patient with aortic insufficiency. The aortic insufficiency is identified by the color flow disturbance that originates from the aortic valve and is directed toward the anterior mitral valve leaflet, creating a convexity in the mitral leaflet.

FIG. 4-57 Transesophageal echocardiogram of the midesophageal aortic valve short-axis view with color flow Doppler in a patient with aortic insufficiency. The origin of the aortic insufficiency is predominantly between the right and left coronary cusps.

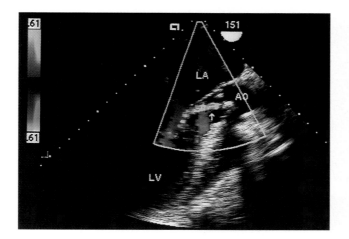

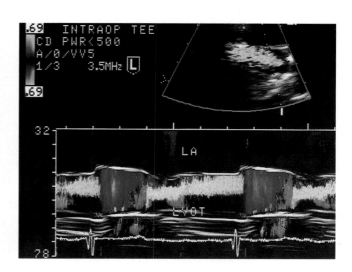

FIG. 4-58 Transesophageal echocardiogram of the midesophageal aortic valve long-axis view with color flow Doppler in a patient with aortic insufficiency *(arrow)*. *AO,* Ascending aorta; *LA,* left atrium; *LV,* left ventricle.

FIG. 4-59 Color M-mode echocardiography of the left ventricular outflow tract *(LVOT)* in a patient with aortic insufficiency. *LA,* Left atrium.

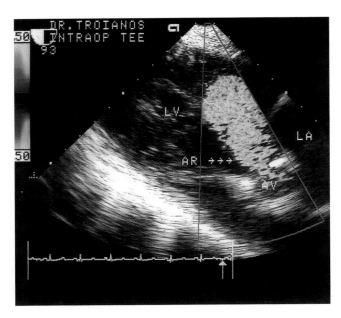

FIG. 4-60 Transesophageal echocardiogram of the transgastric long-axis view with color flow Doppler in a patient with aortic insufficiency (arrows). *AV,* Aortic valve; *LA,* left atrium; *LV,* left ventricle.

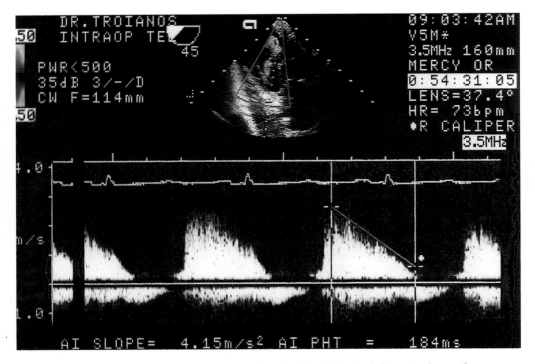

FIG. 4-61 Continuous-wave spectral Doppler velocities within the left ventricular outflow tract in a patient with aortic insufficiency. The slope of the velocity deceleration (AI slope = 4.15 m/sec^2) indicates the severity of the aortic insufficiency.

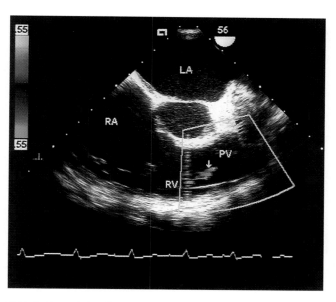

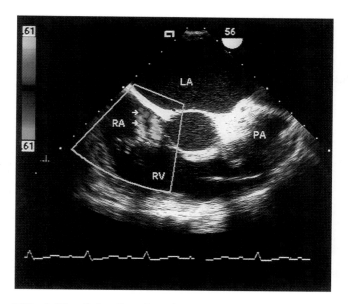

FIG. 4-66 Color flow Doppler applied to the right atrium identifies the flow disturbance *(arrow)* originating from the tricuspid valve and directed into the right atrium *(RA)* as tricuspid regurgitation. *LA,* Left atrium; *PA,* main pulmonary artery; *RV,* right ventricle.

FIG. 4-67 Color flow Doppler applied to the pulmonic valve identifies the flow disturbance *(arrow)* originating from the pulmonic valve and directed into the right ventricle *(RV)* as pulmonic regurgitation. *LA,* Left atrium; *PV,* pulmonic valve; *RA,* right atrium.

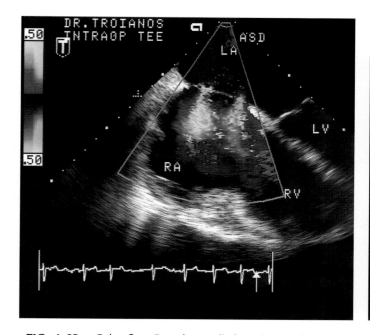

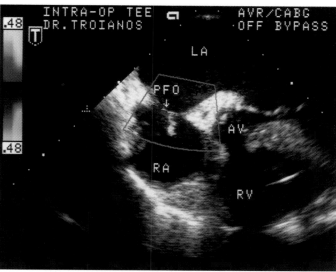

FIG. 4-68 Color flow Doppler applied to the atrial septum identifies two atrial septal defects. The blue jets directed toward the right atrium *(RA)* indicate left-to-right shunting of blood flow. *LA,* Left atrium; *LV,* left ventricle; *RV,* right ventricle.

FIG. 4-70 The small color flow disturbance originating at the atrial septum at the fossa ovalis *(arrow)* and directed toward the right atrium *(RA)* confirms the presence of a patent foramen ovale *(PFO). LA,* Left atrium; *RV,* right ventricle.

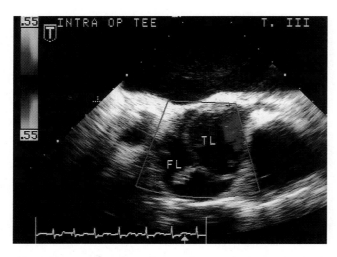

FIG. 4-78 Midesophageal ascending aortic short-axis view in a patient with an aortic dissection. An intimal flap is imaged in the aortic root separating the true lumen *(TL)* and the false lumen *(FL)*. A small high-velocity jet identifies the entry site for the aortic dissection and flow into the false lumen.

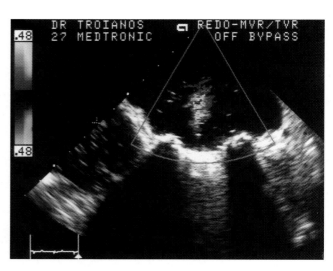

FIG. 4-86 Color flow Doppler echocardiography applied to a tilting disc mechanical mitral valve. A single, trace, central regurgitant jet within the sewing ring is characteristic of this valve.

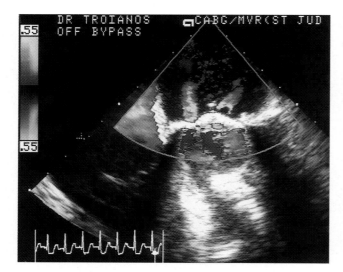

FIG. 4-87 Color flow Doppler echocardiography applied to a bileaflet mechanical mitral valve. Two to five small and symmetric regurgitant jets within the sewing ring are characteristic of this valve.

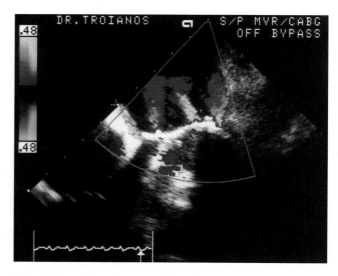

FIG. 4-88 Color flow Doppler echocardiography applied to a bileaflet mechanical mitral valve demonstrates two normal physiologic regurgitant jets within the sewing ring and an additional regurgitant jet outside the sewing ring, indicating a paravalvular leak.

mary chordae from both papillary muscles, so posterior papillary muscle dysfunction is likely to cause bileaflet prolapse at the posterior aspect of the valve (P3 and A3) rather than posterior leaflet prolapse alone.

Mitral Regurgitation

Pathology involving any or all of the structures of the mitral valve apparatus can cause MR. Myxomatous degeneration leading to leaflet prolapse is the most common etiology of MR requiring surgical correction. Chordae tendineae become elongated or rupture. One or both leaflets become redundant and prolapse or flail into the left atrium during systole. Infectious endocarditis causes leaflet perforation or scarring or chordal rupture. A more ominous finding is an annular abscess indicated by an echolucent region or "pocket" adjacent to the annular attachment of the infected leaflets. This finding is a significant problem for the surgeon who needs strong viable tissue in which to sew a prosthetic valve. Paravalvular leaks may occur in the region of an annular abscess after valve replacement. MR as a result of rheumatic endocarditis results from leaflet scarring and retraction and chordal fusion. Annular dilation is another cause of MR. As previously mentioned, the annulus dilates coincidentally with ventricular dilation, except when mitral annular calcification is prominent. The regurgitant jet tends to be centrally directed if annular dilation is the sole reason for valvular incompetence.

Color flow Doppler is used to detect and quantify regurgitant lesions by placing the color sector over the mitral valve and left atrium (Fig. 4-29). Several methods

are used to grade the severity of mitral regurgitation. Spatial area mapping of the color Doppler regurgitant jet provides an estimate of the degree of MR by measuring the regurgitant area or expressing the regurgitant area as a percentage of the left atrial size.[79] Severity is graded as trace, mild (1+), moderate (2+ to 3+), or severe (4+) (Table 4-9). It is important to use multiple imaging planes and approaches to evaluate jet area, particularly if the jet is eccentric or is directed along the left atrial wall. Spatial area mapping of wall-hugging jets (Fig. 4-30) underestimates the severity of regurgitation because, given the same regurgitant orifice size and regurgitant volume, energy is dissipated and

TABLE 4-9
Grading Mitral Regurgitation

DEGREE OF MR	% JET AREA/ LA AREA	JET LENGTH
Trace	0%-10%	<1 cm
1+ (mild)	10%-20%	1-2 cm
2+ (moderate)	20%-30%	1/3 LA anteroposterior distance
3+ (moderate)	30%-40%	1/3 to 2/3 LA antero-posterior distance
4+ (severe)	>40%	>2/3 LA antero-posterior distance

LA, Left atrium; *MR*, mitral regurgitation.

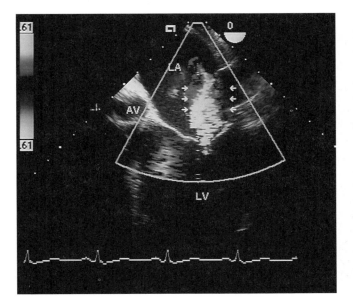

FIG. 4-29 Transesophageal echocardiogram with color flow Doppler. The arrows point to a flow disturbance in the left atrium (LA) that indicates a central mitral regurgitant jet. *LV*, Left ventricle; *AV*, aortic valve.

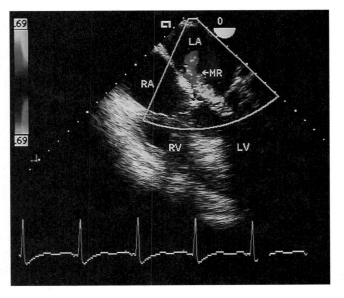

FIG. 4-30 Transesophageal echocardiogram with color flow Doppler. The arrow points to a flow disturbance in the left atrium *(LA)* that indicates an eccentric mitral regurgitant *(MR)* jet directed toward the atrial septum. *LV*, Left ventricle; *RA*, right atrium; *RV*, right ventricle.

TABLE 4-10
Twenty-Two Signs of Severe Mitral Regurgitation

1. Large jet area is a rough guide to severe mitral regurgitation
2. Wall-hugging jets are often associated with severe mitral regurgitation
3. The jet enters the left atrial appendage
4. Color flow jet enters the pulmonary vein or veins
5. The jet circles the left atrium
6. Agitated flow is seen in the left atrium
7. Proximal acceleration signals are proportional to the severity of mitral regurgitation
8. Size of the jet crossing the defect in the mitral valve is proportional to severity
9. Systolic reversal in pulmonary venous pulsed Doppler flow is characteristic
10. Pulsed Doppler signal of mitral inflow is increased
11. Left ventricular outflow tract and transaortic flow velocity are decreased
12. Density of continuous-wave Doppler jet is increased
13. V wave cut-off sign of the mitral regurgitation jet is seen
14. Left atrium is dilated
15. There is exaggerated systolic expansion of the left atrium
16. The interatrial septum bulges from left to right
17. The left ventricle is spherically enlarged
18. Left ventricular contractility appears hyperdynamic
19. There is no spontaneous contrast in the left atrium
20. There is spontaneous contrast in the proximal aorta
21. Mitral valve morphology is abnormal
22. There is right ventricular enlargement

From Schiller NB, Foster E, Redberg RF: *Cardiol Clin* 11:399-408, 1993.

---

velocity is reduced to a greater degree than centrally directed jets. It is common practice to increase the estimated severity of wall-hugging jets by 1 degree from the assessment made by spatial area mapping alone. This limitation emphasizes the need for several methods of assessment. Twenty-two signs of severe mitral regurgitation[80] are listed in Table 4-10.

Pulmonary vein flow interrogation by pulsed-wave Doppler echocardiography is another method of quantifying the degree of MR[81-83] (Fig. 4-31). The absence of valves in pulmonary veins allows transmission of left atrial and MR hemodynamics into the pulmonary venous system (see Fig. 4-15). The A wave, coincident with the "p" wave on the ECG, occurs because the atrial contraction that forces blood into the LV through the mitral valve also forces blood retrograde into the pulmonary veins. With the onset of left ventricular systole, the mitral valve closes, the empty left atrium relaxes and blood travels antegrade in the pulmonary veins from the lungs to the left atrium. This produces the S wave on the spectral Doppler display. The mitral valve opens in early diastole and blood moves from the left atrium to the LV. Blood from the lungs moves antegrade through the pulmonary veins toward the left atrium, producing the D wave on the spectral Doppler display. The S wave is normally larger than the D wave, and both waves are in the same direction from baseline (see Fig. 4-16, *A*). MR changes the appearance of the pulsed-wave Doppler analysis of pulmonary vein flow; the extent of the change depends on the severity of MR. Mild MR causes blunting of the S wave, which becomes equal in height

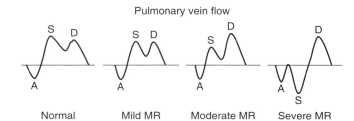

Pulmonary vein flow

Normal   Mild MR   Moderate MR   Severe MR

FIG. 4-31 Illustration of pulmonary vein flow patterns associated with varying degrees of mitral regurgitation *(MR)*. Markings above the horizontal axis indicate flow toward the left atrium, markings below the axis indicate flow toward the lungs. The A wave is flow during atrial contraction; the S wave is flow during systole; and the D wave is flow during early diastole.

to the D wave (Fig. 4-32). Moderate MR causes the S wave to be smaller than the D wave (see Fig. 4-16, *B*). Severe MR causes the S wave to occur in the opposite direction from the D wave (systolic reversal of pulmonary vein flow), as shown in Fig. 4-33.

Calculating regurgitant fraction is another method of quantifying the severity of MR based on the percentage of the left ventricular stroke volume that is ejected into the left atrium during systole. In the absence of aortic regurgitation, left ventricular stroke volume is equal to mitral inflow. Mitral inflow becomes greater than aortic outflow in the presence of MR. The MR volume is the difference between mitral inflow and aortic valve outflow. Regurgitant fraction

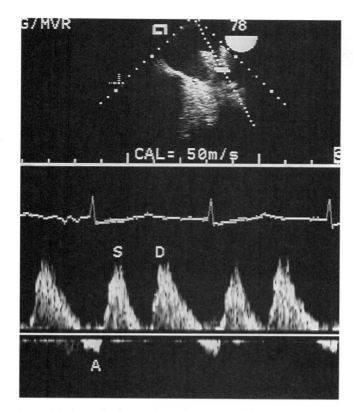

FIG. 4-32 Pulsed-wave Doppler spectral display of pulmonary vein flow in a patient with mild mitral regurgitation. The systolic wave *(S)* is equal to the early diastolic wave *(D)*. The A wave is flow during atrial contraction.

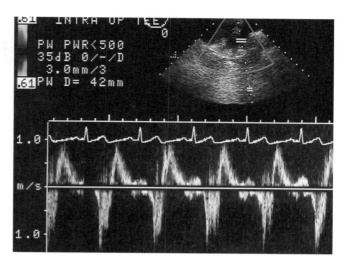

FIG. 4-33 Pulsed-wave spectral Doppler of pulmonary vein flow in a patient with severe mitral regurgitation. The systolic wave occurring after the QRS on the electrocardiogram is directed below the horizontal axis.

TABLE 4-11
Grading Mitral Regurgitation by Regurgitant Fraction and Orifice Size

DEGREE OF MITRAL REGURGITATION	REGURGITANT FRACTION[84]	REGURGITANT ORIFICE SIZE[85]
Mild	<18%	<10 mm²
Moderate	21%-37%	10-25 mm²
Severe	>37%	>25 mm²

is expressed as the proportion of mitral inflow that is regurgitant volume and indicates the severity of MR[84] (Table 4-11).

$$\text{Regurgitant Fraction} = \frac{\text{mitral inflow} - \text{aortic outflow}}{\text{mitral inflow}}$$

Proximal isovelocity surface area (PISA) is a method of quantifying MR by calculating the regurgitant orifice size using the principle of mass conservation. Blood accelerates as it flows toward a small (regurgitant) orifice, passes through multiple isovelocity hemispheres, and ultimately passes through the regurgitant orifice. The principle of mass conservation assumes that the volume of blood in any one isovelocity hemisphere is equal to the volume passing through the regurgitant orifice. Isovelocity hemispheres are identified using color flow Doppler imaging; the color changes as blood converging toward an orifice accelerates beyond the Nyquist limit. The blood velocity at the hemisphere outlined by the change in color is termed the *aliasing velocity* and is equal to the Nyquist limit. Blood flow expressed as the product of the aliasing velocity and area of the isovelocity hemisphere ($2\pi r^2$) is equal to the blood flow through the regurgitant orifice.

The regurgitant orifice velocity allows calculation of the regurgitant orifice area (Fig. 4-34).

$$\text{Regurgitant orifice area} = \frac{2\pi r^2 \times \text{aliasing velocity}}{\text{regurgitant orifice velocity}}$$

Regurgitant orifice area correlates with the severity of MR,[85] as indicated in Table 4-11.

Mitral Stenosis

Mitral stenosis is a reduction in mitral valve orifice area caused by commissural fusion of the leaflets with shortening, calcification, and fusion of the chordae tendineae. Rheumatic endocarditis is the most common cause of mitral stenosis in the United States. The classic manifestation is thickening, localized predominantly at the leaflet tips with varying thickening and calcification at the base and midportion of the leaflets. A compensatory increase in left atrial pressure with restriction of left ventricular inflow creates a pressure gradient between the atrium and ventricle during diastole. Long-standing

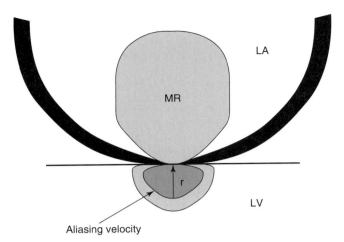

FIG. 4-34   Illustration of proximal flow convergence with mitral regurgitation *(MR)*. The aliasing velocity and the radius *(r)* of the isovelocity hemisphere are used to calculate the regurgitant orifice area. *LA*, Left atrial side of the mitral valve; *LV*, left ventricular side of the mitral valve.

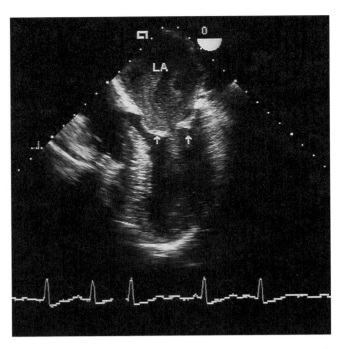

FIG. 4-35   Transesophageal echocardiogram of the midesophageal four-chamber view of the mitral valve in a patient with mitral stenosis. The arrows indicate mitral leaflet doming that creates a "hockey stick" appearance of the leaflets. Spontaneous echocontrast in the left atrium *(LA)* appears as "smoke" and indicates a low-flow state in the left atrium.

mitral stenosis leads to pulmonary hypertension and right heart failure.

Two-dimensional echocardiography is a very important aspect of the TEE evaluation of mitral stenosis. Leaflet doming during diastole creates a "hockey stick" appearance of the anterior leaflet because of localized calcification and restriction at the leaflet tip with relative sparing of the base and midportions of the leaflet. Leaflet doming is best appreciated using long-axis views of the valve (four-chamber, two-chamber, and long-axis) and is a qualitative sign of stenosis (Fig. 4-35). Chordal shortening and fusion is another hallmark of rheumatic mitral stenosis. Two-dimensional echocardiography often reveals the papillary muscle tips in close proximity to the mitral valve leaflets. A classification system for grading mitral stenosis on the basis of two-dimensional echocardiographic features is listed in Table 4-12. A short-axis view of the mitral valve is obtained via a basal transgastric short-axis view of the LV. The stenotic mitral valve in this view appears as a fish mouth because the leaflet edges are thickened and the orifice is small and elliptical. The left atrial cavity is enlarged, whereas the left ventricular cavity is small. Spontaneous echocontrast is often present in the left atrium, particularly if the patient's rhythm is atrial fibrillation, and is indicative of the low-velocity blood flow in the left atrium (Fig. 4-35). The entire left atrium, particularly the left atrial appendage, is carefully examined for thrombus. Discovery of an intracavitary thrombus is immediately communicated to the surgeon to avoid possible dislodgment with surgical manipulation. Right atrial and right ventricular enlargement are observed with right heart failure caused by long-standing mitral stenosis and pulmonary hypertension.

The mitral valve area and transvalvular gradient are used to evaluate the severity of mitral stenosis. It is important to appreciate the dynamic nature of a transvalvular gradient and its dependence on transvalvular flow. Gradient increases as flow increases for a given fixed orifice size. A patient with a low cardiac output will therefore exhibit a lower transvalvular gradient than a patient with the same mitral valve orifice and normal cardiac output. Conversely, a patient with MR or sepsis with increased transvalvular flow will have a higher gradient than a patient with the same orifice and normal transvalvular flow. Transvalvular gradient must be assessed in context of the clinical state of the patient and confounding variables that affect transvalvular flow.

Area determination using planimetry is the easiest concept to understand. A short-axis view of the mitral valve is obtained using the basal transgastric view of the ventricle. The imaging plane is adjusted to obtain a short-axis view of the mitral leaflet tips and a cine loop is reviewed for maximal leaflet opening in diastole. Tracing the area within the leaflet tips determines the area (Fig. 4-36), which indicates the severity of mitral stenosis. This technique has the following limitations: (1) inability to obtain an adequate image of the entire three-dimensional orifice in one two-dimensional imaging plane; (2) heavy calcification, particularly posterior,

TABLE 4-12
Grading Mitral Stenosis by Two-Dimensional Echocardiography

GRADE	LEAFLET MOBILITY	SUBVALVULAR THICKENING	LEAFLET THICKENING	CALCIFICATION
1	Highly mobile valve with only leaflet tips restricted	Minimal thickening just below the mitral leaflets	Leaflets near normal in thickness (4-5 mm)	A single area of increased echo brightness
2	Normal mobility in middle and base portions	Chordal structures thickened up to one third of chordal length	Middle portion of leaflets normal, considerable thickening of margins (5-8 mm)	Scattered area of brightness confined to leaflet margins
3	Valve moves forward during diastole, mainly at the base	Thickening extends to the distal third of the chords	Thickening extends throughout the entire leaflet (5-8 mm)	Brightness extending into the middle portion of the leaflets
4	No or minimal forward movement of the leaflets during diastole	Extensive thickening and shortening of all chordal structures extending down to the papillary muscles	Considerable thickening of all leaflet tissue (>8-10 mm)	Extensive brightness throughout much of the leaflet tissue

From Wilkins GT, Weyman AE, Abascal VM et al: *Br Heart J* 60:299-308, 1988.

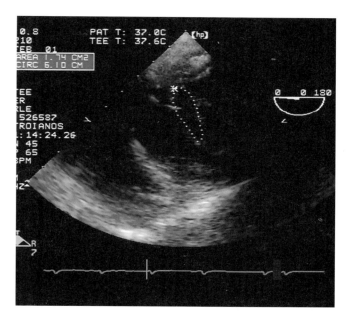

FIG. 4-36   Planimetry of the mitral valve in short axis indicates a reduced orifice size (1.74 cm²) associated with mitral stenosis.

that causes shadowing of the anterior aspect of the valve; (3) the influence of two-dimensional gain control; and (4) the most narrow portion of the valve may not be at the leaflet tips, but subvalvular within the chordal apparatus. Higher gain enhances the thickness of the leaflets

and the orifice appears smaller than with lower, appropriate gain.

Doppler echocardiography is used to determine the severity of mitral stenosis by several methods. Transmitral velocities displayed over time are used to determine the rate of diastolic deceleration, which is a function of the transvalvular pressure gradient. Transvalvular velocity decelerates slower through a more stenotic orifice because the gradient persists for a longer period of time. The rate of deceleration or deceleration slope provides an estimate of mitral valve area (Fig. 4-37). *Pressure half-time* (PHT) is the time required for the peak transmitral pressure gradient to decrease by one half. Because pressure is mathematically related to velocity by the modified Bernoulli equation by $P = 4V^2$, the time required for the pressure gradient to decrease by one half is equivalent to the time required for the peak velocity to decrease 30%.

$$PHT = \frac{P_{MAX}}{2}$$

$$4V^2 = \frac{4V^2_{MAX}}{2}$$

$$V^2 = \frac{V^2_{MAX}}{2}$$

$$V = \frac{V_{MAX}}{\sqrt{2}} = 0.7\, V_{MAX}$$

Studies comparing PHT with mitral valve area using the Gorlin equation determined a linear relationship, such that a PHT of about 220 ms corresponded to a valve area of 1 cm².[86] Mitral valve area is then calculated using PHT, as shown in the following formula.

$$\text{Mitral valve area} = \frac{220}{\text{PHT}}$$

Color Doppler is used to identify the turbulent flow through the narrowed mitral orifice, and the continuous-wave Doppler beam is aligned within the flow disturbance. Transmitral velocities are recorded using continuous-wave Doppler because the peak velocity often exceeds the limits of pulsed-wave Doppler. The deceleration slope is used to determine PHT, and the peak velocity is used to determine the peak gradient using the modified Bernoulli equation. Mean gradient is determined by tracing the spectral Doppler velocity display during diastole.

Methods that use transmitral velocities as a reflection of transvalvular gradients to assess the severity of mitral stenosis assume that the pressure difference between the left atrium and LV is solely because of the stenotic valve. Other determinants of left atrial and left ventricular pressure affect the validity of this assumption. For example, aortic insufficiency and a less compliant LV will lead to a more rapid rise in left ventricular pressure during diastole and allow the pressure between the left atrium and ventricle to equalize more rapidly than would occur with a stenotic mitral valve. Transvalvular velocity measurements in the presence of aortic insufficiency or left ventricular failure will underestimate the severity of mi-

tral stenosis by providing velocity measurements more reflective of a larger orifice than actually exists.

Another method used to calculate mitral valve area involves the continuity equation based on the conservation of mass. This method assumes that blood flow through two consecutive, intact structures is equal. For example, in the absence of pulmonic and mitral insufficiency, the blood flowing through the pulmonary artery and left ventricular outflow tract should equal the flow through the mitral valve. Stroke volume is calculated by measuring the diameter (d) and multiplying the area $[\pi \times (d/2)^2]$ by the VTI of the blood flow in the pulmonary artery or the left ventricular outflow tract. VTI of the mitral valve is obtained from the continuous-wave spectral Doppler display of blood flow velocity through the stenotic mitral orifice (VTI$_{\text{Trans-mitral}}$). Mitral valve area is determined by the following formula:

$$\text{Mitral valve area} = \frac{\text{Stroke volume}}{\text{VTI}_{\text{Trans-mitral}}}$$

The principle of proximal flow convergence described above for determining mitral regurgitant orifice size can also be applied to determine the stenotic mitral orifice. Proximal flow convergence occurs on the left atrial side of the stenotic valve instead of the left ventricular side of the regurgitant valve, and is not affected by planar orifice shape.[87] This principle of proximal flow convergence is an expression of the continuity equation, because blood flowing through an isovelocity sphere proximal to the mitral valve ultimately passes through the valve orifice area. The funnel-shaped angle (α) formed by the mitral leaflets restricts the region of proximal flow and must be incorporated into the equation that describes the flow through the isovelocity surface area (Fig. 4-38). Color Doppler is used to define the isovelocity hemisphere by the aliasing velocity at the border between blue and red bands (Fig. 4-39). The

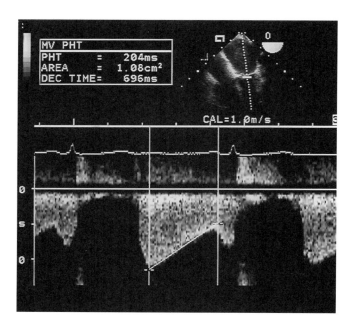

FIG. 4-37 Continuous-wave spectral Doppler velocities through a stenotic mitral valve. The deceleration slope is used to estimate mitral valve area by the pressure half-time method.

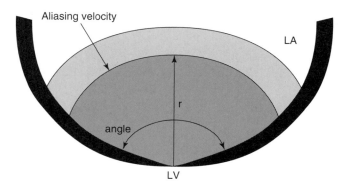

FIG. 4-38 Illustration of proximal flow convergence with mitral stenosis. The aliasing velocity, convergence angle, and the radius (r) of the isovelocity hemisphere are used to calculate the stenotic orifice area. *LA*, Left atrial side of the mitral valve; *LV*, left ventricular side of the mitral valve.

radius (r) is measured from the center of the mitral orifice to the isovelocity hemisphere and the hemispheric velocity is equal to the Nyquist limit for flow away from the ultrasound transducer. The PISA flow is equal to mitral valve orifice flow and is expressed as follows:

$$\text{Mitral orifice flow} = \text{PISA} = 2\pi r^2 \, (\alpha/180) \times \text{hemispheric velocity}$$

Flow through the mitral orifice is the product of mitral valve orifice area and transmitral flow velocity ($VTI_{Trans\text{-}mitral}$). Mitral valve area is then calculated by the following equation:

$$\text{Mitral valve area} = \frac{2\pi r^2 \, (\alpha/180) \times \text{hemispheric velocity}}{VTI_{Trans\text{-}mitral}}$$

Left Atrium

The left atrium is perhaps the most easily imaged structure with TEE because of its close proximity to the esophagus. Left atrial enlargement is common with both chronic MR and mitral stenosis. The left atrium and the left atrial appendage are carefully examined for thrombus formation, particularly in patients with atrial fibrillation and mitral stenosis. The probe is adjusted to image the pulmonary veins by slight turning the probe to the left to image the left pulmonary veins and slightly turning to the right to image the right pulmonary veins. The lower right and left pulmonary veins are imaged by slightly advancing the probe into the esophagus from the position that provided imaging of the upper pulmonary veins. Pulmonary venous flow is evaluated with pulsed-wave Doppler by placing the sample volume in the pulmonary vein. The left upper pulmonary vein is most commonly used because of its parallel orientation in relation to the Doppler beam and the ease by which it is identified.

Aortic Valve

Echocardiographic evaluation of the aortic valve is an important aspect of the perioperative evaluation of surgical patients. The high-resolution images of the aortic valve provided by TEE result from the close proximity of the valve to the esophagus. The application of Doppler echocardiography (pulsed-wave, continuous-wave, and color) with two-dimensional imaging allows for the complete evaluation of stenotic and regurgitant lesions. The increased population of elderly patients needing surgery has increased the prevalence of calcific aortic stenosis. Identifying significant aortic stenosis is important for anesthesia management during noncardiac surgery and for surgical management during non–aortic valve cardiac surgery. Aortic valve replacement after previous coronary artery bypass grafting is associated with higher mortality than combined aortic valve and coronary bypass surgery.[88] It is therefore important to identify even moderate aortic stenosis during coronary bypass surgery and consider combination surgery to avoid the higher mortality associated with reoperation. Certain patients have a rapid progression of aortic stenosis, whereas others have a slower progression. Patients with rapid progression tend to be elderly male smokers with associated coronary artery disease,[89,90] hypercholesterolemia, and elevated serum creatinine levels.[91]

The aortic valve is composed of three cusps that are associated with three bulges or pouchlike dilations in the aortic wall called the *Sinuses of Valsalva* (Fig. 4-40). The anatomic plane of the aortic valve is oblique compared with the plane of the esophagus, which is longitudinal within the body. The right posterior aspect is inferior to the left anterior aspect of the valve. The implication for TEE imaging is that the transducer must be flexed anteriorly and to the left from the transverse plane of the patient, to align the imaging plane with the plane of the aortic valve. Alternatively, a multiplane TEE probe is rotated forward 30° to 60° with anteflexion (Fig. 4-41). This view is important for tracing the aortic valve orifice area using planimetry and for identifying the site of aortic insufficiency using color flow Doppler. The left ventricular outflow tract, proximal to the aortic valve, consists of the inferior surface of the anterior mitral leaflet, the ventricular septum, and the posterior left ventricular free wall. The midesophageal long-axis view (see Fig. 4-26) provides imaging of the left ventricular outflow tract to differentiate valvular from subvalvular stenosis.

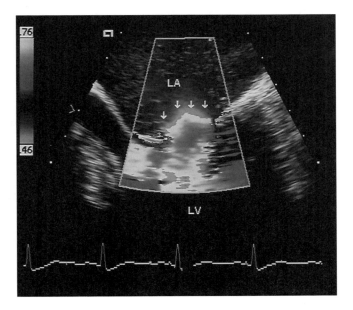

FIG. 4-39 Transesophageal echocardiogram in a patient with mitral stenosis. Color flow Doppler identifies flow convergence on the left atrial *(LA)* side of the mitral valve. The *arrows* indicate the isovelocity hemisphere with an aliasing velocity of 0.46 m/sec (see Nyquist limit on color velocity map).

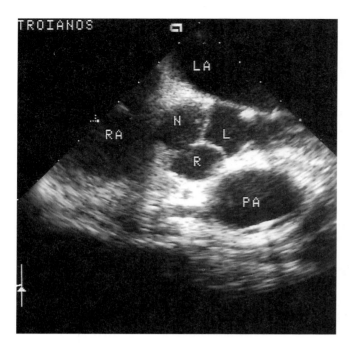

FIG. 4-40   Transesophageal echocardiogram of the mid-esophageal aortic valve short-axis view during diastole. The aortic valve is identified by the right *(R)*, left *(L)*, and non *(N)* coronary cusps. *LA,* Left atrium; *PA,* pulmonary artery/right ventricular outflow tract; *RA,* right atrium.

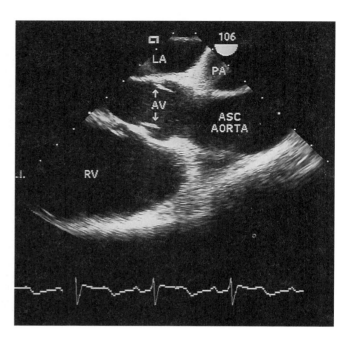

FIG. 4-42   Transesophageal echocardiogram of the mid-esophageal aortic valve long-axis view during systole. This normal aortic valve *(AV)* has leaflets *(arrows)* that open parallel to the aortic walls. The proximal ascending *(ASC)* aorta is also imaged in this view. *LA,* Left atrium; *PA,* pulmonary artery; *RV,* right ventricle.

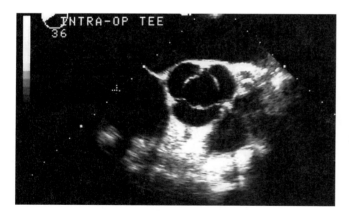

FIG. 4-41   Transesophageal echocardiogram of the mid-esophageal aortic valve short-axis view during systole. A multiplane probe at 36° provided this view in which all three aortic valve cusps are similar in size and appearance, indicating a true short-axis cross section.

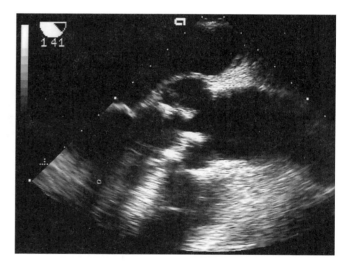

FIG. 4-43   Transesophageal echocardiogram of the mid-esophageal aortic valve long-axis view during systole in a patient with aortic stenosis. The doming of the leaflets is a qualitative sign of aortic stenosis.

Aortic Stenosis

The most common causes of aortic stenosis are calcific stenosis of the elderly, rheumatic, and congenital (bicuspid, rarely unicuspid). Acquired stenosis occurs from calcification of the leaflets (calcific, rheumatic, or congenital) or commissural fusion (usually rheumatic). Subaortic stenosis (subaortic membrane or ridge and asymmetric septal hypertrophy) and supravalvular stenosis (narrowed aortic root) mimic aortic stenosis, but do not represent true valvular stenosis. Many of the echocardiographic techniques used to evaluate the aortic valve, however, can also be used to evaluate subval-

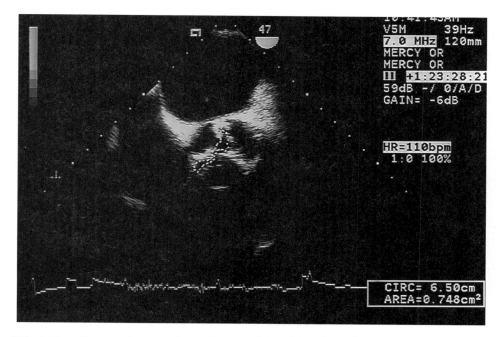

FIG. 4-44   Transesophageal echocardiogram of the midesophageal aortic valve short-axis view during systole in a patient with aortic stenosis. Planimetry of the aortic valve indicates a reduced orifice size (0.748 cm^2) associated with aortic stenosis.

vular and supravalvular pathology. Asymmetric septal hypertrophy or hypertrophic obstructive cardiomyopathy is further discussed in Chapter 11.

The long-axis view of the aortic valve is developed by rotating the multiplane angle forward to 110° to 150° (orthogonal to the short-axis view). A normal aortic valve appears as two thin lines that open parallel to the aortic walls. The ascending aorta is also inspected with this view (Fig. 4-42). An important sign of stenosis is doming of the leaflets during systole (Fig. 4-43). The leaflets are curved toward the midline of the aorta instead of parallel to the aortic wall. Leaflet doming is such an important observation that this finding alone is sufficient for the qualitative diagnosis of aortic stenosis. Coincident with doming is reduced leaflet separation (<15 mm), which is appreciated in both the short- and long-axis views of the aortic valve. The short-axis view of the aortic valve permits evaluation of leaflet motion and calcification, commissural fusion, and leaflet coaptation. This short-axis view (30° to 60°) allows measurement of aortic valve orifice area by two-dimensional planimetry (Fig. 4-44) and provides good correlation with other methods used to assess aortic stenosis.[92] The probe is manipulated to provide the image with the smallest orifice to ensure that the cross section is of the leaflet tips. A cross section that is oblique or inferior to the leaflet tips will overestimate the orifice size (Fig. 4-45). The valve must appear circular and all three cusps must be viewed simultaneously[92] and appear equal in

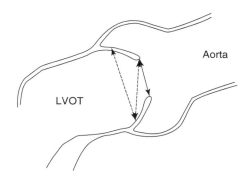

FIG. 4-45   Illustration of various cross sections that may be used to perform planimetry measurements of aortic valve orifice size. The solid line indicates the correct cross section at the tips of the aortic cusps. The two dotted lines indicate an oblique cross section and a cross section that is inferior to the leaflet tips, both of which result in an overestimation of aortic valve orifice size. *LVOT,* Left ventricular outflow tract.

shape to avoid oblique cross sections of the valve that overestimate the orifice size. Multiplane TEE simplifies the location of the actual orifice by imaging the aortic valve, first in long axis, to identify the smallest orifice at the leaflet tips, which is centered on the image display screen. The transducer position is stabilized within the esophagus as the multiplane angle is rotated backward to the short-axis view of the valve. The smallest orifice is traced and the two-dimensional cross-sectional area is displayed. This technique has the following limitations: (1) inability to obtain an adequate short-axis view; (2) heavy calcification, particularly posterior, that causes shadowing of the valve; and (3) the presence of "pin-hole" aortic stenosis, in which the valve orifice cannot be identified. The short-axis view of the aortic valve

identifies congenital abnormalities of the aortic valve, including bicuspid (Fig. 4-46) and unicuspid (Fig. 4-47) valves.

Doppler echocardiography is used to quantitate the severity of aortic stenosis by measuring the transvalvular blood velocity. The peak pressure gradient is estimated from the peak velocity measurement using the modified Bernoulli equation.

$$\text{Aortic Valve Gradient} = 4 \times (\text{Aortic Valve Velocity})^2$$

The midesophageal views of the aortic valve are not suitable for measuring transaortic velocity because accurate Doppler measurements require a parallel alignment of the Doppler beam with the blood flow. The deep apical transgastric view is developed by advancing the probe beyond the transgastric midpapillary and apical short-axis views, maximally anteflexing the probe and flexing it to the left (Fig. 4-48). This places the probe at the left ventricular apex with the ultrasound beam directed toward the base of the heart. The left atrium appears in the far field, to the right of the aortic valve and aortic root. A parallel alignment with blood flow in the left ventricular outflow tract (LVOT) and through the aortic valve is thus achieved. A parallel alignment of the ultrasound beam and aortic valve flow can also be obtained with the transgastric long-axis view. This view is developed from the transgastric mid-

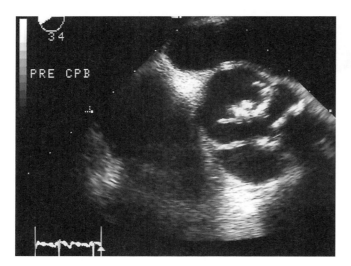

FIG. 4-46 Transesophageal echocardiogram of the midesophageal aortic valve short-axis view in a patient with bicuspid aortic stenosis.

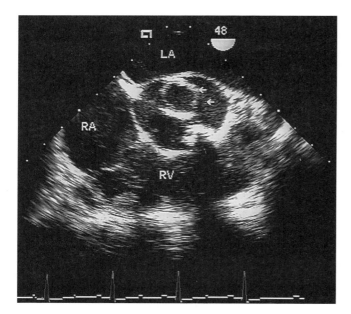

FIG. 4-47 Transesophageal echocardiogram of the midesophageal aortic valve short-axis view in a patient with a unicuspid aortic valve, as indicated by the arrows. *LA*, Left atrium; *RA*, right atrium; *RV*, right ventricle.

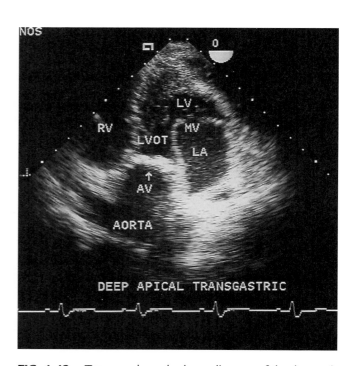

FIG. 4-48 Transesophageal echocardiogram of the deep apical transgastric view. *AV*, Stenotic aortic valve; *LA*, left atrium; *LV*, left ventricle; *LVOT*, left ventricular outflow tract; *MV*, mitral valve; *RV*, right ventricle.

papillary short-axis view by rotating the multiplane angle from zero to about 90°. The left atrium appears on the right side of the screen and the aortic valve is in the far field (Fig. 4-49). These imaging planes are difficult for the novice to obtain, but image acquisition improves with experience.[93]

Color flow Doppler and the audible Doppler signal are useful for identifying the location of the narrow high-velocity jet (Fig. 4-50). The continuous-wave Doppler cursor is placed within the narrow, turbulent jet and the spectral Doppler display is activated. Accurate localization provides a distinctive audible sound and high velocity (>3 m/sec) spectral Doppler recording that exhibits a fine feathery appearance and a midsystolic peak (Fig. 4-51). Normal aortic valves have peak velocities of 0.9 to 1.7 m/sec in adults, and peak in early systole. More dominant and dense lower velocities are also evident on the spectral Doppler display and represent the more laminar, lower velocities in the LVOT. Planimetry of the velocity over time spectral Doppler analysis of transaortic blood flow yields the VTI and an estimate of mean aortic valve gradient.

A gradient across a stenotic orifice is dynamic because of flow dependence. As the flow (or cardiac output) through the valve decreases, the gradient also decreases. Conversely, as flow or the force of contraction increase, the gradient also increases. Pressure gradients obtained

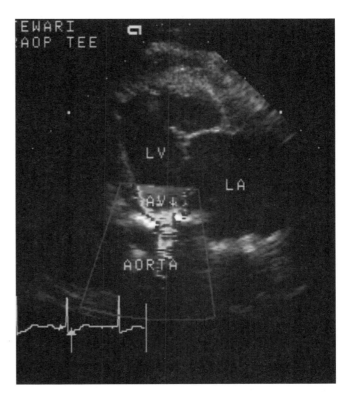

FIG. 4-50   Transesophageal echocardiogram of the deep apical transgastric view with color flow Doppler applied over the stenotic aortic valve. The flow disturbance within the aortic valve *(AV)* identifies the stenotic orifice. *LA,* Left atrium; *LV,* left ventricle.

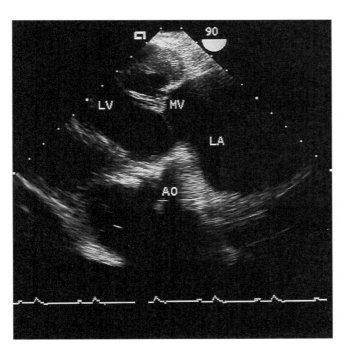

FIG. 4-49   Transesophageal echocardiogram of the transgastric long-axis view. *AO,* Aortic root; *LA,* left atrium; *LV,* left ventricle; *MV,* mitral valve.

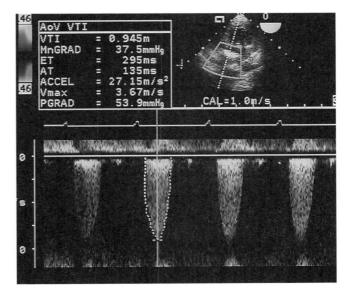

FIG. 4-51   Continuous-wave spectral Doppler velocities through a stenotic aortic valve. The fine feathery appearance of the high (3.67 m/sec) velocities with a midsystolic peak indicates flow through a stenotic aortic valve. The denser lower velocities near the baseline indicate flow through the left ventricular outflow tract.

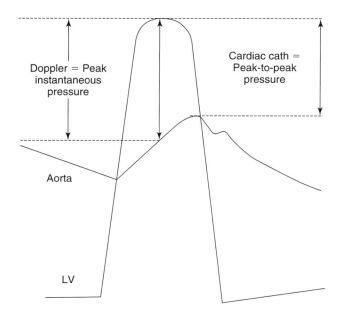

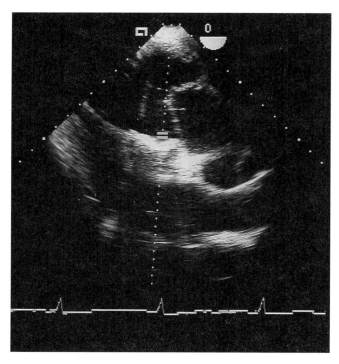

FIG. 4-52   Illustration of the pressure tracings obtained during cardiac catheterization in a patient with aortic stenosis. The pressure gradient obtained with Doppler echocardiography is reflective of the peak instantaneous gradient. The cardiac catheterization gradient is the difference between the peak left ventricular and peak aortic pressures.

FIG. 4-53   Transesophageal echocardiogram of the deep apical transgastric view with the pulsed-wave Doppler sample volume in the left ventricular outflow tract, just inferior to the aortic valve.

preoperatively with TEE use the same principles as intraoperative TEE. However, the intraoperative loading conditions, heart rate, and force of contraction may differ markedly from preoperative conditions, yielding disparate gradient data. Doppler-derived gradients also differ from gradients obtained in the cardiac catheterization laboratory, because of the differing techniques employed for gradient determination. A catheterization-laboratory gradient is usually a "peak-to-peak" gradient, which represents the difference between the peak left ventricular pressure and the peak aortic pressure. A Doppler gradient however, is a "peak instantaneous" gradient, which is greater than the peak-to-peak gradient (Fig. 4-52). It is also important to correctly identify the origin of the gradient between the LV and aorta as either valvular, subvalvular, or supravalvular.

Valve area is considered a more constant and less dynamic assessment of aortic stenosis. Recent evidence, however, indicates that the more pliable (moderately stenotic, nonrheumatic) valves may open more with increased contractility.[94] Determination of aortic valve area with Doppler echocardiography employs the continuity equation, which states that blood flowing through sequential areas of a continuous, intact, vascular system must be equal. Blood flowing through the LVOT is equated with blood flow through the aortic valve.

$$\text{Aortic Valve}_{\text{BLOOD FLOW}} = \text{LVOT}_{\text{BLOOD FLOW}}$$

Substitution of blood flow with the product of velocity (VTI) and cross sectional area yields:

$$\text{Aortic Valve Area} \times \text{Aortic Valve}_{\text{VTI}} = \text{LVOT}_{\text{AREA}} \times \text{LVOT}_{\text{VTI}}$$

Aortic valve area is then calculated as:

$$\text{Aortic Valve Area} = \frac{\text{LVOT}_{\text{AREA}} \times \text{LVOT}_{\text{VTI}}}{\text{Aortic Valve}_{\text{VTI}}}$$

LVOT_{VTI} is measured by placing the pulsed-wave Doppler sample volume in the LVOT just inferior to the aortic valve (Fig. 4-53) and tracing the spectral Doppler velocity over time (Fig. 4-54). Optimal sampling of LVOT velocity is performed by advancing the sample volume toward the aortic valve until aliasing occurs resulting from the high velocity stenotic jet, then moving the sample volume into the LVOT until aliasing no longer occurs. Velocity is thus measured just beneath the aortic valve in the distal LVOT. $\text{LVOT}_{\text{AREA}}$ is determined using the midesophageal long-axis view and measuring the LVOT diameter (d) near the aortic valve

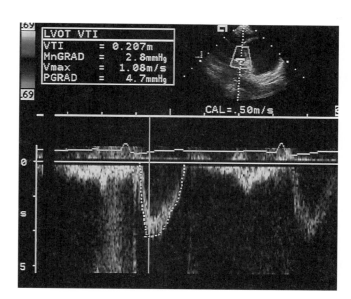

FIG. 4-54   Planimetry of the pulsed-wave spectral Doppler velocities in the left ventricular outflow tract *(LVOT)* provides the velocity time integral *(VTI)* of LVOT flow.

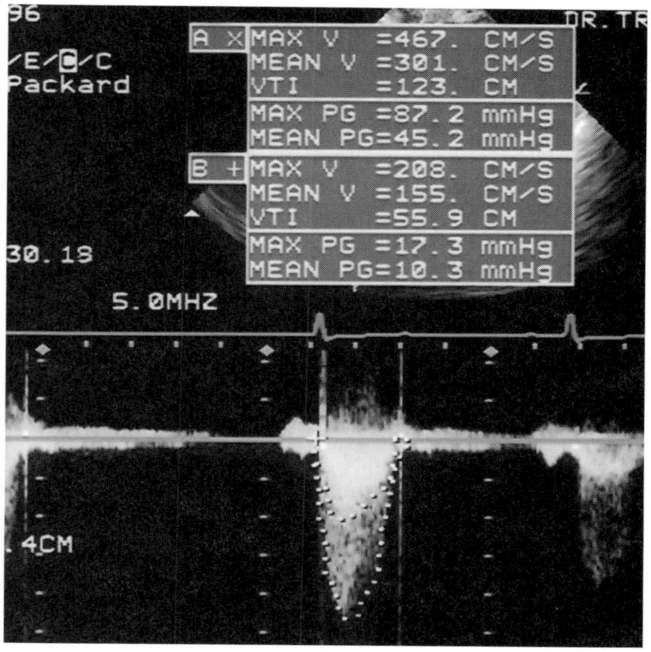

FIG. 4-55   Planimetry of both the aortic valve and left ventricular outflow tract velocities is performed on the same cardiac beat using continuous-wave spectral Doppler.

annulus to correspond to the same anatomic location as the pulsed-wave Doppler recording of LVOT velocity. $LVOT_{AREA}$ is calculated by assuming the LVOT is circular and using the formula: Area $= \pi \times (d/2)^2$. Calculating $LVOT_{AREA}$ is the greatest source of error in the continuity equation for valve area. Erroneously foreshortened measurements of LVOT diameter are squared to significantly underestimate the true $LVOT_{AREA}$. Use of erroneous underestimates of $LVOT_{AREA}$ lead to calculation of smaller than actual aortic valve areas.

Another source of error with using the continuity equation to determine aortic valve area is the patient with an irregular cardiac rhythm, such as atrial fibrillation. The equation is based on the conservation of mass and assumes flow through the LVOT is equal to flow through the aortic valve. Different cardiac beats in a patient with an irregular rhythm have different stroke volumes. It is imperative to measure VTI for both the aortic valve and LVOT using the same cardiac beat. Using the continuous-wave spectral Doppler display of aortic valve flow, the VTI of the aortic valve is traced around the trailing edge of the higher-velocity envelope as previously described. However, instead of using pulsed-wave Doppler to measure LVOT velocity, the $LVOT_{VTI}$ is traced from the same continuous-wave spectral Doppler display as the aortic valve VTI, except that

the denser, lower velocities within the same cardiac beat are traced (Fig. 4-55). This circumvents the problem of different stroke volumes for different beats. This method may also be used for patients with a regular rhythm. The author prefers using pulsed-wave Doppler for $LVOT_{VTI}$ measurements for patients with a regular rhythm, because the continuous-wave Doppler beam used to measure aortic valve VTI may not precisely intercept the aortic valve jet and LVOT flow simultaneously. An alternative to measuring aortic valve and LVOT VTI from the same cardiac beat is to measure aortic valve and LVOT VTI of several (seven or more) cardiac beats and taking the average VTI for each when calculating aortic valve area.

The stroke volume affects calculation of aortic valve area, even in patients with a regular sinus rhythm. Use of dobutamine to induce a larger stroke volume yields a slighter larger area that is related to the continuity equation rather than an actual change in valve area.[95,96]

Aortic Insufficiency

Aortic insufficiency (AI) is caused by either intrinsic disease of the aortic cusps or secondarily from diseases affecting the ascending aorta. Intrinsic valvular problems include rheumatic and calcific and myxomatous valvular disease, endocarditis, traumatic injury, and congenital abnormalities. Conditions affecting the ascending aorta that lead to AI involve annular dilation and include aortic dissection (secondary to blunt trauma or hypertension), mycotic aneurysm, cystic medial necrosis, Marfan's syndrome, and chronic hypertension.

Two-dimensional echocardiography is used to determine the etiology of the AI by identifying structural abnormalities of the leaflets or aortic root. Although two-dimensional echocardiography is not useful for quantifying the severity of AI, there are several useful echocardiographic features associated with AI. The LV is dilated and more spherical in shape with chronic AI, but not necessarily with acute AI. The mitral valve exhibits premature closure and fluttering of the anterior mitral leaflet during diastole. An eccentric AI jet directed toward the anterior mitral valve leaflet may also cause mitral leaflet doming with convexity toward the left atrial side of the valve (Fig. 4-56).

Doppler echocardiography is used to quantitate the severity of AI by several techniques that involve color and pulsed- and continuous-wave Doppler. These techniques are sensitive and reliable, but all have limitations. Color Doppler applied to the short-axis view of the aortic valve (midesophageal 30° to 50°) is useful for localizing the site of regurgitation (Fig. 4-57). Despite the orthogonal relationship between the aortic valve flow and Doppler beam in this short-axis view, the regurgitant orifice is identifiable because the AI jet is usu-

ally not completely orthogonal to the Doppler beam, particularly if the jet is eccentric. The long-axis view of the aortic valve (midesophageal 120° to 150°) is the most useful for quantitating the severity of AI. Color Doppler reveals a flow disturbance in the LVOT originating from the aortic valve and directed into the LV (Fig. 4-58). A central jet is usually caused by aortic root dilation, whereas an eccentric jet usually implies a leaflet

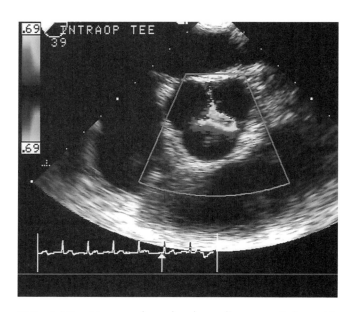

FIG. 4-57 Transesophageal echocardiogram of the midesophageal aortic valve short-axis view with color flow Doppler in a patient with aortic insufficiency. The origin of the aortic insufficiency is predominantly between the right and left coronary cusps.

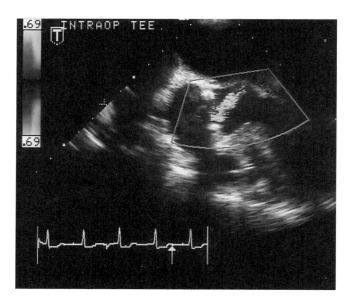

FIG. 4-56 Transesophageal echocardiogram with a color flow Doppler in a patient with aortic insufficiency. The aortic insufficiency is identified by the color flow disturbance that originates from the aortic valve and is directed toward the anterior mitral valve leaflet, creating a convexity in the mitral leaflet.

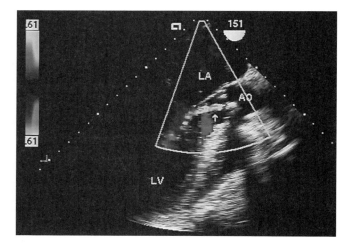

FIG. 4-58 Transesophageal echocardiogram of the midesophageal aortic valve long-axis view with color flow Doppler in a patient with aortic insufficiency *(arrow)*. *AO*, Ascending aorta; *LA*, left atrium; *LV*, left ventricle.

problem. The width of the jet *at the orifice* compared with the width of the LVOT correlates with angiographic determinants of AI[97] (Table 4-13).

A limitation to this technique is that the regurgitant jet orifice and the true LVOT diameter (not foreshortened) may not be in the same imaging plane.[98] This limitation is most apparent if "color M-mode" is used to determine the jet/LVOT ratio. *Color M-mode* refers to the application of M-mode imaging to a color flow Doppler image (Fig. 4-59). M-mode evaluation of the LVOT in the patient with AI is more useful for determining the duration of AI into the diastolic phase than the jet/LVOT ratio. Another limitation to the jet/LVOT ratio method of assessing AI is that the shape of the regurgitant orifice may not be circular or symmetric. An irregularly shaped regurgitant orifice may cause the jet to appear wider in one imaging plane than another;[99] hence the importance of examining multiple imaging planes. The AI jet

may also be eccentric or converge with the mitral valve, rendering the jet particularly difficult to evaluate in patients with mitral stenosis.[100]

If color Doppler cannot be applied to the LVOT from the midesophageal long-axis view because of unusual anatomy or shadowing of the LVOT from a prosthetic mitral or aortic valve, a deep apical transgastric or transgastric long-axis view is used. The AI jet in this view appears as a red or mosaic-colored jet directed away from the aortic valve toward the left ventricular cavity (Fig. 4-60). The length of the jet is not as important as the width of the jet, particularly at the orifice. Multiple imaging planes should be used to appreciate the three-dimensional character of the jet.

Continuous-wave Doppler is also used to determine the severity of AI by measuring the deceleration slope of the regurgitant jet. A deep apical transgastric or transgastric long-axis view aligns the regurgitant jet parallel to the Doppler beam. Color Doppler is useful for identifying the location and direction of the AI jet. The Doppler cursor is placed within the AI jet identified by color flow Doppler and the continuous-wave spectral velocity profile is obtained (Fig. 4-61). The velocity of the regurgitant jet declines more rapidly in patients with severe AI because the larger regurgitant orifice allows a more rapid equilibration of the aortic and left ventricular pressures. In other words, if the pressure difference between the aorta and LV approaches zero rapidly, the regurgitant jet velocity also approaches zero more rapidly, creating a

TABLE 4-13
Grading Aortic Insufficiency

SEVERITY OF AORTIC INSUFFICIENCY	JET WIDTH/ LVOT WIDTH RATIO[97]	AVERAGE REGURGITANT FRACTION[104]
1+	<0.25	28%
2+	0.25-0.46	33%
3+	0.47-0.64	53%
4+	>0.64	62%

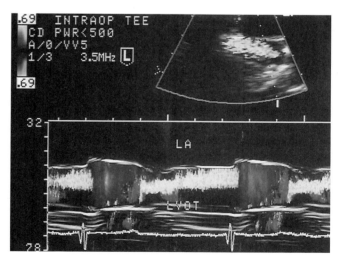

FIG. 4-59   Color M-mode echocardiography of the left ventricular outflow tract *(LVOT)* in a patient with aortic insufficiency. *LA*, Left atrium.

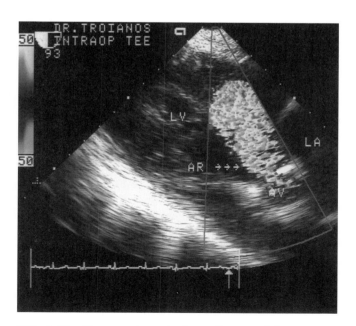

FIG. 4-60   Transesophageal echocardiogram of the transgastric long-axis view with color flow Doppler in a patient with aortic insufficiency (arrows). *AV*, Aortic valve; *LA*, left atrium; *LV*, left ventricle.

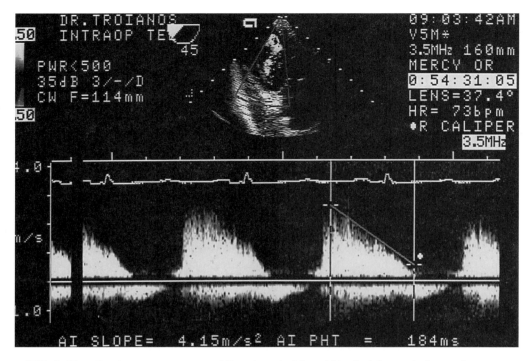

FIG. 4-61 Continuous-wave spectral Doppler velocities within the left ventricular outflow tract in a patient with aortic insufficiency. The slope of the velocity deceleration (AI slope = 4.15 m/sec^2) indicates the severity of the aortic insufficiency.

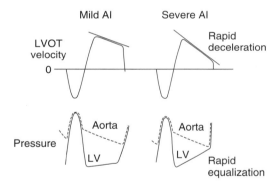

FIG. 4-62 Illustration of the association between the left ventricular outflow tract *(LVOT)* deceleration slope and the pressure difference between the aorta and left ventricle *(LV)* during diastole. The deceleration slope is steeper and approaches zero velocity more rapidly with severe aortic insufficiency *(AI)* because the pressures in the aorta and left ventricle equalize more rapidly.

(Adapted from Feigenbaum H: *Echocardiography*, ed 5, Philadelphia, 1994. Lea & Febiger, p 286.)

steeper slope (Fig. 4-62). A regurgitant velocity slope greater than 3 m/sec^2 is indicative of advanced (3 or 4+) AI.[101]

One limitation to this technique is that factors other than regurgitant orifice size influence the deceleration slope. SVR and left ventricular compliance affect the rate of deceleration, irrespective of the regurgitant orifice size.[102] Decreased SVR (sepsis) and reduced left

ventricular compliance (ischemia, cardiomyopathy, acute AI) cause a steeper deceleration slope because aortic and left ventricular pressures equalize more rapidly with these conditions. Another limitation to this technique is that measurement of regurgitant jet velocity is difficult and unreliable in patients with eccentric jets, because it is difficult to align the Doppler beam with the regurgitant jet.

Pulsed-wave Doppler is used to detect retrograde flow in the aorta during diastole. Holodiastolic flow in the abdominal aorta is both sensitive and specific for *severe* AI. Detection of holodiastolic retrograde flow in the proximal descending thoracic aorta and aortic arch is a sensitive indicator of AI, but is not specific for *severe* AI. Using the short-axis TEE view of the descending thoracic aorta, the pulsed-wave sample volume is placed as distal in the aorta as possible, near the diaphragm. Despite the orthogonal relationship between the aortic flow and Doppler beam in this short-axis view, the flow in the aorta is identifiable because the blood in the aorta tends to swirl as it travels down the aorta. The spectral Doppler display is examined for the duration of diastolic flow. Retrograde flow throughout diastole (holodiastolic) in the distal descending or abdominal aorta (Fig. 4-63) indicates severe AI.[103]

Regurgitant volume and regurgitant fraction can also be used to evaluate the severity of AI. Regurgitant volume is the difference between the systolic flow across the aortic valve and cardiac output. In the absence of

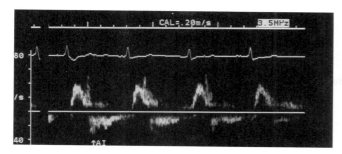

FIG. 4-63 Pulsed-wave Doppler spectral velocity of blood flow in the descending thoracic aorta. The retrograde flow throughout diastole *(arrow)* is termed *holodiastolic* and is associated with severe aortic insufficiency.

intracardiac shunts and MR, flow through the pulmonary artery or mitral valve is equivalent to (net) cardiac output. Pulmonary artery blood flow is reliably measured with TEE by measuring the pulmonary artery diameter (d), calculating its area $[\pi(d/2)^2]$, and multiplying the area by the pulmonary artery VTI and heart rate.[62] Aortic valve systolic flow is the product of aortic valve area and VTI. The aortic regurgitant volume is the difference between aortic valve systolic flow and pulmonary blood flow (cardiac output). Regurgitant fraction is expressed as the proportion of aortic valve systolic flow that is regurgitant volume and indicates the severity of AI[104] (see Table 4-13).

Regurgitant Volume =

$$\text{Aortic Valve Systolic Flow} - \text{Cardiac Output}$$

$$\text{Regurgitant Fraction} = \frac{\text{Regurgitant Volume}}{\text{Aortic Valve Systolic Flow}}$$

The continuity equation could theoretically be used to determine regurgitant orifice size. Diastolic velocities just above the aortic valve (aortic root-VTI) and through the aortic valve (aortic valve-VTI) are determined with Doppler echocardiography and the cross-sectional area of the aortic root is determined with two-dimensional echocardiography.[105,106] This technique, however, has not been widely accepted or validated.

Aortic Valve Regurgitant Orifice =

$$\frac{\text{Aortic Root}_{\text{AREA}} \times \text{Aortic Root Diastolic}_{\text{VTI}}}{\text{Aortic Valve Regurgitant Jet}_{\text{VTI}}}$$

Tricuspid Valve, Right Atrium, and Coronary Sinus

Three leaflets comprise the tricuspid valve: anterior, posterior, and septal. The anterior leaflet is the largest of the three leaflets with chordal attachment to the anterior and medial papillary muscles. It is imaged in the midesophageal four-chamber view (multiplane angle 0° to 20°) as the leaflet located on the left side of the image display (Fig. 4-64). The septal leaflet is also im-

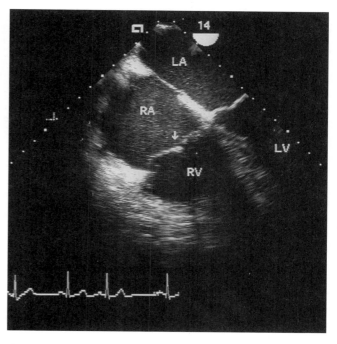

FIG. 4-64 Transesophageal echocardiogram of the midesophageal four-chamber view permits imaging of the anterior *(arrow)* and septal leaflets of the tricuspid valve. *LA*, Left atrium; *LV*, left ventricle; *RA*, right atrium; *RV*, right ventricle.

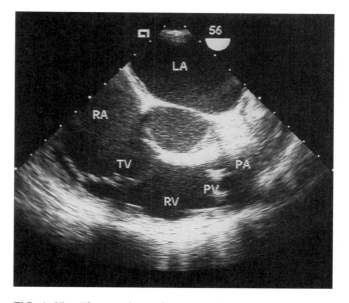

FIG. 4-65 The anterior and posterior leaflets of the tricuspid valve *(TV)* are imaged with this midesophageal right ventricular *(RV)* inflow-outflow view. *LA*, Left atrium; *PA*, main pulmonary artery; *PV*, pulmonic valve; *RA*, right atrium.

aged in the midesophageal four-chamber view. It is attached to the septum and is located on the right side of the image display (Fig. 4-64). In the right ventricular inflow-outflow view at a multiplane angle 60° to 90° (Fig. 4-65), the anterior leaflet is on the right side of the image display.[37] The posterior leaflet is also imaged in this inflow-outflow view (left side of image display)[37] and is the smallest of the three leaflets with chordal attachment to the posterior and anterior papillary muscles. The septal leaflet is slightly larger than the posterior leaflet and has chordal attachment to the posterior and septal papillary muscles.[107]

The right atrium is imaged in the midesophageal four-chamber, right ventricular inflow-outflow, and bicaval views (90° to 110°). The posterior aspect of the right atrial wall is smooth, while the anterior aspect is trabeculated and lined by pectinate muscles that extend into the right atrial appendage. The eustachian valve is imaged at the junction of the inferior vena cava and right atrium. Highly mobile filaments attached to the eustachian valve are termed the *Chiari network* and considered a normal variant.[108] The coronary sinus orifice is located inferiorly within the right atrium along the intraatrial septum. The probe is advanced into the esophagus from the four-chamber view and anteflexed until the image of the right atrium and coronary sinus is developed. Imaging the coronary sinus is important for directing and confirming proper position of the coronary sinus catheter into the coronary sinus to administer retrograde cardioplegia.

Tricuspid Stenosis

Tricuspid stenosis is an obstruction to right ventricular inflow. The etiology of tricuspid stenosis is nearly always rheumatic and associated with rheumatic involvement of the mitral and/or aortic valves. Congenital tricuspid atresia is a rare cause of obstruction. Other causes of right ventricular inflow obstruction include right atrial tumors, endomyocardial fibrosis, tricuspid valve vegetations, extracardiac tumors, and the carcinoid syndrome.[109] Carcinoid syndrome affecting the tricuspid valve is usually accompanied by pulmonic valve disease.

Rheumatic tricuspid stenosis is identified using two-dimensional echocardiography by leaflet doming. Doming is a qualitative sign of stenosis for all stenotic valvular lesions. The leaflets appear thickened with restricted mobility and commissural fusion. These two-dimensional criteria alone are 100% sensitive and 90% specific for the diagnosis of tricuspid stenosis.[110]

Doppler echocardiography is used to quantitate the severity of the tricuspid stenosis by measuring transvalvular velocities. The pulsed-wave Doppler sample volume is placed at the leaflet tips in the RV during diastole. A spectral Doppler pattern resembling that of mitral stenosis is recorded and used to determine the mean gradient and PHT measurements. Mean gradient is determined by planimetry of the spectral Doppler velocities over time, and PHT is obtained from the velocity deceleration slope, as previously described for mitral stenosis. Tricuspid stenosis is considered severe when

the mean gradient exceeds 7 mm Hg and PTH exceeds 190 ms.[111]

Tricuspid Regurgitation

Tricuspid regurgitation is caused by abnormalities of the leaflets, chordae tendineae, papillary muscles, or annulus. The most common cause is annular dilation secondary to right ventricular dilation or failure. Right ventricular hypertension is often a manifestation of mitral valve disease, but is also associated with right ventricular infarction, primary pulmonary hypertension, cor pulmonale, and congenital abnormalities such as pulmonic stenosis or Eisenmenger's syndrome.[109] Leaflet abnormalities are a manifestation of rheumatic endocarditis, myxomatous degeneration, infective endocarditis, and carcinoid syndrome. Other causes of tricuspid regurgitation include trauma, papillary muscle dysfunction, and congenital abnormalities such as Ebstein's anomaly.[109]

Although two-dimensional echocardiography is not used to quantify the severity of tricuspid regurgitation, several echocardiographic findings are associated with tricuspid regurgitation. Myxomatous degeneration, leaflet prolapse, rheumatic valvulitis, and vegetations are structural abnormalities that may be observed in patients with tricuspid regurgitation. Right ventricular, right atrial, and annular dilation are the most common findings. Paradoxical septal motion of the interventricular septum is a manifestation of right ventricular failure or volume overload. Normal septal motion is anterior during diastole and posterior during systole. With volume overload, right ventricular diastolic filling exceeds left ventricular filling resulting in a posterior displacement of the septum in diastole. Although two-dimensional echocardiography provides findings indicative of tricuspid regurgitation, Doppler echocardiography is required for definitive diagnosis and quantification.

Doppler color flow mapping is the most useful method of detecting and quantifying the severity of tricuspid regurgitation, similar to the evaluation of the mitral valve. A systolic flow disturbance is observed originating from the tricuspid valve and directed into the right atrial cavity (Fig. 4-66). Multiple imaging planes are used to appreciate the three-dimensional aspect of the regurgitant jet by moving the probe and adjusting the multiplane angle. Severity of tricuspid regurgitation is assigned based on the size and direction of the color flow disturbance in the right atrium.

Most patients have at least trace tricuspid regurgitation. Continuous-wave Doppler is used to measure the peak velocity of the regurgitant jet. Right ventricular systolic pressure is estimated from this peak velocity using the modified Bernoulli equation ($P = 4V^2$), which represents the systolic pressure gradient between the RV and right atrium. Right atrial pressure (if known, esti-

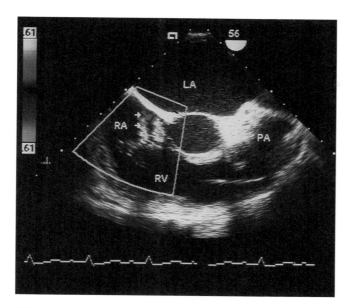

FIG. 4-66   Color flow Doppler applied to the right atrium identifies the flow disturbance *(arrow)* originating from the tricuspid valve and directed into the right atrium *(RA)* as tricuspid regurgitation. *LA,* Left atrium; *PA,* main pulmonary artery; *RV,* right ventricle.

mated if unknown) is added to this pressure gradient to calculate right ventricular systolic pressure.

Hepatic vein flow can also be used to evaluate tricuspid regurgitation. The pulsed-wave sample volume is placed in the hepatic vein from a transgastric imaging site. The spectral Doppler display is examined for systolic flow reversal in a similar manner to evaluating the pulmonary vein for systolic flow reversal with severe MR.

Pulmonic Valve and Pulmonary Artery

The pulmonic valve resembles the aortic valve in structure with three cusps associated with three sinuses in the pulmonary artery. The valve differs from the aortic valve in that the cusps are not as thick and the sinuses lack coronary ostia. The cusps are termed the *left, right,* and *anterior* (or *nonseptal) cusps.*[107] Because the pulmonic valve is located more anterior, it is more difficult to image with TEE than the aortic valve.

Pulmonic Stenosis

The etiology of pulmonic stenosis is usually congenital. Rheumatic valvulitis and the carcinoid syndrome are rare causes of pulmonic stenosis. Rheumatic pulmonic stenosis is usually associated with rheumatic involvement of other cardiac valves. Vegetations or thrombi obstructing flow through the valve cause functional pulmonic stenosis. Subvalvular, infundibular stenosis is usually congenital and mimics pulmonic stenosis.

The right ventricular inflow-outflow view (60° to 90°)

is used to image the pulmonic valve in its long axis, the right ventricular outflow tract, and proximal pulmonary artery (see Fig. 4-66). Thickened leaflets with doming and restricted mobility are the two-dimensional signs of pulmonic stenosis. Poststenotic dilation of the pulmonary artery may be an associated finding. With infundibular stenosis, the leaflets appear normal but the right ventricular outflow tract is narrowed.

Doppler echocardiography is required to determine the severity of valvular stenosis. A parallel alignment between the Doppler beam and the pulmonic valve is obtained using either the ascending aortic short-axis view at the base of the heart, an upper esophageal aortic arch short-axis view, or a deep apical transgastric view. The transvalvular velocity increases as the severity of pulmonic stenosis increases.

Pulmonic Insufficiency

Annular dilation secondary to pulmonary hypertension is the most common cause of pulmonic insufficiency. Less common causes include infective endocarditis, iatrogenic (secondary to surgical treatment of pulmonic stenosis), trauma, carcinoid syndrome, rheumatic valvulitis, myxomatous valve disease, and, rarely, Marfan's syndrome.[109]

Two-dimensional echocardiography is used to detect anatomic abnormalities associated with pulmonic insufficiency. An enlarged pulmonary artery and annular dilation are the most common findings. Leaflet abnormalities associated with myxomatous degeneration, endocarditis, trauma, or congenital deformities may also be observed.

Doppler echocardiography is used to detect and assess the severity of pulmonic insufficiency. A color flow disturbance is observed using the right ventricular inflow-outflow TEE view (60° to 90°), originating from the pulmonic valve and directed into the right ventricular outflow tract (Fig. 4-67). The width of the flow disturbance is indicative of the size of the regurgitant orifice and the severity of the insufficiency. Spectral Doppler can also be used to examine the velocity of the regurgitant jet. The peak regurgitant velocity reflects the pressure gradient between the pulmonary artery (PA) and RV during diastole ($\Delta P = 4V^2$). The PA diastolic pressure is obtained by adding this calculated (PA to RV) pressure gradient (ΔP) to the RV diastolic pressure or CVP.

Atrial Septum

The atrial septum is initially examined with the midesophageal four-chamber view (0° to 20°) as the probe is advanced and withdrawn in the esophagus to image the septum throughout its entire superior-inferior dimension. Continuity of the septum suggests the absence of atrial septal defects, which is confirmed using color flow Doppler. Fig. 4-68 is an example of a patient with

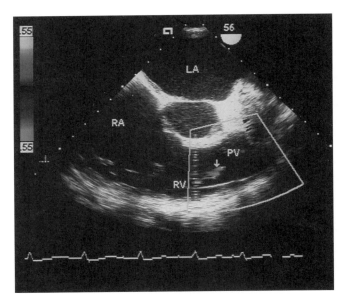

FIG. 4-67 Color flow Doppler applied to the pulmonic valve identifies the flow disturbance *(arrow)* originating from the pulmonic valve and directed into the right ventricle *(RV)* as pulmonic regurgitation. *LA,* Left atrium; *PV,* pulmonic valve; *RA,* right atrium.

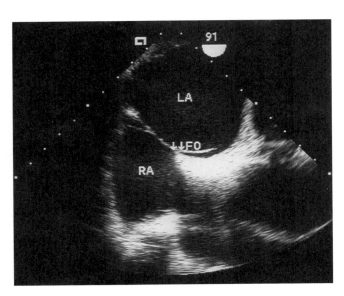

FIG. 4-69 Transesophageal echocardiogram of the atrial septum at 91° multiplane angle. The *arrows* indicate the possibility of a patent foramen ovale *(FO). LA,* Left atrium; *RA,* right atrium.

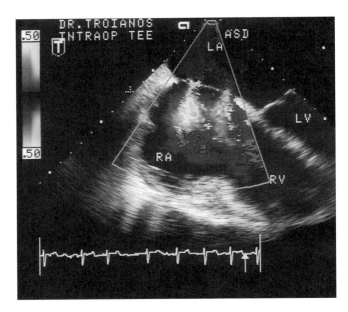

FIG. 4-68 Color flow Doppler applied to the atrial septum identifies two atrial septal defects. The blue jets directed toward the right atrium *(RA)* indicate left-to-right shunting of blood flow. *LA,* Left atrium; *LV,* left ventricle; *RV,* right ventricle.

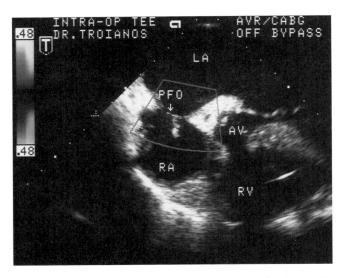

FIG. 4-70 The small color flow disturbance originating at the atrial septum at the fossa ovalis *(arrow)* and directed toward the right atrium *(RA)* confirms the presence of a patent foramen ovale *(PFO). LA,* Left atrium; *RV,* right ventricle.

two atrial septal defects; color flow Doppler indicates the left-to-right flow through both defects. Classification of atrial septal defects is discussed in Chapter 10. The thinnest portion of the septum, the fossa ovalis, is centered in the image display while the multiplane angle is rotated forward to 90° (Fig. 4-69). This view is most useful for detecting a patent foramen ovale (PFO) with

color flow Doppler. Decreasing the Nyquist limit on the color flow Doppler scale aids in detecting low-velocity flow through the PFO (Fig. 4-70). Agitated saline, rapidly injected into the right atrium while 20 cm of continuous positive airway pressure is applied, is also useful for detecting a PFO by the appearance of saline contrast in the left atrium. The 90° view often permits imaging of

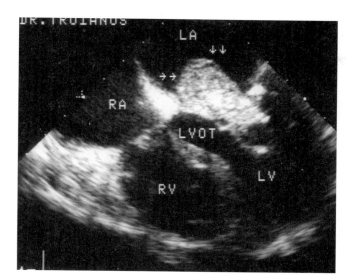

FIG. 4-71 Transesophageal echocardiogram of the mid-esophageal four-chamber view reveals a large atrial myxoma *(arrows)* that abuts the mitral valve during diastole, creating "functional" mitral stenosis. *LA,* Left atrium; *LV,* left ventricle; *LVOT,* left ventricular outflow tract; *RA,* right atrium; *RV,* right ventricle.

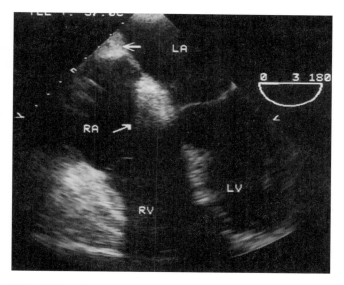

FIG. 4-72 Lipomatous hypertrophy of the atrial septum *(arrows)* may mimic an atrial myxoma or thrombus. *LA,* Left atrium; *LV,* left ventricle; *RA,* right atrium; *RV,* right ventricle.

the saline contrast traversing the atrial septum through the PFO. Potential pathologic consequences of a PFO occur with right-to-left shunting and include paradoxical systemic embolization and hypoxemia.[112]

Myxomas are primary tumors of the heart that most commonly arise from the atrial septum. They usually originate at the fossa ovalis and protrude into the left atrium (75%). These tumors can become so large that they occupy most of the left atrial cavity and create functional mitral stenosis by abutting against the mitral valve during diastole (Fig. 4-71). Other sites of origin include the right atrium (18%), RV (4%), and LV (4%).[113] Careful examination of each cavity for myxomas and thrombi is indicated for the patient with a history of embolic events.

Lipomatous hypertrophy of the atrial septum may have the appearance of a tumor or thrombus, but is merely adipose tissue. This condition typically causes thickening throughout the atrial septum, but spares the fossa ovalis (Fig. 4-72). Computed tomography or magnetic resonance imaging may differentiate lipomatous hypertrophy from other diagnoses, if the echocardiographic diagnosis is unclear.

Aorta

The thoracic aorta consists of three segments (ascending, arch, and descending) and three layers within the aortic wall (intima, media, adventitia). The intima is the

innermost layer, normally a thin layer composed of endothelium. Atherosclerosis develops in the intima, causing thickening and calcification, and leads to the development of plaques that are broad based, protruding, ulcerated, or mobile. The media is the thickest layer, constituting 80% of the aortic wall, and consists of smooth muscle and elastic tissue. Diseases that cause aortic dilation involve the media. The adventitia is the outermost layer and contains the vaso vasorum.

TEE has become the gold standard for evaluating the thoracic aorta. The close proximity between the esophagus and the aorta allows for high-resolution images with considerable definition of pathologic changes. Virtually the entire thoracic aorta can be imaged using TEE, with the exception of the distal ascending aorta and proximal aortic arch. This "blind spot" exists because the trachea or left mainstem bronchus is interpositioned between the aorta and esophagus at this level. The aortic cannulation site for cardiopulmonary bypass, therefore, is not readily imaged with TEE. Konstadt and associates measured the maximal length of ascending aorta in 27 patients using TEE, and compared these measurements to the total length of the ascending aorta and the distance between the aortic valve annulus and the cannulation site as measured by the surgeon.[114] The range of difference between the direct measurement and the TEE measurement was 0.2 to 4.5 cm, representing as much as 42% (4.5 cm of 10.7 cm) of the ascending aorta not imaged by TEE. Furthermore, the aortic cannula was imaged in only 1 of 27 patients. This implies a limited use of TEE for evaluating and detecting pathology in the distal ascending aorta.

Epiaortic ultrasound is used in conjunction with TEE during cardiac surgery to provide a comprehensive echocardiographic evaluation of the thoracic aorta. A high-frequency linear or phased-array probe is placed directly on the ascending aorta to image the potential sites for cannulation, cross-clamping, and vein graft insertion. A linear probe offers the advantage of a wide near field for evaluating the anterior wall of the aorta, but the disadvantage of a larger contact surface or "foot pad." The phased-array probe offers the advantage of a smaller contact surface, but the disadvantage of a smaller, narrow-angled near field (Fig. 4-73). The probe is placed in a sterile sheath containing sterile water or gel. The author prefers water because ultrasonic gel often contains bubbles entrapped within the gel, which distort and interfere with image acquisition. A rubber band is placed on the outside of the sterile sheath to maintain a "stand-off" of fluid over the end of the probe. This provides better visualization of near-field structures and is particularly important with the phased-array probes.

The ascending aorta appears circular when imaged

using the midesophageal ascending aortic short-axis view (Fig. 4-74). This view is useful for positioning the tip of the PA catheter in the proximal right or main pulmonary artery. The ascending aorta is centered on the image display as the multiplane angle is rotated forward to obtain the ascending aortic long-axis view (see Fig. 4-42). This view requires a 100° to 150° multiplane angle, but varies with tortuosity of the aorta. The imaging plane is adjusted to obtain the maximal dimension for measuring the ascending aortic diameter at the sinotubular junction and other specific locations. The near-field aortic wall is the posterior wall of the ascending aorta. The aorta is carefully examined for potentially embolic atherosclerotic plaques, particularly during cardiac surgery that involves manipulation of the ascending aorta. The proximal ascending aorta can also be imaged using the deep apical transgastric view (Fig. 4-75), but is located in the far field, farther from the transducer. The lower image quality of far-field structures does not provide sufficient resolution to detect small atherosclerotic plaques in this view compared with the midesophageal views. The transgastric view is useful when the midesophageal views are obstructed by the tortuosity of the aorta or aortic root pathology.

The descending aorta is examined by turning the probe counterclockwise to the patient's left. The descending aorta appears circular when imaged using the descending aortic short-axis view (Fig. 4-76) and tubular when the multiplane angle is rotated forward to the descending aortic long-axis view. The near-field aortic wall is the anterior wall of the descending aorta when

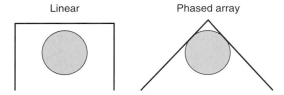

FIG. 4-73 Illustration of the image display of linear and phased-array echocardiography probes. Linear probes offer a wide near field, whereas phased-array probes have a smaller, narrow-angled near field.

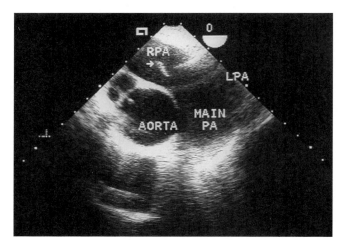

FIG. 4-74 The midesophageal ascending aortic short-axis view provides imaging of the aortic root and pulmonary artery at its bifurcation. The tip of the pulmonary artery catheter *(arrow)* is positioned in the proximal right pulmonary artery *(RPA)* or main pulmonary artery *(PA)* to prevent catheter wedging during cardiopulmonary bypass.

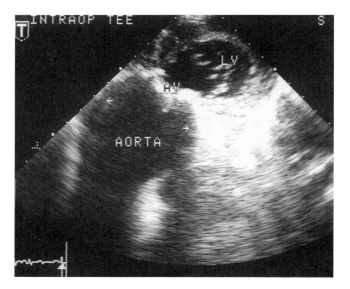

FIG. 4-75 Deep apical transgastric view of the ascending aorta. *AV,* Aortic valve; *LV,* left ventricle.

using these views. These views are also used to identify a left pleural effusion as indicated in Fig. 4-76.

Withdrawing the probe from the descending aortic short-axis view while maintaining the aorta in the center of the image display develops the aortic arch images. The probe is turned to the right in the upper esophagus as the arch comes into view as a tubular structure. Rotating the multiplane angle forward to about 90° develops the aortic arch short-axis view in which the aortic arch appears circular. This view is useful for imaging the origin of the left subclavian artery and occasionally the left carotid artery.

Aortic Dissection

An aortic dissection is a tear in the intima that allows blood to enter into a "false" lumen between the intimal and medial layers of the aortic wall. Aortic dissections are classified on the basis of the extent of the dissection or location of the intimal tear. The pathology and classification of aortic dissections are discussed in Chapter 14. The hallmark of aortic dissection with echocardiography is identification of an intimal flap that divides the true aortic lumen from the false lumen (Fig. 4-77). Several two-dimensional and Doppler echocardiographic characteristics distinguish the true lumen from the false lumen. The true lumen has a higher blood flow velocity profile, whereas the false lumen may contain spontaneous echocontrast, indicative of low-velocity blood flow. The intimal flap moves toward the false lumen as the true lumen expands during systole. The entry site of the dissection will often reveal a small

high-velocity color flow Doppler jet originating at the site of the intimal tear and directed into the false lumen during systole (Fig. 4-78). Aortic dissections involving the ascending aorta commonly cause AI by disrupting the continuity of one or more aortic valve cusps with the aortic annulus. Patients with a congenital bicuspid or unicuspid aortic valve are approximately five times more likely to develop an aortic dissection than normal individuals.[115] Although dissection is more common in the patient with an aortic

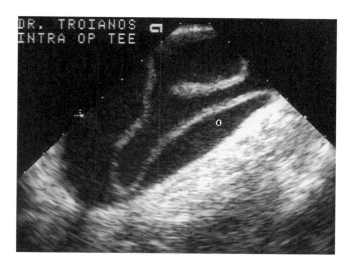

FIG. 4-77   Upper esophageal aortic arch long-axis view demonstrates an aortic dissection with the tear in the aortic arch.

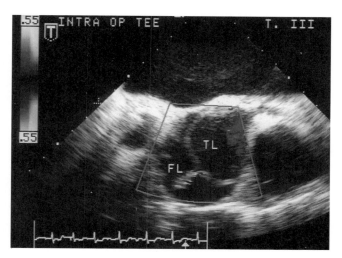

FIG. 4-76   Descending aortic short-axis view provides imaging of the descending thoracic aorta *(DTA)* and is used to identify a pleural effusion surrounding the lung *(arrows)*.

FIG. 4-78   Midesophageal ascending aortic short-axis view in a patient with an aortic dissection. An intimal flap is imaged in the aortic root separating the true lumen *(TL)* and the false lumen *(FL)*. A small high-velocity jet identifies the entry site for the aortic dissection and flow into the false lumen.

aneurysm or Marfan's syndrome, the most prevalent risk factor is chronic hypertension.[115]

Numerous investigators have identified the role of TEE in the diagnosis and evaluation of aortic dissection.[116-118] Erbel and colleagues performed transesophageal and transthoracic echocardiography in 164 consecutive patients with suspected aortic dissection (half of which were subsequently confirmed) to demonstrate a 99% sensitivity and 98% specificity with echocardiography.[116] The one false-negative diagnosis by TEE was also misdiagnosed by aortography. Two false positive diagnoses occurred in patients with aortic ectasia that produced reverberations in the ascending aorta. Neinaber and colleagues demonstrated a 98% sensitivity and 77% specificity using TEE in patients with suspected aortic dissection.[117] In contrast with Erbel's study, these investigators were blinded to the results of the other imaging techniques. Their lower specificity raises concern over the incidence of false-positive results if TEE is used alone to make the diagnosis of aortic dissection. False positive TEE exams are usually caused by ultrasound reverberation from atherosclerotic vessels, a sclerotic root, or calcific aortic disease producing artifacts that resemble intimal flaps.[118] Optimal evaluation of the patient with suspected aortic dissection involves TEE with an additional imaging modality, such as magnetic resonance imaging, aortography, or computed tomography. Additional testing may not always be practical if the patient is hemodynamically unstable or develops an acute aortic dissection intraoperatively. Troianos and colleagues demonstrated the utility of using TEE intraoperatively for patients who develop an acute aortic dissection from surgical manipulation of the aorta.[119] TEE is useful intraoperatively, not only for establishing the diagnosis but also for evaluating the repair of the aorta and the aortic valve.

Atherosclerosis

The high resolution of the aorta produced by TEE reveals striking atherosclerotic changes common in elderly patients (Fig. 4-79). Atherosclerosis occurs in varying degrees that were graded by Hartman and colleagues.[120] The mildest form (Grade I) is a small, thin plaque (<5 mm) with no protrusion or ulceration. A thicker (≥5 mm) nonprotruding plaque is indicative of more severe disease (Grade II). A thin (<5 mm) protruding plaque is Grade III, and a thicker (≥5 mm) protruding plaque is Grade IV. A plaque with mobile components (Grade V) is the most advanced type of atherosclerosis and is a likely source of embolic stroke.[120-124]

The identification of atherosclerotic plaques before surgical manipulation is important because atherosclerosis of the thoracic aorta is an independent predictor of postoperative stroke in patients undergoing cardiac surgery.[121,124] Many surgeons use palpation of the aorta

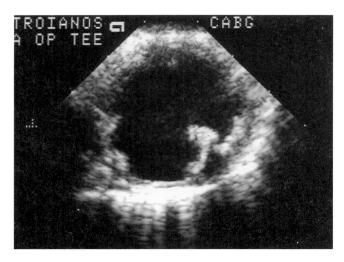

FIG. 4-79 Grade V atheromatous disease in the thoracic aorta. The plaque is greater than 5 mm thick and has protruding and mobile components.

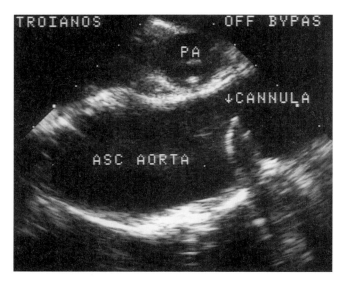

FIG. 4-80 Midesophageal ascending aortic long-axis view images the aortic cannula in the ascending *(asc)* aorta. *PA,* Pulmonary artery.

to guide placement of the aortic cannula, cross-clamp, and proximal vein graft anastomoses. Ascending aortic plaques are often soft and friable, making surgical palpation not only a less reliable indicator of underlying plaques than TEE, but also a potentially dangerous maneuver.[125] TEE is superior to surgical palpation for detecting atherosclerosis, but is limited by the length of ascending aorta that can be imaged by TEE. As previously mentioned, up to 42% of the aorta may not be imaged and the aortic cannulation site is rarely imaged.[114] A TEE image of an aortic cannula in the ascending aorta is shown in Fig. 4-80. Epiaortic ultrasound is superior to TEE for imaging the entire ascending aorta and for detecting atherosclerotic plaques in the ascending aorta.[114,125-127] Minor and major modifications to the surgical procedure based on the discovery of atherosclerotic plaques have the potential to improve patient outcome by reducing the incidence of stroke.[127-129] Major modifications, including deep hypothermic circulatory arrest with atherectomy of the ascending aorta or aortic reconstruction, have been shown to reduce stroke rate despite the more invasive and complicated surgical approach.[125,127,128] Minor modifications, such as using a single aortic cross-clamp, altering the cannulation site, or reducing the number of grafts attached to the aorta, are more readily accepted alternatives that also reduce stroke rate.[127,129] Placement of an intraaortic balloon pump and femoral arterial cannulation for cardiopulmonary bypass are generally avoided if ulcerated, mobile plaques are found in the descending thoracic aorta.

Aneurysms

Aortic dilation is the most common abnormality affecting the aorta. The aortic diameter normally increases with increasing age[38] and body size.[130] *Dilation* refers to an increase in aortic diameter greater than expected for age and body size, and is caused by chronic hypertension, atherosclerosis, or cystic medial necrosis. Dilation is also observed in patients with aortic valve stenosis, referred to as *poststenotic dilation*. The normal narrowing of the aorta at the sinotubular junction and contour of the sinuses of Valsalva are preserved with poststenotic dilation or dilation caused by hypertension or atherosclerosis.[115] The contour of the sinuses of Valsalva is not preserved with dilation resulting from Marfan's syndrome.

Aortic aneurysm refers to a severe dilation of the aortic diameter (Fig. 4-81). Aneurysms may involve more than one segment of the aorta (ascending, arch, descending), are tubular or saccular, and are most often caused by cystic medial necrosis, Marfan's syndrome, hypertension, atherosclerosis, or collagen-vascular or inflammatory diseases.[115] A massively dilated aorta will commonly distort or compress cardiac structures and is prone to dissection or rupture.

Prosthetic Valves

Intraoperative echocardiography is used to determine the feasibility of valve repair and evaluate the success of the surgical repair. If the valve is not repairable or the attempted repair is unsuccessful, TEE is used to estimate the prosthetic valve size and evaluate the function of the prosthetic valve. TEE is also used to evaluate de-airing maneuvers after open chamber procedures. Prosthetic valves are either mechanical or bioprosthetic. Mechanical valves include the caged ball, caged disc, tilting disc, and bileaflet valves. Bioprosthetic valves are porcine, bovine pericardial, stentless, or homograft valves. The

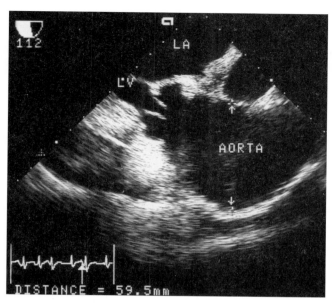

FIG. 4-81   Midesophageal ascending aortic long-axis view identifies an ascending aortic aneurysm measuring 6 cm in diameter. *LA*, Left atrium; *LV*, left ventricle.

hemodynamic, structural, and regurgitant features of each valve are characteristic for that particular valve. To provide meaningful interpretation and reporting of pertinent TEE findings, it is important for the echocardiographer to be familiar with the features of the valve to be implanted. The structural features of the prosthetic valves are summarized in Table 4-14.

The caged ball valve consists of a circular sewing ring with a four-post cage. Within the cage is a spherical silastic ball that occludes the orifice in the closed position and is contained within the cage in the open position. The caged disc valve functions similarly to the caged ball valve. A circular disc occludes the orifice in the closed position and is contained within the cage in the open position. The tilting disc valve consists of a rotatable knitted Teflon sewing ring that is occluded by a circular disc in the closed position. The opening is characterized by a "tilting" of the disc along a central strut creating two unequally sized orifices. The bileaflet mechanical valve consists of two hemicircular hinged discs made from pyrolytic carbon. The leaflets open near perpendicular to the annular plane, creating a smaller central orifice and two larger peripheral orifices.

The porcine bioprosthetic valve is a glutaraldehyde-preserved porcine aortic valve mounted on a polypropylene stent with Dacron fabric and a molded silicone sewing ring. The bovine pericardial valve is a trileaflet valve constructed from bovine pericardium mounted in a support frame with three struts. While these bioprosthetic valves differ in origin, they are similar in appearance, both directly and with echocardiography. There are more options in design and size availability for the

TABLE 4-14
Structural Features of Prosthetic Valves

VALVE TYPE	CLASSIFICATION	EXAMPLES	STRUCTURE
Caged ball	Mechanical	Starr-Edwards	Silastic ball within a 4-strut "cage"
Caged disc	Mechanical	Beall, Kay-Shiley	Silastic disc within a short "cage"
Tilting disc	Mechanical	Medtronic, Bjork-Shiley	Single circular disc opening at oblique angle
Bileaflet	Mechanical	St. Jude, Carbo Medics	Two hemicircular hinged discs
Porcine	Bioprosthesis	Carpentier-Edwards, Hancock	Trileaflet porcine valve mounted on a support with three struts at each commissure
Bovine pericardial	Bioprosthesis	Ionescu-Shiley	Trileaflet valve shaped from bovine pericardium mounted on a support with three struts
Stentless	Bioprosthesis	Toronto-St. Jude, Edwards	Stentless porcine valve
Homograft	Human tissue	Cryopreserved	Human aortic valve
Autograft	Human tissue	Patient's own pulmonic valve	Human pulmonic valve (Ross procedure)

bovine pericardial valve because it is a constructed valve. Both valves open to a circular orifice and provide a laminar flow profile. The porcine bioprosthesis degenerates by leaflet thickening and calcification causing ruptured segments and stenosis. The pericardial valve degenerates by calcification, abrasion, and perforation. The calcification causes stenosis similar to the porcine valve.

Stentless valves, used only in the aortic position, lack the struts within the supporting structure of the valve. This necessitates sewing the supporting structure to the aortic wall and the nonrigid sewing ring within the annulus and is partly responsible for the superior hemodynamic performance.[131] Paravalvular leaks are very unlikely if the surgeon sews both the ring and the supporting structure in an occlusive fashion. Blood would have to penetrate two sutures lines to create a paravalvular leak. Some surgeons may place a few stabilizing sutures in the sewing ring and annulus that are not occlusive. Color flow Doppler after implantation may indicate flow around the annular ring, but this is not considered a paravalvular leak unless the blood crosses the suture line of the supporting structure within the aortic root. Stentless valve dysfunction immediately after implantation occurs because of incorrect valve sizing or a dilated aortic root. Valve sizing is based on the diameter of the sinotubular junction and should not be more than one valve size greater than the aortic annulus[131] (Fig. 4-82). For example, if the aortic annulus measures 23 mm in diameter, the sinotubular junction should not be greater than 25 mm. The correct stentless valve size for this patient is 25 mm. If a 23-mm (too small) stentless valve were used, the supporting structure sewn into a 25-mm aortic root would pull the leaflets apart and cause AI. The same situation occurs when the aortic root is more than one valve size greater than the aortic annulus. If a 25-mm stentless valve were implanted in a 23-mm an-

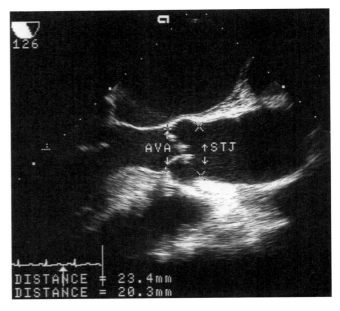

FIG. 4-82 Measurements used for aortic valve surgery are made from the midesophageal aortic valve long-axis view. The stentless valve size is determined by the size of the sinotubular junction *(STJ)* and should not be more than one valve size or approximately 10% greater than the size of the aortic annulus.

nulus (appropriate sizing), but the aortic root measured 27 mm, the valve would leak because the supporting structure sewn into the dilated aortic root would pull the leaflets apart and cause AI. To use a stentless valve for this patient, the annulus would have to be enlarged to accommodate a 27-mm valve or the aortic root downsized to 25 mm.

Human aortic valves (homografts) harvested shortly after death are also used for valve replacement. These are

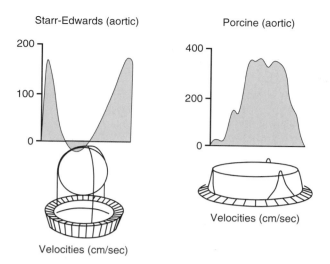

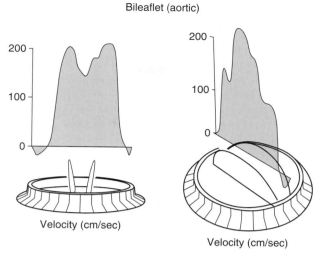

FIG. 4-83 Illustration of the velocity profiles of a Starr-Edwards (ball and cage) aortic valve and a Carpentier-Edwards 2625 porcine aortic valve at peak systole.

(From Yoganathan AP, Heinrich RS, Fontaine AA: Fluid dynamics of prosthetic valves. In Otto CM, editor: *The practice of clinical echocardiography*, Philadelphia, 1997, WB Saunders, pp 790-791.)

FIG. 4-85 Illustration of the velocity profile of a 27-mm St. Jude Medical bileaflet aortic valve at peak systole.

(From Yoganathan AP, Heinrich RS, Fontaine AA: Fluid dynamics of prosthetic valves. In Otto CM, editor: *The practice of clinical echocardiography*, Philadelphia, 1997, WB Saunders, p 788.)

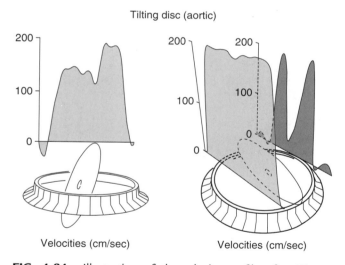

FIG. 4-84 Illustration of the velocity profile of a 27-mm Medtronic-Hall tilting disc aortic valve at peak systole.

(From Yoganathan AP, Heinrich RS, Fontaine AA: Fluid dynamics of prosthetic valves. In Otto CM, editor: *The practice of clinical echocardiography*, Philadelphia, 1997, WB Saunders, p 783.)

bioprosthetic valve is implanted in the pulmonic position, is termed the *Ross procedure*. A homograft is then implanted in the pulmonic position. Advantages to this procedure include an excellent hemodynamic profile for the autograft in the aortic position, tissue viability, and resistance to infection.[134] The pulmonic autograft is nonthrombogenic and has shown growth potential in children.[135-137]

Each prosthetic valve has a characteristic velocity profile based on the physical design of the valve (Figs. 4-83, 4-84, and 4-85). Bioprosthetic valves possess velocity profiles that resemble those of native valves.[138] Blood traverses a bioprosthetic valve through a circular central opening with a typical velocity of 2 to 3 m/sec in the aortic position and 1.5 m/sec in the mitral position. The mechanical valves have a variety of physical designs that produce complicated velocity profiles based on the size and shape of the various orifices[138] (see Figs. 4-83, 4-84, and 4-85). Caution must be exercised when using Doppler velocity measurements as an estimate of mechanical valve gradient. The velocity measurements depend on the location of the Doppler beam within the valve, the orifice through which the Doppler beam is directed, size of the valve, and the site of implantation.

Prosthetic valve evaluation with TEE begins with a complete two-dimensional evaluation using multiple imaging planes. Normal mobility includes appropriate opening and closing of the valve components. The sewing ring is carefully examined for its stability and continuity with the native annulus and surrounding tissue.

commonly implanted as a block with the ascending aorta. TEE is more accurate than transthoracic echocardiography for sizing the aortic annulus, allowing preoperative or pre-bypass selection, and preparation of aortic homografts.[132,133] The patient's own pulmonic valve (autograft), implanted in the aortic position while a

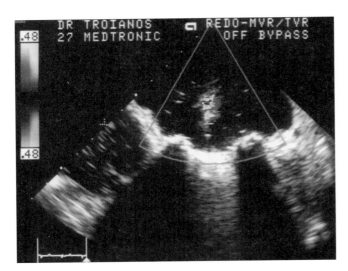

FIG. 4-86 Color flow Doppler echocardiography applied to a tilting disc mechanical mitral valve. A single, trace, central regurgitant jet within the sewing ring is characteristic of this valve.

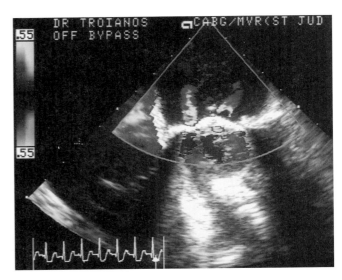

FIG. 4-87 Color flow Doppler echocardiography applied to a bileaflet mechanical mitral valve. Two to five small and symmetric regurgitant jets within the sewing ring are characteristic of this valve.

The presence of extraneous material in the vicinity of the valve is carefully scrutinized. Retained chordae tendineae, leaflet material, calcifications, thrombus, or vegetations may interfere with valve opening, closing, or both. Color flow Doppler is used to evaluate "closing backflow," physiologic regurgitation, and the absence of pathologic regurgitation and paravalvular leaks. "Closing backflow" is observed with color Doppler as the leaflets move toward the annular ring. Regurgitation occurs after valve closure. The trace physiologic regurgitation normally present with all mechanical valves is designed to deter thrombus formation. A single central jet is characteristic of the tilting disc valve (Fig. 4-86), whereas two to five symmetric jets may be observed with the bileaflet mechanical valve (Fig. 4-87). Physiologic jets must be within the sewing ring or annulus and should be symmetric in size and direction. Regurgitant jets that originate outside the sewing ring of the valve are paravalvular leaks (Fig. 4-88). Small paravalvular leaks present immediately after separation from cardiopulmonary bypass may resolve after reversal of anticoagulation.[139] The prognosis of a persistent trace paravalvular leak is unclear. The decision to reoperate and repair the trace paravalvular leak must consider the risk of reoperation and additional cardioplegia versus the risk of developing hemodynamic or hemolytic consequences from the paravalvular leak. Persistent jets that are trace in severity may not exhibit hemodynamic consequences, but may cause hemolysis over time.[140] Larger paravalvular leaks must be carefully assessed for their severity. Paravalvular leaks tend to be eccentric and directed to the atrial wall. Color flow mapping alone may underestimate the severity of these wall-hugging jets.

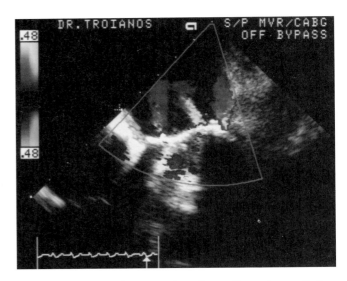

FIG. 4-88 Color flow Doppler echocardiography applied to a bileaflet mechanical mitral valve demonstrates two normal physiologic regurgitant jets within the sewing ring and an additional regurgitant jet outside the sewing ring, indicating a paravalvular leak.

Valves that exhibit more than trace regurgitation or a "rocking" motion of the valve within the annulus warrant reexploration and repair if the patient can tolerate the operation. Multiplane TEE improves classification of prosthetic regurgitation, but has little effect on severity grading.[141]

The author does not routinely determine prosthetic valve gradients or effective orifice area immediately after cardiopulmonary bypass because of the inherent errors involved in measuring velocities through valves with multiple, unevenly sized orifices. Localized gradients and pressure recovery produce discrepancies between Doppler and catheter-derived gradients.[142,143] Doppler velocity data overestimate prosthetic valve gradient, even when pressure recovery is taken into account.[144] Prosthetic valve gradients are more reliably determined by direct pressure measurement on either side of the valve when the valve is open. Gradients immediately following bypass are not reflective of long-term prosthetic valve gradients as the heart undergoes remodeling and the force of contraction, flow, and volume status normalize.

Later complications of prosthetic valves include bioprosthetic leaflet degeneration from calcification or endocarditis. Leaflet perforation, flail segments, leaflet restriction, obstruction, or valve dehiscence can be observed with TEE and indicate the need to replace the bioprosthetic valve. Mechanical valves become dysfunctional from vegetations, thrombus formation, or valve dehiscence. Echocardiographic lucency adjacent to the annular ring of any prosthetic valve with vegetations may indicate abscess formation or fistula. TEE is superior to TTE for the identification of anatomic prosthetic aortic valve lesions (96% vs. 77%) and for localizing the correct origin of the leak (88% vs. 54%).[145]

TEE REPORT AND BILLING

The ability to effectively communicate the TEE examination results to other health care professionals and the medical record is an essential component of performing intraoperative TEE.[146] Many third-party insurers require a complete interpretation and report to be generated by the echocardiographer for payment of professional services. The best way to ensure a complete examination and report is to perform the comprehensive multiplane TEE examination in a routinely consistent manner as described earlier in this chapter, and to document the results of the examination on a standardized reporting form. A task force within the Society of Cardiovascular Anesthesiologists (SCA) is currently working on such a form that may be adopted by a broad spectrum of physicians and practices. The author uses the form in Fig. 4-89 as a starting point to record intraoperative data. The final form is tailored to the individual patient and findings. Key components of this form are a brief patient history that indicates the planned surgical procedure, operation performed, requesting physician, indication for TEE (e.g., evaluate valve repair), probe placement procedure, echocardiographic services performed, and pertinent TEE findings. A summary of the most important findings is listed at the end of the report.

Reimbursement for intraoperative TEE is dependent on whether the echocardiographer is a cardiologist or anesthesiologist, the third-party payer, and the geographic region. The Medicare Report Policy for TEE in Pennsylvania defines reimbursable indications for intraoperative TEE (section H) as follows:

The interpretation of TEE during surgery is covered only when the surgeon or other physician has requested echocardiography for a specific diagnostic reason (e.g., determination of proper valve placement, assessment of the adequacy of valvuloplasty or revascularization, placement of shunts or other devices, assess of vascular integrity, or detection of intravascular air). To be a covered service, TEE must include a complete interpretation/report by the performing physician. When TEE is used for monitoring during a surgical procedure, the placement of the probe (93313) is covered. Coverage for evaluation, however, is not allowed for monitoring, technical trouble shooting, or any other purpose that does not meet the medical necessity criteria for the diagnostic test.

Adhering to the following key points will help ensure reimbursement: (1) document that a surgeon or other physician has requested echocardiography for a specific diagnostic reason, (2) generate a complete interpretation and report, and (3) remember that only probe placement is covered when TEE is used for monitoring. The diagnostic reason for TEE is indicated by the ICD-9 code used to submit the request for reimbursement. Claims submitted without a covered ICD-9 code are denied for not being medically necessary. The author's billing form is shown in Fig. 4-90 and contains only ICD-9 codes deemed reimbursable by the author's local Medicare carrier, which are most commonly used in his practice.

The most common Current Procedural Terminology (CPT) codes of the Health Care Financing Administration Common Procedure Coding System (HCPCS) used for intraoperative TEE with their descriptions are as follows:

93312 Echocardiography, transesophageal, real time with image documentation (2D) (with or without M-mode recording); including probe placement, image acquisition, interpretation, and report

93313 Placement of transesophageal probe only

93314 Image acquisition, interpretation and report only

93315 Transesophageal echocardiography for congenital cardiac anomalies; including probe placement, image acquisition, interpretation and report

93316 Placement of probe only for congenital anomalies

93317 Image acquisition, interpretation and report only for congenital anomalies

93318 Echocardiography, transesophageal (TEE) for monitoring purposes, including probe placement, real time 2-dimensional image acquisition and interpretation leading to ongoing (continuous) assessment of (dynamically changing) cardiac pumping function and to therapeutic measures on an immediate time basis

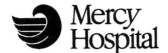

PATIENT NAME:

MR NUMBER:

OPERATOR:

DATE OF SERVICE:

REQUESTING PHYSICIAN:

TEE TAPE NUMBER: **LAP COUNTER -**

CLINICAL HISTORY:

INDICATION FOR TEE: [x] Diagnosis   [ ] Monitoring   [ ] Research

CLINICAL INDICATION:

TEE PROBE PLACEMENT

ECHOCARDIOGRAPHIC SERVICE PERFORMED:

[ ] 2-D TEE, probe placement, image acquistion, interpretation and report (code 93312 – 26 modifier)

[ ] Doppler echocardiography, pulsed wave and/or continuous wave with spectral display (code 93320 – 26)

[ ] Color Doppler flow velocity mapping (code 93325 – 26 modifier)

FINDINGS:

Left ventricle -

Mitral valve -

Left atrium -

Aortic valve -

Inter-atrial septum -

Tricuspid valve -

Aorta -

POSTOP EXAM:

Left ventricle -

Mitral valve -

Aortic valve -

Aorta -

IMPRESSION:

---

cc: Dr.   /Cardiology/XYZ Medical Billing

FIG. 4-89   TEE report form indicates the surgical procedure, clinical history, echocardio-graphic services performed, and echocardiographic findings.

PITTSBURGH ANESTHESIA
ASSOCIATES
TEE BILLING FORM

Hospital: _____ Date of Service: _____

Physician requesting service: _____

Physician Echocardiographer: _____

PROCEDURE CODE

[ ] **TEE used for monitoring only - code 93318**-26   [ ] **TEE probe placement only – code 93313**-26

[ ] **Diagnostic TEE - Check all that apply below:**

[ ] **93312**-26: Echocardiography, transesophageal, real time with image documentation (2D) (with or without M-mode recording) including probe placement, image acquisition, interpretation & report [ ] **93315**-26 for congenital anomalies

[ ] **93320**-26: Doppler echocardiography, pulsed wave and/or continuous wave with spectral display

[ ] **93325**-26: Doppler color flow velocity mapping

ICD-9 CODE (Check all that identify the diagnostic indication for TEE)

LEFT VENTRICLE

[ ] Cardiomegaly	429.3
[ ] Functional disturbance following cardiac surgery	429.4
[ ] Fluid overload	276.6
[ ] Hypertrophic obstructive cardiomyopathy	425.1
[ ] Alcoholic cardiomyopathy	425.5
[ ] Other cardiomyopathy	425.4
[ ] Ventricular septal defect	745.4
[ ] Left ventricular aneurysm	414.10
[ ] Acquired cardiac septal defect	429.71

MITRAL VALVE

[ ] Rheumatic mitral stenosis	394.0
[ ] Rheumatic mitral regurgitation	394.1
[ ] Rheumatic mitral stenosis with regurgitation	394.2
[ ] Mitral regurgitation – non rheumatic	424.0
[ ] Ruptured chordae tendinae	429.5
[ ] Ruptured papillary muscle	429.6
[ ] Other papillary muscle disorders	429.81

AORTIC VALVE

[ ] Rheumatic aortic stenosis	395.0
[ ] Rheumatic aortic insufficiency	395.1
[ ] Rheumatic aortic stenosis with insufficiency	395.2
[ ] Other aortic valve disease with AS or AI	424.1
[ ] Congenital stenosis of aortic valve	746.3
[ ] Congenital insufficiency of aortic valve	746.4

COMBINED AORTIC/MITRAL VALVE DISEASE

[ ] Mitral stenosis with aortic stenosis	396.0
[ ] Mitral stenosis with aortic insufficiency	396.1
[ ] Mitral insufficiency with aortic stenosis	396.2
[ ] Mitral insufficiency with aortic insufficiency	396.3
[ ] MS and/or MI with AS and/or AI	396.8
[ ] Other mitral and aortic	396.9

TRICUSPID VALVE

[ ] Rheumatic disease, stenosis or regurgitation	397.0
[ ] Other, stenosis or regurgitation	424.2

PULMONIC VALVE

[ ] Rheumatic diseases of the pulmonic valve	397.1
[ ] Pulmonary valve disorder, non-rheumatic	424.3

ENDOCARDITIS (any valve)

[ ] Bacterial	421.0
[ ] Endocarditis, not specified as bacterial	424.90

AORTA

[ ] Atherosclerosis	440.0
[ ] Dissection of thoracic aorta	441.01
Thoracic aneurysm:[ ] ruptured 441.1 [ ] unruptured	441.2
[ ] Injury to thoracic aorta	901.0

HYPOTENSION

[ ] Septicemia	038.9
[ ] Volume depletion	276.5
[ ] Cardiogenic shock	785.51
[ ] Traumatic shock	958.4
[ ] Postoperative shock	998.0
[ ] Shock, unspecified	785.50
Hypotension: [ ] specified 458.8 [ ] unspecified	458.9

TUMORS

[ ] Benign neoplasm of the heart	212.7
[ ] Neoplasms of unspecified nature	239.8

CONGENITAL

[ ] Ostium secundum ASD or patent forament ovale	745.5
[ ] Ostium primum	745.61
[ ] Unspecified septal defect	745.9
[ ] Partial anomalous pulmonary venous connection	747.42
[ ] Patent ductus arteriosus	747.0

MISCELLANEOUS

[ ] Air embolism	999.1
[ ] Iatrogenic pulmonary embolism	415.11
[ ] Other pulmonary embolism	415.19
[ ] Atrial fibrillation	427.31
[ ] Atrial flutter	427.32
[ ] OTHER: _____	

FIG. 4-90 TEE billing form indicates the physician requesting the service, procedures performed, and diagnosis code.

93320 Doppler echocardiography, pulsed-wave and/or continuous-wave with spectral display

93321 Follow-up or limited study

93325 Doppler color flow velocity mapping

A "26-modifier" is added to the procedure code to identify the bill as the professional component, whereas a "TC-modifier" identifies the technical component of the bill submitted by the equipment owner (usually the hospital). A "59-modifier" is added if the echocardiographer was also the anesthesiologist for the case to indicate that the TEE procedure was a distinct (independent) procedure from other services performed on the same day to the same patient.

Local carriers may require the physician to demonstrate training and experience specific to the procedure performed and to maintain such documentation for postpayment audit. At a minimum, the echocardiographer is credentialed by the institution in which the TEE is performed. Further demonstration of training and experience may include training documentation, appropriate continuing medical education conference attendance, and successful completion of the "Perioperative Transesophageal Echocardiography Certification Examination" endorsed by the SCA and administered by the National Board of Echocardiography.

DEVELOPING AN INTRAOPERATIVE ECHOCARDIOGRAPHY SERVICE

Intraoperative echocardiography has become an important and necessary component of cardiac surgical care. Many academic and cardiac centers consider TEE and epicardial echocardiography the standards of care for cardiac patients. Some institutions use intraoperative echocardiography for all cardiac surgical procedures, whereas others are more selective based on the patient's medical condition or the planned surgical procedure. New cardiac surgical service programs in community hospitals, more common in recent years, are also faced with the challenge of incorporating intraoperative echocardiography during the planning phase of their development. It is important to consider the issues of developing an intraoperative echocardiography service when caring for patients with cardiac problems.

The first issue to consider is the cost of starting and maintaining an intraoperative echocardiography service. Initial costs are related to purchase of capital equipment and training of personnel. An ultrasound machine capable of typical intraoperative use will cost between $100,000 and $200,000, depending on the features ordered. A multiplane transducer capable of several imaging frequencies will typically cost between $20,000 and $50,000, depending on the manufacturer, other associated purchases, and whether the probe is new or refurbished. Biplane probes may be available at a reduced cost, but will limit the user in terms of ease of use and the views that are possible compared with multiplane probes.

A probe for epicardial or epiaortic ultrasound should also be available. These probes are used for epicardial imaging in the patient in whom TEE views are inadequate or TEE is contraindicated. Epiaortic imaging is routinely used in certain hospitals to evaluate the ascending aorta before instrumentation with aortic cannulae, cross clamps, and proximal vein grafting. These probes can also be used for imaging the internal jugular or subclavian veins for ultrasound-guided cannulation.[147] These higher-frequency (7-10 MHz) phased-array probes are used for pediatric transthoracic echocardiography. Lower frequency probes (2-3 MHz) are used for adult TEE. A full complement of these probes is considered for purchase as a package, especially if the system will be shared with services outside the operating room environment. These transducers generally cost between $5000 and $15,000.

A new intraoperative echocardiography service may operate as a component of an existing cardiology service/echocardiography laboratory or function independently. Arrangements must be made for securing and storing ultrasound equipment, archiving videotapes or digital media, generating reports, establishing service contracts, and maintaining the system. Hospital personnel must be trained to handle the equipment and clean the probes.

An intraoperative echocardiography service requires the availability of physicians with specialized training in intraoperative echocardiography or the training of physicians. An anesthesiologist or cardiologist must possess appropriate training and skills, not only for echocardiography or even TEE, but must be competent in *intraoperative* echocardiography. If an experienced physician is not available to provide this service, recruiting and hiring costs should also be considered as a part of the start-up costs of a new intraoperative service. One experienced echocardiographer with appropriate experience to direct an echocardiography laboratory can provide teaching and on-the-job training to others using a mentoring approach.[148] This is the most cost-effective approach to train anesthesiologists and is a particularly attractive option in private practice settings. The disadvantage is the length of time required to achieve appropriate training and experience, particularly if the caseload is small. Another approach is for an anesthesiologist to spend a dedicated block of time in a more formal educational program.[149] This has traditionally occurred during fellowship training, but is costly and sometimes impractical for the physician already in practice. Savage and colleagues described a 1-year educational program for intraoperative echocardiography that focuses on acquiring the necessary cognitive and technical skills to proficiently perform echocardiography.[149] A summary of requisite cognitive and technical skills is outlined in Table 4-15.

TABLE 4-15
Skills Needed to Perform Transesophageal Echocardiography (TEE)

Cognitive Skills

Knowledge of appropriate indications, contraindications, and risks of TEE

Understanding of differential diagnostic considerations in each clinical case

Knowledge of physical principles of echocardiographic image formation and blood flow velocity measurement

Familiarity with operation of the ultrasound equipment, including the function of all controls affecting the quality of the data displayed

Knowledge of normal cardiovascular anatomy, as visualized tomographically

Knowledge of alterations in cardiovascular hemodynamics and blood flow resulting from acquired and congenital heart diseases

Knowledge of normal cardiovascular hemodynamics and fluid dynamics

Understanding of component techniques for general echocardiography and TEE, including when to use these methods to investigate specific clinical questions

Ability to distinguish adequate from inadequate echocardiographic data and to distinguish an adequate from an inadequate TEE examination

Knowledge of other cardiovascular diagnostic methods for correlation with TEE findings

Ability to communicate examination results to the patient, to other health care professionals, and on the medical record

Technical Skills

Proficiency in performing a complete standard echocardiographic examination using all echocardiographic modalities relevant to the case

Proficiency in safely passing the TEE transducer into the esophagus and stomach and in adjusting probe position to obtain the necessary tomographic images and Doppler data

Proficiency in correctly operating the ultrasound equipment, including all controls affecting the quality of the data displayed

Proficiency in recognizing abnormalities of cardiac structure and function as detected from the transesophageal and transgastric windows, in distinguishing normal from abnormal findings, and in recognizing artifacts

Proficiency in performing qualitative and quantitative analysis of the echocardiographic data

Proficiency in producing a cogent written report of the echocardiographic findings and their clinical implications

From Pearlman AS, Gardin JM, Martin RP et al: *J Am Soc Echocardiogr* 5:187-194, 1992.

KEY POINTS

1. TEE is a valuable clinical tool for evaluating cardiovascular anatomy, myocardial and valvular function, and hemodynamic abnormalities.

2. Intraoperative TEE is used during cardiac surgery to confirm the preoperative diagnosis, evaluate the success of the surgical intervention, and detect complications.

3. Intraoperative TEE is used during noncardiac surgery as a monitor of known cardiac pathology or as a "rescue" monitor for patients suffering unanticipated cardiac decompensation.

4. A new regional wall-motion abnormality detected by TEE is considered the earliest sign of myocardial ischemia.

5. TEE is a sensitive monitor for intracardiac air, but has a more important role in identifying intracardiac defects that predispose patients to paradoxical air embolism to the left heart.

6. Contraindications to TEE are esophageal and gastric disorders manifested by impaired swallowing, hematemesis, melena, or recent gastric or esophageal surgery.

7. Understanding the principles of ultrasound provides the basis for generating optimal images, recognizing artifacts, and interpreting data.

8. Performing an intraoperative TEE examination is a balance between a fastidiously complete comprehensive examination and expedience.

9. The ability to effectively communicate the TEE examination results to other health care professionals and the medical record is an essential component of performing intraoperative TEE.

10. Reimbursement requires documentation that a surgeon or other physician has requested echocardiography for a specific diagnostic reason and generation of a complete interpretation and report.

11. Local carriers may require the physician to demonstrate training and experience specific to the procedure performed and to maintain such documentation for postpayment audit.

KEY REFERENCES

American Society of Anesthesiologists and the Society of Cardiovascular Anesthesiologists Task Force on Transesophageal Echocardiography: Practice guidelines for perioperative transesophageal echocardiography, *Anesthesiology* 84: 986-1006, 1996.

Daniel WG, Erbel R, Kasper W et al: Safety of transesophageal echocardiography. A multicenter survey of 10,419 examinations, *Circulation* 83:817-821, 1991.

Erbel R, Engberding R, Daniel W et al: Echocardiography in diagnosis of aortic dissection, *Lancet* 1:457-461, 1989.

Grayburn PA, Handshoe R, Smith MD et al: Quantitative assessment of the hemodynamic consequences of aortic regurgitation by means of continuous-wave Doppler recordings, *J Am Coll Cardiol* 10:135-141, 1987.

Konstadt SN, Reich DL, Quintana C et al: The ascending aorta: how much does transesophageal echocardiography see? *Anesth Analg* 78:240-244, 1994.

Lambert AS, Miller JP, Merrick SH et al: Improved evaluation of the location and mechanism of mitral valve regurgitation with a systematic transesophageal echocardiography examination, *Anesth Analg* 88:1205-1212, 1999.

Morehead AJ, Firstenberg MS, Shiota T et al: Intraoperative echocardiographic detection of regurgitant jets after valve replacement, *Ann Thorac Surg* 69:135-139, 2000.

Pearlman AS, Gardin JM, Martin RP et al: Guidelines for physician training in transesophageal echocardiography: recommendations of the American Society of Echocardiography Committee for Physician Training in Echocardiography, *Am Soc Echocardiogr* 5:187-194, 1992.

Poortmans G, Schupfer G, Roosens C et al: Transesophageal echocardiographic evaluation of left ventricular function, *J Cardiothorac Vasc Anesth* 14:588-598, 2000.

Ribakove GH, Katz ES, Galloway AC et al: Surgical implications of transesophageal echocardiography to grade the atheromatous aortic arch, *Ann Thorac Surg* 53:758-763, 1992.

Roach GW, Kanchuger M, Mangano CM et al: Adverse cerebral outcomes after coronary bypass surgery, *N Engl J Med* 335:1857-1863, 1996.

Savino JS, Troianos CA, Aukburg S et al: Measurement of pulmonary blood flow with transesophageal two-dimensional and Doppler echocardiography, *Anesthesiology* 75: 445-451, 1991.

Schiller N, Foster E, Redberg RF: Transesophageal echocardiography in the evaluation of mitral regurgitation, *Cardiol Clin* 11:399-408, 1993.

Shanewise JS, Cheung AT, Aronson S et al: ASE/SCA guidelines for performing a comprehensive intraoperative multiplane transesophageal echocardiography examination: recommendations of the American Society of Echocardiography Council for Intraoperative Echocardiography and the Society of Cardiovascular Anesthesiologists Task Force for certification in perioperative transesophageal echocardiography, *Anesth Analg* 89:870-884, 1999.

Shively BK, Charlton GA, Crawford MH et al: Flow dependence of valve area in aortic stenosis: relation to valve morphology, *J Am Coll Cardiol* 31:654-660, 1998.

Smith JS, Cahalan MK, Benefield DJ et al: Intraoperative detection of myocardial ischemia in high-risk patients: electrocardiography versus two-dimensional transesophageal echocardiography, *Circulation* 72:1015-1021, 1985.

Yoganathan AP, Heinrich RS, Fontaine AA: Fluid dynamics of prosthetic valves. In Otto CM, editor: *The practice of clinical echocardiography*, Philadelphia, 1997, WB Saunders.

References*

1. Daniel WG, Mugge A, Martin RP et al: Improvement in the diagnosis of abscesses associated with endocarditis by transesophageal echocardiography, *N Engl J Med* 324:795-800, 1991.

2. Porembka DT, Johnson DJ II, Hoit BD et al: Penetrating cardiac trauma: a perioperative role for transesophageal echocardiography, *Anesth Analg* 77:1275-1277, 1993.

3. Skoularigis J, Essop MR, Sareli P: Usefulness of transesophageal echocardiography in the early diagnosis of penetrating stab wounds to the heart, *Am J Cardiol* 73:407-409, 1994.

4. Practice guidelines for perioperative transesophageal echocardiography. A report by the American Society of Anesthesiologists and the Society of Cardiovascular Anesthesiologists Task Force on Transesophageal Echocardiography, *Anesthesiology* 84:986-1006, 1996.

5. Savage RM, Cosgrove DM: Systematic transesophageal echocardiographic examination in mitral valve repair: the evolution of a discipline into the twenty-first century, *Anesth Analg* 88:1197-1199, 1999.

6. Suriani RJ, Neustein S, Shore-Lesserson L et al: Intraoperative transesophageal echocardiography during noncardiac surgery, *J Cardiothorac Vasc Anesth* 12:274-280, 1998.

7. Marak BA, Wedel DJ, Ammash NM: An unusual presentation of atrial septal defect in a patient undergoing total hip arthroplasty, *Anesth Analg* 91:1134-1136, 2000.

8. Mangano DT, Browner WS, Hollenberg M et al: Association of perioperative myocardial ischemia with cardiac morbidity and mortality in men undergoing noncardiac surgery. The study of perioperative ischemia research group, *N Engl J Med* 323:1781-1788, 1990.

9. Mangano DT, Browner WS, Hollenberg M et al: Long-term cardiac prognosis following noncardiac surgery. The study of perioperative ischemia research group, *JAMA* 268:233-239, 1992.

*The author thanks Peggy Flynn and Barbara Shawhan for their help with the references.

10. Mangano DT, Hollenberg M. Fegert G et al: Perioperative myocardial ischemia in patients undergoing noncardiac surgery—I: Incidence and severity during the 4 day perioperative period. The study of perioperative ischemia (SPI) research group, *J Am Coll Cardiol* 17:843-850, 1991.

11. Mangano DT, Wong MG, London MJ et al: Perioperative myocardial ischemia in patients undergoing noncardiac surgery—II: incidence and severity during the 1st week after surgery. The study of perioperative ischemia (SPI) research group, *J Am Coll Cardiol* 17:851-857, 1991.

12. Fleisher LA: Real-time intraoperative monitoring of myocardial ischemia in noncardiac surgery, *Anesthesiology* 92:1183-1188, 2000.

13. Leung JM, O'Kelly B, Browner WS et al: Prognostic importance of post-bypass regional wall-motion abnormalities in patients undergoing coronary artery bypass graft surgery, *Anesthesiology* 71:16-25.

14. Eisenberg MJ, London MJ, Leung JM et al: Monitoring for myocardial ischemia during noncardiac surgery, *JAMA* 268:210-216, 1992.

15. Reeves ST, Bevis LA, Bailey BN: Positioning a right atrial air aspiration catheter using transesophageal echocardiography, *J Neurosurg Anesthesiol* 8:123-125, 1996.

16. Black S, Muzzi DA, Nishimura RA et al: Preoperative and intraoperative echocardiography to detect right-to-left shunt in patients undergoing neurosurgical procedures in the sitting position, *Anesthesiology* 72:436-438, 1990.

17. Fahy BG, Hasnain JU, Flowers JL et al: Transesophageal echocardiographic detection of gas embolism and cardiac valvular dysfunction during laparoscopic nephrectomy, *Anesth Analg* 88:500-504, 1999.

18. McGrath BJ, Hsia J, Boyd A et al: Venous embolization after deflation of lower extremity tourniquets, *Anesth Analg* 78:349-353, 1994.

19. Aoki N, Soma K, Shindo M et al: Evaluation of potential fat emboli during placement of intramedullary nails after orthopedic fractures, *Chest* 113:178-181, 1998.

20. Takeda K, Sawamura S, Tamai H et al: Reversible tricuspid valve obstruction during removal of renal cell carcinoma with intracardiac tumor extension, *Anesth Analg* 91:1137-1138, 2000.

21. Orihashi K, Matsuura Y, Sueda T et al: Echocardiography-assisted surgery in transaortic endovascular stent grafting: Role of transesophageal echocardiography, *J Thorac Cardiovasc Surg* 120:672-678, 2000.

22. Suriani RJ, Cutrone A, Feierman D et al: Intraoperative transesophageal echocardiography during liver transplantation, *J Cardiothorac Vasc Anesth* 10:699-707, 1996.

23. Huang YC, Cheng YJ, Lin YH et al: Graft failure caused by pulmonary venous obstruction diagnosed by intraoperative transesophageal echocardiography during lung transplantation, *Anesth Analg* 91:558-560, 2000.

24. Canivet JL, Defraigne JO, Demoulin JC et al: Mechanical flow obstruction after heart transplantation diagnosed by TEE, *Ann Thorac Surg* 58:890-891, 1994.

25. Kochar GS, Jacobs LE, Kotler MN: Right atrial compression in postoperative cardiac patients: detection by transesophageal echocardiography, *J Am Coll Cardiol* 16:511-516, 1990.

26. Troianos, CA: Role of anesthesiologists in transesophageal echocardiography, *Advances in anesthesia*, vol 15, St Louis, 1998, Mosby, pp 189-207.

27. Daniel WG, Erbel R, Kasper W et al: Safety of transesophageal echocardiography. A multicenter survey of 10,419 examinations, *Circulation* 83:817-821, 1991.

28. Rousou JA, Tighe DA, Garb JL et al: Risk of dysphagia after transesophageal echocardiography during cardiac operations, *Ann Thorac Surg* 69:486-490, 2000.

29. Kawahito S, Kitahata H, Kimura H et al: Recurrent laryngeal nerve palsy after cardiovascular surgery: relationship to the placement of a transesophageal echocardiographic probe, *J Cardiothorac Vasc Anesth* 13:528-531, 1999.

30. Massey SR, Pitsis A, Mehta D et al: Oesophageal perforation following perioperative transoesophageal echocardiography, *Br J Anaesth* 84:643-646, 2000.

31. Savino JS, Hanson CW 3rd, Bigelow DC et al: Oropharyngeal injury after transesophageal echocardiography, *J Cardiothorac Vasc Anesth* 8:76-78, 1994.

32. Spahn DR, Schmid S, Carrel T et al: Hypopharynx perforation by a transesophageal echocardiography probe, *Anesthesiology* 82:581-583, 1995.

33. Latham P, Hodgins LR: A gastric laceration after transesophageal echocardiography in a patient undergoing aortic valve replacement, *Anesth Analg* 81:641-642, 1995.

34. Kharasch ED, Sivarajan M: Gastroesophageal perforation after intraoperative transesophageal echocardiography, *Anesthesiology* 85:426-428, 1996.

35. Chow MS, Taylor MA, Hanson CW 3rd: Splenic laceration associated with transesophageal echocardiography, *J Cardiothorac Vasc Anesth* 12:314-316, 1998.

36. Gendreau MA, Triner WR, Bartfield J: Complications of transesophageal echocardiography in the ED, *Am J Emerg Med* 17:248-251, 1999.

37. Shanewise JS, Cheung AT, Aronson S et al: ASE/SCA guidelines for performing a comprehensive intraoperative multiplane transesophageal echocardiography examination: recommendations of the American Society of Echocardiography Council for Intraoperative Echocardiography and the Society of Cardiovascular Anesthesiologists Task Force for certification in perioperative transesophageal echocardiography, *Anesth Analg* 89:870-884, 1999.

38. Cohen GI, White M, Sochowski RA et al: Reference values for normal adult transesophageal echocardiographic measurements, *J Am Soc Echocardiogr* 8:221-230, 1995.

39. Troianos CA, Porembka DT: Assessment of left ventricular function and hemodynamics with transesophageal echocardiography, *Crit Care Clin* 12:253-272, 1996.

40. Smith MD, MacPhail B, Harrison MR et al: Value and limitations of transesophageal echocardiography in determination of left ventricular volumes and ejection fraction, *J Am Coll Cardiol* 19:1213-222, 1992.

41. Urbanowicz JH, Shaaban MJ, Cohen NH et al: Comparison of transesophageal echocardiographic and scintigraphic estimates of left ventricular end-diastolic volume index and ejection fraction in patients following coronary artery bypass grafting, *Anesthesiology* 72:607-612, 1990.

42. Clements FM, Harpole DH, Quill T et al: Estimation of left ventricular volume and ejection fraction by two-dimensional transoesophageal echocardiography: Comparison of short axis imaging and simultaneous radionuclide angiography, *Br J Anaesth* 64:331-336, 1990.

43. Harpole DH, Clements FM, Quill T et al: Right and left ventricular performance during and after abdominal aortic aneurysm repair, *Ann Surg* 209:356-362, 1989.

44. Thys D, Hillel Z, Goldman ME et al: A comparison of hemodynamic indices derived by invasive monitoring and two-dimensional echocardiography, *Anesthesiology* 67:630-634, 1987.

45. Leung JM, Levine EH: Left ventricular end-systolic cavity obliteration as an estimate of intraoperative hypovolemia, *Anesthesiology* 81:1102-1109, 1994.

46. Cheung AT, Savino JS, Weiss SJ et al: Echocardiographic and hemodynamic indexes of left ventricular preload in patients with normal and abnormal ventricular function, *Anesthesiology* 81:376-387, 1994.

47. Appleton CP, Galloway JM, Gonzalez MS et al: Estimation of left ventricular filling pressures using two-dimensional and Doppler echocardiography in adult patients with cardiac disease, *J Am Coll Cardiol* 22:1972-1982, 1993.

48. Hoffmann R, Lambertz H, Jutten H et al: Mitral and pulmonary venous flow under influence of positive end-expiratory pressure ventilation analyzed by transesophageal pulsed Doppler echocardiography, *Am J Cardiol* 68:697-701, 1991.

49. Kuecherer HF, Kusumoto F, Muhiudeen IA et al: Pulmonary venous flow patterns by transesophageal pulsed Doppler echocardiography: relation to parameters of left ventricular systolic and diastolic function, *Am Heart J* 122:1683-1693, 1991.

50. Kuecherer HF, Muhiudeen IA, Kusumoto FM et al: Estimation of mean left atrial pressure from transesophageal pulsed Doppler echocardiography of pulmonary venous flow, *Circulation* 82:1127-1139, 1990.

51. Nishimura RA, Abel MD, Hatle LK et al: Relation of pulmonary vein to mitral flow velocities by transesophageal Doppler echocardiography. Effect of different loading conditions, *Circulation* 81:1488-1497, 1990.

52. Kuecherer HF, Foster E: Hemodynamics by transesophageal echocardiography, *Cardiol Clin* 11:475-487, 1993.

53. Hoit BD, Shao Y, Gabel M et al: Influence of loading conditions and contractile state on pulmonary venous flow, *Circulation* 86:651-659, 1992.

54. Porembka DT, Hoit B, Valente J et al: Transesophageal echocardiographic evaluation of left ventricular function in acute sepsis, *Crit Care Med* 21:S129, 1993.

55. Mueller X, Stauffer JC, Jaussi A et al: Subjective visual echocardiographic estimate of left ventricular ejection fraction as an alternative to conventional echocardiographic methods: comparison with contrast angiography, *Cardiol Clin* 14:898-902, 1991.

56. Gorcsan J III, Morita S, Mandarino WA et al: Two-dimensional echocardiographic automated border detection accurately reflects changes in left ventricular volume, *J Am Soc Echocardiogr* 6:482-489, 1993.

57. Cahalan MK, Ionescu P, Melton HJ: Automated real-time analysis of intraoperative transesophageal echocardiograms, *Anesthesiology* 78:477-485, 1993.

58. Thys DM, Hillel Z, Goldman ME et al: A comparison of hemodynamic indices derived by invasive monitoring and two-dimensional echocardiography, *Anesthesiology* 67:630-634, 1987.

59. Otto CM: *Textbook of clinical echocardiography*, ed 2, Philadelphia, 2000, WB Saunders, pp 100-131.

60. Gopal AS, Keller AM, Rigling R et al: Left ventricular volume and endocardial surface area by three-dimensional echocardiography: comparison with two-dimensional echocardiography and nuclear magnetic resonance imaging in normal subjects, *J Am Coll Cardiol* 22:258-270, 1993.

61. Muhiudeen IA, Kuecherer HF, Lee E et al: Intraoperative estimation of cardiac output by transesophageal pulsed Doppler echocardiography, *Anesthesiology* 74:9-14, 1991.

62. Savino JS, Troianos CA, Aukburg S et al: Measurement of pulmonary blood flow with transesophageal two-dimensional and Doppler echocardiography, *Anesthesiology* 75:445-451, 1991.

63. LaMantia K, Harris S, Mortimore K et al: Transesophageal pulse-wave Doppler assessment of cardiac output, *Anesthesiology* 69:A1, 1988.

64. Roewer N, Bednarz F, Schulte am EJ: Continuous measurement of intracardiac and pulmonary blood flow velocities with transesophageal pulsed Doppler echocardiography: technique and initial clinical experience, *J Cardiothorac Anesth* 1:418-428, 1987.

65. Darmon PL, Hillel Z, Mogtader A et al: Cardiac output by transesophageal echocardiography using continuous-wave Doppler across the aortic valve, *Anesthesiology* 80:796-805, 1994.

66. Gorcsan J, Gasior TA, Mandarino WA et al: Assessment of the immediate effects of cardiopulmonary bypass on left ventricular performance by on-line pressure-area relations, *Circulation* 89:180-190, 1994.

67. Tennant R, Wiggers CJ: The effect of coronary occlusion on myocardial contraction, *Am J Physiol* 112:351, 1935.

68. Sutton DC, Cahalan MK: Intraoperative assessment of left ventricular function with transesophageal echocardiography, *Cardiol Clin* 11:389-398, 1993.

69. Smith JS, Cahalan MK, Benefield DJ et al: Intraoperative detection of myocardial ischemia in high-risk patients: electrocardiography versus two-dimensional transesophageal echocardiography, *Circulation* 72:1015-1021, 1985.

70. van Daele MERM, Sutherland GR, Mitchell MM et al: Do changes in pulmonary capillary wedge pressure adequately reflect myocardial ischemia during anesthesia? A correlative preoperative hemodynamic, electrocardiographic, and transesophageal echocardiographic study, *Circulation* 81:865-871, 1990.

71. Shah PM, Kyo S, Matsumura M et al: Utility of biplane transesophageal echocardiography in left ventricular wall motion analysis, *J Cardiothorac Vasc Anesth* 5:316-319, 1991.

72. Tardif JC, Schwartz SL, Vannan MA et al: Clinical usefulness of multiplane transesophageal echocardiography: comparison to biplanar imaging, *Am Heart J* 128:156-166, 1994.

73. Feigenbaum H: *Echocardiography*, Philadelphia, 1994, Lea and Febiger, pp 447-510.

74. Wang XF, Li ZA, Cheng TO et al: Clinical application of three-dimensional transesophageal echocardiography, *Am Heart J* 128:380-388, 1994.

75. Reichek N, Wilson J, St. John Sutton M et al: Noninvasive determination of left ventricular end-systolic stress: validation of the method and initial application, *Circulation* 65:99-108, 1982.

76. Poortmans G, Schupfer G, Roosens C et al: Transesophageal echocardiographic evaluation of left ventricular function, *J Cardiothorac Vasc Anesth* 14:588-598, 2000.

77. Lambert AS, Miller JP, Merrick SH et al: Improved evaluation of the location and mechanism of mitral valve regurgitation with a systematic transesophageal echocardiography examination, *Anesth Analg* 88:1205-1212, 1999.

78. Kumar N, Kumea M, Duran C: A revised terminology for describing surgical findings of the mitral valve, *J Heart Valve Dis* 4:70-75, 1995.

79. Helmcke F, Nanda N, Hsiung M et al: Color Doppler assessment of mitral regurgitation with orthogonal planes, *Circulation* 75:175-183, 1987.

80. Schiller N, Foster E, Redberg RF: Transesophageal echocardiography in the evaluation of mitral regurgitation, *Cardiol Clin* 11:399-408, 1993.

81. Klein AL, Obarski TP, Stewart WJ et al: Transesophageal Doppler echocardiography of pulmonary venous flow; a new marker of mitral regurgitation severity, *J Am Coll Cardiol* 18:518-526, 1991.

82. Klein AL, Stewart WJ, Bartlett J et al: The effects of mitral regurgitation on pulmonary venous flow and left atrial pressure: an intraoperative transesophageal echocardiographic study, *J Am Coll Cardiol* 20:1345-1352, 1992.

83. Castello R, Pearson AC, Lenzen P et al: Effect of mitral regurgitation on pulmonary venous velocities derived from transesophageal echocardiography color-guided pulsed Doppler imaging, *J Am Coll Cardiol* 17:1499-1506, 1991.

84. Allan JJ, Lewis J, Kerber RE: Echocardiographic quantitation of mitral regurgitation: a new Doppler technique, *J Am Soc Echocardiogr* 11:149-154, 1998.

85. Vandervoort PM, Rivera JM, Mele D et al: Application of color Doppler flow mapping to calculate effective regurgitant orifice area, *Circulation* 88:1150-1156, 1993.

86. Otto CM: Valvular stenosis: diagnosis, quantitation, and clinical approach. In Otto CM, editor: *Textbook of clinical echocardiography*, ed 2, Philadelphia, 2000, WB Saunders, pp 229-264.

87. Utsunomiya T, Ogawa T, Doshi R et al: Doppler color flow "proximal isovelocity surface area" method for estimating volume flow rate: Effects of orifice shape and machine factors, *J Am Coll Cardiol* 17:1103-1111, 1991.

88. Odell JA, Mullany CJ, Schaff HV et al: Aortic valve replacement after previous coronary artery bypass grafting, *Ann Thorac Surg* 62:1424-1430, 1996.

89. Peter M, Hoffmann A, Parker C et al: Progression of aortic stenosis, *Chest* 103:1715-1719, 1993.

90. Bahler RC, Desser DR, Finkelhor RS et al: Factors leading to progression of valvular aortic stenosis, *Am J Cardiol* 84:1044-1048, 1999.

91. Palta S, Pai AM, Gill KS et al: New insights into the progression of aortic stenosis: implications for secondary prevention, *Circulation* 101:2497-2502, 2000.

92. Hoffmann R, Flachskampf FA, Hanrath P: Planimetry of orifice area in aortic stenosis using multiplane transesophageal echocardiography, *J Am Coll Cardiol* 22:529-534, 1993.

93. Stoddard MF, Hammons RT, Longaker RA: Doppler transesophageal echocardiographic determination of aortic valve area in adults with aortic stenosis, *Am Heart J* 132:337-342, 1996.

94. Shively BK, Charlton GA, Crawford MH et al: Flow dependence of valve area in aortic stenosis: Relation to valve morphology, *J Am Coll Cardiol* 31:654-660, 1998.

95. Rask LP, Karp KH, Eriksson NP: Flow dependence of the aortic valve area in patients with aortic stenosis: assessment by application of the continuity equation, *J Am Soc Echocardiogr* 9:295-299, 1996.

96. Lin SS, Roger VL, Pascoe R et al: Dobutamine stress Doppler hemodynamics in patients with aortic stenosis: feasibility, safety, and surgical correlations, *Am Heart J* 136:1010-1016, 1998.

97. Perry GJ, Helmcke F, Nanda NC et al: Evaluation of aortic insufficiency by Doppler color flow mapping, *J Am Coll Cardiol* 9:952-959, 1987.

98. Reynolds T, Abate J, Tenney A et al: The JH/LVOH method in the quantification of aortic regurgitation: how the cardiac sonographer may avoid an important potential pitfall, *J Am Soc Echocardiogr* 4:105-108, 1991.

99. Taylor AL, Eichhorn EJ, Brickner ME et al: Aortic valve morphology: An important in vitro determinant of proximal regurgitant jet width by Doppler color flow mapping, *J Am Coll Cardiol* 16:405-412, 1990.

100. Masuyama T, Kitabatake A, Kodama K et al: Semiquantitative evaluation of aortic regurgitation by Doppler echocardiography: Effects of associated mitral stenosis, *Am Heart J* 117:133-139, 1989.

101. Grayburn PA, Handshoe R, Smith MD et al: Quantitative assessment of the hemodynamic consequences of aortic regurgitation by means of continuous-wave Doppler recordings, *J Am Coll Cardiol* 10:135-141, 1987.

102. Griffin BP, Flachskampf FA, Siu S et al: The effects of regurgitant orifice size, chamber compliance, and systemic vascular resistance on aortic regurgitant velocity slope and pressure half-time, *Am Heart J* 122:1049-1056, 1991.

103. Takenaka K, Sakamoto T, Dabestani A et al: Pulsed Doppler echocardiographic detection of regurgitant blood flow in the ascending, descending and abdominal aorta of patients with aortic regurgitation, *J Cardiol* 17:301-309, 1987.

104. Kitabatake A, Ito H, Inoue M et al: A new approach to non-invasive evaluation of aortic regurgitant fraction by two-dimensional Doppler echocardiography, *Circulation* 72:523-529, 1985.

105. Reimold SC, Ganz P, Bittl JA et al: Effective aortic regurgitant orifice area: description of a method based on the conservation of mass, *J Am Coll Cardiol* 18:761-768, 1991.

106. Yeung AC, Plappert T, St. John Sutton MG: Calculation of aortic regurgitation orifice area by Doppler echocardiography: an application of the continuity equation, *Br Heart J* 68:236-240, 1992.

107. Kirklin JW, Barratt-Boyes BG: *Cardiac surgery*, New York, 1993, Churchill Livingstone, pp 589-606.

108. Cujec B, Mycyk T, Khouri M: Identification of Chiari's network with transesophageal echocardiography, *J Am Soc Echocardiogr* 5:96-99, 1992.

109. Braunwald E: Valvular heart disease. In Braunwald E, editor: *Heart disease*, ed 5, Philadelphia, 1997, WB Saunders, pp 1007-1076.

110. Daniels SJ, Mintz GS, Kotler MN: Rheumatic tricuspid valve disease: two-dimensional echocardiographic, hemodynamic, and angiographic correlations, *Am J Cardiol* 51:492-496, 1983.

111. Oh JK, Seward JB, Tajik AJ: *The echo manual*, ed 2, Philadelphia, 1999, Lippincott Williams and Wilkins, pp 103-132.

112. Movsowitz C, Podolsky LA, Meyerowitz CB et al: Patent foramen ovale: A nonfunctional embryological remnant or a potential cause of significant pathology? *J Am Soc Echocardiogr* 5:259-270, 1992.

113. Otto CM: Echocardiographic evaluation of cardiac masses and potential cardiac "source of embolus." In Otto CM, editor: *Textbook of clinical echocardiography*, ed 2, Philadelphia, 2000, WB Saunders, pp 351-372.

114. Konstadt SN, Reich DL, Quintana C et al: The ascending aorta: how much does transesophageal echocardiography see? *Anesth Analg* 78:240-244, 1994.

115. Otto CM: *Textbook of clinical echocardiography*, ed 2, Philadelphia, 2000, WB Saunders, pp 373-394.

116. Erbel R, Engberding R, Daniel W et al: Echocardiography in diagnosis of aortic dissection, *Lancet* 1:457-461, 1989.

117. Nienaber CA, von Kodolitsch Y, Nicolas V et al: The diagnosis of thoracic aortic dissection by noninvasive imaging procedures, *N Engl J Med* 328:1-9, 1993.

118. Cigarroa JE, Isselbacher EM, DeSanctis RW et al: Diagnostic imaging in the evaluation of suspected aortic dissection, *N Engl J Med* 328:35-43, 1993.

119. Troianos CA, Savino JS, Weiss RL: Transesophageal echocardiographic diagnosis of aortic dissection during cardiac surgery, *Anesthesiology* 75:149-153, 1991.

120. Hartman GS, Yao FSF, Bruefach M III et al: Severity of aortic atheromatous disease diagnosed by transesophageal echocardiography predicts stroke and other outcomes associated with coronary artery surgery: a prospective study, *Anesth Analg* 83:701-708, 1996.

121. Katz ES, Tunick PA, Rusinek H et al: Protruding aortic atheromas predict stroke in elderly patients undergoing cardiopulmonary bypass: experience with intraoperative transesophageal echocardiography, *J Am Coll Cardiol* 20:70-77, 1992.

122. Rubin DC, Plotnick GD, Hawke MW: Intraaortic debris as a potential source of embolic stroke, *Am J Cardiol* 69:819-820, 1992.

123. Marschall K, Kanchuger M, Kessler K et al: Superiority of transesophageal echocardiography in detecting aortic arch atheromatous disease: identification of patients at increased risk of stroke during cardiac surgery, *J Cardiothorac Vasc Anesth* 8:5-13, 1994.

124. Roach GW, Kanchuger M, Mangano CM et al: Adverse cerebral outcomes after coronary bypass surgery, *N Engl J Med* 335:1857-1863, 1996.

125. Ribakove GH, Katz ES, Galloway AC et al: Surgical implications of transesophageal echocardiography to grade the atheromatous aortic arch, *Ann Thorac Surg* 53:758-763, 1992.

126. Sylivris S, Calafiore P, Matalanis G et al: The intraoperative assessment of ascending aortic atheroma: epiaortic imaging is superior to both transesophageal echocardiography and direct palpation, *J Cardiothorac Vasc Anesth* 11:704-707, 1997.

127. Davila-Roman VG, Phillips KJ, Daily BB et al: Intraoperative transesophageal echocardiography and epiaortic ultrasound for assessment of atherosclerosis of the thoracic aorta, *J Am Coll Cardiol* 28:942-947, 1996.

128. Kouchoukos NT, Wareing TH, Daily BB et al: Management of the severely atherosclerotic aorta during cardiac operations, *J Card Surg* 9:490-494, 1994.

129. Duda AM, Letwin LB, Sutter FP et al: Does routine use of aortic ultrasonography decrease the stroke rate in coronary artery bypass surgery? *J Vasc Surg* 21:98-109, 1995.

130. Vasan RS, Larson MG, Benjamin EJ et al: Echocardiographic reference values for aortic root size: the Framingham Heart Study, *J Am Soc Echocardiogr* 8:793-800, 1995.

131. Bach DS: Echocardiographic assessment of stentless aortic bioprosthetic valves, *J Am Soc Echocardiogr* 13:941-948, 2000.

132. Abraham TP, Kon ND, Nomeir AM et al: Accuracy of transesophageal echocardiography in preoperative determination of aortic anulus size during valve replacement, *J Am Soc Echocardiogr* 10:149-154, 1997.

133. Oh CC, Click RL, Orszulak TA et al: Role of intraoperative transesophageal echocardiography in determining aortic annulus diameter in homograft insertion, *J Am Soc Echocardiogr* 11:638-462, 1998.

134. Oury JH: Clinical aspects of the Ross procedure: indications and contraindications, *Semin Thorac Cardiovasc Surg* 8:328-335, 1996.

135. Gerosa G, McKay R, Davies J et al: Comparison of the aortic homograft and the pulmonary autograft for aortic valve or root replacement in children, *J Thorac Cardiovasc Surg* 102:51-60, 1991.

136. Walls JT, McDaniel WC, Pope ER et al: Documented growth of autogenous pulmonary valve translocated to the aortic valve position, *J Thorac Cardiovasc Surg* 107:1530-1531, 1994.

137. Elkins RC, Knott CCJ, Razook JD et al: Pulmonary autograft replacement of the aortic valve in the potential parent, *J Card Surg* 9:198-203, 1994.

138. Yoganathan AP, Heinrich RS, Fontaine AA: Fluid dynamics of prosthetic valves. In Otto CM, editor: *The practice of clinical echocardiography*, Philadelphia, 1997, WB Saunders, p 791.

139. Morehead AJ, Firstenberg MS, Shiota T et al: Intraoperative echocardiographic detection of regurgitant jets after valve replacement, *Ann Thorac Surg* 69:135-139, 2000.

140. Garcia MJ, Vandervoort P, Stewart WJ et al: Mechanisms of hemolysis with mitral prosthetic regurgitation, *J Am Coll Cardiol* 27:399-406, 1996.

141. Flachskampf FA, Hoffmann R, Franke A et al: Does multiplane transesophageal echocardiography improve the assessment of prosthetic valve regurgitation? *J Am Soc Echocardiogr* 8:70-78, 1995.

142. Baumgartner H, Khan S, DeRobertis M et al: Discrepancies between Doppler and catheter gradients in aortic prosthetic valves in vitro, *Circulation* 82:1467-1475, 1990.

143. Vandervoort PM, Greenberg NL, Pu M et al: Pressure recovery in bileaflet heart valve prostheses, *Circulation* 92:3464-3472, 1995.

144. Stewart SFC, Nast EP, Arabia FA et al: Errors in pressure gradient measurement by continuous-wave Doppler ultrasound: type, size and age effects in bioprosthetic aortic valves, *J Am Coll Cardiol* 18:769-779, 1991.

145. Mohr-Kahaly S, Kupferwasser I, Erbel R et al: Value and limitations of transesophageal echocardiography in the evaluation of aortic prostheses, *J Am Soc Echocardiogr* 6:12-20, 1993.

146. Pearlman AS, Gardin JM, Martin RP et al: Guidelines for physician training in transesophageal echocardiography: recommendations of the American Society of Echocardiography Committee for physician training in echocardiography, *J Am Soc Echocardiogr* 5:187-194, 1992.

147. Troianos CA, Savino JS: Internal jugular vein cannulation guided by echocardiography, *Anesthesiology* 74:787-789, 1991.

148. Cahalan MK, Foster E: Training in transesophageal echocardiography: In the lab or on the job? *Anesth Analg* 81:217-218, 1995.

149. Savage RM, Licina MG, Koch CG et al: Educational program for intraoperative transesophageal echocardiography, *Anesth Analg* 81:399-403, 1995.

OUTLINE

The plan for anesthetic management of the cardiac patient undergoing surgery must provide for orderly and safe transition to a critical care or postanesthesia care unit (PACU). Important considerations are maintaining hemodynamic stability through appropriate monitoring and pharmacologic intervention and treating pain and awareness. The implications of making the transition from care provided by physicians to that provided by nonphysicians acting on physician orders or protocols are also considered. The plan includes preparing for unexpected events and complications that may arise in the postoperative period. The practitioner who understands the critical importance of these issues is the link that ensures excellence in perioperative anesthesia care. Thoughtful management is as important in the postoperative as in the preoperative and intraoperative phases of surgical treatment. Failure to appreciate this fact may result in complications that lead to significant morbidity or mortality. This chapter reviews the major issues that arise in anesthesia management of the cardiac patient after noncardiac surgery.

INTENSIVE CARE UNIT VERSUS POSTANESTHESIA CARE UNIT

The first decision regarding postoperative care is where that care should take place. The most appropriate setting depends largely on the nature of the surgery and the likelihood of discontinuing mechanical ventilation and hemodynamic monitoring in the short term. Patients undergoing cardiac, pulmonary, or major vascular procedures in the chest or abdomen are generally best managed in a specialized unit where return to normal physiologic function can occur as rapidly as possible. Patients with cardiac disease undergoing other types of surgery may often be managed in the PACU, especially if the PACU is open 24 hours and has sufficient staffing to accommodate short-term weaning from mechanical ventilation and hemodynamic monitoring and support.

Preoperative Variables

Preoperative variables that correlate with adverse patient outcomes are useful in deciding whether the patient with ischemic heart disease who undergoes noncardiac surgery should be admitted to an intensive care unit (ICU).

Many studies have shown that advanced age is a risk factor for perioperative mortality. Fleisher and others[1] demonstrated that 30-day mortality in Medicare beneficiaries undergoing aortic or infrainguinal vascular surgical procedures increased incrementally in different age groups for both types of surgery. The same authors observed improved perioperative and 1-year survival with preoperative stress testing with or without coronary revascularization before vascular surgery.

Previous myocardial infarction (MI) is well recognized as a preoperative variable that increases risk of a surgical procedure. The reported incidence of perioperative MI in patients without evidence of previous infarction ranges from 0.1% to 0.7%.[2] In contrast, the reported incidence of perioperative MI in patients with a previous MI is 6% to 7%, and perioperative MI is associated with a higher mortality than in the general population.

It is unclear which noninvasive cardiac test best predicts negative patient outcome. A metaanalysis of multiple studies involving dipyridamole thallium scintigraphy, ejection fraction estimation by radionuclide ventriculography, ischemia monitoring by ambulatory electrocardiography, and dobutamine stress echocardiography demonstrated that all modalities have predictive value in identifying patients having adverse outcomes after vascular surgery, but one test was not superior to the others.[3]

Cardiac catheterization of 1000 patients undergoing abdominal aneurysm surgery, lower extremity revascularization, or carotid endarterectomy demonstrated significant coronary artery disease (>70% stenosis) involving a single coronary artery in 27%, two coronaries in 19%, and three coronaries in 11% of patients.[4] Routine cardiac catheterization, however, is expensive and associated with morbidity and mortality.

Recent studies have cast serious doubt on the supposition that high-risk cardiac patients who undergo noncardiac surgery generally suffer cardiac complications and demise. A study of 464 men with either documented coronary artery disease (CAD) or at high risk for CAD undergoing noncardiac surgery revealed that noncardiac causes of death were more common. The subgroup with a history of hypertension, severely limited activity, and reduced renal function appeared to be at highest risk for in-hospital mortality.[5]

Intraoperative Variables

Intraoperative events that serve as predictors of morbidity and mortality in patients with cardiac disease are also used to make triage decisions for postoperative care.

In a classic study, Dr. Henry Loeb studied patients with fixed coronary lesions to ascertain the effects of heart rate and increased afterload on myocardial ischemia. CAD patients were stressed by atrial pacing to heart rates of 142 ± 4 beats/min or methoxamine infusion to systolic blood pressure (BP) of 196 ± 5 mm Hg (which resulted in similar myocardial oxygen consumption). Chest pain and ischemic ST-T segment changes were more common in the tachycardia group than the hypertension group.[6]

Several studies in vascular surgery patients have demonstrated the relationship between intraoperative ischemia and adverse cardiac outcome.[7,8] Studies using continuous electrocardiogram (ECG) monitoring with ST segment analysis demonstrated that most ischemic episodes in awake patients are asymptomatic (i.e., without chest pain). The incidence of "silent" ischemia is even higher in elderly patients subjected to general anesthetics, analgesics, and sedatives during the perioperative period.

Tachycardia is common after a surgical procedure and is often associated with ischemia, although many episodes of silent ischemia are not associated with any hemodynamic aberration. Myocardial ischemia is most likely to occur during emergence from general anesthesia.

Studies with continuous ECG monitoring and ST segment analysis demonstrate that preoperative, intraoperative, and postoperative silent ischemic episodes are common. Furthermore, cardiac-related morbidity and mortality is increased in patients with silent myocardial ischemia.[7,8] Perioperative MI correlates with the duration and number of perioperative ischemic episodes and the total perioperative ischemic time. Lack of continuous ECG evidence of myocardial ischemia is associated with an absence of adverse cardiac events in vascular surgical patients.

It is generally reasonable for patients with cardiac disease to recover in the PACU if the nature of the surgical procedure does not require long-term critical care and adequate personnel and resources are available to care for the patient. This decision requires (1) the absence of significant preoperative and intraoperative predictors and (2) anticipated weaning from mechanical ventilation and hemodynamic monitoring within 24 hours. A traditional critical care setting is more appropriate if these criteria are not met.

MONITORING FOR TRANSPORT

The Society for Critical Care Medicine's "Guidelines for Monitoring" suggest the continued monitoring of all parameters monitored in the ICU, emergency room (ER), or operating room (OR) during transport, if at all possible.[9] Although it is never wrong to continue all intraoperative monitoring during transport to the ICU or PACU, it may be desirable from a practical standpoint to reduce the number of monitoring modalities for a relatively brief transport. Selection of minimal monitoring depends on the hemodynamic status of the patient, the nature of the surgical procedure, the occurrence of significant ischemic events during the intraoperative period, and the transport route. If the patient is stable and the destination is adjacent to the OR, electrocardiography and pulse oximetry may suffice. It is advisable to monitor direct arterial pressure to promptly detect and treat hypotension or hypertension during transport. During transport of unstable patients, pulmonary artery pressure and waveform and mixed venous oxygen saturation must all be monitored, if possible. It is particularly important to monitor the pulmonary artery pressure and waveform if the transport route is long or involves elevator rides; such monitoring will help avoid unintentional catheter withdrawal or prolonged wedging. Patient safety is the priority for making these decisions regarding monitoring during transport.

TRANSPORT

Moving a critically ill patient from the OR to the ICU is fraught with hazards. It is mandatory that the clinician be able to rectify all potential mishaps that could occur during transport of the patient. Mishaps of transport can be devastating when the usual standards of high vigilance are relaxed. It is worthwhile for the clinician to consider every patient "critical" during the time of transport and to acknowledge the transport as a high-risk period during the course of a patient's hospitalization.[10] On an institutional level, each hospital should have a formalized plan for intrahospital and interhospital transport; this plan should be multidisciplinary and subject to a quality improvement process.[9]

The anesthesia clinician or OR circulating nurse should call the ICU or PACU to discuss time of arrival and immediate equipment and personnel needs. The surgical procedure and the presence of invasive hemodynamic monitoring, drains, bladder and epidural catheters, nasogastric tube, chest tubes, and pleurevacs should be described. Special airway needs (e.g., face tent, tracheostomy collar, ventilator, T-piece setup) should be addressed.

It is important to make systematic preparations before transport. Elimination of nonessential infusions is useful; essential infusions (e.g., inotropes, nitroglycerin, nitroprusside) should be continued with sufficient fluid volume and battery charge to complete the transport with a large margin of safety. Anesthesia and resuscitative drugs, a working laryngoscope, succinylcholine, a clean endotracheal tube of the proper size, sufficiently full oxygen tank, ECG monitor and defibrillator, pulse oximeter, and a self-refilling breathing bag and mask are essential. Transcutaneous defibrillator and pacemaker

pads should be applied before transporting patients with a disabled implantable defibrillator device and patients with frequent arrhythmias. Implantable defibrillators usually remain inactive during the first 24 to 48 hours postoperatively.

Some clinicians transport the intubated patient with a "Mapleson" or a "Jackson-Rees" circuit. This allows controlled, spontaneous, or assisted ventilation with visual assessment of tidal volumes and tactile assessment of lung compliance by the "trained hand of the anesthetist." The disadvantage of this transport circuit is that because the bag is not self-inflating, the anesthetist is unable to provide positive pressure to the airway should the oxygen supply become exhausted. For this reason, a self-inflating bag, such as the Ambu bag, is essential for every transport, even those using an ancillary breathing circuit.

The transport of a morbidly obese patient with an acknowledged difficult airway represents the greatest potential for catastrophe. Serious consideration is given to transporting the patient asleep and paralyzed, delaying reversal of neuromuscular blockade until the transport is completed. To prevent self-extubation during transport, wrist restraints are applied to the patient emerging from anesthesia with spontaneous ventilation and tolerating the endotracheal tube.

It is useful to remove air from vasoactive infusion bags to reduce entrainment of air and infusion shutdown. An additional safety tip regarding vasoactive medicines administered via "mini-drip" tubing is to include a "dial-a-flow" device in line to reduce the chance of an unintentional full-flowing infusion.

It is important to maintain uninterrupted infusion of pain medicine via an epidural catheter to minimize the incidence of tachycardia and hypertension caused by inadequate pain control. To minimize migration, the catheter can be secured by tunneling it under the skin at time of insertion. A sterile 18-gauge intravenous (IV) catheter over a hollow needle is inserted through the skin several inches lateral to the epidural catheter exit site and tunneled under the skin to exit near the epidural site. The metal needle is then withdrawn from the IV catheter and the sterile epidural catheter is threaded through the IV catheter. The IV catheter is withdrawn, leaving the epidural more snugly secured by two exit sites. The use of a second exit site should be noted on the patient's record. The likelihood of hub disconnection is decreased by taping both the epidural catheter and the hub connector to a tongue blade, thus strengthening the "weakest link" between the epidural infusion and the patient.

Chest tubes are not disconnected from suction until all transport monitors are functional and the patient is ready to leave the OR. The chest tubes are never clamped, but are placed on the transport bed at a lower level than the patient's chest to avoid the drainage of fluid or air into the pleural cavity. Transport of the cardiac patient requires a transport stretcher or bed capable of the Trendelenburg position and height adjustment. The transport bed should be low enough for chest compressions, if necessary, but high enough to allow drainage of chest tubes.

The ability to monitor and maintain the appropriate arterial blood pressure for patient and surgical condition during transport is another important responsibility for the anesthesia clinician. A noninvasive blood pressure measurement obtained after the patient is moved from the operating table to the transport bed verifies the accuracy of the invasive system. A blood pressure cuff attached to an inflating bulb and a manometer is an effective and reliable method of blood pressure measurement that does not rely on battery power and intact pressure tubing. A simple "finger-on-the-pulse" technique is used when transporting a cardiac patient in the absence of invasive arterial line monitoring.

A study examining the efficacy of manual ventilation of critically ill patients demonstrated that most patients become hypotensive and hypocarbic from overzealous manual positive pressure ventilation. Alkalosis increases cardiac irritability and predisposes patients to cardiac rhythm disturbances. Acidosis has a myocardial depressant effect and can also be arrhythmogenic.[10]

The only definitive way to assess the position of the pulmonary catheter during transport is continual visualization of the waveform. Inflation of the pulmonary artery (PA) catheter balloon with the catheter tip in a wedged position may cause rupture of the PA, which carries a 50% mortality. Patients with pulmonary hypertension and mitral regurgitation are of particularly high risk for this dreaded complication. A wedged tracing in patients with severe mitral regurgitation may be misinterpreted as a pulmonary arterial waveform. Failure to recognize a wedged catheter in such a patient can be disastrous if the balloon is inflated. Pulmonary vascular resistance increases as the patient makes the transition from controlled ventilation to spontaneous ventilation. Negative inspiratory pressure may lead to catheter wedging. Rigorous attention must be given to the insertion depth of the pulmonary catheter before and after transport. The PA catheter is easily withdrawn when the patient is moved from the operating table to the transport bed. Vasoactive medications become ineffective if the vasoactive infusion port is withdrawn into the protective sheath. If the PA catheter tip is withdrawn into the right ventricle, the patient will be prone to ventricular arrhythmias, including ventricular fibrillation. For this reason, many clinicians secure the catheters to the shoulder or forehead.

The nasogastric/orogastric (NG/OG) tube and oropharynx should be suctioned immediately before transporting an intubated patient to allow the best visualiza-tion for reintubation should unintentional extubation occur during transport, where suction is usually not immediately available.

TRANSFER OF CARE

The transfer of care occurs after patient assessment and hemodynamic monitoring in the unit confirm acceptable vital signs, adequate respiration, and continuation of all vasoactive infusions. Patient care is commonly transferred to nursing personnel acting by way of physician orders or protocols. The following checklist should be performed to ensure that no details are overlooked:

1. Airway unobstructed; endotracheal tube, if present, properly positioned and free of secretions
2. Appropriate ventilator settings or adequate respiratory rate and tidal volume; acceptable S_pO_2
3. Blood pressure and heart rate satisfactory for the clinical situation
4. Cardiac index > 2 $L/min/m^2$ or optimized
5. Invasive monitoring lines zeroed, transducers appropriately positioned, waveforms appropriate
6. ECG without ischemic changes or arrhythmia; obtain 12-lead if in doubt
7. Report to person assuming responsibility for care to include identification, age, height, weight, medical history, allergies, diagnosis, surgical procedure performed, significant events during intraoperative course, fluid intake and output, pertinent laboratory data, and any other relevant information
8. Appropriate orders for ventilation, fluid and pain management, nausea, and vomiting

MANAGEMENT OF POSTOPERATIVE PROBLEMS
Diagnosis and Treatment of Myocardial Infarction

An accurate diagnosis of postoperative MI is difficult to establish because false-negative and false-positive results occur with all diagnostic techniques. Because of the limitations of each individual test, the detection of perioperative MI is more accurate when a combination of diagnostic criteria is used. The criteria used to diagnose MI in the nonoperative setting may not be directly applicable as criteria for MI (especially non-Q-wave infarction) in the postoperative setting.

Unfortunately, there is no "gold standard" for surgical patients. The diagnosis is based on the preponderance of clinical evidence. Clinical signs and symptoms are not always present. Pathologic confirmation of MI at autopsy represents the "true gold standard." In caring for patients at high risk for myocardial ischemia, the anesthesiologist should be familiar with the pitfalls and controversies described in the literature concerning the various monitoring techniques.

An important publication in 1986 described the frequency of T-wave morphology changes after surgery. Although nonischemic changes in T-wave morphology had been described for a variety of other conditions and procedures (e.g., stress, carbohydrate ingestion, hyperventilation, catecholamine infusion, gallbladder and pancreatic disease, following vagotomy and stellate ganglion block), this was the first study that described these findings in the postoperative setting.[11] The preoperative and postoperative ECGs of a 31-year-old ASA-I patient who underwent parotid gland resection are shown in Fig. 5-1. The authors proposed that T-wave repolarization changes occur with equal frequency in patients with and without CAD, if the repolarization changes are truly nonischemic in nature. This study demonstrated a higher incidence of T-wave changes with abdominal surgeries, as compared with other types of surgery.

Optimal monitoring for myocardial ischemia includes ECG leads II and V_5, based on exercise treadmill testing.[12] Lead V_5 is the single most sensitive lead for intraoperative detection of ischemia. The sensitivity of ischemia detection approaches 100% if leads V_2, V_3, V_4, and V_5 are monitored, indicating the importance of the precordial leads in detecting ischemic changes.

Leads II and V_5 are the recommended choice if 5-lead ECG systems are available in the PACU. ST-segment analysis with alarms based on ST-segment elevation or depression is particularly useful in helping to identify patients with postoperative ischemia. Although the association of prolonged postoperative ischemia and adverse outcome (e.g., MI, death) is well supported in the literature, it is only suspected (not definitively established) that clinical anti-ischemic interventions may reduce risk and improve outcome. The ST-segment monitoring lead is chosen according to the area of myocardium at risk or based on changes noted on the patient's 12-lead ECG during an episode of ischemia. A recent cardiac catheterization or thallium scan are the best sources for identifying which lead should be chosen for ST-segment monitoring, as shown in Table 5-1.[13]

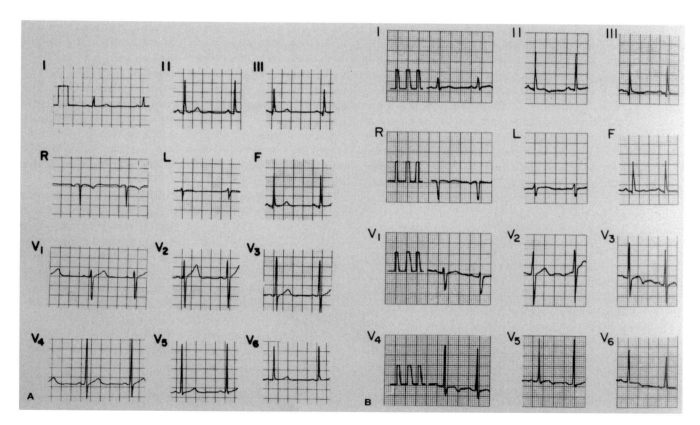

FIG. 5-1 **A,** Preoperative and **B,** postoperative ECGs of a 31-year-old man, ASA 1, who underwent parotid gland resection under morphine-N_2O-ethrane anesthesia. Note flattened T waves in the inferior leads and inverted or biphasic T waves in the anterolateral leads on the postoperative ECG.

(From Breslow MJ, Miller CF, Parker SD et al: *Anesthesiology* 64:400, 1986.)

TABLE 5-1
Location of ECG Changes During Myocardial Infarction

LOCATION OF INFARCTION	ARTERY INVOLVED	LEADS INVOLVED; EGG CHANGES
Anterior wall	LAD	V_{2-4}; Q waves, ST ↑, T ↓
Inferior wall	RCA or LCx	II, III, aVF; Q waves, ST ↑, T ↓
Ventricular septum	LAD	V_{1-2}; Q waves, ST ↑, T ↓
Lateral wall	LCx or LAD	V_{5-6}, I, aVL; Q waves, ST ↑, T ↓
True posterior wall	RCA or LCx	V_{1-3}; tall, upright R; ST ↓; ST ↑ V_{7-9}
Right ventricle	Proximal RCA	V_4R-V_6R; ST ↑

From Love MJ: Cardiovascular diagnostic procedures. In *Critical care nursing*, ed 3, St Louis, 1998, Mosby, p 403.
↑, Elevated; ↓, depressed; *LAD*, left anterior descending; *LCx*, left circumflex; *RCA*, right coronary artery.

Nonsurgical patients have a characteristic rise and fall of serum creatine kinase (CK) when an MI has occurred. CK levels also rise following surgery in the absence of MI. Levels rise during the first and second postoperative day and begin to fall thereafter, usually returning to baseline by the fifth or sixth day. The total amount of CK release is greater in patients with renal insufficiency (creatinine ≥2.5 mg/dl), in patients with hemiplegia or quadriplegia, and in the youngest patients. Although this pattern of CK release occurs with all types of surgical procedures, the total amount is significantly lower in patients who have undergone carotid endarterectomy or other superficial procedures.[14] Thus, CK levels are an inaccurate measure of myocardial injury in the postsurgical patient.

CK-MB levels provide a more specific indication of myocardial injury. Charlson and others analyzed CK-MB fractions in relation to symptoms (e.g., chest pain, signs or symptoms of congestive heart failure, palpitations, arrhythmias, or hypotension) and ECG changes. Fifty-five percent of patients who had both ECG changes and CK-MB levels >3% were asymptomatic. When CK-MB fractions were analyzed in relation to ECG changes, the vast majority of CK-MB positive patients did not have ECG changes. Two thirds of the patients studied had neither ECG changes nor symptoms, whereas 8% had both. Of the patients, 14% were asymptomatic with ECG changes, whereas 11% were symptomatic without ECG changes. These investigators drew the following conclusions based on their study results:

1. If major ECG changes (Q waves, ST elevation, ST depression ≥2 mm, and T-wave inversions) occurred in symptomatic patients, an infarction was usually confirmed with CK-MB isoenzymes.
2. An elevated CK during the first few days after surgery does not necessarily indicate that an MI has

occurred, because this pattern of CK release occurred with all types of surgical procedures, and all types of patients.
3. Some patients with MB levels ≥5%, but without ECG changes or other cardiac complications during their hospitalization, may not have had a postoperative MI.
4. Most patients who experience postoperative myocardial ischemia or infarction are asymptomatic; therefore symptoms should not be required for the diagnosis of postoperative MI.

More recent studies investigated the role of other serum markers and indicators of acute MI in postoperative and nonoperative settings. High postoperative levels of serum troponin T and troponin I are associated with postoperative cardiac complications in high-risk patients undergoing noncardiac surgery.[15-17]

High postoperative troponin levels are associated with increased postoperative release of free and conjugated noradrenaline and adrenaline.[18] Technetium pyrophosphate accumulates in irreversibly injured myocardial cells. A regional uptake of 2+ or more is considered specific for cell necrosis, although false-negative results are not uncommon, especially with nontransmural infarction. When a diffuse pattern is seen, only a 3+ uptake is considered specific enough for a diagnosis of new necrosis. Myocardial scintiscans are most useful in the setting of increased CK-MB liberation in the absence of ECG changes. These scans should be performed within 48 hours of surgery because the uptake becomes normal in a significant proportion of patients by the third day.[19]

Numerous studies address the "symptomatology" of postoperative MI. Clinical presentations of postoperative MI from one study are portrayed in Table 5-2.[20]

The classic presentation of MI with radiating subster-

TABLE 5-2
Clinical Presentation of Postoperative Myocardial Infarction

CLINICAL SIGNS/SYMPTOMS	NUMBER OF PATIENTS (PERCENTAGE)
Hypotension	11 (39%)
Chest pain	11 (39%)
Congestive heart failure	7 (25%)
Cardiopulmonary arrest	1 (4%)
Altered mental status	2 (7%)
Arrhythmia (new onset)	5 (18%)
Nausea, hypertension	1 (4%)

From Becker RC, Underwood DA: *Cleve Clin J Med* 54:27, 1987.

nal chest pain is unusual in the postoperative setting because incisional pain, sedation, and analgesia often mask typical symptoms.[20] Nonanginal modes of presentation, including heart failure, are more common, as are atrial and ventricular arrhythmias. A patient may present with only a brief period of diaphoresis. The presenting symptom may also be unexplained tachycardia or oliguria alone.[21] New ventricular arrhythmias occurring in the postanesthesia care unit are associated with a statistically greater risk of MI. Patients who develop a postoperative MI have ECG evidence of intraoperative or postoperative ischemia associated with atrial and ventricular arrhythmias.[22] The single most important concept to appreciate is that a large proportion of patients who experience a postoperative MI demonstrate no signs or symptoms suggestive of myocardial ischemia and are diagnosed by serial ECG changes.[23]

Although MI can occur at any time during the postoperative period, more than 90% occur within the first 6 days, with a peak incidence on postoperative day three.[20] According to the American College of Cardiology/American Heart Association Task Force Perioperative Cardiovascular Guidelines, it is appropriate (and cost effective) to obtain ECGs preoperatively, immediately after surgery, and for the first 2 days after surgery in patients at risk.[24] The presence of either (1) new ST-segment changes in high-risk patients with or without symptoms, (2) new T-wave abnormalities in association with impaired ventricular function, or (3) ventricular arrhythmias should be presumed to be caused by ischemia.[11] Serial ECGs and a "high index of suspicion" concerning signs and symptoms (acknowledging that a significant portion of patients do not exhibit any symptoms suggestive of MI) guide the therapeutic and consultative decisions in the postoperative period. Postoperative cardiovascular complications

should be managed aggressively, with transfer of the patient to a high-acuity critical care nursing unit and appropriate consultation (cardiology, pulmonary, critical care medicine) provided in a timely fashion. Postoperative congestive heart failure is too often attributed to overly aggressive fluid administration and is empirically treated with diuretics. Evidence in the literature suggests that MI in the perioperative setting is associated with high (50%) mortality and major morbidity. The clinician must have a high index of suspicion, initiate corrective therapy in a timely fashion, and obtain appropriate consultative support to ensure the best possible outcome.

Antman and others reviewed recommendations for treatment of acute MI and performed metaanalyses for effective treatments that improved outcome in patients with acute MI.[25] Statistically significant reductions in mortality were demonstrated with use of thrombolytic agents (t-PA, streptokinase), IV vasodilators (nitroglycerin and nitroprusside), aspirin (ASA), anticoagulants (heparin), IV magnesium salts, and β-blockers. In addition, angiotensin-converting enzyme (ACE) inhibitor therapy in the setting of acute MI (and heart failure) improved outcome in several clinical trials.[26] In contrast, current literature suggests that lidocaine infusions (for prophylactic treatment of potential ventricular arrhythmias) and calcium channel blockers may be potentially harmful.[25] Digoxin administration to patients with congestive heart failure after an acute MI is associated with increased total mortality and increased relative risk for sudden death, presumably from an increased risk of digoxin-induced ventricular tachycardia.[27] Chronic maintenance therapies that reduce mortality following an acute MI (secondary prevention) and improve long-term survival include β-blockers, rehabilitation exercise regimens, antiplatelet drugs, pooled cholesterol-lowering measures (diet, drugs, and ileal bypass surgery), and oral anticoagulants.[25] ACE inhibitors improve survival, but are considerably underutilized. It is estimated that if ACE inhibitors were administered to 1000 patients with moderate left ventricle (LV) dysfunction, 50 deaths and 350 hospitalizations would be prevented.[26] Attempted "secondary prevention" with use of Type I antiarrhythmic drugs is associated with adverse effects, and the beneficial effects of calcium channel blockers have not been consistent.[25]

Acute Interventional Therapy for Perioperative Ischemia
Thrombolytics

The literature during the last two decades demonstrated the importance of timely opening obstructed coronary arteries after acute coronary thrombosis. Nearly all MIs are caused by an acute coronary thrombosis that obstructs blood flow to myocardium supplied by that coronary artery. Multiple thrombolytic drugs are effective in thrombolysis, restoring blood flow and reducing the risk of death. Thrombolytics, however, restore blood flow in only 30% to 60% of patients, and they may be associated with major intracranial hemorrhage. A reopened coronary artery improves survival in patients with acute MI that appears to be independent of improved left ventricular function. Clinical observations suggest that patients with an infarct-related artery that remains occluded 90 minutes after thrombolytic therapy have high subsequent mortality.[29]

Contraindications to thrombolytic therapy in the setting of an acute MI are as follows:

- History of cerebrovascular accident
- Clouded consciousness
- A major bleeding diathesis
- Recent acute internal hemorrhage
- Major surgery or trauma within 10 days
- Uncontrolled hypertension
- A recent arterial or venous puncture in a noncompressible site

The major disadvantage of thrombolytic therapy in general is the risk of stroke, which varies between agents (0.5%-3%).[29] The major disadvantage of thrombolytics in the perioperative period is their contraindication after major surgery.

Angioplasty

Angioplasty with stenting is another modality used to restore flow in an acutely thrombosed coronary artery. The addition of "rescue" angioplasty improves the 30% to 60% effectiveness of thrombolytics in reestablishing blood flow in acute coronary occlusions. The improvement in outcome is less than would be expected, but is explained by logistical delays before reperfusion and by platelet activation associated with angioplasty. Adjunctive therapy with glycoprotein IIb/IIIa antagonists (which block the final common pathway of activated platelet-surface receptors to fibrinogen) may improve the safety and clinical outcomes of rescue angioplasty.[29] Primary angioplasty has the distinct advantage of a lower incidence of bleeding as compared with thrombolytic therapy and is therefore the most appropriate therapy for aggressively treating an acute postoperative MI in a hospital setting that has coronary catheterization/angioplasty capability.

Intraaortic Balloon Pump

The intraaortic balloon pump (IABP) is an adjunct to pharmacologic treatment of myocardial dysfunction and unstable angina. The beneficial hemodynamic effects of the IABP include augmentation of myocardial perfusion during diastole to increase myocardial oxygen delivery, reduction of myocardial oxygen consump-

tion through reduction of left ventricular afterload and wall tension, and modest increase in cardiac output. In the setting of acute coronary occlusion, the IABP causes a redistribution of coronary blood flow to ischemic areas of the myocardium, repleting energy-depleted myocardial cells. The IABP is used to treat reversible ischemia by reducing left ventricular dysfunction before hypotension leads to myocardial necrosis.[30] The incidence of complications is 4% to 12% and mainly involves ischemia to the lower limb, where the IABP is placed. The ischemia is usually reversible with removal of the IABP. Placement of an IABP in high-risk patients decreases mortality in patients undergoing coronary revascularization.

Congestive Heart Failure

The diagnosis of congestive heart failure requires the presence of two major and two minor criteria listed in Table 5-3.[31]

TABLE 5-3
Heart Failure Criteria

Major Criteria
Rales
Neck vein distention
Acute pulmonary edema
Paroxysmal nocturnal dyspnea
Cardiomegaly on chest radiograph
Third heart sound (gallop)
Hepatojugular reflux
Circulation time ≥25 seconds
Increased central venous pressure (>16 cm H_2O at right atrium)
Visceral congestion, cardiomegaly, or pulmonary edema at autopsy
Weight loss >4.5 kg in 5 days in response to CHF treatment

Minor Criteria
Nocturnal cough
Bilateral ankle edema
Dyspnea on ordinary exertion
Pleural effusion
Hepatomegaly
Decrease in vital capacity by 33% from maximal value recorded
Tachycardia >120 beats/min

From Ho KKL, Pinsky JL, Kannel WB et al: *J Am Coll Cardiol* 22 (suppl A):7A, 1993.
CHF, Congestive heart failure.

Fig. 5-2 depicts a pressure-volume loop typical of combined systolic and diastolic heart failure. Any increase in ventricular volume increases left ventricular diastolic pressure in patients with diastolic failure. Both systolic myocardial contraction and diastolic myocardial relaxation are energy (adenosine triphosphate) dependent. Conditions that deplete energy stores, such as increased wall tension and myocardial ischemia, lead to diastolic dysfunction. Left ventricular diastolic dysfunction occurs with decreased elasticity/fibrosis caused by aging and with left ventricular hypertrophy caused by long-standing hypertension or valvular disease, particularly aortic stenosis. Atrial ejection into a stiff, noncompliant left ventricle is responsible for the characteristic abnormalities observed with echocardiography in terms of diastolic relaxation and filling patterns (see Chapter 4). Ventricular dysfunction generally serves as a marker of the severity of coronary artery disease in terms of extensive or multiple MIs. Left ventricular dysfunction or congestive heart failure can also be caused by chronic hypertension, valvular disease or cardiomyopathy. Severe left ventricular dysfunction limits the patient's ability to tolerate the large fluid shifts and volume changes associated with major noncardiac surgery.[32]

The etiology of postoperative congestive heart failure and pulmonary edema is multifactorial. Myocardial ischemia, reduced preoperative left ventricular ejection fraction, postoperative hypertension, hypoxemia, rapid withdrawal of positive pressure ventilation, and discon-

tinuation of previous medical therapy have all been implicated.[33]

Charlson and others evaluated high-risk hypertensive and diabetic patients undergoing elective general surgical procedures to determine predictors of postoperative congestive heart failure. Patients with preoperative cardiac disease (previous MI, valvular disease, or previous history of congestive heart failure), diabetes, and intraoperative increases or decreases of mean arterial blood pressure of 40 mm Hg or more were at highest risk for postoperative congestive heart failure. In contrast, less than 1% of patients without cardiac disease had postoperative congestive heart failure.[34] The significance of substantially depressed left ventricular function or advanced congestive heart failure is that postoperative pulmonary edema is not just an intermediate physiologic aberration, but an independent predictor of adverse outcome and mortality.[32]

Postoperative Arrhythmias

Sinus tachycardia is the most common rhythm disturbance in the postoperative period and should be distinguished from paroxysmal atrial tachycardia. Carotid massage, the classic maneuver used to differentiate the two rhythms, should not be attempted in the patient with known or suspected carotid artery disease. The maneuver may not be effective in patients who have had carotid endarterectomy caused by carotid bulb denervation by surgery. Noncardiac etiologic factors include pain, hypovolemia or hypervolemia, fever, anemia, hypoxemia, anxiety, infection, hypotension, electrolyte abnormalities, mechanical ventilation, and pulmonary emboli.

The Perioperative Ischemia Research Group examined the occurrence of ventricular arrhythmias in men at high risk for coronary artery disease who were undergoing noncardiac surgery.[35] Continuous electrocardiographic recording, using two-channel Holter monitoring of leads CC5 and CM5, was initiated at least 12 hours preoperatively and continued for at least 112 hours postoperatively. A positive occurrence was defined as greater than 30 ventricular ectopic beats per hour or ventricular tachycardia. Twenty-one percent of patients had ventricular arrhythmias or ventricular tachycardia preoperatively. The incidence declined to 15.7% during surgery, but increased to 36.1% in the postoperative period. Factors that predisposed patients to ventricular arrhythmias in the preoperative period included cigarette smoking, history of congestive heart failure, and ECG evidence of myocardial ischemia. The occurrence of intraoperative and postoperative ventricular arrhythmias correlated with the presence of preoperative ventricular arrhythmias. An important finding of this study was that adverse outcomes were NOT as-

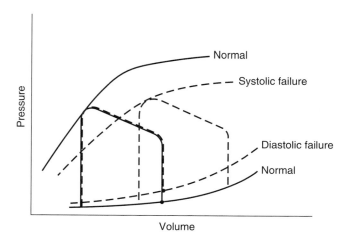

FIG. 5-2 A pressure-volume loop demonstrating combined systolic and diastolic heart failure. With systolic heart failure, the developed pressure is reduced (depressed end-systolic pressure-volume relation) and the heart dilates along a normal diastolic pressure-volume relation. In contrast, with diastolic failure, the end-systolic pressure-volume relation is preserved but the diastolic relation is shifted upward.

(Modified from Grossman W: *Circulation* 81[suppl III]:iii-2, 1990; and Lake CL: Chronic treatment of congestive heart failure. In *Cardiac anesthesia,* ed 4, Philadelphia, 1999, WB Saunders, p 136.)

sociated with arrhythmias in any of the monitoring periods. The authors concluded that nearly half of all high-risk patients undergoing noncardiac surgery had perioperative episodes of ventricular arrhythmias, the vast majority of which were asymptomatic. There were no episodes of sustained ventricular tachycardia or ventricular fibrillation, and ventricular arrhythmias were not associated with adverse ischemic outcomes.

Another important issue is the association of a new ventricular arrhythmia in the postoperative period with postoperative MI. A new ventricular arrhythmia is associated with a greater risk (p < 0.01) of MI.[22] The Perioperative Ischemia Research Group pointed out that arrhythmias can occur after the first symptoms of an acute MI, and that "the possibility of an acute cardiovascular event should be considered before deciding that further monitoring or treatment is unnecessary."[35]

Polanczyk and others examined the occurrence and significance of supraventricular arrhythmias in the perioperative patient.[36] A retrospective study reviewed the records of 4181 patients having noncardiac surgery for new onset atrial fibrillation, atrial flutter, paroxysmal atrial tachycardia, multifocal atrial tachycardia, or supraventricular tachyarrhythmias without discernable P waves. Independent correlates of supraventricular arrhythmias included age greater than 70 years, male sex, history of congestive heart failure, physical exam evidence of significant valvular disease (systolic murmur of grade III or higher), and history of supraventricular arrhythmia. A history of asthma, presence of premature atrial contractions on preoperative ECG, ASA status III or IV, and type of procedure also correlated with the occurrence of supraventricular arrhythmias. Intrathoracic, abdominal (especially aortic aneurysm surgery), and other vascular procedures were independently associated with supraventricular arrhythmias. Intraoperative hypotensive episodes were also independently associated with supraventricular arrhythmias, particularly if the hypotensive episodes lasted longer than 10 minutes. Patients with acute cardiac events (CHF, MI, ischemia without infarction, ventricular tachycardia, or cardiac arrest) had particularly high relative risk for the onset of perioperative supraventricular arrhythmias. Noncardiac events associated with supraventricular arrhythmia included pneumonia, bacteremia, wound infection, urinary tract infection, cerebrovascular accident, pulmonary embolus, and gastrointestinal bleeding. Most cases of supraventricular arrhythmias occur either concurrently or after associated complications, making an interpretation of the association problematic. It may not be clear whether supraventricular arrhythmias cause these complications, are a consequence, or simply a marker for increased incidence of complications. Supraventricular arrhythmias recurred both the day before and day after the diagnosis of postoperative MI, but

always preceded in cases of postoperative cerebrovascular accident. Perioperative supraventricular arrhythmias increase the length and cost of hospital stay.[36]

Although the relationship between digoxin use and perioperative supraventricular arrhythmias is complex, digoxin may be protective in patients undergoing thoracic surgery.[36] Preoperative initiation of digoxin therapy is controversial in these patients. Some clinicians advocate this therapy because of the increased prevalence of intraoperative supraventricular arrhythmias. Digoxin therapy initiated intraoperatively is continued postoperatively with prompt corrections of hypokalemia.[37]

Postoperative atrial fibrillation is often a hemodynamically stable rhythm that does not require treatment.[38] Electrical cardioversion is considered if there is ECG evidence of ischemia, significant mitral or aortic stenosis, or hemodynamic instability. Treatable etiologies of atrial fibrillation (abnormalities of p_aO_2, p_aCO_2, K^+, Mg^{++}, Ca^{++}, temperature, or pH) should be identified and corrected. New-onset atrial fibrillation in an ambulatory surgical patient requires admission to an inpatient facility for evaluation and treatment.

The first priority for treatment of atrial fibrillation is to slow the ventricular rate to decrease myocardial oxygen demand and improve ventricular filling. A diltiazem infusion, or bolus doses of verapamil, a β-blocker, or digoxin loading (500 mcg digoxin IV over 20 minutes, followed by 250 mcg IV every 6 hours times two doses followed by oral dosing) are all accepted treatments. Caution must be exercised when combination therapy is used because the synergy between β-blockers and calcium channel blockers (typically verapamil or diltiazem) can produce profound bradycardia, or even asystole. Anticoagulant therapy must be considered if sinus mechanism is not restored promptly, because some patients with atrial fibrillation develop intraatrial thrombi within a few days. The benefits and risks of anticoagulation in the postoperative period are considered in the context of the type of surgery and the risk of surgical bleeding. Atrial flutter is less stable than atrial fibrillation and demands greater clinical attention, especially if associated with a rapid ventricular response in a patient with coronary artery disease or valvular stenosis.

Hypertension

Systemic hypertension in the postoperative period is a common problem. The practitioner must evaluate and treat any physical factors (fever, pain, bladder distention), psychologic factors (anxiety, abrupt return to consciousness, disorientation), or metabolic abnormalities (hypoxemia, hypercarbia, acidosis) before initiating antihypertensive therapy. Use of pharmacologic therapy is indicated when systemic pressures remain unacceptably high after ensuring adequate oxygenation and ventilation, relieving pain and anxiety, and treating any physical issues. The practitioner should use all available hemodynamic information to choose an effective treatment plan. A variety of medications are available to treat systemic hypertension in the postoperative period.[39] The choice depends on the specific hemodynamic pertubation, pathophysiology of the patient, and preference of the practitioner.

Sodium Nitroprusside

Sodium nitroprusside (SNP) is a potent drug that requires invasive arterial monitoring. SNP is beneficial when cardiac function is marginal, filling pressure is elevated, and systemic vascular resistance (SVR) is high. Both systemic blood pressure and vascular resistance decrease as cardiac output improves. Volume infusion may be required to maintain preload. SNP is avoided during episodes of myocardial ischemia, because it can create a coronary steal syndrome by shunting blood away from ischemic zones and lowering diastolic perfusion pressure.

The adverse effects of SNP are tachyphylaxis, worsening hypoxemia secondary to inhibition of hypoxic pulmonary vasoconstriction, cyanide toxicity, and thiocyanate toxicity.

Cyanide toxicity is manifested by metabolic acidosis and increased mixed venous oxygen saturation. It occurs when large doses are given over several days or in the presence of hepatic dysfunction. Treatment includes administration of sodium bicarbonate to correct metabolic acidosis and sodium thiosulfate (12.5 g in 50 ml 5% dextrose in water over 10 minutes) to convert the cyanide to thiocyanate for excretion by the kidneys. Thiocyanate toxicity is manifest by dyspnea, vomiting, and mental status changes and may develop in patients with impaired renal function. Treatment includes amyl nitrate (inhalation of 1 amp over 15 seconds), infusion of sodium nitrate (5 mg/kg IV push), and sodium thiosulfate (as above).[39]

Nitroglycerin

Nitroglycerin (NTG) can be used postoperatively as a topical ointment or IV infusion. NTG is particularly useful in the setting of hypertension with myocardial ischemia and high filling pressures, because its effects are most predominant on the venous side of the circulation. The starting dose of 0.1 mcg/kg/min (mix of 50 mg in 250 ml) should be administered through non-PVC (polyvinyl chloride) tubing, because as much as 80% of the drug is absorbed by PVC. Methemoglobinemia is rare, but should be suspected in patients who exhibit a low oxygen saturation with an elevated p_aO_2 and "chocolate-brown" blood despite adequate cardiac output. The patient suffering from methe-

moglobinemia appears cyanotic and exhibits progressive weakness and acidosis. Methemoglobin levels can be determined by most clinical laboratories; when the value exceeds 15% to 20% of total hemoglobin, treatment with 1 mg/kg of a 1% solution of methylene blue is appropriate.[39]

Nicardipine

Nicardipine is a titratable IV calcium channel blocker, effective in treating postoperative hypertension in cardiac and noncardiac surgical patients.[40] Nicardipine decreases mean arterial pressure and systemic vascular resistance, and increases cardiac index without increasing heart rate. The drug is a potent coronary vasodilator and causes less inotropic depression than verapamil. Nicardipine is more advantageous than SNP because it causes less venodilation, less reflex tachycardia, and less potential for coronary steal. The drug has a rapid onset of action (1 to 2 minutes) similar to SNP, but has a longer half-life (40 minutes). One potential disadvantage is its ability to worsen hypoxemia by increasing ventilation-perfusion mismatch.[39]

Esmolol

Esmolol is a cardioselective, short-acting β-blocker that is useful in treating hyperdynamic tachycardia during the postoperative period in patients with normal left ventricular function or left ventricular hypertrophy. Esmolol is ideal for treating transient hypertension because of its short duration of action. IV β-blockers should *not* be used in the hypertensive patient with depressed cardiac output.[39]

Labetalol

Labetalol, a combined α-adrenergic and β-adrenergic blocking agent, is a very useful and effective treatment of postoperative hypertension. It is usually administered in small, incremental doses to avoid any untoward side effects, such as hypotension, significant bradycardia, bronchospasm, or ECG changes.[41] It should be used with caution in patients with asthma, recent MI or CHF.

Labetalol has α-adrenoceptor and β-adrenoceptor blocking activity of 1:3 with oral and 1:7 with IV administration. It is devoid of intrinsic sympathomimetic activity at $β_1$-receptors, but may possess intrinsic agonist activity at $β_2$-adrenoceptors. Because the approximate duration of action is 6 hours, labetalol is useful when a longer-acting antihypertensive therapy is required.

Prostaglandin E₁

Prostaglandin E_1 (PGE_1) is a potent direct systemic and pulmonary vasodilator that is useful in treating refractory right heart failure caused by pulmonary hypertension. The medication must be infused into the central venous circulation to minimize systemic hypotension.[39]

Enalaprilat (Vasotec)

Enalaprilat is an ACE inhibitor that may be considered for treatment of postoperative hypertension. Blood pressure reduction is with balanced arterial and venous vasodilation without increasing heart rate. The mechanism of action is inhibition of the conversion of angiotensin I to the vasoconstrictor substance angiotensin II and by decreasing aldosterone secretion. This drug is a good choice when prolonged antihypertensive therapy is required in patients with depressed ventricular function, CHF, or elevated SVR. A dose of 1.25 mg is administered over 5 minutes every 6 hours for patients with a creatinine clearance greater than 30 ml/min. Systemic postural hypotension is uncommon, although it may occur in volume-depleted patients. The onset of action is within 15 minutes, and the maximal effect occurs within 1 to 4 hours. Enalaprilat does not produce hypoxic pulmonary vasoconstriction and therefore has no effect on gas exchange and oxygen delivery.[39]

Hydralazine

Hydralazine is a direct arteriolar dilator that reduces BP but is usually accompanied by compensatory tachycardia. The drug is typically used during the transition from a potent short-acting IV antihypertensive medication for persistent hypertension several days after surgery. The usual dosage is 20 to 40 mg IM every 4 hours or 5 mg IV every 15 minutes until the desired effect is obtained. The drug is difficult to titrate and takes 20 minutes for complete onset, and therefore requires cautious use in the immediate postoperative period.[39]

Fenoldopam

Fenoldopam is a rapidly acting vasodilator that activates D_1 (dopamine) receptors, resulting in peripheral arterial, coronary, mesenteric, and renal vasodilatation. In contrast to dopamine, which activates both D_1 and D_2 receptors and consequently has counteracting effects at the efferent and afferent renal arterioles, fenoldopam markedly increases renal blood flow and has been studied as a renal protective agent. Although mannitol, dopamine, and loop diuretics are commonly used to preserve renal function during cross-clamping of the aorta, double-blind, placebo-controlled studies that demonstrate outcome differences are lacking. Fenoldopam may have a role in this capacity. This agent is useful for the hypertensive patient with severe chronic renal insufficiency for lowering BP and improving renal blood flow and urine output. Fenoldopam is associated with reflex tachycardia and may cause hypokalemia. The drug is administered as a continuous infusion starting at 0.05 to 0.1 mcg/kg/min in a 10 mg/250 ml mix. The dose is increased every 15 minutes in 0.05 to 0.1 mcg/kg/min increments to a maximal rate of 0.3 mcg/kg/min. An infusion of 0.03 mcg/kg/min may improve renal perfusion without causing any hemodynamic effects.[39]

Milrinone

Milrinone is an inotropic vasodilator that selectively inhibits cyclic adenosine monophosphate phosphodiesterase isozyme in cardiac and vascular muscle. Milrinone increases myocardial contractility, improves cardiac index, lowers left ventricular end-diastolic pressure (pulmonary capillary wedge pressure) and SVR, and improves diastolic dysfunction. The typical loading dose of 50 mcg/kg is usually followed by a continuous infusion of 0.25 to 0.75 mcg/kg/min. Milrinone increases ventricular ectopy and increases heart rate in patients with chronic atrial fibrillation. Milrinone is contraindicated in patients with stenotic valvular lesions and hypertrophic obstructive cardiomyopathy.[30]

Sublingual Nifedipine Inappropriate

Sublingual nifedipine is a popular choice for the treatment of hypertensive emergencies. However, serious adverse events with sublingual or oral nifedipine have been reported. Rapid and precipitous lowering of blood pressure combined with peripheral vasodilation produce a steal phenomenon in certain vascular beds, leading to reflex cardioacceleration and excessive catecholamine release. Elderly patients are particularly vulnerable because of vascular disease and target organ impairment.[42] Acute myocardial ischemia and infarction are not uncommon sequelae of this treatment, especially in patients with coronary artery disease or left ventricular hypertrophy.[43] In 1985, the Cardiorenal Advisory Committee of the Food and Drug Administration (FDA) thoroughly reviewed the literature and concluded unanimously that this practice should be abandoned because it was neither safe nor efficacious. Unfortunately, the practicing physician often remains uninformed about FDA decisions and the use of sublingual or oral nifedipine to treat hypertensive emergencies has continued. It is the authors' opinion that sublingual and oral nifedipine should not be used in the postoperative (or emergency) setting for treatment of hypertension, especially because there are better alternatives.

Hypothermia

Hypothermia, which is increasingly recognized as a threat to patients with significant ischemic cardiovascular disease, has detrimental effects on several organ systems. Hypothermia is associated with increased wound infections because of depressed immune function and impaired blood flow and oxygen delivery to the skin. In a study of 200 patients undergoing colorectal surgery, Kutz and others concluded that hypothermia not only increases the incidence of wound infections, but also increases length of hospitalization by an average of 2.6 days.[44] Increased blood loss and transfusion requirements secondary to reduced platelet function and reduced activation of the coagulation cascade are also associated with hypothermia.[45] Coagulopathy, defined as "continuous oozing from small vessels in areolar and fatty tissue that is refractory to stick ties, cautery or packing, the reappearance of bleeding from tissues where hemostasis had been previously achieved, and/or oozing of blood from arterial or venous puncture sites and nasal or oral mucosa," was associated with severe hypothermia in massively transfused trauma patients, and served to differentiate nonsurvivors from survivors.[46] Increased SVR from intense vasoconstriction of the largest organ of the body, the skin, may potentiate myocardial ischemia. In addition, shivering upon emergence from general or regional anesthesia is associated with increased oxygen consumption, especially in elderly patients.[47]

The body contains multiple cold and warmth receptors that transmit sensory information to the posterior hypothalamus to regulate body temperature. Cold receptors are much more prevalent than warmth receptors and are located in the skin, the spinal cord, the abdominal viscera, and in and around the great veins. When the body becomes hypothermic, stimulation of posterior hypothalamic sympathetic centers causes vasoconstriction in the skin and an increase in heat production by shivering, sympathetic "chemical" excitation of heat production, and thyroxine release. Whereas thyroxin takes weeks to increase the rate of cellular metabolism, epinephrine and norepinephrine uncouple cellular oxidative phosphorylation for immediate chemical thermogenesis. General anesthesia lowers the thermoregulatory threshold, rendering the surgical patient poikilothermic (core temperature dependent on ambient temperature) before moderate hypothermia triggers heat-conserving responses. Hypothermia during regional anesthesia occurs by several mechanisms. Afferent neuronal input to the hypothalamus from the anesthetized region is blocked. Shivering is limited to the unanesthetized regions of the body. Heat is redistributed from the core to the periphery and finally to the environment.

A randomized clinical trial comparing normothermic and hypothermic postoperative patients demonstrated more frequent morbid cardiac events (cardiac arrest, unstable angina/ischemia, or MI) in the hypothermic group. There was also a higher incidence of postoperative ventricular tachycardia by Holter monitor in the hypothermic group. The authors concluded that "maintenance of normothermia is associated with a reduction of perioperative morbid events" and "a certain proportion of early postoperative cardiac complications can be prevented by maintaining normothermia."[48]

The most effective strategy for decreasing the incidence of postoperative hypothermia is prevention. No single intraoperative modality is sufficient to prevent postoperative hypothermia. Forced-air convection heating devices are the most effective active warming systems. Mattresses filled with warm water are generally impractical because they are more effective when placed on top rather than underneath the patient. Increasing the OR ambient temperature at the beginning and the end of surgery minimizes patient heat loss during times of maximal skin exposure, and is generally tolerated by the surgical team. Warm prep and irrigating solutions, radiant heaters and passive or active airway heating systems, and active heating of IV fluid and blood products should all be considered. Postoperatively, every attempt must be made to return the hypothermic patient to normothermia as quickly as possible using every appropriate modality.

Some of the worst cases of inadvertent hypothermia in patients with cardiac disease occur in "routine" cases that involve continuous irrigation, such as transurethral prostate or bladder surgery. Irrigation of the bladder with many liters of solution at room temperature can easily cause profound hypothermia, which leads to coagulopathy. The practitioner caring for the elderly patient with heart disease should anticipate the unexpected and maintain core body temperature. It is much easier to maintain proper body temperature than to restore a hypothermic patient to normothermia in the PACU.[22]

KEY POINTS

1. Thoughtful patient management is as important in the postoperative phase as in the preoperative and intraoperative phases of surgical treatment.

2. A decision regarding the most appropriate environment for postoperative care of the cardiac patient depends on a host of patient factors and on individual institutional capabilities.

3. The clinician must plan and carry out monitoring for transport of the postoperative cardiac patient that will ensure hemodynamic stability and allow ongoing therapy during transport.

4. Meticulous planning for transport and appropriate communication with the destination unit will avoid lapses in ongoing care.

5. Early recognition and treatment of myocardial ischemia will afford maximal opportunity for minimizing morbidity and mortality.

6. The occurrence of MI in the perioperative period is an ominous event that must be managed aggressively for the best possible outcome.

7. Congestive heart failure in the perioperative period is an independent predictor of adverse outcome and mortality; the clinician should spare no effort in early diagnosis and aggressive treatment.

8. Arrhythmias are common in the postoperative patient with cardiac disease and may indicate ischemic changes, congestive heart failure, or metabolic abnormalities that need to be addressed before or concurrent with antiarrhythmic therapy.

9. Perioperative hypertension may lead to serious morbidity in the patient with cardiac disease; the clinician should quickly rule out or treat physical factors such as pain or bladder distention before initiating specific antihypertensive therapy.

10. Sublingual nifedipine is not indicated in the management of perioperative hypertension.

11. Hypothermia may lead to a host of negative physiologic and pharmacologic effects. Prevention is the key to management, and aggressive treatment is indicated for hypothermia that occurs despite the clinician's best efforts.

KEY REFERENCES

American Heart Association: 1997-99 Emergency cardiovascular care programs. In *Advanced cardiac life support.* Dallas, 1999, American Heart Association.

Browner WS, Li J, Mangano DT: In-hospital and long-term mortality in male veterans following noncardiac surgery, *JAMA* 268:228-32, 1992.

Fleisher LA, Eagle KA, Shaffer T et al: Preoperative and long-term mortality rates after major vascular surgery: the relationship to preoperative testing in the medicare population, *Anesth Analg* 89:849-855, 1999.

Frank SM, Fleisher LA, Breslow MJ et al: Perioperative maintenance of normothermia reduces the incidence of morbid cardiac events, *JAMA* 277:1127-1134, 1997.

Goldman L: Cardiac risk in noncardiac surgery: an update, *Anesth Analg* 80:810-820, 1995.

Guidelines Committee of the American College of Critical Care Medicine; Society of Critical Care Medicine and American Association of Critical-Care Nurses Transfer Guidelines Task Force: Guidelines for the transfer of critically ill patients, *Crit Care Med* 21:931-937, 1993.

Hines R, Barash PG, Watrous G et al: Complications occurring in the postanesthesia care unit: a survey, *Anesth Analg* 74:503-509, 1992.

Val PG, Pelletier LC, Hernandez MG et al: Diagnostic criteria and prognosis of perioperative myocardial infarction following coronary bypass, *J Thorac Cardiovasc Surg* 86:878-886, 1983.

References

1. Fleisher LA, Eagle KA, Shaffer T et al: Preoperative and long-term mortality rates after major vascular surgery: the relationship to preoperative testing in the medicare population, *Anesth Analg* 89:849-855, 1999.

2. Roberts SL, Tinker JH: Perioperative myocardial infarction. In Gravenstein N, Kirby RR, editors: *Complications in anesthesiology,* ed 2, Philadelphia, 1996, Lippincott-Raven.

3. Mantha S, Roizen MF, Barnard J et al: Relative effectiveness of four preoperative tests for predicting adverse cardiac outcomes after vascular surgery: a meta-analysis, *Anesth Analg* 79:422-433, 1994.

4. Browner WS, Li J, Mangano DT: In-hospital and long-term mortality in male veterans following noncardiac surgery, *JAMA* 268: 228-232, 1992.

5. Hertzer NR, Beven EG, Young JR et al: Coronary artery disease in peripheral vascular patients: a classification of 1000 coronary angiograms and results of surgical management, *Ann Surg* 199: 223-233, 1984.

6. Loeb HS, Saudye A, Croke RP et al: Effects of pharmacologically-induced hypertension on myocardial ischemia and coronary hemodynamics in patients with fixed coronary obstruction, *Circulation* 57:41-46, 1978.

7. McCann RL, Clements FM: Silent myocardial ischemia in patients undergoing peripheral vascular surgery: incidence and association with perioperative cardiac morbidity and mortality, *J Vasc Surg* 9:583-587, 1989.

8. Pasternack PF, Grossi EA, Baumann FG et al: The value of silent myocardial ischemia monitoring in the prediction of perioperative myocardial infarction in patients undergoing peripheral vascular surgery, *J Vasc Surg* 1989;10:617-625, 1992.

9. Guidelines Committee of the American College of Critical Care Medicine; Society of Critical Care Medicine and American Association of Critical-Care Nurses Transfer Guidelines Task Force: Guidelines for the transfer of critically ill patients, *Crit Care Med* 21:931-937, 1993.

10. Braman SS, Dunn SM, Amico CA et al: Complications of intra-hospital transport in critically ill patients, *Ann Intern Med* 107: 469-473, 1987.

11. Breslow MJ, Miller CF, Parker SD et al: Changes in T-wave morphology following anesthesia and surgery: a common recovery-room phenomenon, *Anesthesiology* 64:398-402, 1986.

12. London MJ, Hollenberg M, Wong MG et al: Intraoperative myocardial ischemia: localization by continuous 12-lead electrocardiography, *Anesthesiology* 69:232-241, 1988.

13. Love MJ: Cardiovascular diagnostic procedures. In Thelan LA, Lough ME, Urden LD, Stacy KM, editors: *Critical care nursing*, ed 3, St Louis, 1998, Mosby.

14. Charlson ME, MacKenzie CR, Ales KL et al: The post-operative electrocardiogram and creatine kinase: implications for diagnosis of myocardial infarction after non-cardiac surgery, *J Clin Epidemiol* 42:25-34, 1989.

15. Adams JE, Sigard GA, Allen BT: Diagnosis of perioperative myocardial infarction with measurement of cardiac troponin I, *N Engl J Med* 330:670-674, 1994.

16. Lee TH, Thomas EJ, Ludwig LE. Troponin T as a marker for myocardial ischemia in patients undergoing major non-cardiac surgery, *Am J Cardiol* 77:1031-1036, 1996.

17. Metzler H, Gries M, Rehak P et al: Perioperative myocardial cell injury: the role of troponins, *Br J Anaesth* 78:386-390, 1997.

18. Sametz W, Metzler H, Gries M et al: Perioperative catecholamine changes in cardiac risk patients, *Eur J Clin Invest* 29:582-587, 1999.

19. Val PG, Pelletier LC, Hernandez MG et al: Diagnostic criteria and prognosis of perioperative myocardial infarction following coronary bypass, *J Thorac Cardiovasc Surg* 86:878-886, 1983.

20. Becker RC, Underwood DA: Myocardial infarction in patients undergoing noncardiac surgery, *Cleve Clin J Med* 54:25-28, 1987.

21. Rao TLK, Jacobs KH, El-Etr AA: Reinfarction following anesthesia in patients with myocardial infarction, *Anesthesiology* 59:499-505, 1983.

22. Hines R, Barash PG, Watrous G et al: Complications occurring in the postanesthesia care unit: a survey, *Anesth Analg* 74:503-509, 1992.

23. Baer S, Nakhjavan F, Kajani M: Postoperative myocardial infarction, *Surgery, Gynecology and Obstetrics* 120:315-322, 1965.

24. Report of the American College of Cardiology/American Heart Association Task Force on Practice Guidelines (Committee on Perioperative Cardiovascular Evaluation for Noncardiac Surgery): Executive summary of the ACC/AHA Task Force Report: guidelines for perioperative cardiovascular evaluation for noncardiac surgery, *Anesth Analg* 82:854-860, 1996.

25. Antman EM, Lau J, Kupelnick B et al: A comparison of results of meta-analyses of randomized control trials and recommendations of clinical experts, *JAMA* 268:240-248, 1992.

26. Smith SC. ACE inhibitor therapy: benefits and underuse, *Am Fam Physician* 59:35-38, 1999.

27. Spargias KS, Hall AS, Ball SG: Safety concerns about digoxin after acute myocardial infarction, *Lancet* 354:391-393, 1999.

28. Rutherford JD, Braunwald E: Thrombolytic therapy in acute myocardial infarction, *Chest* 97:136S-145S, 1990.

29. White HD: Future of reperfusion therapy for acute myocardial infarction, *Lancet* 354:695-698, 1999.

30. Christenson JT, Simonet F, Badel P et al: Evaluation of preoperative intra-aortic balloon pump support in high risk coronary patients, *Eur J Cardiothorac Surg* 11:1097-1103, 1997.

31. Lake CL: Chronic treatment of congestive heart failure. In Kaplan JA, Reich OL, Konstadt SN: *Cardiac anesthesia*, ed 4, Philadelphia, 1999, WB Saunders.

32. Goldman L: Cardiac risk in noncardiac surgery: an update, *Anesth Analg* 80:810-820, 1995.

33. Massie BM, Mangano DT: Risk stratification for noncardiac surgery: how (and why)? *Circulation* 87:1752-1755, 1993.

34. Charlson ME, MacKenzie CR, Gold JP et al: Risk for postoperative congestive heart failure, *Surg Gynec Obstet* 172:95-104, 1991.

35. O'Kelly B, Browner WS, Massie B et al: Ventricular arrhythmias in patients undergoing noncardiac surgery, *JAMA* 268:217-221, 1998.

36. Polanczyk CA, Goldman L, Marcantonio ER et al: Supraventricular arrhythmia in patients having noncardiac surgery: clinical correlates and effect on length of stay, *Ann Intern Med* 129:279-285, 1998.

37. Gothard JWW, Kelleher A: Postoperative management. In Gothard JWW, Kelleher A, editors, *Essentials of cardiac and thoracic anaesthesia*, Boston, 1999, Butterworth Heinemann.

38. American Heart Association: 1997-99 Emergency cardiovascular care programs. In *Advanced cardiac life support*. Dallas, 1999, American Heart Association.

39. Bojar RM: *Manual of perioperative care in cardiac surgery*, ed 3, Chicago, 1999, Blackwell Science, pp 264-274.

40. Goldberg ME, Halpern N, Krakoff L et al: Efficacy and safety of intravenous nicardipine in the control of postoperative hypertension, *Chest* 99:393-398, 1991.

41. Leslie JB, Kalayjian RW, Sirgo MA et al: Intravenous labetalol for treatment of postoperative hypertension, *Anesthesiology* 67: 413-416, 1987.

42. Grossman E, Messerli FH, Grodzicki T et al: Should a moratorium be placed on sublingual nifedipine capsules given for hypertensive emergencies and pseudoemergencies? *JAMA* 276: 1328-1331, 1996.

43. O'Mailia JJ, Sander GE, Giles TD: Nifedipine-associated myocardial ischemia or infarction in the treatment of hypertensive urgencies, *Ann Intern Med* 107:185-186, 1987.

44. Kurz A, Sessler DI, Lenhardt R et al: Perioperative normothermia to reduce the incidence of surgical-wound infection and shorten hospitalization, *N Engl J Med* 334:1209-1215, 1996.

45. Schmied H, Kurz A, Sessler DI et al: Mild hypothermia increases blood loss and transfusion requirements during total hip arthroplasty, *Lancet* 47:289-292, 1996.

46. Ferrara A, MacArthur JD, Wright HK et al: Hypothermia and acidosis worsen coagulopathy in the patient requiring massive transfusion, *Am J Surg* 160:515-518, 1990.

47. Frank SM, Fleisher LA, Olson KF et al: Multivariate determinants of early postoperative oxygen consumption in elderly patients, *Anesthesiology* 83:241-249, 1995.

48. Frank SM, Fleisher LA, Breslow MJ et al: Perioperative maintenance of normothermia reduces the incidence of morbid cardiac events, *JAMA* 277:1127-1134, 1997.

CHAPTER 6

Pain Management in the Cardiac Patient: Benefits Beyond Analgesia

Lorin Graef, MD ■ Peter S. Staats, MD

THE NATURE OF PAIN

Building from an accepted definition of pain as a negative emotional experience, the Psychological Behaviorism Theory of Pain recognizes the complexity of the pain experience. The theory delineates seven interrelated aspects of the nature of pain; these aspects are unified by an understanding that an individual's emotional state can modify pain and, in turn, be affected by pain.[1] Thus this theory considers not only the biologic underpinning of the pain experience but also the impact of conditioning, behavior, cognition (e.g., thinking, attention, worry), emotion, personality, and social environment on pain. This unifying approach to pain highlights the importance of following a multidisciplinary approach in our attempt to manage the multidimensional phenomenon we call "pain." Considering pain through this framework also helps us understand that the experience of pain not only signals but also can exacerbate disease. As in the following detailed sections, this adverse impact of pain is particularly important in the cardiac patient.

Despite our heightened awareness of the moral and physiologic imperatives for treating pain, its management in the cardiac patient, especially in the immediate postoperative period, remains inadequate. A recent study, for example, revealed that a significant portion of postoperative cardiac patients could readily provide detailed accounts of the pain they experienced in the intensive care unit.[2] Cardiac pain cannot be viewed simply in terms of the subjective discomfort perceived by the patient; instead, it should be seen as a factor that can seriously compromise a patient's subsequent health and survival. Indeed, surgical stress in conjunction with pain may be responsible for sudden cardiac death in the postoperative period.[3] A consideration of postoperative pain is thus extremely relevant to the cardiac surgery patient.

PERTINENT TYPES OF PAIN

The physician caring for cardiac patients needs to be aware of the different types of pain, including somatic pain, which is mediated by muscles and bones; neuropathic pain, which is nerve related; and visceral pain, which originates in visceral structures. Although the treatment for these syndromes may be similar, each type of pain may also respond to different interventions.

Visceral Pain

Visceral pain (of which cardiac pain is a subset) is often associated with hyperalgesia of overlying tissues and tends to be dull in quality and difficult for patients to localize. This latter feature likely is caused by the convergence of visceral afferents and somatic afferents in similar locations in the spinal cord. Severe visceral pain is often accompanied by nausea, vomiting, sweating, hypotension, and bradycardia.

Visceral pain is sometimes inaccurately considered a variant of somatic pain or confused with neuropathic pain. The fact that visceral pain is "referred pain," radiating away from affected organs, also makes it difficult to diagnose.

Cardiac Pain

The thoracic sympathetic nervous system plays a significant role in the case of cardiac pain, particularly angina.[4] This should come as no surprise, because it has been known for some time that vasoconstriction of cardiac vessels with resultant ischemia produces pain that can be relieved with vasodilators.

The sympathetic nervous system not only modulates blood vessel caliber but also mediates myocardial oxygen supply and demand by affecting hemodynamics. In the normal (healthy) heart, the sympathetic system matches coronary blood flow and myocardial oxygen demand. Such matching may not be possible in the presence of coronary artery disease. A mismatch of supply and demand causes ischemia and arrhythmias.[5] Ischemia provokes a further cardiac sympathetic reflex that increases catecholamine levels and cardiac sympathetic neural discharge.[6] This could lead to complications by several mechanisms (Fig. 6-1).

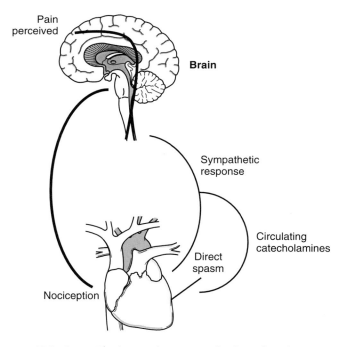

FIG. 6-1 The interactive nature of pain and angina.

In addition to the aforementioned vasoconstriction of vessels by sympathetic stimulation, blood flow may be redistributed away from the endocardium to the epicardium with resulting decreases in coronary blood flow and diastolic perfusion pressure. Neurally decentralized animals given stellate ganglion stimulation develop increased infarct size.[7] Cardiac ischemia may also elicit a vagal response, in addition to the sympathetic reflex. A particularly troublesome consequence of this is the Bezold-Jarisch reflex, which consists of atrioventricular block, prominent bradycardia, peripheral vasodilation, and resultant hypotension. Finally, sympathetic activation may produce a postoperative hypercoagulable state, thereby increasing the likelihood of coronary thrombosis.[8] Strategies to mediate cardiac pain and improve patient outcome are predicated upon improving the myocardial oxygen supply/demand ratio.

Postoperative Pain

The inevitable damage and disruption of tissue during surgery create an inflammatory response. In the peripheral nervous system, activation of high-threshold nociceptors by tissue injury causes the release of several chemicals and mediators, including the prostaglandins, histamine, neuropeptides, cytokines, and leukotrienes that are capable of lowering the threshold of nociceptor activation. Even previously nonnoxious stimuli can elicit pain in this setting.[9] Alterations to the spinal cord may sensitize the central nervous system, causing chronic pain that outlasts the duration of an initiating nociceptive stimulus, such as tissue injury. Postoperative pain management, thus, seeks not only to alleviate pain in the immediate setting, but to prevent a cascade of subsequent adverse events that could lead to chronic pain.[3] Our expanding knowledge about the pathophysiology of pain in the peripheral and central nervous systems has led to a corresponding expansion of analgesic choices and techniques for the delivery of analgesia to appropriate sites in the nervous system to improve postoperative pain control.

PAIN CONTROL METHODS

Many cognitive pain control strategies, such as relaxation techniques, biofeedback, distraction techniques, guided imagery, semantic therapy, and physical rehabilitation, may prove beneficial to postoperative cardiac patients, but a discussion of these is beyond the scope of this chapter. We also will not discuss therapies for neuropathic pain beyond mentioning that these include transcutaneous electrical nerve stimulation (TENS units), oral medications (anticonvulsants, tricyclic antidepressants, opioids, and nonsteroidal anti-inflammatory agents), and topical agents such as the lidocaine patch and capsaicin. Tricyclic antidepressants and anticonvulsants should be used with caution in cardiac surgery patients because these agents can alter hemodynamics.

Preemptive Analgesia

The initiation of analgesics before surgery (preemptive analgesia) is a method of preventing or reducing postoperative pain by impeding the development of central sensitization from the peripheral nociceptor input that arises from operative tissue damage. Without preemptive analgesia, cutting afferent nerve fibers (even without a prior noxious stimulus), may produce long-term facilitation in spinal cord cells that persists even in the absence of input from the transected nerve.[10] Bathing peripheral nerves in a local anesthetic before transsection reduces pain behavior in rats for weeks after neuronectomies.[11]

Despite convincing animal data, the value of using preemptive analgesia in humans remains controversial.[9] Katz and associates compared the administration of pre-incision to postincision epidural opioids in 30 thoracotomy patients. The group treated with preemptive analgesia had significantly reduced visual analogue-scale pain scores 6 hours postoperatively and reduced postoperative morphine requirements.[12] In a study of 40 patients undergoing coronary artery bypass grafting, preemptive treatment with an epidural infusion of local anesthetics, plus ketamine and morphine during surgery, improved postoperative pain relief and the stability of cardiovascular and respiratory functions.[9]

Acute Pain Management

Postoperative pain can be managed by a variety of medications and delivery techniques. Medications include nonsteroidal antiinflammatory drugs (NSAIDs), opioids, and other agents, alone and in combination. Modes of delivery include intramuscular, rectal, intravenous, epidural, and intrathecal routes.

Medications

Nonsteroidal Antiinflammatory Drugs. NSAIDs inhibit the synthesis of prostaglandins by affecting cyclooxygenase and produce analgesic, antiinflammatory, and antipyretic effects. Although many believe that NSAIDs exert their effects peripherally, the reversal of intravenous indomethacin analgesia by intraventricular phentolamine (but not by naloxone) suggests a central mechanism of action as well.[13] NSAIDs may prevent increased concentration of prostaglandins in cerebrospinal fluid (CSF) after N-methyl-D-aspartate receptor activation.[14] Their mild degree of analgesic efficacy has limited the monotherapeutic use of NSAIDs in the acute pain setting. The combination of NSAIDs with opioids decreases the requirement for systemic opioids and thereby decreases opiate-related side effects.[15] Administration of rectal indomethacin in conjunction with morphine after cardiac surgery reduces pain scores and opioid use without increasing side effects.[16] Although NSAIDs are most commonly administered through oral or rectal routes; the advent of ketorolac has allowed intravenous delivery. The previous lack of a parenteral NSAID had also limited the use of this class of drugs in the acute pain setting.

The most common adverse effect of NSAIDs is gastrointestinal (GI) bleeding. This risk is particularly relevant for the elderly, in whom gastrointestinal bleeding accounts for 8,000 to 10,000 deaths annually. The traditional NSAIDs were nonselective in decreasing the production of constitutive prostaglandins (COX 1), which protect the GI mucosa, and inducible prostaglandins (COX 2), which are involved in pain. Newer formulations (celecoxib and rofecoxib) have a reduced risk of gastrointestinal bleeding because they selectively block the production of the COX 2 enzyme.

NSAID use in cardiac surgical patients is limited because of the possible adverse effects on renal function and coagulation. A recent study, however, showed that patients treated with diclofenac exhibited no effect on the postoperative rise in creatinine level and, for unclear reasons, required less morphine than those treated with ketoprofen or indomethacin.[17] Despite the general consensus that NSAIDs prolong bleeding time, there are conflicts in the literature regarding the effect of NSAIDs on coagulation parameters in the perioperative period. For example, diclofenac administered after transurethral prostatectomy[18] and hip replacement[19] showed no significant effect on blood loss compared with placebo, whereas indomethacin was associated with increased blood loss in the perioperative period after abdominal hysterectomy.[20] In contrast, continuous indomethacin infusion during surgery was not associated with increased blood loss in another study.[21] It is not yet clear whether the increased bleeding in the ketorolac studies was related to doses that exceed recently revised dosing standards.[22]

Tramadol. Long available in Europe, tramadol is another agent that has been used in the treatment of postoperative pain. This agent has weak opioid agonist properties that appear to have synergistic effects on serotonergic and noradrenergic neurotransmitter systems. Tramadol is more effective than NSAIDs in controlling postoperative pain and can be administered in reduced doses when combined with NSAIDs. Tramadol can also be administered concomitantly with opioid patient-controlled analgesia (see Delivery Methods). When administered intravenously as a single agent, its effects on postoperative pain are similar to those achieved by morphine or clonidine. The most common side effects of tramadol are nausea and vomiting. There is a low incidence of cardiac depression with this drug.

Nurse-administered analgesia

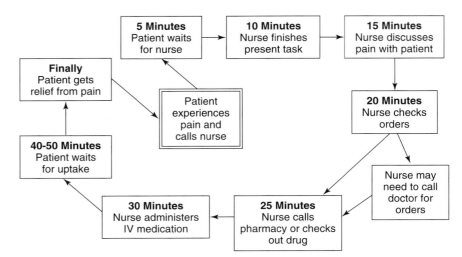

FIG. 6-2 The traditional route from the experience of pain to pain relief for nurse-administered versus patient-controlled analgesia.

Patient-controlled analgesia

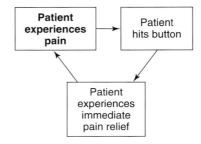

The low abuse potential of tramadol makes it a reasonable choice for long-term therapy.[23]

Opioids. The use of opioids for analgesia is expanding because of new drugs and new modes of delivery. In a study comparing sufentanil, a newer opioid, with intravenous morphine, myocardial ischemia during the first 24 hours after coronary artery bypass grafting was less intense in patients randomized to receive sufentanil. The doses used in this particular study required the patients to receive prolonged mechanical ventilation.[24] Intramuscular injection of opioids, although widely available and requiring a minimum level of expertise, is hindered by lack of patient control and satisfaction and by unpredictable levels of analgesia and pharmacokinetics.[25]

Potent opioid agonists are the mainstay of postoperative pain management. The preferred route of administration is patient-controlled intravenous delivery, which not only gives active control to the patient, but also minimizes dose-associated peaks and troughs. Physicians often underprescribe and nurses underadminister opioids resulting from a concern about side effects or addiction. It is important to note that opioid side effects

are easily controlled and addiction rarely, if ever, occurs in the perioperative setting. Opioids should be used liberally in the critical care setting.

Delivery Methods

Patient-Controlled Analgesia. Patient-controlled analgesia (PCA) allows a patient to operate a microprocessor-controlled infusion pump and self-administer an intravenous, preprogrammed dose of a narcotic. The computerized pump system controls the basal infusion rate and the maximum amount of drug delivered over a given period. Dosing adjustment is facilitated and the timing of administration is recorded by the number of doses and amount of medication consumed.[26] Many different opioids have been used effectively with PCA pumps. Drug choice is based on the desired onset of action, duration of action, and potency.

The lag time between patient need and the delivery of analgesia (e.g., nurse response time, preparation of medication) is eliminated with the PCA system (Fig. 6-2). Side effects arising from the relative overdose associated with the traditional bolus dosing of narcotics are also reduced.[27] The sedation caused by increasing plasma opioid levels renders a patient unable to activate the demand button and prevents further opiate dosing that may cause respiratory compromise.[26] PCA attains a narrower range of plasma drug levels compared with intramuscular bolus dosing. PCA may not be possible in the first few hours postoperatively when patients remain semisedated. Patients can receive unnecessary doses of drugs if well-intentioned family members take it upon themselves to operate the pump, and may receive inappropriately small amounts of a drug if the dosage is not set correctly.

PCA is associated with earlier ambulation, recovery of pulmonary function, toleration of enteral feedings, and hospital discharge compared with intramuscular opioid administration. In a study comparing PCA with a standard (nurse-based) analgesic regimen in 60 postoperative cardiac surgery patients, the postoperative pain score was significantly lower in the PCA group, whereas vital capacity and 1-second forced expiratory volume were significantly lower in the standard group. Because the incidence of side effects was similar in both groups, the investigators concluded that pain management via PCA was superior to nurse-delivered analgesia regimens.[28] These benefits and the resulting increase in patient satisfaction and efficacy of pain control has led to the use of PCA in many settings.

The constant administration of a basal dose of medication in addition to the demand dosages remains controversial. The addition of a basal infusion rate does not alter postoperative pain scores, recovery profiles, patients' ability to sleep, opioid use via patient demands, or supplemental bolus dosages.[29] The basal dose may be set too high, providing patients with unnecessary medication and mitigating their ability to control drug administration.

Intrathecal Injection. Intrathecal injection is also used to deliver perioperative opioids. Intrathecal opioids preferentially inhibit C-fiber nociceptive discharge as compared with Aδ-fiber discharge, thus blocking dull, afferent pain (C-fibers) more effectively than sharp pain (Aδ-fibers).[30] The nature of the chosen drug (lipophilicity) determines the onset and duration of analgesia, the number of dermatomes likely to be affected, and the side effects (Table 6-1). Hydrophilic compounds (morphine) tend to remain in the CSF space, affecting many dermatomes before proceeding with a slow penetration of the spinal cord. Delayed respiratory depression occurs if these drugs slowly spread rostrally into the region of the brainstem. Lipophilic compounds (fentanyl) rapidly clear the CSF space and penetrate the spinal cord, leading to a short duration of action and localized dermatomal level of analgesia.[31]

Combination therapy is administered intrathecally to provide rapid onset and sustained duration of action. The addition of fentanyl and bupivacaine to morphine

TABLE 6-1
The Lipophilicity and Starting Dose of Spinal Opioids for Postoperative Pain

OPIOID	LIPID SOLUBILITY	STARTING DOSE (mg)
Morphine	1.42	0.5-1.0
Hydromorphine	11.36	0.2
Meperidene	38.8	2.0
Methadone	116.0	
Fentanyl	813.0	0.025
Sufentanyl	1778.0	0.01

hastens the onset of analgesia to provide adequate pain relief in the early postoperative period. Patients receiving intrathecal fentanyl, bupivacaine, and morphine have lower average pain scores than patients receiving a combination of intrathecal morphine and fentanyl, with the greatest reduction of pain occurring during the initial 30 minutes postoperatively.[32]

Advantages of the intrathecal method include a minimal systemic effect (a very small amount of drug [<1 mg of morphine] is administered), rapid onset, long duration of action after a single injection, and lack of peak and trough dose effects. The intrathecal method is an easier procedural technique than an epidural infusion and is devoid of possible catheter-related complications. Intrathecal opioids do not affect the sympathetic nervous system or alter hemodynamics.[33] The lack of motor blockade facilitates early ambulation. Intrathecal opioid analgesia can also be used in conjunction with PCA or other analgesic regimens. Disadvantages include the possible need for reinjection, respiratory depression (drug and dose dependent), nausea and vomiting, urinary retention, and pruritus.

Thoracic Epidural Analgesia. Thoracic epidural analgesia (TEA) delivers opioids to treat visceral pain and somatic pain after surgery. TEA affects the sympathetic nervous system at the spinal cord level and provides the equivalent of a sympathectomy without surgery or stellate ganglion blockade. In a comparison of dogs treated with TEA (lidocaine) 1 hour after left anterior descending artery occlusion versus controls treated with intramuscular lidocaine, the TEA group had lower heart rates and cardiac index as well as higher systemic vascular resistance and diastolic filling time, with no change in systemic vascular resistance index. The TEA group also had a higher endocardial-to-epicardial regional myocardial blood flow ratio in the ischemic region, unchanged nonischemic coronary vascular resistance, and lower coronary resistance for collateral flow in the ischemic zone. The extent of myocardial infarction and the arrhythmia score were lower in the TEA group.[34] Another study using TEA in animals with severe coronary artery stenosis showed prevention of sympathetic activation and ischemia.[35]

In humans, TEA has been shown to maintain a stable hemodynamic profile with no change in stroke volume index or stroke work index in healthy patients, and no change in mean arterial pressure, diastolic arterial pressure, coronary perfusion pressure, or peripheral vascular resistance index in patients with unstable angina.[36]

TEA causes a profound redistribution of myocardial blood flow to the endocardium, with the greatest increase in the most compromised hearts, and is associated with a 20% to 25% decrease in coronary vascular resistance for collateral flow into the ischemic myocardium.

TEA produces a significant increase in the diameter of stenotic coronary arteries in patients with coronary artery disease. This is most likely caused by the blockade of α-adrenoreceptor–mediated sympathetic vasoconstriction.[37] The antiischemic effect of sympathectomy may be the result of improved coronary perfusion. There is also a potential for an antiarrhythmic effect, because ventricular ectopy is decreased by TEA in dogs.[34] Similar findings have been obtained in humans. Bromage described a patient with severe refractory angina who had a complete resolution angina and of electrocardiographic abnormalities after a C7-T11 epidural injection.[38] In another human study, inoperable patients with unstable angina who had failed medical therapy obtained relief within 10 to 15 minutes; 26 of 28 patients had no need for nitroglycerin within 3 hours.[39]

TEA is a safe method for producing selective sympathectomy with subsequent physiologic changes likely to be beneficial for a patient with myocardial ischemia. TEA has an advantage over intrathecal administration in that the epidural catheter can be strategically placed to provide pain relief at specific spinal levels. Administration of TEA fentanyl to treat postthoracotomy pain provided better analgesia at a lower dosage than a lumbar epidural catheter.[40]

Thoracic placement has additional advantages, particularly in reference to the postoperative cardiac patient. Early ambulation is not hindered because the lower lumbar and sacral segments are spared. TEA produces relatively less sympathetic blockade than epidural analgesia in other regions of the spinal cord, minimizing the degree of hypotension.[41] However, the sympathetic inhibition that occurs via TEA may be very important for managing chronic pain (such as angina). In contrast with intrathecal administration, TEA eliminates the need for dural puncture and the potential for post–dural puncture headache. This catheter-based delivery system allows continuous epidural infusion and PCA

administration. Continuous epidural infusion allows greater flexibility in the choice of opioids, including those that are shorter acting.

The most common adverse events related to TEA include placement risks such as pain associated with the procedure, direct spinal cord injury, hematoma, and infection, as well as hypotension, headache, and local anesthetic toxicity.[42] Numerous studies involving large numbers of patients have reported a low incidence of such events. The disadvantages of TEA as compared with intrathecal delivery include the necessity of administering larger drug doses to maintain adequate levels in CSF and the spinal cord.

Chronic Pain Management

Thus far, we have emphasized the perioperative pain management of the cardiac surgery patient. Pain states often persist beyond the immediate postoperative period and represent challenging problems for physicians, patients, and patients' families. Besides painful conditions resulting from the surgery itself (such as postthoracotomy pain, pain from wound healing, or nerve damage), many cardiac surgery patients (such as those with coronary artery disease) experience chronic angina despite adequate coronary revascularization. Patients with too high a risk for surgery may have to live with severe debilitating coronary artery disease. There are reasonable alternatives for managing ischemic pain in such patients.

Surgical Sympathectomy

Several methods are available for reducing the potentially deleterious effect of sympathetic activity. Stellectomy was first used by Mayo to treat angina as early as 1913. Percutaneous alcohol neurolysis, thorascopic ganglionectomy, and open surgical sympathectomy were beneficial but associated with operative mortality rates of 5% to 10%. These procedures were replaced by the administration of nitrates and by coronary revascularization procedures.[6] There are several lines of evidence indicating the value of sympathectomy. In 88 patients with severe angina treated with open sympathectomy, one third became symptom free, one third improved significantly, and one third remained unchanged.[43] Bilateral stellate ganglion blocks administered to patients before stress testing, eliminated anginal symptoms and decreased ST-segment depression compared with patients given sham injections.[44] Endoscopic thoracic sympathectomy in 24 patients with unstable angina, resulted in a reduced resting heart rate, no alterations in systolic blood pressure, a decreased frequency of angina (10 patients were free of angina), increased exercise tolerance, and lower ST-segment depression at maximal exercise.[45]

Thoracic Epidural Analgesia

TEA is enjoying increasing popularity as an alternative to surgical sympathectomy. Long-term TEA via an indwelling epidural catheter can be provided for home treatment of inoperable patients with unstable angina, but requires proper vigilance. Twenty patients with severe coronary artery disease, refractory unstable angina, and recent myocardial infarction were treated with TEA (bupivacaine) at home via a tunneled high-thoracic epidural catheter for a mean of 6 months. Most reported satisfaction with the treatment and improved quality of life. The injections provided a rapid onset of complete pain relief with no severe adverse events (except for one case of tachyphylaxis). The frequency of epidural injections decreased over time. This study suggested that long-term TEA treatment in some patients might be equivalent to coronary artery bypass procedures.[46]

Spinal Cord Stimulation

Spinal cord stimulation (SCS) is another method of providing excellent analgesia in a variety of pain syndromes. This technology provides an additional way to improve coronary blood flow in patients with chronic angina.[47] The most likely explanation for the efficacy of SCS lies in its effect on the sympathetic nervous system. Similar to TEA, SCS has benefits and actions beyond that of analgesia. SCS improves exercise tolerance in patients with refractory angina, and reduces anginal attacks and electrocardiographic signs of ischemia. The anti-ischemic action of SCS occurs mostly through myocardial blood flow alterations, as demonstrated by a study of regional myocardial blood flow by positron emission tomography at rest and during a dipyridamole stress test. After 6 weeks of stimulation, the frequency of daily anginal attacks decreased from an average of 3.7 to 1.4. Nitroglycerin use also decreased. Exercise duration and time to the development of angina increased, and mean ST-segment depression was reduced.[48] An ambulatory investigation with Holter monitoring also revealed a lower number and duration of ischemic episodes and a decrease in nitroglycerin consumption.[49]

Concern exists regarding the masking of the warning signals of an impending myocardial infarction in patients with angina treated with analgesia. Several studies have shown that patients treated with SCS continued to experience precordial pain during an acute myocardial infarction.[50,51] Augustinsson and others showed that long-term SCS does not mask ischemia at extreme workloads, nor does it create arrhythmias.[52] Even more importantly, a recent series demonstrated that patients with refractory angina treated with SCS had similar mortality to patients who had coronary artery disease and stable angina pectoris.[53]

CONCLUSION

Care of the cardiac patient must integrate pain management as an imperative. This is especially true in the postoperative setting, whether the operation performed was related to coronary care or to an unrelated ailment. The intersection of the stress response and pain is particularly detrimental to the cardiac patient. In addition to causing unnecessary discomfort, pain increases sympathetic nervous system activity, which has deleterious effects on hemodynamics and myocardial blood flow. Subsequent hypotension, ischemia, and infarction are possible outcomes.

In addition, our evolving insight into the pathophysiology of pain has provided a variety of techniques to treat angina in those cardiac patients who do not respond to or cannot risk surgical management. The pain specialist must work with surgical and intensive care providers to select the most appropriate agents and modalities available for postoperative pain control for each patient.

KEY POINTS

1. Pain is a multidimensional phenomenon that requires a multidisciplinary approach for appropriate management.
2. Management of pain in the cardiac patient remains inadequate.
3. Cardiac pain can seriously compromise a patient's subsequent health, quality of life, and survival.
4. Strategies to mediate cardiac pain and improve patient outcome involve improving the myocardial oxygen supply/demand ratio.
5. The ability to use opioids liberally for postoperative analgesia is benefiting from new agents and new modes of delivery. Any associated side effects can readily be controlled, and in the perioperative setting, addiction rarely, if ever, occurs.
6. PCA offers distinct advantages over traditional delivery methods, including better pain control with a more consistent and appropriate administration of medication.
7. Techniques exist to treat angina in patients who are not candidates for surgical intervention.

KEY REFERENCES

Blomberg S, Emanuelsson H, Kvist H et al: Effects of thoracic epidural anesthesia on coronary arteries and arterioles in patients with coronary artery disease, *Anesthesiology* 73(5): 840-847, 1990.

Cousins MJ, Mather LE: Intrathecal and epidural administration of opioids, *Anesthesiology* 61(3):276-310, 1984.

Davis RF, DeBoer LW, Maroko PR: Thoracic epidural anesthesia reduces myocardial infarct size after coronary artery occlusion in dogs, *Anesth Analg* 65(7):711-717, 1986.

Hautvast RW, Blanksma PK, DeJongste MJ et al: Effects of spinal cord stimulation on myocardial blood flow assessed by positron emission tomography in patients with refractory angina pectoris, *Am J Cardiol* 77(7):462-467, 1996.

Katz J, Kavanaugh BP, Sandler AN et al: Preemptive analgesia: clinical evidence of neuroplasticity contributing to postoperative pain, *Anesthesiology* 77:439-446, 1992.

Mangano DT, Siliciano D, Hollenberg M et al: Postoperative myocardial ischemia. Therapeutic trials using intensive analgesia following surgery. The Study of Perioperative Ischemia (SPI) Research Group, *Anesthesiology* 76(3):342-353, 1992.

Staats PS, Panchal SJ: Thoracic epidural anesthesia for treatment of angina. Pro: the anesthesiologist should provide epidural anesthesia in the coronary care unit for patients with severe angina, *J Cardiothorac Vasc Anesth* 11(1):105-108, 1997.

Tuman KJ, McCarthy RJ, March RJ et al: Effects of epidural anesthesia and analgesia on coagulation and outcome after major vascular surgery, *Anesth Analg* 73(6):696-704, 1991.

References

1. Staats PS, Hekmat H, Staats AW. The psychological behaviorism theory of pain: a basis for unity, *Pain Forum* 5:194-207, 1996.
2. Ferguson JA: Pain following coronary artery bypass grafting: an exploration of contributing factors, *Intensive Crit Care Nurs* 8(3):153-162, 1992.
3. Yung MC, Chang Y, Lai ST et al: Improved postoperative pain relief via preemptive analgesia in relation to heart rate variability for coronary artery bypass grafting: a preliminary report, *Chung Hua I Hsueh Tsa Chin* (Taipei) Jul; 60(1):28-35, 1997.
4. Panchal S, Staats PS: Visceral pain: from physiology to clinical practice, *J Back Musculoskeletal Rehab* 9:233-245, 1997.
5. Moore JM, Liu SS: The role of pain relief in postoperative outcome. In Grass JA, editor: *Problems in anesthesia*, vol 10, Hagerstown, Md, 1998, Lippincott-Raven, pp 91-102.
6. Staats PS, Panchal SJ: Thoracic epidural anesthesia for treatment of angina. Pro: the anesthesiologist should provide epidural anesthesia in the coronary care unit for patients with severe angina, *J Cardiothorac Vasc Anesth* 11(1):105-108, 1997.
7. Flatley KA, DeFily DV, Thomas JX Jr: Effects of cardiac sympathetic nerve stimulation during adrenergic blockade on infarct size in anesthetized dogs, *J Cardiovasc Pharmacol* 7(4):673-679, 1985.
8. Tuman KJ, McCarthy RJ, March RJ et al: Effects of epidural anesthesia and analgesia on coagulation and outcome after major vascular surgery, *Anesth Analg* 73(6):696-704, 1991.
9. Mitchell VD, Raja SN: Preemptive analgesia: pathophysiology. In Benzon HT, Raja SN, Borsook D et al, editors: *Essentials of pain medicine and regional anesthesia*, Philadelphia, 1999, Churchill Livingstone, pp 140-141.
10. Wall PD, Woolf CJ: Muscle but not cutaneous C-afferent input produces prolonged increases in the excitability of the flexion reflex in the rat, *J Physiol* 356:443-458, 1984.
11. Gonzalez-Darder JM, Barbera J, Abellan MJ: Effects of prior anesthesia on autotomy following sciatic transaction in rats, *Pain* 24(1):87-91, 1986.
12. Katz J, Kavanaugh BP, Sandler AN et al: Preemptive analgesia: clinical evidence of neuroplasticity contributing to postoperative pain, *Anesthesiology* 77:439-446, 1992.
13. Hu XH, Tang HW, Li QS et al: Central mechanism of indomethacin analgesia, *Eur J Pharmacol* 263(1-2):53-57, 1994.
14. Sorkin LS: IT ketorolac blocks NMDA-evoked spinal release of prostaglandin E2 (PGE2) and thromboxane B2 (TXB2), *Anesthesiology* 79:A909, 1993.
15. Ready LB, Brown CR, Stahlgren LH et al: Evaluation of intravenous ketorolac administered by bolus or infusion for treatment of postoperative pain: a double-blind placebo-controlled multicenter study, *Anesthesiology*, 80(6):1277-1286, 1994.
16. Rapanos T, Murphy P, Szalai JP et al: Rectal indomethacin reduces postoperative pain and morphine use after cardiac surgery, *Can J Anaesth* 46(8):725-730, 1999.
17. Hynninen MS, Cheng DC, Hossain I et al: Nonsteroidal antiinflammatory drugs in treatment of postoperative pain after cardiac surgery, *Can J Anaesth* 47(12):1182-1187, 2000.
18. Bricker SR, Savage ME, Hanning CD: Peri-operative blood loss and nonsteroidal antiinflammatory drugs: an investigation using diclofenac in patients undergoing transurethral resection of the prostate, *Eur J Anaesthesiol* 4(6):429-434, 1987.
19. Lindgren U, Djupsjo H: Diclofenac for pain after hip surgery, *Acta Orthop Scand* 56(1):28-31, 1985.
20. Engel C, Lund B, Kristensen SS et al: Indomethacin as an analgesic after hysterectomy, *Acta Anaesthesiol Scand* 33(6):498-501, 1989.
21. Taivainen T, Hiller A, Rosenberg PH et al: The effect of continuous intravenous indomethacin infusion on bleeding time and postoperative pain in patients undergoing emergency surgery of the lower extremities, *Acta Anaesthesiol Scand* 33(1):58-60, 1989.
22. Choo V, Lewis S: Ketorolac doses reduced, *Lancet* 342(8863):109, 1993.
23. Lehmann KA: Tramadol in acute pain, *Drugs* 53(suppl 2):25-33, 1997.
24. Mangano DT, Siliciano D, Hollenberg M et al: Postoperative myocardial ischemia. Therapeutic trials using intensive analgesia following surgery. The Study of Perioperative Ischemia (SPI) Research Group, *Anesthesiology* 76(3):342-353, 1992.
25. Austin KL, Stapelton JV, Mather LE: Relationship between blood meperidine concentrations and analgesic response; a preliminary report, *Anesthesiology* 53(6):460-466, 1980.
26. Sherwood ER, Benzon HT: Patient-controlled analgesia. In Benzon HT, Raja SN, Borsook D et al, editors: *Essentials of pain medicine and regional anesthesia*, Philadelphia, 1999, Churchill Livingstone, pp 147-149.

27. Tobias MD, Ferrante FM: Intravenous patient-controlled analgesia. In Grass JA, editor: *Problems in anesthesia*, vol 10, Hagerstown, Md, 1998, Lippincott-Raven, pp 37-44.

28. Boldt J, Thaler E, Lehmann A et al: Pain management in cardiac surgery patients: comparison between standard therapy and patient-controlled analgesia regimen, *J Cardiothorac Vasc Anesth* 12(6):654-658, 1998.

29. Parker RK, Holtmann B, White PF: Effects of a nighttime opioid infusion with PCA therapy on patient comfort and analgesic requirements after abdominal hysterectomy, *Anesthesiology* 76(3): 362-367,1992.

30. Rawal N, Sjostrand UH: Clinical application of epidural and intrathecal opioids for pain mangement, *Int Anesthesiol Clin* 24(2):43-57,1986.

31. Cousins MJ, Mather LE: Intrathecal and epidural administration of opioids, *Anesthesiology* 61(3):276-310, 1984.

32. Gwirtz KH, Peneff G: Intrathecal morphine and fentanyl with and without bupivacaine for the control of postoperative pain after major abdominal surgery, *Anesthesiology* 75(3A):A672, 1991.

33. Wong, CA: Intrathecal opioid injections for postoperative pain. In Benzon HT, Raja SN, Borsook D et al, editors: *Essentials of pain medicine and regional anesthesia*, Philadelphia, 1999, Churchill Livingstone, pp 151-154.

34. Davis RF, DeBoer LW, Maroko PR: Thoracic epidural anesthesia reduces myocardial infarct size after coronary artery occlusion in dogs, *Anesth Analg* 65(7):711-717, 1986.

35. Heusch G, Deussen A: The effects of cardiac sympathetic nerve stimulation on perfusion of stenotic coronary arteries in the dog, *Circ Res* 53:8-15, 1983.

36. Liem TH, Moll JE, Booij LH: Thoracic epidural in a patient with bilateral phaeochromocytoma undergoing coronary artery bypass grafting, *Anaesthesia* 46(8):654-658, 1991.

37. Blomberg S, Emanuelsson H, Kvist H et al: Effects of thoracic epidural anesthesia on coronary arteries and arterioles in patients with coronary artery disease, *Anesthesiology* 73(5):840-847, 1990.

38. Bromage P: *Epidural analgesia*, Philadelphia, 1978, WB Saunders, pp 644-647.

39. Blomberg S, Curelaru I, Emanuelsson H et al: Thoracic epidural anaesthesia in patients with unstable angina pectoris, *Eur Heart J* 10(5):437-444, 1989.

40. Ramsey DH, Olsson GL: Lumbar versus thoracic epidural catheter for post-thoracotomy analgesia, *Anesthesiology* 71:A1146, 1989.

41. Grass, JA: Epidural anesthesia. In Grass JA, editor: *Problems in anesthesia*, vol 10, Hagerstown, Md, 1998, Lippincott-Raven, pp 45-67.

42. Wong HY, Benzon HT: Epidural opioid infusion. In Benzon HT, Raja SN, Borsook D et al, editors: *Essentials of pain medicine and regional anesthesia*, Philadelphia, 1999, Churchill Livingstone, pp 159-163.

43. Lindgren I: Angina pectoris: a clinical study with special reference to neurosurgical treatment. Thesis, *Acta Med Scand*:1-141, 1950.

44. Wiener L, Cox JW: Influence of stellate ganglion block on angina pectoris and the post-exercise electrocardiogram, *Am J Med Sci* 252(3):289-295, 1966.

45. Wettervik C, Claes G, Drott C et al: Endoscopic transthoracic sympathicotomy for severe angina, *Lancet* 345(8942):97-98, 1995.

46. Blomberg S: Long-term home self-treatment with high thoracic epidural anesthesia in patients with severe coronary artery disease, *Anesth Analg* 79(3):413-421, 1994.

47. Chandler MJ, Brennan TJ, Garrison DW et al: A mechanism of cardiac pain suppression by spinal cord stimulation: implications for patients with angina pectoris, *Eur Heart J* 14(1):95-103, 1993.

48. Hautvast RW, Blanksma PK, DeJongste MJ et al: Effects of spinal cord stimulation on myocardial blood flow assessed by positron emission tomography in patients with refractory angina pectoris, *Am J Cardiol* 77(7):462-467, 1996.

49. DeJongste MJ, Haaksma J, Hautvast RW et al: Effects of spinal cord stimulation on myocardial ischemia during daily life in patients with severe coronary artery disease. A prospective ambulatory electrocardiographic study, *Br Heart J* 71(5):413-418, 1994.

50. Andersen C, Hole P, Oxhoj J: Does pain relief with spinal cord stimulation for angina conceal myocardial infarction? *Br Heart J* 71(5):419-421, 1994.

51. Eliasson T, Jern S, Augustinsson LE et al: Safety aspects of spinal cord stimulation in severe angina pectoris, *Coron Artery Dis* 5(10):845-850, 1994.

52. Augustinsson LE, Eliasson T, Mannheimer C: Spinal cord stimulation in severe angina pectoris, *Stereotactic Funct Neurosurg* 65(1-4):136-141, 1995.

53. Jessurun GA, Ten Vaarwerk IA, DeJongste MJ et al: Sequelae of spinal cord stimulation for refractory angina pectoris. Reliability and safety profile of long-term clinical application, *Coron Artery Dis* 8(1):33-38, 1997.

PART II

Anesthetic Management
of Cardiac Disease

CHAPTER 7

Anesthetic Management of the Patient with Coronary Artery Disease

Robert A. Vance, M.D.

OUTLINE

Myocardial ischemia has classically been taught as an imbalance of oxygen supply and demand; however, concepts such as perfusion-contraction matching and the lack of correlation among the various methods for diagnosing myocardial ischemia are often confusing. The purpose of this chapter is to review the basic pathophysiology of myocardial ischemia and the anesthetic management of patients who are potentially at risk for developing myocardial ischemia.

PRACTICAL ANATOMY

Knowledge of cardiac anatomy is of particular importance to the anesthesiologist caring for patients with heart disease. Routine use of transesophageal echocardiography (TEE) and technical advances such as three-dimensional imaging require an understanding of the basic cardiac structures and their spatial relationships. For example, coronary anatomy determines hemodynamic stability during "off pump" coronary ar-

tery bypass surgery. A balanced coronary artery system allows better hemodynamic stability than a right dominant system while the right coronary artery is occluded.

For practical purposes the anatomy of the heart is simply described as the four chambers, myocardium, and coronary arteries. Fig. 7-1 depicts an interior view of the right side of the heart.

Right Atrial Anatomy

The right atrium receives the superior and inferior vena caval blood and coronary venous blood from the coronary sinus. The importance of knowing the anatomic structure of the heart (including the right atrium) is illustrated by the following example. The coronary sinus is often used as a conduit for the delivery of retrograde cardioplegia during cardiac surgery. The coronary sinus catheter balloon can obstruct the small cardiac vein and prevent delivery of cardioplegia solution to the right ventricle. The right heart is subsequently poorly pro-

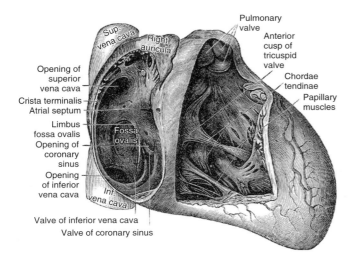

FIG. 7-1   Right side of the heart.

(From Gray H: *Anatomy of the human body*, Philadelphia, 1918, Lea & Febiger, Bartleby.com, 2000.)

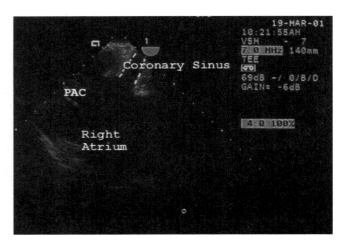

FIG. 7-2   A TEE view of the right atrium. The coronary sinus is highlighted by the dashed lines. A pulmonary artery catheter *(PAC)* is also imaged.

tected from myocardial ischemia during cardiopulmonary bypass.[1] Fig. 7-2 is a TEE view of the coronary sinus emptying into the right atrium.

Left Atrial Anatomy

The left atrium constitutes the majority of the base of the heart (Fig. 7-3). Note the position of the pulmonary venous inflow and the branches of the coronary sinus in Fig. 7-3. Systolic reversal of blood flow from the left atrium into the pulmonary venous system is an indicator of severe mitral regurgitation. Coronary sinus catheters directed into the small or middle cardiac vein may lead to coronary sinus rupture.

Right and Left Ventricular Anatomy

The left anterior descending artery demarcates the right and left ventricle. The right ventricle and pulmonary artery are the most anterior structures. Surgeons must lift the heart out of the pericardial sac to visualize the obtuse marginal branches of the circumflex artery and diagonal branches of the left anterior descending artery. This maneuver may compress the pulmonary outflow tract and result in severe hypotension during "off pump" coronary artery surgery by dramatically reducing preload. In addition, the electrocardiogram (ECG) axis changes during cardiac manipulation, changing the ECG lead/coronary artery anatomy relationship. The left ventricle is located laterally and posteriorly in the surgical field. The cardiac anesthesiologist cannot visually assess left ventricular function during cardiac surgery and must rely on other monitoring modalities such as TEE and pulmonary artery catheterization.

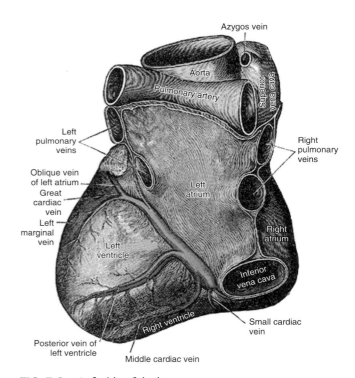

FIG. 7-3   Left side of the heart.

(From Gray H: *Anatomy of the human body*, Philadelphia, 1918, Lea & Febiger, Bartleby.com, 2000.)

Coronary Artery Anatomy

The major coronary arteries arise from two of the three sinuses of Valsalva. These two sinuses always face the pulmonary artery and are thus termed *facing sinuses* or *right and left coronary sinuses*, respectively. The third

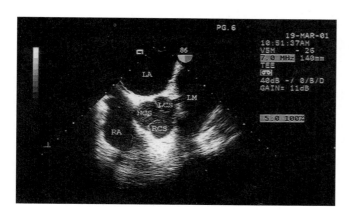

FIG. 7-4 A TEE image of the aortic root demonstrating the left main coronary ostium and left coronary sinus in the lateral and slightly posterior position. The right coronary sinus is anterior. The noncoronary sinus is posterior. *LA,* Left atrium; *LCS,* left coronary sinus; *LM,* left main coronary artery; *NCS,* noncoronary sinus; *RA,* right atrium; *RCS,* right coronary sinus.

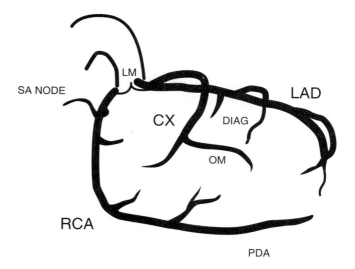

FIG. 7-5 A schematic representation of a right anterior oblique view of the coronary vasculature. *CX,* Circumflex artery; *DIAG,* diagonal branch; *LAD,* left anterior descending artery; *LM,* left main; *OM,* obtuse marginal branch; *PDA,* posterior descending artery; *RCA,* right coronary artery; *SA,* sinoatrial.

sinus is located posterior and is termed the *noncoronary* or *nonfacing sinus.* The right coronary sinus is located anterior, whereas the left coronary sinus is located laterally and slightly posterior. Fig. 7-4 is a TEE image that shows each sinus and the left coronary artery ostium.

The left coronary artery divides into the left anterior descending artery (LAD) and circumflex artery (CIRC). The LAD subsequently gives rise to the diagonal branches. It supplies the anterior wall of the right ventricle, interventricular septum, anterolateral wall of the left ventricle, and ventricular apex. The CIRC and its obtuse marginal branches supply blood to the left atrium, posterior wall of left ventricle, and lateral wall of the left ventricle.

The right coronary artery (RCA) supplies blood to the lateral and posterior walls of the right ventricle and to the inferior wall of the left ventricle. In 85% to 90% of patients, the right coronary artery terminates as the posterior descending artery (PDA). The origin of the PDA determines the pattern of dominance. Most patients have a right-dominant or balanced pattern of blood supply. A balanced pattern exists when there is no particular dominance. The sinoatrial (SA) node receives blood from the RCA in 55% of patients and the atrioventricular node receives blood from the PDA in right-dominant patients.

Fig. 7-5 is a drawing of the coronary arteries, and Fig. 7-6 presents coronary catheterization radiographs of the coronary arteries.

PHYSIOLOGY OF MYOCARDIAL OXYGEN SUPPLY AND DEMAND

The word *ischemia* derives its meaning from the Greek roots *ischein* (to hold back) and *haima* (blood). Medical students are generally taught that ischemia is defined as oxygen delivery (supply) that is inadequate for tissue demand.

Coronary Blood Flow

The physical movement of blood through the coronary arteries must follow the laws of physics. That is,

$$Q = \frac{P}{R}$$

where Q is flow, P is pressure, and R is resistance. Coronary blood flow accounts for approximately 5% (250 ml/min) of cardiac output.

A simple description of coronary blood flow assumes that coronary arteries are nondistensible pipes and that blood is a Newtonian fluid (i.e., a homogeneous fluid). Blood will move from a region of higher pressure (aorta) to one of lower pressure (capillaries). The rate of flow is dependent on the pressure gradient. Moderate pressure gradients will move red blood cells through the coronary arteries in a laminar fashion. The volume of blood per second is described by the Hagen-Poiseuille equation:

$$Q = \frac{\pi(P1 - P2)r4}{8\eta l}$$

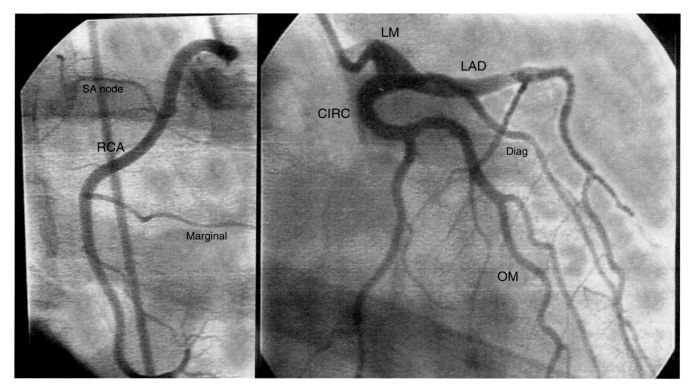

FIG. 7-6 Coronary catheterization views of both the right and left coronary arterial systems. In addition to those arteries seen in Fig. 7-5, a marginal branch of the RCA is annotated. *CIRC,* Circumflex artery; *LAD,* left anterior descending artery; *LM,* left main coronary artery; *OM,* obtuse marginal branch; *RCA,* right coronary artery; *SA,* sinoatrial.

where

Q = volume flow rate
$P1$ = inlet pressure
$P2$ = outlet pressure
r = radius
η = coefficient of viscosity (millipascal second)
l = length

In terms of coronary blood flow, the coronary perfusion pressure (CPP) is expressed by the following formula:

$$CPP = \text{aortic diastolic pressure} - LVEDP$$

where *LVEDP* is left ventricular end-diastolic pressure.

The Poiseuille equation demonstrates that the flow is most dependent on the radius of the blood vessel. Coronary arterioles maximally dilate in response to coronary arterial stenosis.[2] As the radius becomes narrowed and fixed, manipulation of the CPP becomes the most important clinical factor that determines coronary blood flow. During exercise-induced ischemia, the heart rate increases,[3] α_1-adrenergic-induced vasoconstriction occurs, and the left ventricular filling pressure increases. These events reduce coronary blood flow. Maintenance of adequate CPP is one the most important factors in preventing and treating myocardial ischemia.

A second important factor in the Poiseulle equation

is the coefficient of viscosity, η. *Viscosity* is defined by Newton as the ratio of the shear stress to the shear rate of the fluid. Rheologically, blood is a suspension of erythrocytes. Patients with coronary artery disease have rheologic abnormalities (increased shear rates and whole blood viscosities) that are compatible with disturbed blood flow and an enhanced tendency for coronary arterial thrombosis.[5]

Coronary blood flow is phasic, and approximately 70% to 80% of blood flow occurs during diastole. Cardiac contraction impedes myocardial perfusion. The diastolic time must be vigilantly monitored and treated. Boudoulas demonstrated the nonlinear relationship of heart rate and diastolic time.[5] Fig. 7-7 demonstrates the effect of small heart rate changes on diastolic filling time.

The clinical effect of decreasing the heart rate from 70 beats/min to 60 beats/min is more important than decreasing the heart rate from 110 beats/min to 90 beats/min. Anesthetic management of patients with myocardial ischemia or coronary artery disease requires prevention of small increases in heart rate by administering β-blocking drugs and adequate narcotics. β-Blockade therapy that reduces heart rate reduces mortality and improves outcomes.[6]

Heart rate also has an effect on regional coronary

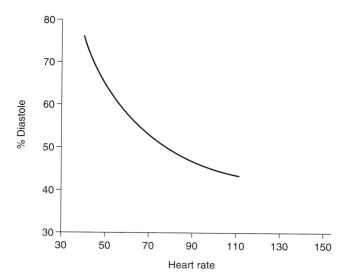

FIG. 7-7   Small increases in heart rate between 50-90 beats/min have a dramatic effect on the percent of time spent in diastole. Because diastolic filling time is a primary determinate of coronary blood flow, low heart rates such as that provided by adequate β-blockade are very effective at increasing oxygen delivery to the myocardium.

(From Boudoulas H, Rittgers SE, Lewis RP et al: *Circulation* 60:164-169, 1979.)

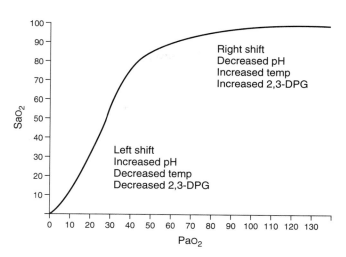

FIG. 7-8   The oxygen-hemoglobin dissociation curve demonstrates that at a PO_2 of 27, hemoglobin oxygen saturation will be 50%. A rightward shift allows the hemoglobin to more readily give up the bound oxygen to the tissues. A leftward shift will cause the oxygen to be more avidly bound by the hemoglobin and therefore less available to the tissues.

blood flow.[7-9] In general, as the heart rate increases subendocardial blood flow decreases. This causes a reduction in regional myocardial contraction. The reduction of perfusion decreases oxygen and nutrient delivery. The reduction of contractile function reduces oxygen and substrate demand. Regional myocardial contraction is coupled to subendocardial blood flow during ischemia. This observation is known as *myocardial perfusion contraction coupling.*[10,11] Recovery of stunned or hibernating myocardium is attributed to improving perfusion and contraction coupling.

Oxygen Content of Blood

The amount of oxygen delivered to the myocardium by coronary blood flow necessarily depends on the concentration of oxygen in the blood. The equation for the oxygen content of the blood is:

$$O_2 \text{ Content} = (1.34)(Hgb)(\%sat) + (0.003)(pO_2)$$

This equation demonstrates that the hemoglobin (Hgb) concentration and the percent saturation (%sat) are much more important than the actual pO_2. The first part of the equation determines the amount of oxygen bound to hemoglobin. The second part of the equation refers to the dissolved component. Clinicians using a conversion factor of 1.39 instead of 1.34 are referring to pure hemoglobin, whereas 1.34 refers to the carrying capacity of unaltered blood.

Fig. 7-8 demonstrates the oxygen hemoglobin dissociation curve and those factors that determine the affinity of hemoglobin for oxygen. P_{50} refers to the point on the curve at which the hemoglobin is 50% saturated with oxygen. Normal P_{50} is 27 torr. A shift of the curve to the left implies decreased oxygen delivery to the cells. Factors that cause a leftward shift of the curve include alkalosis, hypothermia, and decreased 2,3-diphosphoglycerate (2,3-DPG). A shift to the right is caused by acidosis, hyperthermia, and increased 2,3-DPG. Oxygen is more readily available to the cells when the curve is shifted to the right; however, less oxygen will be bound to the hemoglobin as it passes through the lungs. The erythrocyte concentration of 2,3-DPG is the single most important factor that affects oxygen binding. Blood storage rapidly depletes 2,3-DPG, so that a rapid transfusion with a large volume of packed red blood cells may lead to tissue hypoxia despite acceptable levels of oxygen saturation and hemoglobin. The normal level of 2,3-DPG is 12 to 14 μmoles/g Hgb. Stored blood has very low levels of 2,3-DPG, yielding a P_{50} of 16 torr. A normal P_{50} of 27 torr occurs 5 to 24 hours posttransfusion.[11]

The *Bohr effect* describes the effect of hydrogen ions or CO_2 on the affinity of hemoglobin for oxygen. The correct terminology is the *CO_2 Bohr effect* or *hydrogen ion Bohr effect*. Hemoglobin molecules have less affinity for O_2 in the presence of increased H^+ ions or CO_2. The curve therefore shifts to the right.[12]

Clinical studies have not fully elucidated the lowest acceptable level of anemia. In a study of healthy volunteers, isovolemic reduction of hemoglobin to 4.6 to 5.3 mg/dl produced ST-segment changes on Holter monitoring in 2 out of 11 subjects. The authors concluded that reduction of hemoglobin to 5.0 mg/dl infrequently produces myocardial ischemia in healthy patients.[13] In a different study, 3 of 55 subjects developed ECG ST-segment changes suggestive of ischemia during acute reduction of hemoglobin concentrations to 5 g/dl. These authors attributed the imbalance of myocardial oxygen supply and demand to tachycardia.[14] Acute intraoperative, normocarbic, normovolemic hemodilution to 3.0 g/dl in healthy children undergoing scoliosis surgery has been reported without adverse outcomes.[15] In cardiac surgery patients over the age of 75, preoperative systemic oxygen delivery less than 320 ml/min/m[2] and anemia on the second postoperative day is associated with higher postoperative mortality.[16] Brace and colleagues demonstrated no increase in morbidity, mortality, or patient self-assessment of fatigue when the hemoglobin threshold for red cell transfusion after coronary surgery was lowered to 8.0 g/dl.[17] The decision to transfuse a patient must depend on multiple clinical factors such as the ability to maintain adequate perfusion pressure and diagnostic indicators of ischemia.

Factors that affect myocardial oxygen supply (e.g., heart rate, coronary perfusion pressure, O_2 content of the blood) must be adjusted to optimize oxygen delivery. They are of great clinical importance when treating patients with coronary artery disease. Box 7-1 summarizes the determinants of myocardial oxygen supply and methods used to treat supply-induced imbalances.

Factors Affecting Myocardial Oxygen Demand

The basal rate of myocardial oxygen demand is 8 to 10 ml/min/100 gm of heart tissue.[18] The primary determinants of oxygen demand are heart rate, wall tension, and contractility. Perioperative blockade of β-receptors reduces mortality and myocardial infarction in patients undergoing vascular surgery.[19,20] Treatment with atenolol in the perioperative period does not significantly alter the neuroendocrine stress response.[21] However, β-blockade and subsequent heart rate reduction decrease myocardial oxygen consumption and increase supply, even in patients with heart failure. Patients treated with metoprolol in whom ventricular filling pressures are unchanged have a decrease in myocardial oxygen consumption of up to 40%.[6] Metoprolol also improves survival, patient well-being, and New York Heart Association functional class in heart failure patients.[22]

The Pressure-Volume Loop. The relationship of the pressure-volume area to myocardial oxygen consumption is commonly used to examine the effects of different medications on oxygen consumption, preload, afterload, and contractility. Pressure-volume measurements require the simultaneous measurement of pressure and volume. Such measurements are possible using conductance catheters.[23] A conductance catheter uses changing electrical currents caused by blood volume changes to calculate ventricular volume.

A close coupling exists between myocardial oxygen supply and consumption.[24] Myocardial oxygen consumption linearly correlates with the total mechanical energy of cardiac contraction.[25] Total mechanical energy of contraction is represented by ventricular pressure-volume area curves (Fig. 7-9). The components of preload, afterload, and contractility all contribute to myocardial energy consumption. These concepts will be addressed in the following sections.

Preload. Preload is the myocardial fiber length before contraction. Myocardial fiber length determines the force of myocardial fiber contraction. All other factors being equal, the force of contraction varies directly with the end-diastolic fiber length. It is very difficult to separate the effects of preload and afterload on myocardial oxygen consumption ($m\dot{v}O_2$) because end-diastolic fiber length does not influence nonmechanical oxygen consumption.[26,27] The clinical manipulation of preload is an important therapeutic option when caring for pa-

---

BOX 7-1
Myocardial Oxygen Supply Factors Critical for Treatment of Myocardial Ischemia

Heart Rate
Control depth of anesthesia (narcotic bolus, increased volatile agent)
β-Blockade (esmolol intraoperatively, atenolol preoperatively)
Maintain circulatory volume status

Coronary Perfusion Pressure
Maintain systemic vascular resistance (phenylephrine)
Reduce LVEDP (nitroglycerin)

Oxygen Content of Blood
Maintain adequate hematocrit
Maintain proper acid-base balance
Maintain oxygen saturation

LVEDP, Left ventricular end-diastolic pressure.

tients who are at risk for or have developed myocardial ischemia. The primary anti-anginal effect of nitroglycerin is preload reduction by venodilation. Furosemide reduces preload by its diuretic action and by venodilation.[28] Morphine is also useful for treating myocardial ischemia. This drug causes vasodilation (preload reduction) and provides pain relief (heart rate reduction).

Left ventricular end-diastolic myofibril length or preload is determined by end-diastolic volume. Measuring end-diastolic volume is problematic in clinical settings. The pulmonary artery occlusion pressure (PAOP) is useful for inferring left ventricular end-diastolic volume. Multiple assumptions are made when using PAOP to estimate preload. The first consideration is the compliance of the left ventricle. The definition of *compliance* is the unit volume change for each unit pressure change.[29] The left ventricular end-diastolic volume (LVEDV) and the compliance of the myocardium determine the left ventricular end-diastolic pressure (LVEDP). Myocardial ischemia decreases ventricular compliance. LVEDP, therefore, increases during ischemia in the absence of volume changes. This change can be reflected in PAOP measurements. Other factors that affect the relation of PAOP to LVEDP include mitral stenosis, left atrial compliance, and intrathoracic pressures. Box 7-2 summarizes the factors that affect the interpretation of PAOP readings.

Mitral stenosis creates a pressure gradient between the left atrium and the left ventricle. Mitral valve area (MVA) is described by the Gorlin formula:

$$MVA \ (cm^2) = \frac{CO \ (ml/s)}{38(\Delta P)^{1/2}}$$

where CO is cardiac output and ΔP is transvalvular pressure gradient. Overestimation of the transmitral gradient occurs when PAOP is used instead of direct measurement of the left atrial pressure. Because the pressure gradient is in the denominator of the Gorlin formula, there is an underestimation of the MVA when PAOP is used.[30,31] Ischemia monitoring with PAOP requires

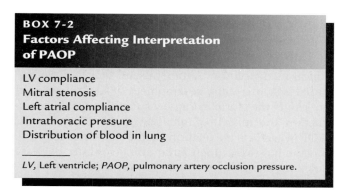

BOX 7-2
Factors Affecting Interpretation of PAOP

LV compliance
Mitral stenosis
Left atrial compliance
Intrathoracic pressure
Distribution of blood in lung

LV, Left ventricle; *PAOP,* pulmonary artery occlusion pressure.

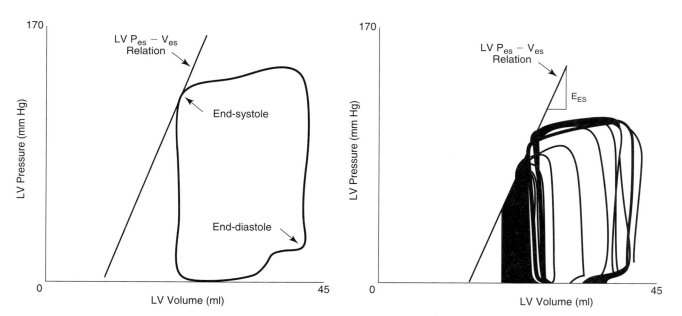

FIG. 7-9 The left panel contains a steady-state pressure-volume loop recorded in a conscious dog. End-systole occurs at the upper left-hand corner of the loop, on the left ventricular end-systolic pressure-volume (P_{es}-V_{es}) relation. The upper left-hand corners fall along the left ventricular end-systolic pressure volume relation whose slope is E_{es}.

(Adapted from Warltier DC, editor: *Ventricular function,* Baltimore, Md., 1995, Williams & Wilkins.)

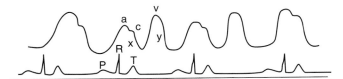

FIG. 7-10 The pulmonary artery occlusion pressure tracing contains three positive deflections and two negative deflections. The a wave follows the ECG P wave by 250 msec. The a wave represents atrial contraction. The c wave follows the a wave by the time period represented by the P-R interval. The c wave represents the upward motion of the mitral valve at the onset of ventricular systole. The x descent represents atrial relaxation. The v wave occurs after the end of the ECG T wave. The v wave represents venous filling of the atrial during ventricular systole when the mitral valve is closed. The y descent is a result of rapid atrial emptying when the mitral valve opens.

the evaluation of trends in pressure changes for correct clinical interpretation. Another useful sign during myocardial ischemia is the development of a large v wave in the PAOP waveform because of papillary muscle dysfunction and mitral regurgitation. Fig. 7-10 shows the PAOP waveform in relation to the electrocardiogram.

Acute increases in left atrial filling volumes decrease the compliance of the left atrium and pulmonary veins.[32] Chronic mitral regurgitation also contributes to the misinterpretation of pulmonary artery pressure. Papillary muscle ischemia may cause acute mitral regurgitation resulting in increased atrial volume and decreased compliance of the left atrium and pulmonary veins.[33]

Finally, the distribution of perfusion of blood in the lung also affects the interpretation of the PAOP. For accurate estimation of the LVEDP by PAOP, a column of blood must exist between the tip of the pulmonary artery catheter (PAC) and the left ventricular cavity. West's Lung Zones (Fig. 7-11) describe the distribution of blood in relation to pulmonary alveolar, pulmonary arterial, and pulmonary venous pressures.

The PAC must be in West Zone III for the PAOP to accurately reflect the left ventricular diastolic pressure. A column of blood between the tip of the catheter and the left ventricle is necessary to accurately estimate LVEDP.

The easiest way to clinically determine whether the PAC tip is in West Zone III is to add 10 cm H_2O positive end-expiratory pressure (PEEP). If the wedge pressure changes by more than 25%, the catheter is most likely not in Zone III. Because most pulmonary blood flow distributes to West Zone III, a flow-directed balloon tip catheter is most likely to be positioned in this zone. Large respiratory excursion of intrathoracic pressure also affects the PAOP. During spontaneous inspiration, the mean wedge pressure declines with the decrease in intra-

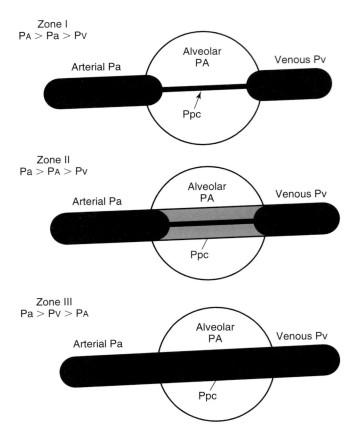

FIG. 7-11 Three zones of the lung in the upright position. Zone III has continuous flow of blood because both the Pa and Pv are greater than PA. *PA*, Pulmonary alveolar pressure; *Pa*, pulmonary arterial pressure; *Pv*, pulmonary venous pressure; *Ppc*, pulmonary capillary pressure.

thoracic pressure. Positive pressure ventilation results in transmission of increased intrathoracic pressure to the pulmonary venous system. More of the lung is likely to have Zone I or II physiology. The measurement of PCWP is always made at the end of expiration and during muscle relaxation because of the confounding physiologic effect associated with inspiration.

Afterload. *Afterload* is physiologically defined as arterial impedance during ventricular ejection.[34] Ventricular and aortic valve geometry (e.g., shape, size, and wall thickness) and aortic impedance to ejection are the primary determinants of afterload. Pressure-volume loops are commonly used to measure afterload. The ratio of the end-systolic pressure to the stroke volume defines the elastance of the arterial tree. Afterload conditions that allow substantial fiber shortening allow greater metabolic efficiency and reduced oxygen consumption.[35] Clinical manipulation of afterload requires a reduction of the size or radius of the left ventricle through preload manipulation, or a reduction of aortic imped-

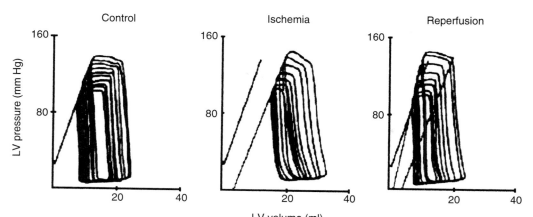

FIG. 7-12   Graphs show changes in end-systolic pressure-volume relations (ESPVR) during control, regional ischemia, and reperfusion periods. The control ESPVR (solid line) is reproduced in each panel. Coronary occlusion shifted the ESPVR rightward with no significant slope change, and reperfusion returned it to the control position with a slight slope increase. This study demonstrates the difficulty of measuring the effects of regional ischemia on global ventricular contractility. *LV*, Left ventricle.

(From Lawrence WE, Maughan L, Kass DA: *Circulation* 85:816-827, 1992.)

ance by decreasing systemic vascular resistance or blood viscosity. While systemic vascular resistance is only one component of afterload, it is the only factor that is easily measured and readily manipulated clinically. Systemic vascular resistance is determined by the following formula:

$$SVR = \frac{MAP - CVP}{CO} \times 80$$

where *MAP* is mean arterial pressure, *CVP* is central venous pressure, and *CO* is cardiac output.

Contractility. Measurement of the ventricular contractile state or inotropy is complex. Pressure-volume loops of the cardiac cycle are typically used to study inotropy. A pressure-volume loop consists of ejection, relaxation, and isovolumic phases. Contractility is measured either during the ejection or isovolumic phase. The end-systolic pressure-volume relationship (ESPVR) isolates the myofibril contractile state from preload or afterload. During regional ischemia, global functional recovery may occur despite persistent regional dysfunction.[36] The mechanism for greater functional benefits beyond that anticipated from regional wall motion analysis remains unclear. Fig. 7-12 illustrates the process of ESPVR determination and is an example of recovery of global myocardial function despite persistent regional dysfunction.

The slope of serial measurements of the ESPVR under differing pharmacologic or load conditions reflects the intrinsic contractile state of the myocardium. Simple clinical models for measuring isolated contractility do not exist. Investigators are evaluating simultaneous pressure and echocardiography area relationships to model measurements of contractile states.[37]

Anesthetic Considerations

Anesthesia for patients with coronary artery disease who require heart surgery includes the same basic considerations as all anesthetized patients. These elements include amnesia, analgesia, hemodynamic stability, maintenance of the integrity of the surgical field, and appropriate intraoperative management to achieve postoperative goals. Thoughtful consideration of these basic requirements demands only a few additional parameters for "cardiac anesthesia." The discussion that follows describes evaluation and treatment of patients with coronary artery disease who require cardiac surgery.

Preoperative Evaluation of Cardiac Surgery Patients.
Patients presenting to the operating room for coronary artery bypass surgery usually undergo extensive preoperative diagnostic testing by their cardiologists. Clinical history and outcome variables are important factors that cardiac anesthesiologists use to develop a thoughtful anesthetic plan. Ischemia most commonly produces chest pain in nondiabetic patients, whereas pump failure produces symptoms of weakness and fatigability. Patients with dyspnea and reduced ejection fraction are more likely to have postoperative complications requiring inotropic support and prolonged hospitalization than patients who present solely with anginal symptoms. Patients and their families should be counseled with realistic expectations concerning critical care issues such as prolonged ventilator support or the use of

an intraaortic balloon pump, based on standard predictors of outcome.

Patient Outcome. Patient outcome following cardiac surgery has been extensively studied. The American College of Cardiology and the American Heart Association have published scientific statements and practice guidelines that suggest management decisions for patients with cardiovascular disease.[38] These statements can be found on the American Heart Association web site at www.americanheart.org. Box 7-3 lists the seven core variables that predict mortality following coronary artery bypass surgery.

Preoperative risk scores and risk tables for mortality, stroke, and mediastinitis are listed in Tables 7-1 and 7-2. Age greater than 80, emergency surgery, and prior coronary artery bypass graft (CABG) are the most common variables associated with mortality. Stroke occurs more commonly in older patients. Chronic obstructive lung disease and severe obesity are strong risk factors for the development of mediastinitis. Renal failure is associated with advanced age, congestive heart failure, and preexisting renal disease.[39,40]

Complications associated with bypass surgery, such as acute posthemorrhagic anemia, atrial fibrillation, and acute myocardial infarction, are routinely reported to the Health Care Financing Administration (HCFA) as diagnosis codes extracted from hospital medical records. Table 7-3 is an example of a risk-adjusted comparison that can be made for Medicare patients. These data allow institutions to identify opportunities for reducing com-

---

BOX 7-3
Core Variables for Predicting Outcome Following CABG Surgery

Priority of operation
Age
Prior heart surgery
Gender
Left ventricular ejection fraction
Left main coronary stenosis
Number of major coronary arteries with significant stenosis

CABG, Coronary artery bypass graft.

TABLE 7-1
Preoperative Estimation of Risk of Mortality, Cerebrovascular Accident, and Mediastinitis

FOR USE ONLY IN ISOLATED CABG SURGERY

Directions: Locate outcome of interest (e.g., mortality). Use the score in that column for each relevant preoperative variable, then sum these scores to get the total score. Take the total score and look up the approximate preoperative risk in the table below.

PATIENT OR DISEASE CHARACTERISTIC	MORTALITY SCORE	CVA SCORE	MEDIASTINITIS SCORE
Age 60-69	2	3.5	
Age 70-79	3	5	
Age ≥80	5	6	
Female sex	1.5		
EF <40%	1.5	1.5	2
Urgent surgery	2	1.5	1.5
Emergency surgery	5	2	3.5
Prior CABG	5	1.5	
PVD	2	2	
Diabetes			1.5
Dialysis or creatinine ≥2	4	2	2.5
COPD	1.5		3.5
Obesity (BMI 31-36)			2.5
Severe obesity (BMI ≥37)			3.5
Total score			

BMI, Body mass index; *CABG*, coronary artery bypass graft; *COPD*, chronic obstructive pulmonary disease; *CVA*, cardiovascular accident; *EF*, ejection fraction; *PVD*, peripheral vascular disease.

plication rates, examine the local factors that contribute to excess complications, and institute practices that improve patient outcome.

Renal dysfunction is a serious complication of heart surgery. It is defined as greater than 2.0 mg/dl serum creatinine or an increase in the baseline creatinine of greater than 0.7 mg/dl. The mortality rate for patients who develop renal dysfunction approaches 20%. Eighteen percent of patients who develop renal dysfunction require dialysis. This is associated with a mortality rate of approximately 66%. Predictors of renal dysfunction include advanced age, history of moderate or severe congestive heart failure, prior bypass surgery, Type I diabetes, and prior renal disease.

Anesthetic Techniques for Coronary Bypass Surgery Requiring Cardiopulmonary Bypass. Multiple techniques have been described for anesthetizing patients undergoing coronary artery bypass surgery. The technique used must attempt to prevent the development of myocardial ischemia and minimize the effect of variables associated with unfavorable outcome. Intraoperative myocardial ischemia occurs in as many as 36% of patients during coronary bypass surgery.[41] Early identification and prompt treatment of intraoperative ischemia may improve outcome in these patients. The anesthetic plan for coronary bypass surgery encompasses monitoring, induction, pre-cardiopulmonary bypass (pre-CPB) considerations, the bypass period, post bypass (post-CPB) management, and transport to the intensive care unit following the completion of surgery.

Monitoring. All patients who undergo bypass surgery require invasive arterial blood pressure monitoring. The location of the arterial catheter varies with anesthesiologist, surgeon, and institution. Consideration must be given to the possibility of radial artery harvesting and

TABLE 7-2
Perioperative Risk

TOTAL SCORE	MORTALITY %	CVA %	MEDIASTINITIS %
0	0.4	0.3	0.4
1	0.5	0.4	0.5
2	0.7	0.7	0.6
3	0.9	0.9	0.7
4	1.3	1.1	1.1
5	1.7	1.5	1.5
6	2.2	1.9	1.9
7	3.3	2.8	3.0
8	3.9	3.5	3.5
9	6.1	4.5	5.8
10	7.7	≥ 6.5	≥ 6.5
11	10.6		
12	13.7		
13	17.7		
14	≥ 28.3		

CVA, Cardiovascular accident.

TABLE 7-3
Institutional Comparison of Complication Rates

This is an example of actual 1996 Medicare Inpatient-HCFA data that compares the rate of complication for a specific DRG to a reference group of selected facilities. These data allow the institution of procedures that can reduce complications and improve patient outcome.

DIAGNOSIS NAME (CODE)	INSTITUTION 898 CASES		REFERENCE GROUP 3363 CASES		
	CASES	RATE (%)	CASES	RATE (%)	EXCESS RATE (%)
Acute posthemorrhagic anemia (2851)	206	22.5	344	10.2	12.7
Surgical complication, heart (9971)	276	30.7	702	20.9	9.8
Hemorrhage complicating a procedure (9981)	77	8.6	202	6.0	2.6
Hyperkalemia (2767)	32	3.5	41	1.2	2.3
Pleural effusion NOS (5119)	47	5.2	101	3.0	2.2
Respiratory complications (9973)	73	8.1	207	6.2	1.9
Atrial fibrillation (42731)	82	9.2	269	8.0	1.2
Congestive heart failure (4280)	50	5.5	166	4.9	0.6

From RA Vance, West Virginia University Hospitals, Inc., unpublished data.
DRG, Diagnosis-related group; *HCFA*, Health Care Financing Administration; *NOS*, not otherwise specified.

TABLE 7-4
Drugs Often Used to Induce General Anesthesia for Patients Undergoing Coronary Bypass Surgery

DRUG	DOSE	EFFECT	CONSIDERATIONS
Fentanyl	2-10 µg/kg	Blunt response to laryngoscopy	Must be used in conjunction with hypnotic (etomidate, Midazolam, thiopental) for amnesia. Combination is likely to produce hypotension.
High dose Fentanyl	50-100 µg/kg	Sole anesthetic, very stable hemodynamics	Disadvantage of awareness, postoperative respiratory depression
High dose Sufentanil	20 µg/kg	As sole anesthetic, very stable hemodynamics	Potential for severe bradycardia/asystole in patients taking calcium channel blockers and β-blockers
Midazolam	0.2-0.3 mg/kg	Lower dose required when given with supplemental narcotic	As sole agent, does not prevent tachycardia or hypertension during intubation
Etomidate	0.3 mg/kg	As sole agent, provides excellent cardiovascular stability	Pain during injection, myoclonus, adrenocortical suppression

the type of retraction used for exposure of the left internal mammary artery. Patients who receive high doses of magnesium from the cardioplegia solution are often vasodilated in the post-bypass period and the radial arterial line tracing may appear damped. In this scenario, a femoral arterial line is preferable because it more closely reflects mean aortic pressure. The intraarterial catheter is placed before or immediately after induction. Placement of the arterial line before induction is preferred in patients with a potentially difficult airway or if rapidly changing hemodynamics are anticipated.

The decision to place a PAC as opposed to only a CVP line is controversial. The information obtained from a PAC is different from that obtained from either a CVP or TEE. Some studies suggest that the use of a PAC does not improve outcome in cardiac surgery.[42] However, prolonged pre-CPB pulmonary hypertension and post-CPB elevation of the pulmonary diastolic pressure predict the development of perioperative myocardial infarction.[43] These hemodynamic variables are only obtained with use of a PAC. It is presumed that early treatment of these hemodynamic abnormalities improves outcome.

Myocardial ischemia decreases left ventricular compliance. This decrease in compliance may increase PAOP for a given left ventricular end-diastolic volume. If the ischemic area includes the papillary muscles, a v wave may develop. Nonischemic factors such as acute increases in afterload or nonischemic mitral valve regurgitation also increase the PAOP.

Standard limb lead and V_5 electrocardiography is one of the most important clinical monitors of ischemia and is routinely used for patients undergoing cardiac surgery. Automated ST-segment trending has moderate sensitivity and specificity (75%) for detecting the same changes found by off-line Holter monitoring.[44] Factors such as left ventricular hypertrophy, cardiac con-

duction, electrolytes abnormalities, and medications (digitalis) produce ST-segment changes in the absence of ischemia.[45]

Core temperature monitoring is accomplished by either rectal or bladder temperature probes. The rate of rewarming affects rectal temperature to a greater degree than bladder temperature.[46]

Induction. Induction of general anesthesia for cardiac surgery patients can be accomplished using many different techniques. Drug effects, titratability, contraindications, and side effects such as myocardial depression or autonomic nervous system effects are factors that must be considered when choosing a particular anesthetic technique. The primary hemodynamic goals during induction are avoiding hypotension (caused by myocardial depressants or vasodilating anesthetic agents) and hypertension or tachycardia (caused by laryngoscopy and intubation). Positive pressure ventilation may cause hypotension in hypovolemic patients or patients with air trapping. Common induction techniques and doses are presented in Table 7-4.

The primary advantages of an opioid induction in patients with cardiac disease are lack of myocardial depression, a tendency for decreased heart rate, and an attenuated response to laryngoscopy and intubation. Fentanyl is probably the most commonly used opioid in cardiac surgery. A nondepolarizing muscle relaxant devoid of cardiovascular side effects is a good choice for facilitating intubation.

Patients were commonly ventilated postoperatively for 24 to 48 hours during the 1960s and 1970s. Prolonged intubation was advocated to decrease the work of breathing.[47,48] Although a high-dose narcotic technique (1 mg/kg morphine sulfate) was thought ideal for cardiac surgery because of the lack of myocardial depression, this assumption was challenged even then. Two studies in 1977 suggested that early extubation follow-

TABLE 7-5
Prebypass Events

EVENT	TECHNIQUES, MONITORING, AND EFFECTS	
Monitor placement	Standard anesthesia monitors	Check isoelectric points for ST-analysis, place intraarterial catheter, central venous or pulmonary artery catheter as indicated
Induction/intubation	Multiple techniques	Monitor for rapidly changing hemodynamics, ischemic episodes
Preparation of surgical field	Begin anesthesia maintenance drugs, obtain appropriate labs (ACT, hematocrit), begin infusion of antifibrinolytics	Blood pressure tends to decrease during period devoid of stimulation
Incision/sternotomy	Bolus doses of narcotic often necessary to treat hypertension	Sternotomy may result in serious hemorrhage (particularly in reoperations)
Aortic cannulation	Surgeons often prefer tight blood pressure control while cannulating the aorta	Hypotension from surgical manipulation of heart, excess bleeding

ACT, Activated clotting time.

ing cardiac surgery was not only feasible, but also possibly beneficial.[49,50] With the development of newer, more potent, and shorter-acting narcotics, high-dose fentanyl (50-100 µg/kg) and sufentanil (10-20 µg/kg) became popular during the 1980s. Early extubation (6 to 8 hours) following cardiac surgery was advocated during the managed care era of the 1990s. Current debate has even focused on extubation immediately following surgery.[51,52]

Because of the desire for early postoperative extubation, reduced doses of opioids are often administered with hypnotic drugs such as benzodiazepines, thiopental, propofol, or etomidate. The administration of hypnotics with opioids must be carried out with extreme caution. The combination of diazepam and fentanyl decreases plasma catecholamines and decreases systemic vascular resistance.[53] The mean arterial pressure can decrease precipitously in hypovolemic patients. Midazolam significantly decreases blood pressure and increases heart rate when used as an induction agent.[54] Propofol causes venodilation and a significant decrease in blood pressure.[55] Vasoactive drugs such as ephedrine or phenylephrine should be readily available to treat hypotensive episodes if a combination of opioids and hypnotics are administered.

The use of remifentanil and sufentanil during induction is associated with a high incidence of bradycardia/asystole in patients treated with β-blockers and calcium channel blockers.[56,57] Patients with coronary artery disease often receive one or both types of these medications. Calcium channel blockers relax vascular smooth muscle by dual mechanisms. In addition to calcium channel inhibition, verapamil and amlodipine also inhibit vascular smooth muscle carbonic anhydrase I

(CA I).[58] Vascular smooth muscle CA I regulates intracellular pH necessary for calcium ion transport. The inhibition of CA I causes vasodilatation and a hypotensive effect. Compensatory increases in heart rate maintain cardiac output. β-Blocking drugs inhibit the compensatory heart rate increase. Potent opioid induction thus produces an even greater reduction in heart rate and mean arterial pressure. Knowledge of the interaction between preoperative medications and anesthetic agents is necessary for planning an appropriate induction regimen.

Prebypass Considerations. Following the induction of anesthesia and intubation of the trachea, anesthesia care is directed toward maintaining stable hemodynamics and preparing the patient for incision. Table 7-5 summarizes prebypass events.

Central venous access for placement of a PAC is usually achieved by a right internal jugular (IJ) approach. A subclavian or left internal jugular approach may be considered when there is difficulty cannulating the right IJ. It is important to consider that the left IJ approach can cause thoracic duct injury, a complication not associated with cannulating the right IJ. Subclavian line placement has been associated with subclavian venous stenosis. It is prudent to avoid subclavian vein puncture in patients with renal disease who may require dialysis. The Trendelenburg position used when obtaining central venous access helps maintain the blood pressure at an acceptable level following the induction of anesthesia. As the operating room table is leveled, blood pressure often declines. A fluid bolus or small dose of a vasoactive drug may be required.

Other activities that take place during the period before incision include antibiotic administration, determination of a baseline-activated clotting time, infusion of antifibrinolytic drugs, and placement of a TEE probe. These multiple activities should not distract anesthesia personnel from vigilant hemodynamic monitoring to maintain optimal heart rate and blood pressure. This author's advice to all residents beginning their "heart room" rotation is to not forget the basic tasks that must be performed for any patient requiring general anesthesia. Placement of intraarterial and pulmonary artery catheters, obtaining baseline coagulation studies, and starting an infusion of antifibrinolytics are only four additional steps that are added to a basic anesthesia care plan. The depth of anesthesia during this time is gradually increased before incision to prevent profound increases in heart rate and blood pressure as the surgery starts. Small doses of short-acting drugs such as esmolol (50-100 mg) or nitroglycerin (50-100 μg) may be given as a supplement to increasing anesthetic depth with additional narcotic or inhalational agent.

The use of volatile anesthetic agents during cardiac surgery has been extensively studied. Isoflurane-fentanyl anesthesia and propofol-fentanyl anesthesia are both acceptable techniques for maintaining anesthesia during CABG surgery.[59] In experimental preparations, isoflurane protects the myocardium during ischemic episodes.[60,61] Isoflurane and other volatile anesthetics mimic the protective effects of a process termed *ischemic preconditioning*.[62] Brief periods of ischemia activate the protein kinase C mediated pathway that confers cardioprotection during subsequently longer periods of ischemia.[63] Halothane and isoflurane provide significant preservation of adenosine triphosphate levels during ischemia, but this preservation does not improve hemodynamic recovery.[64] Although this ability to provide myocardial protection by administering volatile anesthetic agents or via ischemic preconditioning is encouraging, its direct clinical relevance remains unclear.

Other important events during the period before bypass include sternotomy, left internal mammary artery dissection, pericardiotomy, measurement of graft lengths, and aortic and venous cannulation. The lungs are typically deflated during sternotomy to prevent the sternal saw from cutting into the lung parenchyma. A major complication of sternotomy is the accidental tearing of the innominate vein or the right ventricle. Sternotomy is especially hazardous during cardiac reoperations. The need to treat sudden hemorrhage is anticipated by placing large-bore IV catheters before making the incision. Packed red blood cells must be immediately available at the time of sternotomy. Sternal retraction during dissection of the left internal mammary artery may interfere with intravenous or intraarterial catheters in the left arm. Papaverine is commonly injected into the internal mammary artery after its ligation for its vasodilatory effects. Injection of papaverine can cause a sudden drop in mean arterial pressure. This

decrease in blood pressure is usually brief, but may require treatment with a small dose of phenylephrine. A frequent mistake is to treat the brief hypotensive episode caused by papaverine too early and discover that the vasoconstrictor effect predominates to cause an undesirable hypertensive crisis. Hypertension commonly occurs during pericardial incision and manipulation as a result of sympathetic activation. A small bolus of narcotic or esmolol can blunt this hypertensive response.

Heparin is administered before aortic cannulation and internal mammary ligation to prevent thrombus formation. Heparin is a polyanionic mucopolysaccharide that increases the rate of reaction between antithrombin III and Factors II, X, XI, XII, and XIII. A heparin dose of 300 to 400 units/kg is required to achieve an activated clotting time greater than 400 seconds. Adequate anticoagulation must be determined before initiating cardiopulmonary bypass. Heparin is administered into the central venous access after aspirating blood to ensure administration into the central circulation. The heparin bolus must not be injected into intravenous lines that contain vasoactive infusions. The aorta is cannulated after heparin administration.

Atrial manipulation by the surgeon often causes hypotension and atrial arrhythmias and requires hand ventilation to provide better visualization. Atrial fibrillation causing severe hypotension requires cardioversion with internal paddles or rapid initiation of cardiopulmonary bypass. The atrium may tear during placement of the venous cannula. Shed blood is collected into cardiotomy reservoir suction and infused into the aorta from the bypass machine.

Institution of cardiopulmonary bypass is accomplished by unclamping the venous cannula and infusing the pump volume into the patient through the aortic cannula. A list of the clinical tasks during cardiopulmonary bypass is presented in Box 7-4. The surgical field is observed for evidence of venous obstruction, aortic dissection, distention of the heart, spontaneous breathing

---

BOX 7-4
Activities During the Initiation of Cardiopulmonary Bypass

Discontinue mechanical ventilation
Palpate carotids for thrill
Inspect patient's head and eyes for inadequate venous drainage or unilateral cerebral perfusion
Stop intravenous infusions
Inspect surgical field
Maintain anesthesia by pump vaporizer or continuous infusion
Administer additional muscle relaxant to prevent shivering
Monitor hemodynamic pressures
Prepare for weaning from bypass

by the patient, and the conduct of the operation. Intravenous infusions are stopped at this time with the exception of antifibrinolytics. Anesthesia is maintained by volatile anesthetics administered through a vaporizer on the bypass machine or continuous infusion of hypnotic drugs such as propofol. Additional muscle relaxant helps reduce oxygen consumption by subclinical shivering. The ECG, systemic and pulmonary pressures, urine output, and temperature are monitored. Increased pulmonary artery pressure may be caused by catheter migration to more peripheral regions in the lung. The catheter should be pulled back until the pressure decreases. If the pressure remains elevated, the heart should be inspected for left ventricular distention.

Preparation is made for the events after bypass. Most patients do not require inotropic support following successful coronary revascularization. However, patients with a low preoperative ejection fraction, long cross clamp time, or long periods of prebypass ischemia may require inotropic or intraaortic balloon pump support in the period after bypass. Before terminating bypass, atrial and ventricular pacing leads are placed. A pacemaker with a fresh battery should be readily available. The A-V interval is usually set to 150 milliseconds. The heart is paced either synchronously or asynchronously depending on the underlying rhythm and the ability to conduct atrial beats.

Termination of Cardiopulmonary Bypass. Discontinuation of cardiopulmonary bypass requires good communication between the anesthesiologist, surgeon, and perfusionist. As a general rule, oral requests should be orally confirmed by the person to whom the request is directed. The patient is warmed and the surgical sites are checked for bleeding before separation from bypass. Mechanical ventilation is resumed, while delivery of anesthetic agents is continued. Vasoactive infusion drugs are readily available. The venous drainage to the pump is gradually reduced while appropriate volume is delivered from the pump to the patient. Volume therapy is guided by the mean arterial pressure and the pulmonary artery or central venous pressure. Transesophageal echocardiography is a better indicator of volume status because of decreased left ventricular compliance. Cardiac function is evaluated by both visual inspection of the heart and by measuring the cardiac index with a PAC. The venous cannula is removed from the right atrium. Both the surgeon and the perfusionist are notified when the neutralization of heparin with protamine has begun. Cardiotomy suctioning is discontinued when approximately one quarter to one half of the protamine dose has been given. The chest is then closed with adequate hemostasis and the patient is transported to the intensive care unit for postoperative care.

There are a variety of causes leading to poor cardiac function following termination of bypass. Inadequate myocardial protection, preexisting dysfunction, left ventricular distention, and ischemia may all contribute to cardiac failure during the postbypass period. Inotropic support is required to support cardiac function at the expense of increased myocardial work. Epinephrine is an ideal inotrope because of its mixed α and β agonism. Dobutamine is a weaker inotrope, but it is useful for decreasing systemic vascular resistance. Severe cardiac dysfunction is treated with combined infusions of epinephrine and milrinone. Norepinephrine is used in place of epinephrine when systemic vascular resistance is very low following milrinone administration. A combination of epinephrine and dobutamine is not recommended because dobutamine inhibits epinephrine-induced production of cyclic adenosine monophosphate (cAMP) and appears to be clinically subadditive.[65]

Some patients will require placement of an intraaortic balloon pump (IABP). This device is a cylinder-shaped balloon that is placed in the descending aorta. The IABP inflates at the beginning of diastole and deflates before systole. This device dramatically reduces afterload and elevates the diastolic blood pressure, thus reducing myocardial work and improving coronary perfusion, respectively. Proper timing of inflation and deflation are essential for maximizing the benefit of this therapy. The IABP is a very useful tool for treating myocardial ischemia. It is often placed in the cardiac catheterization laboratory during failed angioplasty procedures. The IABP may also be used during noncardiac surgery to prevent ischemia that cannot be controlled by pharmacologic methods. Complications associated with the placement of an IABP include vessel trauma at the insertion site, distal limb ischemia, and thrombosis. An IABP inserted over the original of the left subclavian artery can cause left upper extremity circulatory compromise.

Postoperative myocardial ischemia often occurs in cardiac surgery patients. Leung and colleagues documented a 48% incidence of postoperative ischemia.[66] These investigators found that 38% of ischemic episodes developed during first 2 postoperative days with the peak occurring during the first 2 hours after revascularization. Ischemia detection and treatment are important because postoperative ischemia is related to adverse cardiac outcome. ECG analysis, pulmonary artery pressure data, and segmental wall motion analysis by TEE are all used to detect ischemic changes. Fig. 7-13 demonstrates an example of anterior myocardial wall akinesis detected by TEE.

The treatment of myocardial ischemia is directed at correcting the factors that affect myocardial oxygen supply and demand. Ischemia that develops immediately on separation from bypass may be related to air or particulate emboli in the bypass grafts. Elevation of the mean arterial pressure and incremental increases of a nitroglycerin infusion are effective methods for treating ischemia caused by air in the venous grafts.

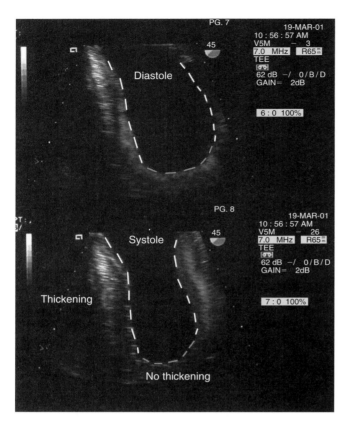

FIG. 7-13 Long axis view LV at end-diastole (*top*) and end-systole (*bottom*). Akinetic anterior segments are identified by a lack of myocardial thickening during systole.

Reinstitution of cardiopulmonary bypass may be necessary because of severe ischemia if pharmacotherapy is ineffective. Graft patency evaluation by the surgeon is accomplished with Doppler flow probes or palpation. Persistent ischemia is treated with placement of an IABP, additional coronary grafts, or both. Ischemia not related to coronary blood flow may be caused by reperfusion injury or intraoperative myocardial infarction. These patients will require support of cardiac function until the myocardial edema resolves and the heart "learns" to function on a new portion of the Starling curve.

Anesthetic Techniques for Patients with Coronary Artery Disease Undergoing Noncardiac Surgery Procedures

Preoperative Evaluation. The clinical challenges of anesthetizing a patient with coronary artery disease are complex. The purpose of the preoperative evaluation is to define the extent of the patient's disease and risk factors and optimize the patient's health to provide the most favorable clinical environment for a good outcome. Consideration is given to risk stratification of patients for a particular procedure, the type of monitoring used to detect ischemia, the anesthetic technique,

and management strategies that reduce cardiac morbidity. Goldman and colleagues published the landmark study "Multifactorial index of cardiac risk in noncardiac surgical procedures" in a 1977 issue of the *New England Journal of Medicine*.[67] This investigation led to other studies that expanded the available knowledge related to the risks associated with noncardiac surgical procedures.

The American Heart Association/American College of Cardiology (AHA/ACC) and the American College of Physicians (ACP) published comprehensive guidelines and algorithms for the preoperative clinical evaluation for patients with coronary artery disease.[68,69] The AHA algorithm is presented in Fig. 7-14. These guidelines are derived from a comprehensive review of the scientific literature on the reported incidence of perioperative cardiac death and nonfatal myocardial infarction risk by patient disease and type of surgery. The AHA guidelines provide an orderly sequence for determining whether a patient is a candidate for surgery and the extent of cardiovascular testing required. The guidelines are based on clinical predictors of increased cardiovascular risk for myocardial infarction, congestive heart failure and cardiac death (Box 7-5), functional capacity of the patient defined by metabolic equivalents (METs) (Table 7-6), and surgical risk (Table 7-7).

The ACP guidelines rely on Detsky's modification of risk factors found in the original Goldman study.[70] The Detsky cardiac risk index assigns a numeric score to various disease states. The ACP guidelines provide an algorithm for necessary presurgery clinical tests. The American Society of Anesthesiologists' patient classification index is predictive of patient outcome, similar to the Detsky Index.[71]

Some patients require coronary angiography and stent placement prompted by the preoperative evaluation. The incidence of death from acute stent thrombosis approaches 20% for patients who have elective surgery within 14 days of stent placement.[72] The incidence of major bleeding is also increased (27%).[72] Elective noncardiac surgery should be postponed 2 to 4 weeks following stent placement to allow for the completion of the mandatory antiplatelet regimen. Because the technology for coronary stenting and antiplatelet therapy is constantly changing, recommendations for postponing elective surgery in these patients may also change.

Monitoring. Intraoperative monitoring for patients with cardiac disease undergoing noncardiac surgery depends on the presence of factors that determine cardiac risk. There is a paucity of clinical studies that provide objective direction for choosing specific monitoring modalities. Monitoring decisions are based on the presence of clinical factors associated with adverse cardiac outcomes. For example, postoperative heart rate control with β-adrenergic blocker therapy reduces myocardial ischemia in patients at risk.[73-76] A reliable

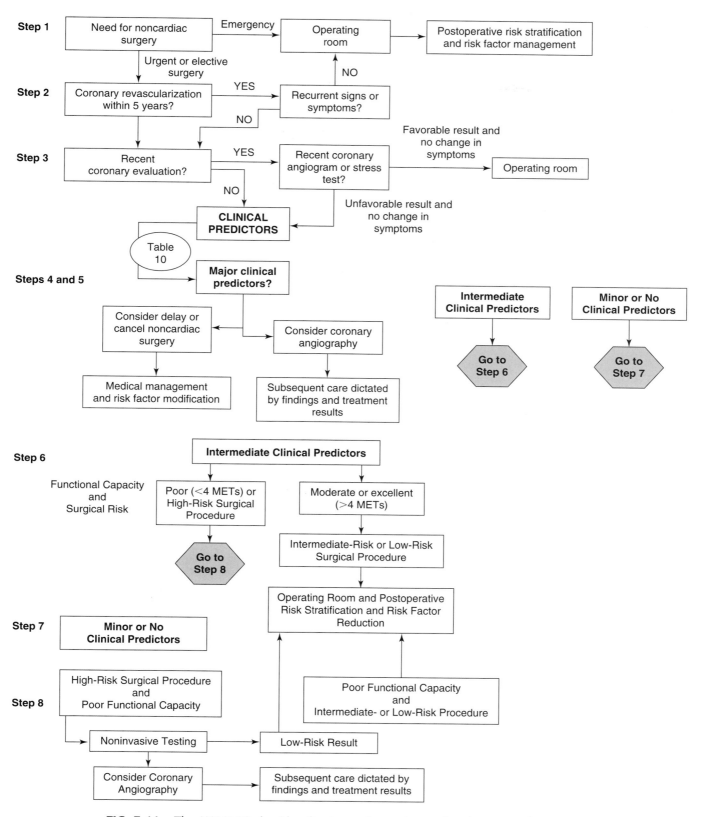

FIG. 7-14   The AHA/ACC algorithm for the cardiac patient undergoing noncardiac surgery demonstrates the patients should be evaluated based on signs and symptoms, clinical predictors, and the risk of the surgical procedure. *MET,* Metabolic equivalent.

(Adapted from Eagle K, Brundage B, Chaitman B et al: *Circulation* 93:1278-1317, 1996.)

BOX 7-5
Clinical Predictors of Increased Perioperative MI, CHF, and Death

Major
Unstable coronary syndrome
Recent MI* with evidence of important ischemic risk by
    clinical symptoms or noninvasive study
Unstable or severe† angina (Canadian Class III or IV) [6]
Decompensated CHF
Significant arrhythmias
High-grade atrioventricular block
Symptomatic ventricular arrhythmias in the presence of
    underlying heart disease
Supraventricular arrhythmias with uncontrolled ventricu-
    lar rate
Severe valvular disease

Intermediate
Mild angina pectoris (Canadian Class I or II)
Prior MI by history or pathologic Q waves
Compensated or prior CHF
Diabetes mellitus

Minor
Advanced age
Abnormal ECG (left ventricular hypertrophy, left bundle
    branch block, ST-T abnormalities)
Rhythm other than sinus (e.g., atrial fibrillation)
Low functional capacity (e.g., inability to climb one flight of
    stairs with a bag of groceries)
History of stroke
Uncontrolled systemic hypertension

From Eagle K, Brundage B, Chaitman B et al: *Circulation* 93:1278-1317, 1996.
CHF, Congestive heart failure; *ECG*, electrocardiogram; *MI*, myocardial infarction.
* The American College of Cardiology National Database Library defines *recent MI* as greater than 7 days but less than or equal to 1 month
(30 days).
† May include "stable" angina in patients who are unusually sedentary.

TABLE 7-6
Estimated Energy Requirements for Various Activities

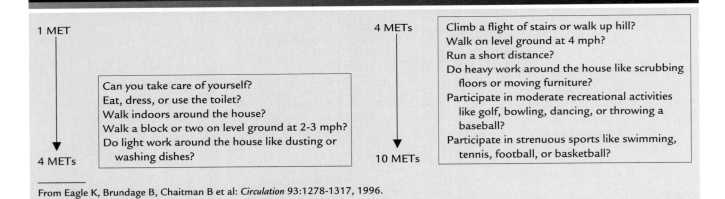

From Eagle K, Brundage B, Chaitman B et al: *Circulation* 93:1278-1317, 1996.
MET, Metabolic equivalent.

method for heart rate detection is standard for all patients during the intraoperative and postoperative periods. Patients who develop myocardial ischemia during the postoperative period are at a significant risk for
cardiac related death, nonfatal myocardial infarction,
or unstable angina.[77] Continuous electrocardiographic

monitoring in the early postoperative period is therefore
recommended.

The decision to use direct intraarterial monitoring of
blood pressure depends primarily on the nature of the
surgery. Major vascular surgery or procedures associated
with extensive blood loss or large fluid shifts require

HIGH Cardiac risk often >5%	INTERMEDIATE Cardiac risk generally <5%	LOW† Cardiac risk generally <1%
Emergent major operations, particularly in the elderly Aortic and other major vascular Peripheral vascular Anticipated prolonged surgical procedures associated with large fluid shifts and/or blood loss	Carotid endarterectomy Head and neck Intraperitoneal and intrathoracic Orthopedic Prostate	Endoscopic procedures Superficial procedure Cataract Cataract Breast

From Eagle K, Brundage B, Chaitman B et al: *Circulation* 93:1278-1317, 1996.
* Combined incidence of cardiac death and nonfatal myocardial infarction.
† Do not generally require further preoperative cardiac testing.

invasive monitoring of blood pressure. Access to the extremities and the ease of obtaining noninvasive blood pressure measurements are considerations for determining whether to place an intraarterial catheter for other types of surgeries. During head and neck procedures, the arms are often tucked at the patient's side. Surgeons may lean on the blood pressure cuff, making frequent determination of blood pressure difficult. For other procedures, such as peripheral vascular surgery, the arms may be readily accessible. Automated noninvasive blood pressure measurements correlate well with central aortic pressure. During noncritical clinical situations, errors of +/− 10 mm Hg occur in approximately 25% of the measurements, whereas errors of +/− 20 mm Hg occur in only 3.2% of measurements.[78]

The decision regarding placement of a pulmonary artery catheter versus a central venous pressure catheter is controversial. Increases in pulmonary artery pressure are not as sensitive for detecting myocardial ischemia as TEE regional wall motion analysis or ECG ST-segment monitoring.[79-80] Pulmonary artery pressure measurement is very useful for management of acute volume changes associated with blood loss. In addition, patients who develop intraoperative ischemia can develop low cardiac output, which requires titration of nitroglycerin or inotropic agents. Low cardiac output is readily detected with a pulmonary artery catheter. Hypotensive episodes of uncertain etiology in patients with only central venous pressure monitoring or no central venous access can be evaluated with a TEE probe placed intraoperatively to assist in the diagnosis and management of the hypotensive episode.

Patients undergoing low-risk procedures such as ophthalmologic procedures, endoscopy, or breast surgery, rarely require invasive monitoring.

Anesthetic Techniques. Multiple investigators have evaluated different anesthetic agents and techniques in cardiac patients undergoing noncardiac surgery. With very few exceptions, most studies do not demonstrate a difference in cardiac morbidity or mortality based on anesthetic technique. Maintenance of stable intraoperative hemodynamics is associated with a lower incidence of intraoperative ischemia.[81] Small oral doses of β-blockers or clonidine blunt sympathetic stimulation and reduce the incidence of intraoperative ischemia.[82-83] Prophylactic nitroglycerin infusion does not reduce the incidence of intraoperative myocardial ischemia.[84]

Patients who develop intraoperative ischemia are treated in the same manner as nonsurgical patients who develop myocardial ischemia. Myocardial supply and demand are optimized in favor of increased supply and decreased demand. Coronary blood flow improves by decreasing heart rate and increasing coronary perfusion pressure (phenylephrine infusion). Anemic patients are transfused with red blood cells to improve oxygen delivery to the myocardium. Volume overload causing increased myocardial wall tension is treated with nitroglycerin. Some patients may even require placement of an intraaortic balloon pump to decrease afterload and increase coronary perfusion pressure.[85]

Although a particular anesthetic technique has not been shown to affect the overall incidence of perioperative myocardial ischemia, some regional techniques have advantages that may improve patient care. Patients undergoing peripheral vascular surgery using epidural have a lower incidence of reoperation because of inadequate tissue perfusion.[86] Elderly patients with hip fractures have a decreased incidence of myocardial ischemia when an epidural infusion of bupivacaine/fentanyl is used for pain control as compared with intramuscular opioids.[87] Patients undergoing upper abdominal surgery have a decreased incidence of postoperative myocardial ischemia when epidural bupivacaine/morphine is used for postoperative pain control as compared to patient-controlled analgesia with morphine.[88] The most likely reason for this finding is less tachycardia in patients with epidural analgesia. Another surgery for which regional anesthesia appears superior to general anesthesia is cataract surgery using a retrobulbar block.[89] Increased intervention by anesthesia personnel improves care of patients undergoing cataract surgery during monitored anesthesia care.[90]

Other factors that decrease the incidence of postoperative myocardial ischemia include the maintenance of normothermia and the prevention of postoperative anemia.[91,92] These physiologic conditions improve myocardial oxygen supply and minimize myocardial oxygen demand.

Roizen has summarized the most important aspect of caring for patients with coronary artery disease who require surgery by stating, "To me, the issue is perhaps best expressed by the thought that, in those least able to tolerate myocardial ischemia, an adequate dose of anesthesia is that which provides the heart with the least stress."[93]

CONCLUSIONS

Myocardial ischemia is an important anesthetic consideration in patients with coronary artery disease undergoing cardiac or noncardiac surgery. Patients who develop intraoperative ischemia are more likely to have postoperative cardiac complications. Myocardial ischemia is detected by electrocardiography, pulmonary artery pressure data, or TEE. Treatment of myocardial ischemia is directed at those factors that favorably influence the supply and demand of oxygen to the myocardium. Anticipation and preparation for treatment of ischemic episodes is essential. The treatment of myocardial ischemia is the same for cardiac and noncardiac surgical patients.

Acknowledgments

Special thanks and deep appreciation to Doctors CM Grande, EH Sinz, and RE Henrickson, for their insightful editorial review and comments pertaining to this manuscript.

KEY POINTS

1. β-Blockade is a very effective way to control heart rate, as a means of decreasing myocardial oxygen demand and increasing supply.
2. It is important to maintain coronary perfusion pressure.
3. Decrease myocardial oxygen demand by preload and afterload reduction.
4. Major morbidity includes mortality, stroke, and renal failure after myocardial infarction.
5. Most types of anesthetic techniques are acceptable as long as myocardial oxygen supply and demand are kept in balance.
6. Use of a PAC is controversial.
7. Patients with coronary artery disease having cardiac surgery require close monitoring and early intervention of myocardial ischemia.
8. Management of acute episodes of myocardial ischemia is the same for surgical and nonsurgical patients.
9. Patients undergoing noncardiac surgery who have intermediate or low risk may not require extensive preoperative testing.

KEY REFERENCES

Boudoulas H, Rittgers SE, Lewis RP et al: Changes in diastolic time with various pharmacologic agents, *Circulation* 60:164-169, 1979.

Eagle K, Brundage B, Chaitman B et al: Guidelines for perioperative cardiovascular evaluation for noncardiac surgery. A report of the American Heart Association/American College of Cardiology Task Force on Assessment of Diagnostic and Therapeutic Cardiovascular Procedures, *Circulation* 93: 1278-1317, 1996.

Eagle KA, Guyton RA, Davidoff R et al: ACC/AHA guidelines for coronary artery bypass graft surgery: executive summary and recommendations: A report of the American College of Cardiology/American Heart Association Task Force on Practice Guidelines (Committee to revise the 1991 guidelines for coronary artery bypass graft surgery), *Circulation* 100: 1464-1480, 1998.

Goto Y, Futaki S, Kawaguchi O et al: Coupling between regional myocardial oxygen consumption and contraction under altered preload and afterload, *J Am Coll of Cardiol* 21(6):1522-1531, 1993.

Indolfi C, Ross JJ: The role of heart rate in myocardial ischemia and infarction. Implications of myocardial perfusion-contraction matching, *Prog Cardiovasc Dis* XXXVI:61-74, 1993.

Klineberg PL, Geer RT, Hirsh RA et al: Early extubation after coronary artery bypass graft surgery, *Crit Care Med* 5:272-274, 1977.

Little WC, Cheng CP: Left ventricular systolic and diastolic performance. In Warltier DC, editor: *Ventricular function*, Baltimore, 1995, Williams & Watkins.

Reich DL, Bodian CA, Krol M et al: Intraoperative predictors of mortality, stroke, and myocardial infarction after coronary artery bypass surgery, *Anesth Analg* 89:814-822, 1999.

Smith RC, Leung JM, Mangano DT: Postoperative myocardial ischemia in patients undergoing coronary artery bypass graft surgery. S.P.I. Research Group, *Anesthesiology* 74:464-473, 1991.

Suga H: Ventricular energetics, *Physiol Rev* 2(70):250, 1990.

Tuman KJ, McCarthy RJ, Spiess BD et al: Effect of pulmonary artery catheterization on outcome in patients undergoing coronary artery surgery, *Anesthesiology* 2:199-206, 1989.

Weiskopf R, Viele M, Feiner J et al: Human cardiovascular and metabolic response to acute, severe isovolemic anemia, *JAMA* 279(3):217-221, 1998.

Zaugg M, Tagliente T, Lucchinetti E et al: Beneficial effects from beta adrenergic blockade in elderly patients undergoing noncardiac surgery, *Anesthesiology* 91(6):1674-1686, 1999.

References

1. Kaukoranta PK, Lepojarvi MV, Kiviluoma KT: Myocardial protection during antegrade versus retrograde cardioplegia, *Ann Thorac Surg* 66:755-761, 1998.

2. Klacke FJ, Mates RE, Canty JM et al: Coronary pressure-flow relationships. Controversial issues and probable implications, *Circ Res* 56:310-323, 1985.

3. Duncker DJ, Van Zon NS, Crampton M et al: Coronary pressure-flow relationship and exercise. Contributions of heart rate, contractility, and α_1-adrenergic tone, *Am J Physiol* H795-H810, 1994.

4. Rainer C, Kawanishi DT, Chardraratna PA et al: Changes in blood rheology in patients with stable angina pectoris as a result of coronary artery disease, *Circulation* 76:15-20, 1987.

5. Boudoulas H, Rittgers SE, Lewis RP et al: Changes in diastolic time with various pharmacologic agents, *Circulation* 60:164-169, 1979.

6. Anderson B, Lomsky M, Waagstein F: The link between acute haemondynamic adrenergic beta-blockade and long-term effects inpatients with heart failure. A study on diastolic function, heart rate, and myocardial metabolism following intravenous metoprolol, *Eur Heart J* 14:1375-1385, 1993.

7. Hongo M, Nakatsuka T, Watanabe N et al: Effects of heart rate on phasic coronary blood flow pattern and flow reserve in patients with normal coronary arteries. A study with an intravascular Doppler catheter and spectral analysis, *Am Heart J* 127:545-551,1994.

8. Dankelman J, Stassen H, Spaan J: System analysis of the dynamic response of the coronary circulation to a sudden change in heart rate, *Med Biol Eng Comp* 28:139-148, 1990.

9. McGinn AL, White CW, Wilson RF: Interstudy variability of coronary flow reserve influence of heart rate, arterial pressure, and ventricular preload, *Circulation* 81:1319-1330, 1990.

10. Indolfi C, Ross JJ: The role of heart rate in myocardial ischemia and infarction. Implications of myocardial perfusion-contraction matching, *Prog Cardiovasc Dis* XXXVI:61-74, 1993.

11. Goto Y, Futaki S, Kawaguchi O et al: Coupling between regional myocardial oxygen consumption and contraction under altered preload and afterload, *J Am Coll Cardiol* 21(6):1522-1531, 1993.

12. Rossi EC, Simon TL, Moss GS, editors: *Principles of transfusion medicine*, Baltimore, 1991, Williams & Watkins.

13. Weiskopf R, Viele M, Feiner J et al: Human cardiovascular and metabolic response to acute, severe isovolemic anemia, *JAMA* 279(3):217-221, 1998.

14. Leung JM, Weiskopf RB, Feiner J et al: Electrocardiographic ST-segment changes during acute, severe isovolemic hemodilution in humans, *Anesthesiology* 93:1004-1010, 2000.

15. Fontana J, Welborn L, Mongan P et al: Oxygen consumption and cardiovascular function in children during profound intraoperative normovolemic hemodilution, *Anesth Analg* 80:219-225, 1995.

16. Rady M, Ryan T, Starr N: Perioperative determinants of morbidity and mortality in elderly patients undergoing cardiac surgery, *Crit Care Med* 26(2):225-235, 1998.

17. Bracey AW, Radovancevic R, Riggs SA et al: Lowering the hemoglobin threshold in coronary artery bypass procedures: effect on patient outcome, *Transfusion* 39:1070-1077, 1999.

18. Weber KT, Janicki JS: The metabolic demand and oxygen supply of the heart: physiologic and clinical considerations, *Am J Cardiol* 44:722-729, 1979.

19. Poldermans D, Boersma E, Bax JJ et al: The effect of bisoprolol on perioperative mortality and myocardial infarction in high-risk patients undergoing vascular surgery. Dutch Echocardiographic Cardiac Risk Evaluation Applying Stress Echocardiography Study Group, *N Engl J Med* 341(24):1789-1794, 1999.

20. Yeager RA, Moneta GL, Ewards JM et al: Reducing perioperative myocardial infarction following vascular surgery. The potential role of beta-blockade, *Arch Surg* 130(8):869-871, 1995.

21. Zaugg M, Tagliente T, Lucchinetti E et al: Beneficial effects from beta adrenergic blockade in elderly patients undergoing noncardiac surgery, *Anesthesiology* 91(6):1674-1686, 1999.

22. Hjalmarson A, Goldstein S, Fagerberg B et al: Effects of controlled-release metoprolol on total mortality, hospitalizations, and well-being in patients with heart failure: the Metoprolol CR/XL Randomized Intervention Trial in congestive heart failure (MERIT-HF), *JAMA* 283(10):1295-1302, 2000.

23. Baan J, Enno T, van der Veld MS et al: Continuous measurement of left ventricular volume in animals and humans by conductance catheter, *Circulation* 70:812-823, 1984.

24. Suga H: Ventricular energetics, *Physiol Rev* 2(70):250, 1990.

25. Shimizu AJ, Mikane T, Mohri S et al: Ventricular pressure-volume area (PVA) accounts for cardiac energy consumption of work production and absorption, *Adv Exp Med Biol* 453:491-497, 1998.

26. Yasumura Y, Nozawa T, Futaki S et al: Minor preload dependence of O_2 consumption of unloaded contraction in dog heart, *Am J Physiol* 256:H1289-1294, 1989.

27. Higashiyama A, Watkins MW, Chen Z et al: Preload does not influence nonmechanical O_2 consumption in isolated rabbit heart, *Am J Physiol* 266:H1047-H1054, 1994.

28. Biddle TL, Yu PN: Effect of furosemide on hemodynamics and lung water in acute pulmonary edema secondary to myocardial infarction, *Am J Cardiol* 43:86-90, 1979.

29. Hill DW: *Physics applied to anaesthesia,* ed 4, London, 1980, Butterworths.

30. Marzocchi A, Piovaccari G, Zimarino M et al: Adjustment of pulmonary capillary wedge pressure for wave delay increase the accuracy of mitral valve area measurement, *J Heart Valve Dis* 4(3):242-246, 1995.

31. Nishimura RA, Rihal CS, Tajik AJ et al: Accurate measurement of transmitral gradient in patients with mitral stenosis: a simultaneous catheterization and Doppler echocardiographic study, *J Am Coll Cardiol* 24:152-158, 1994.

32. Pichard AD, Diaz R, Marchant E et al: Large V waves in the pulmonary capillary wedge pressure tracing without mitral regurgitation: the influence of the pressure/volume relationship on the V wave size, *Clin Cardiol* 6(11):534-541, 1983.

33. West JB, Dollery CT, Naimark A: Distribution of blood flow in isolated lung; relation to vascular and alveolar pressure, *J Appl Physiol* 19:713, 1964.

34. Little WC, Cheng CP: Left Ventricular Systolic and Diastolic Performance. In Warltier DC, editor: *Ventricular function,* Baltimore, 1995, Williams & Watkins.

35. Burkhoff D, de Tombe PP, Hunter WC et al: Contractile strength and mechanical efficiency of left ventricle are enhanced by physiological afterload, *Am J Physiol* 260:H569-H578, 1991.

36. Lawrence WE, Maughan L, Kass DA: Mechanisms of global functional recovery despite sustained postischemic regional stunning, *Circulation* 85:816-827, 1992.

37. Gorcsan J, Shigeki M, Mandarino MS et al: Two-dimensional echocardiographic automated border detection accurately reflects changes in left ventricular volume, *J Am Soc Echocardiogr* 6:482-489, 1993.

38. Eagle KA, Guyton RA, Davidoff R et al: ACC/AHA guidelines for coronary artery bypass graft surgery: executive summary and recommendations: A report of the American College of Cardiology/American Heart Association Task Force on Practice Guidelines (Committee to revise the 1991 guidelines for coronary artery bypass graft surgery), *Circulation* 1000:1464-1480, 1999.

39. Batchelor WB, Anstrom KJ, Muhlbaier LH et al: Contemporary outcome trends in the elderly undergoing percutaneous coronary interventions: results in 7,472 octogenarians. National Cardiovascular Network Collaborations, *J Am Coll Cardiol* 36:723-730, 2000.

40. Suen WS, Mok CK, Chiu SW et al: Risk factors for development of acute renal failure (ARF) requiring dialysis in patients undergoing cardiac surgery, *Angiology* 49:779-800, 1998.

41. Comunale ME, Body SC, Ley C et al: The concordance of intraoperative left ventricular wall motion abnormalities and electrocardiographic S-T segment changes: association with outcome after coronary revascularization. Multicenter Study of Perioperative Ischemia (McSPI) Research Group, *Anesthesiology* 88:945-954, 1998.

42. Tuman KJ, McCarthy RJ, Spiess BD et al: Effect of pulmonary artery catheterization on outcome in patients undergoing coronary artery surgery, *Anesthesiology* 2:199-206, 1989.

43. Reich DL, Bodian CA, Krol M et al: Intraoperative predictors of mortality, stroke, and myocardial infarction after coronary artery bypass surgery, *Anesth Analg* 89:814-822, 1999.

44. Leung JM, Voskanian A, Bellows WH et al: Automated electrocardiograph ST segment trending monitors: accuracy in detecting myocardial ischemia, *Anesth Analg* 87:4-10, 1998.

45. Jain U: Electrocardiographic determination of perioperative myocardial ischemia and stunning, *J Card Surg* 9:413-416, 1994.

46. Brauer A, Weyland W, Fritz U et al: Determination of core body temperature. A comparison of esophageal, bladder, and rectal temperature during postoperative rewarming, *Anaesthesist* 46:683-688, 1997.

47. Cooperman LH, Man EG: Postoperative respiratory care. A review of 65 cases of open heart surgery on the mitral valve, *J Thorac Cardiovasc Surg* 53:504-507, 1967.

48. Zeitlin GL: Artificial respiration after cardiac surgery: some physiological considerations, *Anaesthesia* 20:145-156, 1963.

49. Klineberg PL, Geer RT, Hirsh RA et al: Early extubation after coronary artery bypass graft surgery, *Crit Care Med* 5:272-274, 1977.

50. Prakash O, Jonson B, Meij S et al: Criteria for early extubation after intracardiac surgery in adults, *Anesth Analg* 56:703-708, 1977.

51. Lee TW, Jacobsohn E: Protracheal extubation should occur routinely in the operating room after cardiac surgery, *J Cardiothorac Vasc Anesth* 14:603-610, 2000.

52. Peragallo RA, Cheng DC: Contracheal extubation should not occur routinely in the operating room after cardiac surgery, *J Cardiothorac Vasc Anesth* 14:611-613, 2000.

53. Tomicheck RC, Rosow CE, Philbin DM et al: Diazepam-fentanyl interaction: hemodynamic and hormonal effects in coronary artery surgery, *Anesth Analg* 62:881-884, 1983.

54. Samuleson PN, Reves JG, Kouchoukos NT et al: Hemodynamic responses to anesthetic induction with midazolam or diazepam in patients with ischemic heart disease, *Anesth Analg* 60:802-809, 1981.

55. Muzi M, Berens RA, Kampine JP et al: Venodilation contributes to propofol-mediated hypotension in humans, *Anesth Analg* 74:877-883, 1992.

56. Wang JY, Winship SM, Thomas SD et al: Induction of anesthesia in patients with coronary artery disease: a comparison between sevoflurane-remifentanil and fentanyl-etomidate, *Anaesth Intensive Care* 27:363-368, 1999.

57. Starr NJ, Sethna DH, Estafanous FG: Bradycardia and asystole following the rapid administration of sufentanil with vecuronium, *Anesthesiology* 64:521-523, 1986.

58. Puscas L, Gilau L, Coltau M et al: Calcium channel blockers reduce blood pressure in part by inhibiting vascular smooth muscle carbonic anhydrase I, *Cardiovasc Drug Ther* 14:523-528, 2000.

59. Phillips AS, McMurray TJ, Mirakhur RK et al: Propofol-fentanyl anesthesia: a comparison with isoflurane-fentanyl anesthesia in coronary artery bypass grafting and valve replacement surgery, *J Cardiothorac Vasc Anesth* 8:289-296,1994.

60. Kersten JR, Schmeling TJ, Pagel PS et al: Isoflurane-enhanced recovery of canine stunned myocardium: a role for protein kinase C? *Anesthesiology* 87:699-709, 1997.

61. Ismaeil MS, Tkachenko I, Gamperl AK et al: Mechanisms of isoflurane-induced myocardial preconditioning in rabbits, *Anesthesiology* 90:812-821, 1999.

62. Toller WG, Kersten JR, Gross ER et al: Isoflurane preconditions myocardium against infarction via activation of inhibitory guanine nucleotide binding proteins, *Anesthesiology* 92:1400-1407, 2000.

63. Belhomme D, Peynet J, Florens E et al: Is adenosine preconditioning truly cardioprotective in coronary artery bypass surgery? *Ann Thorac Surg* 70:590-594, 2000.

64. Boutros A, Wang J, Capuano C: Isoflurane and halothane increase adenosine triphosphate preservation, but do not provide additive recovery of function after ischemia, in preconditioned rat hearts, *Anesthesiology* 86:109-117, 1997.

65. Prielipp RC, MacGregor DA, Royster R: Dobutamine antagonizes epinephrine's biochemical and cardiotonic effects: results of an in vitro model using human lymphocytes and a clinical study in patients recovering from cardiac surgery, *Anesthesiology* 89:49-57, 1998.

66. Smith RC, Leung JM, Mangano DT: Postoperative myocardial ischemia in patients undergoing coronary artery bypass graft surgery. S.P.I. Research Group, *Anesthesiology* 74:464-473, 1991.

67. Goldman L, Caldera DL, Nussbaum SR et al: Multifactorial index of cardiac risk in noncardiac surgical procedures, *N Engl J Med* 297:845-850, 1977.

68. Eagle K, Brundage B, Chaitman B et al: Guidelines for perioperative cardiovascular evaluation for noncardiac surgery. A report of the American Heart Association/American College of Cardiology Task Force on Assessment of Diagnostic and Therapeutic Cardiovascular Procedures, *Circulation* 93:1278-1317, 1996.

69. Palda VA, Desky AS: Guidelines for assessing and managing the perioperative risk from coronary artery disease associated with major noncardiac surgery, *Ann Intern Med* 79:661-669, 1997.

70. Detsky A, Abrams H, McLaughlin J et al: Predicting cardiac complications in patients undergoing non-cardiac surgery, *J Gen Intern Med* 1:211-219, 1986.

71. Gilbert K, Larocque BJ, Patrick LT: Prospective evaluation of cardiac risk indices for patients undergoing noncardiac surgery, *Ann Intern Med* 133:384-386, 2000.

72. Kaluza GL, Joseph J, Lee JR et al: Catastrophic outcomes of noncardiac surgery soon after coronary stenting, *J Am Coll Cardiol* 35:1288-1294, 2000.

73. Wallace A, Layug B, Tateo I et al: Prophylactic atenolol reduces postoperative myocardial ischemia. McSPI Research, *Anesthesiology* 88:7-17, 1998.

74. Zaugg M, Tagliente T, Lucchinetti E et al: Beneficial effects from beta-adrenergic blockade in elderly patients undergoing noncardiac surgery, *Anesthesiology* 91:1674-1686, 1999.

75. Urban MK, Markowitz SM, Gordon MA et al: Postoperative prophylactic administration of beta-adrenergic blockers in patients at risk for myocardial ischemia, *Anesth Analg* 90:1257-1261, 2000.

76. Poldermans D, Boersma E, Bax J et al: The effect of bisoprolol on perioperative mortality and myocardial infarction in high-risk patients undergoing vascular surgery, *N Engl J Med* 341:1789-1794, 1999.

77. Mangano D, Browner W, Hollenberg M et al: Association of perioperative myocardial ischemia with cardiac morbidity and mortality in men undergoing noncardiac surgery, *N Engl J Med* 323:1781-1788, 1990.

78. Lehmann KG, Gelman JA, Weber MA et al: Comparative accuracy of three automatic techniques in the noninvasive estimate of central blood pressure in men, *Am J Cardiol* 81:1004-1012, 1998.

79. van Daele M, Sutherland G, Mitchell M et al: Do changes in pulmonary capillary wedge pressure adequately reflect myocardial ischemia during anesthesia? A correlative preoperative hemodynamic electrocardiographic, and transesophageal echocardiographic study, *Circulation* 81:865-871, 1990.

80. Leung J, O'Kelly M, Browner W et al: Are regional wall motion abnormalities detected by transesophageal echocardiography triggered by acute changes in supply and demand? *Anesthesiology* 69:A901, 1988.

81. Christopherson R, Glavan N, Norris E et al: Control of blood pressure and heart rate in patients randomized to epidural or general anesthesia for lower extremity vascular surgery. Perioperative Ischemia Randomized Anesthesia Trial (PIRAT) Study Group, *J Clin Anesth* 8:578-584, 1996.

82. Stone J, Foëx P, Sear J et al: Myocardial ischemia in untreated hypertensive patients: effect of a single small oral dose of a beta-adrenergic blocking agent, *Anesthesiology* 68:495-500, 1988.

83. Stuhmeier K, Mainzer B, Cierpka J et al: Small, oral dose of clonidine reduces the incidence of intraoperative myocardial ischemia in patients having vascular surgery, *Anesthesiology* 85:706-712, 1996.

84. Dodd TM, Stone JG, Cormilas J et al: Prophylactic nitroglycerin infusion during noncardiac surgery does not reduce perioperative ischemia, *Anesth Analg* 76:705-713, 1993.

85. Masaki E, Takinami M, Kurata Y et al: Anesthetic management of high-risk cardiac patients undergoing noncardiac surgery under the support of intraaortic balloon pump, *J Clin Anesth* 11:342-345, 1999.

86. Christopherson R, Beattie C, Frank SM et al: Perioperative morbidity in patients randomized to epidural or general anesthesia for lower extremity vascular surgery. Perioperative Ischemia Randomized Anesthesia Trial Study Group, *Anesthesiology* 79:422-434, 1993.

87. Scheini H, Virtanen T, Kentala E et al: Epidural infusion of bupivacaine and fentanyl reduces perioperative myocardial ischemia in elderly patients with hip fractures—a randomized controlled trial, *Acta Anaesthesiol Scand* 44:1061-1070, 2000.

88. de Leon-Casasola OA, Lema MJ, Karabella D et al: Postoperative myocardial ischemia: epidural versus intravenous patient-controlled analgesia. A pilot project, *Reg Anesth* 20:105-112, 1995.

89. Glantz L, Drenger B, Gozal Y: Perioperative myocardial ischemia in cataract surgery patients: general versus local anesthesia, *Anesth Analg* 91:1415-1419, 2000.

90. Rosenfeld SI, Litinsky SM, Snyder DA et al: Effectiveness of monitored anesthesia care in cataract surgery, *Ophthalmology* 106:1256-1260, 1999.

91. Frank SM, Fleisher LA, Breslow MJ et al: Perioperative maintenance of normothermia reduces the incidence of morbid cardiac events. A randomized clinical trial, *JAMA* 277:1127-1134, 1997.

92. Nelson AH, Fleisher LA, Rosenbaum SH: Relationship between postoperative anemia and cardiac morbidity in high-risk vascular patients in the intensive care unit, *Crit Care Med* 21:860-866, 1993.

93. Roizen MF: Should we all have a sympathectomy at birth? Or at least preoperatively? *Anesthesiology* 68:482-484, 1988.

CHAPTER 8

Valvular Heart Disease

Ashraf M. Ghobashy, M.D. ■ Paul G. Barash, M.D.

OUTLINE

Continued

Tissue (bioprosthetic) valves
  Heterografts
  Homografts

Autografts

Valvular heart disease (VHD) presents as either a congenital or acquired disease. The most common congenital valvular lesion in adults is a bicuspid aortic valve. Acquired valvular heart lesions can be considered the "mirror" image of coronary artery disease (CAD). In patients with CAD, the coronary lesion leads to myocardial structural abnormalities such as a dysfunctional or ruptured papillary muscle secondary to ischemia; these abnormalities in turn lead to valvular dysfunction such as mitral regurgitation (MR). In contrast, patients with VHD have valvular lesions that lead to myocardial hypertrophy and, subsequently, left ventricular hypertrophy (LVH) with resultant myocardial ischemia (e.g., aortic stenosis [AS]). CAD may also coexist with valvular disease.

Knowledge of the etiology and pathophysiology of VHD is important to anesthesiologists. Patients with these lesions can require extensive preoperative evaluation, special intraoperative management, and possible postoperative intensive care. Even in an ambulatory surgical setting, management of the patient with VHD requires extensive preparation to avoid complications and subsequent hospital admission.

PATHOPHYSIOLOGY OF VALVULAR HEART DISEASE

Management of patients with VHD requires an understanding of the pressure and volume loads imposed on the heart by these lesions and the compensatory mechanisms that adapt to these changes (Fig. 8-1). Failure of these compensatory mechanisms provides important clinical signs that must be recognized to manage them and to avoid serious complications.

Valvular lesions that produce an increased afterload, that is, the load against which the ventricle contracts during systole, result in concentric ventricular hypertrophy. This concentric increase in myofibrils becomes the main compensatory mechanism that distributes the pressure or wall stress over a greater mass of myocardium. The consequence of this hypertrophy is increased oxygen demand beyond the coronary supply. This makes the myocardium, particularly the subendocardium, vulnerable to myocardial ischemia. A typical example of this situation is AS.

Valvular lesions that produce an increased preload lead to ventricular dilation. An increase in the initial myocardial fiber length before ventricular contraction is the main compensatory mechanism. Ventricular func-

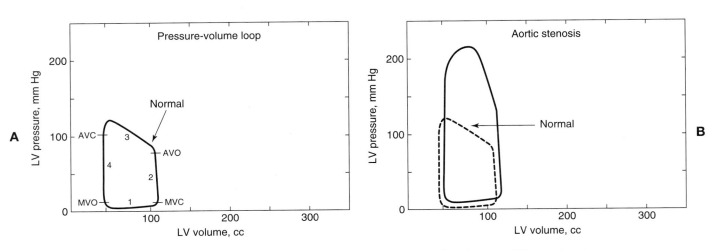

FIG. 8-1 **A,** Normal pressure-volume loop. *AVC,* Aortic valve closure; *AVO,* aortic valve opening; *MVC,* mitral valve closure; *MVO,* mitral valve opening. **B,** Pressure-volume loop for aortic stenosis. *LV,* Left ventricle.

(From Jackson JM, Thomas SJ, Lowenstein E: *Semin Anesth* 1:239, 1982.)

tion deteriorates over time with the development of ventricular failure. Aortic regurgitation and MR are classic examples.

Most valvular lesions lead to pulmonary vascular complications by increasing the left atrial pressure. This in turn is reflected on the pulmonary vasculature by the development of pulmonary venous congestion, interstitial lung edema, and pulmonary arterial hypertension. This leads to right ventricular pressure overload and subsequent right ventricular failure. The decision to manage these lesions surgically must be made in a timely fashion before pulmonary hypertension becomes irreversible.

PREOPERATIVE EVALUATION OF PATIENTS WITH VALVULAR HEART DISEASE

A preoperative workup of the patient with VHD is required to avoid perioperative complications. The extent of this evaluation is tailored to the proposed surgical procedure and the patient's physical status. Accurately defining the goals of the preoperative workup avoids unnecessary and expensive preoperative testing, particularly if the results will not change the perioperative management of the patient (Box 8-1).

History

Patient history will reveal the duration of symptoms related to a specific valvular lesion. Patients subconsciously modify their level of activity to match the limitation imposed by the valvular lesion. Special attention is given to the duration and degree of any change in activity level. The anesthesiologist must elucidate the presence of hemodynamic derangements, failing compensatory mechanisms, and the presence of complica-

tions related to the valvular lesion (e.g., atrial fibrillation, infective endocarditis, or congestive heart failure [CHF]). Symptoms of dyspnea (exertional dyspnea, paroxysmal nocturnal dyspnea, and orthopnea), the presence of CHF, the presence of arrhythmias (atrial fibrillation and/or ventricular arrhythmias), and symptoms of pulmonary vascular congestion are all evaluated preoperatively.

Angina pectoris is an important symptom of CAD but is also a symptom of valvular disease. AS with the resultant LVH leads to angina because of the imbalance between the increased muscle mass and lack of coronary perfusion to the subendocardium. Patients with aortic insufficiency (AI) experience angina because of the low diastolic aortic pressure combined with elevated left ventricular end-diastolic pressure (LVEDP). Decreased coronary perfusion leads to symptoms of angina. $\downarrow$ Coronary perfusion $\Rightarrow$ $\downarrow$ aortic diastolic pressure and $\uparrow$ LVEDP.

Concomitant systemic diseases, especially diabetes mellitus and hypertension, contribute to coronary vascular disease and are important to identify and manage preoperatively. Uncontrolled hypertension leads to large swings in blood pressure intraoperatively. Elevated blood pressure is deleterious to regurgitant lesions and worsens the regurgitant fraction. Low blood pressure is common after anesthetic induction in hypertensive patients. This leads to decreased coronary perfusion and myocardial ischemia.

The nature of the proposed surgery is important information because of the predictable effect on patient outcome in VHD patients. Patients who have had multiple valve replacements, combined valve and coronary artery bypass graft (CABG) procedures, and major abdominal or vascular surgeries have a higher risk of morbidity and mortality. Minor surgeries such as ophthalmologic or distal extremity surgery carry less risk and require less preoperative testing.

Physical Examination

Physical examination should focus on assessment of the cardiac murmur caused by the valvular lesion and its timing, site, intensity, radiation, and characteristics. In addition, systemic manifestations secondary to the valvular lesion (e.g., CHF, infective endocarditis) should also be sought.

Laboratory Workup

A complete blood count is obtained on all patients. The hemoglobin level indicates the degree of cardiorespiratory reserve. Patients with stenotic lesions cannot increase oxygen delivery by increasing cardiac output (CO) and are dependent on adequate oxygen-carrying

---

BOX 8-1
Goals of the Preoperative Workup in Patients with Valvular Heart Disease (VHD)

Determine a specific anatomic diagnosis
Detect the severity of valvular stenosis and/or regurgitation
Determine the pathophysiologic effects of VHD
  Pulmonary (e.g., pulmonary edema)
  Cerebral (e.g., embolization)
  Cardiac (e.g., arrhythmias, such as atrial fibrillation)
  Hepatic (e.g., chronic congestion)
Determine the functional status of the myocardium
  (ejection fraction)
Diagnose concomitant coronary artery disease

capacity. An elevated white blood cell count may differentiate endocarditis from other causes of valvular regurgitation. Serum electrolyte determination is particularly important for patients receiving diuretic medications. Creatinine level is an important indicator of renal function. Arterial blood gas determination reveals acid-base status and indicates the level of cardiorespiratory reserve.

Electrocardiogram

The electrocardiogram (ECG) is important for evaluating the patient's baseline rate, rhythm, and arrhythmias necessitating preoperative treatment, control, optimization, or cardiology consultation. The ECG may demonstrate LVH that requires special attention perioperatively to the myocardial oxygen supply-demand balance and myocardial preservation. Patients with ischemic changes on ECG before and during surgery are vulnerable to increased cardiac morbidity in the postoperative period.[1,2] The preoperative ECG can serve as a baseline for comparison both intraoperatively and postoperatively. The presence of a left bundle-branch block may preclude placement of a pulmonary artery (PA) catheter without myocardial pacing capability.

Chest X-Ray

A chest X-ray (CXR) is essential before surgery for patients with known VHD. The presence of cardiac chamber enlargement (left atrium [LA] in mitral heart disease; left ventricle [LV] in AS, AI, and MR; right ventricle [RV] in tricuspid regurgitation [TR] and pulmonic valvular disease) is easily diagnosed with a CXR. Increased pulmonary vascular markings and cardiomegaly are indicators of pulmonary venous congestion. Pulmonary vascular engorgement represents a redistribution of pulmonary blood flow from the base to the apex of lung fields.

A lateral CXR is beneficial for reoperative procedures by indicating the proximity of the RV to the back of the sternum. An alternative to median sternotomy may be required for cardiac procedures in which the RV is adherent to the sternum. One example is a right thoracotomy approach to mitral valve replacement (MVR).

Echocardiography

Preoperative echocardiography is useful for both anatomic and physiologic evaluation of patients with VHD. Two-dimensional echocardiography provides detailed images of anatomic structure of valve leaflets, such as leaflet thickening, calcification, restriction, mobility and vegetations, and lack of leaflet coaptation. Left ventricular wall thickness and chamber size are indicators of ventricular function and performance.

Color flow Doppler is useful for estimating the degree of valvular regurgitation and identifying coexisting cardiac defects and abnormal blood flow patterns. Pulsed-wave and continuous-wave Doppler echocardiography allow for the measurement of flow velocities across stenotic valves, estimation of gradients, calculation of valve area, and evaluation of regurgitant severity.

Echocardiography is applicable preoperatively by using both the transthoracic and the transesophageal approach, if required. The latter approach has gained much popularity as an intraoperative diagnostic tool capable of providing important data on cardiac performance, valve anatomy and function, intraoperative assessment of valve repair or replacement, cardiac function, and intraoperative hemodynamics. This is especially valuable in patients with VHD, and does not interfere with the conduct of cardiac surgery procedures.

Cardiac Catheterization

Cardiac catheterization is indicated in patients with VHD if there is a discrepancy between the clinical assessment and the results of noninvasive testing. Coronary angiography is recommended before any open heart procedures involving cardiac valve surgery to evaluate the coronary vasculature for possible concomitant intervention. Patients with VHD often have risk factors for CAD such as advanced age, hypercholesterolemia, and hypertension. Patients with known CAD, and patients in whom CAD is suspected to be an etiologic factor in their valve disease (e.g., patients with MR), must have coronary angiography. Combined left- and right-sided cardiac catheterization is beneficial in assessment of patients with left ventricular dysfunction, pulmonary hypertension, or impaired right ventricular function.

In patients with regurgitant valvular lesions, cardiac catheterization provides a qualitative assessment of the degree of regurgitation by visual determination of the washout of dye from the LA in cases of MR, or from the LV in cases of AI. The degree of regurgitation is then expressed on a relative scale of 1+ to 4+, with 4+ representing severe regurgitation.

The regurgitant fraction is calculated during cardiac catheterization as the fraction of the total CO that regurgitates into the receiving chamber (i.e., LA in MR and LV in AI):

$$\text{Regurgitant fraction} = \frac{\text{Total SV} - \text{Forward SV}}{\text{Total SV}}$$

The angiographically measured CO is used to calculate the total stroke volume (SV), by dividing CO by the heart rate. In the presence of valve regurgitation, the angiographic CO is always more than the net forward CO.

The Gorlin equation[3] is used to calculate the stenotic valve area by measuring the pressure gradient across the valve and the CO during ventricular systolic ejection (in the case of the aortic valve), or ventricular diastolic filling (in the case of the mitral valve).

INFECTIVE ENDOCARDITIS PROPHYLAXIS

Infective endocarditis (subacute bacterial endocarditis [SBE]) is an inflammation of the endocardium that is caused by microorganisms and primarily affects heart valves. Prosthetic and intracardiac structures are affected to a lesser degree.

Classification of the disease into acute and subacute has largely been abandoned. At present, SBE is classified on the basis of etiology (organisms involved) and/or the anatomic structures affected by the disease (native or prosthetic valve endocarditis; right- or left-sided endocarditis).

Small thrombi are formed on diseased valve surfaces and on the sewing ring of prosthetic valves. In the setting of bacteremia, these thrombi become infected and a vegetation is formed. The process results in valve tissue destruction and embolization of infected vegetation particles with systemic effects. Vegetations occur most frequently on the ventricular surface of a diseased aortic valve followed by the atrial surface of the mitral and the tricuspid valves.

Once formed, infected vegetations are extremely difficult to eradicate or "sterilize" because fibrin and white blood cells form a barrier around the infective organism, making it difficult for even potent antibiotics to reach the infected nidus of the vegetation. Thus, it is very important to administer prophylactic antibiotics before, during, and after an invasive procedure for any susceptible patient with VHD or a prosthetic valve in place. Guidelines for the latest recommendations of infective endocarditis prophylaxis by the American Heart Association are included in Boxes 8-2 and 8-3 and Tables 8-1 and 8-2.

AORTIC VALVE DISEASE

The aortic valve separates the LV and the ascending aorta. It is composed of three semilunar cusps without a surrounding fibrous ring. The cusps are related to the three sinuses of Valsalva, after which they are named: left coronary (posterior) cusp, right coronary (anterior) cusp, and noncoronary cusp. The main function of the aortic valve is to prevent regurgitation of the left ventricular SV back to the LV during diastole. At the same time, a normal aortic valve offers no resistance to LV systolic ejection; that is, there is no gradient across a normal aortic valve.

BOX 8-2
Cardiac Conditions Associated with Endocarditis

Endocarditis Prophylaxis Recommended
High-risk category
  Prosthetic cardiac valves, including bioprosthetic and homograft valves
  Previous bacterial endocarditis
  Complex cyanotic congenital heart disease (e.g., single ventricle states, transposition of the great arteries, tetralogy of Fallot)
  Surgically constructed systemic pulmonary shunts or conduits
Moderate-risk category
  Most other congenital cardiac malformations (other than above and below)
  Acquired valvular dysfunction (e.g., rheumatic heart disease)
  Hypertrophic cardiomyopathy
  Mitral valve prolapse with valvular regurgitation and/or thickened leaflets

Endocarditis Prophylaxis Not Recommended
Negligible-risk category (no greater risk than the general population)
  Isolated secundum atrial septal defect
  Surgical repair of atrial septal defect, ventricular septal defect, or patent ductus arteriosus (without residual beyond 6 months)
  Previous coronary artery bypass graft surgery
  Mitral valve prolapse without valvular regurgitation
  Physiologic, functional, or innocent heart murmurs
  Previous Kawasaki disease without valvular dysfunction
  Previous rheumatic fever without valvular dysfunction
  Cardiac pacemakers (intravascular and epicardial) and implanted defibrillators

From Dajani AS, Taubert KA, Wilson W et al: *Circulation* 96:358,1997.

Aortic Stenosis

AS is the most common valve disease state encountered by anesthesiologists in the elderly population. The prevalence of aortic valve sclerosis is 29%, and that of AS is 2%. Both states are risk factors for increased mortality in patients older than 65 years.[4]

Of the 54,000 surgical valve procedures performed in the United States in 1994, more than half were aortic valve replacements (AVRs).[5]

Etiology

Calcific AS is the most common cause of patients requiring AVR in the United States and accounts for 51% of cases. Secondary calcification of a bicuspid aor-

with a trileaflet valve.[9] Rheumatic involvement of the aortic valve is characterized by commissural fusion of the valve leaflets and is almost always accompanied by rheumatic mitral valve disease (Fig. 8-2). Obstruction to left ventricular outflow can be caused by aortic valve stenosis, supravalvular stenosis, subvalvular obstruction (e.g., hypertrophic obstructive cardiomyopathy), or subaortic membrane.

Pathophysiology

Obstruction at the **aortic valve** level causes an increased flow velocity across the valve and creates a pressure gradient between the LV and the ascending aorta. In patients with left ventricular dysfunction, both flow velocity across the aortic valve and pressure gradient are lower than expected for a given degree of stenosis. A decreased force of left ventricular contractility cannot generate a high transaortic velocity and pressure gradient.

Left ventricular outflow obstruction leads to chronic left ventricular **pressure overload**. The response of the LV myocardium to progressive pressure overload is concentric hypertrophy. LVH is the adaptive mechanism for maintaining normal wall stress. Increased wall thickness in response to increases in left ventricular pressure distributes wall stress over greater myocardial mass. Contractility is maintained and ejection fraction is preserved until late in the disease course. Diastolic dysfunction is a manifestation of inadequate relaxation in response to increased intraventricular pressure and wall tension and is more common in the elderly patient (>70 years). Doppler echocardiography is useful for evaluating systolic and diastolic dysfunction. A normal transmitral Doppler interrogation is shown in Fig. 8-3. With diastolic dysfunction, the left ventricular Doppler inflow velocity curve shows reduced early diastolic filling velocity (E-velocity), prolonged early diastolic deceleration time, increased time from flow onset to the E-velocity peak, and an increased late diastolic filling velocity with atrial contraction (A-velocity); that is, the E:A ratio is less than 1. With severe systolic dysfunction and an elevated LVEDP, the filling pattern reverses (increased E-velocity, rapid deceleration slope, and reduced A-velocity), reflecting reduced diastolic compliance and an elevated end-diastolic ventricular pressure (restrictive pattern).

Inadequate **coronary blood flow** in the absence of significant coronary atherosclerosis, accounts for the clinical presentation of angina in patients with AS. This limited coronary blood flow results from increased left ventricular mass without a corresponding increase in coronary vessel proliferation to the ventricular muscle. There is an imbalance in the myocardial oxygen demand/supply ratio as left ventricular wall stress and oxygen demands increase out of proportion to the increase in coronary blood flow. Subendocardial blood

tic valve accounts for 36% of cases, and rheumatic disease accounts for no more than 9% of cases.[6]

Contrary to the belief that calcific AS is an age-related process, recent studies suggest that calcification is caused by an active disease process.[7] A congenital bicuspid aortic valve occurs in 1% to 2% of the population,[8] and presents as calcific AS two decades earlier than calcific AS

TABLE 8-1

American Heart Association Recommended Antibiotic Prophylaxis for Dental, Oral, Respiratory Tract, and Esophageal Procedures

	DRUG	DOSING REGIMEN
Standard general prophylaxis	Amoxicillin	Adult: 2.0 g; child: 50 mg/kg PO 1 hr before procedure
Unable to take oral medications	Ampicillin	Adult: 2.0 g IM or IV; child: 50 mg/kg IM or IV 30 min before procedure
Allergic to penicillin	Clindamycin **or**	Adult: 600 mg; child: 20 mg/kg PO 1 hr before procedure
	Cephalexin or cefadroxil **or**	Adult: 2.0 g; child: 50 mg/kg PO 1 hr before procedure
	Azithromycin or clarithromycin	Adult: 500 mg; child: 15 mg/kg PO 1 hr before procedure
Allergic to penicillin and unable to take PO	Clindamycin or cefazolin	Adult: 600 mg; child: 20 mg/kg IV within ½ hr before procedure
		Adult: 1.0 g; child: 25 mg/kg IM or IV within ½ hr before procedure

From Dajani AS, Taubert KA, Wilson W et al: *Circulation* 96:358, 1997.
IM, Intramuscular; *IV,* intravenous; *PO,* by mouth.

TABLE 8-2

Prophylactic Regimens for Genitourinary/Gastrointestinal (Excluding Esophageal) Procedures[22]

SITUATION	AGENTS*	REGIMEN†
High-risk patients	Ampicillin plus gentamicin	Adult: ampicillin 2.0 g IM or IV plus gentamicin 1.5 mg/kg (not to exceed 120 mg) within 30 min of starting procedure; 6 hr later, ampicillin 1 g IM/IV or amoxicillin 1 g orally
		Child: ampicillin 50 mg/kg IM or IV (not to exceed 2.0 g) plus gentamicin 1.5 mg/kg within 30 min of starting the procedure; 6 hr later, ampicillin 25 mg/kg IM/I or amoxicillin 25 mg/kg orally
High-risk patients allergic to ampicillin/amoxicillin	Vancomycin plus gentamicin	Adult: vancomycin 1.0 g IV over 1-2 hr plus gentamicin 1.5 mg/kg IV/IM (not to exceed 120 mg); complete injection/infusion within 30 min of starting procedure
		Child: vancomycin 20 mg/kg IV over 1-2 hr plus gentamicin 1.5 mg/kg IV/IM; complete injection/infusion within 30 min of starting procedure
Moderate-risk patients	Amoxicillin or ampicillin	Adult: amoxicillin 2.0 orally 1 hr before procedure, or ampicillin 2.0 g IM/IV within 30 min of starting procedure
		Child: amoxicillin 50 mg/kg orally 1 hr before procedure, or ampicillin 50 mg/kg IM/IV within 30 min of starting procedure
Moderate-risk patients allergic to ampicillin/amoxicillin	Vancomycin	Adult: vancomycin 1.0 g IV over 1-2 hr; complete infusion within 30 min of starting procedure
		Child: vancomycin 20 mg/kg IV over 1-2 hr; complete infusion within 30 min of starting procedure

From Dajani AS, Taubert KA, Wilson W et al: *Circulation* 96:358, 1997.
IM, Intramuscular; *IV,* intravenous.
*Total children's dose should not exceed adult dose.
†No second dose of vancomycin or gentamicin is recommended.

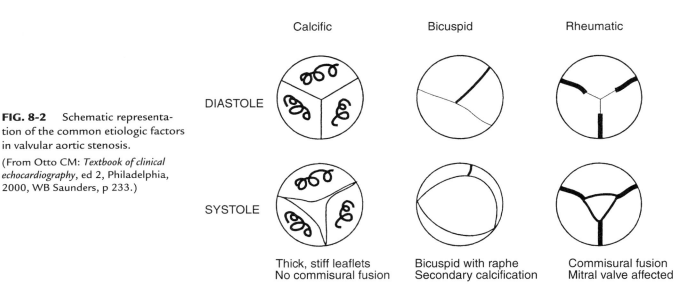

Calcific   Bicuspid   Rheumatic

DIASTOLE

SYSTOLE

Thick, stiff leaflets
No commisural fusion

Bicuspid with raphe
Secondary calcification

Commisural fusion
Mitral valve affected

FIG. 8-2 Schematic representation of the common etiologic factors in valvular aortic stenosis.

(From Otto CM: *Textbook of clinical echocardiography*, ed 2, Philadelphia, 2000, WB Saunders, p 233.)

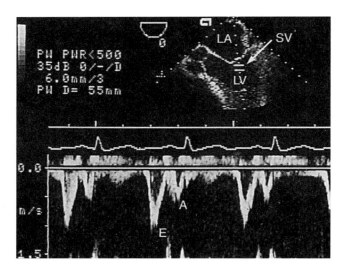

FIG. 8-3 Pulsed-wave Doppler image of a normal left ventricular inflow pattern. *LA,* Left atrium; *LV,* left ventricle; *SV,* sampling volume.

(From Otto CM: *Textbook of clinical echocardiography*, ed 2, Philadelphia, 2000, WB Saunders, p 73.)

flow is further decreased because of impaired early diastolic relaxation and increased diastolic wall stress.

Chronically elevated LVEDP leads to **pulmonary hypertension** in patients with isolated AS. Concurrent pulmonary disease and impaired left ventricular systolic function exacerbates the pulmonary hypertension in these patients. Although pulmonary hypertension increases risk for cardiac surgery, the pulmonary pressure usually returns to normal after AVR.

Asymptomatic patients with AS have slightly decreased **exercise tolerance**. Normal patients increase their CO in response to exercise. Patients with AS have a fixed SV, limiting their exercise tolerance. Increases in

CO must occur by increasing heart rate. This, however, comes at the expense of increased myocardial oxygen demand and decreased supply.

Classification

The normal adult aortic valve orifice is 3.0 to 4.0 cm^2. The degree of AS is graded by aortic valve area as mild (>1.5-2.0 cm^2), moderate (1.0-1.5 cm^2), or severe (<1.0 cm^2). The degree of AS based on mean pressure gradient is graded as mild (<25 mm Hg), moderate (25-50 mm Hg), or severe (>50 mm Hg). As mentioned previously, aortic value gradient is dependent on both CO and aortic valve area. Use of these values for grading the degree of stenosis is predicated on a normal CO.

Aortic valve area is calculated from Doppler echocardiographic data by using the continuity equation, or from cardiac catheterization data by using the Gorlin equation, on the basis of transaortic flow rate and the systolic pressure gradient across the valve.[3] Doppler valve area represents the physiologic orifice area (i.e., cross-sectional area of flow), whereas Gorlin formula valve area represents the anatomic orifice area. Both valve area measurements reflect the same underlying physiologic parameter, and both provide reliable data for clinical decision making when performed correctly and evaluated in context.

Because of its dependence on left ventricular function, the classification of AS based on transvalvular pressure gradient is less reliable than that based on valve area. Patient size and level of activity play an important role in surgical management decisions. A valve area of 1.0 cm^2 in a patient with a large body surface area may be severely debilitating, whereas a valve area of 0.7 cm^2 in a patient with a small body surface area may be well tolerated.

Patients present with different symptomatology irrespective of the severity of their stenosis. Therapeutic corrective surgery is based on the presence or absence of symptoms. Consequently, neither the absolute valve area nor the transvalvular pressure gradient is the primary determinant for AVR.

Symptoms/Clinical Picture

The natural history of AS in the adult consists of a prolonged latent period during which time morbidity and mortality are very low. The latency period for calcific AS is 54 to 78 years, for bicuspid AS is 42 to 54 years, and for rheumatic AS is 21 to 57 years.[10]

The rate of progression of the stenotic lesion in patients with moderate AS, assessed using cardiac catheterization and Doppler echocardiographic studies, is in the range of 0.1 to 0.3 cm^2 per year. Although the systolic pressure gradient across the valve may increase by 6 to 7 mm Hg per year, it is not possible to predict the rate of progression in an individual patient.

Once the symptoms of angina, syncope, or heart failure develop, a critical point in the natural history of AS ensues. Patients' longevity is 3 to 5 years (45 ± 13 months) after the onset of anginal symptoms, 1 to 3 years (27 ± 15 months) after the onset of exertional syncope, and less than 1 to 2 years (11 ± 10 months) after the appearance of CHF.[10] Patients with severe AS require careful monitoring for development of symptoms and disease progression.

Decreased **exercise tolerance** due to exertional dyspnea or fatigue is the most common initial symptom of valvular AS. This symptom occurs because of elevated LVEDP. The sudden onset of heart failure or pulmonary edema can be initiated by an acute infectious process, anemia, or any other hemodynamic stress that leads to acute decompensation in a previously asymptomatic patient.

Exertional angina is another common initial symptom in adults with valvular AS because of an increased oxygen demand by the hypertrophied myocardium.

The third classic symptom of AS is **exertional syncope**. Potential mechanisms of syncope in AS include ventricular arrhythmias and left ventricular systolic dysfunction. Recent evidence supports an acute decrease in blood pressure because of an inappropriate left ventricular baroreceptor response. The elevated ventricular pressure activates baroreceptors that mediate peripheral vasodilation. This in turn leads to severe hypotension in the presence of AS with a fixed CO, and the patient loses conciousness.[11]

Sudden death is known to occur in patients with severe AS. This is most likely because of ventricular arrhythmias. Although sudden death is rare in asymptomatic patients with AS (<2%), it can be as frequent as 10% in symptomatic patients with known severe AS.

The systolic murmur of AS is loudest at the base, over the right second intercostal space. In general, the loudness of the murmur correlates with jet velocity or pres-

sure gradient. The murmur has a crescendo-decrescendo pattern of amplitude and radiates to the carotid arteries in most patients. The second heart sound in severe AS is typically single (not split) because the aortic component is inaudible as a result of impaired motion of the thickened valve leaflets. An S_4 gallop reflects an increased atrial contribution to ventricular filling.

Palpation of carotid and radial pulses reveals slow rise and low amplitude.

Treatment

Medical. Medical therapy is beneficial in the asymptomatic patient with known AS for preventing complications. It is important to recognize the onset of symptoms early, because once symptoms develop, surgical intervention is recommended to relieve symptoms and improve longevity and lifestyle. Patients who are not surgical candidates can benefit from pharmacologic therapy by improvement of symptoms.[11]

Because the timing of surgical intervention is based on symptom onset, the most important parameters to follow are the patient's symptoms and functional status. Repeat echocardiographic examination is indicated before major noncardiac procedures or events. In the absence of new symptoms, routine evaluation at annual intervals is appropriate for patients with moderate or severe stenosis (aortic jet velocity >3.0 m/s). With mild AS (jet velocity 2.0 to 3.0 m/s), evaluation every 2 to 3 years is reasonable in the absence of any change in clinical status or physical examination findings. Asymptomatic patients are referred to surgery if the left ventricular function begins to exhibit deterioration.[12]

Appropriate antibiotic prophylaxis is recommended for all patients with AS undergoing both cardiac and noncardiac procedures. The risk of endocarditis is especially high for patients with a bicuspid aortic valve.

Interventional. Aortic balloon valvuloplasty has a role in the treatment of adolescents and young adults with AS but has a very limited role in older adults with calcific lesions. Immediate hemodynamic improvement includes a moderate reduction (60%) in the transvalvular pressure gradient, but the postvalvotomy valve area is rarely greater than 1.0 cm^2. Serious complications occur with a frequency of greater than 10%, and restenosis and clinical deterioration occur within 6 to 12 months in most patients. For these reasons, balloon valvotomy is not a substitute for AVR in adult patients with AS.

Balloon valvuloplasty has a temporary role in the management of symptomatic patients who are not candidates for AVR. Patients with severe AS and refractory pulmonary edema or cardiogenic shock may benefit from aortic valvuloplasty as a "bridge" to surgery. An improved hemodynamic state will reduce the risks of subsequent AVR. Asymptomatic patients with severe AS who require urgent noncardiac surgery may be candidates for valvuloplasty, but most patients are successfully treated with more conservative measures.[12]

Surgical. The noticeable decrease in the operative mortality of AVR procedures in recent years is related to earlier recognition of symptoms and hence better patient selection. Surgical techniques and myocardial preservation have also improved. Recent studies indicate an operative mortality rate of 2.7% to 8.3% for adults younger than 70 years with isolated AS. Older adults have an operative mortality rate of 2.7% to 16% for isolated AS. Operative mortality rates for AVR are related to age, ejection fraction, coexisting CAD and previous myocardial infarction, baseline functional class, atrial fibrillation, hypertension, emergency surgery, and concomitant mitral valve surgery.

If CABG is performed during the same operative session, operative mortality is 4.4% to 12.8% for younger patients and 8% to 21% for the elderly. The operative mortality is doubled in patients with CAD that is not corrected during the same operative session. This is most likely because of inadequate myocardial preservation of the hypertrophied ventricle.[13] Most surgeons prefer to perform concurrent coronary bypass grafting in adults with valvular AS if angiography demonstrates significant coronary artery narrowing.[11]

The question of performing AVR in the patient undergoing coronary bypass grafting with mild to moderate AS is even more controversial. Without surgery, the gradient would be expected to increase by an average rate of 6 to 8 mm Hg per year. One fourth of these patients will require future AVR. The operative mortality of AVR in the setting of previous CABG is 14% to 24%. It is therefore recommended that if the aortic valve gradient is greater than 20 to 25 mm Hg in a patient requiring CABG surgery, AVR should be considered.[14] The operative mortality from an initial AVR/CABG is significantly less than the mortality of AVR with previous CABG. The patient with mild to moderate AS will most likely develop symptoms from AS before reaching the end of expected benefit from CABG.[14]

Anesthesia Management

Preoperative Evaluation. Patients with the physical findings of AS should have selected preoperative testing, including an ECG, a CXR, and an echocardiogram. The ECG reveals LVH in 70% to 80% of patients with severe AS, and left atrial enlargement in 80%. The CXR may be normal, or may reveal increased cardiac silhouette, left ventricular enlargement, left atrial enlargement, manifestations of CHF, poststenotic dilation of the ascending aorta, or aortic valve calcification. The preoperative two-dimensional echocardiogram is valuable for confirming the severity of aortic valve disease and for determining LV size and function, degree of hypertrophy, and presence of other associated valve disease. Doppler echocardiography is useful for measurement of the transvalvular pressure gradient and calculation of valve area. Some patients will require cardiac catheterization and coronary angiography at the time of initial evaluation. This is appropriate if there is a discrepancy between the clinical and echocardiographic examinations or if the patient has angina symptoms and AVR is planned.[12]

Exercise testing in adults with AS is discouraged mainly because of safety concerns. The test has limited diagnostic accuracy when used to assess the presence or absence of CAD in the setting of AS. Exercise testing should not be performed in symptomatic patients. Exercise testing is safe in asymptomatic patients and may provide information not discovered during the initial clinical evaluation. Exercise testing in asymptomatic patients with AS should be performed only under the direct supervision of an experienced physician, with close monitoring of blood pressure and the ECG. Such testing identifies patients who have limited exercise capacity or exercise-induced symptoms despite a negative medical history. An abnormal hemodynamic response (e.g., hypotension) in a patient with severe AS is sufficient reason to consider AVR.[12]

Intraoperative Management (Table 8-3). Anesthetic goals for patients with AS undergoing surgery include maintenance of preload for the noncompliant ventricle, a high afterload in the face of a reduced or fixed CO, a slow (but not too slow) heart rate, and optimal left ventricular contractility. The increased oxygen demands of the hypertrophic ventricle are managed by avoiding ischemia and controlling the autonomic response to surgical stimulation.

Noncardiac surgery. Acute decompensation in the asymptomatic patient with known moderate or severe AS can occur during noncardiac surgery, particularly in the setting of major changes in blood volume or fluid shifts. Preoperative echocardiographic assessment of AS severity and left ventricular function provides the clini-

---

TABLE 8-3
Hemodynamic Management Goals of Patients with Aortic Stenosis

PARAMETER	HEMODYNAMIC GOAL
Preload	Increase to distend the stiff ventricle
Afterload	Avoid decreases in SVR
Rate	Maintain 60-80 beats/min
Contractility	Avoid myocaradial depressants
O$_2$ demand	Increased because of increased LV mass
Rhythm	Maintain sinus rhythm

LV, Left ventricular; *SVR,* systemic vascular resistance.

cian with knowledge of cardiac reserve. Judicious use of invasive intraoperative monitoring is recommended to optimize loading conditions and thus avoid preventable complications of decompensation in these patients. It is especially important to continue monitoring postoperatively until fluid shifts have stabilized.

The CO of patients with moderate to severe AS is described as "fixed" because valve obstruction limits SV. Hypotension caused by afterload reduction cannot be compensated by an increase in CO. Uncompensated arterial vasodilation leads to myocardial ischemia and further decreases in CO. This has led to the avoidance of major conduction anesthesia for noncardiac surgery in patients with AS. Spinal and epidural anesthesia also cause venodilation that reduces effective preload, leading to greater reductions in CO and hypotension. Spinal and epidural anesthesia may be used for specific settings, provided that preload is effectively monitored and maintained, sympathetic blockade is minimized, and hypotension is treated aggressively. Epidural techniques may be preferable to spinal techniques because of the slower onset of sympathetic blockade in the former. Similar to spinal anesthesia, hypotension with epidural anesthesia must be treated aggressively.[15]

Premedication is tailored to left ventricular function and should avoid reduction in systemic vascular resistance (SVR). Prophylactic antibiotics, supplemental oxygen, and the patient's usual medications should all be included in premedication. Intraoperative invasive monitoring depends on the nature of the planned surgery and whether major fluid shifts are expected. The use of PA catheter data is helpful to differentiate hypovolemia from cardiac failure.

General anesthesia induction is accomplished with an agent that neither reduces SVR nor produces myocardial depression. Patients with poor left ventricular function benefit from a narcotic-based anesthetic. Bradycardia, however, reduces CO as a result of the fixed SV and may lead to left ventricular distention. Tachycardia reduces the time for ventricular filling and predisposes the patient to myocardial ischemia by increasing myocardial oxygen demand. The choice of muscle relaxant is important for mediation of the desired hemodynamic effect. Vecuronium is an appropriate choice for a patient with a normal to high heart rate, whereas pancuronium would be appropriate to counteract the bradycardiac effects of a narcotic induction for a patient receiving β-blockers.

Maintenance of anesthesia for patients with normal left ventricular function is accomplished with a low concentration of a volatile anesthetic (to avoid both severe myocardial depression and significant peripheral vasodilatation). Patients with poor left ventricular function may not tolerate even low concentrations of a volatile anesthetic and they will benefit from a narcotic-based anesthetic.

It is essential to maintain sinus rhythm in patients with AS because of the dependence of the CO on left ventricular preload. Bradycardia or nodal rhythm is promptly treated with atropine or a β agonist, depending on the origin of the bradycardia. Care must be taken not to "overtreat" the bradycardia. Tachycardia could be disastrous because of its deleterious effects. Persistent tachycardia should be treated with a β antagonist such as esmolol. β-Blockers should be used with extreme caution. These patients are dependent on endogenous β-adrenergic activity to maintain SV through a stenotic valve. A defibrillator should be available whenever anesthesia is administered to the patient with AS. Atrial fibrillation or flutter severely impairs preload. A rapid ventricular response further compounds the hypotension leading to myocardial ischemia. Should cardiac arrest occur, external cardiac massage is not likely to be effective in these patients.[16]

Cardiac surgery. The choice of premedication is dependent on the patient's preoperative ventricular function, anxiety level, and postoperative extubation planning (i.e., whether the patient is a candidate for "fast tracking").

Arterial cannulation and a central venous introducer are necessities before aortic valve surgery. The benefit of a PA catheter is debatable and depends on ventricular function, institutional bias, surgical preference, and nursing care in the postoperative intensive care unit. The central venous pressure underestimates the LVEDP because of the change in left ventricular compliance associated with LVH. In addition, the pulmonary capillary wedge pressure (PCWP) may also underestimate the LVEDP (premature closure of the mitral valve).

Anesthesia induction is accomplished by using either a narcotic-only technique or a balanced anesthetic technique. Because narcotics have no myocardial depressant action, they can be safely administered as a "sole" anesthetic in patients with poor left ventricular function. Fentanyl (50-75 mcg/kg) or sufentanil (10-15 mcg/kg) can be used safely in this subset of patients. However, because of potential problems with awareness and the need for prolonged postoperative ventilatory support, a balanced anesthetic is preferable. Fentanyl (10-15 mcg/kg) or sufentanil (1-3 mcg/kg) combined with a benzodiazepine and/or a nonopioid induction agent (e.g., etomidate) also provide for a smooth induction. Anesthesia is maintained with repeated narcotic doses or a continuous infusion of sufentanil (1 mcg/kg/hr) and midazolam (0.2 mcg/kg/min) without marked afterload reduction or hemodynamic aberrations. Sufentanil is more effective than fentanyl in blocking the response to surgical stimulation (sternotomy, sternal retraction, and aortic manipulation).[17]

Choice of a neuromuscular blocking agent depends on the resting heart rate and the expected change with induction of anesthesia.[18] In presence of β-blockade, the combination of vecuronium and a narcotic may lead to bradycardia. Pancuronium is a better choice in this situation.

In patients with AS, adequate **preload** is essential to maintain CO. Decreased left ventricular compliance secondary to concentric hypertrophy and increased LVEDP make preload augmentation extremely important in managing these patients. In spite of its limitations, a PA catheter is essential for anesthesia management. Maintenance of **afterload** is necessary to compensate for a "fixed" CO, avoiding the downward spiral of hypotension, decreased coronary perfusion, myocardial ischemia, and further hypotension.

An optimal heart **rate** for the patient with AS is low but not too low (60-80 beats/min), thus avoiding bradycardia in a patient whose fixed SV makes CO "rate dependent." Tachycardia is also deleterious because of its effects on duration of diastole, coronary perfusion, and increased oxygen demand.

CO is maintained to ensure adequate coronary and vital organ perfusion. Myocardial depressants, either anesthetics or negative inotropic drugs, should be used with caution. The use of a β-blocker to control heart rate or treat a supraventricular arrhythmia could be detrimental in patients with left ventricular dysfunction and AS. Coincidentally, these drugs have benefits by reducing tachycardia, protecting against ischemia, and improving diastolic relaxation in these patients.

Adequate **oxygen** supply to the myocardium at risk, particularly in the subendocardial areas, is essential if myocardial ischemia is to be avoided. Hypotension is treated promptly with volume expansion and an α agonist. Phenylephrine is preferable to ephedrine because of the associated bradycardia and tachycardia, respectively.

The atrial "kick" contributes 20% to left ventricular preload and hence CO in patients without AS and normal LV compliance. In patients with advanced AS and secondary reduced left ventricular compliance, this contribution increases to 35% to 40%. This obviates the necessity of maintaining a sinus **rhythm** in patients with AS. Thus, supraventricular arrhythmias, especially atrial fibrillation and flutter, require aggressive treatment with synchronized DC cardioversion.

Surgical protection of the myocardium in the severely hypertrophied ventricle can be challenging. Difficulties in cardioplegia administration in these patients result from the concentric LVH. This is further compromised by concomitant AI that often accompanies the stenotic lesion. Cardioplegic solution is delivered either directly into the coronary ostia or retrogradely via the coronary sinus, should anterograde aortic root delivery be inadequate. If AI coexists with the stenotic lesion, a vent is placed via a pulmonary vein to the LA through the mitral valve and into the LV to avoid its distention during cardiopulmonary bypass (CPB).

Following valve replacement and hypothermic CPB, reduction in the transvalvular gradient leads to a reduction of end-systolic volume and therefore increased ejection fraction and CO. Patients with preserved left ventricular function exhibit a mild improvement in ejection fraction, and those with poor baseline LV systolic function exhibit a dramatic increase in ejection fraction.[19] Vasodilator therapy improves CO in patients with increased afterload following CPB. Systolic dysfunction may exist before CPB or may occur intraoperatively because of inadequate myocardial protection during CPB. Inotropic drugs are used following CPB to augment SV and CO.[15]

Patients with preserved LV function, increased LV wall thickness, and small LV chamber size exhibit a 25% incidence of dynamic midchamber LV outflow obstruction after AVR. These patients have marked hypotension and dyspnea secondary to the impaired outflow that resembles hypertrophic obstructive cardiomyopathy. Systolic anterior mitral valve motion is seen on echo with a small, hyperdynamic LV. Management consists of increasing preload, augmenting afterload, and discontinuing inotropic support. The condition improves during the early postoperative period. However, these patients have a prolonged postoperative course compared with patients without obstruction.[20]

Most patients with normal preoperative LV function exhibit gradual regression of LVH over several years after AVR. However, patients with an ejection fraction less than 50% show less regression of their LVH postoperatively.[21] Hypertension is common after AVR in patients with preserved preoperative left ventricular function. Vasodilators are required postoperatively for treatment of this increase in blood pressure.

Aortic Insufficiency

From 20% to 30% of patients undergoing aortic valve surgery have isolated AI, and another 12% to 30% have combined AS and AI.[22,23] Aortic root dilation and degenerative valve leaflet changes account for the increasing recognition of AI in the aging population.[24]

Etiology

One half of patients undergoing surgery for treatment of AI have aortic root dilation; the other half have a valve leaflet abnormality. Congenital anomalies of the aortic valve associated with AI include bicuspid, monocuspid, quadricuspid, and fenestrated valve. The most common anomaly among these is a bicuspid aortic valve, which in turn is frequently associated with coarctation of the aorta or aortic root dilation.

Rheumatic aortic valve disease is invariably accompanied by mitral valve involvement and is characterized by leaflet thickening and commissural fusion. Isolated rheumatic aortic valve disease is rare. Infective endocar-

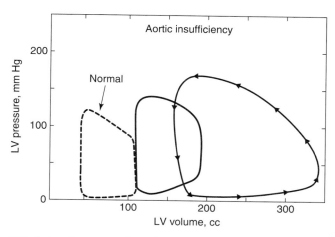

FIG. 8-4 Pressure-volume loop for aortic insufficiency (AI). The middle loop represents acute AI; the far right loop represents chronic AI. *LV,* Left ventricular.

(From Jackson JM, Thomas SJ, Lowenstein E: *Semin Anesth* 1:239, 1982.)

ditis leading to leaflet destruction is another cause of acquired AI.

Aortic root dilation may be congenital, as in sinus of Valsalva aneurysm or Marfan syndrome, or acquired secondary to hypertension, aortic atherosclerotic disease, or cystic medial necrosis. Less common causes of aortic root dilation include syphilitic aortitis, rheumatic arthritis, and ankylosing spondilitis.

Acute AI is less common and accompanies aortic dissection, infective endocarditis with leaflet perforation, or trauma.

Pathophysiology (Fig. 8-4)

Chronic AI is characterized by LV volume overload that is invariably accompanied by pressure overload. This culminates in LV dilation with wall thickening in an attempt to maintain forward SV in compensation for the diastolic regurgitant volume.

Early in the disease process, the LV dilates and thickens with preserved function. Later, with severe AI, dilation becomes more prominent than hypertrophy and the LV systolic function begins to deteriorate. The mitral annulus dilates as the LV dilates, with resultant MR.

AI is characterized by a wide pulse pressure. This occurs because of an increased SV with increased systolic pressure but with a sudden pressure collapse during diastole secondary to the "run off" of regurgitant blood back to the LV through the incompetent valve. The SVR decreases secondary to an increased SV, which in turn decreases the diastolic pressure further. Decreased diastolic pressure decreases coronary perfusion pressure. Myocardial ischemia is worsened by increased O_2 demand secondary to ventricular hypertrophy. This latter effect is not prominent until later in the disease process

when growth of the coronary vasculature is unable to keep up with LV dilation and hypertrophy.

In acute AI, the LV does not compensate for an acute increase in LVEDV by dilation or hypertrophy. Thus the LVEDP rises acutely with development of LV failure and acute pulmonary edema. The LV cannot acutely compensate for the sudden onset of regurgitant SV, reducing both the forward CO and diastolic blood pressure. Myocardial ischemia develops with the acute rise in LVEDP and the decreased coronary perfusion. The low forward SV is partially compensated by tachycardia. The presentation of acute AI is markedly different from chronic AI where physiologic compensatory mechanisms have enough time to develop.

Classification

AI is classified on the basis of acuity (acute vs. chronic) and severity of regurgitation. The severity of AI is quantified by using color flow Doppler echocardiography. The proximal regurgitant jet width is expressed as a percentage of the left ventricular outflow tract (LVOT) width. AI is mild if jet width is less than 25% of LVOT diameter, moderate if jet width is 25% to 65% of LVOT diameter, or severe if jet width is greater than 65% of LVOT diameter.[25] Further echocardiographic evaluation is described in Chapter 4.

AI is also quantified by using cardiac catheterization: Contrast dye is injected into the ascending aorta and the clearance of dye from the LVOT is noted.

Symptoms/Clinical Picture

Most patients with chronic AI are asymptomatic and are diagnosed incidentally during a routine physical examination. Patients remain asymptomatic for years, even after the diagnosis of moderate or severe AI is made. Symptoms develop insidiously and are often unnoticeable to the patient. Careful history taking and physical examination are pivotal in making this diagnosis. Patients develop LV dysfunction or symptoms requiring surgical intervention at an annual rate of 5%. Risk stratification correlates well with end-systolic dimension (<40 mm or >50 mm).[26]

Patients with chronic AI exhibit symptoms only after LV function deteriorates. The earliest symptom of chronic AI is exertional dyspnea caused by elevation of LVEDP with exercise. Angina occurs with decreases in diastolic blood pressure in presence of LVH. Angina is also a symptom of coexisting CAD, particularly in the elderly patient. Symptoms of LV dysfunction include dyspnea at rest, paroxysmal nocturnal dyspnea, and orthopnea. Syncope and sudden death are rare with chronic AI.

Physical examination of a patient with chronic AI reveals a widened pulse pressure with associated peripheral hemodynamic signs. These include a "water hammer" pulse (Corrigan's sign), finger nail bed systolic pulsations with gentle pressure (Quincke's pulse), head nodding, and a systolic-diastolic bruit over the femoral artery with application of gentle pressure using a stethoscope (Duroziez's sign). The left ventricular apex is laterally displaced and auscultation reveals a normal first heart sound, an exaggerated aortic component of the second sound, and a holodiastolic high pitch murmur at the lower left sternal border. In severe AI, auscultation may reveal a relative AS murmur resulting from increased flow through the aortic valve in the absence of organic AS. Austin Flint murmur is a diastolic rumbling murmur resulting from undulations of the anterior mitral leaflet by the regurgitant jet of AI.

Patients with acute AI usually present with tachycardia, tachypnea, and pulmonary edema. The murmur is characteristically low pitched and present only in early diastole. There are no accompanying peripheral hemodynamic signs or signs of LV apical displacement.

Treatment

Medical. Many patients with chronic AI are asymptomatic even after the early onset of LV dysfunction. Patients with a diagnosis of AI should be evaluated at regular intervals for early detection of LV systolic function deterioration and timely surgical intervention. Endocarditis prophylaxis is recommended for all patients with AI of rheumatic origin, patients with audible murmurs, patients with 2+ or greater regurgitation by Doppler, and patients with a bicuspid aortic valve.

Therapeutic measures that reduce LV afterload are used to reduce LV end-systolic wall stress and reduce the regurgitant fraction. This may reduce the rate of progression of aortic regurgitation and/or LV systolic function deterioration.

Patients with aortic root dilatation warrant surgical intervention on the basis of the extent of the dilatation rather than on the degree of LV function deterioration. An example is the patient with Marfan syndrome in whom surgery is indicated when the aortic root diameter exceeds 1.5 times the normal diameter expected for age.[27] Interim medical therapy in patients with aortic root dilation is β-blocker medication rather than afterload reduction. Negative inotropes decrease the force of systolic contraction and minimize sheer force, thus avoiding expansion of the aortic root.

Surgical. Surgical intervention is the treatment of choice for symptomatic patients with severe AI and LV dysfunction. The decision to operate is more difficult in the asymptomatic patient with moderate to severe disease. The optimal timing of surgery should occur before LV dysfunction becomes irreversible.

Aortic valve repair is advantageous when possible. Examples include resuspension of cusps involved in aortic dissection, and repair of a perforated leaflet or a congenitally fenestrated valve. The Ross procedure is considered for younger patients and provides good hemodynamic outcomes. The procedure consists of an AVR with a pulmonic autograft and a bioprosthetic valve placed in the pulmonic position. It obviates long-term anticoagulation from a mechanical valve but is considered to have increased longevity over a bioprosthetic valve in the aortic position. The procedure has yet to stand the test of time.[28,29]

Stentless bioprosthetic valves and homografts also provide better alternatives in terms of longevity and hemodynamics over conventional tissue valves.[30,31]

Anesthesia Management

Preoperative Evaluation. Besides history and physical examination, preoperative workup includes CXR, ECG, and echocardiography. Cardiac catheterization is performed depending on the symptoms, degree of LV dysfunction, and the nature of the planned surgery (e.g., cardiac surgery necessitates catheterization in all patients).

The ECG demonstrates LVH with strain pattern. ST-T changes can be present even in absence of CAD. A left bundle-branch block is usually associated with left ventricular dysfunction.

CXR reveals an enlarged cardiac silhouette with or without ascending aortic dilation. Both the ECG and CXR manifestations of LV enlargement are expected to regress after surgical correction of AI.

Echocardiography is used to examine the anatomic structure of the aortic valve and the aortic root, assess the severity of AI, and evaluate left ventricular function.

Cardiac catheterization is used to evaluate patients undergoing cardiac surgery. It is used to assess the severity of AI, measure intracardiac pressures, and determine the presence of CAD.

Intraoperative Management (Table 8-4). The anesthetic goals for patients with chronic AI are to maintain LV preload, reduce resistance to forward SV by reduction

TABLE 8-4

Hemodynamic Management Goals in Patients with Chronic Aortic Insufficiency

PARAMETER	HEMODYNAMIC GOAL
Preload	Increase
Afterload	Vasodilators are beneficial
Rate	Avoid slow rate; faster desirable
Contractility	Avoid myocardial depressants
O$_2$ demand	Increased because of increased LV mass
Rhythm	Maintain sinus rhythm

LV, Left ventricular.

of afterload (SVR), avoid slower heart rates that increase diastolic time for regurgitation, and maintain or improve LV contractility. Optimal oxygen supply is important in terms of coronary perfusion pressure and oxygen-carrying capacity because LVH increases oxygen demand.

Noncardiac surgery. Neuraxial regional techniques, either alone or combined with general anesthesia, are usually beneficial for reducing afterload and favoring forward flow. LV preload must be maintained to avoid reduction in CO.

Myocardial depressants are avoided, especially in the patient with severe AI and LV function deterioration. A narcotic-based anesthetic is favored in these patients because of the lack of myocardial depression. However, bradycardia may worsen regurgitation, and could precipitate ventricular distention and elevated LVEDP.

Cardiac surgery. Premedication is administered to avoid anxiety-induced afterload augmentation. Medications that increase venous capacitance with preload reduction or cause bradycardia with prolongation of diastole and worsening of regurgitation are avoided.

Invasive monitoring with arterial and pulmonary arterial catheterization and intraoperative transesophageal echocardiography (TEE) are commonly used for these cases. The PA catheter may underestimate LVEDP in patients with severe AI and markedly elevated LVEDP or acute AI with lack of ventricular compensation. If LV dilation causes MR, the PCWP will overestimate the LVEDP.[15]

Intraoperative TEE provides a baseline examination of the aortic valve and the aortic root anatomy. TEE also provides a baseline assessment of left ventricular function, wall thickness, and end-systolic dimension before CPB. After AVR, TEE is used for evaluation of the prosthetic valve and for detecting paravalvular leaks. After aortic valve repair, TEE provides an immediate assessment of the success of repair intraoperatively.

A narcotic-based technique for both induction and maintenance of anesthesia is preferred for the patient with left ventricular dysfunction. The use of pancuronium as a muscle relaxant is preferred because of its effect on increasing the heart rate, thus reducing the diastolic time during which regurgitation occurs. Increasing the heart rate from 60 to 90 beats/min can reduce LVEDP by reducing regurgitation, thus improving diastolic coronary filling and avoiding subendocardial ischemia.

The use of intraaortic balloon counter pulsation (IABP) is contraindicated in the presence of AI because diastolic augmentation worsens AI and increases LVEDP. With resolution of AI by surgical correction, successful weaning from CPB in patients with LV decompensation may necessitate the use of positive inotropes with IABP.

Immediately following corrective surgery, LVEDP

and LVEDV decrease before resolution of LVH and dilatation. If LV function does not improve within 6 months after AVR, irreversible LV dysfunction is present. The 5-year survival rate reflects these changes after surgery. Survival is 85% to 90% if the LV size returns to normal after surgery but as low as 43% if LVEDP and LVEDV remain elevated.

MITRAL VALVE DISEASE

The mitral valve (MV) is a bileaflet valve that separates the LA and the LV. A normal valve has a surface area of 4 to 6 cm^2. The two leaflets are attached to a fibrous ring. The anterior leaflet comprises two thirds of the surface area and one third of the annular attachment. The posterior leaflet comprises one third of the surface area and is attached to two thirds of the annulus. The leaflets are attached to papillary muscles by the chordae tendinae. There are two papillary muscles, a smaller posterior-medial muscle, and a larger anterior-lateral muscle. The subvalvular apparatus prevents the MV from prolapsing into the LA during ventricular systole. Its role in maintaining the geometry of the LV is important for left ventricular contractility.

Mitral Stenosis

The incidence of rheumatic mitral stenosis (MS) has markedly decreased in the western world over the last four decades. In a European study, MS accounted for 43% of all VHD cases in 1960 as opposed to only 9% in 1985.[32]

Etiology

Rheumatic MS is the most common pathologic form of the disease in 99% of excised stenotic mitral valves.[33] However, 40% of patients with rheumatic MS are asymptomatic. Rheumatic involvement of multiple cardiac valves occurs in 38% of patients with MS, with the aortic valve being most frequently involved.[34] Calcific MS as an extension of severe mitral annular calcification in the elderly is rare (3%)[35] and congenital MS is responsible for the disease in less than 1% of patients.

Pathophysiology (Fig. 8-5)

Rheumatic MS is characterized by commissural fusion; thickening and fibrosis of the valve leaflets; and shortening, thickening, and fusion of the chordae tendinae. With disease progression, superimposed calcification of the valvular and subvalvular apparatus ensues. MS results in mechanical obstruction to blood flow from the LA to the LV. A pressure gradient between the LA and the LV occurs during diastole. As obstruction to flow increases, the mean transmitral pressure gradient rises to 10 to 25 mm Hg (normally <5 mm Hg). The gradient increases with the stress of exercise, ane-

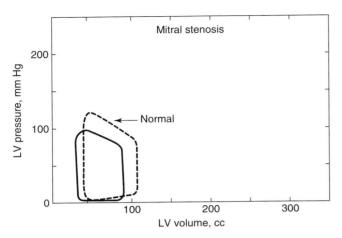

FIG. 8-5 Pressure-volume loop for mitral stenosis. *LV*, Left ventricular.

(From Jackson JM, Thomas SJ, Lowenstein E: *Semin Anesth* 1:239, 1982.)

mia, fever, pregnancy, or MR. Increased flow volume across the valve in diastole leads to hemodynamic decompensation.

Left atrial pressure rises in an attempt to overcome the obstruction and leads to left atrial enlargement and pulmonary venous engorgement.

Left atrial enlargement is complicated by thrombus formation and/or atrial fibrillation. Even with sinus rhythm, left atrial enlargement is accompanied by reduced blood flow velocity that predisposes the patient to atrial thrombus formation. Left atrial dilation often leads to atrial dysrhythmias, most commonly atrial fibrillation.[36] With the development of atrial fibrillation, a multidirectional pattern of blood flow further predisposes to thrombus formation. A left atrial thrombus is found in 17% of patients undergoing surgery for MS; one third of these thrombi are found in the left atrial appendage.[37]

Pulmonary hypertension develops by transmission of pulmonary venous pressure to pulmonary arterial pressure from the high-pressure LA. Pulmonary edema occurs when the pulmonary venous pressure exceeds the plasma oncotic pressure. Increased transudation of fluid into the pulmonary interstitium (i.e., pulmonary edema) leads to decreased lung compliance and increased work of breathing. Clinically, the patient presents with dyspnea on exertion. Patients with MS also exhibit reactive pulmonary arterial vasoconstriction, which also contributes to pulmonary hypertension. Initially, pulmonary hypertension is reversible with relief of the mitral valve obstruction, but once aneurysmal dilation of the arterial wall ensues, the disease state becomes irreversible. Pulmonary hypertension is rare with left atrial pressures less than 20 mm Hg.[38]

Chronic pulmonary hypertension increases with in-creased right ventricular afterload and leads to right ventricular hypertrophy, right ventricular dilation, and eventually right heart failure. Tricuspid valve regurgitation occurs because of tricuspid annular dilation secondary to right ventricular dilation, or because of rheumatic involvement of the tricuspid valve.

Left ventricular function abnormalities are observed in patients with MS.[39] Left ventricular ejection fraction is frequently decreased. The etiology of this ventricular dysfunction is not clear. Left ventricular geometry is distorted by fusion and shortening of the chordae tendineae. Distorted LV geometry can also be the result of the accompanying right ventricular dysfunction and the effects on the interventricular septum.[40] Other etiologic factors include abnormal diastolic filling of the LV, particularly in presence of atrial fibrillation, and a decreased left ventricular preload due to the stenotic valve. Left ventricular function remains depressed in a number of patients, even after successful MV surgery or balloon valvuloplasty.

Classification

The normal MV area is 4.0 to 6.0 cm². Narrowing of the valve area to less than 2.5 cm² must occur before symptoms develop, even with exertion. Mild MS, defined as a valve area greater than 1.5 cm² and a mean gradient less than 5 mm Hg, usually does not produce symptoms at rest. However, severe MS, defined as a valve area less than 1.0 cm² and a mean gradient greater than 25 mm Hg, places the patient in New York Heart Association (NYHA) class III or IV, especially when pulmonary hypertension develops.[12]

Symptoms/Clinical Picture

MS has a long latent period before symptoms appear. The latent period from the onset of rheumatic fever to the development of symptoms ranges from 20 to 40 years. Even after the initial onset of symptoms, 10 years elapse before the symptoms become disabling. The 10-year survival rate, therefore, depends on the severity of symptoms. The 10-year survival rate for asymptomatic patients is 80%. Symptomatic untreated patients have a 50% to 60% 10-year survival rate, and patients with significant symptoms have a 0% to 15% survival rate. The mean survival of patients with severe pulmonary hypertension is less than 3 years.[12] The leading causes of mortality in patients with MS are CHF (60%-70%), systemic embolization (20%-30%), pulmonary embolism (10%), and intercurrent infection (1%-5%).[12]

Patients with mild MS are usually asymptomatic. **Dyspnea** in patients with mild MS is usually precipitated by exercise, emotional stress, infection, pregnancy, or atrial fibrillation with a rapid ventricular response. From 30% to 40% of patients with symptomatic MS develop atrial fibrillation. This complication is more common in older patients and is associated with a worse prognosis. The 10-year survival rate of patients with atrial fibrillation is 25% compared with 46% in patients who remain in sinus rhythm.[12] Loss of atrial contribution to the left ventricular preload and the accompanying rapid ventricular rate are the main causes of hemodynamic decompensation when atrial fibrillation develops in patients with MS. The risk of arterial embolization, especially stroke, is another consequence that significantly increases in patients with atrial fibrillation.

Treatment

Medical. Prophylaxis against rheumatic fever is recommended in patients with MS. Antibiotic endocarditis prophylaxis is also strongly recommended. Patients with moderate or severe MS are advised to avoid physical stress that causes tachycardia. **Negative chronotropic** agents, such as β-blockers or calcium channel blockers, may be of benefit in patients with sinus rhythm who have exertional symptoms with tachycardia. **Diuretics** are useful if there is evidence of pulmonary vascular congestion. **Digitalis** is mainly beneficial in controlling the ventricular response to atrial fibrillation and it may also be of benefit in patients with left and/or right ventricular dysfunction.

Treatment of an acute episode of rapid **atrial fibrillation** consists of anticoagulation with heparin and control of the ventricular response. The ventricular response is controlled with intravenous digoxin, calcium channel blockers, or β-blockers. Hemodynamic instability is an indication for heparin infusion and urgent electrical cardioversion. Atrial fibrillation for more than 24 to 48 hours without anticoagulation places the patient at an increased risk for embolic events after cardioversion. The decision to electively cardiovert depends on the duration of atrial fibrillation, the hemodynamic response to atrial fibrillation, history of prior episodes of atrial fibrillation, and history of prior embolic events. If the patient has been in atrial fibrillation for more than 24 to 48 hours without long-term anticoagulation, one of two approaches is recommended. The first is anticoagulation with warfarin for 3 weeks, followed by elective cardioversion. The second is anticoagulation with heparin and use of TEE to exclude the presence of a left atrial thrombus. Cardioversion is then performed with an intravenous heparin infusion administered before, during, and after the procedure. It is important to continue anticoagulation after cardioversion to prevent thrombus formation caused by atrial mechanical inactivity and then to maintain long-term warfarin therapy unless there is a strong contraindication to anticoagulation.[12]

An embolic event may be the initial manifestation of MS. One third of embolic events occur 1 month after the onset of atrial fibrillation, and two thirds occur within 1 year. Prevention of systemic embolization is essential for patients with rheumatic atrial fibrillation. Systemic embolization occurs in 10% to 20% of patients with MS. Risk factors for embolization in patients with MS are age, atrial fibrillation, and history of previous embolic events. The frequency of embolic events is not related to the severity of MS, CO, size of the LA, or the presence of symptoms.[12]

Interventional. Patients with NYHA functional class II symptoms and moderate or severe stenosis (mitral valve area <1.5 cm^2 or mean gradient >5 mm Hg) are considered for mitral balloon valvotomy if they have suitable mitral valve morphology. Patients with NYHA functional class III or IV symptoms and evidence of severe MS have a poor prognosis if left untreated, and intervention with either balloon valvotomy or surgery is indicated.[12]

Percutaneous mitral balloon valvotomy was initially performed in the mid-1980s. The procedure soon became an accepted alternative to surgical approaches in selected patients (as mentioned earlier). The immediate results of percutaneous mitral valvotomy are comparable to those of mitral commissurotomy. The mean valve area usually doubles (from 1.0 to 2.0 cm^2), and the transmitral gradient decreases by 50% to 60%. The overall success rate is 80% to 95%. Success is defined as a postvalvotomy mitral valve area greater than 1.5 cm^2 and a decrease in left atrial pressure to less than or equal to 18 mm Hg in the absence of complications. Acute complications of the procedure include severe MR (2%-10%) and a residual atrial septal defect. Long-term follow-up studies at 3 to 7 years indicate more favorable hemodynamic and symptomatic results with percutaneous balloon valvotomy than with closed commissurotomy, and results equivalent to those of open commissurotomy. Patients with valvular calcification, thickened fibrotic leaflets with decreased mobility, and subvalvular fusion have a higher incidence of acute complications and a higher rate of recurrent stenosis on follow-up. Patients with noncalcified pliable valves and no calcium in the commissures have a high success rate (>90%), low complication rate (<2%-3%), and sustained improvement in 80% to 90% of patients over a 3- to 7-year period. Relative contraindications to percutaneous balloon valvotomy include left atrial thrombus and significant (3+ to 4+) MR.[12] TEE is a useful test to determine the presence of left atrial thrombus, specifically in the left atrial appendage.

The current recommendations of the ACC/AHA *Task Force on Management of Patients with Valvular Heart Disease*[12] states that in centers with skilled, experienced operators, percutaneous balloon valvotomy should be considered as the initial procedure of choice for symptomatic patients with moderate to severe MS who have a favorable valve morphology in the absence of significant MR or a left atrial thrombus.

Surgical. With the development of CPB in the 1960s, open mitral commissurotomy and replacement of the MV became the surgical procedures of choice for treatment of MS.

The long-term results of open mitral commissurotomy are poor and most patients ultimately require MVR, although the lag time between commissurotomy and valve replacement may be substantial. Open MV commissurotomy is recommended for patients with NYHA functional class III or IV with moderate or severe MS (valve area ≤1.5 cm^2) if percutaneous mitral balloon valvotomy is not available, the patient has a left atrial thrombus despite anticoagulant therapy, or the valve is nonpliable. The decision to repair or replace the valve is made intraoperatively. Significant calcification, fibrosis, and subvalvular fusion of the MV apparatus will prompt an MVR rather than repair.

For the patient with NYHA functional class III symptoms resulting from severe MS or combined MS/MR, MVR provides excellent symptomatic improvement. Postponing surgery until the patient reaches the functional class IV symptomatic state is avoided because operative mortality is high and long-term outcome is suboptimal. Surgery should not be denied if a patient presents in NYHA functional class IV heart failure, because the outlook without surgical intervention is grave. There is controversy about whether asymptomatic or mildly symptomatic patients with severe MS (valve area <1 cm^2) and severe pulmonary hypertension (PA systolic pressure >60-80 mm Hg) should undergo MVR to prevent right ventricular failure, but surgery is generally recommended in such patients. It is recognized that patients with such severe pulmonary hypertension are rarely asymptomatic.[12]

Anesthesia Management

Preoperative Evaluation. The diagnosis of MS is based on history, physical examination, CXR, ECG, and two-dimensional and Doppler echocardiography.

A preoperative **CXR** usually reveals left atrial enlargement with mitralization of the left cardiac border with or without widening of the carinal angle. Manifestations of pulmonary vascular congestion with or without pulmonary edema may also be imaged with redistribution of pulmonary blood flow to the upper lung fields.

A preoperative **ECG** may show P-mitral with or without atrial fibrillation and/or right axis deviation.

The diagnostic tool of choice in the evaluation of a patient with MS is two-dimensional and Doppler **echocardiography.** The morphologic appearance of the MV apparatus is assessed by two-dimensional echocardiography, including leaflet mobility, leaflet thickness, leaflet calcification, subvalvular fusion, and appearance of the commissures. These features may be important when considering the timing and intervention to be performed. Chamber size and function and other structural valvular, myocardial, and pericardial abnormalities should also be assessed.

The hemodynamic severity of the obstruction is assessed with Doppler echocardiography. The transmitral velocity is accurately and reproducibly measured by continuous-wave Doppler. The mean gradient is calculated from the velocity measurements by the modified Bernoulli equation. MV area can be measured by either the diastolic pressure half-time method, the continuity equation, or two-dimensional planimetry.

The pressure half-time method may provide inaccurate estimates of MV area in patients with abnormalities of left atrial or LV compliance, AI, and previous mitral valvotomy.

PA systolic pressure is estimated by using Doppler echocardiographic velocity measurement of a TR jet. Formal hemodynamic exercise testing by supine bicycle or upright treadmill is performed with Doppler interrogation of transmitral and tricuspid velocities. This allows measurement of both the transmitral gradient and PA systolic pressure at rest and with exercise. Dobutamine stress testing is performed in a similar manner.

Cardiac **catheterization** is indicated when there is a discrepancy between Doppler-derived measurements and the clinical status of a symptomatic patient, there is a suspicion of CAD, or the patient is to undergo mitral valve surgery. Absolute left- and right-sided pressure measurements should be obtained during catheterization when there is elevation of PA pressure out of proportion to mean gradient and valve area. Catheterization, including left ventriculography (to evaluate the severity of MR), is indicated when there is a discrepancy between Doppler-derived mean gradient and valve area.

Intraoperative Management (Table 8-5). Anesthetic goals for patients with MS undergoing surgery are main-

TABLE 8-5
Hemodynamic Management Goals in Patients with Mitral and/or Tricuspid Stenosis

PARAMETER	HEMODYNAMIC GOAL
Preload	Maintain
Afterload	Decreased SVR is poorly tolerated; keep high
Rate	Maintain at 60-80 beats/min
Contractility	Maintain within normal
O$_2$ demand	Usually normal
Rhythm	Usually atrial fibrillation; must control ventricular response

SVR, Systemic vascular resistance.

tenance of LV preload without precipitating pulmonary edema, avoiding decreases in SVR in the setting of a "fixed" CO, and maintaining a slower heart rate. Biventricular function and oxygen delivery are maintained while exacerbation of pulmonary hypertension is avoided. The pulmonary vascular resistance increases in response to hypoxia or hypercarbia. A slightly hypocarbic state is preferred. Maintenance of sinus rhythm or a slow ventricular response in patients with atrial fibrillation is also important.

Although maintenance of left ventricular preload is important, avoiding volume overload will reduce the likelihood of pulmonary edema. Central venous or pulmonary pressure monitoring is essential for guiding intravascular volume management.

A slower heart rate provides more time for diastolic filling through the stenotic valve. If the patient is in sinus rhythm, the heart rate should be monitored between 60 and 80 beats/min, using a negative chronotropic agent if necessary. Acute atrial fibrillation and severe hypotension are immediately treated with electrical cardioversion. Atrial fibrillation with mild hypotension can be treated pharmacologically with phenylephrine to support blood pressure and an intravenous β-blocker, a calcium channel blocker, or IV digoxin (see section on treatment).

Noncardiac surgery. Premedication should avoid pharmacologic agents that cause respiratory depression that result in hypoxemia and/or hypercarbia with worsening of pulmonary hypertension. Supplemental oxygen is administered with premedication to avoid hypoxemia. Scopolamine and glycopyrrolate are preferred over atropine because they are less chronotropic. Antibiotic prophylaxis against bacterial endocarditis is essential for these patients (see section on treatment). Digitalis is administered perioperatively if the indication is control of ventricular response to atrial fibrillation. Intraoperative anticoagulant therapy is controversial and must be discussed with the surgeon and cardiologist (see section on anticoagulants). The effect of preoperative diuretic therapy on intravascular volume and serum potassium level should be assessed and adjusted preoperatively.

Anesthesia induction is accomplished with any agent that fulfills the hemodynamic goals of avoiding tachycardia and marked afterload reduction. Ketamine is avoided because of its tachycardiac effects, and propofol may cause deleterious vasodilation. Etomidate is a good choice. Although tachycardia should be avoided, severe bradycardia may cause decreased CO because of the fixed SV. A muscle relaxant with a positive chronotropic effect, such as pancuronium, can balance the bradycardia that can be produced by a narcotic technique. Pancuronium administered without negative chronotropic drugs can increase the ventricular response rate in patients with rapid atrial fibrillation by facilitating conduc-

tion at the atrioventricular node. Tachycardia in the setting of atrial fibrillation may have profound deleterious hemodynamic consequences.

Anesthesia is maintained with either a narcotic-based anesthetic and/or a low concentration of a volatile anesthetic. The use of nitrous oxide (N_2O) in patients with MS is controversial. N_2O may be safe in asymptomatic patients or in those with mild pulmonary hypertension. However, N_2O can worsen pulmonary hypertension in patients with baseline severe pulmonary hypertension.[41] The effects of N_2O on pulmonary pressure should be monitored with a PA catheter in symptomatic patients with profound pulmonary hypertension.

Intraoperative fluid management is challenging given the need to optimize left ventricular preload without overloading the pulmonary circulation. Right ventricular failure secondary to intraoperative pulmonary hypertension will require the use of inotropic drugs, pulmonary vasodilators, or phosphodiesterase inhibitors (i.e., milrinone) on the basis of the pattern of hemodynamic deterioration.

The decision to extubate the patient with MS at the end of a noncardiac procedure should be considered in the anesthetic management plan. This decision is based on baseline cardiorespiratory function and the nature and duration of the operative procedure. Anticholinesterase medications combined with glycopyrrolate are not contraindicated. Extubation is postponed and ventilation supported after major abdominal or thoracic surgical procedures to avoid postoperative hypoventilation that will exacerbate pulmonary hypertension. Appropriate postoperative pain management is important to avoid the associated deleterious tachycardia and hyperdynamic cardiovascular effects.

Cardiac surgery. Premedication should be "light" to avoid respiratory depression (hypercarbia and/or hypoxemia) that will exacerbate pulmonary hypertension. Once premedication is given, supplemental oxygen is administered as part of the premedication. Tachycardia should also be avoided. Digitalis should be continued on the morning of surgery if used for rate control.

Arterial and pulmonary arterial monitoring are necessary for intraoperative management. The PA wave form contains a large "A" wave, which is absent with atrial fibrillation. A prominent "V" wave may be present with concomitant MR. Many clinicians will advance the PA catheter into the PA, but not to a wedge position if pulmonary hypertension is severe. These patients are vulnerable to PA rupture so that unnecessary wedging should be avoided.

Intraoperative TEE is very useful for intraoperative diagnosis and management of patients with MS undergoing corrective MV surgery. The initial intraoperative echocardiographic examination verifies the diagnosis of MS and estimates the MV area and gradient. The pressure half-time method is commonly used to estimate area in the absence of AI. The presence of mitral annular calcification and atrial size are important in guiding the appropriate surgical technique. Baseline assessment of left ventricular function is helpful in anticipating the need for inotropes during weaning from CPB.

MR after mitral commissurotomy is readily detected intraoperatively, allowing early intervention and surgical correction before the patient leaves the operating room. Paravalvular leaks or prosthetic valve dysfunction after MVR is also easily diagnosed and managed within the same operating session.

Ventricular dysfunction during weaning from CPB requires the administration of positive inotropes. Inodilators are particularly beneficial with coexisting pulmonary hypertension. After MVR, pulmonary hypertension should improve over the first few postoperative days. Irreversible pulmonary hypertension with or without LV dysfunction is a poor prognostic sign.

Some patients with preoperative atrial fibrillation revert to sinus rhythm after MVR. Every attempt should be made to keep the patient in sinus rhythm during weaning from CPB and postoperatively. Atrial contraction improves left ventricular preload, and hence CO is optimized during the critical immediate postoperative period.

Mitral Regurgitation

Minimal MR is present in as many as 40% to 80% of the population. The incidence of MR in the general population increases with age.[42] The exact prevalence of MR is difficult to estimate.

Etiology

The most common causes of severe MR requiring surgical intervention are myxomatous MV disease (62%), ischemic dysfunction of the papillary muscle (30%), bacterial endocarditis (5%), and rheumatic heart disease (3%).[43]

Mitral valve prolapse (MVP) was first described as a syndrome in 1966.[44] The condition is present in 5% to 15% of the population. Thus, MVP is estimated to be the most common VHD in the United States. However, a recent report that uses specific echocardiographic criteria in a community-based sample of the population found the prevalence to be a low 2.4%.[45] Complications of MVP are atrial fibrillation, cerebrovascular disease, syncope, heart failure, and MR requiring surgery.

MR can originate from abnormalities of the valve leaflets, chordae tendinae, papillary muscles, or annulus (secondary to left ventricular distention).

Myxomatous degeneration affects the MV **leaflets**, which is most commonly manifested by posterior mitral leaflet thickening with or without chordal

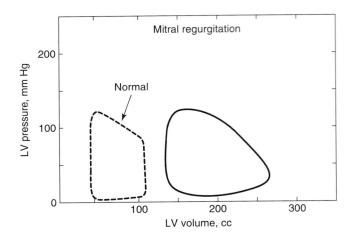

FIG. 8-6   Pressure-volume loop for mitral regurgitation. *LV,* Left ventricular.

(From Jackson JM, Thomas SJ, Lowenstein E: *Semin Anesth* 1:239, 1982.)

rupture. Endocarditis primarily affects the MV leaflets and may cause perforation and probable chordal rupture.

Congenital diseases causing MR include cleft anterior mitral leaflet and Marfan syndrome. Cleft anterior mitral leaflet is commonly associated with primum atrial septal defects. Marfan syndrome involvement of the MV is characterized by anterior mitral leaflet lengthening without thickening or involvement of the subvalvular apparatus, but rarely requires surgical correction.

Mitral **annular** calcification in the elderly is another cause of MR, because of the loss of mitral annular flexibility. This is more common in females and is usually accompanied by AS, hypertension, renal failure, and diabetes mellitus.[46,47]

Mitral annular dilation, with secondary MR, results from left ventricular dilation/failure or dilated cardiomyopathy.

Acute MR carries a poor prognosis if it is not treated surgically. Acute MR is caused by myocardial infarction, trauma, or mitral endocarditis. Posterior papillary muscle dysfunction is more common than anterior papillary muscle dysfunction. The anterior papillary muscle receives blood supply from two coronary arteries, whereas the posterior muscle has a single coronary artery supply. Mitral endocarditis can result in acute MR by leaflet perforation or destruction of the subvalvular apparatus by the infective process.

Pathophysiology (Fig. 8-6)

Chronic Mitral Regurgitation. *Chronic* MR results in left ventricular volume overload, which in turn leads to eccentric hypertrophy and left ventricular dilation. This response, in the early stages of the disease,

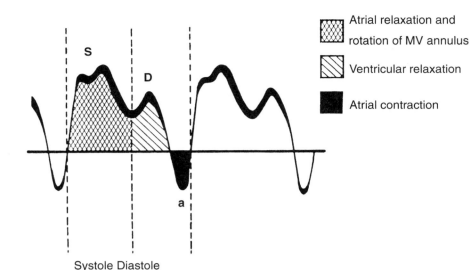

Atrial relaxation and
rotation of MV annulus

Ventricular relaxation

Atrial contraction

Systole Diastole

FIG. 8-7   Schematic representation of a normal pulsed-wave Doppler tracing of pulmonary vein flow. The timing of the systolic (*S*), diastolic (*D*), and atrial contraction (*a*) waveforms are presented. *MV*, Mitral valve.

(From Rafferty TD: *Basics of transesophageal echocardiography*, New York, 1995, Churchill Livingstone, p 86.)

maintains a normal LVEDP with volume overload, that is, elevated LVEDV. The total LV SV increases to compensate for the regurgitant flow. The LA dilates, and as a result, protects the pulmonary vasculature from developing pulmonary hypertension early in the disease process. The consequence of LA distention is atrial fibrillation.

As the degree of MR worsens, LV hypertrophy and dilation are inadequate to maintain a normal forward SV. Left atrial enlargement becomes inadequate in preserving the pulmonary vascular pressure and avoiding pulmonary hypertension. The MV annulus dilates with left ventricular dilation.

Left ventricular dysfunction is masked because the regurgitant SV is directed toward the relatively lower pressure LA. The LA acts as a "pop-off" valve or low afterload for ventricular ejection. As LV function deteriorates and forward SV decreases, reflex pulmonary hypertension ensues with resultant RV failure.

Acute Mitral Regurgitation. *Acute* MR results in a sudden, severe increase in left atrial pressure because of a noncompliant LA. This sudden increase in LA pressure is immediately reflected into the pulmonary circulation with development of pulmonary edema. Left ventricular preload is markedly increased by the regurgitant volume. Reflex sympathetic stimulation causes tachycardia and increased contractility, with an inevitable increase in myocardial O_2 demand and decreased supply (shorter diastole resulting from tachycardia and decreased CO resulting from MR). This adverse myocardial oxygen balance is further complicated if the cause of the acute MR is ischemic in origin (papillary muscle dysfunction or rupture).

Classification
The severity of MR is based on the regurgitant fraction, that is, regurgitant LV SV. MR is considered mild

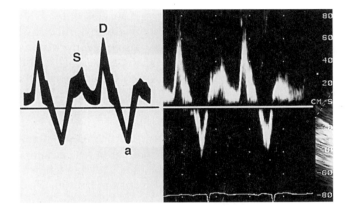

FIG. 8-8   Pulsed-wave Doppler tracing of pulmonary vein flow showing blunting of the systolic wave (*S*) in cases of moderate mitral regurgitation. *a*, Atrial contraction wave; *D*, diastolic wave.

(From Rafferty TD: *Basics of transesophageal echocardiography*, New York, 1995, Churchill Livingstone, p 91.)

(regurgitant fraction <30%), moderate (between 30% and 60%), or severe (>60%).

Qualitative assessment of MR is performed during cardiac catheterization, and is based on the amount of dye that regurgitates to the LA during systole in comparison with forward ejection to the ascending aorta.

Quantitatively, the degree of MR is estimated by using color flow and pulsed-wave Doppler echocardiographic evaluation of the LA and the pulmonary vein flow pattern (Figs. 8-7, 8-8, and 8-9).

Symptoms/Clinical Picture
Patients with myxomatous or rheumatic disease remain asymptomatic for years after the onset of their disease process. Patients with MR secondary to CAD or LV dysfunction present with symptoms of MR with manifestation of the primary disease.

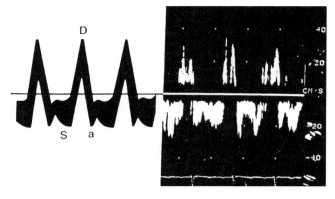

FIG. 8-9 Pulsed-wave Doppler tracing of pulmonary vein flow showing systolic wave (*S*) reversal in severe mitral regurgitation. *a*, Atrial contraction wave; *D*, diastolic wave.

(From Rafferty TD: *Basics of transesophageal echocardiography*, New York, 1995, Churchill Livingstone, p 92.)

Symptoms include easy fatigability, exertional dyspnea, orthopnea, pulmonary congestion, and symptoms of right heart failure (i.e., distended neck veins, hepatic congestion, ankle edema, and ascites). The onset of symptoms in some patients will coincide with the onset of atrial fibrillation. The development of atrial fibrillation in patients with MV disease generally worsens their survival rate.[48]

Atrial fibrillation is present in two thirds of patients with long-standing MR. Cardiac palpation reveals lateral and inferior displacement of the apex. The characteristic MR murmur is holosystolic with maximal intensity at the cardiac apex, and radiation to the left axilla. A midsystolic click with or without a late systolic murmur is auscultated in patients with MVP. Patients with acute MR present with the sudden onset of pulmonary edema and CHF, and occasionally systemic hypotension with cardiovascular collapse.

Treatment
Medical. The therapeutic goal of medical therapy in acute MR is to stabilize the patient by diminishing the degree of MR, increasing forward CO, and reducing pulmonary congestion. Vasodilating drugs (nitroprusside) are useful in the normotensive patient, and may effectively accomplish all three goals. Nitroprusside should not be administered alone to hypotensive patients because of the risk of decreasing diastolic blood pressure and coronary perfusion. Combination therapy with an inotropic agent (e.g., dobutamine) or an inodilator (e.g., milrinone) is beneficial. Aortic balloon counter pulsation is also useful in hypotensive patients with MR because of increases in forward output and mean arterial pressure while regurgitant volume and LV filling pressure are decreased. These measures are used to stabilize the patient while preparing for surgery. Patients with infective endocarditis as the cause of acute MR

benefit from identification and treatment of the infectious organism.

The role of medical therapy in patients with *chronic* symptomatic MR is controversial. These patients need to be managed surgically before deterioration of LV function. The ventricular response rate to atrial fibrillation is controlled with digitalis, calcium channel blockers, β-blockers, or amiodarone. The risk of embolism in patients with MR and atrial fibrillation is less than that of MS and atrial fibrillation. International normalized ratio (INR) should be maintained between 2 and 3 in patients with MR who develop atrial fibrillation.

Patients with MVP who experience palpitations, chest pain, anxiety, or fatigue often respond to β-blocker therapy. First-line therapy is the cessation of stimulants such as caffeine, alcohol, and cigarettes. This may be sufficient to control symptoms.

Daily aspirin therapy (80-325 mg/day) is recommended for patients with MVP and documented focal neurologic events, who are in sinus rhythm without atrial thrombi. Such patients should also avoid smoking cigarettes and using oral contraceptives. Long-term anticoagulation therapy with warfarin (INR 2-3) is recommended for patients who suffer stroke and recurrent transient ischemic attacks while receiving aspirin therapy. Warfarin therapy (INR 2-3) is indicated in patients older than 65 years with MVP and atrial fibrillation and those with MR, hypertension, or a history of heart failure. Aspirin therapy is satisfactory in patients with atrial fibrillation who are younger than 65 years, without MR, hypertension, or heart failure. Daily aspirin therapy is often recommended for patients with high-risk echocardiographic characteristics.[12]

Surgical. There are three surgical approaches to treat MR: mitral valve repair, MVR with preservation of the subvalvular apparatus, and MVR with removal of the subvalvular apparatus.

Mitral valve repair preserves the native MV, preserves LV function by not removing the subvalvular apparatus, and avoids long-term anticoagulation. The procedure is technically demanding. Successful repair is dependent on the skill and experience of the surgeon, particularly if the anterior mitral leaflet is involved. The success rate is lower for repairs involving the anterior mitral leaflet as compared with the posterior leaflet.

MVR with preservation of chordae and papillary muscles helps maintain the LV geometry. The disadvantages of MVR are valve deterioration if a bioprosthetic valve is used and long-term anticoagulation if a mechanical prosthetic valve is used.

MVR with removal of the chordae and papillary muscles is not performed unless the subvalvular apparatus is completely distorted and/or calcified (e.g., rheumatic mitral disease).

Patients with severe MR and symptoms of CHF despite normal LV function with echocardiography (ejection fraction >60% and end-systolic dimension <45 mm) require surgery. The feasibility of MV repair is dependent on several factors, including valve anatomy and surgical expertise. Successful surgical repair improves symptoms, preserves LV function, and avoids problems associated with prosthetic valves. When a repair is not feasible, MV replacement with chordal preservation is the best alternative to relieve symptoms and maintain LV function.[12]

The timing of surgery in asymptomatic patients is more controversial. There seems to be agreement that MV surgery is appropriate with the onset of echocardiographic indicators of LV dysfunction. These indicators include LV ejection fraction less than or equal to 60% and/or LV end-systolic dimension greater than or equal to 45 mm (AHA). Patients with NYHA class III/IV symptoms display excess mortality and morbidity after surgery compared with patients with class I/II symptoms, independent of age or LV function. The recommendation is that early surgery should be considered even when no or minimal symptoms are present to benefit from the better postoperative outcome observed at that stage.[49]

Symptomatic patients with severe MR because of MVP and impaired LV systolic function require cardiac catheterization and evaluation for MV surgery. The thickened, redundant MV can often be repaired rather than replaced, providing lower operative mortality and excellent short- and long-term results.

Management of MVP may require valve surgery, particularly for those who develop a flail mitral leaflet as a result of chordal rupture or marked chordal elongation. Such valves can be successfully repaired by surgeons experienced with MV repair, particularly when the posterior leaflet of the MV is the leaflet that is predominantly affected. Symptoms of heart failure, severity of MR, the presence of atrial fibrillation, LV systolic function, LV end-diastolic and end-systolic volumes, and PA pressure (at rest and during exercise) all influence the decision to recommend MV surgery.

Anesthesia Management

Preoperative Evaluation. History and physical examination focus on abnormalities in the cardiorespiratory system and right heart failure. CXR reveals signs of left atrial enlargement. LV enlargement is observed with advanced disease with or without pulmonary congestion. A preoperative ECG may show atrial fibrillation, left atrial enlargement, and LVH in severe cases.

Preoperative echocardiography is very helpful for both anatomic and functional diagnosis. MV leaflet thickening and doming is characteristic of MS that accompanies MR in rheumatic disease. Thickened, redundant, and prolapsing leaflets with loss of leaflet coaptation, is characteristic of myxomatous disease. A ruptured chord (or chordae) is common in patients

---

TABLE 8-6
Hemodynamic Management Goals of Patients with Mitral Regurgitation

PARAMETER	HEMODYNAMIC GOAL
Preload	Maintain, but do not "overfill"
Afterload	Vasodilators are beneficial
Rate	Avoid slow rate; faster is better except with ischemic MR
Contractility	Avoid myocardial depressants
O_2 demand	Increased because of increased ventricular mass
Rhythm	Usually atrial fibrillation

MR, Mitral regurgitation.

---

presenting for surgery. The echocardiographic criteria for diagnosis of classic MVP are superior displacement of the mitral leaflets of more than 2 mm during systole with a maximal leaflet thickness of at least 5 mm during diastasis. Nonclassic prolapse is defined as displacement of more than 2 mm, with a maximal thickness of less than 5 mm.[45] Left atrial enlargement with left and/or right ventricular enlargement is also observed with an echocardiographic examination.

The severity of MR is assessed by using color and pulsed-wave Doppler echocardiography. Assessment of right and left ventricular function is also important. Preoperative ejection fraction and LV end-systolic diameter predict perioperative outcome in patients with chronic MR undergoing MVR.[50]

Cardiac catheterization is not required for the diagnosis of MVP or MR but is helpful in evaluating associated conditions (e.g., CAD and atrial septal defect). Cardiac catheterization also provides hemodynamic assessment of severe MR, which is important information before MV repair or replacement is considered.

Intraoperative Management (Table 8-6). Anesthetic goals for MR are keeping the patient "full, fast, and vasodilated." These goals include maintenance of left ventricular preload without worsening pulmonary hypertension, reduction of LV afterload to promote forward SV, and a faster heart rate that reduces the regurgitant fraction. Left ventricular contractility is maintained with adequate oxygen supply for the increased myocardial O_2 demand, and therapy to maintain sinus rhythm or an appropriate ventricular response to atrial fibrillation is instituted.

Noncardiac surgery. Antibiotic prophylaxis is an integral part of surgical premedication for all patients with MR undergoing surgery. Preoperative sedation is tailored to the patient's preoperative left ventricular function. The use of invasive intraoperative monitoring is based on the nature of the surgery, the severity of MR, and the baseline LV function. PA catheter data are beneficial for guiding the perioperative use of vasoactive drugs (vasodilators and inotropic drugs), estimating CO, and monitoring ventricular filling pressures. The presence of a "giant V wave" in a PCWP tracing is diagnostic of MR. The size of the "V wave" does not correlate with the severity of MR. Some patients with severe MR may not have a V wave on their PCWP tracing. The presence and size of the V wave depends on the compliance of the LA and the direction of the MR jet. A jet directed toward the left pulmonary venous system may not yield as large a V wave as a jet directed toward the right pulmonary veins if the tip of the PA catheter is in the right lung.

Regional anesthesia with reduction of SVR may be a tempting option for patients with MR. However, regional anesthesia causes acute reduction of both preload and afterload. If regional anesthesia is to be used, the better choice would be epidural anesthesia over spinal anesthesia because of the more controlled and gradual sympathectomy. Sedation administered with regional anesthesia must be titrated carefully to avoid hypoxemia and hypercarbia that may worsen pulmonary hypertension.

General anesthesia requires the selection of an induction agent with minimal myocardial depression. Pancuronium, with its modest tachycardiac effects, is an attractive choice for a muscle relaxant. Anesthesia can be maintained with narcotics and a potent inhalational agent such as isoflurane that possesses the favorable hemodynamic characteristics of mild tachycardia, SVR reduction, and mild myocardial depression.

Postoperative management is equally important for maintaining oxygenation and avoiding hypercarbia, acidosis, and hypothermia. Appropriate pain control avoids the associated hazard of worsening pulmonary hypertension and/or precipitation of CHF because of unwanted increases in afterload secondary to pain or hypercarbia from overzealous analgesic control.

Cardiac surgery. The goals in premedication for cardiac surgery are the same as for noncardiac surgery. Respiratory depressant drugs are used cautiously to avoid hypoxemia and hypercarbia. Supplemental oxygen is part of the premedication.

Intraoperative monitoring includes intraarterial and pulmonary arterial catheterization. A prominent V wave on the PA trace (in the wedged position) is commonly observed in patients with acute MR because of lack of left atrial and pulmonary vascular compliance. The V wave is less prominent in patients with chronic MR.

Anesthetic agents with myocardial depressant properties are avoided. A narcotic-based general anesthetic is preferable, especially in the patient with poor left ventricular function.

Intraoperative TEE provides prebypass evaluation of myocardial contractility, preload, and MV anatomy and function. This information is the basis for surgical decision-making processes about whether to repair or replace the valve and guides the type of repair that would be most suitable for the patient (see earlier section on surgical treatment). A systematic TEE examination, using multiple views, identifies the type and location of the lesion causing MV dysfunction by examination of the different segments of the MV. This precise localization of pathology establishes the mechanism of MR.[51] Intraoperative TEE also guides the perioperative pharmacologic management of hemodynamics in patients with MR. One example is the reduction of the regurgitant fraction with the institution of a systemic vasodilator (e.g., nitroprusside), as observed on the midesophageal four-chamber view by using color flow Doppler imaging. TEE is useful in post-CPB evaluation of MV repair or replacement, with early detection of significant MR or systolic anterior motion after repair or paravalvular leakage after replacement. Left ventricular preload is optimized without overtreating and risking the development of pulmonary hypertension or CHF. Heart rate is maintained in the normal to high range to limit ventricular distention leading to mitral annular dilatation, thus reducing the regurgitant fraction.

Positive inotropic agents may be necessary both before and after the repair. Hemodynamic goals after separation from CPB are optimization of LV loading conditions and contractility. After valve replacement or repair, the LV does not have the low pressure "pop off" in the LA and must eject the entire SV into the aorta, effectively creating a marked increase in afterload for the LV. This can lead to LV strain and/or failure, despite the presence of a reduced LV preload. Positive inotropes are used alone (dobutamine) or in combination with vasodilators (epinephrine and nitroglycerin) to optimize preload, afterload, and contractility. Phosphodiesterase-III inhibitors are useful in patients with preoperative pulmonary hypertension as both positive inotropes and pulmonary vasodilators (inodilators). Nitric oxide as a specific pulmonary vascular dilator is used in patients not responding to isoproterenol or inodilators.

Most patients with atrial fibrillation revert to sinus rhythm immediately after MV repair/replacement. This is usually short lived, and patients remain in sinus rhythm for only a few hours before reverting back to atrial fibrillation. Preservation of the subvalvular apparatus during surgery helps preserve LV function postoperatively. Mortality after mitral valve repair is much lower compared with replacement because of the durability of the repair, lack of postoperative anticoagulation, lower incidence of thromboembolic complications and infective endocarditis, and preservation of LV function. Although some results vary among different studies, most studies indicate a lower mortality with

MV repair. The need for mechanical support of the circulation with an IABP is negligible in patients undergoing MV repair as compared with patients undergoing MVR.[52-55]

TRICUSPID VALVE DISEASE

The tricuspid valve separates the right atrium (RA) and the RV and has a surface area of 7 to 9 cm^2. The tricuspid valve is composed of three leaflets: anterior (the largest), posterior, and septal.[56] The leaflets arise from a fibrous annulus. The leaflet tips are attached by chordae tendinae to two papillary muscles that prevent the valve leaflets from prolapsing into the RA during ventricular systole. Right ventricular dilation is inevitably accompanied by tricuspid valve annular dilation that results in TR.[57]

Tricuspid Regurgitation
Etiology

Functional TR secondary to right ventricular dilation is the most common form of the disease. The RV dilates as a consequence of left-sided failure, pulmonary hypertension, or rheumatic mitral disease. Endocarditis and chest trauma are the main causes of primary TR in adults. Primary congenital TR can be caused by Ebstein's anomaly or carcinoid syndrome. Trace TR is detectable by echocardiography in up to 80% of the population without any ill consequences. Thus, mild TR is considered normal.[58]

Pathophysiology

The RV dilates in response to chronic volume overload caused by TR. Dilation occurs predominately in the short-axis dimension.[59] Initially, the right ventricular function is preserved since the RV is able to compensate for volume overload. Right ventricular systolic dysfunction occurs earlier than left ventricular dysfunction for similar volume overload conditions. The patient enters a vicious cycle of volume overload that leads to right ventricular and annular dilation that leads to worsening TR and more volume overload.

The RV is even less tolerant of pressure overload. Significant right ventricular functional and clinical deterioration occur much earlier when associated with increased pulmonary vascular resistance. Atrial fibrillation complicates right atrial dilation if TR is long standing.

Classification

The degree of TR is classified by noninvasive preoperative echocardiography. The severity of TR is determined by the absolute length of the regurgitant jet or the jet area relative to that of the RA. Pulsed-wave Doppler examination of the hepatic vein flow plays a role in assessing severity of TR that is similar to the pulmonary vein evaluation for MR.

Symptoms/Clinical Picture

Patients with TR present with manifestations of systemic vascular congestion including anorexia, sense of fullness, and lower limb edema. Physical signs include jugular venous congestion with a prominent V wave (also appreciable on a CVP tracing), hepatomegaly, and hepatic dysfunction. The pansystolic murmur of TR is best auscultated at the right sternal border. Patients with secondary TR may also have signs and symptoms of left heart failure.

Treatment

Medical therapy includes salt restriction, diuretics, and digitalis. Surgical management includes annuloplasty, leaflet plication, or valve replacement. Valve replacement is indicated in the setting of valvular destruction (endocarditis) or subvalvular fusion (rheumatic).

Anesthesia Management (Table 8-7)

The anesthetic management of patients with TR includes optimization of right ventricular preload to preserve the RV SV without increasing central venous congestion, maintaining a higher heart rate to decrease annular dilatation, preserving RV contractility, and decreasing pulmonary vascular resistance. Decreasing pulmonary vascular resistance is achieved by avoiding hypoxia, hypercarbia, and N$_2$O.

Positive inotropes with pulmonary vasculature dilating effects are most beneficial in patients with TR and pulmonary hypertension. The inodilators amrinone and milrinone also improve forward SV in these patients. Inhaled N$_2$O is beneficial because of its pulmonary vasodilator action that reduces right ventricular afterload.

Termination of CPB can be challenging after tricuspid valve replacement for TR because of reduced inflow area and elimination of the RV "pop off" into the RA. This serves to place increased strain on the RV, which must eject its entire SV forward against a relatively increased afterload. Preload augmentation and management of RV strain with positive inotropes and/or inodilators are

TABLE 8-7
Hemodynamic Management Goals in Patients with Tricuspid Regurgitation

PARAMETER	HEMODYNAMIC GOAL
Preload	Increase
Afterload	Vasodilators beneficial
Rate	Keep >80 beats/min
Contractility	Avoid myocardial depressants
O$_2$ demand	Increased demand because of increased mass
Rhythm	Usually atrial fibrillation

essential during this critical period. Further options for managing right ventricular failure are a right ventricular assist device or PA balloon counter pulsation if drug therapy is ineffective for separating the patient from CPB. These relatively heroic measures emphasize the importance of pharmacologic therapy in these patients before these options are considered.

Tricuspid Stenosis

Etiology

Tricuspid stenosis (TS) is primarily caused by rheumatic heart disease. Involvement of the tricuspid valve in carcinoid syndrome or systemic lupus erythematosus are causes of TS.

Classification

The normal tricuspid valve area is 7 to 9 cm^2 and the normal gradient across the valve is 1 mm Hg. Valve area reduction below 1.5 cm^2 leads to symptoms of systemic vascular congestion and produces a transvalvular gradient up to 3 mm Hg. Severe stenosis is defined by a valve area less than or equal to 1.0 cm^2 with a gradient of greater than or equal to 5 mm Hg.

Symptoms/Clinical Picture

TS resulting from rheumatic valvulitis is almost always accompanied by MS. The clinical picture in combined MS and TS predominantly resembles MS. TS is manifested by symptoms and signs of systemic venous congestion. These include jugular venous congestion with a prominent A wave, peripheral edema, hepatomegaly, and ascites.

A rumbling murmur is auscultated along the right sternal border.

Treatment

Salt restriction, diuretics, and digitalis serve to optimize the patient's condition before surgery by reducing hepatic congestion, thus improving hepatic function.

Surgical management consists of tricuspid commissurotomy. Tricuspid valve replacement is performed if there is significant valvular calcification or subvalvular stenosis.

Anesthesia Management

PA catheterization is challenging because floatation of a PA catheter through the stenotic tricuspid valve may be difficult. The PA catheter is withdrawn into the RA before the surgeon begins the valve replacement. Alternatively, the PA catheter is not inserted initially. TEE is used for volume and contractility monitoring intraoperatively. The surgeon can also direct a PA catheter through the prosthetic valve before closing the RA or can insert a left atrial catheter.

Anesthetic goals for TS include maintenance of right

ventricular preload without increasing systemic venous congestion, maintaining a slower sinus rhythm for optimal right ventricular diastolic filling, and a normal to higher SVR to maintain the blood pressure with fixed CO.

When TS coexists with MV disease, management of the patient is based on the MV lesion.

ARTIFICIAL CARDIAC VALVES

The decreasing morbidity and mortality of patients with VHD is the result of earlier diagnosis, improved medical management, optimizing the time of intervention, better surgical technique, and sophisticated prosthetic valve designs. The ideal artificial heart valve possesses characteristics and hemodynamics similar to those of the native valve.[60] The availability of multiple artificial valve designs in the market suggests that the ideal heart valve has not been designed yet (Box 8-4).

Artificial heart valves are either mechanical or tissue valves. **Mechanical valves** are classified as *single-disc* valves, *bileaflet* valves, and *ball-cage* valves (Fig. 8-10 and Table 8-8). The major advantage of mechanical valves is durability, and the major disadvantage is thrombogenicity necessitating lifelong anticoagulation.

Tissue valves areas follow: (1) nonhuman or made of pericardial tissue (*heterograft*), (2) harvested from a human at the time of death (*homograft or allograft*), or (3) *autografts* transferred from one position in the heart to another (e.g., pulmonary valve used in the aortic position). The major advantage of tissue valves is their lack of thrombogenicity and the major disadvantage is limited durability.

Mechanical Valves

Mechanical valves are known for their durability, with 10-year survival rates in the 92% to 96% range for the St. Jude valve, 9-year survival rates of 82% to 88% for

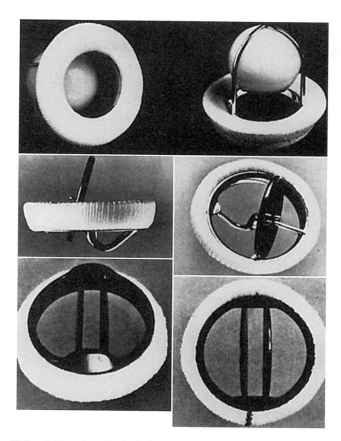

FIG. 8-10 Mechanical heart valves: Starr-Edwards (*top*), Medtronic-Hall (*middle*), and St. Jude Medical (*bottom*).

(From Nottestad SY, Zabalgiotia M: Echocardiographic recognition and quantitation of prosthetic valve dysfunction. In Otto CM, editor: *The practice of clinical echocardiography*, Philadelphia, 1997, WB Saunders, p 798.)

TABLE 8-8
Characteristics of Mechanical Valves

	TILTING DISC	BILEAFLET	BALL-CAGE
Opening angle	60°-80°	75°-90°	N/A
Peak velocity	2 m/sec	Ao: 2.2-3.8 m/s MV: 1.3-1.9 m/s	2 m/sec
Physiologic regurgitation	5-9 ml/ beat	5-10 ml/ beat	2-5 ml/ beat

Modified from Otto CM: *Valvular heart disease*, Philadelphia, 1999, WB Saunders, pp 380-416.
Ao, Aortic valve; *MV*, mitral valve.

the Omnicarbon valve, and 10-year survival rates of 60% to 70% for the Starr-Edwards valve. These valves require lifelong anticoagulation for the patient. Even with appropriate anticoagulant therapy, bileaflet valves have a thromboembolism rate of 0.6% to 1.8% per patient-year and bleeding complications as low as 0.8% to 1.2% per patient-year.

Tilting Disc
Tilting disc mechanical valves include Omniscience, Medtronic-Hall, and Bjork-Shiley prosthetic valves.

A tilting disc valve is composed of a circular disc that is secured within a rigid annulus and hinged with lateral or central metal struts. The disc opens at an angle of 60° to 80°, yielding in two unequal semilunar orifices. Blood velocity through the valve is in the range of 2 m/sec, generating a pressure gradient of 5 to 25 mm Hg in the aortic position and 5 to 10 mm Hg in the mitral position.

A physiologic regurgitant volume of 5 to 9 ml/beat is designed into the valve to reduce thrombogenicity. Frequent thromboembolic complications and strut failure

led to the removal of the Bjork-Shiley valve from the market. The Medtronic-Hall valve is one of the most commonly used prosthetic valves today.

Bileaflet
Bileaflet mechanical valves include St. Jude Medical and CarboMedics valves. A bileaflet valve is composed of two semilunar discs attached to the valve ring by small hinges. The leaflets open at an angle of 75° to 90° with the annular plane, creating a central slitlike opening between the two leaflets and two larger, semicircular openings laterally between the leaflets and the ring.

The peak velocity through these valves ranges between 2.2 and 3.8 m/sec in the aortic position and 1.3 and 1.9 m/sec in the mitral position. A physiologic regurgitant volume of 5 to 10 ml/beat is also designed into these valves and yields three to five regurgitant jets with color flow Doppler echocardiography.

Ball-Cage
The Starr-Edwards valve is the typical example of a ball-cage prosthetic valve, and is the only ball-cage valve in clinical use. The transvalvular velocity is typically 2 m/sec. The disadvantage to this valve design is the associated high shear forces leading to blood and endothelial damage, a high incidence of thrombogenicity, and poor hemodynamic performance. A 2 to 5 ml/beat physiologic regurgitant volume is produced during valve closure.

Tissue (Bioprosthetic) Valves
Heterografts (Fig. 8-11)

Heterografts include porcine and pericardial valves. A native porcine aortic valve is composed of two fibrous leaflets and one muscular leaflet. The muscular leaflet is replaced by a fibrous leaflet from another native valve during manufacturing. Heterograft valves are produced

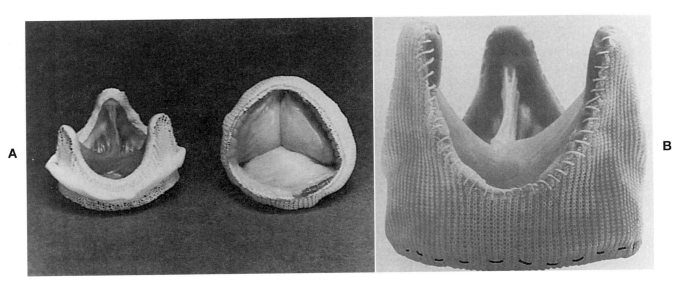

FIG. 8-11 Heterograft tissue valves. **A,** Carpentier-Edwards aortic valve. **B,** Toronto Stentless porcine valve.
(Courtesy St. Jude Medical Heart Valve Division, St Paul, Minn.)

as either *stented* or *stentless*. *Stented heterograft valves* are composed of three fibrous porcine leaflets mounted on a semirigid stent or wires that are conformed to the shape of the annular ring. Stented porcine valves offer suboptimal hemodynamics, in comparison with native valves, resulting from the presence of the rigid sewing ring and stents. The stents maintain the geometry of the valve and facilitate its implantation, but they also decrease hemodynamic efficiency and accelerate valve deterioration and calcification. The peak velocity of a stented porcine aortic valve is 2 to 3 m/sec, with a pressure gradient of 10 to 15 mm Hg. The peak velocity in the mitral position is 1.5 to 2 m/sec, with a peak gradient of 4 to 7 mm Hg. The physiologic regurgitation present in mechanical valves is absent in bioprosthetic valves, although minimal regurgitation is present in up to 10% of normally functioning tissue valves.

Stented porcine valves begin to deteriorate after 5 to 7 years. The rate of deterioration is 3.3% per patient-year, but increases dramatically after 10 years.[61]

Stentless heterograft valves are available for implantation only in the aortic position. The stentless design in these valves improves the hemodynamic profile and reduces valve deterioration over time. Types of prosthetic stentless valves include the Toronto SPV valve, the Edwards stentless valve, the Medtronic *freestyle* valve, and the Cryolife-O'Brien valve. These valves are manufactured from treated porcine valves with the addition of Dacron fabric around the sewing ring. They are either implanted in a subcoronary position, as a miniroot or as total root replacement, where reimplantation of the coronaries is required.

Choosing the appropriate valve size is of significant importance. Implantation of an undersized valve results in overstretching of the leaflets and marked AI. Sizing of

the valve is performed before CPB by using TEE.[62,63] Confirmation of the annular and sinotubular junction diameters is performed by the surgeon with a sizer. The sinotubular junction should not exceed 10% in excess of the diameter of the aortic annulus to avoid stretching of the leaflets and a loss of valve coaptation during diastole, resulting in AI.[30]

More than 95% of patients have minimal or no AI following valve implantation.[64,65] The mean transvalvular gradient is initially 15 mm Hg,[66,67] but decreases by 30% after 6 months, with remodeling of the aortic root and regression of LV hypertrophy.[30,68]

Homografts
Homografts are available for the more commonly used aortic and mostly experimental mitral positions. *Aortic valve homografts* are preferably harvested within 24 hours of the donor's death, and are sterilized with antibiotics and/or cryopreserved. The rationale in preparation is to preserve some viable cells that respond to hemodynamic stress by producing collagen and elastin, thus maintaining valve integrity. Neither donor-recipient matching nor immunosuppression is required with this implantation procedure.

The aortic homograft may be implanted in the subcoronary position by using the valve tissue alone, as an inclusion cylinder inside the native aorta, or preferably as a complete root replacement necessitating reimplantation of the coronaries. The choice of the homograft is based on measurement of both aortic annulus and sinotubular junction diameters either with preoperative angiography or echocardiography.[69] The durability of aortic homografts is yet to be determined, but preliminary data suggest valve failure increasing after 10 years, with a higher rate of deterioration.

Implantation of *mitral homografts* is largely experimental in major academic centers. The homograft is harvested from a human at the time of death and is cryopreserved at $-150°$ C. The homograft is composed of the MV annulus, leaflets, chordae, and papillary muscles.

Mitral homograft implantation is indicated in cases in which reconstructive surgery of the MV is not feasible (i.e., advanced rheumatic mitral disease with calcification and acute infective endocarditis with extensive destruction of the MV leaflets). Advantages of mitral homografts are the lack of lifelong anticoagulation and preservation of the subvalvular apparatus and LV geometry.

Difficulties with MV homografts emerge from either inappropriate tissue conservation (before cryopreservation became the standard practice), or technical difficulties with papillary muscle implantation.[70]

The use of a prosthetic mitral ring annuloplasty is an essential part of the procedure. The ring is required for remodeling a dilated ring (to the size of the graft), alleviation of traction on the circumferential suture line, and reduction of tension on the subvalvular apparatus (by increasing the coaptation surface of the leaflets).[70]

Autografts

The Ross procedure refers to harvesting the pulmonic valve, annulus, and proximal ascending PA, implanting this into the aortic position as a complete aortic root replacement, then reconstruction of the right ventricular outflow tract by using a pulmonary homograft conduit.

Advantages of the Ross procedure include the potential for growth when applied to children, near native hemodynamics, lack of thrombogenicity, and resistance to infection.

Disadvantages include technical difficulties with a double graft valve procedure, limited applicability to children and young adults, and size discrepancy between the aortic and pulmonary roots.[71,72] The discrepancy in size should not be more than 2 to 3 mm. The aortic root should not be greater than 29 mm in diameter, otherwise aortic root reduction is required.[73]

Late pulmonary homograft failure has been reported up to 20 years, necessitating reoperation in 15% to 29% of survivors. Early autograft failure is caused by technical faults or persistent endocarditis. Late autograft failure is caused by aortic annular dilation, valve degeneration, or infective endocarditis.[74]

PERIOPERATIVE MANAGEMENT OF ANTICOAGULATION

Continuous effective anticoagulation is essential for patients with mechanical valves. The increased use of the INR has improved the management of anticoagulation

in patients with VHD. Even with appropriate anticoagulant therapy, bileaflet valves have a thromboembolism rate of 0.6% to 1.8% per patient-year. Single tilting leaflet valves have a thromboembolic frequency of 0.4% to 1.0% in the aortic position[75,76] and 1.5% to 4.6% in the mitral position.[77]

With current therapeutic warfarin dosing and monitoring of effect, bleeding complications are as low as 0.8% to 1.2% per patient-year. On the other hand, the incidence of thromboembolism in patients with heterograft aortic porcine valves is as low as 1.6% per patient-year in the absence of chronic anticoagulation.

Appropriate perioperative anticoagulation management is of particular importance in the patient with a mechanical valve who is undergoing anesthesia and surgery. Anticoagulation should be more aggressive for patients with mechanical valves in the mitral position than in the aortic position because of the higher incidence of thromboembolic accidents. On the other hand, there is a risk of significant bleeding if anticoagulation is maintained perioperatively.[78]

Perioperative therapeutic options for a patient with a mechanical valve in the aortic position are as follows[79]:

1. Discontinue oral anticoagulants several days before the procedure to allow the INR to return to near normal (INR = 1) and reinstitute therapy shortly after surgery.
2. Reduce the anticoagulant dose to maintain a lower subtherapeutic INR during the procedure (INR <1.5).
3. Discontinue oral anticoagulants 3 to 5 days before surgery and institute heparin therapy aimed at prolonging the partial thromboplastin time (PTT) to at least twice the control level. Heparin is then discontinued 2 to 4 hours before surgery and resumed after the surgical procedure when it is considered safe to do so. Thereafter, the oral anticoagulant is reinstituted.[78]

Tinker and Tarhan did not observe any thromboembolic events in 105 patients with mechanical valves in the aortic position when oral anticoagulants were discontinued 1 to 3 days before surgery and resumed 1 to 3 days afterward.[80] The third therapeutic option listed earlier is most suitable for patients with a history of thromboembolic events while receiving oral anticoagulants and for patients with a mechanical valve in the mitral position.[79] Small parenteral doses of vitamin K_1 (0.5-1.0 mg IV) are recommended for use during emergency surgery when the need for rapid reversal of anticoagulants is required.[81] This also allows for reinstitution of postoperative therapeutic anticoagulation.

This approach markedly reduces the INR within 12 to 24 hours without creating a state of relative resistance to oral anticoagulants postoperatively, as would be the case if high-dose vitamin K is given. It is worth mentioning that, to avoid cardiovascular collapse, intravenous vitamin K should not be administered rapidly.[82]

KEY POINTS

1. Knowledge of the etiology and pathophysiology of VHD is important to anesthesiologists because these lesions require extensive preoperative evaluation, special intraoperative management, and possible postoperative intensive-care management.

2. Management of patients with VHD requires an understanding of the pressure and volume loads imposed on the heart by these lesions and the compensatory mechanisms observed in the clinical setting.

3. The normal adult aortic valve orifice is 3.0 to 4.0 cm^2. In terms of the aortic valve area, the degree of AS is graded as mild (area >1.5 cm^2) moderate (area of 1.0-1.5 cm^2), or severe (area <1.0 cm^2). In terms of pressure gradient across the aortic valve, AS is graded as mild (mean gradient <25 mm Hg), moderate (mean gradient of 25-50 mm Hg), or severe (mean gradient >50 mm Hg), provided the CO is normal. These values are used in context of the patient's size and level of activity for surgical management decisions. Therapeutic interventions for corrective surgery are largely based on the presence or absence of symptoms. Once the symptoms of angina, syncope, or heart failure develop, a critical point in the natural history of AS ensues. Sudden death is known to occur in patients with severe AS.

4. Anesthetic goals for patients with AS undergoing surgery are maintaining adequate preload for the noncompliant ventricle, maintaining a high afterload to preserve blood pressure in the setting of a reduced/fixed CO, maintaining a slow heart rate, preserving left ventricular contractility, and fulfilling the increased oxygen demands of the hypertrophic ventricle by avoiding ischemia and controlling the autonomic responses to surgical stimulation.

5. Spinal and epidural anesthesia for patients with AS undergoing noncardiac surgery results in venodilation that reduces effective preload and causes a resultant reduction in CO and hypotension. Spinal and epidural anesthesia may be used in these patients in the appropriate surgical setting, provided that preload is effectively monitored and maintained and the lysis of sympathetic tone is minimized to lower segments. Epidural techniques may be preferable to spinal techniques because of the slower onset of sympatholysis and better control of the anesthetic level.

6. For patients with AS undergoing cardiac surgery, protecting the myocardium of the severely hypertrophied ventricle can be challenging. Lack of adequate myocardial preservation during CPB necessitates the use of positive inotropic drugs to facilitate weaning and separation from CPB. Patients with adequate myocardial protection usually show LV function improvement and regression of LVH after relief of the aortic valve obstruction.

7. One half of patients undergoing surgical treatment of AI have aortic root dilation; the other half have a valve leaflet abnormality. The onset of AI may be acute or chronic. Acute AI does not allow the LV to compensate for the sudden increase in LVEDV.

8. Anesthetic goals for patients with chronic AI are to increase LV preload, reduce resistance to forward SV by reduction of afterload (SVR), avoid slower heart rates that provide increased time for regurgitation, and maintain or improve LV contractility and oxygen supply in the presence of LVH with increased oxygen demand.

9. Whenever applicable, neuraxial regional techniques, either alone or combined with general anesthesia, are usually beneficial for patients with AI undergoing noncardiac surgery by reducing the afterload and favoring forward flow. LV preload must be maintained to avoid a reduction in CO.

10. The use of IABP is contraindicated in the presence of AI because diastolic augmentation will increase AI and LVEDP. Delivery of the cardioplegia solution during cardiac surgery necessitates using direct infusion into the coronary ostia or the retrograde route through a coronary sinus cannula for proper myocardial preservation.

11. After surgical correction of AI, successful weaning from CPB might necessitate the use of positive inotropes and/or IABP, especially in patients with LV dysfunction. LVEDP and LVEDV decrease immediately following corrective surgery, earlier than LVH and dilation.

12. Rheumatic MS is the most common pathologic form of the disease. Obstruction to flow from the LA to the LV results in increased pulmonary venous pressure followed by increased pulmonary arterial pressure and reduced LV filling, particularly when the patient develops atrial fibrillation.

13. The normal MV area is 4.0 to 6.0 cm^2. Mild MS (valve area >1.5 cm^2 and mean gradient <5 mm Hg) usually does not produce symptoms at rest. Severe MS (valve area <1.0 cm^2 and pressure gradient >25 mm Hg) places the patient in NYHA class III or IV when pulmonary hypertension develops.

14. Anesthetic goals for patients with MS undergoing surgery are maintenance of LV preload without producing pulmonary edema, avoidance of decreased SVR because of the "fixed" CO, maintenance of a slower heart rate, maintenance of biventricular contractility and oxygen supply, avoiding exacerbation of pulmonary hypertension, and maintenance of

sinus rhythm or a slow ventricular response in patients with atrial fibrillation.

15. Premedication in patients with MS should avoid respiratory depressant drugs that result in hypoxemia and/or hypercarbia with worsening of pulmonary hypertension. Patients with MS are treated as having a "fixed" CO when considering regional versus general anesthesia for noncardiac surgery. Regional techniques, accompanied by acute, marked afterload reduction (e.g., spinal anesthesia), are used cautiously. Epidural techniques are preferred over spinal techniques because of the better control of the level of sympatholysis.

16. Myxomatous mitral valve disease (MVP) is the most common cause of MR requiring surgical intervention. MVP is present in 2.4% of the population.

17. Acute MR presents with sudden onset of pulmonary edema and CHF, and occasionally with hypotension and cardiovascular collapse. The goals of nonsurgical therapy are to diminish the amount of MR, increase forward CO, and reduce pulmonary congestion. These goals are accomplished with the administration of an arterial vasodilator (e.g., nitroprusside) and by avoiding a reduction in coronary perfusion.

18. MV repair is beneficial by preserving the native MV, preserving LV geometry by retaining the subvalvular apparatus, and avoidance of long-term anticoagulation.

19. Anesthetic goals for patients with MR include maintenance of left ventricular preload without worsening pulmonary hypertension, reduction of LV afterload to promote forward SV, a faster heart rate to help reduce the regurgitant fraction, maintenance of left ventricular contractility with adequate oxygen supply for the increased myocardial O_2 demand, and maintenance of sinus rhythm or a controlled ventricular response with atrial fibrillation.

20. Regional anesthesia, with reduction of SVR, is a good consideration for patients with MR undergoing noncardiac surgery.

21. The use of positive inotropic agents may be necessary both before and after MV repair/replacement for MR. After valve replacement or repair, the LV does not have the low-pressure pulmonary system for systolic ejection. The LV afterload has a higher systemic pressure (SVR). This can lead to LV strain, LV failure and hypotension, and reduced CO and coronary perfusion.

22. Artificial heart valves are either mechanical or tissue valves. The major advantage of mechanical valves is durability and the major disadvantage is thrombogenicity necessitating lifelong anticoagulation. The major advantage of tissue valves is their lack of thrombogenicity and their major disadvantage is limited durability.

23. Tissue valves are nonhuman or made of pericardial tissue (*heterograft*), harvested from a human at the time of death (*homograft or allograft*), or transferred from one position in the heart to another (*autograft*; e.g., pulmonary valve used in the aortic position).

KEY REFERENCES

Bonow RO, Carabello B, de Leon AC Jr et al: ACC/AHA guidelines for the management of patients with valvular heart disease. A report of the American College of Cardiology/American Heart Association Task Force on Practice Guidelines (Committee on Management of Patients with Valvular Heart Disease), *Circulation* 98:1949, 1998.

Carabello BA, Crawford FA Jr: Valvular heart disease, *N Engl J Med* 337:32, 1997.

Dajani AS, Taubert KA, Wilson W et al: Prevention of bacterial endocarditis: recommendations by the American Heart Association, *Circulation* 96:358, 1997.

Freed LA, Levy D, Levine RA et al: Prevalence and clinical outcome of mitral-valve prolapse, *N Engl J Med* 341:1, 1999.

Kearon C, Hirsch J: Management of anticoagulation before and after elective surgery, *N Engl J Med* 336:1506, 1997.

Lambert A-S, Miller JP, Merrick SH et al: Improved evaluation of the location and mechanism of mitral valve regurgitation with a systematic transesophageal echocardiography examination, *Anesth Analg* 88:1205, 1999.

Otto CM: *Valvular heart disease*, ed 1, Philadelphia, 1999, WB Saunders.

Waller BF: *Pathology of the heart and great vessels*, New York, 1988, Churchill Livingstone.

Wells FC, Shapiro LM: *Mitral valve disease*, ed 2, London, 1996, Butterworth-Heinemann.

Willerson JT, Cohn JN, McAllister Jr. HA et al: *Atlas of valvular heart disease: clinical and pathologic aspects*, New York, 1998, Churchill Livingstone.

References

1. Slogoff S, Keats AS: Does perioperative myocardial ischemia lead to postoperative myocardial infarction? *Anesthesiology* 62:107, 1985.

2. Mangano DT, Browner WS, Hollenberg M et al: Association of perioperative myocardial ischemia with cardiac morbidity and mortality in men undergoing non-cardiac surgery, *N Engl J Med* 323:1781, 1990.

3. Gorlin R, Gorlin SG: Hydraulic formula for calculation of the area of the stenotic mitral valve, other cardiac valves, and central circulatory shunts, *Am Heart J* 41:1, 1951.

4. Otto CM, Lind BK, Kitzman DW et al: Association of aortic-valve sclerosis with cardiovascular mortality and morbidity in the elderly, *N Engl J Med* 341:142, 1999.

5. Vital and health statistics, series 13, vol 127, 1995, National Center for Health Statistics.

6. Dare AJ, Veinot JP, Edwards WD et al: New observations on the etiology of aortic valve disease: a surgical pathologic study of 236 cases from 1990, *Hum Pathol* 24:1330, 1993.

7. Otto CM, Kuusisto J, Reichenbach DD et al: Characterization of the early lesion of "degenerative" valvular aortic stenosis: histologic and immunohistochemical studies, *Circulation* 90:844, 1994.

8. Roberts WC: The congenitally bicuspid aortic valve: a study of 85 autopsy cases, *Am J Cardiol* 26:72, 1970.

9. Beppu S, Suzuki S, Matsuda H et al: Rapidity of progression of aortic stenosis in patients with congenital bicuspid aortic valves, *Am J Cardiol* 71:322, 1993.

10. Horstekotte D, Loogen F: The natural history of aortic valve stenosis, *Eur Heart J* 9(suppl E):57, 1988.

11. Otto CM: Aortic stenosis. In Otto CM, editor: *Valvular heart disease*, Philadelphia, 1999, WB Saunders.

12. Bonow RO, Carabello B, de Leon AC Jr et al: ACC/AHA guidelines for the management of patients with valvular heart disease. A report of the American College of Cardiology/American Heart Association Task Force on Practice Guidelines (Committee on Management of Patients With Valvular Heart Disease), *Circulation* 98:1949, 1998.

13. Fremes SE, Goldman BS, Ivanov J et al: Valvular surgery in the elderly, *Circulation* 80(suppl I):177, 1989.

14. Hilton TC: Aortic valve replacement for patients with mild to moderate aortic stenosis undergoing coronary artery bypass surgery, *Clin Cardiol* 23:141, 2000.

15. Frasco P, deBruijn NP: Valvular heart disease. In Estafanous FG, Barash PG, Reves JG, editors: *Cardiac anesthesia-principles and clinical practice*, Philadelphia, 1994, Lippincott.

16. Stoelting RK, Dierdorf SF: *Anesthesia and co-existing disease*, New York, 1993, Churchill Livingstone.

17. Bovill J, Sebel P, Fiolet J et al: The influence of sufentanil on endocrine and metabolic responses to cardiac surgery, *Anesth Analg* 62:391, 1983.

18. Larach D, Hensley FJ, Martin D et al: Hemodynamic effects of muscle relaxant drugs during anesthetic induction in patients with mitral or aortic valvular heart disease, *J Cardiothorac Vasc Anesth* 5:126, 1991.

19. Harpole DH, Jones RH: Serial assessment of ventricular performance after valve replacement for aortic stenosis, *J Thorac Cardiovasc Surg* 99:645, 1990.

20. Bartunek J, Sys SU, Rodrigues AC et al: Abnormal systolic intraventricular flow velocities after valve replacement for aortic stenosis: mechanisms, predictive factors, and prognostic significance, *Circulation* 93:712, 1996.

21. Krayenbuehl HP, Hess OM, Monrad ES et al: Left ventricular myocardial structure in aortic valve disease before, intermediate, and late after aortic valve replacement, *Circulation* 79:744, 1989.

22. Edwards WD: Surgical pathology of the aortic valve. In Waller BF, editor: *Pathology of the heart and great vessels*, New York, 1988, Churchill Livingstone.

23. Fermes SE, Goldman BS, Ivanov J et al: Valvular surgery in the elderly, *Circulation* 80(suppl I):77, 1989.

24. Seder JD, Burke JF, Pauletto FJ: Prevalence of aortic regurgitation by color flow Doppler in relation to aortic root size, *J Am Soc Echocardiogr* 3:316, 1990.

25. Switzer D, Yoganathan A, Nanda N et al: Calibration of color flow Doppler mapping during extreme hemodynamic conditions in vitro: a foundation for a reliable quantitative grading system for aortic incompetence, *Circulation* 75:837, 1987.

26. Bonow RO, Lakatos E, Maron BJ et al: Serial long-term assessment of the natural history of asymptomatic patients with chronic aortic regurgitation and normal left ventricular systolic function, *Circulation* 84:1625, 1991.

27. Legget ME, Unger TA, O'Sullivan CK et al: Aortic root complications in Marfan's syndrome: identification of a lower risk group, *Heart* 75:389, 1996.

28. Sievers HH, Leyh R, Loose R et al: Time course of dimension and function of the autologous pulmonary root in the aortic position, *J Thorac Cardiovasc Surg* 105:775, 1993.

29. Elkins RC, Knott Craig CJ, Razook JD et al: Pulmonary autograft replacement of the aortic valve in the potential parent, *J Card Surg* 9:198, 1994.

30. Del Rizzo DF, Goldman BS, David TE: Aortic valve replacement with a stenless porcine bioprosthesis: multicentre trial. Canadian Investigators of the Toronto SPV Valve Trial, *Can J Cardiol* 11:597, 1995.

31. Knott Craig CJ, Elkins RC, Stelzer PL et al: Homograft replacement of the aortic valve and root as a functional unit, *Ann Thorac Surg* 57:1501, 1994.

32. Horstkotte D, Niehues R, Strauer BE: Pathomorphological aspects, aetiology and natural history of acquired mitral valve stenosis, *Eur Heart J* 12(supp):55, 1991.

33. Olson LJ, Subramanian R, Ackerman DM et al: Surgical pathology of the mitral valve: a study of 712 cases spanning 21 years, *Mayo Clin Proc* 62:34, 1987.

34. Waller BF: Morphological aspects of valvular heart disease. II. *Curr Probl Cardiol* 9:1, 1984.

35. Hammer WJ, Roberts WC, deLeon AC: "Mitral stenosis" secondary to combined "massive" mitral anular calcific deposits and small, hypertrophied left ventricles: hemodynamic documentation in four patients, *Am J Med* 38:814, 1965.

36. Bailey G, Braniff B, Hancock E et al: Relation of left atrial pathology to atrial fibrillation in mitral valvular disease, *Ann Intern Med* 69:13, 1968.

37. Waller BF: Etiology of mitral stenosis and pure mitral regurgitation. In Waller BF, editor: *Pathology of the heart and great vessels*, New York, 1988, Churchill Livingstone.

38. Otto CM: Mitral stenosis. In Otto CM, editor: *Valvular heart disease*, Philadelphia, 1999, WB Saunders.

39. Heller S, Carlton R: Abnormal left ventricular contraction in patients with mitral stenosis, *Circulation* 42:1099, 1970.

40. Gaasch WH, Folland ED: Left ventricular function in rheumatic mitral stenosis, *Eur Heart J* 12(suppl B):66, 1991.

41. Schulte-Sasse U, Hess W, Tarnow J: Pulmonary vascular responses to nitrous oxide in patients with normal and high pulmonary vascular resistance, *Anesthesiology* 57:9, 1982.

42. Yoshida K, Yoshikawa J, Shakudo M et al: Color Doppler evaluation of valvular regurgitation in normal subjects, *Circulation* 78:840, 1988.

43. Waller BF, Morrow AG, Maron BJ et al: Etiology of clinically isolated, severe, chronic, pure mitral regurgitation: analysis of 97 patients over 30 years of age having mitral valve replacement, *Am Heart J* 104:276, 1982.

44. Barlow JB, Bosman CK: Aneurysmal protrusion of the posterior leaflet of the mitral valve: an auscultatory-electrocardiographic syndrome, *Am Heart J* 71:166, 1966.

45. Freed LA, Levy D, Levine RA et al: Prevalence and clinical outcome of mitral-valve prolapse, *N Engl J Med* 341:1, 1999.

46. Korn D, DeSanctis RW, Sell S: Massive calcification of the mitral annulus, *N Engl J Med* 267:900, 1962.

47. Fenster MS, Feldman MD: Mitral regurgitation: an overview, *Curr Probl Cardiol* 20:193, 1995.
48. Cohn LH: Surgery for mitral regurgitation, *JAMA* 260:2883, 1988.
49. Tribouilloy CM, Enriquez-Sarano M, Schaff HV et al: Impact of preoperative symptoms on survival after surgical correction of organic mitral regurgitation: rationale for optimizing surgical indications, *Circulation* 99:400, 1999.
50. Treasure T: Timing of surgery in chronic mitral regurgitation. In Wells FC, Shapiro LM, editors: *Mitral valve disease*, ed 2, London, 1996, Butterworth-Heinemann.
51. Lambert A-S, Miller JP, Merrick SH et al: Improved evaluation of the location and mechanism of mitral valve regurgitation with a systematic transesophageal echocardiography examination, *Anesth Analg* 88:1205, 1999.
52. Dalby A, Firth B, Forman R: Preoperative factors affecting the outcome of isolated mitral valve replacement: a 10 year review, *Am J Cardiol* 47:826, 1981.
53. Yacoub M, Halim M, Radley-Smith R et al: Surgical treatment of mitral regurgitation caused by floppy valves: repair versus replacement, *Circulation* 64(S2):11, 1981.
54. Cohn L, Allred E, Cohn L et al: Early and late risk of mitral valve replacement: a 12 year concomitant comparison of the porcine bioprosthetic and prosthetic disc mitral valves, *J Thorac Cardiovasc Surg* 90:872, 1985.
55. Kawachi Y, Oe M, Asou T et al: Comparative study between valve repair and replacement for pure mitral regurgitation-early and late postoperative results, *Jpn Circ J* 55:443, 1991.
56. Hauck A, Freeman D, Ackerman D et al: Surgical pathology of the tricuspid valve: a study of 363 cases spanning 25 years, *Mayo Clin Proc* 63:851, 1988.
57. Wooley C: Rediscovery of the tricuspid valve, *Curr Probl Cardiol* 6:1, 1981.
58. Otto CM: Etiology and prevalence of valvular heart disease. In Otto CM, editor: *Valvular heart disease*, Philadelphia, 1999, WB Saunders.
59. Bommer W, Weinert L, Neumann A et al: Determination of right atrial and right ventricular size by two-dimensional echocardiography, *Circulation* 60:91, 1979.
60. Cohn LH, Lipson W: Selection and complications of cardiac valvular prostheses. In Baue AE, Geha AS, Hammond GL et al, editors: *Glenn's thoracic and cardiovascular surgery*, Stamford, Conn, 1996, Appleton and Lange.
61. Fann JI, Miller DC, Moore KA et al: Twenty-year clinical experience with porcine bioprostheses, *Ann Thorac Surg* 62:1301, 1996.
62. Walther T, Falk V, Autschbach R et al: Hemodynamic assessment of the stentless Toronto SPV bioprosthesis by echocardiography, *J Heart Valve Dis* 3:657, 1994.
63. Walther T, Autschbach R, Falk V et al: The stentless Toronto SPV bioprosthesis for aortic valve replacement, *Cardiovasc Surg* 4:536, 1996.
64. Goldman BS, David TE, Del Rizzo DF et al: Stentless porcine bioprosthesis for aortic valve replacement, *J Cardiovasc Surg* 35(suppl 1):105, 1994.
65. Wong K, Shad S, Waterworth PD et al: Early experience with the Toronto stentless porcine valve, *Ann Thorac Surg* 60(suppl 2): S402, 1995.
66. Mohr FW, Walther T, Baryalei M et al: The Toronto SPV bioprosthesis: one-year results in 100 patients, *Ann Thorac Surg* 60:171, 1995.
67. Casabona R, De Paulis R, Zattera GF et al: Stentless porcine and pericardial valve in aortic position, *Ann Thorac Surg* 54:681, 1992.
68. Westaby S, Amarasena N, Long V et al: Time related hemodynamic changes after aortic replacement with the freestyle stentless xenograft, *Ann Thocac Surg* 60:1633, 1995.
69. Bartzokis T, St Goar F, DiBiase A et al: Freehand allograft aortic valve replacement and aortic root replacement: utility of intraoperative echocardiography and Doppler color flow mapping, *J Thorac Cardiovasc Surg* 101:545, 1991.
70. Acar C, Tolan M, Berrebi A et al: Homograft replacement of the mitral valve-graft selection, technique of implantation, and results in forty three patients, *J Thorac Cardiovasc Surg* 111:367, 1996.
71. Ross DN: Replacement of aortic and mitral valves with a pulmonary autograft, *Lancet* 2:956, 1967.
72. Ross DN: Aortic root replacement with a pulmonary autograft-current trends, *J Heart Valve Dis* 3:358, 1994.
73. David TE, Omran A, Webb G et al: Geometric mismatch of the aortic and pulmonary roots causes aortic insufficiency after the Ross procedure, *J Thorac Cardiovasc Surg* 112:1231, 1996.
74. Oury JH, Eddy AC, Cleveland JC: The Ross procedure: a progress report, *J Heart Valve Dis* 3:361, 1994.
75. Bjork VO, Henze A: Management of thromboembolism after aortic valve replacement with the Bjork-Shiley tilting disc valve: medicamental prevention with dicumarol in comparison with dipyidamole-acetylsalicylic acid: surgical treatment of prosthetic thrombosis, *Scand J Thorac Cardiovasc Surg* 9:183, 1975.
76. Bloomfield P, Wheatley DJ, Prescott RJ et al: Twelve-year comparison of a Bjork-Shiley mechanical heart valve with porcine prostheses, *N Engl J Med* 324:573, 1991.
77. Tavel ME, Stein PD: Management of anticoagulants in a patient requiring major surgery, *Chest* 114:1756, 1998.
78. Katholi RE, Nolan SP, McGuire LB: Living with prosthetic heart valves: subsequent noncardiac operations and the risk of thromboembolism or hemorrhage, *Am Heart J* 92:162, 1976.
79. Stein PD, Alpert JS, Copeland J et al: Antithrombotic therapy in patients with mechanical and biological prosthetic heart valves, *Chest* 108:371S, 1995.
80. Tinker JH, Tarhan S: Discontinuing anticoagulant therapy in surgical patients with cardiac valve prostheses, *JAMA* 239:738, 1978.
81. Shetty HGM, Backhouse G, Bentley DP et al: Effective reversal of warfarin-induced excessive anticoagulation with low dose vitamin K_1, *Thromb Haemost* 67:13, 1992.
82. Barash P, Kitahata LM, Mandel S: Acute cardiovascular collapse after intravenous phytonadione, *Anesth Analg* 55(2):304, 1976.

OUTLINE

Cardiac electrophysiologic problems for anesthesiologists include (1) rationale selection of drugs for the management of patients with chronic or new cardiac arrhythmias, and (2) strategies for the care of patients with rhythm-management devices (i.e., pacemakers, internal cardioverterdefibrillator [ICD]). However, before these problems are discussed, we must first consider concepts of arrhythmogenesis that are fundamental to effective arrhythmia prevention and management.

CONCEPTS OF ARRHYTHMOGENESIS
Substrates and Imbalance

The heart's function is to generate sufficient cardiac output to meet changing body needs. To accomplish this, the specialized cardiac conducting system is responsible for the generation and propagation of electrical impulses—action potentials (APs), which initiate orderly contraction of atrial and ventricular muscle. The timing and speed of impulse generation and propagation are regulated by the autonomic nervous system. If this process occurs at an inappropriate rate or is disrupted, an arrhythmia is present. Inherent stability of this system is normally well preserved.

However, cardiovascular and systemic disease may alter the structure of the heart through remodeling. Myocardial remodeling includes replacement microfibrosis and reduction in the number of gap junctions (intercellular connections) after cell loss between surviving fibers, producing a "substrate" that is conducive to discontinuous conduction phenomena, functional reentry, and arrhythmias. However, this might be insufficient to sustain arrhythmias without an additional insult, such as physiologic imbalance resulting from drug toxicity, hypoxia, myocardial ischemia, electrolyte disturbances, or a catecholamine surge. Such imbalance would appreciably alter normal electrophysiologic properties or generate new "abnormal" phenomena (see the following sections). The latter might be the mechanism for extrasystoles that initiate tachyarrhythmias. Accordingly, the effects of imbalance would not act as triggers for arrhythmias, but, rather, would compliment those of myocardial remodeling to sustain arrhythmias. Hence, the concept of substrates and imbalance is fundamental to effective prevention and management of arrhythmias.

Normal Cardiac Electrophysiology

Ion Channels, Currents, and Gating. Ion channels are large glycoproteins that span the cell membrane bilayer. With appropriate stimulation (propagating AP), they form pores that permit ions to cross the membrane rapidly, thereby creating ion currents responsible for AP generation and propagation. Some ion channels open only after a delay following the stimulus, whereas others rectify (notably, potassium [K^+] channels) after stimulation. Rectification is the voltage dependence of resistance to inward or outward ion flow. Stimuli for ion-channel opening include membrane voltage changes, chemical mediators (which act directly or via second messenger receptors), and mechanical deformation. Gating is the process whereby ion-channel proteins change their conformation in response to external stimuli. Gating is the process responsible for channel opening and closing. Gating characteristics can be rapid (≤ 1 ms), or slow (seconds). Once the channel is open, the proteins may remain open until closed by another stimulus. Alternatively, they may close despite a maintained stimulus (i.e., inactivate). Inactivated ion chan-

nels usually do not open again until they have recovered from inactivation, which is a time-dependent or, often, a voltage-dependent process. Ion channels share considerable homology, especially in the segments, which span the membrane. Consequently, some channel-active drugs interact with more than one ion channel in heart tissue (e.g., amiodarone), or with the same channel in other tissues (local anesthetics).

Cardiac Resting and Action Potential. The resting membrane potential (phase 4 of the AP) is normally -80 to -90 mV in *fast-response* fibers. Examples are atrial and ventricular muscle and Purkinje fibers, whose AP upstrokes (phase 0) are largely dependent on the rapid influx of sodium (Na^+) (Fig. 9-1). Resting membrane potential (phase 4) is kept fairly stable by K^+ current (inward rectifier, I_{K1}), and both active and passive ion-exchange mechanisms (see Fig. 9-1). The former uses energy from adenosine triphosphate. Vagal stimulation (acetylcholine) can also activate a hyperpolarizing K^+ current (I_{KACh}) during phase 4. With the arrival of propagating AP or external depolarizing

FIG. 9-1 Representation of the action potential *(AP)* and resting membrane potential *(RMP)* in a quiescent Purkinje fiber, with typical intracellular and extracellular ion concentrations during AP phase 4 (RMP). Inward depolarizing currents are shown in black, and outward repolarizing currents are shown in gray. Also shown are the active and passive ion exchangers that restore intracellular ion concentrations during phase 4. The adenosine 5-triphosphate *(ATP)*-dependent sodium/potassium (Na/K) pump maintains steep outward- and inward-directed gradients *(arrows)* for K^+ and Na^+, respectively, and generates a small net outward current. The passive Na/Ca exchanger generates a small net inward current. A small, inward "leak" of Na^+ keeps the RMP slightly positive to the K equilibrium potential (-96 mV). Phase 1 is initial rapid repolarization, phase 2 is the plateau, and phase 3 is the final repolarization. The cell is unresponsive to propagating AP or external stimuli during the absolute refractory period *(ARP)*. A small electronic potential "a" occurs in response to a propagating AP or external stimulus during the relative refractory period *(RRP)*. A normal AP is generated at "b" (end of RRP), when the Na channels have recovered from inactivation. Note that threshold potential *(TP)* is more positive during the RRP. See text for further discussion.

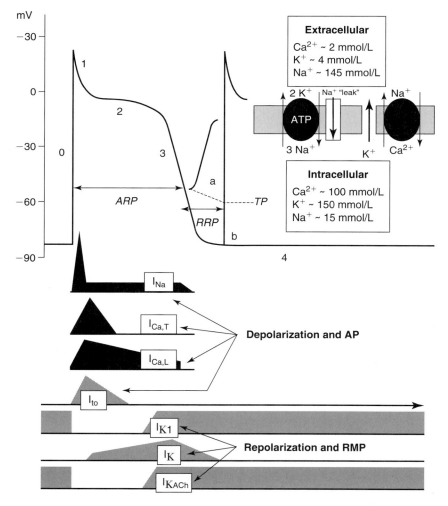

stimuli, there is a rapid reversal of transmembrane potential during AP phase 0 to +20 to +30 mV (see Fig. 9-1). Transient outward K^+ current (I_{to}) causes early rapid repolarization (AP phase 1, Fig. 9-1). This is soon balanced by the increased calcium (Ca^{2+}) influx and the late inactivating I_{Na}, which cause the AP plateau (phase 2). During phase 2, another outward K^+ current—the delayed rectifier (I_K)—activates to initiate final AP repolarization (phase 3), as shown in Fig. 9-1. Active and passive ion-exchange pumps, Na^+ "leak" current, and outward K^+ current help maintain the resting membrane potential during phase 4 (see Fig. 9-1).

Automaticity. Primary pacemaker cells of the sinuatrial (SA) node and latent pacemaker cells found along the sulcus terminalis, and within the coronary sinus ostium, atrioventricular (AV) junction, and His-Purkinje system, do not have a stable transmembrane potential during phase 4. Instead, they slowly depolarize during diastole (phase 4 depolarization or automaticity) to threshold potential (about −55 mV) for regenerative Na^+ influx and phase 0 depolarization. The maximum level of transmembrane potential achieved early during phase 4 depolarization is the maximum diastolic potential. Normally, the SA node overdrives latent pacemakers. However, they may escape through default or usurpation to cause ectopic rhythms (e.g., wandering atrial pacemaker, junctional or ventricular escape rhythms).

Automaticity must be the result of a net gain in intracellular positive charges (depolarizing current) during diastole (phase 4 depolarization). The mechanism varies among fiber types, depending most on maximum diastolic potential. Critical to the pacemaker potential is the absence or presence of distinct ionic conductances. For example, in contrast to working atrial or ventricular muscle, pacemaker cells have almost no resting I_{K1} conductance (see Fig. 9-1) to fix resting membrane potential near the K^+ equilibrium potential. Thus, diastolic membrane potential is more unstable, so that modest inward currents can depolarize these fibers. Contributing to this change in SA node fibers is a voltage-dependent channel activated at membrane potentials negative to −50 to −60 mV, with a reversal potential of around −20 mV. This pacemaker current (I_f) for the most part is carried by monovalent cations (Na^+, K^+). Other currents involved are I_K, $I_{Ca,L}$, $I_{Ca,T}$, and a background current (I_b). I_b is carried mainly by Na^+, but differs from I_{Na}. Since repolarization results in closure or deactivation of channels carrying I_K, this causes a decline in K^+ conductance, which contributes to the net depolarizing current during phase 4. $I_{Ca,L}$ and $I_{Ca,T}$ contribute to phase 4 depolarization and the AP upstroke at membrane potentials positive to −55 mV. Activation of K^+ current by acetylcholine or adenosine (I_{KACh}) will oppose spontaneous phase 4 depolarization.

Conduction. AP propagation is very fast in fast-response fibers (see earlier discussion). However, in SA and AV node cells, with maximum diastolic potentials in the range of −60 to −70 mV, the AP upstrokes are more dependent on the inward movement of Ca^{2+}. As a result, the AP upstroke velocity and propagation are much slower, so that these fibers are termed *slow-response* fibers. Conduction of AP within and between the atria, and to the AV node, occurs over preferential conducting pathways. These are electrophysiologically, but not anatomically, distinct pathways when compared with surrounding working atrial myocardium. Further, there appear to be fast and slow atrial inputs to the AV node. The AV node normally provides sufficient conduction delay for adequate ventricular filling. The ventricular specialized conducting system consists of the His (common) bundle, the left bundle branch (with anterior, posterior, and septal divisions) and right bundle branch, and branching Purkinje fibers that terminate on ventricular muscle. The ventricular conducting system provides for orderly, rapid, synchronized contraction of both ventricles.

Electrophysiologic Mechanisms for Arrhythmias

Depressed Fast Response and Abnormal Automaticity. Many abnormal electrophysiologic phenomena occur in partially depolarized fast-response fibers (see preceding section), termed the *depressed fast response* (DFR). Cellular depolarization responsible for the DFR has a number of potential causes, including ischemia, hypoxia, myocardial injury, and hyperkalemia. Reduced AP upstroke velocity and slow conduction in DFR fibers are consequent to incomplete recovery from inactivation of Na^+ channels. Membrane depolarization to −50 mV inactivates all of the Na^+ channels. At potentials positive to −55 mV, $I_{Ca,L}$ and $I_{Ca,T}$ are activated to generate the AP upstroke (as in SA and AV node cells). With the DFR, electrophysiologic changes are likely to be heterogeneous because of varying degrees of Na^+ channel inactivation among fibers. This causes variable impairment of conduction and uneven refractoriness in affected portions of the heart, changes conducive to reentry of excitation (see the following sections). Further, DFR fibers (working atrial or ventricular muscle, Purkinje fibers), can exhibit abnormal automaticity, the probable cause for escape rhythms and slow monomorphic ventricular tachycardia with acute myocardial infarction.

Afterdepolarizations and Triggered Arrhythmias. Under pathologic circumstances, there may be small depolarizing potentials before (early afterdepolarization, EAD) or after full AP repolarization (delayed afterdepolarization, DAD). If these reach threshold for regenerative depolarization, they may initiate supraventricular tachycardia (SVT) or ventricular tachycardia (VT) due to triggered activity. DAD results from the oscillatory release of Ca^{2+} from overloaded sarcoplasmic reticulum, and may be the cause for ventricular arrhythmias with acute myocardial infarction and for atrial or ventricular arrhythmias with digitalis excess. EADs are associated with acquired or congenital QT interval prolongation, involve defects in the genes encoding Na^+ and K^+ channels involved in repolarization, and are believed to be the inciting mechanism for torsades de pointes VT (polymorphic VT *in association with* QT interval prolongation).

Reentry of Excitation. The impulse originating in the SA node continues until the entire heart has been activated and becomes completely refractory. If some fibers are not activated, and the propagating impulse returns by another pathway to excite them, this is reentry of excitation. The basic criteria for ascribing abnormal beats or rhythm to reentry were first formulated by Mines in 1913: (1) there must be an area of unidirectional conduction block; (2) the reentrant pathway must be defined; namely, the movement of the excitatory wavefront should be observed to progress through the pathway, return to its point of origin, and then return to reexcite the same pathway; and (3) it must be possible to terminate reentry by interrupting the circuit at some point to rule out a focal (automatic or triggered) origin. These criteria have been satisfied for many clinical tachyarrhythmias, since it is now possible to map tachycardia circuits during electrophysiologic studies and to interrupt reentry circuits by surgical or catheter ablation techniques.

Slow conduction is a basic requirement for reentry. That is, there must be sufficient delay of the propagating impulse in an alternate pathway to permit tissue proximal to a site of unidirectional block to recover from refractoriness. If so, reentry would be facilitated by conduction that was slower than normal. There is a reduction in the amplitude and upstroke velocities of premature beats that are initiated before full repolarization (Fig. 9-2) and a reduction in their speed of propagation. Since the speed of conduction depends on the magnitude of I_{Na} during phase 0, which is in turn dependent on the resting membrane potential and Na^+ channel availability, the speed of conduction is also slowed in depressed fast-response fibers. Also, the coupling resistance between adjacent fibers (i.e., the gap junctions) is another factor that may influence the speed of conduction. As this is increased (e.g., due to aging or disease), the speed of conduction decreases.

Unidirectional block of conduction is another requirement for reentry. It may occur as the result of nonuniform recovery of excitability due to regional differences in refractoriness or to geometric factors. For example, the way in which myocardial cells are connected to one another influences the speed of conduction, with longi-

tudinal conduction velocity about three times that of transverse conduction velocity.

There are several types of reentry. *Anatomical reentry* requires a fixed, anatomically defined circuit. Such circuits might occur in fibrotic regions of the atria or ventricles, or in surviving muscle fibers with healed infarctions. Anatomically defined circuits are also involved in VT because of bundle-branch reentry, atrial flutter caused by reentry confined to the right atrium, and paroxysmal SVT caused by AV node and accessory conduction pathway reentry (see the following section). *Functional reentry* does not require an anatomically defined circuit. It takes place in contiguous fibers with discordant electrophysiologic properties. Dispersed excitability or refractoriness, and anisotropic distribution of intercellular resistance allow initiation and maintenance of reentry. Examples of functional reentry are *leading circle* reentry and *random reentry*, both important mechanisms for clinical atrial fibrillation. With leading circle reentry, the propagating tachycardia wavefront circulates around a central core that is kept refractory by impulses propagating toward it from all sides of the circuit. Random reentry occurs when impulses propagate randomly and continuously, reexciting areas that were excited shortly before by another wavelet.

Atrioventricular Node "Fast-Slow" and Accessory Atrioventricular Pathways. "Fast-slow pathway" AV node reentry and "concealed" accessory AV conduction pathway reentry account for 80% to 85% of paroxysmal SVT (PSVT). Accessory AV pathways or connections are working atrial fibers that bridge the AV groove at any location along the mitral or tricuspid annulus, except where the mitral annulus is contiguous with the aorta. They provide the anatomical substrate for ventricular preexcitation (electrocardiogram [ECG] δ wave) and AV reciprocating tachycardia in the Wolff-Parkinson-White (WPW) syndrome. These connections are said to be "concealed" if they do not conduct impulses to the ventricles during sinus rhythm to produce preexcitation, but do conduct from the ventricles to atria during PSVT. In approximately 60% of patients *without* evidence of ventricular preexcitation in sinus rhythm who have PSVT, the mechanism for tachycardia is AV nodal reentry. In 30% of these patients, the mechanism for tachycardia involves the AV node and accessory pathways. In the remainder, the mechanism for tachycardia involves SA node or intraatrial reentry.

PSVT due to fast-slow pathway AV nodal reentry does not, as formerly believed, involve functional dissociation of the AV node into two pathways. Results of clinical electrophysiologic investigation and radiofrequency catheter and surgical ablation are conclusive: the slow and fast AV nodal pathways have their origins well outside the limits of the compact AV node, and they consist of ordinary atrial muscle fibers. Target sites for ablation

A   **AV NODE REENTRY TACHYCARDIA**
(common form)

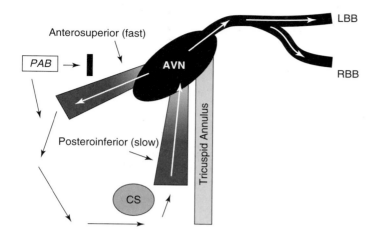

B   **AV RECIPROCATING TACHYCARDIA**
(orthodromic)

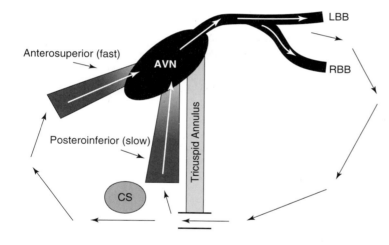

FIG. 9-2   Mechanisms for paroxysmal (reentrant) supraventricular tachycardia. **A,** Common form of atrioventricular *(AV)* node reentry tachycardia (AVNRT). The reentry loop involves the AV node, atria, and anterosuperior (fast pathway) and posteroinferior atrial (slow pathway) approaches to the AV node. The atrial premature beat *(PAB)* that initiates tachycardia blocks in the fast pathway with longer refractoriness than in the slow pathway. However, it conducts to the ventricles by the slow pathway, which is no longer refractory. During AVNRT, antegrade conduction occurs via the posteroinferior (slow) pathway, and retrograde conduction via the anterosuperior (fast) pathway. During the *uncommon form* of AVNRT (not shown), a ventricular premature beat penetrates the slow pathway to initiate reentry. Antegrade conduction is via the fast pathway. **B,** AV reciprocating tachycardia (AVRT) involving an accessory AV pathway. AVRT can be orthodromic (shown) or antidromic (not shown), depending on the direction of impulse propagation in the accessory pathway. With the former, activation of the ventricles during tachycardia is by the normal pathway (atrial approaches → AV node → His bundle). The impulse returns to the atria via the accessory pathway and gives rise to a narrow QRS tachycardia. With antidromic tachycardia (≤10% of AVRT), the ventricles are activated via the accessory pathway, giving rise to a wide QRS, preexcited tachycardia (see text). *AVN,* Atrioventricular node; *CS,* coronary sinus; *LBB,* left bundle branch; *RBB,* right bundle branch.

of the *fast pathway* in PSVT due to AV nodal reentry are located along the anterosuperior portion of the interatrial septum near the tricuspid annulus, just proximal to the compact AV node (see Fig. 9-2). Target sites for ablation of the *slow pathway* in PSVT due to AV nodal reentry are found more posteriorly along the tricuspid annulus, close to the ostium of the coronary sinus (see Fig. 9-2).

PSVT due to accessory pathway reentry is known as AV reciprocating tachycardia (AVRT), since both the atria and ventricles are required for reentry (see Fig. 9-2). The orthodromic variety of AVRT (see Fig. 9-2) is by far most common. It is important to note that ventricular activation during AVRT is by the normal pathway (AV node → His bundle), so that the result is a narrow QRS tachycardia. In contrast, with antidromic AVRT (≤10% of AVRT), impulses are conducted to the ventricle over the accessory pathway. This produces a wide QRS tachycardia, which is easily misdiagnosed as VT. However,

whenever confronted with wide QRS tachycardia in a patient with WPW, it is worth remembering that VT is rare without other overt heart disease.

Mechanisms for Clinical Arrhythmias. Clinical arrhythmias result from abnormal cellular and macroscopic electrophysiologic phenomena, as discussed earlier. However, ascribing one or another mechanism to a clinical rhythm disturbance may be problematical, especially in the critical care and perioperative arena. Indeed, because of the effects of multiple drugs and physiologic imbalance, along with underlying myocardial disease (the "substrate"), two or more mechanisms may be operational. For example, consider the origin of paroxysmal atrial fibrillation following cardiopulmonary bypass in a patient with hypertension and chronic pulmonary disease. Either of these systemic conditions may be associated with atrial remodeling, which provides the "substrate" for functional reentry. The inciting factor for

MECHANISM	ARRHYTHMIAS
Altered normal automaticity	Sinus bradycardia and tachycardia, sinus arrhythmia, wandering atrial pacemaker, AV junctional and ventricular escape rhythms
Abnormal automaticity	Slow monomorphic VT, accelerated junctional or ventricular rhythm with acute myocardial infarction, some ectopic atrial tachycardia
Triggered activity (DAD)	Some VT first 24 hours after myocardial infarction, atrial or ventricular tachycardias with digitalis toxicity, VT mediated by catecholamines
Triggered activity (EAD)	Polymorphic VT in the setting of QT interval prolongation (torsades de pointes)
Anatomic reentry	Paroxysmal SVT to SA node, atrial or AV node reentry; AV reciprocating tachycardia; VT with healed infarction; atrial flutter (possibly anatomic and functional)
Functional reentry	Atrial fibrillation; monomorphic and polymorphic VT with acute myocardial infarction; ventricular fibrillation

AV, Atrioventricular; *DAD*, delayed afterdepolarization; *EAD*, early afterdepolarization; *SA*, sinuatrial; *SVT*, supraventricular tachycardia; *VT*, ventricular tachycardia.

atrial fibrillation might be atrial extrasystoles triggered by delayed afterdepolarizations. In turn, these might result from intracellular Ca^{2+} overload resulting from elevated catecholamines. Alternatively, inadequate myocardial protection (especially the right atrium) might partially depolarize some fibers. If so, abnormal automaticity might be the cause for atrial extrasystoles. Confirmed or postulated mechanisms for specific clinical arrhythmias are given in Table 9-1.

THERAPY OF ARRHYTHMIAS

There can be no doubt that the emphasis on therapy for arrhythmias, especially ventricular arrhythmias with coronary artery disease, has moved from drugs to "electricity" (implanted pacemakers, cardioverter-defibrillators) or catheter-surgical ablation. While antiarrhythmic drugs have proved safe and effective when the heart is structurally normal, in abnormal heart (myocardial remodeling consequent to disease), drug efficacy has been modest. Indeed, use of drugs in this circumstance has been associated with increased mortality due to proarrhythmia (see the following sections). Nonetheless, drugs are an important adjunct to electrical therapy for management of ventricular tachyarrhythmias and are the mainstay of treatment for atrial fibrillation.

Antiarrhythmic Drugs

Antiarrhythmic Drug Action. Ion channels and neurohormonal receptors modulating their function, not electrophysiologic phenomena per se, are now primary

TABLE 9-2
Properties of the Ideal Antiarrhythmic Drug

Specificity	The drug should interact with the specific ion channel(s) involved in the genesis of the arrhythmia.
Pharmacodynamics	The kinetics of association and dissociation should be such that effects (e.g., slowing of conduction, prolongation of refractoriness) are maximal during tachycardia.
Pharmacokinetics	Brief onset and duration of action after parenteral administration. High bioavailability, rapid onset of action, and infrequent dosing after oral administration.

targets for antiarrhythmic drug action. The goal of therapy is, as far as possible, to restore normal impulse initiation and propagation, or to slow the effective ventricular rate with chronic atrial fibrillation. Desirable properties of an antiarrhythmic drug are listed in Table 9-2. Specific targets for antiarrhythmic action include ion currents responsible for automaticity, depolarization, the AP plateau, and AP repolarization.

Automaticity. The pacemaker current (If) helps initiate automaticity in SA node cells and subsidiary pacemaker fibers. While specific blockers of this current have been identified, their use is limited because sinus tachycardia is usually a compensatory rhythm disturbance.

Both T-type and L-type Ca^{2+} current also contribute to the pacemaker potential and conduction in SA node and subsidiary pacemakers, but clinically effective antagonists (verapamil, diltiazem) block only L-type current. Either is effective for slowing AV conduction with atrial fibrillation-flutter and for terminating SA and AV node reentry. Dihydropyridine Ca^{2+} antagonists (nifedipine, nicardipine) are not effective blockers of L-type current in heart.

Depolarization. Block of fast Na^+ inward current (I_{Na}) by Class I drugs is useful against reentrant arrhythmias in atrial, ventricular, and Purkinje fibers, since their AP upstrokes are largely dependent on I_{Na}. However, there is recognized potential for proarrhythmia with Class IC Na^+ channel blockers (see the following sections). The antiarrhythmic efficacy of Na^+ channel blockers is determined in large part by how they interact with the multiple states of the Na^+ channel (open, closed, inactivated). This has clinical ramifications. For example, compared with primary open-state blockers (Class IA, disopyramide, quinidine), drugs that block both open and inactivated Na^+ channels (Class IB, lidocaine, mexiletine) depress AP phase 0 and conduction more in partially depolarized fibers. Consequently, Class IB blockers are effective against reentrant VT with acute myocardial infarction and ischemia, but not necessarily in patients with healed infarcts. In contrast, open-state blockers (quinidine, disopyramide) prolong AP duration. This increases the time that Na^+ channels are inactivated. If so, they may enhance the blocking action of inactivated state (IB) blockers, which is the rationale for combining class IA and IB drugs.

Action Potential Plateau. Both the Na^+ and Ca^{2+} channels contribute inward current during the AP plateau (see Fig. 9-1). Increasing either current component will prolong AP duration and directly (Ca^{2+}) or indirectly (Na^+) cause positive inotropy. However, there is a down side. If Na^+ or Ca^{2+} activators bind during the AP plateau, AP plateau prolongation could lead to regenerative depolarization and EADs, with EAD-triggered activity the result. EADs have been implicated as the triggering mechanism for torsade de pointes in the setting of prolonged repolarization. If so, drugs that block inward Na^+ or Ca^{2+} current (cardiac calcium channel blockers: verapamil, diltiazem) might be effective against resulting arrhythmias.

Action Potential Repolarization. The emphasis of antiarrhythmic drug research and development has shifted to Class III drugs that prolong AP duration and refractoriness by blocking voltage-gated K^+ channels. The basis of this shift is multifactorial: (1) evidence of relative inefficacy and increased proarrhythmia with Class I agents; (2) the Class III action is particularly effective against anatomical reentry in the atria (atrial flutter) or ventricles (monomorphic VT); (3) Class III drugs appear more effective than Class I drugs for initial treatment

and prevention of lethal ventricular tachyarrhythmias; (4) Class IA and IC drugs depress myocardial contractility, whereas Class III drugs either do not affect it or slightly increase it (attributed to increased Ca^{2+} current during AP plateau, which enhances Ca^{2+} release from the sarcoplasmic reticulum); and (5) Class III drugs are reported to reduce defibrillation thresholds, which should enhance ICD shock efficacy.

The K^+ channel blockers are a diverse group of compounds that share the property of prolonging AP duration and refractoriness in atrial and ventricular muscle and in Purkinje fibers. They include Class IA, IC, and III drugs in the modified Vaughan-Williams classification. The degree of AP duration prolongation is variable among Class IA and IC drugs, despite the fact that all block the delayed rectifier (I_K), and some (quinidine, disopyramide) also block the inward rectifier (I_{K1}) and the transient outward current (Ito) as well (see Fig. 9-1). This effect is due to the attendant influence of these drugs on I_{Na}, particularly the slowly inactivating or late component. For example, potent block of this late component by flecainide shortens AP duration, countering its effect to block I_K. Quinidine and disopyramide (Class IA) are nonspecific K^+ current blockers, blocking all three components (see Fig. 9-1). Procainamide (Class IA) and flecainide (Class IC) are selective blockers of I_K. The Class III drugs (sotolol, amiodarone, and bretylium) are relatively nonselective K^+ blockers. Sotolol is also a nonselective β-blocker. Initially, bretylium causes catecholamine release. Amiodarone exhibits all four class actions: it blocks I_K and I_{K1}, Na^+ and Ca^{2+} channels, and $α_1$- and $β_1$-adrenergic receptors. This nonspecificity, in addition to its high selectivity for the slowly inactivating component of I_K (I_{Ks}), is now believed to explain the lower proarrhythmic potential with amiodarone compared with other antiarrhythmic agents (see the following sections).

Most Na^+ channel blockers, especially in higher concentrations, cause use-dependent block. Depression of Na^+ current and conduction velocity is greater at faster heart rates. While "ideal" K^+ channel blockers should do the same, *behavior* of most (except, amiodarone, flecainide) is just the opposite. Prolongation of AP duration and refractoriness is maximal at slow heart rates, with progressively reduced effects at faster rates. While such reverse rate-dependent behavior* is expected to

---

*Technically, it is not "reverse use-dependence." Most K^+ channel blocking drugs (including amiodarone and flecainide) block I_K in a use-dependent fashion. Furthermore, block is increased at depolarized potentials, when channels are in the open state. Accordingly, drug *block* (what occurs at the K^+ channel level, the conventional meaning for "use-dependence") shows normal use-dependence. If so, the term *reverse rate-dependence* may be the more appropriate way to describe K^+ channel blocker behavior.

limit the efficacy of most K$^+$ blockers for terminating sustained tachyarrhythmias, as a group K$^+$ blockers are moderately effective.

Several mechanisms have been proposed to explain reverse rate-dependent behavior with K$^+$ channel blockers. First, at faster heart rates, the relative contribution of other ionic processes (e.g., the inactivation of I$_{Ca,L}$) may exceed that of I$_K$. Second, at fast heart rates, the slowly activating component of I$_K$ (I$_{Ks}$) is more important than its faster component (I$_{Kr}$) in mediating AP repolarization. Since most selective I$_K$ blockers target I$_{Kr}$ and have little affinity for I$_{Ks}$, they should be less effective at fast heart rates. In this regard, it is notable that amiodarone primarily blocks I$_{Ks}$, which may in part explain why it prolongs AP duration over a range of heart rates. Finally, preferential block of open K$^+$ channels does not necessarily result in conspicuous use-dependent block, especially if recovery from block is slow (dofetilide) or onset of block is very rapid (quinidine). This is because, as for Na$^+$ channel blockers, the onset/offset kinetics of K$^+$ channel block are key determinants of use-dependent block. Thus, if the onset of block is rapid, steady-state block could be achieved during a single AP, with little additional block at fast rates. Conversely, with slow offset of block, there would be little dissipation of block between beats, and steady-state block would be achieved at relatively slow heart rates.

Proarrhythmia. Proarrhythmia is the aggravation of arrhythmias or provocation of new arrhythmias by antiarrhythmic drugs. Life-threatening polymorphic VT in association with QT interval prolongation (torsade de pointes) is the manifestation with antiarrhythmic drugs that prolong the QT interval (Class IA, IC, and III drugs). Factors or conditions that predispose or contribute to proarrhythmia are listed in Table 9-3. For patients receiving oral therapy with Class IA and III drugs, the estimated annual incidence of proarrhythmia is less than 5%. With amiodarone, the annual incidence may be less than 2%. However, when Class IC drugs were used for suppression of chronic, asymptomatic, nonsustained ventricular arrhythmias in CAST (Cardiac Arrhythmia Suppression Trial), patients experienced up to a 20% incidence of proarrhythmia and twofold to threefold increase in expected mortality. Explanations for the lower incidence of proarrhythmia with amiodarone compared with other drugs that prolong AP duration and refractoriness are as follows: (1) its potent Class I and IV activity (i.e., block of inward depolarizing current) would inhibit EADs possibly the triggering mechanism for torsade de pointes (as discussed earlier); and (2) it has enhanced selectivity for K$^+$ channels that activate slowly during repolarization (I$_{Ks}$). Most other antiarrhythmic drugs that prolong the QT interval selectively suppress the rapidly activating component of I$_K$ (I$_{Kr}$). Indeed, there is now interest in developing Class

---

TABLE 9-3
Factors and Conditions That Predispose or Contribute to Proarrhythmia

- Structural heart disease
- Left ventricular dysfunction
- Bradycardia with QT interval prolongation
- T-wave alternans
- Female gender
- Ventricular preexcitation (WPW)
- Atrial flutter-fibrillation
- Electrolyte imbalance (especially ↓ K$^+$, ↓ Mg^{2+})
- Digitalis and diuretic therapy
- Tricyclic antidepressants

K$^+$, Potassium; *Mg^{2+}*, magnesium; *WPW*, Wolff-Parkinson-White syndrome.

III drugs that are selective for I$_{Ks}$ because there should be reduced propensity for proarrhythmia.

Drug Therapy for Specific Arrhythmias. Hemodynamically disadvantageous bradycardia and escape rhythms consequent to sinus node dysfunction or heart block, especially in the setting of cardiac surgery, are best managed by temporary pacing. Anticholinergic drugs (atropine) are often ineffective, produce untoward tachycardia, or may cause worse arrhythmias. In addition to excess tachycardia, catecholamines may contribute to DAD- or EAD-triggered activity (see earlier discussion) and associated arrhythmias (see Table 9-1), especially with ischemia or myocardial remodeling consequent to cardiovascular or other systemic disease. Antiarrhythmic drugs are used for the management of tachyarrhythmias. Table 9-4 lists the likely mechanism, desired ("target") antiarrhythmic effect, and useful drugs, both for parenteral (intravenous), and oral therapy.

Rhythm Management Devices

Cardiac pacing and direct current (DC) cardioversion and defibrillation have undergone significant evolution and growth since the first asynchronous transvenous antibradycardia pacemaker was implanted in 1958. Today, more than 500,000 patients in the United States have permanent pacemakers. Based on industry estimates, 115,000 pacemaker systems and 40,000 ICDs are implanted each year (U.S.). Modern pacemakers pace in one or both chambers, and can adapt the rate of pacing to meet changing body needs (adaptive-rate pacing). Modern ICDs provide antitachycardia pacing and, when needed, shocks to terminate atrial or ventricular tach-

TABLE 9-4
Antiarrhythmic Drugs Used for the Management of Specific Tachyarrhythmias

ARRHYTHMIA	MECHANISM	TARGET EFFECT	DRUGS
Paroxysmal supraventricular tachycardia (PSVT)	Reentry involving SA or AV nodes, or "concealed" AP	↑ SA or AV node refractoriness	*IV*: adenosine, BB, CCB, edrophonium *Oral*: BB, CCB, DIG, amiodarone
AV reciprocating tachycardia (PSVT in WPW patient)	Reentry involving AV node and AP (the AP is "manifest" as delta wave—preexcitation)	↑ SA or AV node refractoriness; ↑ atrial (AP) refractoriness	*IV*: same as PSVT; Class IA and IC *Oral*: same as PSVT; Class IA and IC (not DIG)
Atrial flutter and fibrillation	Atrial reentry	Rate—AV node Rhythm—↑ atrial refractoriness	*IV*: BB, CCB, DIG, ibutilide, amiodarone? *Oral*: Class IA and IC, III, BB, CCB, DIG
Atrial flutter and fibrillation (WPW)	Atrial reentry with possible dangerous ventricular rates	Rate—AV node + AP Rhythm—↑ AP and atrial refractoriness	*IV*: *Not* CCB or DIG alone; amiodarone *Oral*: Class IA, IC and III; BB
Ventricular tachycardia (VT), monomorphic or polymorphic (not with long QT)	Anatomic and/or functional ventricular reentry	↑ Refractoriness and conduction time in ventricles	*IV*: lidocaine, amiodarone, procainamide *Oral*: Class IA and III (not IC) + ICD
Polymorphic VT with long QT (torsade de pointes)	Triggered by EADs; triggered activity or functional reentry	Abolish EADs, shorten action potential duration	*IV*: Mg, amiodarone, BB; ↑ heart rate* *Oral*: amiodarone, K-channel openers†; ↑ heart rate*
Ventricular fibrillation	Functional reentry	↑ Refractoriness and conduction time in ventricles	*IV*: amiodarone (?)‡, lidocaine, bretylium *Oral*: Class IA and III (not IC) + ICD

↑, Increase; *AP*, accessory pathway; *AV*, atrioventricular; *BB*, β-blockers; *CCB*, calcium channel blockers; *DIG*, digitalis; *EAD*, early afterdepolarization; *ICD*, internal cardioverter-defibrillator; *IV*, intravenous; *K*, potassium; *Mg*, magnesium; *SA*, sinoatrial; *WPW*, Wolff-Parkinson-White.
*Temporary pacing (*not* isoproterenol) or permanent pacing.
†Chromokalin, pinacidil, nicorandil (investigational drugs).
‡Recent data suggest amiodarone may be initial drug of choice (vs. lidocaine).

yarrhythmias. Contemporary devices provide dual-chamber bradycardia and adaptive rate pacing as well.

Pacing and DC cardioversion or defibrillation have advantages over drugs for the treatment of tachyarrhythmias. The therapeutic effect is immediate and the "dose" (i.e., pacing mode, rate, current) is easier to titrate than it is with drugs. Also, drugs may not produce the desired effect or cause proarrhythmia. There are also side effects with drugs and the effects may last longer than desired. However, there are also disadvantages with device therapy, including risk of sepsis, hemorrhage or direct myocardial injury with invasive methods, stimulation of tachyarrhythmias, and inability to achieve the desired therapeutic effect in some patients.

Pacemaker Design and Function. Most pacemakers now implanted in the United States pace and sense in the right atrium, the right ventricle, or both, and can adapt the pacing rate to meet changing metabolic demands (adaptive-rate pacing). They automatically mod-

ify other behavior aspects in response to changing physiologic circumstances by altering timing intervals, stimulus amplitudes or durations, and other operating characteristics. Devices with programmable antitachycardia functions may be prescribed in addition to drugs for patients with reentrant SVT. However, the increasing application of catheter or surgical ablation has reduced the prevalence of SVT as an indication for pacing.

Pacemakers are powered by lithium-iodine batteries, and have an expected service life of 5 to 12 years, depending on the desired therapeutic capability (single- or dual-chamber pacing, adaptive-rate pacing, etc.). Most pacemaker lead systems are inserted transvenously by invasive cardiologists or cardiac electrophysiologists. The electrode may be *unipolar* (with part or all of the metal housing of the pulse generator serving as an anode), but is more often *bipolar* (with two electrodes in close proximity at the endocardial surface). With many newer devices, lead polarity is programmed. While most patients have one lead for ventricular pacing or two for dual-chamber pacing, there is increasing interest in multisite pacing, which requires more electrodes, for optimizing chamber-contraction timing or discouraging paroxysmal atrial fibrillation.

In essence, the pacemaker is like a battery with a switch that can be closed momentarily, allowing electric current to flow from the battery through myocardial tissue and back again, inducing depolarization of the atria or ventricles when current flows during their physiologic nonrefractory periods. In addition, by sensing intrinsic atrial or ventricular depolarizations, pacemakers can be *inhibited* from providing unnecessary or inappropriate stimuli. With dual-chamber devices, sensed intrinsic atrial depolarizations may *trigger* ventricular stimulation to maintain AV synchrony and an optimal, uniform cardiac output.

Despite the simplicity of fundamental operation, modern pacemakers can be programmed to modify the settings of many operating parameters, including stimulus amplitudes and durations, lower rate limits, maximum atrial tracking rates, refractory-period durations, and many others. Moreover, pacemaker telemetry often provides invaluable assistance in diagnosis by allowing intracardiac electrograms and associated timing diagrams to be plotted, event histories to be explored, operating variables to be measured, and programmed settings to be verified.

Pacemaker Timing Intervals. All contemporary pacemakers sense in at least one chamber, so that there is the possibility that they may sense extraneous signals (electromagnetic or mechanical interference) or potentials emanating from the other chamber ("AV crosstalk": pacing stimuli, depolarizations). This could lead to inappropriate stimulation or failure to deliver stimulation, the potential of which can be understood as a result of familiarity with basic pacemaker timing design. As shorthand for this discussion, we will use a simplified version of the North American Society for Pacing and Electrophysiology, British Electrophysiology Group (NASPE-BPEG) three-letter code to designate pacing modes (Table 9-5). Single-chamber pacing modes (AAI, VVI) have a single basic timing interval: the interval between pacemaker stimuli in the absence of sensed events. This interval is equivalent to the pacemaker's "escape interval," inversely proportional to the pacing rate:

$$\text{Interval (ms)} = 60{,}000/\text{rate (ppm)}$$

$$\text{Rate (ppm)} = 60{,}000/\text{interval (ms)}$$

where *ms* is milliseconds and *ppm* is pulses (paced) per minute.

In the VVI mode, as shown in Fig. 9-3, pacing occurs at the programmed escape interval VV unless a spontaneous event is sensed. This resets the escape inter-

val (VV), thus inhibiting the pending atrial stimulus, because pacing can occur only if the interval is allowed to complete itself ("time out"). Fig. 9-4 illustrates the basic timing design of a DDD pacemaker (see Table 9-5), which is capable of pacing and sensing in both the atrium and the ventricle. Dual-chamber pacemakers

CHAMBER PACED	CHAMBER SENSED	RESPONSE TO SENSING
A—atrium	A—atrium	I—inhibition stimulus output*
V—ventricle	V—ventricle	T—trigger stimulus output†
D—dual (atrium and ventricle)	D—dual (atrium and ventricle)	D—both I and T‡

TABLE 9-5
Simplified Version of NASPE-BPEG Three-Letter Code to Designate Pacing Mode

NASPE-BPEG, North American Society for Pacing and Electrophysiology, British Electrophysiology Group.
*Sensing in one chamber will lead to inhibition of stimulation in that chamber.
†Sensing in the atrium will trigger stimulation in the ventricle.
‡Sensing in the atrium will trigger stimulation in the ventricle, if spontaneous ventricular depolarization does not occur within preset AV interval, causing inhibition of stimulus output.

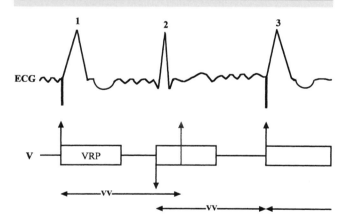

FIG. 9-3 VVI pacing, which might be prescribed for a patient with fixed atrial fibrillation and atrioventricular heart block. In the first beat, the ventricle *(V)* is paced *(arrow* toward electrocardiogram *[ECG]).* This resets the programmed escape interval *(VV)* and initiates the pacemaker's ventricular refractory period *(VRP).* The VRP prevents the resulting T wave from being interpreted by the device as an R wave, which would reset the timing inappropriately. A sensed spontaneous beat (beat 2, *arrow* away from ECG) occurs before VV times out, resetting the escape interval *without* pacing. It also inhibits the stimulus that would otherwise have occurred *(hatched arrow* in VRP). Without further sensing, the second VV interval times with delivery of a pacing stimulus (beat 3).

have *two* fundamental timing intervals, whose sum is the programmed escape interval. The first of these is the AV interval, which begins with an atrial pacing stimulus or a sensed atrial event and ends with the subsequent ventricular stimulus. The second component is the ventriculoatrial (VA) interval, which is the interval between a ventricular stimulus or sensed R wave and the subsequent atrial stimulus. During the pacemaker's atrial and ventricular *refractory periods,* shown as rectangles in the timing overlays (see Fig. 9-4), sensed events do not reset the pacemaker's escape timing. During the ventricular-channel *blanking period* (see Fig. 9-4), ventricular sensing is disabled altogether to prevent saturation of the ventricular sensing amplifier by the relatively high voltage generated by the atrial stimulus. This al-

lows the ventricular-channel sensing circuit to be available for sensing sooner after an atrial stimulus ("alert period"). When sensing occurs in either pacemaker channel outside the refractory or blanking periods (not shown), the interval currently in effect (AV or VA) is terminated before it can time out and produce a stimulus, and the other timing interval begins immediately. Thus when an R wave is sensed during the AV interval, the VA interval is initiated without pacing, and when a P wave is sensed during the VA interval, the AV interval is initiated without pacing.

Pacemaker-Mediated Tachycardia, Crosstalk, and Interference. Pacemaker sensing is accomplished by measuring voltages that appear across the pacing-sensing

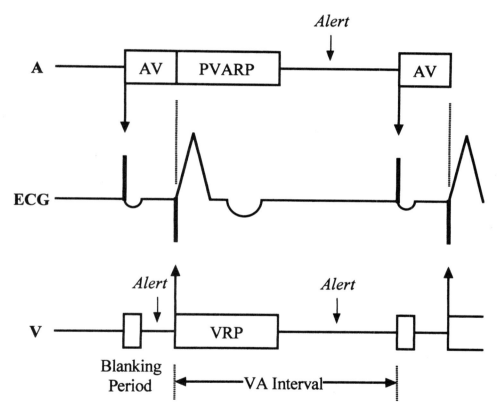

FIG. 9-4 DDD pacing, as might be prescribed for a patient with intermittent sinus node dysfunction and atrioventricular *(AV)* heart block. The programmed AV interval between atrial and ventricular pacing stimuli *(arrows* from above and below, respectively, pointing toward the electrocardiogram *[ECG])* allows time for ventricular filling. The atrial sensing channel is refractory from the atrial stimulus to the end of the postventricular atrial refractory period *(PVARP),* preventing sensing from resetting the escape timing. The ventricular sensing channel has a programmable blanking period, during which time the ventricular sensing amplifier is turned off to prevent its being saturated by the relatively high voltage generated by the atrial stimulus. Sensing resumes immediately thereafter (first "Alert" period). This enables the ventricular channel to sense a conducted R wave, reset the timing, and inhibit a ventricular pacing stimulus. However, as shown, this does not occur. The AV interval times out with delivery of a ventricular stimulus. The ventricular-channel refractory period *(VRP)* prevents sensing of the T wave, which could inappropriately reset the timing. Sensing during the "Alert" period after the PVARP or VRP *will* reset basic timing, initiating a new AV or ventriculoatrial *(VA)* interval, respectively.

electrodes when a spontaneous depolarization occurs. A degree of selectivity is achieved by attenuating low-frequency (T waves) and high-frequency (myopotentials) components, and by requiring that the sensed signal exceed a programmable amplitude threshold. Particularly with unipolar electrode systems, however, spurious interference signals can be detected and treated like P waves or R waves, producing inappropriate triggering or inhibition of pacemaker stimuli. Moreover, a DDD pacemaker usually cannot distinguish between spontaneous atrial depolarizations that result from antegrade or retrograde conduction. *Pacemaker-reentrant tachycardia* (PRT) is a form of pacemaker-mediated tachycardia (PMT) in which a retrograde P wave sensed by the atrial channel of a DDD pacemaker resets (i.e., initiates) the AV interval. Ventricular pacing takes place when this interval times out, producing retrograde VA conduction and another retrograde P wave, which is sensed by the pacemaker, and so on. PRT can be terminated temporarily by placing a magnet over the pulse generator. This action disables the sensing function in most devices and produces asynchronous (DOO) pacing as long as the magnet is in place. The device can also be reprogrammed in various ways, but these methods are beyond the scope of this discussion. A second form of PMT is the *inappropriate tracking of sensed atrial events*. These can be physiologic in origin, as in atrial flutter or fibrillation, or can originate from extrinsic noise (e.g., electrocautery interference). The resulting synchronous ventricular pacing at an inappropriately high rate may be hemodynamically undesirable. Again, the device can be reprogrammed or manufacturers can use various methods to reduce this problem. However, as with PRT, a magnet placed over the pulse generator will temporarily remove the problem. *Crosstalk* is an engineering term that refers to the unwanted appearance of signals in one channel or circuit that are also present in another channel or circuit. Particularly in unipolar atrial pacing, the afterpotential that follows an atrial stimulus may be sensed in the ventricular channel of a dual-chamber pacemaker. This may be misinterpreted as a spontaneous ventricular depolarization, leading to inhibition of output and asystole. A similar problem may arise with atrial-channel "oversensing" of electrical interference signals from an electrocautery device. Methods exist to deal with this problem, either through the manufacturers or through reprogramming, but a magnet suffices in emergencies. Finally, when continuous electrocautery noise or other electromagnetic interference signals are sensed repeatedly by an implanted pacemaker, this generally invokes a form of "noise reversion." The noise reversion feature (the methods used may vary) provides temporary asynchronous pacing with no inhibition by any cardiac or extrinsic signal. Both single- and dual-chamber pacemakers incorporate this feature. Although it has recently

been learned that the ultrasonic scalpel does not produce interference with pacemakers, it is premature to suggest that this device be used routinely in place of conventional electrocautery in patients with pacemakers or ICDs. Readers are encouraged to keep abreast of developments in this arena.

Temporary Pacing. Epicardial, transvenous, transcutaneous, and transesophageal routes are used for temporary pacing. Because of their proximity to myocardium, epicardial, endocardial, or transesophageal leads are also useful for ECG diagnosis. Epicardial atrial, ventricular, or dual-chamber pacing is used in cardiac surgery to increase heart rate, suppress bradycardia-dependent tachycardia, overdrive junctional or ventricular escape rhythms, suppress atrial or ventricular extrasystoles, and terminate reentrant SVT or atrial flutter. Atrial or dual-chamber pacing is preferred to ventricular pacing for preservation of atrial transport function. Transvenous atrial, ventricular, or dual-chamber pacing is used for most other temporary pacing. Pacing pulmonary artery or balloon-floatation catheter electrodes that do not require fluoroscopy for positioning are used by many anesthesiologists and intensivists. Noninvasive transcutaneous pacing (TCP) is used if invasive pacing is not feasible or is impractical. While current adult advanced cardiac life-support guidelines emphasize use of TCP in out-of-hospital arrest, results are discouraging when TCP is not instituted early after cardiac arrest. Limitations of TCP in the perioperative setting are (1) nonphysiologic (ventricular) pacing, (2) inability to capture in some patients, (3) access (sterile fields, patient position), and (4) discomfort in conscious patients. Stethoscope, pill, and catheter electrodes are available for transesophageal (TE) pacing. TE ventricular pacing and electroversion are feasible, but remain under investigation. TE atrial pacing has been used to treat bradycardia and escape rhythms in adults, to treat bradycardia and tachyarrhythmias in neonates and children, and to terminate reentrant SVT and atrial flutter.

Indications for Pacing. Today, about one half of pacemakers are prescribed to treat bradycardia that is due to sinus node dysfunction, with most of the remaining pacemakers prescribed for AV heart block, hypersensitive carotid sinus syndrome, and neurogenic syncope. A joint task force of the American Heart Association and American College of Cardiology last published their recommendations for implantation of permanent pacemakers in 1998. Indications for implantation were grouped as Class I, II, or III. A Class I indication was a condition for which there was evidence or general agreement that a pacemaker would be useful and effective. A Class II indication was a condition for which there was conflicting evidence and/or a divergence of opinion as to the usefulness or efficacy of device implantation. An indication was Class III if there was evidence or general agreement that a device was not useful or effective, and possibly harmful. Evidence was "level A" if data supporting the recommendation were derived from multiple randomized clinical trials involving a large number of patients. If evidence was "level B," data were derived from a limited number of trials with comparatively small numbers of patients, or from well-designed retrospective analysis of nonrandomized trials. If evidence was "level C," consensus expert opinion or favorable clinical experience was the source for the recommendation. In general, a pacemaker is indicated (Class I) when symptoms are clearly related to bradycardia. The current guidelines include indications for pacemaker implantation in patients with bradycardia due to sinus node dysfunction, AV heart block, hypersensitive carotid sinus syndrome or neurally mediated syncope; patients with fascicular heart block after the acute phase of myocardial infarction; and in children and adolescents.

Internal Cardioverter-Defibrillator. ICDs are prescribed for patients considered at high risk for sudden death due to VT or ventricular fibrillation (VF). ICDs have undergone explosive evolution since they were first implanted in 1980. First- and second-generation ICDs used epicardial patch electrodes implanted at median sternotomy or open left thoracotomy, and delivered only shocks. Contemporary devices use transvenous lead systems for sensing, pacing for bradycardia or to terminate tachycardia, and shock delivery. Currently, at least three types of lead systems are in use. The first has a single right-ventricular (RV) lead with two spring electrodes, one in the RV and the other in the superior vena cava (SVC). A second tip electrode in the RV is used for pacing and sensing. The second lead system has a single RV lead, with one spring electrode and a distal electrode for pacing and sensing. A separate spring electrode resides in the right atrium or SVC. The third system has a single RV spring electrode, with the titanium housing of the pulse generator serving as the anode. Subcutaneous patches in various configurations may be used, together with the housing of a subpectorally implanted pulse generator, to achieve a lower defibrillation threshold.

ICDs are powered by lithium-silver vanadium pentoxide cells and have a service life of 6 to 8 years. The evolution of new designs has reduced mass and volume from 250 to 280 g and 150 cm³ to 132 g and 83 cm³, respectively. Future devices will be even smaller. ICDs use one or more capacitors to store electric charge and deliver high-voltage, biphasic shocks when needed. They incorporate integrated circuitry that regulates the strength and timing of impulses or shocks. Like pacemakers, modern ICDs are also programmable for shock strength; "backup" antibradycardia pacing for postshock asystole or bradycardia; and algorithms for the detection, diagnosis, and treatment of tachycardia. ICD algo-

rithms consider both rate and rate stability to distinguish tachycardia from fibrillation. Often ICDs are programmed to provide tiered therapy, which begins with antitachycardia pacing, followed by a series of progressively stronger shocks as long as the arrhythmia persists.

Management of Patients with a Pacemaker or ICD. Most patients with implanted devices have myocardial dysfunction and many other systemic diseases. A complete history and physical examination should be recorded, with special attention to functional status, progression of disease, current medications, and compliance with treatment. The results of a recent 12-lead ECG and any other indicated diagnostic and laboratory tests should be available.

At the time of device implantation, patients receive a card that identifies the model and serial numbers of the pacemaker or ICD, the date of implantation, and the implanting physician. If the device can be identified, the manufacturer also has this information in its registry. The device may often be identified from the operative report or from a chest radiograph of the pulse generator that allows identification of the manufacturer from a unique radiopaque marker. A guidebook for pacemaker and ICD pulse generators and leads is compiled and periodically updated by each of the U.S. manufacturers (Table 9-6). It lists the identifying radiopaque markers for all models of pacemaker and ICD devices that might be encountered in patients. Once the manufacturer and device have been identified, the manufacturer can be contacted for further information through its Web site or telephone hotline (see Table 9-6).

Not uncommonly, patients with pacemakers have adequate spontaneous rhythm. Thus, the functional status of the device will be unknown to the casual observer. Ideally, the pacemaker clinic staff should be called on for device evaluation and reprogramming as indicated. The indications for implantation and the programmable-parameter settings should be noted, together with recommendations for perioperative management. If this is impossible, the basic function of a pacemaker whose output is inhibited by the patient's spontaneous rhythm can be determined by applying a magnet to convert the device to asynchronous operation. Cholinergic stimulation (e.g., the Valsalva maneuver, carotid sinus massage, IV adenosine 6-12 mg, or IV edrophonium 5-10 mg) can also be used to reduce the intrinsic heart rate below the pacemaker's programmed lower rate limit, resulting in the release of pacing stimuli.

Management of Pacemaker or ICD System Implantation or Revision. As earlier noted, modern pacemaker and ICDs systems use transvenous leads. A thoracotomy

TABLE 9-6
U.S. Pacemaker and ICD Manufacturers, with 24-Hour Hotlines and Web Sites

MANUFACTURER	HOTLINE & WEB SITE	PRODUCTS
Biotronik, Inc. 6024 Jean Road Lake Oswego, OR 97035-5369	1-800-547-9001 1-503-635-9936 (fax) www.biotronik.com	Single- and dual-chamber pacemakers; single-chamber ICD
Guidant Corporation* 4100 Hamline Avenue North St. Paul, MN 55112-5798 (CPI, Intermedics)	1-800-CARDIAC (227-3422) 1-800-474-3245 (fax) www.guidant.com	Single- and dual-chamber pacemakers (Intermedics); single- and dual-chamber ICDs (CPI)
Medtronic Corporation 7000 Central Avenue NE Minneapolis, MN 55432	1-800-328-2518 1-800-824-2362 (fax) www.medtronic.com	Single- and dual-chamber pacemakers; single- and dual-chamber ICDs
St. Jude Medical* Cardiac Rhythm Management Division 15900 Valley View Court Sylmar, CA 91342 (Pacesetter, Ventritex)	1-800-777-2237 1-800-756-7223 (fax) www.sjm.com	Single- and dual-chamber pacemakers (Pacesetter); single-chamber ICD (Ventritex)

ICD, Internal cardioverter-defibrillator.
*Parent company, including recent acquired or merged companies.

is not required for system implantation or revision. Both the pulse generator and leads are implanted by using local anesthesia and conscious sedation. Nonetheless, monitored anesthesia care or general anesthesia may be requested for ICD system implantation or revision, especially if the procedure involves repeated induction of VT or VF with painful shocks. However, a thoracotomy is required in neonates, infants, and small children, for whom epicardial lead systems are still used most of the time.

The following recommendations apply to the intraoperative management of ICD implantation:

1. Consider temporary pacing with disadvantageous bradycardia for any cause. Chronotropic drugs and backup transcutaneous pacing should be available.
2. Establish a reliable means for pulse monitoring (arterial pressure or pulse oximetry waveform).
3. Select the best ECG leads for ischemia detection and arrhythmia diagnosis.
4. Pulmonary artery catheters are no longer advised, and may interfere with ICD lead positioning.
5. Techniques and agents for monitored anesthesia care or general anesthesia vary, with patient tolerance and effects on the ability to induce and terminate VT or VF of primary importance. IV anesthesia, with propofol, etomidate, or midazolam and a short-acting opiate, is reasonable. The airway should be secured if there is to be repeated induc-

tion of destabilizing tachycardia during testing of cardioversion or defibrillation thresholds. Primary reliance on volatile agents is discouraged because of potentially unfavorable hemodynamic actions (increased heart rate, negative inotropy, and preload reduction). Also, some older agents (halothane, enflurane) have been shown in animal models to reduce inducibility of ventricular tachycardia. These properties of desflurane and sevoflurane are unknown.

6. Since antiarrhythmic drugs affect the induction of tachyarrhythmias and increase cardioversion and defibrillation thresholds, their use is discouraged unless needed for patient stability. It is unlikely that infiltration of small amounts of local anesthesia for venous or arterial access would affect electrophysiologic testing or defibrillation thresholds, but larger amounts with regional anesthesia (field blocks) might do so.
7. An external cardioverter-defibrillator must be available and functioning, with pads properly positioned. Apex and posterior pad electrodes should be used. Alternatively, paddles should be applied so that the vector of the applied voltage is roughly perpendicular to an imaginary line connecting the pulse generator and the ventricular electrodes.
8. Program the ICD off if electrocautery is used during system implantation or revision.

TABLE 9-7
Suggested Management for Patients with Pacemakers or ICD Having Unrelated Surgery

Elective Surgery*

- Contact pacemaker/ICD clinic or manufacturer during the preoperative evaluation. Identify and interrogate the device, and reprogram if necessary (i.e., nature and/or location of planned surgery, unipolar cautery, etc.).
- With a pacemaker-dependent patient, reprogram the device to a triggered or asynchronous mode. Program magnet-activated testing and adaptive-rate pacing off.
- With ICD, program tachycardia sensing off. Do not use magnet to disable sensing unless you know what the programmed response is. Have an external cardioverter-defibrillator available.
- If possible, locate the cautery grounding plate so that the pulse generator and leads are not in the current pathway between it and the bovie tool. Also, the grounding plate should be located as far as possible from the pulse generator and leads. Use the lowest possible cautery energy and short bursts to minimize adverse effects of EMI.
- Monitor arterial pulse waveform and heart sounds to detect EMI-related hemodynamic instability, which is unlikely. But, should this occur, proceed as during urgent or emergent surgery (below).
- If external defibrillation is required, locate defibrillation pads or paddles at least 10 cm from the pulse generator and implanted electrodes. Use apex- (anterior-) posterior position if possible. As near as possible, current flow between the paddles should be perpendicular to the major lead axis.
- After surgery, arrange to have device function tested by pacemaker/ICD clinic, and reprogram or replace the device if necessary.

Urgent or Emergent Surgery

- If time permits, identify the implanted device from the patient's medical record, identification card, or "x-ray signature." Contact the manufacturer (see Table 9-6) and follow their recommendations.
- Institute ECG, arterial pulse waveform and heart sounds monitoring. If no pacing artifacts are seen, and the device is a pacemaker, place a magnet over the pulse generator to determine whether the device is functional. Alternatively, consider vagal maneuver or drug to slow intrinsic rate.
- If EMI-related pacemaker malfunction is hemodynamically destabilizing, program the device to a triggered or asynchronous mode. If this is not possible, a magnet over the pulse generator will convert many (but not all) devices to an asynchronous pacing mode.
- If the device is an ICD, without knowing how it is programmed, or what the magnet response is, it is generally advised not to place a magnet over the pulse generator to disable tachycardia sensing. This should be considered, however, if repeated shocks or antitachycardia pacing in response to sensed EMI are hemodynamically destabilizing.
- After surgery, arrange to have device function tested by pacemaker/ICD clinic and reprogram or replace the device if necessary.

ECG, Electrocardiogram; *EMI,* electromagnetic interference; *ICD,* internal cardioverter-defibrillator.
*It is assumed that for patients having elective surgery and at risk for related device malfunction, the pacemaker/ICD clinic or manufacturer will have been contacted regarding appropriate perioperative management, including device interrogation and reprogramming if necessary.

KEY POINTS

1. Arrhythmias continue to be a problem in cardiac surgical patients. Acute atrial fibrillation and VT are most troublesome. These disturbances can arise due to effects of atrial and ventricular *remodeling,* consequent to aging, hypertension, chronic pulmonary disease, and ischemic heart disease. Myocardial remodeling, by altering electrophysiologic properties, provides a *substrate* that is capable of sustaining arrhythmias (often, functional reentry), provided an imposed *physiologic imbalance* triggers the disturbance. Hence, fundamental to prevention and management of arrhythmias are optimal management for underlying heart disease and correction of untoward physiologic imbalance.

2. *Proarrhythmia* is a condition whereby antiarrhythmic drugs paradoxically aggravate arrhythmias or create new arrhythmias. Drug therapy is no longer empiric. Instead, it is targeted at specific ion channels and currents believed to be responsible for triggering and sustaining arrhythmias. Current interest is in the development of drugs that produce use-dependent prolongation of cardiac repolarization with reduced risk of proarrhythmia, specifically, by block of the slowly activating component of the delayed rectifier K^+ current (I_{Ks}). Amiodarone, for example, may supplant lidocaine as the initial drug of choice for treatment of destabilizing or life-threatening ventricular arrhythmias. It is also effective against supraventricular tach-

yarrhythmias, but its use in perioperative settings for this indication requires further study.

3. Perioperative management for the patient with a pacemaker or ICD remains a challenge for anesthesiologists and intensivists, given the increasing sophistication of these devices and the potential for adverse effects with exposure to electromagnetic or electromechanical interference, especially surgical electrocautery. However, this problem can be addressed with more complete understanding of implanted-device function, especially pacemaker timing cycles. This allows the practitioner to comprehend and even predict inappropriate device function, and to make the necessary adjustments in patient management.

As a rule, if interference is likely to be a problem for a pacemaker-dependent patient, the device should be programmed to an asynchronous mode. The response to magnet application is not uniform for all devices. Similarly, tachycardia therapies with ICDs should be programmed off. A magnet should be used only if a programmer is not available and interference causes repeated, unnecessary shocks. Finally, device function must be checked after the procedure, and pacing or ICD therapy reprogrammed if required. Recommendations for the perioperative management of patients with pacemakers or ICDs are summarized in Table 9-7.

KEY REFERENCES

Atlee JL: Cardiac electrophysiology. In Priebe H-J, Skarvan K, editors: *Cardiovascular physiology*, ed 2, London, 2000, BMJ Books, pp 73-118.

Atlee JL, Bernstein AD: Cardiac rhythm management devices. Part 1. Indications, device selection and function. *Anesthesiology*, 2001 (in press).

Atlee JL, Bernstein AD: Cardiac rhythm management devices. Part 2. Perioperative management. *Anesthesiology*, 2001 (in press).

Balser JR: The rationale use of intravenous amiodarone in the perioperative period, *Anesthesiology* 86:974-987, 1997.

Epstein MR, Mayer, Jr, JE, Duncan BW: Use of an ultrasonic scalpel as an alternative to electrocautery in patients with pacemakers, *Ann Thorac Surg* 65:1802-1804, 1998.

Grant AO: Mechanisms of action of antiarrhythmic drugs: from ion channel blockage to arrhythmia termination, *Pacing Clin Electrophysiol* 20:432-434, 1997.

Gregoratos G, Cheitlin M, Conill A, et al: ACC/AHA guidelines for implantation of cardiac pacemakers and antiarrhythmia devices: a report of the ACC/AHA Task Force on Practice Guidelines (Committee on Pacemaker Implantation), *J Am Coll Cardiol* 31:1175-1206, 1998.

Kudenchuk PJ, Cobb LA, Copass MK et al: Amiodarone for resuscitation after out-of-hospital cardiac arrest due to ventricular fibrillation.

Mines GR: On dynamic equilibrium in the heart, *J Physiol (Lond)* 46:349-383, 1913.

Morganroth J: Proarrhythmic effects of antiarrhythmic drugs: evolving concepts, *Am Heart J* 123:1137-1139, 1992.

Spach MS, Boineau JP: Microfibrosis produces electrical load variations due to loss of side-to-side cell connections, *Pacing Clin Electrophysiol* 20:397-413, 1997.

Task Force of the Working Group on Arrhythmias of the European Society of Cardiology: The Sicilian Gambit. A new approach to the classification of antiarrhythmic drugs based on their actions on arrhythmogenic mechanisms, *Circulation* 84:1831-1851, 1991.

Waldo A, Wells J, Cooper T et al: Temporary cardiac pacing: applications and techniques in the treatment of cardiac arrhythmias, *Prog Cardiovasc Dis* 23:451-474, 1981.

Whalley DW, Wendt DJ, Grant AO: Basic concepts in cellular cardiac electrophysiology. Part II. Block of ion channels by antiarrhythmic drugs, *Pacing Clin Electrophysiol* 18:1686-1704, 1995.

CHAPTER 10

Congenital Heart Disease

Ingrid Hollinger, M.D. ■ David L. Reich, M.D. ■ David Moskowitz, M.D.

OUTLINE

Safe anesthetic management for patients with congenital heart disease (CHD) requires a careful and thorough preoperative evaluation. Formulating an anesthetic plan requires an in-depth understanding of the specific car-diac lesion, its pathophysiologic consequences, and the effects of anesthetic agents on these consequences. Likewise, the requirements of the proposed surgery need to be considered.

TABLE 10-1
Syndromes with Congenital Cardiac Defects[31,32]

ETIOLOGY	INCIDENCE OF CONGENITAL HEART DISEASE (% OF PATIENTS)	CARDIAC LESIONS IN ORDER OF FREQUENCY
Chromosomal Anomalies		
Trisomy 21	40	ECD, ASD, TOF, PDA
Trisomy 18	90	VSD, PDA, ASD, bicuspid PV, CoA, bicuspid AV
Trisomy 13	80	PDA, VSD, ASD, abnormal valves, CoA
5p⁻ (cri du chat)	25	VSD, PDA, ASD, PS
4p⁻ (Wolf's)	50	VSD, ASD, PDA, PS
XO (Turner)	10-30	CoA, AS, VSD, ASD
Genetic or Unknown Etiology		
Ellis-van-Creveld	50-60	Single atrium, ECD, PDA
Holt-Oram	50	ASD, VSD, TOF, PS, PDA
VATER	25	VSD
Rubinstein-Taybi	15-20	ECD, ASD
Noonan	50	PS, ASD
DiGeorge	90-100	Interrupted aortic arch type B, aberrant right subclavian artery, right aortic arch, truncus arteriosus, TOF
Goldenhar's (hemifacial microsomia)	50	TOF, VSD, PDA, CoA
William's Elfin Face	80	Supravalvar AS, peripheral AS, peripheral PS, interrupted arch
Teratogenic		
Alcohol	25-30	VSD, PDA, ASD
Trimethadione	15-30	TGA, TOF, HLHS
Rubella	35	Peripheral PS, PDA, VSD, ASD

AS, Aortic stenosis; *ASD,* atrial septal defect; *AV,* aortic valve; *CoA,* coarctation of the aorta; *ECD,* endocardial cushion defect; *HLHS,* hypoplastic left heart syndrome; *PDA,* patent ductus arteriosus; *PS,* pulmonic stenosis; *PV,* pulmonary valve; *TGA,* transposition of the great arteries; *TOF,* tetralogy of Fallot; *VSD,* ventricular septal defect.

The incidence of CHD is approximately 6 to 8 infants of every 1000 live births. Once considered rare, the incidence of CHD has increased secondary to improvements in diagnostic testing, increased awareness, and improved medical treatments of the critically ill. As a result, 40,000 children are born each year with CHD.[1] The incidence is two to three times higher in premature infants, even if persistent patent ductus arteriosus (PDA) is excluded.

Associated extracardiac defects are present in 5% to 50% of children with CHD.[2] The defect is part of a syndrome or chromosomal anomaly in 17% to 18% (Table 10-1). Genitourinary tract anomalies are among the most common lesions, and are present in 4% to 15% of patients with CHD.[3] In addition, approximately half of all infants with CHD require hospital admission for either medical or surgical therapy during the first year of life, the majority within the first 2 months.[4] This further stresses the importance of a thorough preoperative evaluation.

There are many ways to classify CHD. One method is to divide CHD into cyanotic and acyanotic lesions, which is a clinical categorization. These divisions are then further subdivided according to a lesion's effects on pulmonary blood flow. Alternatively, CHD can be categorized according to the physiologic alterations produced by the lesion (Table 10-2). Chapter 10 uses the latter method to classify congenital heart defects and reviews the current management of CHD, the results of therapy, and implications for anesthetic management in cardiac and noncardiac surgery.

GENERAL PRINCIPLES

Blood flow is the volume of blood passing through a structure per unit of time. Examples of structures include blood vessels, heart valves, abnormal communications between heart chambers, and stenotic lesions. Blood flows from an area of higher pressure to an area of lower pressure. The flow rate is directly related to the pressure

**TABLE 10-2
Congenital Heart Defects (CHDs)
Classified by Physiology**

Left-to-Right Shunts (Increased Pulmonary Blood Flow [Congestive Heart Failure/Acyanotic])
• Atrial septal defect (15% of CHD)
• Ventricular septal defect (20%-25% of CHD)
• Single ventricle (1%-1.5% of CHD)
• L-Transposition of the great vessels (1.5% of CHD)
• Patent ductus arteriosus (5%-10% of CHD)
• Endocardial cushion defect (3%-4% of CHD)

Right-to-Left Shunts (Decreased Pulmonary Blood Flow [Cyanotic])
• Tetralogy of Fallot (10% of CHD)
• Pulmonary atresia (1% of CHD)
• Tricuspid atresia (2%-3% of CHD)
• Ebstein's anomaly (1% of CHD)

Complex Shunts (Mixing of Pulmonary and Systemic Circulation)
• Truncus arteriosus (4% of CHD)
• Transposition of the great vessels (5% of CHD)
• Total anomalous pulmonary venous return (1.5% of CHD)
• Double outlet right ventricle (0.5% of CHD)
• Hypoplastic left heart syndrome (7%-9% of CHD)
• Heterotaxy syndromes (1% of CHD)

Obstructive Lesions
• Coarctation of the aorta (6%-7% of CHD)
• Interrupted aortic arch (1%-2% of CHD)
• Aortic stenosis (8%-10% of CHD)
• Pulmonic stenosis (10% of CHD)
• Mitral stenosis (0.2%-0.6% of CHD)
• Supravalvular mitral ring
• Shone syndrome
• Cor triatriatum (0.5% of CHD)

Miscellaneous
• Vascular ring
• Anomalous origin of the left coronary artery
• Kawasaki disease

differential across a structure and indirectly related to the resistance across the structure. This is analogous to Ohm's law of electrical current across a circuit:

$$V = I \times R,$$

where the voltage (V) is equivalent to the pressure differential, current (I) is equivalent to blood flow, and resistance (R) is the resistance to flow within the circuit.

There are three major determinants of resistance to blood flow across a structure: (1) the viscosity of the blood, (2) the length of the structure, and (3) its radius. The radius of the lumen that the blood traverses is the most important determinant of resistance. The Hagen-Poiseuille law of laminar flow through a pipe indicates that decreasing the radius by 50% increases the resistance to flow sixteenfold, because resistance is inversely proportionate to radius to the fourth power. Flow across congenital heart lesions, however, is often turbulent, the lesions may be irregular in shape, and they may more closely resemble orifices than tubes. Nevertheless, the physical principles mentioned earlier are important.

Although these seem like simple concepts, using anesthetics, vasoactive drugs, and other techniques to manipulate these variables are the keys to mastering pediatric cardiac anesthesia. Alterations in systemic vascular resistance (SVR), pulmonary vascular resistance (PVR), preload, and heart rate may lead to dramatic changes in the patient's hemodynamic and respiratory status by redistributing blood flow between the lungs and the systemic circulation. PVR must not further decrease in patients with high Qp/Qs (excessive pulmonary blood flow) to avoid congestive heart failure and poor peripheral perfusion. Conversely, patients with a low Qp/Qs (inadequate pulmonary blood flow) are dependent on a low PVR and high SVR to maintain pulmonary blood flow and adequate arterial oxygen tension (Pa_{O_2}). Factors that influence PVR are listed in Table 10-3. Rapid changes in the cardiopulmonary status occur in patients with CHD during the perioperative period. By applying the preceding concepts, the anesthesiologist can avoid detrimental physiologic changes to the patient.

Effect of Intracardiac Shunts on Anesthetic Update and Distribution

The uptake of inhalational anesthetic agents is only minimally influenced by a left-to-right shunt unless peripheral perfusion is poorly maintained. Under these circumstances, induction with a poorly soluble agent may be accelerated.[5] Induction with intravenous agents, however, may be delayed, since a considerable portion of the drug is recirculated through the lung. If the amount of drug injected is increased to achieve the desired effect more rapidly, side effects of overdose may appear when peak drug level finally reaches the brain and the peripheral circulation.

LEFT-TO-RIGHT SHUNTS

Simple left-to-right shunts result in increased pulmonary blood flow. Congenital heart defects that fall under this classification include (1) atrial septal defects (ASDs), (2) ventricular septal defects (VSDs), (3) PDA, (4) endocardial cushion defects, and (5) aortopulmonary windows. Patients with a small shunt may have minimal or no symptoms, and only present with a murmur. Patients with a large left-to-right shunt may exhibit signs of right-sided heart failure from the increased pulmonary blood flow (ascites and edema) and left-sided heart failure from the excessive preload and diminished systemic blood flow (dyspnea and fatigue). Patients with these congenital heart defects are usually acyanotic because there is no obstruction to pulmonary blood flow. Cyanosis occurs when there is massive mixing of arterial and venous blood (e.g., truncus arteriosus) or congestive heart failure severe enough to impair oxygen diffusion. Patients with long-standing, uncorrected left-to-right shunts may develop pulmonary hypertension secondary to pulmonary artery smooth muscle hyperplasia from increased pulmonary blood flow (see below).

TABLE 10-3
Factors that Influence Pulmonary Vascular Resistance (PVR)

Increase PVR
- Sympathetic stimulation
  - Pain
  - Light anesthesia
- Decreasing pH
- Increasing $Paco_2$
- Decreasing Pao_2
- Hypothermia
- Increased intrathoracic pressure
  - Controlled ventilation
  - PEEP
  - Atelectasis
- Mechanical compression

Decrease PVR
- Block sympathetic stimulation
  - Anesthesia
- Increasing pH
- Decreasing $Paco_2$
- Increasing Pao_2
- Minimizing intrathoracic pressure
  - Spontaneous ventilation
  - Normal lung volumes
  - High frequency jet ventilation
- Pharmacological agents
  - Phosphodiesterase inhibitors
  - Isoproterenol
  - Prostaglandin E_1
  - Prostacyclin (PGI_2)
  - Nitric oxide

$Paco_2$, Arterial carbon dioxide tension; Pao_2, arterial oxygen tension; *PEEP*, positive end-expiratory pressure.

Atrial Septal Defects

There are four major types of ASD (Fig. 10-1). These include (1) ostium primum defects, (2) ostium secundum defects, (3) patent foramen ovale, and (4) sinus venosus defects. Rarer entities, such as an unroofed coronary sinus or single atrium (cor triloculare biventriculare), should also be considered in the same class.

Ostium primum ASDs occur low in the inferior atrial septum and result from failure of the septum primum to fuse with the endocardial cushions. Because many structures are dependent on the endocardial cushion for normal growth, ostium primum ASDs may be associated with abnormalities of the interventricular septum, the mitral and tricuspid valves, and the papillary muscles. Ostium primum accounts for approximately 20% of ASDs.

Ostium secundum ASDs are located in the middle of the atrial septum at the fossa ovalis. Excessive resorption of septum primum leaves very little septum remaining at the site of the foramen ovale. These lesions represent a spectrum from a small defect caused by an abnormally large ("stretched") patent foramen ovale to large defects that encompass the entire foramen ovale. Ostium secundum ASDs account for 75% of all ASDs. These defects are more common in females, with a male-to-female ratio of 1:2. The main cause of clinical deterioration of patients with secundum ASD in adult life is atrial arrhythmias, particularly atrial fibrillation and flutter. Children with secundum ASD are usually asymptomatic.

Functional closure of the foramen ovale occurs after birth, but anatomic closure is not complete until 2 to 3 months of age. Unlike the septum primum, the septum secundum does not migrate all the way down to the

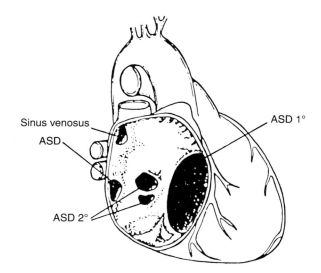

FIG. 10-1   The atrial septum showing several types of atrial septal defects as seen from the right atrium. *ASD*, Atrial septal defect; *1°*, primum; *2°*, secundum.

endocardial cushions. Therefore, its free edge may not fuse with the septum primum. Patency of the foramen ovale on probing persists in 50% of children up to 5 years of age and in 20% to 40% of the adult population. There is usually no shunting across the patent foramen ovale because the flaplike structure is closed in the normal situation in which the left atrial pressure exceeds the right atrial pressure. Right-to-left shunting can occur, however, with transient or persistent increases in right atrial pressure. Left-to-right shunting across a patent foramen ovale may occur if it is stretched by a distended atrium or if the flap valve is deficient.

Sinus venosus ASDs account for about 10% of all ASDs. The defect lies posterior to the fossa ovalis in the upper atrial septum. This type of ASD is frequently associated with partial anomalous pulmonary venous return from the right upper pulmonary vein, which is "unroofed" by the defect. The right upper pulmonary vein drains into the right atrium or the superior vena cava.

Coronary sinus ASD is the least common type of ASD and lies at the site of the anticipated coronary sinus ostium. It is usually associated with absence of the coronary sinus and a persistent left superior vena cava draining into the roof of the left atrium. It may be associated with a complete atrioventricular (AV) canal defect and heterotaxy syndromes.

Common atrium is characterized by complete absence of the atrial septum. It is frequently combined with other cardiac anomalies, such as transposition, double-outlet right ventricle (DORV), univentricular heart, and anomalous pulmonary venous connection in association with heterotaxy syndromes. Nearly complete mixing of systemic and pulmonary blood occurs, but pulmonary blood flow exceeds systemic blood flow. Cyanosis may be constantly present or apparent only during exercise. Surgical repair is performed early in life to prevent development of pulmonary vascular disease.

Ventricular Septal Defects

Ventricular septal defects (VSDs) are the most common congenital heart defects, occurring in 2 per 1000 live births (20%-25% of all patients with CHD). They are slightly more common in females (56%) than in males (44%). There are multiple classifications of VSDs. For simplification, Becu et al[6] and Kirklin et al[7] divided the right ventricle into two portions (right ventricular outflow tract and inflow tract) as a tool for identifying the anatomic locations of VSDs.[8] The outflow tract lies between the pulmonic valve above and the tricuspid valve below, and is part of the membranous portion of the interventricular septum. The crista supraventricularis is located within the right ventricular outflow tract and overlies a portion of the aortic root. This explains why VSDs located in the pulmonary outflow tract can be associated with portions of the aortic valve.

VSDs that form above the crista supraventricularis are called *supracristal*. Defects located here form just below the pulmonic valve and lie in the outflow tract. Defects below the crista supraventricularis within the right ventricular outflow tract are also membranous defects and account for approximately 80% of VSDs. Typically, these defects extend into the muscular portion of the interventricular septum. VSDs located in the inflow tract appear either posteriorly under the septal leaflet of the tricuspid valve (membranous type), or in the mid-to-apical region of the muscular septum (muscular type). Defects under the septal leaflet of the tricuspid valve are also called *posterior defects* and are commonly termed *AV canal defects* because of the close association of this region to the endocardial cushion and left ventricle. Defects located in the muscular septum are frequently multiple in nature (Fig. 10-2).

Small VSDs restrict the amount of left-to-right shunting and limit the hemodynamic consequences. With a large defect (approximating the size of the normal age-appropriate aortic orifice or larger), there is no restriction to flow, and shunting depends largely on the relative ratio of pulmonary to systemic vascular resistance. In the early neonatal period, the PVR is high, and the patient may have no signs or symptoms relating to the VSD. As the PVR declines during the second and third week of life, congestive heart failure may ensue due to volume overload on the left ventricle as the left-to-right shunting increases. This presentation may be delayed 2 to 3 months postnatally because exposure of the pulmonary circulation to systemic pressure delays the normal decline in the PVR, limiting the severity of the left-to-right shunting.

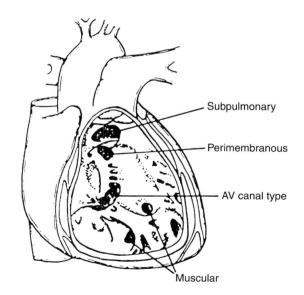

FIG. 10-2   The ventricular septum, showing several types of ventricular septal defects as seen from the right ventricle. *AV,* Atrioventricular.

An estimated 25% to 50% of all small to moderate-sized VSDs close spontaneously—generally during the first year of life. Many become smaller throughout life and remain benign. Probably fewer than 5% of large VSDs undergo spontaneous closure. Surgery is indicated for primary closure of the defect during the first year of life only in infants with congestive heart failure and failure to thrive despite medical therapy. Surgical mortality rate should be 5% or less. If infants with large VSDs are only treated medically, high pulmonary artery pressures lead to progressive pulmonary vascular obstructive disease, particularly after the second year of life. In the past, pulmonary artery banding was performed in small infants to protect the pulmonary vasculature from exposure to systemic pressures. The combined mortality rate of the initial procedure and of the subsequent repair of the VSD with debanding, however, was higher than that for primary surgical closure. Moderate-size defects with only mild elevation of pulmonary artery pressures can be managed medically during infancy. The defect should be closed surgically if a large left-to-right shunt (Qp:Qs >2) persists, and if there is evidence that pulmonary artery pressures are greater than one third of systemic pressures. Surgery is not recommended for small VSDs.

Patients who have VSD closure during infancy show normal growth and development. Pulmonary artery pressures return to normal, as does left ventricular function. In patients operated on during childhood, left ventricular function may remain mildly depressed and exhibit dysfunction with intense exercise, despite lack of clinical symptoms at rest. Patients may have conduction defects after surgical closure, most commonly right bundle-branch block or a combination of right bundle-branch block with left anterior hemiblock. Complete heart block is, fortunately, rare.

Ventricular Septal Defect with Infundibular Pulmonic Stenosis. Hypertrophy of the infundibulum of the right ventricle may occur in patients with large VSDs (particularly those with right aortic arch). This obstruction leads to a progressive decrease in left-to-right shunting and protection of the pulmonary vascular bed from systemic pressures. If the muscle hypertrophy becomes severe, right-to-left shunting may eventually occur, initially only during exercise. These patients may develop the same clinical features as in tetralogy of Fallot. Pulmonary stenosis rarely becomes prominent before 4 to 5 years of age. Treatment is surgical repair during childhood with closure of the septal defect and resection of the infundibular muscle bands.

Ventricular Septal Defect with Aortic Insufficiency. Approximately 5% of patients with VSD (more commonly males) develop signs of aortic valve incompetence, which may become the predominant problem.

Supracristal VSD is especially prone to this complication. The right coronary cusp tends to herniate through the VSD in these patients and may cause a degree of right ventricular outflow obstruction. Aortic insufficiency in infracristal VSD is rare and usually is associated with anomalies of the aortic commissures and infundibular pulmonic stenosis. Mild aortic insufficiency may be treated by closure of the VSD alone. With more severe insufficiency, aortic valvuloplasty is performed at the time of VSD closure. The aortic insufficiency does not appear to progress after repair. Surgery is performed when leaflet prolapse is recognized with angiography or if signs of aortic insufficiency occur.

Left Ventricular to Right Atrial Shunt

Communications between the left ventricle and right atrium constitute fewer than 1% of all congenital cardiac defects. There is a slight female preponderance. Approximately one third of the defects are located above the tricuspid valve, and the remainder are below and in association with malformation of the septal leaflet. The shunt is always large, because of the marked pressure difference between the left ventricle and right atrium during systole, which is present from birth. Volume overload of the right ventricle and enlargement of the pulmonary artery occur. The increased pulmonary circulation leads to volume overload of the left side, and heart failure may occur in the first few months of life. There is always marked enlargement of the right atrium. The lesion may decrease in size, but spontaneous closure has not been observed.

There is a high incidence of endocarditis (6% of recorded cases) and atrial dysrhythmias (5% of recorded cases). Because of the large shunt and high endocarditis risk, surgical correction should be performed in early childhood. Long-term postoperative complications include complete heart block (4%) and atrial dysrhythmias (3%).

Single Ventricle

Connection of both atria, usually via two AV valves to a single ventricular chamber, is a rare anomaly, accounting for approximately 1% to 1.5% of all CHD. There is a slight male preponderance. The single ventricle is a morphologic left ventricle in nearly 80% of cases and the relationship of the great vessels is either d-transposed or l-transposed. All patients with d-transposition have a degree of subaortic stenosis, and more than 50% of those with l-transposition tend to have subaortic and subpulmonary obstruction. Half of the patients present within the first month of life and close to 90% within the first 6 months. Without surgical intervention, 75% of these infants die within this period.

Patients without obstruction to pulmonary blood

flow have signs in early infancy of a large left-to-right shunt with congestive heart failure, growth retardation, and frequent respiratory infections. Despite nearly complete mixing of systemic and pulmonary venous blood in the systemic ventricle, cyanosis is not prominent in these children. Cyanosis is present and heart failure rare in patients with obstruction to pulmonary outflow. With pulmonary atresia, pulmonary blood flow may be ductus dependent.

Palliative procedures performed during infancy consist of pulmonary artery banding in patients without pulmonary stenosis who have unremitting congestive heart failure. Banding may lead to the development of subaortic stenosis. Unfavorable anatomy may require that the pulmonary artery be interrupted and a shunt inserted for pulmonary blood flow. In patients with pulmonary outflow obstruction, a systemic-to-pulmonary shunt is created. Long-term survival is poor with palliative operations because of progressive myocardial fibrosis, secondary subaortic obstruction, or insufficient pulmonary blood flow. Patients at present undergo bidirectional cava-pulmonary anastomosis at approximately 6 months of age and a modified Fontan procedure between 2 and 3 years of age.

Although during the 1970s and 1980s patients with favorable anatomy had a septation procedure performed between 4 and 5 years of age, progressive cardiovascular deterioration and late mortality led to abandonment of this procedure.[9] Only half of patients are asymptomatic after the Fontan operation and many patients continue to receive digitalis or diuretics and afterload reducing agents. While described here for anatomic reasons, single ventricle physiology and its anesthetic management are discussed under the section on hypoplastic left heart syndrome (HLHS), as are the anesthetic management issues following bidirectional cava-pulmonary anastomosis and modified Fontan procedure.

L-Transposition of the Great Arteries

Abnormal rotation of the bulboventricular loop results in ventricular inversion and transposition of the great arteries. The anatomic left ventricle receives the systemic venous return and ejects into the pulmonary artery, and the anatomic right ventricle receives the pulmonary venous return and ejects into the aorta (Fig. 10-3). If no additional anomalies exist, a hemodynamically normal heart is the result; hence the name "corrected transposition."

This malfunction is rare, occurring in fewer than 1.5% of all CHD, with slight male preponderance. Only 1% of patients have physiologically normal hearts. Because of the ventricular inversion, the AV valves, the coronary arteries, and the conduction system are also inverted. The left-sided tricuspid valve is frequently in-

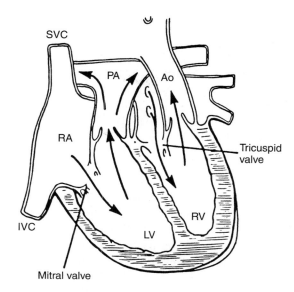

FIG. 10-3 Circulation in corrected transposition. *Ao,* Aorta; *IVC,* inferior vena cava; *LV,* left ventricle; *PA,* pulmonary artery; *RA,* right atrium; *RV,* right ventricle; *SVC,* superior vena cava.

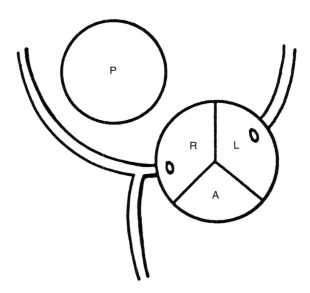

FIG. 10-4 Coronary anatomy in corrected transposition. The right coronary artery gives off the left anterior descending coronary artery and the left coronary artery has only the circumflex distribution. *A,* Anterior; *L,* left; *P,* pulmonary artery; *R,* right.

sufficient. The left anterior descending coronary artery, originating on the right, traverses the pulmonary outflow tract (Fig. 10-4). The bundle of His has a much longer course, which may explain the very high incidence of heart block, both spontaneously and following surgery. Eighty percent of patients have a large VSD and 70% of patients have pulmonary outflow obstruction. Malposition of the heart (dextrocardia or mesocardia) is frequently present.

The majority of patients in the first month of life have signs reflective of the predominant physiology. There is congestive failure in the presence of a large left-to-right shunt through the VSD, or cyanosis and hypercyanotic spells if pulmonary outflow obstruction is prominent. Prognosis depends on the degree of hemodynamic abnormality. Patients with a large VSD and no pulmonary stenosis have a higher mortality rate (35%) during the first year of life than those with pulmonary outflow obstruction (20%).

Heart failure is initially treated with digitalis and diuretics, and if this is unsuccessful, banding of the pulmonary artery may be performed to relieve failure and protect the pulmonary vascular bed. Nearly 50% of children with pulmonary obstruction require a systemic-to-pulmonary shunt for palliation of cyanosis. Total correction in corrected transposition (the double-switch procedure) is surgically difficult and carries a high mortality rate (40%). Because of the abnormal coronary arterial anatomy, a conduit repair is required for correction of severe pulmonic stenosis. Systemic AV valve insufficiency may require repair or replacement at the time of VSD closure. Conduction disturbance is present in 40% to 50% of patients postoperatively. Patients may develop sudden complete heart block after the age of 20 years.

Patent Ductus Arteriosus

The ductus arteriosus is a communication from the main pulmonary to the proximal descending aorta. Its main role in the fetus is to allow deoxygenated blood returning to the right side of the heart to bypass recirculation to the left heart and head vessels by entering the descending aorta. Eventually, this blood is oxygenated when it flows through the placenta before returning to the heart. During the first day of extrauterine existence, oxygenated blood flowing through the ductus chemically induces constriction. Anatomic closure takes place a few weeks later. Persistent patency of this conduit is abnormal but may be lifesaving to the infant with obstruction to flow into either the systemic or pulmonary system (i.e., HLHS or pulmonary valve atresia, respectively). Certain conditions and pharmacologic agents prevent the ductus from constricting (Table 10-4). Other agents promote closure of the ductus (e.g., indomethacin). Patency of the ductus beyond 3 months of age is abnormal. Premature infants exhibit delayed closure of the ductus arteriosus because of immaturity of the ductal musculature, and if ductal closure cannot be achieved pharmacologically, surgical ligation is performed to treat ventilator dependence and congestive heart failure.

Shunting through a PDA is mainly left to right. The amount of shunting depends on the size of the ductus and the SVR:PVR ratio. A small PDA may cause an in-

---

TABLE 10-4
Conditions and Agents that Affect the Ductus Arteriosus

Conditions and Agents that Prevent Constriction
- Hypoxia
- Acidosis
- Pharmacological agents
  - Prostaglandin E_1

Conditions and Agents that Cause Closure
- Indomethacin
- Hyperoxia

---

crease in pulmonary blood flow but not affect pulmonary artery pressures. A large PDA leads to congestive heart failure within the first year of life from left-to-right shunting. A large PDA may also result in pulmonary hypertension, leading to obstructive pulmonary vascular disease. Severe pulmonary hypertension due to a pulmonary hypertensive crisis (e.g., persistent fetal circulation of the newborn) or obstructive pulmonary vascular disease, may reverse shunting through the PDA. This leads to "differential" cyanosis that is more pronounced in the lower extremities.

Endocardial Cushion Defects

Endocardial cushion defects have a wide range of presentations ranging from simple isolated ASDs and VSDs with a form of AV valve involvement to complete AV canal defects. This section only describes complete AV canals. Complete AV canals consist of an ostium primary ASD, a large VSD, and a wide spectrum of anatomic abnormalities of the AV valves (Fig. 10-5). Classification of complete AV canals is based on the configuration, relationships, and attachments of the abnormal AV valve.[10] Complete AV canal defects result from failure of fusion of the endocardial cushions. Because the cushions do not fuse, the atrial and ventricular septa have defects. The ASD lies inferiorly and posteriorly, is adjacent to the AV valve, and is known as an *ostium primum defect.* The VSD is in the posterior (inflow) portion of the membranous septum.

Typically, complete AV canal defects are associated with large left-to-right shunts at the atrial and ventricular levels, along with a moderate amount of common AV valve insufficiency. These patients almost always have severe congestive heart failure during infancy. The mortality rate is high for medical therapy alone, related to the rapid development of pulmonary vascular occlusive disease. Complete surgical correction is the recom-

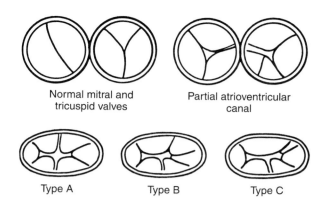

FIG. 10-5 Classification of atrioventricular canal defects according to Rastelli.

mended therapy because these patients are usually refractory to medical therapy.

Anesthetic Considerations for Patients with Left-to-Right Shunts

The anesthetic considerations in ASD repairs typify those of patients with predominantly left-to-right shunting. Because of the uncertainty regarding the presence of transient right-to-left shunting at the defect, it is important to avoid the injection of air in the intravenous lines to prevent the small risk of paradoxic embolization. Antibiotic prophylaxis is another consideration; it is almost universally applied in cardiac surgery and is mandatory in most noncardiac surgery for endocarditis prophylaxis. In secundum ASDs, prerepair and postrepair, and repaired simple VSDs and PDAs, prophylaxis for prevention of bacterial endocarditis is not required except for the 6 months following surgical closure.[11]

The third, and by far the most important consideration, is the use of physiologic maneuvers to minimize excessive pulmonary blood flow by increasing PVR. The minimum fractional inspired oxygen concentration (Fio_2) consistent with adequate oxygenation should be used. The patient should be ventilated with adequate tidal volume, but with a ventilatory rate slow enough to maintain normocarbia or slight hypercarbia (arterial carbon dioxide tension [$Paco_2$] of 40-50 mm Hg). While hypothermia and metabolic acidosis may also reduce pulmonary blood flow, they should not necessarily be therapeutic goals of anesthetic and ventilatory management. Nevertheless, they may be tolerated within reason (base deficits of 3-5 mEq/L and core temperatures of 34° C-35° C) when they occur unintentionally. These principles for limiting excessive pulmonary blood flow apply to all left-to-right shunts, and are referred to throughout this chapter. In many other lesions that may or may not be present in patients with left-to-right shunts, preload, afterload, heart rate, and contractility may need to be manipulated to optimize

the hemodynamic situation. While these parameters must be kept within normal limits, there are no specific goals for these parameters in the management of the left-to-right shunt per se.

In most cases, the anesthetic management of VSDs is identical to that for all left-to-right shunts. In large VSDs, however, manipulation of afterload may also affect the hemodynamic situation. Many infants receive angiotensin-converting enzyme inhibitors to decrease the impedance to forward flow through the aortic valve. While there are no data to support this, vasodilating anesthetic agents, such as isoflurane, or vasodilators, such as sodium nitroprusside, may be advantageous for this reason. Excessive systemic vasodilation, however, is undesirable, because it could induce right-to-left shunting across a large VSD, with concomitant cyanosis and hypotension, especially if there is obstruction to right ventricular outflow.

Following cardiopulmonary bypass (CPB), the situation is reversed. Patients tend to have pulmonary vasoconstriction in the early postbypass period. Also, the hemodynamic consequences of high Fio_2 are no longer present after the defect has been repaired. A higher Fio_2 and avoidance of hypercarbia are the general rule following CPB. Modified ultrahemofiltration following CPB appears to improve the hemodynamic situation.[12] Most anesthetic agents are well tolerated in patients with left-to-right shunts. There are certain caveats. Potent inhalational anesthetics may be poorly tolerated by a failing myocardium and can cause severe hypotension. Opioid-relaxant techniques are better for such patients coming for repair of their cardiac lesion, but may still induce hypotension if there is high resting sympathetic tone. Nitrous oxide increases PVR and may decrease flow through the defect, but is harmful if paradoxic air embolization occurs. High-dose narcotics and ketamine appear to blunt the stress response in the pulmonary vascular bed. Ketamine, because of its indirect sympathomimetic effect, is well tolerated by patients with borderline myocardial reserve.[13]

EISENMENGER COMPLEX AND SYNDROME

The development of a markedly elevated PVR with reversal of the shunt in the presence of a large VSD, first described by Victor Eisenmenger in 1897, has been termed the *Eisenmenger complex*. The designation *Eisenmenger syndrome* describes a pathophysiologic entity in which pulmonary hypertension due to a high PVR leads to a bidirectional or predominantly right-to-left shunt at the aortopulmonary, atrial, or ventricular level. As the PVR exceeds the SVR, this leads to a reversal of the shunting (i.e., tardive cyanosis due to right-to-left shunt).

Fewer than 10% of children with a large VSD develop this problem, but it is present in more than 50% of adults with large aortopulmonary or ventricular communications. Because the underlying defect must allow for equalization of pressures between the ventricles, there is usually a history of congestive heart failure in infancy that improves as PVR increases. Obstructive pulmonary vascular disease may be present after the age of 2 years, and presence of a fixed elevation in PVR renders the underlying defect inoperable. Children usually exhibit few symptoms except for occasional exertional dyspnea and fatigue. Cyanosis and failure are rare. Symptoms become increasingly prominent during the late twenties and early thirties. Death frequently occurs suddenly in these patients, usually in their thirties.

Anesthetic Management of Eisenmenger Complex and Syndrome

These patients usually present for noncardiac surgery, labor and delivery, or heart-lung transplantation. Perioperative dehydration is avoided in patients who are cyanotic because increased blood viscosity may result in pulmonary and systemic vascular bed thrombosis. Meticulous attention is given to avoid air and particulates in the intravenous lines to prevent paradoxic embolization of air or clot to the systemic circulation. Since the PVR is fixed, shunting is largely determined by SVR. A fall in SVR causes increased cyanosis due to increased right-to-left shunting. High ventilation pressure may cause further reduction in pulmonary blood flow. Pulmonary function in these patients is abnormal, with reduction in total lung capacity, vital capacity, and compliance. Residual and closing volumes are increased.

Various reports of anesthetic management of patients with Eisenmenger syndrome have been published.[14,15] Recommendations include sedation to reduce preoperative anxiety and oxygen consumption, use of anesthetic agents with minimal effect on peripheral vascular resistance and myocardial contractility (narcotic or ketamine), prevention of hypoxia and hypoventilation intraoperatively and postoperatively, and prevention of bradycardia by the use of anticholinergics. Regional anesthesia with attendant sympathetic blockade is relatively contraindicated in these patients. All patients require endocarditis prophylaxis. Anticoagulation that is appropriate to the surgical procedure may improve outcome by prevention of thromboembolic complications.

In noncardiac procedures, postoperative and postpartum mortality rates are high. Invasive hemodynamic monitoring and intensive care unit observation may be warranted on this basis. Heart-lung transplantation, which "cures" the Eisenmenger syndrome, is not discussed in this chapter.

PREDOMINANT RIGHT-TO-LEFT SHUNT LESIONS WITH DECREASED PULMONARY BLOOD FLOW
Tetralogy of Fallot

The combination of VSD, pulmonary valvular and/or right ventricular infundibular stenosis, right ventricular hypertrophy, and a large overriding aorta is known as *tetralogy of Fallot*. It is the most common cyanotic defect seen after the first year of life, contributing to 10% of all congenital cardiac lesions. Males are more often affected than females by a 3:2 ratio, and 25% to 30% of patients have a right-sided aortic arch.

The degree of right ventricular outflow or pulmonic obstruction determines the onset and severity of cyanosis. With severe obstruction, cyanosis appears with closure of the ductus arteriosus in the neonatal period. Prostaglandin E_1 maintains ductal patency and is thus used to clinically stabilize the patient before surgical intervention. Many infants do not develop symptoms until 3 to 6 months of age and even then may not appear cyanotic at rest. However, episodes of severe cyanosis with hyperventilation and acidosis, known as *hypercyanotic spells* (or "tet" spells), may occur. They are caused by severe infundibular spasm, probably induced by changes in venous return and PVR. Reduction in peripheral vascular tone leads to decreased pulmonary blood flow because more blood is shunted to the systemic circulation. Decreased venous return further decreases pulmonary blood flow. In older children, squatting posture may improve symptoms by increasing venous return from the lower extremities and by increasing peripheral vascular resistance. The treatment of hypercyanotic spells is described in the section on the anesthetic management of tetralogy of Fallot and cyanotic lesions.

In tetralogy of Fallot, both ventricles work at systemic pressure, but volume overload does not occur and congestive heart failure is rare. If pulmonary stenosis is moderate, the patient may be acyanotic and have signs of left-to-right shunt. With progression of infundibular stenosis, cyanosis becomes apparent. Chronic hypoxemia leads to polycythemia and the development of collateral circulation to the lungs.

The mortality rate of untreated patients with tetralogy of Fallot approaches 50% by 5 years of age and 70% by the age of 10 years. Only 3% to 5% of patients survive to adulthood. Complications occurring early in patients with tetralogy of Fallot are cerebrovascular accidents, probably due to venous thrombosis from polycythemia, cerebral abscesses due to the loss of the filtering effect of the lungs, and subacute bacterial endocarditis. Early corrective surgery is presently advocated and associated with a low operative mortality rate (<10%). Infants with hypoplasia of the pulmonary arteries are not candidates for early correction, and a systemic-to-pulmonary artery shunt is created to improve pulmonary blood flow and allow growth of the pulmonary vasculature. The modified Blalock-Taussig operation is preferred if vessel size is adequate.

In complete repair of tetralogy of Fallot, the right ventricular obstruction has to be completely relieved. A patch is placed to close the VSD and another is placed in the right ventricular outflow tract. If necessary, the patch crosses the pulmonary valve annulus and extends into the main pulmonary artery. In surgery requiring a transannular patch, the resulting pulmonary insufficiency appears to be well tolerated in the short term. Complications of reparative surgery include residual pulmonic stenosis (10%–20%), residual VSD (5%), and, rarely, complete heart block. Right bundle-branch block is commonly observed after right ventriculotomy. Between 8% and 11% of patients develop supraventricular tachycardia postoperatively. Up to 23% of patients develop exercise-induced ventricular ectopy.[16,17] The majority of these patients have elevated right ventricular pressure postoperatively. In one series, 38% of patients with premature ventricular contractions on a resting electrocardiogram (ECG) died suddenly within 3 months to 8 years postoperatively. Approximately 7% of patients died within 15 years after complete repair. Postoperative ventricular ectopy should be treated aggressively with pharmacologic therapy or implantable cardioverter-defibrillator devices.

Residual biventricular dysfunction has been observed after complete repair of tetralogy of Fallot, even in the absence of hemodynamic abnormalities. Response to maximal exercise is abnormal, with reduction in maximal oxygen uptake and a reduced cardiac index. Repair before the age of 2 years appears to be associated with better preservation of myocardial function. The anesthetic management of tetralogy of Fallot and pulmonary atresia with VSD is discussed in the section on anesthetic management of tetralogy of Fallot and cyanotic lesions.

Pulmonary Atresia with Ventricular Septal Defect

Pulmonary atresia with VSD may be considered an extreme form of tetralogy of Fallot. The majority of infants born with this anomaly become cyanotic shortly after birth and may die within hours after the ductus arteriosus closes. They require clinical stabilization with prostaglandin E_1, which maintains ductal patency, and a surgical shunt within the first few days of life. The remainder of patients in this group have large and multiple aortopulmonary collaterals and may not exhibit cyanosis until after infancy, when the collateral vessels become inadequate or stenotic. With very large collateral vessels, obstructive pulmonary vascular disease may develop.

Definitive repair for these children consists of a valved prosthetic conduit or homograft placed between the right ventricle and pulmonary artery and closure of the VSD (Fig. 10-6). Large collateral vessels are ligated. Currently available conduits develop obstruction within several years following the procedure and become inadequate as the child grows. Multiple reoperations may be required.

A number of anatomically different congenital cardiac lesions have clinical features similar to those of tetralogy of Fallot. These include DORV with subaortic VSD and pulmonary stenosis, and single ventricle with pulmonic stenosis. The physiologic considerations for anesthetic management are similar.

Pulmonary Atresia with Intact Ventricular Septum

Absence of the pulmonary valve with an intact ventricular septum and varying degrees of right ventricular hypoplasia account for about 1% of all CHD. Pulmonary blood flow is completely dependent on the ductus arteriosus, which is frequently hypoplastic. Symptoms appear shortly after birth with cyanosis and tachypnea. Metabolic acidosis and signs of heart failure develop rapidly. Patients require palliation or correction within the first few days of life. The patency of the ductus arteriosus is maintained with prostaglandin E_1.

If the right ventricle is normal, an open or closed pulmonary valvotomy is performed, and the patient is maintained on a prostaglandin infusion for several days until the right ventricle adapts to increasing forward flow. In patients with right ventricular hypoplasia, a systemic-to-pulmonary shunt may be required in addition to valvotomy to maintain pulmonary perfusion and systemic oxygenation.

Patients with severe hypoplasia of the right ventricle may develop coronary cavitary fistulae—also known as *coronary sinusoids*. These sinusoids preclude a biventricular repair because decompression of the right ventricle would lead to myocardial ischemia and death. In these patients, a palliative shunt is performed in the neonatal period. Later therapy consists of cavopulmonary anastomoses (see section on hypoplastic left heart syndrome).

Tricuspid Atresia

Atresia of the tricuspid valve is always associated with an ASD (usually a patent foramen ovale). The mitral valve and left ventricle are hyperplastic and the right ventricle is hypoplastic or absent. Tricuspid atresia occurs in 1.5%

to 3% of all patients with CHD and is slightly more common in males.

Tricuspid atresia is divided into three different types (I, II, and III), depending on the relationship of the great vessel (normal, d-transposed, or l-transposed). Further subclassification relates to the presence of pulmonic stenosis or a VSD. Fifty percent of all patients with tricuspid atresia have normally related great vessels, a small VSD, and pulmonary atresia and stenosis. Only 10% to 15% have no obstruction to pulmonary blood flow.

Cyanosis often occurs on the first day of life and is due to the obligatory right-to-left shunt across the ASD.

Patients with transposition and a large VSD may have only mild cyanosis and present with congestive heart failure in the first few months. The diagnosis of tricuspid atresia is suspected in the presence of cyanosis with left-axis deviation on the ECG and a left ventricular hypertrophy pattern in the precordial leads.

Tricuspid atresia is not a correctable lesion, and the series of palliative operations is typical of all single-ventricle repairs. A systemic-to-pulmonary shunt is created in infancy. A bidirectional Glenn shunt is created at 4 to 6 months of age, and a Fontan procedure is performed at 2 to 4 years of age (Fig. 10-7). Even with optimal surgical management, only 50% of pa-

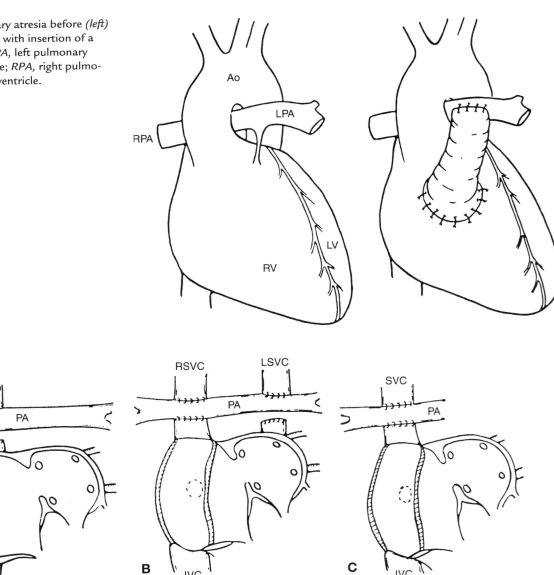

FIG. 10-6 Pulmonary atresia before *(left)* and after *(right)* repair with insertion of a conduit. *Ao,* Aorta; *LPA,* left pulmonary artery; *LV,* left ventricle; *RPA,* right pulmonary artery; *RV,* right ventricle.

FIG. 10-7 Cavopulmonary anastomoses and modified Fontan procedure. **A,** Bidirectional Glenn shunt. **B** and **C,** Total cavopulmonary anastomoses with one or two superior venae cavae. *IVC,* Inferior vena cava; *LSVC,* left superior vena cava; *PA,* pulmonary artery; *RSVC,* right superior vena cava; *SVC,* superior vena cava.

tients survive past the second decade of life. A complete description of anesthetic considerations following cavopulmonary anastomoses is discussed in the section on HLHS.

Ebstein's Anomaly of the Tricuspid Valve

Ebstein's anomaly consists of malformation of the posterior and septal leaflets of the tricuspid valve, which are adherent to the right ventricular wall, resulting in downward displacement of the free edge of the valves into the right ventricle away from the AV junction. The portion of the right ventricle above the downwardly displaced valve is thin-walled ("atrialized") and functionally becomes a common chamber with the right atrium. The right ventricle below the displaced valve is normal but markedly reduced in size, with a patent foramen ovale present in 75% of cases. The malformation is rare, with an incidence of 0.5% of all CHD, and affects both sexes equally. Familial occurrence has been reported.

Tricuspid valve stenosis and insufficiency coexist in most cases. Cyanosis due to shunting at the atrial level may be present in varying severity and tends to become more pronounced with age. With severe tricuspid malformation, cyanosis may be present in the neonate, but improves with the fall in PVR postnatally. Tachycardia causes increased cyanosis because of impaired right ventricular filling. Atrial emptying is delayed and results in the shunting of blood back and forth between the right atrium and the atrialized portion of the right ventricle between atrial and ventricular systole (ping-pong effect). Paroxysmal atrial tachycardia occurs in 25% of patients and may cause syncope. Death during childhood is due to congestive heart failure or cardiac arrhythmias. About one third of patients die before the age of 10 years, and fewer than 20% survive beyond adolescence without surgery.

Surgical intervention should be considered if exercise intolerance, heart failure, and progressive cyanosis appear in patients with this anomaly. The abnormal valve may be replaced, or the atrialized portion of the ventricle plicated with tricuspid annuloplasty. The latter procedure appears to have better results.

Anesthetic Management of Tetralogy of Fallot and Cyanotic Lesions with Decreased Pulmonary Blood Flow

The patient should arrive in the operating room well sedated. Preoperative fluid restriction is minimized with maintenance fluid given intravenously to prevent hemoconcentration and hypovolemia. Wide variations in hemodynamics are avoided during induction to prevent increases in oxygen demand or hypercyanotic spells. The anesthetic agents used should have minimal peripheral vasodilating effects. For example,

halothane is theoretically preferable to isoflurane or sevoflurane for this purpose. Mild myocardial depression may relieve infundibular obstruction and is therefore desirable. If intravenous agents are used, they should be carefully titrated to prevent relative overdose. Intravenous barbiturate requirements are reduced. This induction effect of intravenous drugs is probably related to a partial bypassing of the pulmonary circulation. A right-to-left shunt prolongs induction with poorly soluble inhalational anesthetics. This is offset by a surgically created systemic-to-pulmonary shunt. Induction time with highly soluble agents is nearly normal because these patients usually hyperventilate to maintain a normal arterial partial pressure of carbon dioxide ($Paco_2$).

Ketamine should theoretically be problematic in tetralogy of Fallot. The associated tachycardia and the inotropic effects associated with catecholamine release should incite or worsen infundibular spasm. Nevertheless, years of clinical experience and one study[18] demonstrate that arterial oxygen saturation generally increases on induction of anesthesia in cyanotic patients. The reasons for this paradox are probably related to the reduction in oxygen consumption that occurs in the anesthetized state and the maintenance of SVR. Ketamine is therefore an acceptable agent for induction and maintenance of anesthesia in patients with tetralogy of Fallot physiology.

While PVR is not the primary determinant of decreased pulmonary blood flow, maneuvers to minimize PVR are prudent. Oxygenation is frequently improved under general anesthesia by using any number of agents. This is probably related to relaxation of the infundibular muscle with lower catecholamine levels, pulmonary vasodilation from higher oxygen concentration, and reduced peripheral oxygen demands.

Monitoring blood pressure is problematic in patients with previous shunting procedures that have used the subclavian arteries. The contralateral arm should be used for invasive or noninvasive monitoring. For major surgery, intraarterial and central venous pressures are measured directly. This allows blood sampling for blood gas and acid-base measurements. Because the major stress for these patients is on the right ventricle, central venous pressure is used to assess cardiac performance. Transesophageal echocardiography is indicated to evaluate the results of corrective surgery.

The obstruction to pulmonary outflow may be fixed or dynamic in nature. With fixed obstruction, right-to-left shunting is influenced by changes in peripheral vascular resistance. A decline in SVR may lead to increasing cyanosis, acidosis, and myocardial depression, creating a vicious circle. In patients with dynamic infundibular stenosis, severe infundibular spasm may be triggered intraoperatively by hypovolemia, relative anemia, manipulation of intracardiac monitoring lines, inotropic agents, and surgical manipulation. Prompt treatment is essential.

Perioperative therapy of hypercyanotic spells includes decreasing infundibular spasm with myocardial depression, decreasing heart rate, and increasing preload. Another goal (especially in fixed right ventricular outflow obstruction) is to increase SVR to decrease right-to-left shunting across the VSD. Modalities that decrease infundibular spasm include β-adrenergic blockers, sedative medications, halothane, and intravenous fluid administration. Modalities that increase SVR include phenylephrine administration, and physical maneuvers, such as abdominal aortic compression and squatting posture. The classic treatment of hypercyanotic spells with morphine is counterintuitive in that histamine release would tend to decrease preload. The sedative effects of morphine are the major benefit. The resultant decrease in intrinsic catecholamine levels is the probable mechanism of the relief of the infundibular spasm. Higher oxygen concentrations may have little effect in improving systemic oxygenation. Acidosis should be corrected and venous return improved by administration of fluids.

Maintenance of cardiac output is essential since the oxygen content of the blood is low. Bradycardia is very poorly tolerated for this reason. In patients with systemic-to-pulmonary shunts, adequate systemic blood pressure is necessary to maintain pulmonary perfusion.

All patients with right-to-left shunts are at an increased risk of systemic embolization of air or particulates from intravenous lines. In older cyanotic patients with severe polycythemia, hemodilution to a hematocrit of 55% to 60% should be performed before elective surgery. This improves cardiac output, peripheral perfusion, and oxygen transport. It may also improve the coagulation defects commonly found in polycythemic patients. Hemodilution to normal levels may be very dangerous, however, as oxygen transport becomes seriously limited.

Patients with cyanosis have a blunted response to hypoxia, which may persist after correction of the underlying lesion.[19] In patients with reduced pulmonary blood flow, marked ventilation/perfusion inequalities exist. Positive-pressure ventilation may worsen this problem, leading to an increase in dead-space ventilation and arterial $Paco_2$. A moderate degree of hyperventilation is required to maintain normal $Paco_2$ with severely reduced pulmonary blood flow.

Patients who have undergone surgical correction present less of an anesthetic problem for subsequent noncardiac surgery. They may, however, have some impairment of right and left ventricular function with a tendency to develop arrhythmias. Ventricular ectopy should be treated, since it has been implicated in sudden death. Patients require endocarditis prophylaxis for life. The presence of residual defects should be determined before elective surgery.

COMPLEX SHUNTS
Truncus Arteriosus

Truncus arteriosus is an uncommon congenital anomaly in which a single great vessel originates from both ventricles above a large VSD, giving rise to the pulmonary arteries, coronary arteries, and the continuation of the aorta. This malformation represents 4% of congenital cardiac lesions. At present, three forms of truncus are recognized[20] (Fig. 10-8). In type I, a short pulmonary trunk arises from the truncus and divides into both pulmonary arteries; in type II the pulmonary arteries arise separately but in close proximity to each other from the posterior aspect of the truncus; and in type III, both pulmonary arteries arise

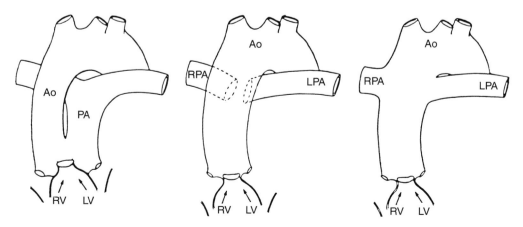

FIG. 10-8 Truncus arteriosus. Classification according to Colett and Edwards. *Ao*, Aorta; *LPA*, left pulmonary artery; *LV*, left ventricle; *PA*, pulmonary artery; *RPA*, right pulmonary artery; *RV*, right ventricle.

separately from the respective lateral aspects of the truncal artery.

Patients show signs of congestive heart failure and pulmonary overperfusion in early infancy. Truncal valve insufficiency may also be present. Heart failure is severe and resistant to therapy. Unless surgical correction is performed, death occurs in the first year of life in more than 80% of patients. Survivors develop obstructive pulmonary vascular disease, rendering them inoperable. These patients all deteriorate progressively with pulmonary hypertension and right heart failure.

Because of the dismal natural history of this disease, correction is generally performed before 3 months of age. It consists of VSD closure with diversion of left ventricular output to the truncal artery and placement of a valved graft between the right ventricle and pulmonary circulation. Since only a small conduit can be used during infancy, at least one additional operation is necessary as the patient outgrows the initial conduit. Currently available conduits deteriorate over time, and further replacements of the conduit become necessary. Truncal valve insufficiency necessitates valve replacement at either the initial or subsequent surgery.

Anesthetic Considerations for Truncus Arteriosus

Elective surgery is unlikely to be performed before the correction of the cardiac lesion. At the time of the cardiac repair, the management follows the principles outlined in massive left-to-right shunts as described earlier. Limited Fio_2, hypoventilation, and mild hypothermia are beneficial before CPB. An arterial oxygen saturation of about 80% is ideal. Many patients require inotropic therapy due to severe congestive heart failure. Following

CPB, patients are at risk for pulmonary hypertensive crisis and myocardial failure. Prolonged ventilation with an opioid infusion is recommended in the early postoperative period. Anesthetic agents are chosen for minimal cardiovascular side effects. The authors prefer ketamine before CPB, and high-dose opioids thereafter.

For noncardiac surgery after correction, patients may appear asymptomatic but may have a considerable pressure gradient across the right ventricular-to-pulmonary-artery conduit. Right ventricular failure and ventricular arrhythmias may develop with stress or large, rapid, fluid shifts. Central venous monitoring is essential under these circumstances to assess right ventricular function. Increased PVR worsens right ventricular function, and acute preload reduction may lead to systemic cardiovascular collapse. Selection of anesthetic agents is based on using drugs with minimal effect on vasomotor tone and myocardial performance. Maintenance of heart rate is essential, as is endocarditis prophylaxis. Use of invasive monitoring should be considered early in the course of extensive surgery. Pulmonary artery catheters are contraindicated because of the presence of a prosthetic valve in the pulmonary outflow tract.

D-Transposition of the Great Arteries

In d-transposition of the great arteries, the aorta arises from the right ventricle and the pulmonary artery from the left ventricle (Fig. 10-9). The pulmonary and systemic circulations therefore are "in parallel" rather than "in series," and systemic arterial oxygenation depends on mixing between the circulations through anatomic communications (i.e., ductus arteriosus, ASD, or VSD).

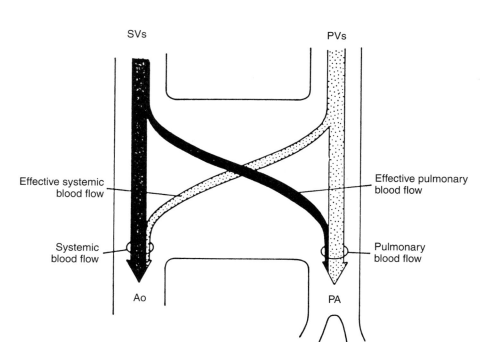

FIG. 10-9 Circulation in d-transposition of the great vessels. *Ao,* Aorta; *PA,* pulmonary artery; *PVs,* pulmonary veins; *SVs,* systemic veins.

(From Kidd BSL: Transposition of the great arteries. In Keith JD et al, editors: *Heart disease in infancy and childhood,* ed 3, New York, 1978, Macmillan.)

This is a common malformation. The overall incidence is 5% of all CHD but it is the most common lesion (17%) seen during the first week of life. Without treatment, 50% die within the first 6 months, and 90% within the first year of life. There is a marked male preponderance (60%-70%).[21]

Blood shunted anatomically from left to right constitutes the effective systemic blood flow and blood shunted right to left constitutes the effective pulmonary blood flow, and the very large blood volume that is being recirculated does not contribute to effective gas exchange. Patients with d-transposition are divided into groups depending on the presence of a VSD or restriction to pulmonary blood flow. Transposition with an intact ventricular septum is the most common lesion (50%), followed by transposition with VSD (30%).

Patients with d-transposition have hypoxemia, acidosis, and/or congestive heart failure in the newborn period or early infancy. If pulmonic stenosis is significant, signs of pulmonary hypoperfusion are present. Initiation of therapy with prostaglandin E_1 maintains the patency of the ductus arteriosus and stabilizes the oxygen saturation. At many centers, a balloon atrial septostomy (Rashkind procedure) is done in the catheterization laboratory to allow mixing between the two circulations. These therapies permit survival until surgery can be performed. Patients with an intact septum and a large PDA may be less cyanotic.

Infants with a large VSD have adequate mixing despite the transposition and are usually only mildly cyanotic. They do, however, develop severe congestive heart failure between 2 and 6 weeks of age, which is often resistant to medical management, and they require pulmonary artery banding or early correction for survival. Pulmonary artery banding is only performed when the VSD is not amenable to surgical repair.

Previously, the most commonly performed operations were the Mustard and Senning procedures (Fig. 10-10). These are only physiologic corrections, directing systemic venous return through the mitral valve into the left ventricle and pulmonary artery and pulmonary venous return through the tricuspid valve into the right ventricle and aorta via placement of an intraatrial baffle. An elective Mustard or Senning repair was commonly performed between 6 and 12 months to prevent pulmonary vascular disease. The mortality rate for this procedure ranged from 5% to 20% in patients during the first few weeks and months of life. The use of the right ventricle as the systemic pump is a shortcoming of these procedures, and ventricular dysfunction and tricuspid insufficiency are prominent in later life. Severe dysrhythmias and obstruction of the systemic or pulmonary venous return at the atrial level frequently develop several years postoperatively. These patients may present for noncardiac surgery or heart transplantation.

The current standard therapy is anatomic correction by switching of the great arteries with coronary reim-

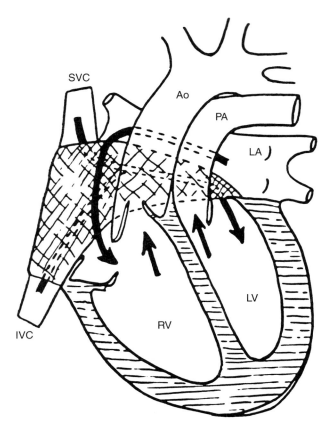

FIG. 10-10 Transposition of the great vessels: blood flow after a Mustard or Senning procedure. *Ao,* Aorta; *IVC,* inferior vena cava; *LA,* left atrium; *LV,* left ventricle; *PA,* pulmonary artery; *RV,* right ventricle; *SVC,* superior vena cava.

plantation (Fig. 10-11), as described by Jatene et al.[22] This surgery is performed in neonates. In patients with a large VSD, a pulmonary banding procedure may be performed to postpone the definitive repair beyond the neonatal period.

Anesthetic Management for d-Transposition of the Great Arteries

The arterial switch (Jatene) procedure is commonly performed within the first 2 weeks of life. Some patients are stable with prostaglandin E_1 infusions after balloon atrial septostomy, but others are quite ill with respiratory insufficiency. Many anesthetic techniques are possible, but high-dose opioid anesthesia is associated with improved survival in comparison with halothane-morphine anesthesia.[23] The authors typically find that high-dose opioid anesthesia leads to refractory hypotension in the pre-CPB period, and often use ketamine as the primary anesthetic agent initially. High-dose opioid anesthesia is instituted during CPB. The post-CPB period is occasionally complicated by "coronary stretch"—a syndrome with ST-segment depression, prominent v waves on the left atrial waveform (with or without mitral regurgitation), and depressed left ventricular function. The etiology of the syndrome is related to

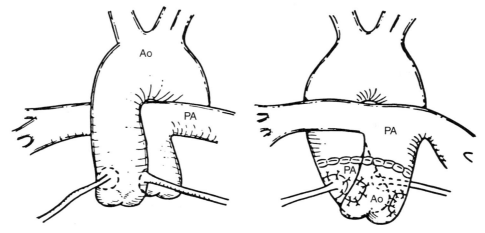

FIG. 10-11   Repair of transposition of the great vessels by the arterial switch operation. *Left,* Before operation. *Right,* After operation. *Ao,* Aorta; *PA,* pulmonary artery. (From Jatene AD, Iontes VF, Paulista PP: *J Thorac Cardiovasc Surg* 72:364, 1976.)

overfilling of the left ventricle, causing stretching of the reimplanted coronary arteries, with kinking of the vessels leading to coronary artery obstruction.

Because of the low effective pulmonary blood flow, induction of anesthesia with inhalational agents is prolonged and adverse side effects may linger after the anesthetic is discontinued. Intravenous agents must be used with caution; they have a rapid onset of action since most of the venous return enters the aorta.

Some children or adults who have survived Mustard and Senning procedures present for noncardiac surgery in later years. Although they may appear clinically normal without evidence of cyanosis or failure, they may not tolerate anesthesia and surgery well. Atrial dysrhythmias are common after intraatrial repairs and may become more frequent with time. The most serious of these is sick sinus syndrome, which may necessitate placement of a temporary pacemaker for surgery if a permanent pacemaker is not already in place. There may be systemic venous obstruction at the baffle site, leading to signs of venous congestion. Significant baffle obstruction usually requires reoperation. Left-sided baffle obstruction (more common after the Senning procedure) may lead to pulmonary hypertension. Increases in peripheral vascular resistance worsen the condition of the patient under these circumstances.

Insertion of pulmonary artery catheters in these patients is technically difficult because of the tortuous pathway of the venous blood flow and may cause arrhythmias or baffle disruption. The right ventricle, carrying the systemic load, has limited reserve and may fail if stressed by rapid fluid shifts or with use of myocardial depressant agents. Patients are still at risk for endocarditis, and patients with conduits are at a higher risk after repair than before. The arterial switch procedure is still

relatively new and, therefore, little is known about the long-term effects of this procedure, but obstructions above the semilunar valves have been reported.[24] It is prudent to assume that coronary artery disease may be present. The ECG is carefully monitored for ischemia. An anesthetic technique that reduces myocardial oxygen demand is a reasonable choice.

Total Anomalous Pulmonary Venous Return

Connection of all pulmonary veins to either the right atrium or one of the systemic veins is a relatively rare congenital anomaly present in fewer than 1.5% of all patients with CHD, but is the twelfth most common lesion seen during the first year of life. It is seen more frequently in males. Four anatomic sites of anomalous vein insertion are identified: (1) supracardiac, into either a left or right superior vena cava; (2) cardiac, into the coronary sinus or right atrium; (3) infracardiac, into the portal vein, hepatic veins, or ductus venosus; and (4) mixed, with insertion at more than one level (Fig. 10-12). Drainage into a left superior vena cava is seen most frequently. From 25% to 30% of patients have associated cardiac anomalies, particularly of the heterotaxy (asplenia) type. Presence of an intraatrial communication is necessary for survival, and an ASD or patent foramen ovale is part of the complex.

The right heart has an increased volume load from the large left-to-right shunt, similar to the physiology of a secundum ASD. Systemic saturation and output depend on the degree of mixing at the atrial level, but many patients are mildly cyanotic. Excessive pulmonary blood flow is present in the majority of supracardiac and cardiac connections, which may be associated with reduced forward cardiac output.

Pulmonary venous hypertension and congestive heart failure are present in most infradiaphragmatic connections because of obstruction of pulmonary venous return. Congestive heart failure symptoms are present early in life. Tachypnea, frequent respiratory infections, and failure to thrive are common presenting features. Without surgical treatment, the mortality of these infants approaches 80% by 1 year of life.

Anesthetic Considerations for Total Anomalous Pulmonary Venous Return

For patients with supracardiac drainage, the excessive pulmonary blood flow is managed as described for patients with large left-to-right shunts. The patients with infracardiac drainage are more of a challenge because of pulmonary venous hypertension with congestive heart failure. In these patients, the lungs are noncompliant,

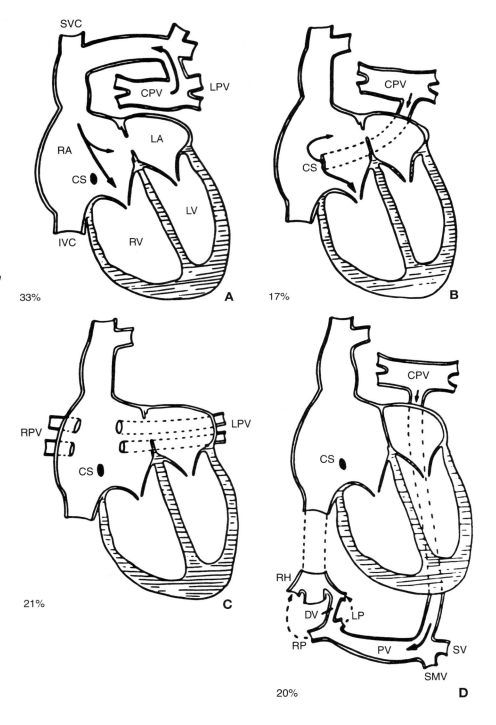

FIG. 10-12   Total anomalous pulmonary venous return. **A,** To left innominate vein. **B,** To coronary sinus. **C,** To right atrium. **D,** Infradiaphragmatic to portal vein. *Ao,* Aorta; *CPV,* common pulmonary vein; *CS,* coronary sinus; *DV,* ductus venosus; *IVC,* inferior vena cava; *LA,* left atrium; *LP,* left portal vein; *LPV,* left pulmonary vein; *LV,* left ventricle; *PV,* portal vein; *RA,* right atrium; *RH,* right hepatic vein; *RP,* right portal vein; *RPV,* right pulmonary vein; *RV,* right ventricle; *SMV,* superior mesenteric vein; *SV,* splenic vein; *SVC,* superior vena cava.

(From Lucas RV: Anomalous venous connections. In Adams FH, Emmanouilides GC, editors: *Heart disease in infants, children and adolescents,* ed 3, Baltimore, 1983, Williams & Wilkins.)

and positive end-expiratory pressure may be beneficial. Nevertheless, the PVR should be maintained somewhat high before CPB to reduce pulmonary blood flow. Inotropic support is often needed if there are signs of low cardiac output. The anesthetic agents used should have minimal myocardial depressant effects.

PVR may remain high following CPB, especially in patients with infracardiac drainage. Strategies to reduce PVR after CPB include hyperventilation, high Fio_2, normothermia, normal acid-base status, and high-dose opioid anesthesia. In addition, pulmonary vasodilation by using inhaled nitric oxide may be helpful. Postoperatively, mechanical ventilation and continued opioid infusion are accepted means of preventing pulmonary hypertensive crises. Patients presenting for later noncardiac surgery should be relatively normal if the reparative surgery was successful. A preoperative pediatric cardiology consultation should assess the quality of the repair and any residual pulmonary venous obstruction.

Double-Outlet Right Ventricle

In DORV, both great vessels arise from the morphologic right ventricle. There is always an associated VSD. This malformation accounts for fewer than 0.5% of all CHD and shows no predilection for either sex or race. Prematurity is common, as is the presence of coarctation and mitral valve disease. Clinical presentation is largely determined by the location of the VSD in relation to the great vessels and the presence or absence of pulmonic stenosis.

Patients with subaortic VSD without pulmonary outflow obstruction are clinically similar to patients with large VSDs and follow a similar clinical course with early congestive heart failure and late cyanosis when pulmonary vascular disease develops. The majority of these patients, however, have associated pulmonic stenosis, and their clinical presentation is similar to that in tetralogy of Fallot. Patients with subpulmonic VSDs compose the "Taussig-Bing group" of DORV, which is rarely associated with pulmonic stenosis. Clinically, they are cyanotic due to mixing of systemic and pulmonary venous blood in the ventricles, but have increased pulmonary blood flow with congestive heart failure due to the anatomy of the lesion.

Medical therapy for patients with volume and pressure overload consists of treating congestive heart failure by using digoxin, diuretics, and afterload reduction. Repairs are now commonly performed in infancy. Palliative operations are performed only in very small infants or those in whom a two-ventricle repair is impossible. Palliative procedures include pulmonary artery banding to treat congestive heart failure and prevent development of pulmonary vascular obstructive disease in patients with excessive pulmonary blood flow, or creation of a systemic-to-pulmonary shunt in patients with insufficient pulmonary blood flow. Complete surgical correction consists of diverting the left ventricular output via an intracardiac tunnel to the aorta, which may necessitate enlargement of the VSD. Blood from the right ventricle flows around the tunnel to the pulmonary artery. Enlargement of the right ventricular outflow tract or interposition of a prosthesis may be necessary in patients with right ventricular outflow obstruction.

Anesthetic management also follows the principles outlined earlier, depending on the degree of limitation or excess of pulmonary blood flow.

Hypoplastic Left Heart Syndrome

Atresia of the aortic valve, associated with atresia or severe stenosis of the mitral valve, hypoplasia or absence of the left ventricle, and hypoplasia of the ascending aorta or interrupted aortic arch constitute the HLHS. It is more common in males and affects 7% to 9% of all infants with cardiac disease. Systemic perfusion is dependent on a PDA and an ASD. Pulmonary overperfusion and low systemic output are always present. Without surgery, the mortality rate approaches 95% within the first month as the ductus closes.

Surgical palliation is conducted in three stages[25] (Fig. 10-13). In the Norwood stage I, a neo-aorta is created

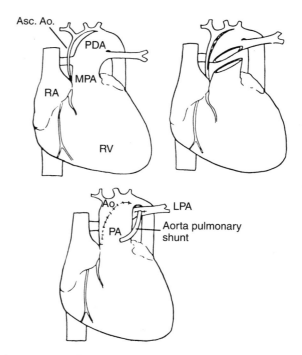

FIG. 10-13   Palliation of hypoplastic left heart syndrome. *Asc Ao,* Ascending aorta; *LPA,* left pulmonary artery; *MPA,* main pulmonary artery; *PDA,* patent ductus arteriosus; *RA,* right atrium; *RV,* right ventricle.

(From Norwood WI, Lang P: *N Engl J Med* 308:23, 1983.)

of pulmonary artery, native aortic, and homograft tissue. The neo-aorta arises from the right ventricle. A small central shunt is connected to the confluence of the pulmonary arteries as the sole source of pulmonary blood flow. At 4 to 6 months of age, a bidirectional Glenn shunt connects the superior vena cava to the pulmonary arteries and the central shunt is ligated. Finally, at 2 to 4 years of age, a Fontan procedure completes the third stage.

In all patients with post-Fontan physiology, the systemic venous pressure drives blood flow across the pulmonary vascular bed. Blood flow is dependent on a pressure difference between the systemic veins and the left atrium. Systemic venous pressures are therefore mild to moderately elevated postoperatively. Chronic liver congestion and ascites may be present and patients may be unable to increase cardiac output appropriately. Maintenance of sinus rhythm is important to maintain pulmonary blood flow and low systemic venous pressures.

Anesthetic Considerations for Hypoplastic Left Heart Syndrome

Norwood Stage I Procedure. The relative balance of pulmonary and systemic blood flow is the key to managing any patient with univentricular physiology, of which HLHS is a prototypical case. With complete mixing of pulmonary and systemic venous blood in the single ventricle, the optimal situation for tissue oxygen delivery is achieved with a 1:1 systemic-to-pulmonary blood-flow ratio. This generally correlates with arterial oxygen saturation in the range of 75% to 80%, but requires mixed venous oxygen saturation monitoring for adequate calculations.[26]

In the preoperative and pre-CPB periods, neonates with HLHS are prone to pulmonary steal. In pulmonary steal, the lungs are overperfused at the expense of systemic circulation. Relatively high oxygen saturation, poor peripheral perfusion, and metabolic acidosis characterize the steal syndrome. Therapy consists of limiting the inspired oxygen concentration and mild hypoventilation to increase the $Paco_2$. During surgery for the Norwood stage I, the surgeon can snare one of the pulmonary arteries to diminish pulmonary flow before CPB. After CPB, the situation is dynamic. The relative SVRs and PVRs, as well as the size of the central shunt, interact to determine the relative pulmonary-to-systemic blood-flow ratio. The saturation is maintained in the 70% to 80% range by using variable Fio_2 and hypercapnia or hypocapnia as appropriate.

Although many techniques are possible, the authors prefer ketamine before CPB. Induction with high-dose opioid is associated with ablation of sympathetic tone, resulting in excessive pulmonary blood flow with profound hypotension requiring inotropic therapy. High-dose opioid anesthesia is used during CPB. A landmark article by Anand and Hickey[23] demonstrated improved outcome in neonates with CHD by using high-dose opioid anesthesia as compared with halothane-morphine anesthesia. We therefore induce high-dose opioid anesthesia during the CPB period and maintain this technique into the early postoperative period. Lower levels of stress hormones and prophylaxis against pulmonary hypertensive crises are the likely causes of the improved outcomes found by Anand and Hickey.

Patients with Norwood stage I physiology who require surgery before the bidirectional Glenn shunt are treated as typical infants with cyanotic CHD and shunt dependence. The pulmonary blood flow is balanced with physiologic maneuvers, and prophylactic measures to prevent endocarditis and air embolism are performed.

Bidirectional Glenn Shunts and Modified Fontan Procedures (Norwood Stages II and III). The later management of patients with HLHS is less complicated and follows the principles outlined earlier for patients with diminished pulmonary blood flow. The single right ventricle has reduced reserve as a systemic pump. These patients are therefore more sensitive to myocardial depressant anesthetics. After cavopulmonary anastomoses, patients need sufficient venous pressure to maintain pulmonary perfusion and ventricular return. The PVR is minimized with hyperventilation, high Fio_2, and normothermia. Excessive intrathoracic pressures are poorly tolerated because of the absence of a right-sided pump.

In noncardiac surgery, adequate preload and prevention of increases in PVR and intrathoracic pressure are the key points. Patients have limited cardiac reserve since the single right ventricle is more prone to myocardial failure. Anesthetic agents are chosen to minimize myocardial depression. Patients with intracardiac suture lines are prone to life-threatening atrial arrhythmias.

Heterotaxy (Asplenia and Polysplenia) Syndromes

Agenesis of the spleen is associated with malposition of the abdominal viscera and complex cyanotic CHD (Ivemark syndrome). A combination of the following defects is usually present: l- or d-transpositions of the great vessels, pulmonary atresia or severe stenosis, large defects or absence of the atrial and ventricular septa, AV canal, total anomalous pulmonary venous return, persistence of the left superior vena cava, and absence of the coronary sinus. In the majority of cases there are bilateral trilobed lungs. Dextrocardia is present in 50% of cases.

The condition is extremely rare (0.1% of CHD) and palliative procedures are performed on the basis of the predominant lesions. Males are affected more frequently, by a 2:1 ratio. Two thirds of patients die within the first 2 months of life. Survivors undergo palliative surgery to improve pulmonary blood flow. These patients are extremely susceptible to overwhelming infection, and prophylactic antibiotics and bacterial vaccines are used. Patients have Howell-Jolly bodies in the peripheral blood smear.

Polysplenia is the presence of two or more spleens of nearly equal size and is nearly always associated with complex cardiac malformation. This syndrome is also extremely rare. The lesions most commonly associated with polysplenia are total anomalous venous return, absence of the hepatic portion of the inferior vena cava with azygous continuation, ASD, and situs inversus. The lungs are bilaterally bilobed. Symptoms of heart failure usually develop in infancy. Cyanosis is uncommon. The prognosis depends on the underlying defect, but prognosis in general is better than in asplenia. The lesions are frequently operable and the patients do not appear to be more susceptible to infection.

Anesthetic Management for Heterotaxy Syndromes

The choice of anesthetic technique and degree of monitoring depends on the dominant cardiac lesion(s) and the proposed procedure. The preceding sections describe the approach to patients with excessive or diminished pulmonary blood flow. Prevention of embolization and prophylaxis against endocarditis is essential.

OBSTRUCTIVE LESIONS
Coarctation of the Aorta

Isolated coarctation of the aorta is the fifth or sixth most common congenital cardiac defect, accounting for 6% to 7% of all CHD. Coarctation affects males twice as frequently as females and is the lesion most commonly associated with the Turner syndrome of XO karyotype. A bicuspid aortic valve is found in 50% to 80% of patients with coarctation.

The coarctation is a constriction of the aorta, at or near the junction of the ductus arteriosus and the aortic arch, and distal to the left subclavian artery. The involved segment may be discrete or of significant length. The narrowing of the aorta may occur proximal to the entrance of the ductus (preductal or infantile type of coarctation), usually as a long segmental narrowing. The constriction may also occur at or below the ductus (postductal or adult type of coarctation), usually as a localized narrowing (Fig. 10-14). Forty percent of patients with preductal coarctation have associated severe intracardiac anomalies, compared with only 14% of patients with postductal coarctation. Prostaglandin E_1 is administered to patients with ductal-dependent distal circulation as soon as the diagnosis is established.

The physiologic problem in coarctation is maintenance of blood flow to the lower half of the body in the

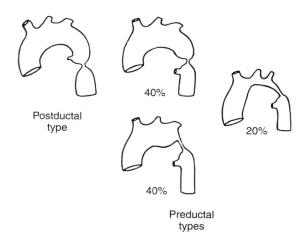

FIG. 10-14   Coarctation of the aorta. Preductal and postductal anatomic variants.

(From Keith JD: Coarctation of the aorta. In Keith JD et al, editors, *Heart disease in infancy and childhood*, ed 3, New York, 1978, Macmillan.)

presence of an aortic obstruction. Adaptive mechanisms cause elevation of the systolic blood pressure in the proximal aorta to increase the pressure gradient, arteriolar constriction to maintain diastolic pressure, and development of collateral vessels that bypass the obstruction. In the preductal form of coarctation, blood flow to the lower half of the body occurs via a PDA.

Coarctation of the aorta is the second most common cause of congestive heart failure in infancy and childhood, with more than half of patients becoming symptomatic within the first years of life. Eighty percent of these patients have an associated defect, most commonly PDA (two thirds) or VSD (30%-35%). The coarctation is preductal in two thirds of these infants.

The systolic blood pressure in the upper extremity, particularly the right arm, is greater than the systolic pressure in the lower extremity, except in patients with a low output state or a large ductus supplying blood flow to the lower extremity. The latter is frequently associated with a VSD and high systemic pressures in the pulmonary artery.

Medical therapy and balloon dilatation are frequently unsuccessful, necessitating surgical repair of the coarctation by resection and end-to-end anastomosis. Older techniques included patch aortoplasty and subclavian flap angioplasty (Fig. 10-15). Reduction of left ventricular afterload by coarctation repair generally leads to improvement in patients with associated VSD. Repair of these VSDs can be postponed, since 50% become smaller or close spontaneously. Pulmonary artery banding is performed at the time of coarctation repair in patients with complex lesions, not amenable to correction in infancy, that could result in pulmonary hypertension. The PDA is always ligated.

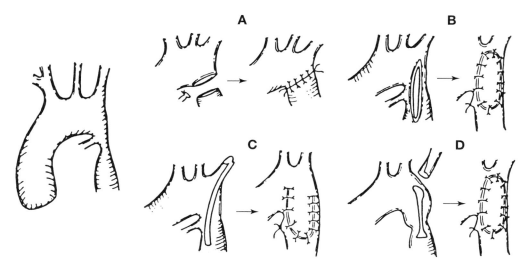

FIG. 10-15 Surgical procedures for repair of coarctation. **A,** Resection and end-to-end anastomosis. **B,** Patch aortoplasty. **C,** Subclavian flap repair. **D,** Subclavian flap repair with repositioning of the left subclavian artery.

FIG. 10-16 Interrupted aortic arch: classification after Celoria and Patton. *LCC,* Left common carotid artery; *LPA,* left pulmonary artery; *LS,* left subclavian artery; *MPA,* main pulmonary artery; *PDA,* patent ductus arteriosus; *RCC,* right common carotid artery; *RPA,* right pulmonary artery; *RS,* right subclavian artery.

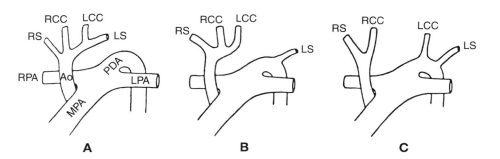

The majority of patients with isolated postductal coarctation are not diagnosed until later in life, most commonly because of the incidental finding of a heart murmur or systolic hypertension between 4 and 5 years of age. Systolic pressure is markedly higher in the upper extremities in 90% of patients. The children are otherwise normal, without signs of congestive failure.

Surgical repair is performed shortly after the diagnosis is established. Repairs in later childhood and adolescence are associated with a 10% to 20% incidence of persistent hypertension despite adequate relief of the obstruction. This may lead to premature death from cardiovascular disease.

Patients with coarctation have an increased incidence of cerebral aneurysm, which may lead to cerebrovascular accidents, even in the presence of a normal postoperative blood pressure. The risk of endocarditis is not eliminated with coarctation repair. Infection may occur at the anastomotic site, with mycotic aneurysm formation and aortic rupture, or at the aortic or mitral valve; these valves are frequently abnormal (bicuspid aortic valve, mitral valve prolapse). Aneurysmal dilatation of the site of the coarctation repair is a long-term sequela of patch aortoplasty. Only patients with hypertension develop this aneurysmal dilatation during childhood. A

very rare but catastrophic sequela of coarctation repair is spinal cord injury with paraplegia. The prognosis for unrepaired coarctation is poor. Twenty percent die in the second decade of life and ninety percent before the age of 50 years as a consequence of severe hypertension.

Two percent of patients with coarctation have associated coarctation of the abdominal aorta. This is most commonly seen in females. Hypertension is usually pronounced, and renal involvement is common. Corrective surgery is usually performed after childhood, with resection of the lesions or interposition of a graft.

Interrupted Aortic Arch

Interrupted aortic arch is an uncommon congenital lesion accounting for approximately 1.4% of all infants seen with CHD. A segment of the aortic arch is absent or atretic, leading to complete aortic discontinuity. The embryogenetic basis is failure of fusion of the fourth and sixth aortic arches. The defect may be located distal to the left subclavian artery (type A), between the left carotid and left subclavian arteries (type B), or distal to the innominate and proximal to the left carotid arteries (type C)[27] (Fig. 10-16). The lesion is commonly associated with VSD and PDA, the latter supplying the blood flow to the distal aorta. Type B interruption is the most common defect. Symptoms of a large left-to-right shunt with heart failure and pulmonary hyperperfusion are present shortly after birth. Physiologic closure of the ductus leads to systemic underperfusion with metabolic acidosis and renal failure. Without surgical intervention, death occurs in 90% of patients within the first month of life. Bypassing the interruption by using the carotid or subclavian artery, tube graft interposition, and direct anastomosis have been used. Pulmonary artery banding or primary repair of an associated VSD has been performed simultaneously.

Prostaglandin E_1 is used preoperatively to maintain patency of the ductus and systemic perfusion.[28] Surgical mortality rate is fewer than 10%. Only intermediate-term follow-up of survivors has been reported.[29,30] Subaortic stenosis appears to be more common in these patients, requiring further surgery. With growth, relative coarctation at the graft site may occur, necessitating surgical revision. Aortic interruption may be associated with DiGeorge syndrome and patients may develop severe hypocalcemia. Calcium levels should be monitored perioperatively.

Anesthetic Considerations for Coarctation of the Aorta and Interrupted Aortic Arch
Symptomatic infants usually undergo repair before any elective noncardiac surgery. The anesthetic agents are usually chosen to minimize myocardial depression; however, high-dose opioids are usually avoided to facilitate more rapid extubation. The procedure is performed via a left thoracotomy and monitoring lines are placed accordingly. Mild hypothermia to 32° C to 34° C is used to protect the spinal cord from the ischemic insult during aortic cross-clamping. Blood pressure must be measured in the right upper extremity. The authors use neuraxial opiates (preservative-free morphine 70-100 μg/kg via the caudal foramen) to facilitate postoperative analgesia.

The hypertensive response to aortic cross-clamping may be more marked in older patients. Antihypertensive medications, such as sodium nitroprusside, may be required to control acute hypertension. The anesthetic management includes a double-lumen endotracheal tube if the patient is large enough.

Even after repair, patients presenting for noncardiac surgery may have an exaggerated blood pressure response to stress and require sufficient anesthetic depth to blunt this response. Inhalation anesthetics and muscle relaxants without sympathomimetic side effects are good choices. Associated cardiac defects and their physiologic consequences are taken into consideration. Patients with associated Turner syndrome may be difficult to intubate. Hypertension is commonly present in many patients postoperatively. Two thirds of patients after coarctation repair exhibit marked systolic hypertension with stress. Since cerebral aneurysms are more common

in these patients, subarachnoid hemorrhage may occur. All patients require endocarditis prophylaxis preoperatively and postoperatively.

Supravalvular Aortic Stenosis

Supravalvular aortic stenosis is a narrowing of the aorta locally or diffusely above the level of the coronary arteries. This is most commonly associated with Williams syndrome—idiopathic infantile hypercalcemia. Patients are often retarded. Since the coronary arteries are located proximal to the obstruction, they are subjected to the high pressures of the left ventricle, are frequently tortuous, and may develop premature coronary atherosclerosis. Clinical symptoms are similar to those of valvular aortic stenosis. Surgical treatment for localized stenosis consists of patch enlargement of the narrowed segment.

Discrete Subvalvular Aortic Stenosis

Discrete subvalvular aortic stenosis is a membranous diaphragm or ring encircling the left ventricular outflow tract. The malformation accounts for 8% to 10% of all cases of congenital aortic stenosis. Jet lesions of the aortic cusps develop, causing valve degeneration and aortic insufficiency. There is a very high risk of infective endocarditis. Clinical presentation is similar to that of valvular aortic stenosis and depends on the severity of obstruction. Surgery is recommended even for mild-to-moderate stenosis, because of the likelihood of developing progressive obstruction and aortic insufficiency. The membranous or fibrous ridge is excised. The existing jet lesion and scarring following manipulation of the valve during surgery may require children with this malformation to undergo valve replacement. Heart block is a recognized complication due to the proximity of the conduction system to the membrane.

Anesthetic Considerations in Aortic Stenosis
The anesthetic management of pediatric patients with aortic stenosis mirrors that in adults. Preload, afterload, and contractility must be maintained. Tachycardia should be avoided and sinus rhythm maintained whenever possible.

Pulmonic Stenosis

A pressure gradient between the right ventricle and the pulmonary artery constitutes the main physiologic derangement in pulmonic stenosis. It is present as a secondary defect in 25% to 30% of congenital cardiac lesions but occurs as an isolated defect in about 10% of patients with CHD. Pulmonic stenosis is the lesion most commonly associated with Noonan syndrome. The stenosis is most commonly at the valve level with fusion of the leaflets, producing a dome-shaped valve with a small central opening. The severity of clinical symptoms depends on the degree of right ventricular outflow obstruction. Patients with mild-to-moderate obstruction are generally asymptomatic, and the stenosis is usually discovered during a routine examination because of the presence of a systolic murmur. Secondary changes include hypertrophy of the right ventricle (which may produce infundibular stenosis) and poststenotic dilatation of the pulmonary trunk.

Right ventricular pressure may exceed the pressure in the left ventricle with severe stenosis. Right atrial pressure is elevated and right-to-left shunting occurs across a patent foramen ovale or ASD. If no communication between the right and left heart exists, syncope may occur during exercise because of the inability to increase cardiac output. Right ventricular ischemic changes with myocardial fibrosis and coronary artery occlusions may develop in these patients, leading to right ventricular failure.

All symptomatic patients, or those with right ventricular-to-pulmonary artery gradients exceeding 70 mm Hg, require relief of their obstruction. Gradients of less than 50 mm Hg usually do not progress over time. Obstruction may be relieved by open or closed valvotomy or percutaneous valvuloplasty. Percutaneous procedures have become the treatment of choice, but are not recommended for patients with associated infundibular stenosis. Successful valvotomy or valvuloplasty decreases right ventricular pressure to half of preprocedure values or lower. Infundibular stenosis usually resolves with time.

Infants with critical pulmonic stenosis usually present 24 to 48 hours after birth with cyanosis and metabolic acidosis. Pulmonary blood flow is ductus dependent and patency of the ductus arteriosus is maintained with prostaglandin E_1. These patients frequently have hypoplasia of the right ventricle associated with endomyocardial fibrosis. Relief of the right ventricular outflow obstruction is performed emergently and frequently combined with a systemic-to-pulmonary shunt, since pulmonary blood flow may be inadequate. Invasive monitoring is used for major surgery. Endocarditis prophylaxis is of utmost importance. Patients who have undergone valvuloplasty usually have a residual defect that should be assessed before elective surgery. They are still at high risk for endocarditis. Patients with critical stenosis should not undergo elective noncardiac surgery.

Anesthetic Considerations for Pulmonic Stenosis

All patients with pulmonic stenosis (prerepair or postrepair) require endocarditis prophylaxis. Patients with mild degrees of obstruction should otherwise experience no anesthetic problems. Patients with moderate degrees of obstruction who appear clinically normal may have limited myocardial reserve and are prone to

right heart failure. Cardiac output is potentially limited by the stenotic lesion. Anesthetic management consists of selection of appropriate anesthetic agents with minimal cardiovascular and peripheral vasodilatory side effects and right-sided pressure monitoring.

Critically ill neonates with ductal-dependent circulation are managed by optimizing oxygenation and altering PVR to maintain a single ventricle physiology with balanced pulmonary and systemic blood flow. They are prone to hemodynamic collapse, therefore necessitating the use of anesthetic agents with minimal myocardial depression.

Peripheral Pulmonic Stenosis

Stenosis of the pulmonary arteries, either proximal or distal, occurs in 2% to 3% of all patients with CHD. This lesion and PDA are the lesions most commonly associated with the congenital rubella syndrome. Patients with mild to moderate bilateral stenosis or unilateral disease are usually asymptomatic. Patients with severe obstruction present with dyspnea, fatigue, and signs of right heart failure. Treatment is surgical if the obstruction is located proximally. Multiple distal stenoses may improve with growth of the patient; otherwise, death occurs during infancy or early childhood. The anesthetic management is the same as described earlier for pulmonic stenosis.

LESIONS CAUSING LEFT VENTRICULAR INFLOW OBSTRUCTION
Mitral Stenosis

Isolated mitral stenosis is one of the rarest forms of CHD, occurring in 0.6% of autopsied and 0.2% to 0.4% of clinically diagnosed patients with CHD. It is more common in males.

Developmental abnormalities of the mitral valve leaflets, commissures, chordae tendineae, annulus, supravalvular area, or papillary muscles lead to obstruction of left ventricular filling. Left atrial pressure rises as a compensatory mechanism to maintain blood flow across the stenotic area. With further reduction in valve orifice, blood flow becomes turbulent, which increases resistance to total flow and leads to a higher pressure gradient. Pulmonary venous pressure becomes secondarily elevated, eventually leading to elevation of pulmonary artery and right ventricular pressures. The vascular congestion results in a decrease in static and dynamic compliance. Bronchial venous congestion leads to edema of the bronchial mucosa and increased airway resistance. The work of breathing is increased and abnormalities in gas exchange are common with significant disease.

Left ventricular filling depends on the size of the valve orifice and diastolic filling time. Tachycardia causes marked elevation in atrial pressure and reduction in cardiac output. Left ventricular dysfunction from ischemia and fibrosis frequently complicates severe stenosis. Approximately 50% of patients with congenital mitral stenosis have other congenital cardiac anomalies.

Patients commonly present with exertional dyspnea and recurrent pulmonary infections. Infants exhibit failure to thrive, and episodes of congestive heart failure may occur. The diagnosis is frequently established late.

Patients with intractable congestive failure, pulmonary edema, or pulmonary artery hypertension to systemic levels require surgical intervention. Unrelieved left atrial hypertension causes progressive obstructive pulmonary vascular disease. Mitral valvotomy or fenestration of the mitral valve is generally performed in infants or small children. With severely deformed valves, radical valvuloplasty is recommended to avoid replacement. These procedures are palliative for these patients to allow for growth and development and relief of clinical symptoms. Eventually mitral valve replacement becomes necessary in the majority of cases.

Prognosis of symptomatic infants is poor. Forty percent die within the first 6 months irrespective of therapy. Surgical mortality rate is between 30% and 40%, with 50% of patients surviving beyond 5 to 10 years. Presently fewer than 20% of patients survive to adulthood.

Supravalvular Mitral Ring

Accumulation of connective tissue arising from the atrial surface of the mitral valve produces a supravalvular ring, reducing the effective mitral orifice. This rarely occurs as an isolated malformation but is usually associated with a degree of valvular mitral stenosis. The clinical presentation is indistinguishable from valvular stenosis. Treatment consists of surgical excision of the ring tissue.

Parachute Mitral Valve (Shone Syndrome)

Insertion of all chordae tendineae into a single papillary muscle causes a parachute deformity of the mitral valve. Blood flow from the left atrium must pass through interchordal spaces, and various degrees of functional mitral stenosis result. The lesion is commonly associated with other forms of left-sided obstruction, such as supravalvular mitral ring, subvalvular or valvular aortic stenosis, and coarctation of the aorta. Presence of all four obstructive lesions together constitutes the Shone syndrome. Median survival approaches 10 years of age and correlates best with left ventricular size. Patients are managed medically with control of heart failure and pulmonary infections throughout childhood, since relief of the obstruction requires mitral valve replacement. Surgical approaches are directed toward alleviating the obstructions to flow.

Cor Triatriatum

The left atrium of patients with cor triatriatum is abnormally partitioned into two chambers, the upper one (smooth walled) receiving the pulmonary veins and the lower one (trabeculated) bordering the mitral valve. Communication between the two chambers is through fenestrations in the dividing membrane. The hemodynamic consequence is pulmonary venous obstruction similar to that of mitral stenosis. The malformation occurs in about 0.5% of all CHD. Males are affected more commonly.

In classic cor triatriatum, no communication exists between the two left atrial chambers and the right atrium. Consequent to the obstruction of pulmonary venous return, pulmonary artery hypertension develops with right ventricular hypertrophy. Onset of symptoms is usually within the first few years of life, characterized by breathlessness and frequent respiratory infections. Patients with severe obstruction present with pulmonary edema and right heart failure and are often considered to have primary pulmonary disease. Death occurs within months if the obstruction is not relieved by surgical excision of the membrane dividing the atrium. The pulmonary vascular changes appear to be reversible with surgical correction.

Anesthetic Considerations for Left Ventricular Inflow Obstruction

All patients coming for cardiac surgery and the majority of postoperative patients have a pressure gradient across the mitral valve. Flow though the valve occurs during diastole, and shortening diastole decreases ventricular filling. Therefore, tachycardia must be avoided. Hypovolemia and vasodilators that reduce preload also impair blood flow across the stenotic lesion. The heart is unable to compensate for a reduction in afterload by increasing stroke volume or cardiac output, since both are limited by the amount of blood that passes through the stenotic area. Overzealous administration of fluids or alterations in position may increase central blood volume and cause a rapid rise in left atrial pressure; this may lead to pulmonary edema. Patients are at risk for bacterial endocarditis. Patients may have marked alterations in gas exchange due to chronic pulmonary congestion.

The anesthetic techniques and agents are chosen to avoid tachycardia, minimize vasodilatation, and avoid depression of myocardial function. Preload must be maintained. Tachycardia requires prompt treatment, preferably with a short-acting β-blocker such as esmolol. Atrial fibrillation and systemic embolization are extremely uncommon in children with mitral stenosis. Congestive failure is treated with caution to avoid excessive depletion of intravascular volume, since induction of anesthesia may cause severe hypotension under these circumstances. Hypotension due to peripheral vasodilatation is treated with judicious use of a vasoconstrictor such as phenylephrine.

Disturbances in pulmonary gas exchange are common. Ventilatory management should minimize PVR. Positive end-expiratory pressure is beneficial for preventing and treating pulmonary edema. Hypoxia may lead to acute right heart failure by increasing PVR. Most patients therefore require higher inspired oxygen concentrations. Patients frequently require prolonged mechanical ventilation following cardiac surgery.

Intravascular volume status for any major noncardiac surgery is managed with invasive monitoring. Electrolyte abnormalities caused by diuretic therapy should be normalized before elective surgery. Pulmonary artery pressures reflect only the filling status of the left atrium, with left ventricular end-diastolic pressure dependent on the gradient across the lesion. Acute elevations in left atrial pressure are treated with increased positive-pressure ventilation, venodilating drugs (nitroglycerin, low-dose nitroprusside), and reverse Trendelenburg position. Patients with hemodynamic decompensation during surgery may need inotropic support.

An opioid-relaxant anesthetic technique is a prudent choice to minimize tachycardia, myocardial depression, and vasodilatation. Induction of anesthesia may be markedly prolonged secondary to low cardiac output. Ketamine causes less tachycardia in infants and children and maintains vascular tone. Inhalation anesthetics are poorly tolerated in the presence of a low, fixed cardiac output.

VASCULAR RING ANOMALIES

Anomalies in the development of the aortic arch system may be associated with anomalous vascular structures compressing the trachea or esophagus (Fig. 10-17). The incidence of aortic arch malformation is not known. Symptomatic patients comprise approximately 1.5% of patients with CHD.

The heart is generally normal in these patients and symptoms usually relate to the degree of respiratory obstruction. Patients with severe tracheal compression exhibit stridor, wheezing, recurrent pneumonia, and emphysematous pulmonary changes within the first few months of life. Respiratory distress is aggravated by feeding and lessened by hyperextension of the head. Severely affected infants show failure to thrive. Other causes of stridor or frequent pneumonia (e.g., laryngeal web, tracheomalacia, tracheoesophageal fistula, gastric reflux, Pierre-Robin anomaly, choanal atresia) must be excluded. The airway obstruction may be life threatening. The compressed area is frequently located in the lower trachea but may be located distally in one of the main bronchi. Esophageal obstruction may occur, with swallowing difficulties and frequent

vomiting. However, symptoms are generally less severe and the condition may remain undiagnosed for many years.

Medical management consists of careful positioning to minimize tracheal compression, feeding with liquids or soft foods, and prompt treatment of pulmonary infections. The trachea becomes stiffer and less easily compressed as the infant grows. Patients with severe symptoms and significant tracheal narrowing require surgery to relieve the vascular obstruction.

Anesthetic Considerations for Vascular Ring Anomalies

Patients require a thoracotomy for repair. Monitoring lines should be placed in such a way that surgical manipulation does not interfere with their functioning. Patients may have significant tracheomalacia and require postoperative ventilation for that reason. Since cardiac function is normal in these patients, no specific anesthetic technique is recommended. Transesophageal echocardiography is avoided to prevent airway compression and obstruction of the airway.

ANOMALOUS ORIGIN OF THE LEFT CORONARY ARTERY

Anomalous origin of the left coronary artery from the right sinus of Valsalva causes the vessel to course between the aorta and right ventricular outflow tract or pulmonary trunk. Compression of the vessel may occur during exercise and has been implicated as a cause of death in young healthy athletes. The anomaly is rare.

Origin of the left coronary artery from the pulmonary trunk (ALCAPA) is a rare but frequently lethal anomaly. It is usually referred to as *Bland-White-Garland syndrome*. From 80% to 90% of patients become symptomatic in infancy and the majority die from congestive heart failure. The physiologic derangement consists of hypoperfusion of the left coronary artery by a low-pressure system with reduced oxygen saturation. The development of coronary collaterals results in left-to-right shunting into the pulmonary artery and coronary steal, causing left-sided myocardial ischemia. These events occur as the pulmonary pressure decreases in the postnatal period, although pulmonary artery pressure may remain elevated subsequent to poor left ventricular output and elevated left atrial pressures with secondary pulmonary hypertension. Endocardial and transmural myocardial ischemia and infarction result from the decreased left myocardial perfusion, leading to papillary muscle dysfunction and mitral regurgitation. Infants may have signs of anginal attacks during feeding. The ECG resembles that of an adult with coronary artery disease. Infants with ischemic attacks require urgent surgery because of the risk of sudden death, and patients

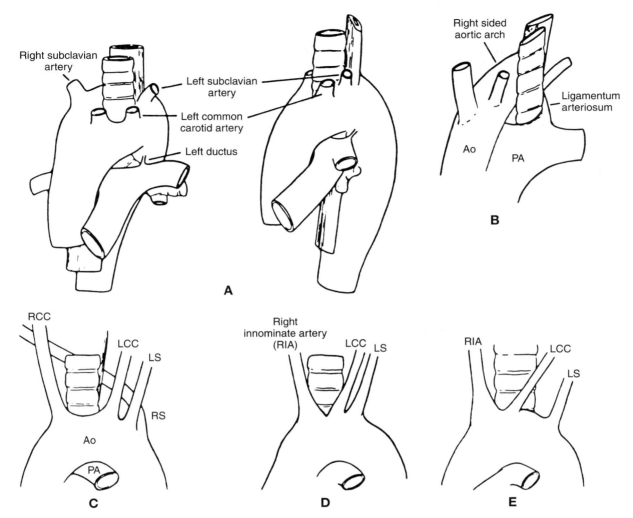

FIG. 10-17 Vascular ring anomalies (after Gross[33]). **A,** Double aortic arch. **B,** Right aortic arch with left ligamentum arteriosum. **C,** Anomalous right subclavian artery. **D,** Anomalous right innominate artery. **E,** Anomalous left common carotid artery. *Ao,* Aorta; *LCC,* left common carotid artery; *LS,* left subclavian artery; *PA,* pulmonary artery; *RCC,* right common carotid artery; *RS,* right subclavian artery.

with heart failure are managed conservatively with the expectation that collateral circulation will develop and myocardial function will improve.

Eventually all patients with this anomaly require correction to prevent sudden death. Various surgical approaches have been advocated. Simple ligation of the vessel in cases with left-to-right shunting and good collaterals may effect cure, but the result is unpredictable and leaves the patient with a single coronary artery. Procedures that are favored presently preserve a "two-coronary-artery" system. This may be accomplished by anastomosing either a systemic artery or a vein graft to the anomalous vessel, redirecting aortic blood flow to the anomalous coronary ostium via transpulmonary arterial baffle, or reimplanting the

anomalous vessel into the aorta by using a cuff of pulmonary trunk. Surgery results in resolution of ischemic attacks and improved myocardial performance.

Anesthetic Considerations for Anomalous Origin of the Left Coronary Artery

Patients with Bland-White-Garland syndrome require early surgical correction. The patients are usually in a low cardiac output state with congestive heart failure and mitral regurgitation. Anesthetic agents that cause minimal myocardial depression, afterload reduction, and maintenance of an adequate heart rate are important. Patients may require increased Fio_2 and positive end-expiratory pressure to maintain adequate gas exchange. Patients frequently require inotropic support before and after CPB, because the ischemic myocardium recovers function slowly. There may be permanent loss of myocardial reserve due to infarction. For noncardiac surgery, management depends on the degree of residual cardiovascular abnormality. Patients may have reduced cardiac reserve because of myocardial scarring or residual mitral insufficiency. Use of anesthetic agents that cause minimal myocardial depression, maintenance of heart rate, and direct monitoring of systemic arterial and venous pressures for major surgery are indicated.

In older patients with the uncorrected anomaly, care should be taken to avoid increases in myocardial oxygen demand (tachycardia, hypertension) or decreases in myocardial oxygen supply (low diastolic pressure, high left ventricular end-diastolic pressure). Patients are at risk for bacterial endocarditis after corrective surgery.

KAWASAKI DISEASE

Mucocutaneous lymph node syndrome or Kawasaki disease is an acute febrile erythematous disease with desquamative conjunctivitis, stomatitis, and nonsuppurative lymphadenitis, accompanied by myocarditis in 25% to 50% of cases. The disease is most common between 6 months and 5 years of age, with a median age of 2.3 years, and occurs primarily in Asian males. It is most prevalent in Japan.

The pathologic basis for the disease consists of widespread microvasculitis. Involvement of the coronary vessels results in development of coronary aneurysms, coronary artery stenoses, thromboses, or rupture. A coronary artery lesion occurs in about 17% of affected patients. Involvement of the heart accounts for the 1.2% to 2.5% mortality rate reported for this disease. The coronary arteritis is usually silent until infarction or angina occurs.

Treatment consists of therapy with aspirin until all symptoms have subsided. In patients with coronary aneurysms, aspirin therapy should be continued for at least 12 months. The aneurysms usually regress spontaneously. If no improvement occurs and severe coronary artery disease persists, bypass grafting or coronary aneurysmectomy must be performed. Prognosis for patency of bypass grafts appears to be less favorable in this young group of patients.

Anesthetic Considerations for Kawasaki Disease

Anesthetic management should consider the predominant cardiac derangements. Heart failure or arrhythmias may be present. Maintenance of myocardial oxygen balance is paramount in significant coronary artery disease. Monitoring for arrhythmias and myocardial ischemia is essential.

CONCLUSIONS

CHD creates significant challenges for the anesthesiologist. Safe clinical care requires an adequate knowledge of the underlying pathophysiology of the congenital heart lesion, the use of anesthetic agents and techniques to optimize the patient's condition, and the effects of the surgical procedure. Close collaboration with pediatric cardiologists and surgeons is the best method of ensuring the highest level of care for patients with CHD.

KEY POINTS

1. Optimize SVR and PVR to balance pulmonary and systemic blood flow by using respiratory maneuvers and pharmacology.
2. Determine the presence and significance of associated congenital anomalies.
3. Endocarditis prophylaxis may be required even after lesions are repaired.
4. Meticulously remove all air bubbles from intravenous lines to prevent paradoxic embolization.
5. Atrial and ventricular arrhythmias may occur even after lesions are repaired. The risk of arrhythmia may increase with age.

KEY REFERENCES

Anand KJS, Hickey PR: Halothane-morphine compared with high-dose sufentanil for anesthesia and postoperative analgesia in neonatal cardiac surgery, *New Engl J Med* 326:1, 1992.
Benson DW: Changing profile of congenital heart disease, *Pediatrics* 83:790, 1998.
Dajani AS, Taubert KA, Wilson W et al: Prevention of bacterial endocarditis. Recommendations by the American Heart Association, *JAMA* 277:1794, 1997.
Elliott M: Modified ultrafiltration and open heart surgery in children, *Paediatr Anesth* 9:1, 1999.

Laishley RS, Burrows FA, Lerman J et al: Effect of anesthetic induction regimens on oxygen saturation in cyanotic congenital heart disease, *Anesthesiology* 65:673, 1986.

Rossi AF, Sommer RJ, Lotvin A et al: Usefulness of intermittent monitoring of mixed venous oxygen saturation after stage I palliation for hypoplastic left heart syndrome, *Am J Cardiol* 73:1118, 1994.

Tanner GE, Anger DG, Barash PG et al: Effects of left-to-right, mixed left-to-right and right-to-left shunts on inhalational anesthetic induction in children, *Anesth Analg* 64:101, 1985.

References

1. *American Heart Association 2001 heart and stroke statistical update.* Dallas: American Heart Association, 2000.
2. Zahka KG: Associated abnormalities in children with congenital heart disease. In Emmanouilides GC, Riemenschneider TA, Allen HD, Gutgesell HP, editors: *Moss and Adams heart disease in infants, children and adolescents,* Baltimore, 1995, Williams and Wilkins.
3. Sparks RS, Perloff JK: Genetics, epidemiology, counseling and prevention. In Perloff JK, Child JS, editors: *Congenital heart disease in adults,* Philadelphia, 1991, WB Saunders.
4. Benson DW: Changing profile of congenital heart disease, *Pediatrics* 83:790, 1998.
5. Tanner GE, Anger DG, Barash PG et al: Effects of left-to-right, mixed left-to-right and right-to-left shunts on inhalational anesthetic induction in children, *Anesth Analg* 64:101, 1985.
6. Becu LM, Fontana RS, DuShane JW et al: Anatomic and pathologic studies in ventricular septal defect, *Circulation* 14:349, 1956.
7. Kirklin JW, Harshbarger HG, Donald DE et al: Surgical correction of ventricular septal defect: anatomic and technical considerations, *J Thorac Surg* 33:45, 1957.
8. Harlan BJ, Starr A, Harwin FM: Ventricular septal defects. In Harlan BJ, Starr A, Harvin FM, editors: *Illustrated handbook of cardiac surgery.* New York, 1996, Springer, pp 237-246.
9. Cetta F, Mair DD, Feldt RH et al: Improved early mortality after modified Fontan operation for complex congenital heart disease, *Am J Cardiol* 72:499, 1993.
10. Rastelli GC, Kirklin JW, Titus JL: Anatomic observations on complete form of persistent common atrioventricular canal with special reference to atrioventricular valves, *Mayo Clin Proc* 41:299, 1968.
11. Dajani AS, Taubert KA, Wilson W et al: Prevention of bacterial endocarditis. Recommendations by the American Heart Association, *JAMA* 277:1794, 1997.
12. Elliott M: Modified ultrafiltration and open heart surgery in children, *Paediatr Anesth* 9:1, 1999.
13. Reich DL, Silvay G: Ketamine: an update on the first 25 years of clinical experience, *Can J Anaesth* 36:186, 1989.
14. Lyons B, Motherway C, Casey W et al: The anaesthetic management of the child with Eisenmenger's syndrome, *Can J Anaesth* 42:904, 1995.
15. Ammash NM, Connolly HM, Abel MD et al: Noncardiac surgery in Eisenmenger syndrome, *J Am Coll Cardiol* 33:222, 1999.
16. Dunnigan A, Pritzker MR, Benditt DG et al: Life threatening ventricular tachycardias in late survivors of surgically corrected tetralogy of Fallot, *Br Heart J* 52:198, 1984.
17. Gatzoulis MA, Balaji S, Webber SA et al: Risk factors for arrhythmia and sudden cardiac death late after repair of tetralogy of Fallot: a multicentre study, *Lancet* 356:975, 2000.
18. Laishley RS, Burrows FA, Lerman J et al: Effect of anesthetic induction regimens on oxygen saturation in cyanotic congenital heart disease, *Anesthesiology* 65:673, 1986.
19. Lister G, Pitt BR: Cardiopulmonary interactions in the infant with congenital heart disease, *Clin Chest Med* 4:219, 1983.
20. Colett RW, Edwards JE: Persistent truncus arteriosus: a classification according to anatomic types, *Surg Clin North Am* 29:1245, 1949.
21. Report of the New England Regional Cardiac Program, *Pediatrics* 65(suppl 2), 1980.
22. Jatene AD, Iontes VF, Paulista PP: Anatomic correction of transposition of the great vessels, *J Thorac Cardiovasc Surg* 73:363, 1976.
23. Anand KJS, Hickey PR: Halothane-morphine compared with high-dose sufentanil for anesthesia and postoperative analgesia in neonatal cardiac surgery, *New Engl J Med* 326:1, 1992.
24. Massin MM: Midterm results of the neonatal arterial switch operation: a review, *J Cardiovasc Surg (Torino)* 40:517, 1999.
25. Norwood WI, Lang P: Physiologic repair of aortic atresia-hypoplastic left heart syndrome, *N Engl J Med* 308:23, 1983.
26. Rossi AF, Sommer RJ, Lotvin A et al: Usefulness of intermittent monitoring of mixed venous oxygen saturation after stage I palliation for hypoplastic left heart syndrome, *Am J Cardiol* 73:1118, 1994.
27. Celoria GC, Patton RB: Congenital absence of the aortic arch, *Am Heart J* 58:407, 1959.
28. Radford DJ, Bloom KR, Coceani F et al: Prostaglandin E1 for interrupted aortic arch, *Lancet* 2:95, 1976.
29. Menahem S, Rahayoe AU, Brwan WJ et al: Interrupted aortic arch in infancy: a 10 year experience, *Pediatr Cardiol* 13:214, 1992.
30. Jahangiri M, Zurakowski D, Mayer JE et al: Repair of the truncal valve and associated interrupted arch in neonates with truncus arteriosus, *J Thorac Cardiovasc Surg* 119:508, 2000.
31. Steinberg AG, bearn AG, Motulsky AG et al: Genetics of cardiovascular disease. In *Progress in medical genetics,* vol 5, Philadelphia, 1983, WB Saunders.
32. Noonan JA: Association of congenital heart disease with syndromes and their defects, *Pediatr Clin North Am* 25:797, 1978.
33. Gross RE: *The surgery of infancy and childhood,* Philadelphia, 1953, WB Saunders.

CHAPTER 11

Less Common Cardiac Problems

Elizabeth Herrera, M.D. ∎ Jack S. Shanewise, M.D.

OUTLINE

CARDIAC TAMPONADE
Definition/Pathophysiology

Cardiac tamponade is a pathophysiologic continuum occurring when there is compression of the heart within the pericardial sac from effusion fluid, blood, clots, or purulence, causing progressive increases in intrapericardial pressure.[1] The pressure is transmitted to the cardiac chambers and causes elevation of intracardiac pressures with eventual limitation of ventricular filling, resulting in reduction of stroke volume and cardiac output. Initially, rises in intrapericardial pressure cause collapse of the right atrium and ventricle in early diastole, limiting filling only during this part of the cardiac cycle. During this time, cardiac output may be maintained by compensatory increases in adrenergic tone, causing tachycardia, increased contractility, and venoconstriction. Eventually, this compensation is overwhelmed by progressive increments in intrapericardial pressure, stimulating the release of the neurohumoral mediators, renin,

angiotensin II, aldosterone, and arginine vasopressin, similar to the situation seen with decreased cardiac output from congestive heart failure. This results in further stimulation of the sympathetic nervous system, vasoconstriction, and retention of sodium and water by the kidneys.[2] Serum levels of atrial natriuretic factor do not increase, unlike in congestive heart failure, because there is no atrial stretch.

The filling of each cardiac chamber is dependent on its transmural pressure, which is the intracardiac pressure minus pericardial pressure. Right atrial (RA) mean pressure and right ventricular (RV) diastolic pressure, though somewhat lower than the corresponding left-sided chambers, are normally higher than intrapericardial pressure.[4] When intrapericardial pressure rises to the level of RA and RV diastolic pressures, the transmural pressure distending these chambers declines to nearly zero and may actually become negative. Cardiac output becomes severely compromised because these chambers are compressed during the entire phase of diastole and can no longer fill effectively. When fluid accumulation is acute, hemodynamic compromise can be rapid, as in the setting of trauma with the accumulation of blood in the pericardial sac. Chronic pericardial effusions result from fluid accumulating slowly over time and may occur from various disease states, including uremia, myxedema, idiopathic pericarditis, or malignancy. Large amounts of fluid may be present in the pericardial space and the progression to hemodynamic compromise is slower. Without the proper diagnosis and management, however, chronic effusions may result in severe reductions in stroke volume and cardiac output, as in the setting of acute cardiac tamponade.

Variations Induced by Respiration

Normally, intrathoracic and intracardiac pressures are coupled, with inspiration resulting in negative intrathoracic pressure and increased venous return to the right side of the heart in a spontaneously breathing patient. Systemic arterial pressure and left ventricular (LV) stroke volume decrease with inspiration, secondary to ventricular interdependence and other conditions that decrease LV filling. These conditions include (1) increased venous return to the right heart resulting from a fall in intrathoracic and intrapericardial pressures with leftward shift of the interventricular septum, (2) increased venous capacitance in the pulmonary vascular bed, and (3) increased LV transmural pressure resulting from negative inspiratory thoracic pressure.[5] Normal respiratory variation is a decrease of 10 mm Hg or less of systolic arterial pressure during the inspiratory phase of the respiratory cycle. The opposite changes occur during expiration when the filling of the left heart chambers becomes augmented, causing an increase in systemic arterial pressure and LV stroke volume (Fig. 11-1). For patients with controlled, positive pressure ventilation, right heart filling is decreased and left heart filling is augmented during inspiration.

With tamponade physiology, the respiratory variation in systemic arterial pressure becomes more pronounced (Fig. 11-2). Because diastolic compliance of the right ventricle is greater than that of the left ventricle, similar changes in pericardial pressure have a more pronounced effect on the right heart. The slight decrease in this pressure with spontaneous inspiration allows for increased venous return preferentially to the right side of the heart. The leftward shift of the interventricular septum can become more pronounced and further compromise left heart filling. This is responsible for *pulsus paradoxus*, the decrease in systemic arterial pressure with inspiration of greater than 10 mm Hg, which is an exaggeration of the normal response. The apparent paradox, as described by Dr. Kussmaul in 1873, is the

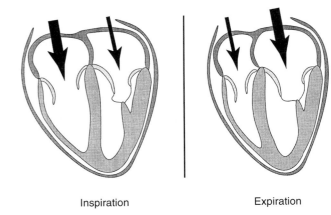

FIG. 11-1 Normal respiratory variation in flow through the right and left hearts. During spontaneous inspiration (*left*) the systemic venous return to the right atrium is somewhat increased because of slightly negative intrathoracic pressure, whereas the pulmonary venous return to the left heart is decreased. During expiration (*right*), opposite changes occur. Systemic stroke volume and blood pressure change in response to the pulmonary venous return.

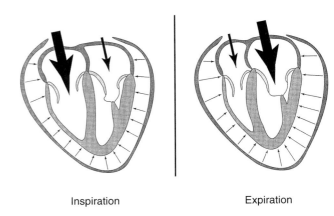

FIG. 11-2 Respiratory variation in flow through the right and left sides of the heart is increased with cardiac tamponade. As a result, systemic stroke volume and blood pressure decrease dramatically during spontaneous inspiration, producing pulsus paradoxus.

disappearance of the pulse on inspiration despite the persistence of the heartbeat.[6]

The introduction of positive intrathoracic pressure by mechanical ventilation decreases RV filling during inspiration as a result of increased pleural pressure. In normal patients and in those with compromised LV function, LV stroke volume may increase with positive pressure inspiration because of a decrease in LV afterload. While this may be beneficial in patients with congestive heart failure, it may worsen tamponade physiology by compromising RV filling and overwhelming compensatory mechanisms that maintain hemodynamics.[7]

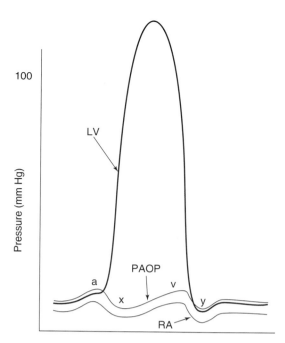

FIG. 11-3   Normal pressure waveforms. Pulmonary artery occlusion pressure (*PAOP*) is slightly higher than right atrial pressure (*RA*). Both have normal positive a and v waves and negative x and y descents. *LV*, Left ventricular pressure.

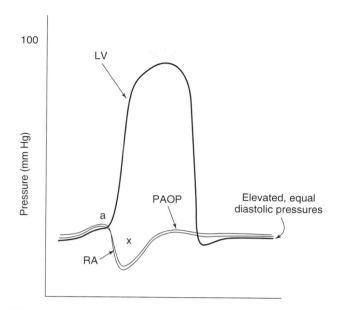

FIG. 11-4   Pressure waveforms with cardiac tamponade. Pulmonary artery occlusion pressure (*PAOP*) and right atrial pressure (*RA*) are increased and equalized as a result of elevated intrapericardial pressure. The x descent is prominent and the y descent is decreased. *LV*, Left ventricular pressure.

Pressure Waveforms

The events occurring during the cardiac cycle are demonstrated by a series of waves and descents on the central venous pressure and pulmonary artery (PA) occlusion pressure waveforms in the right and left atria, respectively (Fig. 11-3). The positive waves reflect positive pressure in the atrial chambers from either atrial contraction (a wave) or filling during ventricular systole (v wave), and the descents reflect negative pressure occurring from atrial relaxation (x descent) or emptying during ventricular diastole (y descent). The tracing of the pressure waveform may vary depending on factors influencing the events of the cardiac cycle. Tamponade physiology produces a characteristic waveform reflecting compression of the cardiac chambers (Fig. 11-4). The compressive effect of the pericardial fluid is most influential when the pressure is lowest in a particular cardiac chamber, which occurs during ventricular systole for the atria and during diastole for the ventricles. When intrapericardial pressures exceed those of the RA in systole and the RV in diastole, RA systolic collapse and RV diastolic collapse may occur (Fig. 11-5). This is seen as a loss of the y descent because this waveform reflects passive atrial emptying and early ventricular diastolic filling. As intracardiac volume decreases during ventricular ejection, there is a transient decrease in both RA and intrapericardial pressures manifested by a prominent x descent, representing this fall in RA pressure during atrial relaxation.

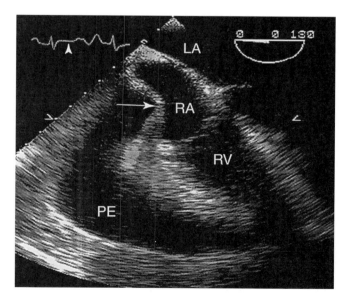

FIG. 11-5   Transesophageal echocardiogram of a patient with cardiac tamponade. There is collapse of the right atrium (*arrow*) during systole (*arrowhead*) because the intrapericardial pressure exceeds the right atrial pressure at this point in the cardiac cycle. Dots along the edge of the image are separated by 1 cm. *LA*, Left atrium; *PE*, pericardial effusion; *RA*, right atrium; *RV*, right ventricle.

When the RA (central venous) and left atrial (LA) pressure waveforms are superimposed on the corresponding waveforms of the RV and LV, pressures in all four cardiac chambers become nearly equal during the time of ventricular diastole. This equalization of pressures occurs early in diastole because intracardiac pressures are lowest at this time in the cardiac cycle. Gradually these pressures rise throughout diastole with tamponade physiology, as the ventricles eventually receive preload volume.

Diastolic Filling Patterns

Doppler echocardiography can be used to obtain information regarding inflow to both the atria and the ventricles. Because cardiac tamponade characteristically affects diastole, one would expect alterations in diastolic atrial and ventricular inflow patterns. Many variables can affect these patterns, including patient age, heart rate, respiration, atrial contractile function, and ventricular systolic and diastolic function. Tamponade physiology, however, produces marked changes from the normal flow patterns. By using echocardiography, Doppler examination of LA and LV inflow velocities can be obtained by either continuous- or pulsed-wave modalities. Normally, pulmonary venous inflow to the atrium occurs throughout the cardiac cycle, whereas LV inflow only takes place during diastole. Rapid ventricular filling in early diastole corresponds to the E velocity, followed in late diastole by the A velocity corresponding to atrial contraction. The E velocity is normally slightly higher than the A velocity. In tamponade physiology, the E velocity is decreased initially, then as the disease progresses, the A velocity also decreases. Respiratory variation becomes more marked with further decrease of the E velocity during spontaneous inspiration; the opposite changes occur during positive pressure ventilation (Fig. 11-6).

Preoperative Evaluation

Common Causes. The development of pericardial inflammation and effusion can occur with various medical disease states, including malignancy, idiopathic or viral pericarditis, uremia, or, less commonly, pericarditis associated with myocardial infarction, invasive diagnostic cardiac procedures, purulent bacterial infection, and tuberculosis. In the surgical patient population, pericardial tamponade may arise from blood in the pericardial space following cardiac surgery or central venous catheter placement, or as a complication of aortic dissection, ruptured aortic or ventricular aneurysm, or penetrating cardiac trauma[6,8,9] (Box 11-1). In the case of medical pericarditis, large serous or serosanguinous effusions accumulated gradually may be present before the occurrence of clinical signs of tamponade. Rapidly accumu-

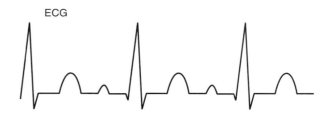

ECG

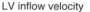

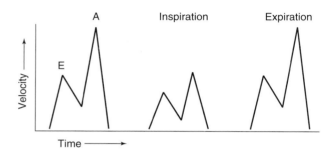

LV inflow velocity

FIG. 11-6 Changes in left ventricular (*LV*) diastolic inflow velocity pattern with cardiac tamponade as measured with Doppler echocardiography. As tamponade worsens, the size of the early (*E*) filling wave decreases relative to the atrial (*A*) filling wave. There is marked decrease in both E and A waves during spontaneous inspiration. The electrocardiogram (*ECG*) is shown to demonstrate time in the cardiac cycle.

BOX 11-1
Causes of Cardiac Tamponade

Common medical causes
  Malignancy, idiopathic pericarditis, viral pericarditis, uremia
Less common causes
  Myocardial infarction, cardiac catheterization, purulent pericarditis, tuberculosis
Surgical conditions
  Aortic dissection, ascending aortic aneurysm rupture, ventricular rupture, penetrating heart wound, blunt chest trauma, cardiac surgery, central venous cannulation

---

lating blood or clot, though smaller in volume, may produce tamponade physiology with sufficient hemodynamic compromise to warrant surgical intervention. Also, if thrombus is present, the cardiac chambers affected depend on the location of the clot. Thus tamponade may be regional, especially following cardiac surgery, and may not always follow the pattern of all cardiac chamber involvement[10] (Fig. 11-7). Such cases may not have equalization of right and left heart filling pressures and may cause isolated LA collapse.

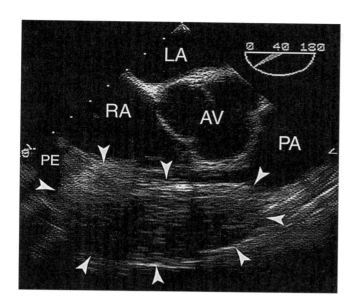

FIG. 11-7 Transesophageal echocardiogram of a patient with localized cardiac tamponade shortly after cardiac surgery. A large clot (*arrowheads*) in the anterior pericardial space has produced localized compression of the right ventricle between the right atrium (*RA*) and the main pulmonary artery (*PA*). A small amount of pericardial fluid (*PE*) is visible, but no collapse or compression of the right atrium or left atrium (*LA*) is seen. Dots along the edge of the image are separated by 1 cm. *AV*, Aortic valve.

Related Pathology. Patients who come to the operating room with blood in the pericardial cavity from trauma-related injuries are at risk for other potentially life-threatening injuries, including cervical spine instability, pneumothorax, and head injury. Acute aortic dissections and ruptured ascending aortic aneurysms may extend proximally to involve the aortic valve (AV) or the coronary arteries, causing acute aortic insufficiency or myocardial ischemia, respectively. Suspicion of lung carcinoma or other malignancy, uremia, or infection must be present for all patients who have large pericardial effusions. For patients who develop cardiac tamponade from mediastinal bleeding following cardiac surgery, medical coagulopathy may be present as well as surgical bleeding.

Differential Diagnosis. Any disease state in which signs and symptoms of acute or chronic right heart failure occur can mimic the presentation of cardiac tamponade. These states include RV dysfunction from ischemia, infarction, massive pulmonary embolism, severe chronic obstructive pulmonary disease, or pulmonary hypertension. Other disease entities that may have similar presentations include effusive constrictive pericardi-

BOX 11-2
Clinical Manifestations of Cardiac Tamponade

Symptoms
  Shortness of breath, orthopnea, anxiety, agitation
Signs
  Tachycardia, hypotension, jugular venous distention, decreased heart sounds, pulsus paradoxus, pulsus alternans

tis, superior vena cava syndrome, tension pneumopericardium, and restrictive cardiomyopathy. Patient history and diagnostic evaluation by laboratory studies, electrocardiogram (ECG), chest radiograph, and echocardiography supplement the physical findings to aid in diagnosis.

Clinical Manifestations. As mentioned earlier, the physiologic consequences of a pericardial effusion depend on the rapidity of its accumulation. The clinical manifestations of cardiac tamponade are caused by compression of the cardiac chambers impeding blood entry into both the right and left heart, causing venous pooling in both the systemic and pulmonary circulations (Box 11-2). Jugular venous distention and pulmonary venous congestion result in distended neck veins and shortness of breath, even in the sitting position. Decreased preload into the LV results in diminished stroke volume and profound systemic hypotension with compromised end organ perfusion, causing agitation or restlessness, myocardial ischemia, cool extremities, and decreased urine output. Large effusions may mask heart sounds, though a pericardial friction rub may be present. Patients with chronic pericardial effusions have more time to develop these clinical manifestations, and physical findings may resemble those of right heart failure, including hepatomegaly and ascites. Conditions causing acute hemorrhage into the pericardial space are more likely to cause the classical findings of Beck's triad, as described by Dr. Claude S. Beck in 1935: (1) decreased systemic arterial pressure, (2) elevation of systemic venous pressure, and (3) a small, quiet heart.[11] The hallmark of cardiac tamponade is an inspiratory decline in systolic blood pressure of greater than 10 mm Hg or pulsus paradoxus, though this finding is neither completely sensitive nor specific. Patients with regional tamponade, LV dysfunction, atrial septal defect, or aortic insufficiency, or those on positive pressure ventilation may not demonstrate a pulsus paradoxus.[12] In addition, other conditions that may cause a pulsus paradoxus in the absence of cardiac tamponade include chronic obstructive pulmonary disease and severe hypovolemia. Tachycardia and *pulsus alternans* are additional possible hemodynamic manifestations of cardiac tamponade. Pulsus alternans is a change in the blood pressure as felt by the pulse as a consequence of the heart changing its axis with every beat while it swings like a pendulum in the large effusion (Fig. 11-8). The change in axis essentially changes the loading conditions of the heart and is responsible for the change in blood pressure. On the ECG it is seen as *electrical alternans* as the heart changes axis from beat to beat.

Electrocardiogram. Large pericardial effusions isolate the heart from the chest wall, reducing the amplitude of the QRS complexes, which is interpreted as low voltage on the ECG. Findings suggestive of pericardial inflammation may be present, including elevation of ST- and T-wave segments, usually in all leads. Electrical alternans on the ECG in a patient with known pericardial effusion is suggestive of cardiac tamponade; however, it can be present following a myocardial infarction and in other conditions, including tension pneumothorax and constrictive pericarditis.[13]

Chest Radiograph. There is no specific chest radiograph that is diagnostic for this condition. Larger effusions may enlarge the cardiac silhouette, whereas the heart may appear normal in size with smaller effusions. Patients with aortic dissections or ruptured ascending aneurysms may present with a widened mediastinum on chest radiograph, and those with pneumopericardium may have a layer of air surrounding the cardiac silhouette, extending to the aorta.

Echocardiography. The diagnosis of cardiac tamponade is made on the basis of physiology; echocardiography is therefore the diagnostic tool of choice because it provides physiologic as well as anatomic information.[12] Echocardiographic signs of cardiac tamponade include pericardial effusion, systolic collapse on the right atrium, diastolic collapse of the right ventricle,

increased respiratory variation of peak ventricular inflow velocities, and paradoxical motion of the ventricular septum during diastole (Box 11-3). With acute hemopericardium, especially immediately after cardiac surgery, there may be localized compression by clot of a cardiac chamber. The mere presence of a pericardial effusion without other clinical and echocardiographic signs does not confirm the diagnosis of tamponade. On the other hand, the absence of any of the other signs does not exclude the possibility of cardiac tamponade. Suggestive clinical and echocardiographic evidence can be present in a patient without a large effusion, but with one sufficient to produce compression.[14]

Anesthetic Management

Preoperative Optimization. Forward flow through the heart depends on four variables: preload, afterload, heart rate, and contractility. Because the underlying problem with cardiac tamponade is a deficiency in preload, despite the presence of neck vein distention and shortness of breath, establishment of large-bore intravenous access and subsequent fluid administration is vital. In normal physiology, slowing the heart rate augments diastolic filling. With tamponade physiology, however, anatomic compression of the cardiac chambers limits filling so that increasing diastolic filling time does not increase stroke volume. Thus, the major determinant of cardiac output becomes the heart rate. Any medications that slow the heart rate would be detrimental in this situation. Forward flow is optimized by both volume resuscitation and sympathomimetics that increase heart rate and contractility, such as epinephrine.

Monitoring. Patients coming to the operating room for removal of a pericardial effusion may be at different points on the continuum of physiologic compromise. All patients can potentially worsen after the induction of general anesthesia and initiation of positive pressure ventilation. For this reason and for diagnostic purposes, invasive monitoring by systemic arterial and PA catheters is warranted before induction, in addition to standard monitors. It may be difficult to obtain central ve-

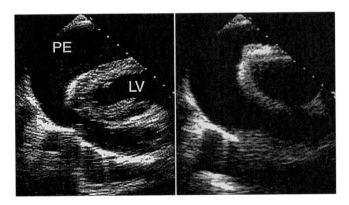

FIG. 11-8 Transesophageal echocardiogram of a patient with a large pericardial effusion (*PE*) showing large shifts in the position of the left ventricle (*LV*) at different stages of the cardiac cycle. Such changes can produce pulsus alternans and/or electrical alternans. The echo transducer is located in the stomach so that the diaphragm is located at the vertex (*top*) of the image. Dots along the edge of the image are separated by 1 cm.

BOX 11-3
Echocardiographic Signs of Cardiac Tamponade

Pericardial effusion
Systolic collapse of right atrium
Diastolic collapse of right ventricle
Increased respiratory variation of peak ventricular inflow velocities
Paradoxical motion of ventricular septum in diastole
Localized compression of cardiac chamber

nous access in an awake patient with severe shortness of breath when supine. In these cases, the anesthesiologist must be aware of possible hemodynamic compromise and secure large-bore intravenous access for resuscitation fluids and medications before induction. Pulsus paradoxus may be evident on the systemic arterial waveform while the patient is spontaneously ventilating.

Induction. Important considerations for the anesthesiologist include the effects of sedatives, general anesthetics, and positive pressure ventilation on preload, afterload, heart rate, and contractility. As mentioned previously, patients with cardiac tamponade benefit from sympathomimetics. Induction agents such as thiopental have opposite effects, causing sympatholysis. The loss of sympathetic tone results in vasodilation, including venodilation, decreased heart rate, and mild myocardial depression. Venous return is decreased by positive pressure ventilation. For these reasons, induction of general anesthesia may be accompanied by severe hypotension and subsequent hemodynamic decompensation. Induction agents that preserve sympathetic tone (etomidate) or have sympathomimetic effects (ketamine) are preferred. The surgical team should be prepared to intervene immediately after induction to relieve the tamponade in the event of hemodynamic decompensation. This includes prepping and draping the patient before induction. In extreme situations when a patient is not intubated and is too severely short of breath for the supine position, some pericardial fluid may be removed via a small pericardial window by using local anesthesia and sedation before the induction of anesthesia for the more definitive surgical procedure. Another option to consider is to temporarily decrease the tamponade by pericardiocentesis before induction of anesthesia. Many patients, especially trauma victims, come to surgery for pericardial tamponade as an emergency, but have full stomachs requiring rapid sequence induction, further complicating the anesthetic management. Awake fiberoptic intubation has been reported as another option to consider in managing these challenging cases.[15]

Cardiac Surgical Corrective Procedures

Invasive procedures for evacuation of pericardial fluid under pressure include percutaneous pericardiocentesis, subxiphoid pericardiotomy, and partial or extensive pericardiectomy. The choice of procedure will depend on the nature and severity of the pericardial effusion and the availability of personnel and equipment to perform them. Hemopericardium following acute trauma or cardiac surgical procedures requires definitive mediastinal exploration to evaluate the cause of bleeding and to evacuate fresh blood and hematoma. The operating room is the preferred environment for this procedure.

This therapy can, however, be initiated at the bedside if necessary. Surgical drainage is also preferred in the setting of posterior, loculated, or purulent effusions. Emergent drainage of a pericardial effusion can be performed at the bedside by needle aspiration with or without the use of echocardiography. Serous effusions are more amenable to this procedure.

Most pericardial effusions of clinical significance are detected during the preoperative evaluation. Patients may, however, come to the operating room for various surgical procedures with undiagnosed pericardial effusions or with effusions that were previously diagnosed as clinically insignificant. These patients may become hemodynamically unstable during the induction of general anesthesia or with vasodilation associated with regional anesthesia. Resuscitation efforts are directed at the restoration of cardiac output by the administration of intravenous fluids and sympathomimetics. A high index of suspicion for tamponade is necessary to make the diagnosis. Diagnoses other than cardiac tamponade need to be considered if the hemodynamics do not improve with removal of pericardial fluid.

CONSTRICTIVE PERICARDITIS
Definition/Pathophysiology

Constrictive pericarditis is an uncommon disease associated with pericardial inflammation that progresses to fibrosis or calcification. The heart becomes encased within a noncompliant, "constrictive" pericardial shell. The condition was first described over 300 years ago as *concretio cordis,* an appropriate term to describe the condition.[16] The inflammatory process is usually symmetrical but may be localized, resulting in scarring of the affected pericardium, obliteration of the pericardial space, and adherence of the fibrous pericardium to the epicardium. If symmetrically fibrotic, all cardiac chambers are equally affected. The pathophysiology of constrictive pericarditis includes impaired diastolic filling, exaggerated ventricular interdependence, and dissociation of intracardiac pressures from intrathoracic pressures during respiration.[17] Late diastolic filling is restricted, in contrast to tamponade physiology in which early diastolic filling is affected. Stroke volume becomes relatively fixed. As in tamponade physiology, cardiac output is maintained initially by an increase in adrenergic tone, resulting in increased heart rate, vasoconstriction, and contractility. The renin-angiotensin-aldosterone system becomes activated with retention of sodium and water supplementing preload to the right heart. Despite high atrial pressures, atrial natriuretic factor is not activated until after pericardiectomy because of the lack of atrial stretch.[18] Early diastolic filling is unimpeded and occurs abnormally rapidly until the ventricular volume reaches the capacity determined by the surrounding densely adherent pericardium. Eventually, the fibrous scarring can become so severe that compensatory mechanisms can no longer maintain cardiac output, epicardial arteries become obliterated in the dense scar tissue compromising myocardial perfusion, and myocardial systolic function can worsen from ischemia or atrophy.[19] This usually requires years to develop following the clinical or subclinical episode of acute pericarditis. Subacute noncalcific pericarditis takes less time to manifest and is characterized by a pericardial fibrin layer that is not rigid. Compression of the heart occurs under an elastic fibrin layer described as "rubber bands around the heart."[20] This form of effusive pericarditis resembles cardiac tamponade in that the compression occurs throughout the cardiac cycle. Early diastolic filling is impeded initially, with eventual restriction of filling throughout the cardiac cycle as the disease progresses.

Variations Induced by Respiration

The normal decrease of 10 mm Hg or less in systolic arterial pressure with negative inspiratory pressure occurs from (1) increased venous return to the right heart, causing leftward displacement of the ventricular septum, (2) increased capacitance of the pulmonary vascular bed, and (3) increased LV transmural pressure. This normal decrease of less than 10 mm Hg in systolic arterial pressure is maintained in pure constrictive pericarditis. The rigid pericardial shell completely isolates the heart from pressure changes occurring in the thorax, dissociating intracardiac pressure from intrathoracic pressure. There may be minimal or no increase in venous return to the right heart during inspiration. Because pulmonary venous capacitance vessels are intrathoracic and still dilate during inspiration, there is still decreased flow into the left atrium, decreasing pulmonary venous and mitral valve (MV) flow velocities. Kussmaul's sign is observed in chronic constrictive pericarditis, as a normal, small decrease in systolic arterial pressure associated with normal or elevated central venous pressure or during negative inspiratory pressure.[21] The opposite changes occur with expiration. The subacute form of pericarditis can manifest as pericardial tamponade with an exaggeration of right heart filling during inspiration and subsequent pulsus paradoxus, if the pericardium must be sufficiently compliant to allow transmission of intrathoracic pressure to intracardiac pressure.[22]

Pressure Waveforms

The pathophysiology of constrictive pericarditis produces characteristic findings on pressure waveforms. Early diastolic filling of the right and left ventricles, representing passive atrial emptying, occurs during the y descent on the central venous pressure and PA occlusion

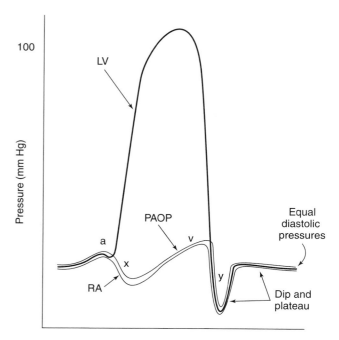

FIG. 11-9 Pressure waveforms with constrictive pericarditis. Pulmonary artery occlusion pressure (*PAOP*) and right atrial pressure (*RA*) are increased and equalized. There is a characteristic rapid fall of these pressures in early diastole followed by an abrupt increase, the "dip and plateau" sign. *LV*, Left ventricular pressure.

pressure waveforms, respectively. The steep y descent in constrictive pericarditis occurs because of abnormally rapid ventricular filling during this time. The rapid fall in atrial pressure represents the rapid movement of blood into the ventricles. Filling abruptly ceases as the limits of ventricular expansion are reached. The pressures associated with the noncompliant pericardium are reflected as a rise and plateau on the pressure waveforms. This produces the characteristic "dip and plateau" or "square root" waveform pattern (Fig. 11-9). As volume is ejected from the ventricle during systole, negative pressure within the pericardium is reflected as a sharp x descent of atrial relaxation. Other medical conditions such as the cardiomyopathies produce similar patterns and are characterized by restriction of filling.[23]

Diastolic Filling Patterns

Rapid early diastolic filling of both the right and left ventricles is reflected on Doppler interrogation of ventricular inflow velocities as a high early diastolic (E) velocity with a short deceleration time. The late diastolic (A) velocity is decreased because of the reduced ventricular inflow during atrial contraction (Fig. 11-10). There is characteristically a decrease in transmitral flow velocities during spontaneous inspiration in constrictive pericarditis because of vasodilation of the pulmonary bed. Maneuvers that decrease preload, such as squatting or

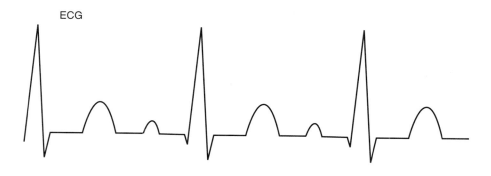

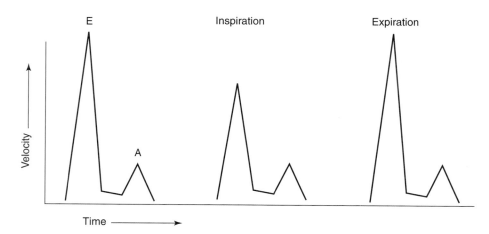

FIG. 11-10   Changes in left ventricular diastolic inflow velocity pattern with constrictive peri-carditis as measured with Doppler echocardiography. The early (*E*) filling wave is prominent and has a rapid deceleration compared with the atrial (*A*) filling wave as the pericardium limits ventricular expansion. The peak E-wave velocity decreases somewhat during spontaneous inspiration because of increased pulmonary venous capacitance. The electrocardiogram (*ECG*) is shown to demonstrate time in the cardiac cycle.

the reverse Trendelenburg position, exaggerate this pattern.[24] Table 11-1 compares constrictive pericarditis with cardiac tamponade.

Preoperative Evaluation

Common Causes. Chronic constrictive pericarditis develops following any inflammatory process involving the pericardium, though in most cases the cause is unknown. Inflammation may arise from medical conditions such as viral, tuberculous, fungal, or parasitic infections, connective tissue disorders such as rheumatoid arthritis and systemic lupus erythematosus, malignancy, mediastinal radiation, uremia, or following a myocardial infarction. Pericarditis may also occur after cardiac surgery or mediastinal trauma. Tuberculosis, historically a leading cause throughout the world, remains the lead-

ing cause in developing countries.[25] The three most common identifiable causes from a recent series of 135 patients undergoing pericardiectomy at the Mayo Clinic were cardiac surgery, inflammatory pericarditis, and mediastinal radiation.[26]

The development of constrictive pericarditis is usually gradual, often delayed for several years following the episode of acute pericarditis. It occurs rarely in a shorter time frame after a period of only weeks to months following traumatic pericardial injury. The average duration of symptoms before pericardiectomy ranges from 11.7 to 23.4 months.[26,27]

Clinical Manifestations. The most important clinical finding of constrictive pericarditis is an elevation of jugular venous pressure.[28] Peripheral edema, hepatic congestion, and ascites develop with chronicity and

TABLE 11-1
Comparison of Cardiac Tamponade with Constrictive Pericarditis

	TAMPONADE	CONSTRICTION
Right atrial pressure	Increased	Increased
Ventricular filling pressures	Right = left	Right = left
Diastolic pressure waveforms	Prominent x descent Absent y decent	"Dip and plateau" sign
Two-dimensional echo	Pericardial effusion	Pericardial thickening
Doppler echo	Decreased E wave Increased respiratory Variation of E wave	Rapid E-wave deceleration

mimic right heart failure. Pulmonary congestion develops from left heart pressure elevation and is manifested by dyspnea, orthopnea, and productive cough. Patients undergoing pericardiectomy commonly exhibit most of these symptoms of congestive heart failure.[21,26] Patients become severely debilitated with cardiac cachexia, muscle wasting, and chronic fatigue without surgical intervention.

Physical examination reveals neck vein distention with diastolic collapse during the steep y descent (Friedreich's sign). Increased neck vein distention during inspiration (Kussmaul's sign), is difficult to appreciate. A loud diastolic pericardial knock is auscultated along the left sternal border with chronic constrictive pericarditis and corresponds to the abrupt cessation of early ventricular filling. Hepatomegaly and liver dysfunction may be present, with physical findings of ascites, spider angiomas, and palmar erythema. Angina, pericardial friction rub, and pulsus paradoxus are uncommon manifestations in this disease.[29]

Preoperative Considerations. Constrictive pericarditis impedes cardiac output mainly by limiting preload. Of the other three variables responsible for cardiac output, afterload, heart rate, and contractility, only an increase in heart rate can effectively improve cardiac output. This pathophysiology was demonstrated in a series of patients atrially paced before and after pericardiectomy. The maximal cardiac output achieved preoperatively was during a heart rate of 140 beats/min, whereas postoperatively, stroke volume index doubled without augmentation of the heart rate.[30] As in tamponade

physiology, medications that cause bradycardia are detrimental.

Large-bore intravenous access is essential because of the potential for large blood loss. Available blood products should include cryoprecipitate, fresh frozen plasma, and platelets, in addition to packed red blood cells, particularly if preoperative liver dysfunction is present. Cardiac output is optimized by judicious volume administration and increasing the heart rate by medications or atrial pacing.

Related Pathology. Chronic passive hepatic congestion produces varying degrees of liver dysfunction and is primarily responsible for the medical problems associated with constrictive pericarditis. These include coagulopathy, hypoalbuminemia, elevated serum bilirubin, pleural effusions, and anemia. The underlying medical condition leading to constrictive pericarditis, either directly or indirectly through treatment, should be considered and includes malignancy, connective tissue disorder, renal failure, coronary artery disease, or infection.

Differential Diagnosis. Constrictive pericarditis does not present as an acute problem; thus patients arriving at the operating room for pericardiectomy are considered to be undergoing elective surgery. The disease is differentiated from restrictive cardiomyopathy by radiographic imaging such as computerized tomography and magnetic resonance imaging (MRI). The most sensitive imaging technique is MRI because of its ability to accurately detect the degree and extent of pericardial thickening and calcification. MRI also allows for the identification of other mediastinal structures that can potentially compress the pericardium and the cardiac structures.[31,32]

Electrocardiographic findings include low QRS voltage, inverted T waves, and large or biphasic P waves. Atrial fibrillation may also be present. Chest radiography identifies calcium in the pericardium, pleural effusions, and prominent right superior mediastinum from engorgement of the superior vena cava.[33] Echocardiography demonstrates pericardial thickening and constraint in both M-mode and two-dimensional (2D) imaging.

Anesthetic Management

Monitoring. The three most important considerations for anesthetic management of patients undergoing pericardiectomy for constriction are (1) the pathophysiology of the disease, which may not immediately improve with pericardial stripping, (2) the potential for massive blood loss, and (3) rapid hemodynamic changes associated with surgical manipulation of the heart. Standard American Society of Anesthesiologists (ASA) monitoring with ST segment analysis on the ECG facilitates detection of myocardial ischemia. Invasive monitoring with arterial and PA catheters allows for continuous recognition of hemodynamic changes, cardiac output measurements, and mixed venous oxygen saturation determinations. Transesophageal echocardiography (TEE) provides real-time imaging of loading conditions, regional wall-motion abnormalities, and biventricular function, and is thus a valuable diagnostic tool in the hemodynamic assessment of patients undergoing pericardiectomy.

Induction. Patients undergoing pericardiectomy exhibit varying degrees of congestive heart failure. The principles of hemodynamic optimization previously described for cardiac tamponade pertain to the induction and maintenance of general anesthesia for patients with constrictive pericarditis. The cardiovascular depressant effects of induction agents and volatile anesthetics may require treatment with sympathomimetics such as epinephrine. Avoidance of bradycardia through medication or electrical pacing is paramount. The effect of positive pressure ventilation on hemodynamics is minimal because of the dissociation of intracardiac pressure from intrathoracic pressure. One-lung ventilation is required if an anterolateral thoracotomy is the chosen surgical approach.

Surgical Corrective Procedure

Radical pericardiectomy is the definitive treatment for constrictive pericarditis and involves the surgical removal of pericardium anteriorly between the two phrenic nerves, great vessels superiorly and the diaphragm inferiorly. Posteriorly, the pericardium is removed from the ventricular surfaces and, if possible, from the atria and the venae cavae.[26,34] This wide excision establishes a surgical plane between the epicardium and pericardium. Careful, tedious stripping of the pericardium is a surgical challenge, particularly in the setting of previous mediastinal irradiation. The surgical approach is through a median sternotomy or left anterolateral thoracotomy, and performed with or without the use of cardiopulmonary bypass (CPB). Adequate preparation necessitates the availability of emergent institution of CPB, should the patient become hemodynamically unstable, such as from the unintentional entry into a cardiac chamber. Preoperative femoral artery cannulation saves valuable time if access becomes necessary for emergent initiation of CPB or intraaortic balloon pump counterpulsation. Active intraoperative communication is essential during acute hemodynamic changes with cardiac manipulation, as ventricular filling is impaired and atrial or ventricular arrhythmias become malignant. Inotropic and antiarrhythmic medications, blood products, and perfusion services for cell saver and CPB should be readily available throughout the surgery. Following the procedure, patients are transferred to an intensive care unit setting for close observa-

tion of mediastinal drainage and hemodynamics before extubation.

Constrictive pericarditis may coexist with other causes of ventricular dysfunction such as active myocarditis or postradiation cardiomyopathy. These patients may not demonstrate significant improvement in diastolic filling immediately following pericardiectomy.[33] Echocardiographic exams performed greater than 3 months postoperatively in a series of 35 patients revealed similar ejection fractions to the preoperative period but with increased LV end-diastolic diameter, and diastolic filling patterns ranging from normal in 57% of patients, to restrictive in 34% of patients, to constrictive in 9% of patients.[35] Despite the complexity of both the procedure and the disease, in-hospital mortality ranges from 0% to 10% in modern series. Long-term survival is high, and functional status improves significantly in most patients.

SYSTOLIC ANTERIOR MOTION OF THE MITRAL VALVE

Systolic anterior motion (SAM) of the MV is an uncommon but important pathophysiologic phenomenon with significant implications for anesthesiologists. Sir Russell Brock, a pioneer cardiac surgeon, noticed this clinical entity in the 1950s when he encountered several patients with the symptoms and signs of valvular aortic stenosis (AS) but who were found to have normal AVs at surgery.[36] He noticed an abnormally thick ventricular septum in these patients and hypothesized that they had "functional" aortic subvalvular stenosis similar to that of the pulmonary outflow obstruction caused by the muscular RV outflow tract of tetralogy of Fallot. This condition has come to be known as *hypertrophic obstructive cardiomyopathy* (HOCM) and is the most common cause of mitral SAM.[37] Angiographic data in the 1960s suggested that abnormal motion of the MV, rather than simple narrowing of the left ventricular outflow tract (LVOT) with hypertrophied myocardium, caused the LV outflow obstruction along with the mitral regurgitation (MR) associated with HOCM.[38] Abnormal SAM with ventricular septal contact of the MV was demonstrated in 1969 by echocardiography in patients with HOCM.[39] By 1973, quantification of the gradient across the LVOT by echocardiography was reported, thus providing a safe and simple means of evaluating these patients.[40]

No single, simple explanation has been proposed that adequately accounts for the pathophysiology encountered with mitral SAM. Early theories included the Venturi mechanism, which theorizes that the anterior leaflet of the MV is pulled anteriorly to the septum because of elevated systolic flow velocity resulting from narrowing of the LVOT or hyperdynamic contractility of the base of the ventricular septum. The high-flow velocity on the LVOT side of the MV would lower the pressure by the Bernoulli effect and displace the leaflet toward the septum. This does not explain, however, why some patients with HOCM, a narrow LVOT, and elevated flow velocity do not develop mitral SAM, or why others without hypertrophic cardiomyopathy do. Also, studies in which the flow velocity in the LVOT is carefully measured have shown that the MV begins its motion anteriorly *before* the velocity in the LVOT increases.[41] More recently, a mechanism involving abnormal positioning of the papillary muscles has been proposed and supported with animal models of the disease.[42] This theory states that abnormal displacement of the papillary muscles anteriorly and toward the center of the LV with redundancy of the chordae tendineae may initiate the anterior motion of the MV, which is then drawn further toward the septum by the Venturi mechanism (Fig. 11-11). Echocardiographic studies of patients with HOCM have found abnormally

long MV leaflets compared with those of normal patients.[43] It is important to remember that, although mitral SAM is most commonly associated with hypertrophic cardiomyopathy, asymmetrical hypertrophy of the ventricular septum is not a necessary or sufficient prerequisite for this pathophysiology to develop.

There are two adverse hemodynamic consequences of mitral SAM: (1) LVOT obstruction producing functional AS, and (2) MR, both of which are a result of the abnormal motion of the MV (Box 11-4). The dynamic LVOT obstruction caused by mitral SAM is due to the narrowing of the LVOT by the abnormal motion and position of the MV leaflets. This motion also tends to pull the anterior leaflet from the posterior, producing MR, which typically is directed posteriorly in the opposite direction of the leaflet displacement. Secondary hemodynamic consequences of the LVOT outflow obstruction and MR are elevated LA pressures, pulmonary vascular congestion, and low cardiac output. The LVOT obstruction may be severe, producing gradients across the LVOT over 100 mm Hg. The other important characteristic of the LVOT obstruction and MR produced by SAM is their dynamic nature, literally varying on a beat-to-beat basis.[44] Hemodynamic changes that tend to decrease the size of the LV tend to worsen mitral SAM and its consequences (Box 11-5). On the other hand, changes that

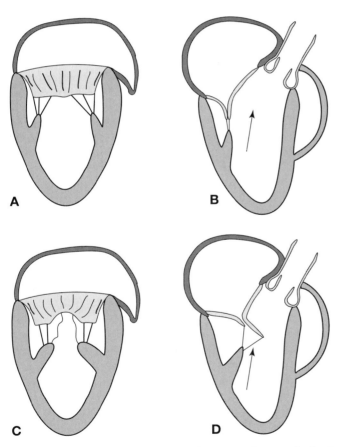

FIG. 11-11 Papillary muscle displacement theory of mitral systolic anterior motion. **A** and **B,** Normal papillary muscle position and support of the mitral valve. **C,** Convergent displacement of the papillary muscles causes laxness of support for the central portion of the mitral valve. **D,** Anterior displacement of the papillary muscle places the mitral valve in the path of outflow from the left ventricle.

(From Cape EG, Simons D, Jimoh A et al: *J Am Coll Cardiol* 13: 1438-1448, 1989.)

BOX 11-4
Consequences of Mitral Systolic Anterior Motion

Primary consequences
    Dynamic LVOT obstruction: functional aortic stenosis
    Dynamic mitral regurgitation
Secondary consequences
    Increased LAP, pulmonary vascular congestion
    Low cardiac output
    Systemic hypotension

LAP, Left atrial pressure; *LVOT,* left ventricular outflow tract.

BOX 11-5
Factors Aggravating Mitral Systolic Anterior Motion

Decreased LV end-diastolic volume resulting from any of the following:
    Hypovolemia
    Decreased systemic vascular resistance
    Increased myocardial contractility
    Tachycardia

LV, Left ventricular.

increase the size of the LV decrease SAM and the LVOT obstruction and MR that it causes. Mitral SAM can cause sudden and dramatic swings in hemodynamics. Thus, a patient with the propensity for SAM may not develop significant outflow obstruction or MR until reaching a certain degree of hypovolemia. For example, mitral SAM may suddenly begin after induction of anesthesia and result in rapid deterioration in blood pressure with elevation of left-sided filling pressures. Conversely, this patient's hemodynamics will suddenly and dramatically improve after appropriate treatment aimed at increasing the size of the LV to the point where the septal-leaflet contact ceases.

Preoperative Evaluation

Mitral SAM is most commonly associated with HOCM, but patients with significant outflow obstruction represent only a small subset of all patients with hypertrophic cardiomyopathy. Symptoms of this condition are often vague and nonspecific, including transient episodes of lightheadedness, near syncope and syncope, chest pain, fatigue, and shortness of breath (Box 11-6). There is poor correlation between the extent of hypertrophy and severity of symptoms. HOCM produces three characteristic findings on physical examination: (1) a harsh systolic murmur heard best along the left sternal border and apex, often radiating to the axilla if MR is present, (2) an abrupt arterial pulse that falls off rapidly in midsystole (pulsus bisferiens), and (3) an initially powerful apical impulse that may be bifid as well. Provocative interventions that decrease the size of the LV, such as the Valsalva maneuver or inhalation of amyl nitrate, will increase the obstruction and gradient and make the murmur louder. The ECG shows changes consistent with LV hypertrophy in virtually all patients. Because the hypertrophy is usually concentric in HOCM, the cardiac

silhouette in standard chest roentgenograms is often normal. If present, signs of pulmonary vascular congestion are not specific for HOCM.

Echocardiography is the best way to diagnose HOCM and can be used to assess its severity as well as the response to treatment.[45] Two-dimensional images of the LV reveal abnormally thick walls, usually worse in the septum. Evidence of diastolic dysfunction of the hypertrophied myocardium can be obtained by examining the pulmonary venous and transmitral inflow velocity profiles with pulsed-wave Doppler. Real-time 2D imaging clearly shows SAM and septal contact of the MV (Fig. 11-12), and color flow Doppler (CFD) shows MR and high-velocity, turbulent flow in the LVOT during systole (Fig. 11-13). M-mode tracings of the AV show midsystolic closure of the leaflets. Finally, spectral Doppler measurements of the blood velocity of the LV outflow show a characteristic late peak during systole and allow calculation of the peak gradient and localization of the point of outflow obstruction of the LVOT (Box 11-7). Provocative maneuvers such as the Valsalva maneuver or inhalation of amyl nitrate may be used to increase the obstruction and the gradient and demonstrate their dynamic nature.

There are a number of conditions other than HOCM in which mitral SAM has been reported (Box 11-8). In 1976, Bulkley and Fortuin[46] documented mitral SAM by echocardiography in a septic patient with a variable

---

BOX 11-6
Clinical Aspects of Hypertropic Obstructive Cardiomyopathy

Symptoms
  Episodic lightheadedness
  Syncope and near syncope
  Fatigue
  Shortness of breath
  Chest pain
Signs
  Systolic ejection murmur along left sternal border
  Apical murmur of mitral regurgitation
  Pulsus biciferens
  Powerful apical impulse
Symptoms and signs dynamic and increased by Valsalva maneuver or inhalation of amyl nitrate

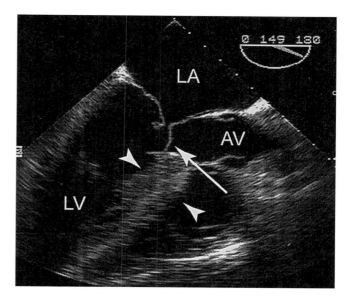

FIG. 11-12 Transesophageal echocardiogram of a patient with hypertrophic obstructive cardiomyopathy. This midesophageal long-axis view made during systole shows mitral systolic anterior motion with the anterior mitral leaflet (*arrow*) in contact with the ventricular septum, obstructing the left ventricular outflow tract. The gap between the leaflets is also visible. The ventricular septum is abnormally thick (*arrowheads*). *AV*, Aortic valve; *LA*, left atrium; *LV*, left ventricle.

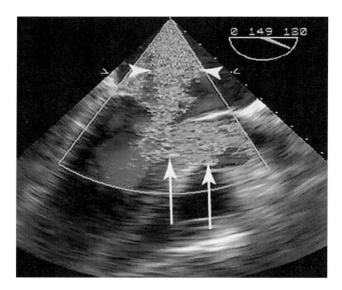

FIG. 11-13 Transesophageal echocardiogram with color flow Doppler of the same patient and image orientation as in Fig. 11-12. The image shows high-velocity, turbulent flow in the left ventricular outflow tract (*arrows*) and severe mitral regurgitation (*arrowheads*).

BOX 11-8
Conditions Associated with Mitral Systolic Anterior Motion

Most common associations
   Hypertrophic obstructive cardiomyopathy
   Mitral valve repair surgery
Rare, reported associations
   Aortic valve replacement surgery
   Acute myocardial infarction
   Mitral annular calcification
   Mitral valve prolapse
   Anemia
   Cardiac surgery after cardiopulmonary bypass

BOX 11-7
Echocardiographic Signs of HOCM

Two-dimensional echocardiography
   Hypertrophy of the LV, usually asymmetrical
   Mitral SAM
Color flow Doppler
   Dynamic mitral regurgitation
   High-velocity, turbulent LV outflow
Spectral Doppler
   High-velocity flow in LVOT with late peak
   Peak velocity localized to LVOT
M-mode echocardiography
   Midsystolic closure of aortic valve leaflets

_____
HOCM, Hypertropic obstructive cardiomyopathy; *LV*, left ventricle; *LVOT*, left ventricular outflow tract; *SAM*, systolic anterior motion.

---

systolic murmur who was shown to have a structurally normal heart at autopsy. Since then, SAM of the MV has been reported in a number of situations other than HOCM, including anemia,[47] MV repair surgery,[48] AV replacement surgery,[49] acute myocardial infarction,[50] mitral annular calcification,[51] and MV prolapse.[52] More recently, Krenz et al[53] documented with epicardial echocardiography acute LVOT obstruction secondary to mitral SAM during cardiac surgery in four patients without HOCM.

Perhaps the most common and best-recognized cause of mitral SAM other than HOCM is MV repair surgery. Mitral SAM has been reported to be responsible for many of the immediate failures of MV repairs.[54] This causes both LVOT outflow obstruction and MR. It is usually associated with repair of a myxomatous MV with redundant leaflets in which a large segment of the posterior leaflet has been resected, necessitating a large decrease in the size of the MV annulus. Careful measurements of the MV in these patients has shown that mitral SAM is likely to occur when the point of coaptation of the anterior and posterior leaflets is displaced too far toward the base of the leaflet as a result of reduction in annular size.[55] The extra leaflet tissue distal to the point of coaptation is prone to anterior displacement, leading to significant mitral SAM (Fig. 11-14). A surgical technique called the *sliding leaflet repair* has been developed as an attempt to avoid mitral SAM.[56] It permits resection of a large portion of the posterior MV leaflet with less reduction in the size of the annulus. Another important point to remember is that mitral SAM is most likely to occur with a hyperdynamic, relatively empty LV, conditions often present immediately after CPB. Immediately after CPB for mitral repair, many patients with mitral SAM improve with appropriate medical management in the operating room, such as increasing intravascular volume, avoidance of vasodilators and inotropic drugs, and administration of pure α agonists such as phenylephrine. Patients with persistent, severe mitral SAM, or who require unreasonable doses of vasoactive medications to reduce SAM, may require reinstitution of CPB for revision of the repair or prosthetic valve replacement.

Mitral SAM may be easily confused with other conditions causing hypotension, low cardiac output, and elevated left-heart filling pressures (Box 11-9). As mentioned earlier, Brock's experience with this entity was due to his confusion of HOCM with valvular AS. Both can produce similar symptoms and findings with cardiac catheterization, that is, a pressure gradient between the LV and the aorta. The gradient with HOCM, however, is usually very dynamic and variable, depending on the volume status of the cardiovascular system and

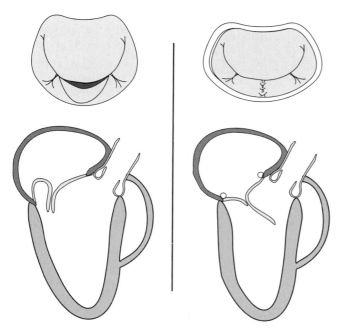

FIG. 11-14   Mitral systolic anterior motion (SAM) after mitral valve repair. Prolapse of the middle scallop of the posterior leaflet of the mitral valve is illustrated on the left. The result of a quadrangular resection and ring annuloplasty is shown on the right. There is reduction in the size of the annulus with displacement of the point of leaflet coaptation toward the base of the anterior mitral leaflet, resulting in SAM.

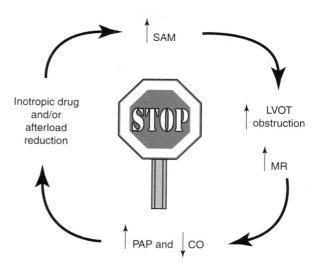

FIG. 11-15   The vicious cycle caused by inappropriate treatment of mitral systolic anterior motion (*SAM*) on the basis of a misdiagnosis of myocardial failure from pulmonary artery catheter data. Mitral SAM should be suspected when such patients worsen with inotropic or afterload reduction therapy. The diagnosis can be easily made with echocardiography. *CO*, Cardiac output; *LVOT*, left ventricular outflow tract; *MR*, mitral regurgitation; *PAP*, pulmonary artery pressure.

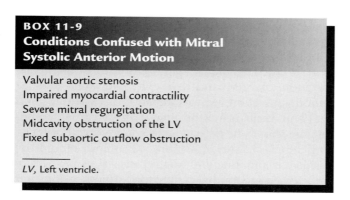

BOX 11-9
Conditions Confused with Mitral Systolic Anterior Motion

Valvular aortic stenosis
Impaired myocardial contractility
Severe mitral regurgitation
Midcavity obstruction of the LV
Fixed subaortic outflow obstruction

LV, Left ventricle.

the systemic vascular resistance. Valvular AS produces a more stable, fixed gradient. HOCM and valvular AS are easily distinguished, however, with echocardiography, which directly visualizes the abnormal mitral motion in HOCM and the thickened immobile leaflets in AS.

The hemodynamic picture caused by mitral SAM, high left-heart filling pressures and low cardiac output, may be confused with impaired myocardial contractility when one is considering the hemodynamic parameters alone. This may lead to afterload reduction or positive inotropic therapy, both of which will aggravate SAM and its hemodynamic consequences. This may lead to a downward spiral wherein as the patient's hemodynamics worsen, treatment is increased, further worsening

SAM and its adverse effects, prompting even further increase of inappropriate treatment (Fig. 11-15). One should consider the possibility of mitral SAM in patients with apparent impairment of myocardial contractility as assessed by hemodynamic data if the response to therapy is unexpected or inappropriate.

Another important differential diagnosis in the patient with high PA pressure and low cardiac output is severe MR not due to mitral SAM. Patients with ischemic heart disease or dilated LV can develop dynamic, central MR resulting from distortion of the normal geometry of the MV resulting from enlargement of the LV.[57] Significant MR can also be due to structural abnormalities of the valve as with myxomatous degeneration, rheumatic disease, or endocarditis. Distinction of these more common forms of MR from that resulting from mitral SAM is important because the treatments are diametrically opposed: interventions typically used to treat MR, afterload reduction, inotropic therapy, and intraaortic ballooncounterpulsation will aggravate rather than improve the hemodynamics with mitral SAM. The distinction between these entities is most easily made with echocardiography, which provides accurate information about the severity and mechanism of MR, allowing appropriate therapeutic interventions and assessment of the response.

Another condition that may be confused with mitral SAM is midcavity obstruction of the LV.[58] In this variant of hypertrophic cardiomyopathy, complete obliteration of the LV cavity at its midlevel during systole causes obstruction to outflow from the LV to the aorta. The clinical picture may be similar to HOCM with SAM, but the distinction between the two can usually be made by careful echocardiographic examination, which can detect the presence or absence of mitral SAM and localize the level of obstruction to LV outflow. Medical management of the two entities is similar, with the obstruction of both improving with volume administration, α agonists, and negative inotropic drugs. It is important to distinguish midcavity obstruction from mitral SAM, however, in patients with persistent significant symptoms despite optimal medical management because the former condition is not amenable to surgery while the latter is. Also, some patients with a presumed diagnosis of HOCM and isolated dynamic LVOT obstruction have been found to have a fixed subaortic outflow obstruction not due to mitral SAM.[59] Careful 2D and Doppler echocardiography is the best way to distinguish these patients from those with true HOCM.

Treatment

Most patients with HOCM gain significant relief with medical management. β-Adrenergic antagonists and calcium channel blockers are effective in decreasing symptoms and increasing exercise tolerance in HOCM as well as in decreasing LVOT gradients. Dual-chamber pacing improves symptoms and diminishes LVOT obstruction in some HOCM patients. The improvement is probably from asynchronous contraction of the LV with paradoxical motion of the septum enlarging the LVOT.[60] Surgery is indicated for a small group of patients with HOCM that remain significantly symptomatic despite these therapies.[61]

Surgery for HOCM was first performed in 1958, and most commonly consists of resection of a portion of the hypertrophied ventricular septum through the AV in a procedure referred to as *septal myectomy*.[62] This results in widening of the LVOT with decrease in mitral SAM, LVOT obstruction, and MR. MV replacement, the other surgical approach to this disease, is considered less desirable than myectomy because of the risks of prosthetic valve thromboembolism and long-term anticoagulation, but is used for specific indications, which are discussed in the following section. Hospital mortality for septal myectomy is about 5%, with good, persistent symptomatic relief reported by most patients.[63,64] Improved long-term survival over medical management has not been clearly demonstrated. Surgery is reserved for patients with significantly impaired symptoms in whom an LVOT gradient of 50 mm Hg or more has been documented despite optimal medical therapy. A more

recent catheter-based treatment for HOCM, involving injection of ethanol through the first septal perforator artery to ablate the proximal portion of the ventricular septum, is being applied with success in some centers.[65]

Anesthetic Considerations for Hypertrophic Obstructive Cardiomyopathy Surgery

Providing anesthesia for a patient undergoing surgical repair for HOCM can be challenging and requires some significant variations from the care provided for more "routine" cardiac surgery, such as coronary artery bypass graft surgery. HOCM is uncommon and these procedures are performed infrequently even at busy referral centers. Patients are susceptible to subendocardial ischemia because of hypertrophy, and should be monitored with at least one precordial ECG lead. Invasive monitoring devices should include an indwelling arterial cannula to monitor blood pressure continuously. A pulmonary artery catheter (PAC) should be inserted even with good systolic ventricular function because diastolic dysfunction is usually present with significantly elevated left-heart filling pressures as a result of the hypertrophic cardiomyopathy. A PAC provides monitoring of these pressures and the ability to measure cardiac output. This important measure of cardiac performance is critical postoperatively. The ability to sample mixed venous blood with a PAC is useful for evaluating the presence or degree of an interventricular shunt should a ventricular septal defect (VSD) occur during the septal myectomy.

Induction of anesthesia of a patient with HOCM must proceed gradually and cautiously to avoid aggravation of SAM and severe hypotension. Keys to smooth induction are maintenance of LV filling (and size) and avoidance of positive inotropic drugs. Hypovolemia should be detected and corrected with intravenous fluid before induction. Ketamine should be avoided as an induction drug because of its propensity to increased myocardial contractility. Hypotension after induction should be treated by placing the patient in Trendelenburg position and using volume infusion to increase venous return to the heart. Pure α-agonist agents such as phenylephrine should be used to treat more severe hypotension. If a patient develops tachycardia, β-antagonist drugs such as esmolol should be given. Adequate depth of anesthesia should be assured before intubation and incision to avoid tachycardia from sympathetic nervous system stimulation.

Drugs that produce myocardial depression with minimal vasodilation are preferred for maintenance of anesthesia. Halothane has been advocated because its predominant hemodynamic effect is negative inotropy with less vasodilation and tachycardia than isoflurane.[66] Blood loss is treated aggressively because hypovolemia can cause sudden, severe hypotension in patients with HOCM as mitral SAM suddenly worsens. Such hypotension, on the other hand, can suddenly improve when the volume is replaced and the end-diastolic volume of the LV reaches a size at which the SAM improves.

Intraoperative Echocardiography during Hypertrophic Obstructive Cardiomyopathy Surgery

Intraoperative echocardiography (IOE) has become an almost indispensable part of surgery for HOCM, providing crucial anatomic information to the surgeon as to the size and location of the myectomy. The results of the procedure, assessed immediately after CPB, indicate whether there is a need for further corrective surgery. IOE can also detect complications such as VSD and aortic regurgitation, permitting timely surgical intervention when indicated.[44,67] The first step in the prebypass assessment of a patient undergoing HOCM surgery is to measure the thickness of the septum in the region of the planned myectomy. Most patients have a relatively thin septum close to the AV that increases in thickness toward the apex. Measurements should be made at end diastole, most easily defined as the onset of the QRS complex. Occasionally, the surgeon may choose to replace the MV rather than perform a myectomy if the septum is not particularly thick, usually less than 1.8 cm. Next, the presence and severity of mitral SAM should be assessed. Most patients needing surgery will have septal contact; that is, the MV leaflets will move anteriorly across the LVOT in systole and touch the septum. The distance of the point of septal contact from the AV should be measured to ensure that the myectomy will extend beyond that point. The clinician should carefully examine the MV in multiple imaging planes, looking for additional pathologic conditions such as prolapse, ruptured chordae tendineae, and flail segments that may necessitate valve repair or replacement. HOCM patients have abnormally long mitral leaflets with the point of coaptation of the anterior and posterior leaflets occurring more proximally than that of normal patients.[44] CFD should next be used to assess the severity and direction of MR. Most patients with MR resulting from HOCM have a posterolaterally directed jet because the SAM pulls the anterior leaflet away from the posterior leaflet. Another echo finding of HOCM is fluttering of the AV leaflets during systole because of the turbulent ejection through the LVOT. This tends to be most prominent on the right and left coronary cusps and is best demonstrated with the increased temporal resolution of M-mode echocardiography. Finally, the gradient across the LVOT should be measured by using continuous-wave Doppler (CWD) with the transgastric long-axis view. This gradient is quite dynamic and should be assessed multiple times as the hemodynamics vary.

Doppler echo will underestimate the gradient unless the ultrasound beam is parallel to the flow being measured. The velocity profile of LV outflow in HOCM has a characteristic appearance with a more gradual initial upstroke and later peak than normal and has been described as a "dagger-like" appearance. Pulsed-wave Doppler is helpful in locating the exact location of the obstruction, which is usually at the point of contact of the MV with the septum, but can also occur at the midventricular level or at the AV.

After bypass for HOCM surgery, IOE truly becomes indispensable by providing the most effective and expeditious means of assessing the adequacy of the myectomy and the presence or absence of complications. The size and the location and extent of the myectomy should be evaluated with 2D echo in multiple imaging planes and transducer positions. The width and depth of the myectomy is often best seen in the transgastric short-axis view obtained at the level of the MV. Keep in mind that the myectomy often results in a narrow trench only a centimeter or so wide and will not be apparent in many of the views. Careful examination with CFD of the right ventricle adjacent to the myectomy should be performed to check for high-velocity flow from the LV to RV, indicating a VSD. Next, attention should be turned to the MV and the effect that the myectomy has had on SAM. Ideally, there will be no residual SAM, but some residual SAM is usually present, especially early after CPB if the LV is underfilled and hyperdynamic. In general, though, the SAM should not be severe enough to cause septal contact of the MV. SAM after septal myectomy can be improved in many cases by proper hemodynamic management, such as volume administration, β-antagonist drugs, and α-agonist drugs. What may initially appear to be an inadequate result may become acceptable with appropriate therapy. The next major issue to be addressed with echo is the amount of residual MR present, which is evaluated with CFD after a careful 2D exam of the mitral anatomy. This is usually mild (1+) or less, but should be no more than moderate (2+). As with SAM, MR may be quite variable, depending on the hemodynamic conditions. MR is usually directly related to the amount of residual SAM present and may improve significantly with appropriate treatment. Other causes of MR, such as ruptured chordae and flail leaflet, may indicate the need for valve replacement. The AV should be carefully examined with 2D echo and aortic regurgitation assessed with CFD because surgical access to the septum is through the AV and this may be damaged by retraction.[68] Finally, the gradient across the LVOT should be measured again with CWD. Again, no residual gradient is ideal, but some residual gradient is often present; more than 50 mm Hg would be clearly unacceptable and an indication for revision of the myectomy or MV replacement. Some clinicians will try to provoke latent obstruction with a small bolus of isoproterenol (2-4 μmg) or clamping the inferior vena cava and consider revision if the provocable gradient exceeds 50 mm Hg. These criteria are essentially arbitrary and based only on personal experience. In contrast, others assess the results of the myectomy only under ideal hemodynamic circumstances, believing that these conditions can be maintained postoperatively long term in most patients. Obviously, decisions regarding the need for further resection of septum are difficult. The likelihood of gaining significant improvement is balanced against the risk of creating complications such as VSD. Additional, often helpful information may be obtained by assessing the LV-to-aorta gradient with direct pressure measurements. This option should be considered when adequate CWD measurements across the LVOT cannot be made. Also, epicardial echocardiography may be used when transesophageal windows do not provide the needed information.[68]

On occasion, CFD reveals a small jet of flow into the ventricular chamber from the region of the myectomy. This flow undoubtedly is due to a severed septal-perforating coronary artery and does not appear to be of any significant consequence.

Anesthetic Management of Hypertrophic Obstructive Cardiomyopathy for Noncardiac Surgery

Patients with HOCM appear to have an increased incidence of perioperative cardiac complications, most commonly congestive heart failure and arrhythmias. The incidence of significant, persistent adverse outcome is very low.[69,70] The following recommendations for management, while based on anecdotal reports and personal experience, rely on knowledge of and are consistent with the pathophysiologic principles of mitral SAM discussed earlier.

There should be a low threshold for inserting an arterial cannula in patients with HOCM undergoing surgery, especially if the procedure is prolonged or likely to involve significant shifts in fluid. The ability to monitor blood pressure continuously is critical in managing these patients with extremely dynamic lesions. Assessing preload by measuring CVP and pulmonary artery occlusion pressure (PAOP) may be difficult because of the diastolic dysfunction caused by hypertrophied myocardium. These monitors may be useful when interpreted with the understanding of the pathophysiology of mitral SAM, especially in the postoperative period. Elevated left-heart filling pressures occurring acutely may be due to SAM and its adverse consequences associated with hypovolemia. The most effective way to monitor cardiac status in patients with HOCM undergoing general anesthesia is with TEE. This permits direct visualization of the MV and the severity of SAM, LVOT obstruction, and MR. TEE also provides

images of the LV chamber size, a direct measure of preload.

Most consider spinal anesthesia relatively contraindicated in patients with HOCM because of the potential for sudden, uncontrolled decreases in preload and systemic vascular resistance.[71] Epidural anesthesia for labor and delivery has been used in patients with HOCM, but should be dosed gradually with careful attention paid to maintenance of adequate intravascular volume.[72] General anesthesia can be safely used in most patients with HOCM by understanding the pathophysiology and its implications for therapy.

Preexisting fluid deficits should be diagnosed and treated before induction. The specific drugs used for an anesthetic are less important than is their careful application with an understanding of the pathophysiology of mitral SAM. Induction of anesthesia should be gradual to avoid sudden decreases in preload or vascular resistance or increases in inotropic state. Ketamine should not be used because it increases heart rate and contractility. β-Antagonist drugs such as esmolol may be used to attenuate surges in sympathetic tone caused by intubation or incision. Halothane has been recommended for maintenance of anesthesia because of its ability to decrease heart rate and contractility,[67] but other agents and total intravenous techniques have been used successfully in HOCM patients.[73]

Proper treatment of hypotension in patients with HOCM is critical because certain common drugs, such as ephedrine or epinephrine, may make these patients worse (Box 11-10). Increased intravascular volume improves mitral SAM and the attendant hypotension. Hypotension should be treated first by placing the patient in Trendelenburg position (head down) and rapidly infusing intravenous fluid. Any surgical maneuvers that decrease venous return should be stopped immediately. Pure α agonists such as phenylephrine should be given if hypotension does not promptly re-

---

BOX 11-10
Treatment of Hypotension Associated with Mitral Systolic Anterior Motion

Increase LV end-diastolic volume
   Trendelenburg position (head down)
   Infuse intravascular volume
Increase systemic vascular resistance
   Pure α-agonist drugs
      Phenylephrine, metaraminol
Decrease myocardial contractility and heart rate
   β-Antagonist drugs
      Esmolol, metoprolol, propranolol

LV, Left ventricle.

spond to volume. Drugs that increase contractility such as ephedrine and epinephrine should be avoided because they may increase SAM and aggravate rather than ameliorate hypotension. β-Antagonist drugs such as esmolol may be helpful if the patient has tachycardia, good systolic LV function, and hypotension resulting from mitral SAM. When available, assessment with TEE is the most expedient and accurate way to diagnose suspected mitral SAM and monitor responses to therapeutic interventions.

Treatment of low cardiac output in patients with HOCM requires the careful assessment of a number of critical hemodynamic factors: LV end-diastolic volume, global LV systolic function (contractility), the presence and severity of mitral SAM and its adverse consequences, LVOT obstruction, and MR. This is usually best accomplished in the operating room with TEE. There is usually significant diastolic dysfunction from myocardial hypertrophy, necessitating higher left-sided filling pressures than normal to achieve adequate LV end diastolic volume. A low LV end-diastolic volume tends to worsen mitral SAM and hence LVOT obstruction and MR in patients with HOCM. Thus, rapid infusion of intravascular volume is usually the mainstay of therapy for low cardiac output in these patients. If severe SAM is suspected or documented with TEE, α agonists may be administered in an attempt to reverse this pathophysiology. If tachycardia and mitral SAM accompany good contractility of the myocardium, negative inotropic drugs such as esmolol may increase cardiac output by decreasing mitral SAM and its adverse consequences. It is expected that vasodilator drugs and positive inotropic drugs would aggravate rather than improve the hemodynamics in these situations and should generally be avoided. Drugs that combine these hemodynamic effects such as isoproterenol, dobutamine, amrinone, and milrinone may be particularly harmful. Similarly, the hemodynamic effects of balloon counterpulsation, lowered afterload, and LV end-diastolic volume, aggravate mitral SAM, making the insertion of an intraaortic balloon pump harmful rather than helpful in most of these patients.[74] Occasionally, a patient with HOCM may simultaneously have impaired myocardial contractility and significant mitral SAM, especially after CPB. Such patients are quite difficult to manage. The best course of action is to provide a complete and ongoing assessment with TEE to determine the relative contribution of each factor to the low cardiac output state. Because responses may be unpredictable, interventions based on this complete assessment should be as short acting and easily reversible as possible. A carefully balanced combination of volume administration, vasoconstriction, and positive inotropic drug therapy may be needed to achieve satisfactory hemodynamics. The key is to monitor continuously and tailor therapy to the combination of hemodynamic lesions present in a particular patient, being ready to change course quickly should the hemodynamic condition deteriorate.

KEY POINTS

Cardiac Tamponade
1. A rapid accumulation of a small amount of fluid is more likely to cause tamponade than a slow accumulation of a large amount of fluid.
2. Tamponade after cardiac surgery may be due to localized compression of the heart and great vessels.
3. Establish large-bore IV access and hemodynamic monitors *before* induction of anesthesia.
4. Tamponade physiology can be aggravated by positive pressure ventilation.
5. Induction of anesthesia with drugs that cause sympatholysis can cause hemodynamic collapse. Etomidate and ketamine are preferred drugs for induction.
6. The surgical team should be ready to rapidly intervene before induction of anesthesia. Prepare and drape the patient *before* induction.
7. Consider relieving tamponade physiology with pericardiocentesis *before* induction of anesthesia.
8. Treat hypotension with volume infusion and sympathomimetics.

Constrictive Pericarditis
1. Constrictive pericarditis causes impaired ventricular filling and elevation of CVP and PAOP.
2. It is often associated with impaired ventricular function, especially after pericardiectomy.
3. Establish large-bore IV access and hemodynamic monitors *before* induction of anesthesia.
4. Pericardiectomy may be associated with rapid blood loss.
5. Manipulation of the heart during pericardiectomy may cause hemodynamic instability.
6. Treat hypotension with volume infusion and sympathomimetics.

Mitral Systolic Anterior Motion

1. Mitral systolic anterior motion is most commonly associated with HOCM.
2. It can cause acute failure of an MV repair.
3. It is best diagnosed and assessed with echocardiography.
4. It causes LVOT obstruction and MR.
5. It is easily confused with impaired myocardial function by PAC data.
6. It is aggravated by hypovolemia, vasodilation, tachycardia, and increased myocardial contractility.
7. Treat hypotension with volume infusion, pure α-agonist drugs, and negative inotropic drugs.

KEY REFERENCES

Cardiac Tamponade

Bommer WJ, Follette D, Pollock M et al: Tamponade in patients undergoing cardiac surgery: a clinical-echocardiographic diagnosis, *Am Heart J* 130(6):1216-1223, 1995.

Fowler NO: Cardiac tamponade: a clinical or an echocardiographic diagnosis? *Circulation* 87(5):1738-1741, 1993.

Merce J, Sagrista-Sauleda J, Permanyer-Miralda G et al: Correlation between clinical and Doppler echocardiographic findings in patients with moderate and large pericardial effusion: implications for the diagnosis of cardiac tamponade, *Am Heart J* 138(4 Pt 1):759-764, 1999.

Spodick DH: Pathophysiology of cardiac tamponade, *Chest* 113(5):1372-1378, 1998.

Constrictive Pericarditis

Ling LH, Oh JK, Schaff HV et al: Constrictive pericarditis in the modern era: evolving clinical spectrum and impact on outcome after pericardiectomy, *Circulation* 100(13): 1380-1386, 1999.

Myers RB, Spodick DH: Constrictive pericarditis: clinical and pathophysiologic characteristics, *Am Heart J* 138(2 Pt 1): 219-232, 1999.

Senni M, Redfield MM, Ling LH et al: Left ventricular systolic and diastolic function after pericardiectomy in patients with constrictive pericarditis: Doppler echocardiographic findings and correlation with clinical status, *J Am Coll Cardiol* 33(5):1182-1188, 1999.

Takata M, Harasawa Y, Beloucif S et al: Coupled vs. uncoupled pericardial constraint: effects on cardiac chamber interactions, *J Appl Physiol* 83(6):1799-1813, 1997.

Mitral Systolic Anterior Motion

Grigg LE, Wigle ED, Williams WG et al: Transesophageal Doppler echocardiography in obstructive hypertrophic cardiomyopathy: clarification of pathophysiology and importance in intraoperative decision making, *J Am Coll Cardiol* 20(1):42-52, 1992.

Haering JM, Comunale ME, Parker RA et al: Cardiac risk of noncardiac surgery in patients with asymmetric septal hypertrophy, *Anesthesiology* 85(2):254-259, 1996.

Maron BJ, Bonow RO, Cannon RO et al: Hypertrophic cardiomyopathy: interrelations of clinical manifestations, pathophysiology, and therapy, *N Engl J Med* 316:780-789, 1987.

Marwick TH, Stewart WJ, Currie PJ et al: Mechanisms of failure of mitral valve repair: an echocardiographic study, *Am Heart J* 122:149-156, 1991.

McCully RB, Nishimura RA, Tajik AJ et al: Extent of clinical improvement after surgical treatment of hypertrophic obstructive cardiomyopathy, *Circulation* 94(3):467-471, 1996.

References

1. Spodick DH: Pathophysiology of cardiac tamponade, *Chest* 113(5):1372-1378, 1998.
2. Hirsch AT, Dzau VJ, Creager MA: Baroreceptor function in congestive heart failure: effect on neurohumoral activation and regional vascular resistance, *Circulation* 75(5 Pt 2):IV36-48, 1987.
3. Spodick DH: Low atrial natriuretic factor levels and absent pulmonary edema in pericardial compression of the heart, *Am J Cardiol* 63(17):1271-1272, 1989.
4. Spodick DH: The normal and diseased pericardium: current concepts of pericardial physiology, diagnosis and treatment, *J Am Coll Cardiol* 1(1):240-251, 1983.
5. Otto CM: *Textbook of clinical echocardiography*, ed 2, Philadelphia, 2000, WB Saunders, pp 213-228.
6. Lorell BH: Pericardial diseases. In E. Braunwald, editor: *Heart disease: a textbook of cardiovascular medicine*, ed 5, Saunders Philadelphia, 1997, WB Saunders, pp 1486-1490.
7. Miro AM, Pinsky MR: Heart-lung interactions. In M. J. Tobin, editor: *Principles and practice of mechanical ventilation*, New York, 1994, McGraw-Hill, pp 647-667.
8. Atar S, Chiu J, Forrester JS et al: Bloody pericardial effusion in patients with cardiac tamponade: is the cause cancerous, tuberculous, or iatrogenic in the 1990s? *Chest* 116(6):1564-1569, 1999.
9. Baumgartner FJ, Rayhanabad J, Bongard FS et al: Central venous injuries of the subclavian-jugular and innominate-caval confluences, *Texas Heart Inst J* 26(3):177-181, 1999.
10. Bommer WJ, Follette D, Pollock M et al: Tamponade in patients undergoing cardiac surgery: a clinical-echocardiographic diagnosis, *Am Heart J* 130(6):1216-1223, 1995.
11. Beck CS: Two cardiac compression triads, *JAMA* 104:714, 1935.
12. Fowler NO: Cardiac tamponade: a clinical or an echocardiographic diagnosis? *Circulation* 87(5):1738-1741, 1993.

13. Eisenberg MJ, de Romeral LM, Heidenreich PA et al: The diagnosis of pericardial effusion and cardiac tamponade by 12-lead ECG: a technology assessment, *Chest* 110(2):318-324, 1996.

14. Merce J, Sagrista-Sauleda J, Permanyer-Miralda G et al: Correlation between clinical and Doppler echocardiographic findings in patients with moderate and large pericardial effusion: implications for the diagnosis of cardiac tamponade, *Am Heart J* 138(4 Pt 1):759-764, 1999.

15. Breen PH, MacVay MA: Pericardial tamponade: a case for awake endotracheal intubation [letter], *Anesth Analg* 83(3):658, 1996.

16. McCaughan BC, Schaff HV, Piehler JM et al: Early and late results of pericardiectomy for constrictive pericarditis, *J Thorac Cardiovasc Surg* 89(3):340-350, 1985.

17. Myers RB, Spodick DH: Constrictive pericarditis: clinical and pathophysiologic characteristics, *Am Heart J* 138(2 Pt 1):219-232, 1999.

18. Wolozin MW, Ortola FV, Spodick DH et al: Release of atrial natriuretic factor after pericardiectomy for chronic constrictive pericarditis, *Am J Cardiol* 62(17):1323-1325, 1988.

19. Levine HD: Myocardial fibrosis in constrictive pericarditis: electrocardiographic and pathologic observations, *Circulation* 48(6):1268-1281, 1973.

20. Hancock EW: On the elastic and rigid forms of constrictive pericarditis, *Am Heart J* 100(6 Pt 1):917-923, 1980.

21. Meyer TE, Sareli P, Marcus RH et al: Mechanism underlying Kussmaul's sign in chronic constrictive pericarditis, *Am J Cardiol* 64(16):1069-1072, 1989.

22. Takata M, Harasawa Y, Beloucif S et al: Coupled vs. uncoupled pericardial constraint: effects on cardiac chamber interactions, *J Appl Physiol* 83(6):1799-1813, 1997.

23. Wynne J, Braunwald E: The cardiomyopathies and myocarditises. In A. S. Fauci et al, editors: *Harrison's principals of internal medicine,* ed 14, 1998, New York, McGraw-Hill, p 1339.

24. Oh JK, Tajik AJ, Appleton CP et al: Preload reduction to unmask the characteristic Doppler features of constrictive pericarditis: a new observation, *Circulation* 95(4):796-799, 1997.

25. Pedreira Perez M, Virgos Lamela A, Crespo Mancebo FJ et al: 40 years' experience in the surgical treatment of constrictive pericarditis, *Arch Inst Cardiol Mex* 57(5):363-373, 1987.

26. Ling LH, Oh JK, Schaff HV et al: Constrictive pericarditis in the modern era: evolving clinical spectrum and impact on outcome after pericardiectomy, *Circulation* 100(13):1380-1386, 1999.

27. Nataf P, Cacoub P, Dorent R et al: Results of subtotal pericardiectomy for constrictive pericarditis, *Eur J Cardiothorac Surg* 7(5):252-255, 1993.

28. Lorell BH: Pericardial diseases. In E. Braunwald, editor: *Heart disease: a textbook of cardiovascular medicine,* ed 5, Philadelphia, 1997, WB Saunders, p. 1497.

29. Lange RL, Botticelli JT, Tsagaris TJ et al: Diagnostic signs in compressive cardiac disorders: constrictive pericarditis, pericardial effusion, and tamponade, *Circulation* 33(5):763-777, 1966.

30. Chandrashekhar Y, Anand IS, Kalra GS et al: Rate-dependent hemodynamic responses during incremental atrial pacing in chronic constrictive pericarditis before and after surgery, *Am J Cardiol* 72(7):615-619, 1993.

31. Masui T, Finck S, Higgins CB et al: Constrictive pericarditis and restrictive cardiomyopathy: evaluation with MR imaging, *Radiology* 182(2):369-373, 1992.

32. Goldstein JA: Differentiation of constrictive pericarditis and restrictive cardiomyopathy, *ACC Educational Highlights,* pp 14-22, Fall 1998.

33. Lorell BH: Pericardial diseases. In E. Braunwald, editor: *Heart disease: a textbook of cardiovascular medicine,* ed 5, Philadelphia, 1997, Saunders, pp 1499-1501.

34. Arsan S, Mercan S, Sarigul A et al: Long-term experience with pericardiectomy: analysis of 105 consecutive patients, *Thorac Cardiovasc Surg* 42(6):340-344, 1994.

35. Senni M, Redfield MM, Ling LH et al: Left ventricular systolic and diastolic function after pericardiectomy in patients with constrictive pericarditis: Doppler echocardiographic findings and correlation with clinical status, *J Am Coll Cardiol* 33(5):1182-1188, 1999.

36. Brock R: Functional obstruction of the left ventricle, *Guys Hospital Reports* 106:221-238, 1957.

37. Maron BJ, Bonow RO, Cannon RO et al: Hypertrophic cardiomyopathy: interrelations of clinical manifestations, pathophysiology, and therapy, *N Engl J Med* 316:780-789, 1987.

38. Fix P, Moberg A, Soderberg H et al: Muscular subvalvular aortic stenosis: abnormal anterior mitral leaflet possibly the primary factor, *Acta Radiol* 2:177-193, 1964.

39. Shah PM, Gramiak R, Kramer DH: Ultrasound localization of left ventricular outflow tract obstruction in hypertrophic obstructive cardiomyopathy, *Circulation* 40:3-11, 1969.

40. Henry WL, Clark CE, Glancy DL et al: Echocardiographic measurement of the left ventricular outflow gradient in idiopathic hypertrophic subaortic stenosis, *N Engl J Med* 288:989-993, 1973.

41. Gardin JM, Dabestani A, Glasgow GA et al: Echocardiographic and Doppler flow observations in obstructed and nonobstructed hypertrophic cardiomyopathy, *Am J Cardiol* 56:614-621, 1985.

42. Cape EG, Simons D, Jimoh A et al: Chordal geometry determines the shape and extent of systolic anterior mitral motion: in vitro studies, *J Am Coll Cardiol* 13:1438-1448, 1989.

43. Grigg LE, Wigle ED, Williams WG et al: Transesophageal Doppler echocardiography in obstructive hypertrophic cardiomyopathy: clarification of pathophysiology and importance in intraoperative decision making, *J Am Coll Cardiol* 20(1):42-52, 1992.

44. Kizilbash AM, Heinle SK, Grayburn PA: Spontaneous variability of left ventricular outflow tract gradient in hypertrophic obstructive cardiomyopathy, *Circulation* 97(5):461-466, 1998.

45. Levine RA: Echocardiographic assessment of the cardiomyopathies. In Weyman AE, editor: *Principles and practice of echocardiography,* ed 2, . Philadelphia, 1994, Lea & Febiger, pp 798-804.

46. Bulkley BH, Fortuin NJ: Systolic anterior motion of the mitral valve without asymmetric septal hypertrophy, *Chest* 69(5):694-696, 1976.

47. Levisman JA: Systolic anterior motion of the mitral valve due to hypovolemia and anemia (letter), *Chest* 70:687-688, 1976.

48. Termini BA, Jackson PA, Williams CD: Systolic anterior motion of the mitral valve following annuloplasty, *Vasc Surg* 11:55-60, 1977.

49. Cutrone F, Coyle JP, Novoa R: Severe dynamic left ventricular outflow tract obstruction following aortic valve replacement diagnosed by intraoperative echocardiography, *Anesthesiology* 72:563-566, 1990.

50. Haley JH, Sinak LJ, Tajik AJ et al: Dynamic left ventricular outflow tract obstruction in acute coronary syndromes: an important cause of new systolic murmur and cardiogenic shock, *Mayo Clin Proc* 74(9):901-906, 1999.

51. Lindvall K, Herrlin B: Mitral annulus calcification, systolic anterior motion of the anterior mitral leaflet and outflow obstruction in two patients without hypertrophic cardiomyopathy, *Acta Med Scand* 209:513-518, 1981.

52. Kessler KM, Anzola E, Sequeira R et al: Mitral valve prolapse and systolic anterior motion: a dynamic spectrum, *Am Heart J* 105:685-688, 1983.

53. Krenz HK, Mindich BP, Guarino T et al: Sudden development of intraoperative left ventricular outflow obstruction: differential and mechanism. An intraoperative two-dimensional echocardiographic study, *J Cardiac Surg* 5:93-101, 1990.

54. Marwick TH, Stewart WJ, Currie PJ et al: Mechanisms of failure of mitral valve repair: an echocardiographic study, *Am Heart J* 122:149-156, 1991.

55. Lee KS, Stewart WJ, Lever HM et al: Mechanism of outflow tract obstruction causing failed mitral valve repair: anterior displacement of leaflet coaptation, *Circulation* 88 [5 Pt 2]:II24-29, 1993.

56. Jebara VA, Mihaileanu S, Acar C et al: Left ventricular outflow tract obstruction after mitral valve repair: results of the sliding leaflet technique, *Circulation* 88(5 Pt 2):II30-34, 1993.

57. He S, Fontaine AA, Schwammenthal E et al: Integrated mechanism for functional mitral regurgitation: leaflet restriction versus coapting force: in vitro studies, *Circulation* 96(6):1826-1834, 1997.

58. Harrison MR, Grigsby CG, Souther SK et al: Midventricular obstruction associated with chronic systemic hypertension and severe left ventricular hypertrophy, *Am J Cardiol* 68(8):761-765, 1991.

59. Bruce CJ, Nishimura RA, Tajik AJ et al: Fixed left ventricular outflow tract obstruction in presumed hypertrophic obstructive cardiomyopathy: implications for therapy, *Ann Thorac Surg* 68(1): 100-104, 1999.

60. Gadler F, Linde C, Juhlin-Dannfeldt A et al: Influence of right ventricular pacing site on left ventricular outflow tract obstruction in patients with hypertrophic obstructive cardiomyopathy, *J Am Coll Cardiol* 27(5):1219-1224, 1996.

61. Fananapazir L, McAreavey D: Therapeutic options in patients with obstructive hypertrophic cardiomyopathy and severe drug-refractory symptoms, *J Am Coll Cardiol* 31(2):259-264, 1998.

62. McIntosh CL, Maron BJ: Current operative treatment of obstructive hypertrophic cardiomyopathy, *Circulation* 78(3):487-495, 1988.

63. McCully RB, Nishimura RA, Tajik AJ et al: Extent of clinical improvement after surgical treatment of hypertrophic obstructive cardiomyopathy, *Circulation* 94(3):467-471, 1996.

64. Williams WG, Wigle ED, Rakowski H et al: Results of surgery for hypertrophic obstructive cardiomyopathy, *Circulation* 76(5 Pt 2): V104-108, 1987.

65. Faber L, Meissner A, Ziemssen P et al: Percutaneous transluminal septal myocardial ablation for hypertrophic obstructive cardiomyopathy: long term follow up of the first series of 25 patients, *Heart* 83(3):326-331, 2000.

66. Reitan JA, Wright RG: The use of halothane in a patient with asymmetrical septal hypertrophy: a case report, *Canadian Anaesthetists' Society Journal* 29(2):154-157, 1982.

67. Marwick TH, Stewart WJ, Lever HM et al: Benefits of intraoperative echocardiography in the surgical management of hypertrophic cardiomyopathy, *J Am Coll Cardiol* 20(5):1066-1072, 1992.

68. Sasson Z, Prieur T, Skrobik Y et al: Aortic regurgitation: a common complication after surgery for hypertrophic obstructive cardiomyopathy, *J Am CollCardiol* 13(1):63-67, 1989.

69. Thompson RC, Liberthson RR, Lowenstein E: Perioperative anesthetic risk of noncardiac surgery in hypertrophic obstructive cardiomyopathy, *JAMA* 254(17):2419-2421, 1985.

70. Haering JM, Comunale ME, Parker RA et al: Cardiac risk of noncardiac surgery in patients with asymmetric septal hypertrophy, *Anesthesiology* 85(2):254-259, 1996.

71. Loubser P, Suh K, Cohen S: Adverse effects of spinal anesthesia in a patient with idiopathic hypertrophic subaortic stenosis, *Anesthesiology* 60(3):228-230, 1984.

72. Tessler MJ, Hudson R, Naugler-Colville M et al: Pulmonary oedema in two parturients with hypertrophic obstructive cardiomyopathy (HOCM), *Can J Anaesth* 37(4 Pt 1):469-473, 1990.

73. Bell MD, Goodchild CS: Hypertrophic obstructive cardiomyopathy in combination with a prolapsing mitral valve: anaesthesia for surgical correction with propofol, *Anaesthesia* 44(5):409-411, 1989.

74. Morewood GH, Weiss SJ: Intra-aortic balloon pump associated with dynamic left ventricular outflow tract obstruction after valve replacement for aortic stenosis, *J Am Soc Echocardiogr* 13(3): 229-231, 2000.

PART III

Specific Cardiothoracic Surgical Procedures

CHAPTER 12

Cardiopulmonary Bypass

Heather E. Manspeizer, M.D. ■ Linda Shore-Lesserson, M.D.

OUTLINE

Cardiopulmonary bypass (CPB) has become an integral component of cardiac surgery as we know it today. CPB creates a bloodless surgical field by allowing blood to bypass the heart and the lungs during cardiac procedures while maintaining oxygenation, ventilation, and systemic perfusion pressure. In addition to cardiac surgery, CPB has been used during periods of asystole, inadequate cardiac output, and when the lungs cannot maintain appropriate physiologic gas exchange resulting from insufficient pulmonary perfusion.

Total CPB is a condition in which all systemic venous drainage to the heart is diverted into the CPB circuit. The diverted blood passes through an external oxygenator, heat exchanger, external pump, and arterial filter before reentering the arterial systemic circulation. The pump generates the flow that returns blood to the patient and maintains systemic arterial pressure.

In partial CPB, only a portion of systemic venous return is diverted from the right heart to the CPB circuit. During partial bypass, the undiverted blood continues to the right atrium (RA), into the right ventricle (RV) and the pulmonary circulation. The oxygenated blood continues to the left atrium (LA) and left ventricle (LV), where it is ejected into the systemic circulation. For partial CPB to be effective, the heart must continue to beat and the lungs must be ventilated.

COMPONENTS OF THE CARDIOPULMONARY BYPASS CIRCUIT

CPB diverts blood away from the surgical field, creates a bloodless surgical field, and provides optimal surgical exposure for procedures on the heart, lungs, and great vessels. There are several integral components essential to CPB, as illustrated in Fig. 12-1.

Venous Drainage

Blood from the venous circulation passively drains from the patient by gravity and is collected in a venous reservoir bag positioned below the patient. When blood is appropriately drained from the superior vena cava (SVC) and inferior vena cava (IVC), RA pressure approaches zero.[1] Drainage of the right heart is best accomplished by either direct cannulation of the SVC and IVC (bicaval cannulation) or by the use of a two-staged cannula in the RA. Bicaval cannulation with snares provides better venous decompression of the right heart than bicaval cannulation without snares, although the Sarns 51F two-staged RA cannula has been shown to be equally effective as bicaval cannulation.[1]

Although the more effective cannulation sites are the SVC/IVC (bicaval) or RA (two-staged), femoral venous cannulation is particularly useful during reoperations or when CPB must commence emergently. The femoral cannula is inserted into the femoral vein and advanced into the IVC and RA. The major advantage of femoral venous cannulation is that it can be performed emergently without sternotomy. However, typically a smaller

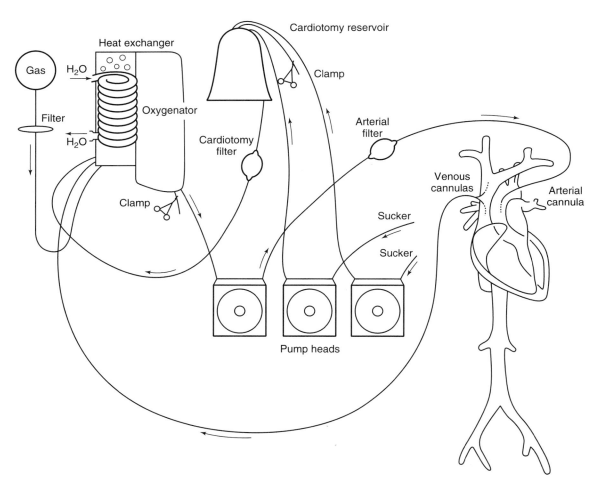

FIG. 12-1 Cardiopulmonary bypass diverts blood away from the surgical field, creates a bloodless surgical field, and provides optimal surgical exposure for procedures on the heart, lungs, and the great vessels. The integral components essential of the extracorporeal circuit are shown in this figure.

(From Lake CL: *Pediatric cardiac anesthesia*, Norwalk, Conn, 1988, Appleton and Lange, p 157.)

cannula (20 French) must be employed because of the limited diameter of the femoral vein. Unfortunately, because of its smaller size, the main disadvantage of the femoral cannulation site is that cardiac drainage and decompression are less effective than with either bicaval cannulation or the two-staged cannula.

Reservoir

The venous reservoir bag collects blood from the venous drainage and the cardiotomy suction drain. From the reservoir bag, blood is pumped through the membrane oxygenator and heat exchanger, and then returns to the patient after passing through an arterial filter. To prevent massive gas emboli, the volume in the reservoir bag should not be allowed to empty.

Pumps

The roller and the centrifugal are two types of CPB pumps used in clinical practice. The roller pump, otherwise known as the *peristaltic pump*, propagates continuous nonpulsatile blood flow by compressing plastic tubing between the roller and the backing plate. The blood flow generated is related to pump speed. Newer roller pumps are advantageous because they are capable of generating pulsatile flow. A disadvantage of the roller pump is that it can pump large volumes of air indiscriminately if an air alarm is not placed in the circuit. Centrifugal pumps consist of a series of cones that spin and propel blood flow forward by centrifugal force. These pumps are incapable of any type of pulsatile flow, however, and will not pump air when air is entrained.

Centrifugal pumping techniques have been shown to reduce blood loss,[2] improve renal function, and protect against neurologic complications[3] when compared with roller pumps. However, attenuation of the inflammatory response has not been uniformly demonstrated with centrifugal pumps. Recent comparisons between centrifugal and roller pumps have shown no difference in the generation of microemboli,[4] neutrophil activation,[5] or the rates of hemolysis.[6] Some reports have even suggested that centrifugal pumps generate a greater systemic inflammatory response than the standard roller pump.[7] However, others note that although centrifugal pumps result in greater intraoperative complement and neutrophil activation, the two pumps result in similar postoperative inflammation.[8] Furthermore, less thrombin and subsequent fibrin deposition is produced with a centrifugal pump, which suggests that there may be less microvascular coagulation during CPB when using a centrifugal pump instead of a roller pump.[9,10] In the pediatric literature, centrifugal pumps have been associated with less blood trauma, reduced platelet activation, less systemic inflammation, and improved postoperative renal function.[11]

Pump Prime

The pump prime is made of a balanced salt solution. Colloids (albumin, hetastarch), mannitol, bicarbonate, heparin, and other electrolytes are routinely included in the pump prime. Although the ideal priming solution is unknown, colloid may be more beneficial than crystalloid because it increases oncotic pressure. However, the clinical benefits in terms of outcome have not been proven.[12-14] Recently, another colloid with a short intravascular half-life, pentastarch, has been found as safe as albumin or Ringer's solution during CPB.[15]

Exogenous blood is commonly avoided in the pump prime because an asanguinous pump prime has been shown to improve intraoperative and postoperative hemostasis and renal function.[16] However, in children and neonates, and in adults with significant preoperative anemia, an asanguinous pump prime will result in hemodilution that potentially decreases oxygen-carrying capacity to detrimental levels. These patients require blood in the prime.

Recently, retrograde autologous blood priming has been proposed and used for CPB. The technique of retrograde autologous priming (RAP) involves draining the arterial line, venous reservoir and oxygenator, and venous lines into a recirculation bag until the venous line becomes sanguineous. During this time, the systolic arterial pressure is maintained greater than 100 mm Hg (Fig. 12-2). When CPB is initiated, autologous blood

RAP Circuit

- 1. Drain arterial line (350 ml)
- 2. Drain venous reservoir and oxygenator (400 ml)
- 3. Drain venous line (350 ml)
- Total: 1100 ml

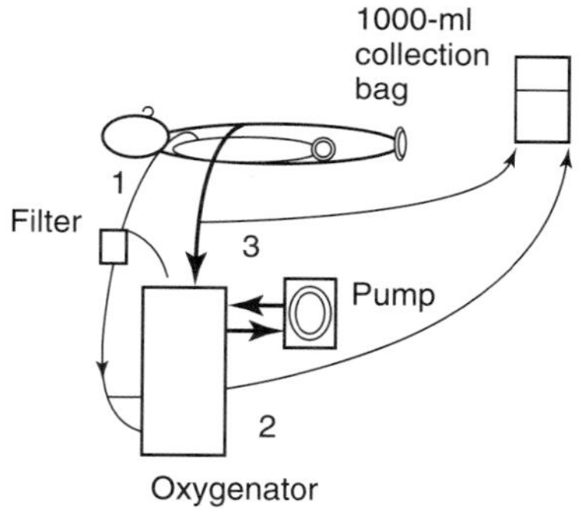

Schema of the RAP technique. 1. Arterial line drainage. While systolic arterial blood pressure is being maintained greater than 100 mm Hg, the recirculation line clamp is slowly released and blood travels through the pump arterial line from the aorta through the filter, into the recirculation line, and up into a 1000 ml transfer bag. 2. Venous reservoir and oxygenator drainage. The line between the oxygenator and arterial line filter is clamped and the recirculation line is unclamped. The arterial pump is slowly advanced until the venous reservoir volume drops to 200 ml. At this time, the arterial line filter purge is opened and the arterial pump is again advanced until the fluid exiting the oxygenator outlet becomes sanguineous. The arterial pump is stopped and the pump outlet and recirculation lines are clamped. The recirculation line is then removed from the 1000 ml bag and attached to the recirculation port on the oxygenator reservoir. 3. Venous line drainage. As bypass is commenced, the venous line prime is drained into the recirculation bag, and this 1/4-inch line is clamped once the venous line fluid becomes sanguineous. The recirculation bag is rehung to allow for crystalloid transfusion as necessary.

FIG. 12-2 A retrograde autologous priming (RAP) circuit.

(From Rosengart TK, DeBois W, O'Hara M et al: *J Thorac Cardiovasc Surg* 115:427, 1998.)

has primed the circuit and is returned to the patient. The introduction of RAP into clinical practice has significantly reduced the extent of hemodilution and the number of patients requiring red cell transfusion during cardiac surgery.[17]

Oxygenators

The CPB oxygenator performs the gas exchange functions of the lungs in the CPB circuit. Although blood is pumped under pressure, the gas exchange occurs at atmospheric pressure because the oxygenator is vented to the atmosphere. Two types of oxygenators, bubble and membrane, are used in clinical practice.

Bubble Oxygenators. Bubble oxygenators deliver oxygen and remove carbon dioxide via a gas bubble–blood interface. Gas is bubbled through the oxygenator so that gas exchange can occur, and subsequently the gas bubble–blood mixture passes through a defoamer/debubbler. Using the bubble oxygenator, CO_2 exchange is proportional to gas flow, whereas O_2 transfer is proportional to bubble size. Unfortunately, this gas bubble–blood interface is not physiologic and may potentially result in blood trauma. Once blood trauma and hemolysis develop, organ damage and capillary plugging become a genuine concern. Other problems associated with the bubble oxygenator include the activation of complement,[18] abnormal hemostasis,[19,20] and the formation of particulate and gaseous microemboli.[21]

Membrane Oxygenators. Membrane oxygenators permit gas exchange across a thin membrane, which eliminates the gas bubble–blood contact and the need for a defoamer. Hemolysis occurs less often with the membrane oxygenator, but the impact this has on clinical outcome and transfusion requirements remains controversial.[22-24] Another advantage of the membrane oxygenator is that oxygen and carbon dioxide can be adjusted independently. The Fio_2 of the inspired gas controls oxygen tension, whereas CO_2 is regulated by total gas flow. A membrane oxygenator can thus deliver air-oxygen mixtures, whereas bubble oxygenators can administer only 100% oxygen.

Heat Exchangers

The heat exchanger is an essential component of CPB when hypothermic techniques for cerebral and myocardial protection are employed. Water of a predetermined temperature is pumped into spiral coils and the patient's blood flows through the adjacent tubing in the opposite direction using a countercurrent mechanism. The heat exchanger relies on the efficiency of the countercurrent system to warm or cool the blood.

Arterial Inflow

The arterial cannula is commonly positioned in the ascending aorta, proximal to the innominate artery, to allow perfusion of the head vessels, distal aorta, and coronary ostia. However, the femoral artery may be used as an alternative arterial cannulation site. When the femoral artery is cannulated, the proximal aorta and the coronary ostia are perfused by retrograde flow. Like femoral venous cannulation, femoral arterial cannulation is useful for emergency CPB and for reoperations where the risk of hemorrhage during sternotomy is great. However, the necessity for smaller cannulae and the increased risk for aortic dissection and lower extremity neurologic deficits limit its routine use.[25]

Cardiotomy Suction

The cardiotomy suction removes shed blood from the surgical field so it can be processed and retransfused to the patient. A roller pump provides the suction for this system, which is used for blood conservation during CPB. The collected blood can flow directly into a reservoir bag that contains a filter, or through a filtered cardiotomy suction, before returning to the venous reservoir. To prevent clot formation in the cardiotomy suction or the venous reservoir, the cardiotomy suction can be used only after complete heparinization. Unfortunately, the cardiotomy suction is a potential source of blood traumatization[19] during CPB because the simultaneous aspiration of air and blood causes blood trauma.[26] For this reason, the cardiotomy pump should run slowly to avoid air aspiration.

Ventricular Venting

Because blood return to the RV, from the coronary sinus and the vena cavae, is usually successfully collected with either the two-stage cannula or bicaval cannulation, an RV vent is rarely necessary. More commonly, however, an LV vent may be necessary to avoid distention of the LV upon initiation and maintenance of CPB. Distention of the LV may cause myocardial warming and subsequent ischemia resulting from increased myocardial oxygen consumption. Surgical exposure may also be compromised. Blood return to the LV may occur from the thebesian veins, bronchial veins, aortic valve incompetence, or from an extracardiac left-to-right shunt. Access to the LV may be gained through the following techniques: (1) the right superior pulmonary vein to LA to LV, (2) direct LA cannulation, or (3) direct LV cannulation. Blood collected from the LV vent drains into either a filtered cardiotomy reservoir and then into the venous reservoir, or directly into the venous reservoir. Active venting of the LV should be avoided to prevent air entrainment.

Micropore Filters

The cardiotomy and arterial lines contain microporous filters. These filters remove particulate matter (bone, tissue, fat, blood clots, and pieces of foreign material) and air. The pore size of these filters varies, but is usually between 30 and 40 microns.

Ultrafiltration

Ultrafiltration, or hemofiltration, devices are similar to the devices used in hemodialysis. They are interposed into the CPB circuit when it is necessary to remove excess fluid and hemoconcentrate. An ultrafiltrate is formed across a semipermeable membrane, which is collected by suction. The hematocrit of the remaining blood in the CPB circuit increases. In children, modified ultrafiltration (MUF) is performed after weaning the patient from CPB. MUF has been shown to improve hemodynamics and early postoperative oxygenation, reduce postoperative blood loss, and shorten the duration of mechanical ventilation in pediatric patients.[27,28] Cytokines, complement, and other early inflammatory mediators may also be reduced during MUF.[29-31]

Heparin-Bonded Circuits

Heparin-bonded CPB circuits have been developed in which heparin can be ionically or covalently bonded to the CPB circuit. Because of its stronger bond, covalently bound heparin dissociates into the systemic circulation to a lesser degree. Covalent bonding also allows heparin to be bound to the circuit with its active site exposed to blood flow. These heparin-bonded circuits are thought to have two advantages. First, there is less activation of complement and other inflammatory processes.[32-34] Second, the systemic concentration of heparin can be lowered, which may potentially reduce blood loss during surgery and reduce the need for blood products at the end of the procedure.[35] The literature also suggests that the use of heparin-bonded circuits may lessen the inflammatory component of cerebral injury,[36] resulting in less atrial fibrillation and a reduced incidence of postoperative cerebral dysfunction.[37]

PREPARING FOR CARDIOPULMONARY BYPASS
Anticoagulation

CPB could not be accomplished safely without using anticoagulants to prepare blood for its contact with the extracorporeal circuit. An ideal anticoagulant should be easy to administer, rapid in onset, titratable, predictable, measurable in a timely fashion, and reversible. The most commonly used anticoagulant, heparin, was discovered serendipitously in 1913 by a medical student experi-

menting with extracts from bovine liver. He found that this particular heparinlike substrate had anticoagulant properties. The first clinical use of heparin for CPB in humans did not occur until 1953. Heparin use during CPB has continued until the present time, most likely because of its rapid onset, ease of measurement, and ease of reversibility. The consistent use of heparin is either a testimonial to its effectiveness or demonstrative of our inability to find a more suitable alternative.

Unfractionated heparin is a highly sulfated glycosaminoglycan composed of alternating subunits of substituted D-glucosamine and uronic acid moieties. Its molecular weight ranges from 3000 to 30,000 daltons, with an average molecular weight of 15,000 daltons. A specific pentasaccharide-glucosamine sequence is required for its binding to antithrombin III (ATIII), which was discovered to be the "heparin cofactor" in 1939. Under normal circumstances, ATIII binds to thrombin at a rate proportional to the concentration of the reactants present. However, the reaction rate is greatly accelerated in the presence of heparin. In the absence of ATIII, heparin is clinically ineffective as an anticoagulant; thus adequate ATIII activity is necessary in patients about to undergo heparinization for cardiac surgical procedures. The endogenous activities of ATIII that are enhanced by heparin include the inhibition of factors IIa (thrombin), IXa, Xa, XIa, and XIIa.[38] In decreasing order of sensitivity, the unfractionated heparin-ATIII complex inhibits factors IIa, Xa, IXa, XIa, and XIIa with respectively decreasing rates of reaction.[39]

Heparin is the endogenous proteoglycan of the mast cell and is purified from porcine intestinal mucosa or bovine lung, tissues that have a rich mast cell population. Heparin derived from porcine intestinal mucosa has a different molecular weight, structure, and physiologic activity than heparin derived from bovine lung sources. These differences may account for some of the variability in patient responses to heparin and have implications for dosing and reversal strategies.[40]

Pharmacology

Intravenous heparin has a peak effect 1 minute after injection, followed by a redistribution phase approximately 10 minutes after its peak effect.[41] Redistribution outside of the plasma compartment does occur, because it is known that heparin binds endothelial cells and many plasma proteins found in association with endothelial cells. Endothelial cells bind and depolymerize heparin via PF4. Uptake into the cells of the reticuloendothelial system, vascular smooth muscle, and extracellular fluid may account for the phenomenon referred to as *heparin rebound*.

The half-life of heparin is not linear with increasing doses of heparin, probably as a result of saturation of heparin binding sites.[42] At a dose of 100 U/kg, the half-life of heparin is approximately 60 minutes; at 200 U/kg the half-life is approximately 93 minutes; and at 400 U/kg the half-life is approximately 125 minutes. Heparin elimination most likely results from endothelial cell uptake, absorption by body tissues, a small amount of metabolism, and renal elimination. During CPB, heparin decay varies substantially; because hemodilution and hypothermia alter the metabolism of heparin, it is difficult to measure its decay. In a CPB study, Mabry and associates[43] found that the consumption of heparin varied from 0.01 to 3.86 U/kg/min and that there was no correlation between the initial sensitivity to heparin and the rate of heparin decay. In the pediatric population, the consumption of heparin is increased above that of adult levels.[44]

The differences between porcine intestinal and bovine lung heparin likely result from the tissue source of origin, not from the animal source. Both mucosal and lung-derived heparin have been used successfully for anticoagulation for CPB. Heparin derived from porcine mucosal sources has a lower molecular weight and a shorter saccharide chain sequence than heparin derived from lung sources. This short-chain, or lower-molecular-weight, heparin is an effective anticoagulant as a result of its factor Xa inhibitory activity. Long-chain, or higher-molecular-weight, heparins have a greater effect in their thrombin inhibitory activity, but are also able to inhibit factor Xa. At least an 18-saccharide unit chain is required for thrombin inhibition because heparin must be large enough to bind to ATIII and thrombin binding sites simultaneously. For factor Xa inhibition, heparin binding to ATIII is required, but simultaneous heparin binding to factor Xa does not occur.

Monitoring Anticoagulation

The activated clotting time (ACT) is the most commonly used confirmatory test for assessing heparin-induced anticoagulation. ACT is often criticized for its propensity to overestimate the anticoagulant response under conditions of hypothermia, hemodilution, or aprotinin therapy. Using ACT alone, patients may be potentially susceptible to a consumptive coagulopathy marked by thrombin-antithrombin III complexes, fibrinopeptide A, and prothrombin fragment 1.2 complexes. In 1978, Young and associates determined in monkeys that an ACT of 400 seconds or greater was needed to inhibit production of fibrin monomer during CPB.[45] Thus it is current practice in many institutions to administer a weight-based single bolus of heparin to achieve ACT of 400 seconds or greater. The protamine dose is then calculated based on the heparin dose given or by an in vitro protamine titration assay. Dosing schema for heparin and protamine that are based on patient weight do

not account for interpatient variability and may result in a relative overdose or underdose of either or both drugs. A number of different heparin and protamine management strategies have been reported with varying effects on microvascular coagulation and perioperative bleeding.

Heparin Concentration Monitoring

Heparin concentration monitoring can be performed with the Hepcon instrument (Medtronic Hemotec, Parker, Colo.), which measures ACT and calculates heparin concentration using an automated protamine titration. The measure of heparin concentration has been shown to better correlate with the anti-factor Xa activity on CPB than the Hemochron ACT,[46] because ACT increases in response to hypothermia and hemodilution. Despotis and associates have shown a reduction in chest closure time and reduced transfusion requirements when using Hepcon heparin management in association with a transfusion algorithm.[47] Individual heparin sensitivity can also be measured using this system by constructing heparin dose response curves using the ACT response to known in vitro concentrations of heparin. This allows for calculation of the required heparin dose based on each patient's sensitivity.

Hemochron RxDx

The Hemochron RxDx system is another point of care assay, whereby the baseline ACT, ACT in response to a known quantity of heparin (heparin response time), and an estimate of the patient's blood volume yield the dose-response relationship needed to calculate the heparin dose required to achieve a predetermined ACT. Similarly, using the patient's ACT and the ACT response to a known quantity of protamine (protamine response time), the protamine titration estimates the protamine dose needed to neutralize only the circulating heparin. The success of the RxDx system in predicting individual heparin and protamine doses has been reported by Jobes and associates,[48] who found less mediastinal tube drainage and a reduced incidence of transfusion. No differences in bleeding were reported in a subsequent study, possibly owing to tight control of post-CPB protamine administration.[49]

Antifibrinolytics Agents

There has been extensive interest in the use of antifibrinolytic agents to reduce bleeding in cardiovascular surgical procedures. The most widely used antifibrinolytic agents are epsilon aminocaproic acid (EACA), tranexamic acid (TA), and aprotinin. Aprotinin has unique antiprotease properties that will be summarized.

Aprotinin is a high-molecular-weight proteinase inhibitor of bovine origin that specifically inhibits trypsin, chymotrypsin, plasmin, and kallikrein in a dose dependent fashion. Because of its action on the latter two enzymes, aprotinin is effective in minimizing activation of the hematologic system during CPB and in preventing fibrinolysis.

Efficacy of Antifibrinolytic Activity

When administered in the full Hammersmith regimen, aprotinin has been shown to reduce perioperative blood loss and transfusion requirements in patients undergoing primary and repeat cardiac surgery, in patients with endocarditis, and in those with aspirin pretreatment.[50,51] The "high-dose" administered in this regimen is 2 million kallikrein-inhibiting units (KIU) as a loading dose, 2 million KIU added to the pump priming solution, and 500,000 KIU/hr as an infusion. Beneficial effects have also been documented using "low-dose" aprotinin (half and quarter Hammersmith doses) and a single pump prime dose. The use of aprotinin in high or low dose has been shown superior to placebo in reducing chest tube drainage, limiting transfusion requirements, and creating a dry surgical field.

The cost of high-dose aprotinin (approximately $1000 per patient) has stimulated interest in the use of lower-dose regimens and in the use of synthetic antifibrinolytic agents, which are considerably less expensive and potentially adequately efficacious in reducing transfusions. These agents are EACA and TA, which act as lysine analogs and bind to the lysine binding sites of plasmin and plasminogen, thereby preventing their activity. Plasmin and fibrin degradation products have adverse effects on platelet function and are associated with hydrolysis of the platelet glycoprotein 1b (GP1b) receptor. Plasmin inhibition may therefore contribute to some form of indirect platelet protection; however, the major mechanism whereby these agents reduce bleeding in cardiac surgery is through direct inhibition of fibrinolysis. Standard-dose regimens include EACA 150 mg/kg followed by 15 mg/kg/hr, although other dose schedules have been used successfully (10 g × 3 doses). TA has a wide variation in dosing applications. Some investigators have administered large doses of 5 to 10 g and have shown efficacy without adverse sequelae.[52] Horrow studied the dose response of TA and found 10 mg/kg followed by 1 mg/kg/hr to be the minimum effective dose.[53]

Compared with placebo, the synthetic antifibrinolytic agents effectively attenuate markers of fibrinolysis and have blood-sparing properties that are most apparent during higher-risk surgical procedures.[54] When the synthetic agents are compared with aprotinin, aprotinin reduces blood loss to a greater degree; however, differences in transfusion requirements are much more difficult to elicit.

Antiinflammatory Activity

The *whole-body inflammatory response* to CPB is a constellation of cascades that become activated as a result of contact of blood with the nonendothelial surfaces of the extracorporeal circuit. The activated cascades include the coagulation system, the fibrinolytic system, and the complement cascade. This is marked by an increase in cytokine levels and leukocyte activation markers. Cytokines that increase during the systemic inflammatory response include tumor necrosis factor α, interleukin (IL)-1, IL-6, IL-8, and others. Antiinflammatory cytokines decrease during CPB. Leukocyte activation markers and cytokine levels are increased after CPB for up to 24 hours postoperatively.

Many technologic and pharmacologic interventions have been investigated for their ability to reduce the inflammatory response to CPB. As mentioned, the widespread use of membrane oxygenators has reduced overall cellular activation during CPB in comparison with the older bubble oxygenators. Pharmacologic interventions are also widely used as antiinflammatory measures. Steroids are well known for their antiinflammatory effects. Concerns of increased risk of infection caused a reduction in the use of steroids in the last decade, but recent interest in attenuating the inflammatory response has caused a renewed interest in their use. As a result of aprotinin's antikallikrein activity, the use of high-dose aprotinin attenuates the inflammatory response to CPB, and minimizes elevations of IL-6 and leukocyte elastase. In a randomized prospective study in 20 patients, aprotinin therapy reduced airway nitric oxide (NO) production and reduced the in vitro expression of messenger RNA for NO synthesis.[55] Aprotinin has also been shown to increase the concentration of the antiinflammatory cytokine IL-10[56] (Fig. 12-3). Hill and associates elegantly demonstrated that these antiinflammatory effects are not achieved with the synthetic antifibrinolytic agents.[57]

Antiinflammatory effects of aprotinin are achieved at concentrations greater than 200 to 400 KIU/ml. These plasma levels are reliably obtained after treatment with the high-dose regimen. Clinical studies comparing the antiinflammatory potency of high-dose aprotinin with that of methylprednisolone reveal comparable degrees of attenuated inflammatory markers[58] (Fig. 12-4). In dogs, a randomized comparison of aprotinin versus placebo was undertaken in a coronary occlusion and reperfusion model. Animals that received high-dose aprotinin demonstrated preserved regional myocardial contractility and systolic shortening compared with pla-

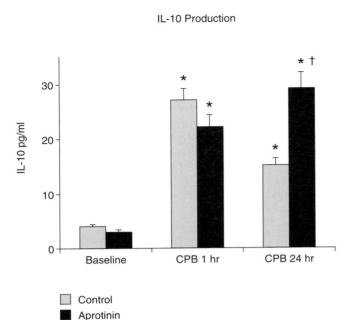

IL-10 Production

FIG. 12-3 Twenty patients were randomized to receive high-dose aprotinin or placebo (control) for cardiopulmonary bypass. At 24 hours postoperatively, aprotinin enhanced the release of the antiinflammatory cytokine interleukin (IL)-10 (*p < 0.05 vs. baseline; †p < 0.05 vs. control).

(Modified from Hill GE, Diego RP, Stammers AH et al: *Ann Thorac Surg* 65:66-69, 1998.)

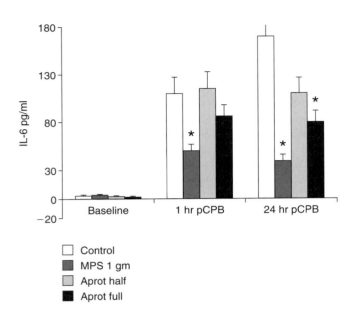

Aprotinin and Methylprednisolone: Antiinflammatory effects

FIG. 12-4 Forty adult cardiac surgical patients were randomized to receive placebo (control), low-dose aprotinin, high-dose aprotinin, or methylprednisolone. Only high-dose aprotinin and methylprednisolone successfully reduced the expression of the proinflammatory cytokine interleukin (IL)-6 (*p < 0.05).

(Modified from Diego RP, Mihalakakos PJ, Hexum TD et al: *J Cardiothorac Vasc Anesth* 11:29-31, 1997.)

cebo. The mechanism of this protection was not studied, but was postulated as an antiinflammatory effect.[59]

Outcome has been shown to be significantly improved by aprotinin therapy in the pediatric population.[60] Whether this is a result of an attenuation of the inflammatory response or just a result of reduced transfusions has yet to be determined.

Thrombotic Complications of Antifibrinolytic Therapy

Agents that promote hemostasis impose the theoretic risk of thrombotic complications. Although reports and case studies exist that document thrombotic complications of these agents, the documentation is largely anecdotal and fails to account for other preexisting thrombosis risks. At one large institution, the incidence of stroke after cardiac surgery does not appear to have increased since the widespread pervasive use of EACA.[61]

Thrombosis is less likely to occur using high-dose aprotinin therapy because the plasma levels achieved cause kallikrein inhibition, which induces a mild anticoagulant effect. Nevertheless, an increased incidence of

myocardial infarction (MI), which was corroborated by intracoronary thromboses seen on autopsy evaluation, was found in cardiac reoperation patients.[62] However, the patients in this study were likely to have received subtherapeutic heparin doses because of prolongation of the celite-ACT measurements by aprotinin. Because the celite ACT is synergistically prolonged in the presence of aprotinin and heparin, it is necessary to maintain celite ACT of more than 800 seconds or to use another method of anticoagulation monitoring (kaolin ACT, heparin concentration, high-dose thrombin time). In a prospective multinational study, graft patency and MI rates were compared in placebo and aprotinin therapy groups. Although there was no difference in the incidence of MI between groups, there was a slight increased risk of graft nonpatency in the aprotinin group; this increase disappeared when the data were adjusted for surgical risk factors[63] (Fig. 12-5).

Vascular Cannulation

Vascular cannulation can be initiated once appropriate anticoagulation has been achieved. The venous cannula

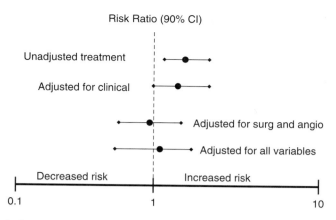

FIG. 12-5 Graft patency relative risk ratio and 90% confidence interval *(CI)* for aprotinin versus placebo in a multicenter randomized controlled trial. Unadjusted data showed slight increase in risk. When data were adjusted for clinical variables, surgical *(surg)* and angiographic *(angio)* risk factors, and all risk factors, the statistical significance of the risk ratio disappeared. (Modified from Alderman EL, Levy JH, Rich JB et al: *J Thorac Cardiovasc Surg* 116:716-730, 1998.)

diverts blood from the patient at low venous pressures to the CPB pump, while the arterial cannula returns oxygenated blood back to the arterial circulation at sufficient pressures and flows necessary to maintain vital organ perfusion.

Arterial Cannulation

Arterial cannulation is routinely achieved before venous cannulation for a number of reasons. First, once arterial cannulation is established, transfusion is possible, and this becomes particularly useful when venous cannulation is associated with massive hemorrhage. Second, arterial cannulation allows transfusion of oxygenated blood if cardiac decompensation occurs before venous cannulation. In the situation when only the arterial cannula has been positioned, emergency CPB (or sucker-bypass) takes place. The cardiotomy suckers provide the venous return and the arterial cannula provides systemic perfusion.

Arterial cannulation is ordinarily accomplished through the ascending aorta; the femoral artery remains a necessary alternative location. The ascending aorta is usually preferred because it allows placement of a larger cannula, positioned proximal to the innominate artery but distal to the proposed sites for the proximal anastomoses of coronary bypass grafts. The ascending aorta is also more favorable than the femoral artery because the risk of dissection and lower-extremity neurologic deficits are reduced when compared with the femoral artery.[25] Complications of arterial cannulation include malposition, dissection, embolism, and hemorrhage.

The femoral artery is an appropriate alternative when massive hemorrhage is anticipated during sternotomy or mediastinal dissections (i.e., during reoperations). It is also one of the recommended cannulation sites for patients with severe atherosclerosis, an ascending aortic aneurysm or dissection, or known cystic medial necrosis.[64] Unfortunately, the risk of arterial dissection is greater with femoral cannulation (0.5%-0.9%)[25] compared with proximal aortic cannulation (0.02%-0.35%).[25,65,66] Although a higher number of surgical complications may occur with femoral cannulation, cerebral perfusion, as determined by electroencephalogram monitoring, is not different than with aortic cannulation.[67]

Venous Cannulation

Venous cannulation is typically established via the RA. Usually, a two-staged single cannula is placed into the right atrial appendage. The single cannula has fenestrations at two locations. When properly positioned, this allows for drainage of the RA/SVC and IVC. All blood, including blood entering the RA via coronary sinus, is diverted from the heart. One major advantage of the single cannula is that only one cannulation site is required. However, the limitation of the single cannula is that access to the RA is restricted because of the size and position of the cannula itself. Any malposition of the cannula is detected by a reduction in venous return back to the pump.

Bicaval cannulation is necessary for many open-heart procedures that require access to the atria or atrioventricular valves. For these procedures, one cannula is necessary to cannulate the SVC and another to cannulate the IVC. All blood is diverted away from the heart. Malposition of either cannula results in obstruction of venous return. IVC obstruction is typically detected only by decreased venous drainage, whereas SVC obstruction can be detected by venous engorgement of the head and neck, edema of the conjunctiva, and an elevation in the measured central venous pressure (CVP). CVP should be measured from the sideport of the pulmonary artery (PA) catheter introducer to monitor SVC pressure.

Femoral venous cannulation is advantageous during emergent CPB and reoperations because it does not require sternotomy. The femoral cannula is inserted into the femoral vein and advanced into the IVC and RA. Femoral venous cannulation is advantageous because it may be performed emergently without sternotomy. However, it is less effective than either bicaval cannulation or the two-staged cannula because of its smaller size and flow limitations.

Complications of Vascular Cannulation

Safety of CPB requires vigilance on the part of the anesthesiologist, perfusionist, and surgeon. Problems must be identified and diagnosed early, and treatment should be prompt. Most of the following problems are likely to occur as CPB is initiated. However, they may occur at any time during CPB.

Aortic Dissection. Aortic dissection occurs during the cannulation process when the cannula causes a separation of the intimal wall from the media and adventitia, thereby creating a false lumen for blood flow. Diagnosis is made when a low or zero blood pressure is measured in the radial or femoral arterial line. In addition, the perfusionist detects a high "arterial line pressure," and myocardial ischemia or aortic insufficiency may occur. Transesophageal echocardiography is useful in the visualization of aortic dissection (Fig. 12-6).

Prevention of aortic dissection is primarily surgical. However, the degree of damage is minimized by the vigilance of the anesthesiologist and perfusionist. It is common practice to decrease arterial pressure during cannulation and removal of the aortic cannula. A very effective and readily reversible technique is to temporarily clamp the IVC for aortic cannulation as a means of lowering aortic wall tension (R. F. DiMarco, Jr., personal communication to editor). Treatment of aortic dissection begins with the discontinuation of pump flow, repositioning and replacement of the arterial cannula, and repair of the dissection.

Arterial Cannula Malposition. Malposition of the arterial cannula may result in carotid or innominate artery hyperperfusion.[68-71] Essentially all the pump outflow is directed into a carotid artery, typically the right. Complications include cerebral edema and arterial rupture. Ipsilateral blanching of the face, or ipsilateral pupil dilation, in the presence of low radial or femoral arterial pressures may also occur. A right radial artery may reveal hypertension resulting from innominate artery hyperperfusion. Presence of a thrill with neck palpation over both carotid arteries may indicate aortic cannula malposition.

Cannula Reversal. If the CPB circuitry were accidentally reversed, the results would be catastrophic. The venous drainage would be connected to the arterial cannula and the arterial inflow would be connected to the RA or vena cava. Ultimately, blood would be drained from the aorta, resulting in systemic arterial hypotension. Blood would be returned through the venous system at high pressure, causing the rupture of veins. Arterial hypotension, facial edema, and severe venous congestion provide the diagnosis of cannula reversal. CVP pressures would be elevated, and surgical palpation would reveal a flaccid aorta and tense vena cava. Although some organs can be perfused in a retrograde fashion, cannula reversal is clearly catastrophic. Surgical vigilance is the primary prevention.

If cannula reversal has been identified, immediate termination of CPB is essential. The patient should be placed in a steep Trendelenburg position to maintain cerebral perfusion. The cannulas and tubing should be inspected for air, and appropriately de-aired. Once the tubing is properly connected, CPB should resume.

Massive Gas Embolism. Massive gas embolism is a major catastrophic event, resulting in stroke, MI, end organ damage, or death. Gas emboli consist of either air or oxygen. Causes of massive gas emboli in-

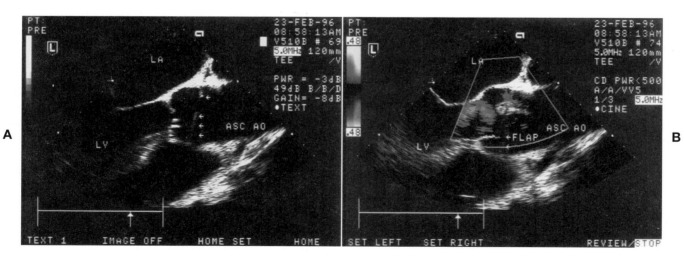

FIG. 12-6   **A,** Aortic dissection can occur during the cannulation process when the cannula causes a separation of the intimal wall from the media and adventitia, creating a false lumen for blood flow. **B,** Doppler illustrates the flow of blood across the intimal tear.

clude pumping air through an empty reservoir, low reservoir level, disconnection within the CPB circuit, reversal of pump-head tubing, reversal of pump-head rotational direction, and a clotted oxygenator. Additional causes include ejection of blood before de-airing after open-chamber procedures, inadequate air removal after cardiotomy, PA suctioning that entrains air, a pressurized cardiotomy reservoir, and an aortic line not clamped at the end of CPB. A vented arterial-line filter on the pump is a recommended safety device that reduces embolization.

In an 8-year study comprising 3620 CPB operations from multiple centers, Mills and associates reported 13 instances of massive air embolism. Emergency air-embolism protocol was followed. Four patients died instantaneously. Three patients experienced cerebral injury that resolved within 2 months. The remaining patients did not develop neurologic sequelae.[72] Mills and associates stated that "prevention includes a systematic check of pump suckers and perfusion lines before bypass, a sensing device on the oxygenator reservoir, secure fixation of the oxygenator and avoidance of traffic around pump equipment."[72] They also recommended "immediate cessation of pump flow and inspection for abnormal noise, use of standard maneuvers to remove air from the heart, and carotid compression with resumption of heartbeat."[72]

An emergency air-embolism protocol involves placing the patient in steep Trendelenburg and creating an aortotomy in the ascending aorta for retrograde drainage from the cerebrovascular bed. The aortic cannula is removed and the air vented from the cannulation site. Temporary retrograde perfusion through the SVC may also be used. Subsequent steps include resuming CPB with hypothermia, elevating perfusion pressure, administering systemic steroids, ventilating with 100% oxygen, and initiating deep barbiturate anesthesia[72] (Table 12-1).

Venous Air Lock. An *air lock* occurs when air enters the venous outflow line, resulting in slowing or complete cessation of venous blood flow to the CPB reservoir. The volume of blood that can be delivered to the patient's arterial circulation becomes limited. Once a venous air lock is discovered, CPB should be discontinued, if possible, until the source of the venous line air is identified. CPB may resume when the problem has been corrected.

Other Preparations

Before initiating CPB, the patient is appropriately anesthetized. CPB causes a dilution of anesthetics and muscle relaxants. Supplemental intravenous anesthetics and muscle relaxants should be administered with the initiation of CPB.

There is a tendency for the PA catheter to migrate in the pulmonary arterial system as a result of redundant catheter length, manipulation of the heart, and intracardiac volume depletion. The catheter should be pulled back approximately 3 to 5 cm before initiating CPB to prevent advancement of the PA catheter into the wedge position that may lead to PA rupture.[73] If transesophageal echocardiography (TEE) is used for surgery, it should be placed into the "freeze" mode and in a neutral position to avoid thermal and physical injury to the esophagus during hypothermic CPB.

MANAGEMENT OF CARDIOPULMONARY BYPASS
Initiation

The perfusionist, anesthesiologist, and surgeon must work in a coordinated fashion to ensure that CPB is smoothly initiated. The clamps are removed from the venous line and venous blood is drained from the patient into the CPB circuit. Mechanical obstruction, SVC engorgement, and venous air lock must be identified and promptly treated. Oxygenation of the blood and perfusion of vital organs are assessed. The arterial blood should be bright red, whereas the venous blood is darker. The surgeon and perfusionist should be notified immediately if the arterial blood is not a brighter red. A malfunctioning oxygenator or cannula reversal may be the cause.

Arterial inflow must be assessed as bypass is initiated. Systemic hypotension commonly occurs because of an acute reduction in blood viscosity because of hemodilution. A mean arterial pressure less than 30 mm Hg may indicate an aortic dissection, which must be diagnosed immediately. A high arterial-line pressure or a carotid thrill may indicate malposition of the arterial cannula. This must also be recognized and treated promptly.

Once complete CPB is achieved, ventilation is discontinued. Complete collapse of the lungs provides optimal surgical exposure and a still surgical field. No beneficial effects have been demonstrated by ventilating the lungs during CPB. Ventilation of nonperfused lungs in an attempt to prevent postoperative atelectasis may increase intrapulmonary shunting.[74]

CVP and pulmonary artery pressure (PAP) should be near zero during complete CPB. Cannulation sites, venous drainage, PA catheter position, and CPB tubing should be inspected. The arterial waveform will become nonpulsatile when the aorta is cross-clamped.

Pump Flow

CPB pump flow must be adequate to meet the demands of oxygen consumption, which varies with temperature. Pump flow is adjusted to maintain adequate oxygen delivery at various temperatures. Nomograms

TABLE 12-1
Protocol for Treating Massive Gas Embolism

1. Stop CPB immediately.
2. Place patient in steep Trendelenburg position.
3. Remove aortic cannula; vent air from aortic cannulation site.
4. De-air arterial cannula and pump line.
5. Institute hypothermic retrograde SVC perfusion by connecting arterial pump line to the SVC cannula with caval tape tightened. Blood at 20°-24° C is injected into the SVC at 1-2 L/min or more, and air plus blood is drained from the aortic root cannulation site to the pump.
6. Carotid compression is performed intermittently during retrograde SVC perfusion to allow retrograde purging of air from the vertebral arteries.
7. Maintain retrograde SVC perfusion for at least 1-2 min. Continue for an additional 1-2 min if air continues to exit from aorta.
8. In extensive systemic air injection accidents in which emboli to splanchnic, renal, or femoral circulation are suspected, retrograde IVC perfusion may be performed after head de-airing procedures are completed. This is performed while the carotid arteries are clamped and the patient is in head-up position to facilitate removal of air through the aortic root vent but prevent reembolization of the brain.
9. When no additional air can be expelled, resume anterograde CPB, maintaining hypothermia at 20° C for at least 40-45 min. Lowering patient temperature is important because increased gas solubility helps to resorb bubbles and because decreased metabolic demands may limit ischemic damage before bubble resorption.
10. Induce hypertension with vasoconstrictor drugs. Hydrostatic pressure shrinks bubbles; also, bubbles occluding arterial bifurcations are pushed into one vessel, opening the other branch.
11. Express coronary air by massage and needle venting.
12. Steroids may be administered, although this is controversial. The usual dose of methylprednisolone is 30 mg/kg.
13. Barbiturate coma should be considered if the embolism occurred during warm CPB and if the myocardium will be able to tolerate the significant negative inotropy. Thiopental, 10 mg/kg loading dose plus infusion of 1-3 mg/kg/hr, may be used empirically. If EEG monitoring is available, titration of barbiturate to an EEG burst-suppression (1 burst/min) pattern is preferable.
14. Patient is weaned from CPB.
15. Continue ventilating the patient with 100% O_2 for at least 6 hr to maximize the blood-alveolar gradient for elimination of N_2.
16. A hyperbaric chamber (if locally available) can accelerate resorption of residual bubbles. However, the risk of moving a critically ill patient must be weighed against the potential benefits.

Modified from Mills NL, Ochsner JL: *J Thorac Cardiovasc Surg* 80:712, 1980.
CPB, Cardiopulmonary bypass; *EEG*, electroencephalogram; *IVC*, inferior vena cava; *SVC*, superior vena cava.
Note: This protocol should be reviewed together by all members of the cardiac team every 3 months.

exist for adjusting perfusion flow based on temperature (Fig. 12-7).

Temperature, hemodilution, and arterial resistance determine the relationship between pump flow and pressure during CPB. During hypothermic CPB, pump flows of 1.2 L/min/m^2 perfuse the majority of the microcirculation when the hematocrit is 22%. Cerebral blood flow autoregulation remains intact at 20° C, and flows of 1.2 L/min/m^2 have been shown to be adequate despite limited reserves.[75]

Fifty percent hemodilution during CPB is considered safe. In the presence of cyanotic heart disease, hemodilution should be less than 40%, even in the presence of polycythemia.[77] Adequate perfusion is monitored by the mixed venous oxygen saturation, which should be maintained greater than 70%. This does not guarantee

appropriate perfusion to all tissues during CPB.[78] An important sign of adequate renal perfusion is urinary output. Low urine output does not always indicate renal hypoperfusion, but elevating the mean arterial pressure (MAP) with vasoconstrictors or volume is appropriate in an attempt to increase the urine output. Interestingly, MAP during CPB has not been shown to predict postoperative renal dysfunction. Instead, important predictors of renal dysfunction and acute renal failure following CPB are preoperative left ventricular dysfunction and prolonged cardiopulmonary bypass.[76]

Blood Pressure

The management of blood pressure during CPB depends on pump flow and systemic vascular resistance

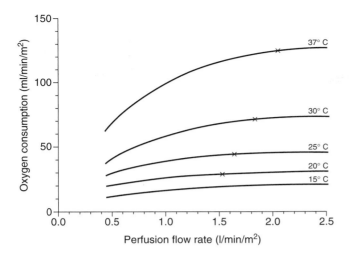

FIG. 12-7 A nomogram for perfusion flow based on temperature, illustrating the relationship of temperature, perfusion flow rates, and oxygen consumption.

(From Kirklin JW, Baratt-Boyes BG: *Cardiac surgery*, New York, 1986, Wiley, p 35.)

(SVR). For patients with unaltered cerebral autoregulation, the MAP is usually maintained above 40 to 50 mm Hg. However, patients with impaired organ flow (i.e., carotid stenosis) or altered autoregulation (i.e., hypertension) typically require higher MAP during CPB.

Blood pressure can be adjusted by varying pump flow or SVR. Pump pressure is determined by temperature and oxygen consumption, which is seen in the nomogram (see Fig. 12-7). Although the pump flow can be altered to change blood pressure, this maneuver should be limited. For example, increasing pump flow to accommodate a low SVR may increase blood cell trauma, and decreasing the pump flow to compensate for a high SVR may result in inadequate tissue perfusion and metabolic acidosis. Once pump flow is determined, further adjustments in blood pressure should be accomplished by altering the SVR.

Increasing SVR is the primary means of increasing blood pressure during CPB. α-Adrenergic agonists are most commonly used in this situation. Phenylephrine boluses (80-200 μg) are used first, and may be repeated to maintain blood pressure. Patients who are refractory to phenylephrine may require boluses of methoxamine (1-5 mg). Norepinephrine is another alternative, which is commonly administered through an infusion pump into the venous reservoir or central venous catheter.

Blood pressure is decreased primarily by lowering SVR. Intravenous anesthetics such as narcotics and benzodiazepines are used to ensure hypnosis and may serve to lower SVR as well. Benzodiazepines are particularly useful in situations where awareness is a concern. Volatile anesthetics may be administered through a calibrated vaporizer in the oxygenator gas-inlet line. Isoflu-

rane reliably produces peripheral vasodilation, is safe for coronary artery bypass graft (CABG)[79] and valvular surgery,[80] and diminishes the cortisol response to CPB.[81] Volatile anesthetics are usually discontinued when the aortic cross-clamp is removed to ensure sufficient washout time before separation from CPB. Propofol infusions (50-100 μg/kg/min) and direct-acting vasodilators, such as sodium nitroprusside infusion (1-5 μg/kg/min) or trimethaphan boluses (1-5 mg), may also be used. α-Adrenergic blockers and calcium channel blockers may also be useful, though some calcium channel blockers may cause cardiac depression.

Nonpulsatile versus Pulsatile Flow

There is considerable controversy in the literature regarding pulsatile versus nonpulsatile pump flow. Many studies support the benefits of pulsatile flow,[82-86,88-93] whereas others do not.[87,94] Those in support have shown that pulsatile flow is more physiologic because it attenuates the hormonal stress response to CPB,[88] reduces vasopressin levels,[89-91] and maintains thyroid hormone metabolism.[92] Pulsatile flow diminishes fluid overloading,[95] protects pulmonary function,[96] and may reduce the incidence of postoperative hypertension following CPB.[82] However, others have noted that routine CPB does not alter adrenocortical function and that the addition of pulsatile flow produces little improvement.[97] Studies have demonstrated no difference in hemodynamics,[98] neurologic outcome,[36,99-101] or renal function[102] with pulsatile flow. Pulsatile perfusion for core cooling and rewarming of infants is considered safe and more physiologic than nonpulsatile perfusion.[83]

Acid-Base

Acid-base management during CPB is the subject of another controversial debate in the cardiac surgery literature.[36,103-110] The two strategies for managing acid-base status during hypothermia during CPB are the α-stat and pH-stat methods. Gas solubility for oxygen and carbon dioxide is inversely proportional to temperature. The blood gas instrument calculates pH, Pao_2 and $Paco_2$ for a range of hypothermic temperatures using an internal nomogram, but the arterial blood gas is normally reported at body temperature (37° C).

The cerebral vasculature and cerebral blood flow are sensitive to $Paco_2$. For example, an increase in $Paco_2$ decreases cerebral vascular resistance, which increases cerebral blood flow. Conversely, decreases in $Paco_2$ increase cerebral vascular resistance, which decreases cerebral blood flow. During hypothermic conditions, more CO_2 dissolves in the blood, which results in a decrease in (gaseous) $Paco_2$ and a respiratory alkalosis.

With the α-stat management method, no correction of CO_2 is made for the patient's actual temperature.

Despite hypothermia, the blood gas is determined at 37° C and reported at 37° C. pH is maintained at 7.4 with a $Paco_2$ of 40 mm Hg, and the patient has a relative alkalosis (lower $Paco_2$)at actual body temperature. Oxygenator and gas flows are adjusted to maintain a "normothermic" blood gas pH of 7.4 and $Paco_2$ of 40 mm Hg. The α-stat strategy is considered more physiologic than the pH-stat method because the ionization state of histidine remains constant throughout all temperature ranges, which preserves protein structure and function.

During pH-stat acid-base management strategy, the reported blood gases are adjusted for the patient's actual blood temperature. The pH-stat method maintains a pH of 7.4 and a $Paco_2$ of 40 mm Hg after correction for body temperature. To maintain normal temperature-adjusted pH and $Paco_2$, CO_2 gas must be added to oxygenator gas mixture, because the $Paco_2$ measured values are lower for a given volume of CO_2 in the blood.

The pH-stat blood gas strategy was once considered advantageous because the cerebral dilatory effects of CO_2 increase cerebral blood flow and ultimately decrease the risk of cerebral ischemia.[103] This increase in cerebral blood flow may actually increase the risk of embolization, produce a "steal" phenomenon,[104] and impair autoregulation of the cerebral vasculature.[105]

The α-stat strategy decreases cerebral blood flow and metabolism, whereas pH-stat strategy results in uncoupling by increasing cerebral blood flow and decreasing metabolism. Stephan and associates compared both strategies and found no statistically significant differences between the metabolic variables. Cerebral blood flow and cerebral metabolism normalized after rewarming independently of acid-base management during hypothermia. However, postoperative neurologic dysfunction occurred more often in the pH-stat group.[106] Other investigators have found that the α-stat management preserves cerebral blood flow and metabolism.[107,108]

Unfortunately, the outcome studies in the literature have conflicting results.[36,106,109,110] Although Murkin and associates found that α-stat management is associated with a decreased incidence of postoperative cognitive dysfunction in patients undergoing prolonged CPB,[36] others have suggested that at moderate hypothermia neither pH management strategy has any clinically significant effect on neurologic or cardiac outcomes.[110] For patients with normal preoperative renal function, the method of pH management does not affect perioperative renal function,[102] and during moderate hypothermic CPB oxygen delivery is not affected by the pH-stat strategy used.[109]

Temperature

Thermoregulation is impaired during anesthesia for cardiac surgery. Traditionally, CPB was performed with

hypothermia because cerebral metabolism and cerebral blood flow are reduced and the brain is protected from hypoxic injury.[78,111] Unfortunately, hypothermia also results in coagulopathies, poor wound healing, delayed awakening, and decreased metabolism of most anesthetic drugs and muscle relaxants. Normothermic ("warm") bypass techniques have been proposed, although normothermia during CPB may however decrease the brain's tolerance to the ischemic injury. Active warming during cardiopulmonary bypass (≥35° C) has been shown to increase the risk of perioperative neurologic injury in patients undergoing elective coronary artery revascularization.[112] However, maintenance of normothermia may facilitate early tracheal extubation.

It has been suggested that a compromise of mild hypothermia (34° C) may be the optimal condition for fast-track patients.[113] Mild hypothermia is potentially beneficial to the patient, providing protection from cerebral ischemia and hypoxemia.

Nevertheless, whole-body rewarming should occur evenly to prevent subsequent decreases in core body temperature. In addition to the esophageal temperature probe, peripheral temperature should be monitored with a rectal, bladder, or cutaneous probe.[114,115]

Cardioplegia Solutions

Cardioplegia is a dextrose solution necessary for myocardial preservation during CPB. In addition to many homeostatic electrolytes, it contains bicarbonate, mannitol, insulin, and a high concentration of potassium. After the aortic cross-clamp is placed, the heart is arrested in diastole with anterograde and/or retrograde cardioplegia.

Anterograde cardioplegia is administered into the aorta or coronary ostia, whereas retrograde cardioplegia is delivered into the coronary sinus. Typically, anterograde cardioplegia is administered at a rate of 200 to 300 ml/min with aortic root pressures between 60 and 100 mm Hg. A flow rate of 200 ml/min is optimal for preservation of ventricular function.[116] Patients with atherosclerosis or aortic insufficiency may have inadequate delivery of anterograde cardioplegia. Retrograde cardioplegia, which preserves left ventricular function better than anterograde cardioplegia, is considered a superior technique.[117]

Coronary collateral flow may actually impede cardioplegic myocardial protection in patients with extensive disease because it warms the myocardium and increases metabolism.[118]

Blood cardioplegia protects the myocardium and allows quick recovery of cardiac contractility with reperfusion.[119] Cold and warm continuous blood cardioplegia appear to preserve myocardial function, but cold cardioplegia is preferred by some because of the known benefit of hypothermia.[120] The use of intermittent warm-blood cardioplegia may not be as beneficial as continuous warm-blood cardioplegia. Intermittent warm-blood cardioplegia was compared with continuous warm-blood cardioplegia in porcine hearts exposed to global ischemia. Continuous warm-blood cardioplegia preserved left ventricular function better than intermittent warm-blood cardioplegia.[121] RV function is also protected using continuous warm cardioplegia.[122] One study found that retrograde warm-blood cardioplegia may be safer than anterograde cardioplegia.[123]

SEPARATION FROM CARDIOPULMANARY BYPASS
Preparation

The first step toward separation from CPB is rewarming, which occurs after removal of the aortic cross-clamp. Normothermia must be restored gradually. Skin surface warming preserves perioperative thermal balance and reduces bleeding following cardiac surgery.[124] Cerebral temperatures above 37° C may result in neurologic injury.[125] SVR decreases during rewarming because of vasodilation. Vasopressors are often necessary to maintain adequate perfusion pressure. The brain equilibrates with blood temperature very rapidly during rewarming so that intraoperative awareness becomes a real possibility. Additional intravenous anesthesia and muscle relaxation are commonly administered.

Spontaneous myocardial activity commences during rewarming. Occasionally, ventricular fibrillation, heart block, or other dysrhythmias may occur. Direct current countershock is usually effective in converting ventricular fibrillation to an organized rhythm, and heart block often resolves spontaneously. Ventricular and/or atrial pacing may be necessary.

Before terminating the bypass, an arterial blood gas (ABG) sample is analyzed for pH, Pao_2, $Paco_2$, hemoglobin, and hematocrit. Electrolytes, including, Na^{++}, K^+, and ionized Ca^{++}, are also measured. Any abnormality in ABG, electrolytes, or hematocrit should be corrected before separating from CPB.

Separation from CPB cannot occur without the restoration of lung ventilation. Initially sustained positive pressure (20-40 cm H_2O) breaths are provided to reinflate areas of atelectasis. Mechanical ventilation is resumed with 100% oxygen, and all monitors and alarms are reactivated.

Intracardiac air is introduced in all open cardiac procedures, and may also be present in closed procedures. Removal of air is believed to prevent cerebral emboli, although the presence of intracardiac air is not predictive of neurologic injury.[126] The patient is placed in the Trendelenburg position until most of the intracardiac air has been eliminated, as evidenced by direct surgical inspection or TEE. A variety of de-airing techniques

TABLE 12-2
Vasoactive Medications for Separation from Cardiopulmonary Bypass

DRUG	DOSE
Amrinone	0.75-1.5 mg/kg loading dose
	5-10 µg/kg/min
Dobutamine	2.5-10 µg/kg/min
Dopamine	2-20 µg/kg/min
Epinephrine	0.05-0.2 µg/kg/min
Esmolol	0.50 mg/kg loading dose
	100 µg/kg/min
Isoproterenol	0.01-0.05 µg/kg/min
Milrinone	50 µg/kg loading dose
	0.375-0.75 µg/kg/min
Nitroglycerin	0.5-5.0 µg/kg/min
Nitroprusside	0.1-5.0 µg/kg/min
Norepinephrine	0.05-0.2 µg/kg/min
Phenylephrine	0.1-5.0 µg/kg/min
Vasopressin	1.0-8.0 units/hr

have been used, but no one technique has been shown superior.[127]

Strategies for Weaning

The beating heart is examined before weaning CPB. If the heart appears vigorous and ejects blood, difficulty in separating from CPB is unlikely. A poorly contracting heart indicates difficulty in separating from CPB. Inotropic agents such as dobutamine, dopamine, and epinephrine should be administered to improve contractility (Table 12-2). In addition to assessing ventricular function, early assessment of SVR is important for selecting the appropriate vasopressor, vasodilator, or vasoactive combination (see Table 12-2). LV volume status is optimized during and immediately following separation from CPB.

Termination of CPB

Termination of CPB requires communication between the surgeon, perfusionist, and anesthesiologist. As the patient meets criteria for separation from bypass, the perfusionist gradually clamps the venous tubing, which decreases blood flow to the CPB reservoir and increases venous return to the heart. At the same time, the arterial pump head is slowed, and blood is gradually transfused to the patient via the arterial cannula. Appropriate preload is established and a pulsatile arterial waveform resumes. Adequate biventricular function is determined by visual and TEE evaluation of the heart, systemic blood pressure, PA catheter waveform, and CVP, allowing discontinuation of the arterial transfusion and termination of CPB.

Mechanical Assist Devices

Inadequate myocardial protection or severely compromised prebypass ventricular function may make weaning from CPB difficult and challenging. Indications for mechanical assist devices include left or right ventricular failure despite maximal intravenous inotropic therapy (Tables 12-3 and 12-4). Several ventricular assist devices are currently used in cardiac surgical practice (Table 12-5). Some devices provide temporary circulatory support, whereas others are more permanent.

TABLE 12-3
Post-CPB Maximal Inotropic Support: The Use of Two or More Intravenous Inotropic Agents Listed in Table 12-2

Amrinone >10 μg/kg/min (after loading dose 0.75-1.5 mg/kg)
Dobutamine >10 μg/kg/min
Dopamine >10 μg/kg/min
Epinephrine >0.2 μg/kg/min
Milrinone >0.75 μg/kg/min (after loading dose 50 μg/kg)

_____
CPB, Cardiopulmonary bypass.

TABLE 12-4
Post-CPB Ventricular Failure (may be left and/or right ventricular failure)

LEFT VENTRICULAR FAILURE	RIGHT VENTRICULAR FAILURE
Cardiac index <1.8-2.0 L/min/m^2 SBP <90 mm Hg' MAP <70 mm Hg LAP >18-25 mm Hg	Cardiac index <1.8-2.0 L/min/m^2 SBP <90 mm Hg' MAP <70 mm Hg RAP >18-25 mm Hg

_____
CPB, Cardiopulmonary bypass; LAP, left atrial pressure; MAP, mean arterial pressure; RAP, right atrial pressure; SBP, systolic blood pressure.

TABLE 12-5
Mechanical Circulatory Assist Devices

CLASSIFICATION	SUBTYPES	INDICATIONS	CONTRAINDICATIONS
Intraaortic balloon pump		Refractory myocardial ischemia Cardiogenic shock Stabilization before surgery (i.e., left main disease) Postcardiac surgery (reversible LV dysfunction, intraoperative MI)	Aortic insufficiency Aortic dissection Aortic aneurysm
Centrifugal pumps	Bio-Medicus Centramed Medtronic Terumo	LVS, RVS, BVS Short term or intermediate	Long term (i.e., mobile patient)
Ventricular assist devices	Thoratec TCI (Heartmate) Novacor Abiomed BVS 5000	All LVAD, RVAD, BVAD except Novacor (LVAD only) Short term: Abiomed Intermediate or long term: Thoratec Long term: TCI and Novacor (bridge to cardiac transplant)	Mechanical aortic valve Severe aortic insufficiency
Total artificial heart	Cardiowest artificial heart	Bridge to cardiac transplant	Patients not suitable for transplant

_____
BVAD, Biventricular assist device; BVS, biventricular support; LVAD, left ventricular assist device; LVS, left ventricular support; RVAD, right ventricular assist device; RVS, right ventricular support.

MANAGEMENT FOLLOWING CARDIOPULMONARY BYPASS
Reversal of Anticoagulation

Heparin-induced anticoagulation is most commonly reversed with protamine. Protamine is a highly basic, arginine-rich protein with a molecular weight of 4300 Daltons. As a highly negatively charged molecule, protamine binds to the highly positively charged sulfate groups on the heparin molecule with an ionic linkage. The resultant complex renders heparin inactive. Protamine has been isolated from sperm heads in many species, including vertebrates. The protamine source for commercial preparation is the salmon sperm head. Protamine also binds to positively charged groups such as phosphate groups and may have important biologic properties in angiogenesis and immune function.[128,129] Protamine is mixed with insulin in neutral protamine Hagedorn and protamine-zinc insulin preparations to delay absorption and thus prolong the half-life of insulin. Protamine mixed with heparin causes crystallization or precipitation. This observation led to the discovery that protamine is a heparin antidote. Protamine is available as a sulfate or a chloride salt. There appears to be no clinical advantage to using one particular formulation of protamine.[130] The sulfate salt form is used more extensively throughout the United States.

Protamine is rapidly distributed throughout the extracellular space after intravenous injection. Bound and unbound protamine is inactivated and degraded by circulating proteases. Because protamine is eliminated from plasma considerably faster than the heparin, free protamine is unlikely to be present longer than free heparin. Heparin-protamine complexes are eliminated primarily by the reticuloendothelial system and may also be cleared by macrophages in the pulmonary circulation. If bound protamine is degraded by proteases, free heparin will remain. The recommended dose of protamine for heparin reversal is 1 to 1.3 mg protamine per 100 units of heparin; however, this dose often results in a protamine excess.

Protamine injection causes adverse hemodynamic effects, which have been classified into three types.[131-133] The Type I reaction is most common. It is characterized by hypotension and usually occurs during rapid administration of the drug. It is thought to be the result of the release of nitric oxide-related substances, inhibition of vasoactive substances, or release of histamine from mast cells. Type I reactions occur in the presence of protamine alone, and do not rely on the presence of heparin-protamine complexes. Type II reactions are categorized as IIA (anaphylaxis), IIB (anaphylactoid), and IIC (noncardiogenic pulmonary edema). True anaphylaxis is the result of a specific antiprotamine immunoglobulin E antibody produced during a prior exposure to protamine. Anaphylactoid reactions are characterized by complement activation, which is a result of the heparin-protamine complex.

Type III reactions are heralded by hypotension and catastrophic pulmonary hypertension leading to right heart failure.[134] The Type III reaction is idiosyncratic and is not associated with histamine release. It is presumably the result of large heparin-protamine complexes that form when heparin is neutralized by protamine,[135] and is associated with increased expression of thromboxane B2 and C5a.[136-138] Pretreatment with a thromboxane synthesis inhibitor or a thromboxane receptor blocker can prevent the reaction.[139]

Protamine excess has adverse effects on coagulation. Large doses prolong the whole blood clotting time (WBCT) and ACT, possibly via thrombin inhibition.[140,141] Protamine has also been associated with thrombocytopenia, inhibition of platelet aggregation, alteration in the platelet surface membrane, and depression of the platelet response to various agonists.[142,143]

Because protamine has such a vast array of adverse hemodynamic and hemostatic effects, there is considerable ongoing investigation in search of a suitable alternative. Hexadimethrine, a synthetic agent, has many of the same adverse effects as protamine and was withdrawn from clinical use because of renal toxicity.

Platelet Factor 4

Platelet factor 4 (PF4), a component of the α granule of platelets, binds to and inactivates heparin. Because it is a naturally occurring peptide, it is likely that PF4 has less immunogenicity than protamine. Animal data suggest that PF4 is devoid of adverse hemodynamic effects and may be infused more rapidly.[144] The PF4-heparin complexes are not associated with alterations in cardiac filling pressures and do not result in the liberation of free heparin or heparin rebound. Heparin reversal has been documented by WBCT, ACT, and heparin concentration at a PF4 concentration of 40 μ/ml, approximately twice the reversal dose of protamine.[145] Levy and associates[146] reported the reversal dose of PF4 to be approximately 60 μ/ml, and documented similar ACT and viscoelastic measurements of clot formation when compared with protamine. PF4 has not yet been approved by the U.S. Food and Drug Administration for reversal of heparin anticoagulation.

Heparinase

Heparinase (Neutralase, IBEX, Montreal, Calif.) is an enzyme that specifically degrades heparin by catalyzing cleavage of the saccharide bonds found in the heparin molecule. This enzyme has a molecular weight of 42,500 Daltons and is produced by the bacterium *Flavobacterium heparinum*. Each heparinase molecule can cleave approximately 70 saccharide bonds, yielding smaller oligosaccharides with reduced anticoagulant properties compared with the parent molecule.[147,148]

Heparinase I in a dose of 5 µg/kg successfully neutralized heparin in healthy volunteers and in patients who had undergone CPB.[149] Adverse hemodynamic effects are lacking because of the different method of heparin neutralization. Doses sufficient to neutralize a dose of 300 units/kg have no significant hemodynamic[150] or antiplatelet effects.[142]

Heparin Rebound

Heparin rebound describes the reestablishment of a heparinized state after heparin neutralization with protamine. Various explanations for heparin rebound have been proposed. The most commonly accepted is that rapid distribution and clearance of protamine occurs, leaving unbound heparin remaining after protamine clearance. Also possible is the release of heparin from tissues considered heparin storage sites (endothelium, connective tissues).[151] Variations in the timing and dosage of protamine and increased awareness of heparin rebound have led to a reduction in the incidence of untreated heparin rebound as a cause for excessive bleeding after CPB. Residual low levels of heparin are detected by sensitive heparin-concentration monitoring in the first hour after protamine reversal,[152,153] and may be present for up to 6 hours postoperatively.

Management of Postbypass Bleeding

The etiology of post-bypass bleeding includes platelet dysfunction, thrombocytopenia, dilution of serum procoagulants, fibrinolysis, residual heparin effect, and surgical causes.[154] Increased awareness of the risks of blood-product transfusion has focused attention on the prevention of bleeding and the judicious use of allogeneic blood products. Various pharmacologic and technologic advances have greatly reduced the incidence of transfusion during routine CPB.[35,37,47] Increased use of bedside coagulation monitoring as a part of a transfusion algorithm also reduces transfusions.[155] These algorithms stress the importance of bedside coagulation testing in preventing indiscriminate transfusion therapy. Ideally a test of platelet function would be an important component of a transfusion algorithm for blood conservation. Despotis and associates published an algorithm in 1994 that did not incorporate a test of platelet function, but did use platelet count to divide patients into

treatment groups.[156] These investigators demonstrated a reduction in transfusion therapy despite the lack of a platelet function test. Available technology for measuring platelet function includes the thromboelastograph (Haemoscope, Skokie, Ill.), Hemostatus (Medtronics, Parker, Colo.), Ultegra (Accumetrics, San Diego, Calif.), Platelet Function Analyzer-100 (Dade Behring, Deerfield, Ill.), and whole-blood aggregometry (Chronolog, Havertown, Pa.).

Thromboelastography (TEG) is a viscoelastic test of blood clotting that correlates with bleeding after cardiac surgery.[157,158] Transfusion algorithms that use TEG reduce exposure to allogeneic blood products in liver transplantation[159-161] and cardiac surgery.[162] Hemostatus also correlates with post-CPB blood loss and is useful in a comprehensive blood conservation program.[163,164]

Most CPB procedures are performed without routine transfusion. Patients undergoing high-risk cardiac surgery are more likely to require platelet and coagulation factor transfusions[165] because of prolonged CPB times and dilutional effects. Valvular surgery is associated with a moderate to high risk of perioperative transfusion. Reoperative cardiac surgical patients have prominent inflammatory responses resulting from their thromboplastin-rich scar tissue and prolonged exposure to the extracorporeal circuit.[62] Patients undergoing deep hypothermic circulatory arrest compose another subgroup of high-risk patients in whom the benefits of transfusion-sparing strategies are most useful.

SUMMARY

CPB is an essential component of cardiac surgery as we know it today. Complex surgical repairs, requiring asystole and a bloodless surgical field, would be impossible without the use of CPB. In this chapter we reviewed the elements of CPB and discussed how CPB works. Problems encountered during and after CPB, including hemodynamic variability, coronary and cerebral ischemia, and coagulopathy, were also discussed. These techniques of oxygenation, ventilation, and perfusion have been improved over the past 35 years and allow the repair of increasingly more complex cardiac lesions. Clearly, the benefits outweigh the risks to the cardiac surgical patient when CPB is used appropriately.

KEY POINTS

1. CPB, which is comprised of many elements (e.g., reservoir, pump, pump prime, oxygenator, heat exchanger, arterial inflow, cardiotomy suction, ventricular vent, micropore filters, circuitry), is an essential and integral part of successful cardiac surgery.
2. Preparation for CPB includes anticoagulation and vascular cannulation.

3. Oxygenation, ventilation, and perfusion of the cardiac patient determine appropriate management of CPB.
4. Separation from CPB is accomplished using weaning strategies that understand hemodynamic variability and cardiac function.

5. The goals following CPB are to achieve hemodynamic stability, reverse the anticoagulation, and to manage postbypass bleeding.

KEY REFERENCES

Despotis GJ, Santoro SA, Spitznagel E et al: Prospective evaluation and clinical utility of on-site monitoring of coagulation in patients undergoing cardiac operation, *J Thorac Cardiovasc Surg* 107:271-279, 1994.

Mills NL, Ochsner JL: Massive air embolism during cardiopulmonary bypass. Causes, prevention, and management, *J Thorac Cardiovasc Surg* 80:708-717, 1980.

Murkin JM, Martzke JS, Buchan AM et al: A randomized study of the influence of perfusion technique and pH management strategy in 316 patients undergoing coronary artery bypass surgery. II. Neurologic and cognitive outcomes, *J Thorac Cardiovasc Surg* 110:349-362, 1995.

Shore-Lesserson L, Manspeizer HE, DePerio M et al: Thromboelastography-guided transfusion algorithm reduces transfusions in complex cardiac surgery, *Anesth Analg* 88:312-319, 1999.

References

1. Bennett EV Jr, Fewel JG, Ybarra J et al: Comparison of flow differences among venous cannulas, *Ann Thorac Surg* 36:59-65, 1983.
2. Curtis JJ, Walls JT, Wagner-Mann CC et al: Centrifugal pumps: description of devices and surgical techniques, *Ann Thorac Surg* 68:666-671, 1999.
3. Klein M, Dauben HP, Schulte HD et al: Centrifugal pumping during routine open heart surgery improves clinical outcome, *Artif Organs* 22:326-336, 1998.
4. Mullges W, Berg D, Jorge Babin-Ebel J et al: Cerebral microembolus generation in different extracorporeal circulation systems, *Cerebrovasc Dis* 9:265-269, 1999.
5. Macey MG, McCarthy DA, Trivedi UR et al: Neutrophil adhesion molecule expression during cardiopulmonary bypass: a comparative study of roller and centrifugal pumps, *Perfusion* 12:293-301, 1997.
6. Hansbro SD, Sharpe DA, Catchpole R et al: Haemolysis during cardiopulmonary bypass: an in vivo comparison of standard roller pumps, nonocclusive roller pumps and centrifugal pumps, *Perfusion* 14:3-10, 1999.
7. Ashraf S, Butler J, Tian Y et al: Inflammatory mediators in adults undergoing cardiopulmonary bypass: comparison of centrifugal and roller pumps, *Ann Thorac Surg* 65:480-484, 1998.
8. Baufreton C, Intrator L, Jansen PG et al: Inflammatory response to cardiopulmonary bypass using roller or centrifugal pumps, *Ann Thorac Surg* 67:972-977, 1999.
9. Brister SJ, Pelletier A, Fedorshyn J et al: Cardiopulmonary bypass pumps and thrombin generation: what goes around comes around, *ASAIO J* 44:794-798, 1998.
10. Yoshikai M, Hamada M, Takarabe K et al: Clinical use of centrifugal pumps and the roller pump in open heart surgery: a comparative evaluation, *Artif Organs* 20:704-706, 1996.
11. Morgan IS, Codispoti M, Sanger K et al: Superiority of centrifugal pump over roller pump in paediatric cardiac surgery: prospective randomised trial, *Eur J Cardiothorac Surg* 13:526-532, 1998.
12. Marelli D, Paul A, Samson R et al: Does the addition of albumin to the prime solution in cardiopulmonary bypass affect clinical outcome? A prospective randomized study, *J Thorac Cardiovasc Surg* 98:751-756, 1989.
13. Sade RM, Stroud MR, Crawford FA Jr et al: A prospective randomized study of hydroxyethyl starch, albumin, and lactated Ringer's solution as priming fluid for cardiopulmonary bypass, *J Thorac Cardiovasc Surg* 89:713-722, 1985.
14. Hoeft A, Korb H, Mehlhorn U et al: Priming of cardiopulmonary bypass with human albumin or Ringer lactate: effect on colloid osmotic pressure and extravascular lung water, *Br J Anaesth* 66:73-80, 1991.
15. London MJ, Franks M, Verrier ED et al: The safety and efficacy of ten percent pentastarch as a cardiopulmonary bypass priming solution. A randomized clinical trial, *J Thorac Cardiovasc Surg* 104:284-296, 1992.
16. Verska JJ, Ludington LG, Brewer LA 3d: A comparative study of cardiopulmonary bypass with nonblood and blood prime, *Ann Thorac Surg* 18:72-80, 1974.
17. Rosengart TK, DeBois W, O'Hara M et al: Retrograde autologous priming for cardiopulmonary bypass: a safe and effective means of decreasing hemodilution and transfusion requirements, *J Thorac Cardiovasc Surg* 115:426-38; discussion 438-439, 1998.
18. Cavarocchi NC, Pluth JR, Schaff HV et al: Complement activation during cardiopulmonary bypass. Comparison of bubble and membrane oxygenators, *J Thorac Cardiovasc Surg* 91:252-258, 1986.
19. van den Dungen JJ, Karliczek GF, Brenken U et al: Clinical study of blood trauma during perfusion with membrane and bubble oxygenators, *J Thorac Cardiovasc Surg* 83:108-116, 1982.
20. van Oeveren W, Kazatchkine MD, Descamps-Latscha B et al: Deleterious effects of cardiopulmonary bypass. A prospective study of bubble versus membrane oxygenation, *J Thorac Cardiovasc Surg* 89:888-899, 1985.
21. Padayachee TS, Parsons S, Theobold R et al: The detection of microemboli in the middle cerebral artery during cardiopulmonary bypass: a transcranial Doppler ultrasound investigation using membrane and bubble oxygenators, *Ann Thorac Surg* 44:298-302, 1987.
22. Sade RM, Bartles DM, Dearing JP et al: A prospective randomized study of membrane versus bubble oxygenators in children. *Ann Thorac Surg* 29:502-511, 1980.
23. Hessel EA 2d, Johnson DD, Ivey TD et al: Membrane versus bubble oxygenator for cardiac operations. A prospective randomized study, *J Thorac Cardiovasc Surg* 80:111-122, 1980.

24. Clark RE, Beauchamp RA, Magrath RA et al: Comparison of bubble and membrane oxygenators in short and long perfusions, *J Thorac Cardiovasc Surg* 78:655-666, 1979.

25. Serry C, Najafi H, Dye WS et al: Superiority of aortic over femoral cannulation for cardiopulmonary bypass, with specific attention to lower extremity neuropathy, *J Cardiovasc Surg (Torino)* 19:277-279, 1978.

26. Wright G, Sanderson JM: Cellular aggregation and trauma in cardiotomy suction systems, *Thorax* 34:621-628, 1979.

27. Journois D, Pouard P, Greeley WJ et al: Hemofiltration during cardiopulmonary bypass in pediatric cardiac surgery. Effects on hemostasis, cytokines, and complement components, *Anesthesiology* 81:1181-1189; discussion 26A-27A, 1994.

28. Walpoth BH, Amport T, Schmid R et al: Hemofiltration during cardiopulmonary bypass: quality assessment of hemoconcentrated blood, *Thorac Cardiovasc Surg* 42:162-169, 1994.

29. Andreasson S, Gothberg S, Berggren H et al: Hemofiltration modifies complement activation after extracorporeal circulation in infants, *Ann Thorac Surg* 56:1515-1517, 1993.

30. Journois D, Israel-Biet D, Pouard P et al: High-volume, zero-balanced hemofiltration to reduce delayed inflammatory response to cardiopulmonary bypass in children [see comments], *Anesthesiology* 85:965-976, 1996.

31. Millar AB, Armstrong L, van der Linden J et al: Cytokine production and hemofiltration in children undergoing cardiopulmonary bypass, *Ann Thorac Surg* 56:1499-1502, 1993.

32. Schreurs HH, Wijers MJ, Gu YJ et al: Heparin-coated bypass circuits: effects on inflammatory response in pediatric cardiac operations, *Ann Thorac Surg* 66:166-171, 1998.

33. Videm V, Svennevig JL, Fosse E et al: Reduced complement activation with heparin-coated oxygenator and tubings in coronary bypass operations, *J Thorac Cardiovasc Surg* 103:806-813, 1992.

34. Baufreton C, Moczar M, Intrator L et al: Inflammatory response to cardiopulmonary bypass using two different types of heparin-coated extracorporeal circuits, *Perfusion* 13:419-427, 1998.

35. Aldea GS, Zhang X, Memmolo CA et al: Enhanced blood conservation in primary coronary artery bypass surgery using heparin-bonded circuits with lower anticoagulation, *J Card Surg* 11:85-95, 1996.

36. Murkin JM, Martzke JS, Buchan AM et al: A randomized study of the influence of perfusion technique and pH management strategy in 316 patients undergoing coronary artery bypass surgery. II. Neurologic and cognitive outcomes, *J Thorac Cardiovasc Surg* 110:349-362, 1995.

37. Aldea GS, O'Gara P, Shapira OM et al: Effect of anticoagulation protocol on outcome in patients undergoing CABG with heparin-bonded cardiopulmonary bypass circuits, *Ann Thorac Surg* 65:425-433, 1998.

38. Hirsh J, Raschke R, Warkentin TE et al: Heparin: mechanism of action, pharmacokinetics, dosing considerations, monitoring, efficacy, and safety, *Chest* 108:258S-275S, 1995.

39. Pixley RA, Schapira M, Colman RW: Effect of heparin on the inactivation rate of human activated factor XII by antithrombin III, *Blood* 66:198-203, 1985.

40. Boldt J, Zickmann B, Ballesteros M et al: Does the preparation of heparin influence anticoagulation during cardiopulmonary bypass? *J Cardiothorac Vasc Anesth* 5:449-453, 1991.

41. Gravlee GP, Angert KC, Tucker WY et al: Early anticoagulation peak and rapid distribution after intravenous heparin, *Anesthesiology* 68:126-129, 1988.

42. de Swart CA, Nijmeyer B, Roelofs JM et al: Kinetics of intravenously administered heparin in normal humans, *Blood* 60:1251-1258, 1982.

43. Mabry CD, Read RC, Thompson BW et al: Identification of heparin resistance during cardiac and vascular surgery, *Arch Surg* 114:129-134, 1979.

44. Horkay F, Martin P, Rajah SM et al: Response to heparinization in adults and children undergoing cardiac operations, *Ann Thorac Surg* 53:822-826, 1992.

45. Young JA, Kisker CT, Doty DB: Adequate anticoagulation during cardiopulmonary bypass determined by activated clotting time and the appearance of fibrin monomer, *Ann Thorac Surg* 26:231-240, 1978.

46. Despotis GJ, Summerfield AL, Joist JH et al: Comparison of activated coagulation time and whole blood heparin measurements with laboratory plasma anti-Xa heparin concentration in patients having cardiac operations, *J Thorac Cardiovasc Surg* 108:1076-1082, 1994.

47. Despotis GJ, Grishaber JE, Goodnough LT: The effect of an intraoperative treatment algorithm on physicians' transfusion practice in cardiac surgery [see comments], *Transfusion* 34:290-296, 1994.

48. Jobes DR, Aitken GL, Shaffer GW: Increased accuracy and precision of heparin and protamine dosing reduces blood loss and transfusion in patients undergoing primary cardiac operations, *J Thorac Cardiovasc Surg* 110:36-45, 1995.

49. Shore-Lesserson L, Reich DL, DePerio M: Heparin and protamine titration do not improve haemostasis in cardiac surgical patients [see comments], *Can J Anaesth* 45:10-18, 1998.

50. Murkin JM: Cardiopulmonary bypass and the inflammatory response: a role for serine protease inhibitors? *J Cardiothorac Vasc Anesth* 11:19-23; discussion 24-25, 1997.

51. Royston D: Aprotinin in patients having coronary artery bypass graft surgery, *Curr Opin Cardiol* 10:591-596, 1995.

52. Karski JM, Teasdale SJ, Norman PH et al: Prevention of postbypass bleeding with tranexamic acid and epsilon-aminocaproic acid, *J Cardiothorac Vasc Anesth* 7:431-435, 1993.

53. Horrow JC, Van Riper DF, Strong MD et al: The dose-response relationship of tranexamic acid, *Anesthesiology* 82:383-392, 1995.

54. Blauhut B, Gross C, Necek S et al: Effects of high-dose aprotinin on blood loss, platelet function, fibrinolysis, complement, and renal function after cardiopulmonary bypass [see comments], *J Thorac Cardiovasc Surg* 101:958-967, 1991.

55. Hill GE, Springall DR, Robbins RA: Aprotinin is associated with a decrease in nitric oxide production during cardiopulmonary bypass, *Surgery* 121:449-455, 1997.

56. Hill GE, Diego RP, Stammers AH et al: Aprotinin enhances the endogenous release of interleukin-10 after cardiac operations, *Ann Thorac Surg* 65:66-69, 1998.

57. Hill GE, Robbins RA: Aprotinin but not tranexamic acid inhibits cytokine-induced inducible nitric oxide synthase expression, *Anesth Analg* 84:1198-1202, 1997.

58. Hill GE, Alonso A, Spurzem JR et al: Aprotinin and methylprednisolone equally blunt cardiopulmonary bypass-induced inflammation in humans, *J Thorac Cardiovasc Surg* 110:1658-1662, 1995.

59. McCarthy RJ, Tuman KJ, O'Connor C et al: Aprotinin pretreatment diminishes postischemic myocardial contractile dysfunction in dogs, *Anesth Analg* 89:1096-1100, 1999.

60. D'Errico CC, Shayevitz JR, Martindale SJ et al: The efficacy and cost of aprotinin in children undergoing reoperative open heart surgery, *Anesth Analg* 83:1193-1199, 1996.

61. Bennett-Guerrero E, Spillane WF, White WD et al: Epsilon-aminocaproic acid administration and stroke following coronary artery bypass graft surgery, *Ann Thorac Surg* 67:1283-1287, 1999.

62. Cosgrove DM 3d, Heric B, Lytle BW et al: Aprotinin therapy for reoperative myocardial revascularization: a placebo-controlled study [see comments], *Ann Thorac Surg* 54:1031-1036; discussion 1036-1038, 1992.

63. Alderman EL, Levy JH, Rich JB et al: Analyses of coronary graft patency after aprotinin use: results from the International Multicenter Aprotinin Graft Patency Experience (IMAGE) trial, *J Thorac Cardiovasc Surg* 116:716-730, 1998.

64. Pillai R, Venn G, Lennox S et al: Elective femoro-femoral bypass for operations on the heart and great vessels, *J Thorac Cardiovasc Surg* 88:635-637, 1984.

65. Murphy DA, Craver JM, Jones EL et al: Recognition and management of ascending aortic dissection complicating cardiac surgical operations, *J Thorac Cardiovasc Surg* 85:247-256, 1983.

66. Taylor PC, Groves LK, Loop FD et al: Cannulation of the ascending aorta for cardiopulmonary bypass. Experience with 9,000 cases, *J Thorac Cardiovasc Surg* 71:255-258, 1976.

67. Salerno TA, Lince DP, White DN et al: Arch versus femoral artery perfusion during cardiopulmonary bypass, *J Thorac Cardiovasc Surg* 76:681-684, 1978.

68. Dalal FY, Patel KD: Another sign of inadvertent carotid cannulation [letter], *Anesthesiology* 55:487, 1981.

69. Ross WT Jr., Lake CL, Wellons HA: Cardiopulmonary bypass complicated by inadvertent carotid cannulation, *Anesthesiology* 54:85-86, 1981.

70. Sudhaman DA: Accidental hyperperfusion of the left carotid artery during CPB [letter], *J Cardiothorac Vasc Anesth* 5:100-101, 1991.

71. McLeskey CH, Cheney FW: A correctable complication of cardiopulmonary bypass, *Anesthesiology* 56:214-216, 1982.

72. Mills NL, Ochsner JL: Massive air embolism during cardiopulmonary bypass. Causes, prevention, and management, *J Thorac Cardiovasc Surg* 80:708-717, 1980.

73. Johnston WE, Royster RL, Choplin RH et al: Pulmonary artery catheter migration during cardiac surgery, *Anesthesiology* 64:258-262, 1986.

74. Svennevig JL, Lindberg H, Geiran O et al: Should the lungs be ventilated during cardiopulmonary bypass? Clinical, hemodynamic, and metabolic changes in patients undergoing elective coronary artery surgery, *Ann Thorac Surg* 37:295-300, 1984.

75. Fox LS, Blackstone EH, Kirklin JW et al: Relationship of whole body oxygen consumption to perfusion flow rate during hypothermic cardiopulmonary bypass, *J Thorac Cardiovasc Surg* 83:239-248, 1982.

76. Hilberman M, Myers BD, Carrie BJ et al: Acute renal failure following cardiac surgery, *J Thorac Cardiovasc Surg* 77:880-888, 1979.

77. Kawamura M, Minamikawa O, Yokochi H et al: Safe limit of hemodilution in cardiopulmonary bypass—comparative analysis between cyanotic and acyanotic congenital heart disease, *Jpn J Surg* 10:206-211, 1980.

78. Michenfelder JD, Theye RA: Hypothermia: effect on canine brain and whole-body metabolism, *Anesthesiology* 29:1107-1112, 1968.

79. Driessen JJ, Giart M: Comparison of isoflurane and midazolam as hypnotic supplementation to moderately high-dose fentanyl during coronary artery bypass grafting: effects on systemic hemodynamics and early postoperative recovery profile, *J Cardiothorac Vasc Anesth* 11:740-745, 1997.

80. Howie MB, Black HA, Romanelli VA et al: A comparison of isoflurane versus fentanyl as primary anesthetics for mitral valve surgery, *Anesth Analg* 83:941-948, 1996.

81. Flezzani P, Croughwell ND, McIntyre RW et al: Isoflurane decreases the cortisol response to cardiopulmonary bypass, *Anesth Analg* 65:1117-1122, 1986.

82. Philbin DM, Levine FH, Kono K et al: Attenuation of the stress response to cardiopulmonary bypass by the addition of pulsatile flow, *Circulation* 64:808-812, 1981.

83. Williams GD, Seifen AB, Lawson NW et al: Pulsatile perfusion versus conventional high-flow nonpulsatile perfusion for rapid core cooling and rewarming of infants for circulatory arrest in cardiac operation, *J Thorac Cardiovasc Surg* 78:667-677, 1979.

84. Jacobs LA, Klopp EH, Seamone W et al: Improved organ function during cardiac bypass with a roller pump modified to deliver pulsatile flow, *J Thorac Cardiovasc Surg* 58:703-712, 1969.

85. Dunn J, Kirsh MM, Harness J et al: Hemodynamic, metabolic, and hematologic effects of pulsatile cardiopulmonary bypass, *J Thorac Cardiovasc Surg* 68:138-147, 1974.

86. Shepard RB, Kirklin JW: Relation of pulsatile flow to oxygen consumption and other variables during cardiopulmonary bypass, *J Thorac Cardiovasc Surg* 58:694-702, 1969.

87. Boucher JK, Rudy LW, Edmunds LH: Organ blood flow during pulsatile cardiopulmonary bypass, *J Appl Physiol* 36:86-90, 1974.

88. Kaul TK, Swaminathan R, Chatrath RR et al: Vasoactive pressure hormones during and after cardiopulmonary bypass, *Int J Artif Organs* 13:293-299, 1990.

89. Philbin DM, Levine FH, Emerson CW et al: Plasma vasopressin levels and urinary flow during cardiopulmonary bypass in patients with valvular heart disease: effect of pulsatile flow, *J Thorac Cardiovasc Surg* 78:779-783, 1979.

90. Taylor KM, Brannan JJ, Bain WH et al: Role of angiotensin II in the development of peripheral vasoconstriction during cardiopulmonary bypass, *Cardiovasc Res* 13:269-273, 1979.

91. Taylor KM, Bain WH, Russell M et al: Peripheral vascular resistance and angiotensin II levels during pulsatile and no-pulsatile cardiopulmonary bypass, *Thorax* 34:594-598, 1979.

92. Buket S, Alayunt A, Ozbaran M et al: Effect of pulsatile flow during cardiopulmonary bypass on thyroid hormone metabolism, *Ann Thorac Surg* 58:93-96, 1994.

93. Song Z, Wang C, Stammers AH: Clinical comparison of pulsatile and nonpulsatile perfusion during cardiopulmonary bypass, *J Extra Corpor Technol* 29:170-175, 1997.

94. Salerno TA, Henderson M, Keith FM et al: Hypertension after coronary operation. Can it be prevented by pulsatile perfusion? *J Thorac Cardiovasc Surg* 81:396-399, 1981.

95. Thompson T, Minami K, Dramburg W et al: The influence of pulsatile and nonpulsatile extracorporeal circulation on fluid retention following coronary artery bypass grafting, *Perfusion* 7:201-211, 1992.

96. Konishi H, Sohara Y, Endo S et al: Pulmonary microcirculation during pulsatile and non pulsatile perfusion, *ASAIO J* 43:M657-M659, 1997.

97. Kono K, Philbin DM, Coggins CH et al: Adrenocortical hormone levels during cardiopulmonary bypass with and without pulsatile flow, *J Thorac Cardiovasc Surg* 85:129-133, 1983.

98. Frater RW, Wakayama S, Oka Y et al: Pulsatile cardiopulmonary bypass: failure to influence hemodynamics or hormones, *Circulation* 62:I19-I25, 1980.

99. Shaw PJ, Bates D, Cartlidge NE et al: An analysis of factors predisposing to neurological injury in patients undergoing coronary bypass operations, *Q J Med* 72:633-646, 1989.

100. Hindman BJ, Dexter F, Ryu KH et al: Pulsatile versus nonpulsatile cardiopulmonary bypass. No difference in brain blood flow or metabolism at 27 degrees C, *Anesthesiology* 80:1137-1147, 1994.

101. Hindman B: Cerebral physiology during cardiopulmonary bypass: pulsatile versus nonpulsatile flow, *Adv Pharmacol* 31:607-616, 1994.

102. Badner NH, Murkin JM, Lok P: Differences in pH management and pulsatile/nonpulsatile perfusion during cardiopulmonary bypass do not influence renal function, *Anesth Analg* 75:696-701, 1992.

103. Wollman H, Stephen GW, Clement AJ et al: Cerebral blood flow in man during extracorporeal circulation, *J Thorac Cardiovasc Surg* 52:558-564, 1966.

104. Prough DS, Stump DA, Roy RC et al: Response of cerebral blood flow to changes in carbon dioxide tension during hypothermic cardiopulmonary bypass, *Anesthesiology* 64:576-581, 1986.

105. Henriksen L: Brain luxury perfusion during cardiopulmonary bypass in humans. A study of the cerebral blood flow response to changes in CO_2, O_2, and blood pressure, *J Cereb Blood Flow Metab* 6:366-378, 1986.

106. Stephan H, Weyland A, Kazmaier S et al: Acid-base management during hypothermic cardiopulmonary bypass does not affect cerebral metabolism but does affect blood flow and neurological outcome, *Br J Anaesth* 69:51-57, 1992.

107. Murkin JM, Farrar JK, Tweed WA et al: Cerebral autoregulation and flow/metabolism coupling during cardiopulmonary bypass: the influence of $Paco_2$, *Anesth Analg* 66:825-832, 1987.

108. Govier AV, Reves JG, McKay RD et al: Factors and their influence on regional cerebral blood flow during nonpulsatile cardiopulmonary bypass, *Ann Thorac Surg* 38:592-600, 1984.

109. Baraka AS, Baroody MA, Haroun ST et al: Effect of α-stat versus pH-stat strategy on oxyhemoglobin dissociation and whole-body oxygen consumption during hypothermic cardiopulmonary bypass, *Anesth Analg* 74:32-37, 1992.

110. Bashein G, Townes BD, Nessly ML et al: A randomized study of carbon dioxide management during hypothermic cardiopulmonary bypass [see comments], *Anesthesiology* 72:7-15, 1990.

111. Kramer RS, Sanders AP, Lesage AM et al: The effect profound hypothermia on preservation of cerebral ATP content during circulatory arrest, *J Thorac Cardiovasc Surg* 56:699-709, 1968.

112. Mora CT, Henson MB, Weintraub WS et al: The effect of temperature management during cardiopulmonary bypass on neurologic and neuropsychologic outcomes in patients undergoing coronary revascularization, *J Thorac Cardiovasc Surg* 112:514-522, 1996.

113. Leslie K, Sessler DI: The implications of hypothermia for early tracheal extubation following cardiac surgery, *J Cardiothorac Vasc Anesth* 12:30-34; discussion 41-44, 1998.

114. Bone ME, Feneck RO: Bladder temperature as an estimate of body temperature during cardiopulmonary bypass, *Anaesthesia* 43:181-185, 1988.

115. Horrow JC, Rosenberg H: Does urinary catheter temperature reflect core temperature during cardiac surgery? *Anesthesiology* 69:986-989, 1988.

116. Rao V, Cohen G, Weisel RD et al: Optimal flow rates for integrated cardioplegia, *J Thorac Cardiovasc Surg* 115:226-235, 1998.

117. Iannettoni MD, Rohs TJ Jr, Gallagher KP et al: The regional effect of retrograde cardioplegia in areas of evolving ischemia, *Chest* 108:1353-1357, 1995.

118. Olinger GN, Bonchek LI, Geiss DM: Noncoronary collateral distribution in coronary artery disease, *Ann Thorac Surg* 32:554-557, 1981.

119. Schlensak C, Doenst T, Beyersdorf F: Clinical experience with blood cardioplegia, *Thorac Cardiovasc Surg* 46(suppl 2):282-285; discussion 286-287, 1998.

120. Ericsson AB, Takeshima S, Vaage J: Warm or cold continuous blood cardioplegia provides similar myocardial protection, *Ann Thorac Surg* 68:454-459, 1999.

121. Ericsson AB, Kawakami T, Vaage J: Intermittent warm blood cardioplegia does not provide adequate myocardial resuscitation after global ischaemia, *Eur J Cardiothorac Surg* 16:233-239, 1999.

122. Iguidbashian JP, Follette DM, Pollock ME et al: Advantages of continuous noncardioplegic warm blood retrograde perfusion over antegrade perfusion during proximal coronary anastomoses [see comments], *J Card Surg* 10:27-31, 1995.

123. Honkonen EL, Kaukinen L, Pehkonen EJ et al: Right ventricle is protected better by warm continuous than by cold intermittent retrograde blood cardioplegia in patients with obstructed right coronary artery, *Thorac Cardiovasc Surg* 45:182-189, 1997.

124. Hohn L, Schweizer A, Kalangos A et al: Benefits of intraoperative skin surface warming in cardiac surgical patients, *Br J Anaesth* 80:318-323, 1998.

125. Grocott HP, Newman MF, Croughwell ND et al: Continuous jugular venous versus nasopharyngeal temperature monitoring during hypothermic cardiopulmonary bypass for cardiac surgery, *J Clin Anesth* 9:312-316, 1997.

126. Topol EJ, Humphrey LS, Borkon AM et al: Value of intraoperative left ventricular microbubbles detected by transesophageal two-dimensional echocardiography in predicting neurologic outcome after cardiac operations, *Am J Cardiol* 56:773-775, 1985.

127. Oka Y, Moriwaki KM, Hong Y et al: Detection of air emboli in the left heart by M-mode transesophageal echocardiography following cardiopulmonary bypass, *Anesthesiology* 63:109-113, 1985.

128. Taylor S, Folkman J: Protamine is an inhibitor of angiogenesis, *Nature* 297:307-312, 1982.

129. Folkman J, Langer R, Linhardt RJ et al: Angiogenesis inhibition and tumor regression caused by heparin or a heparin fragment in the presence of cortisone, *Science* 221:719-725, 1983.

130. Benayahu D, Aronson M: Comparative study of protamine chloride and sulphate in relation to the heparin rebound phenomenon, *Thromb Res* 32:109-114, 1983.

131. Horrow JC: Protamine: a review of its toxicity, *Anesth Analg* 64:348-361, 1985.

132. Horrow JC: Adverse reactions to protamine, *Int Anesthesiol Clin* 23:133-144, 1985.

133. Horrow JC: Thrombocytopenia accompanying a reaction to protamine sulfate, *Can Anaesth Soc J* 132:49-52, 1985.

134. Lowenstein E, Johnston WE, Lappas DG et al: Catastrophic pulmonary vasoconstriction associated with protamine reversal of heparin, *Anesthesiology* 59:470-473, 1983.

135. Shanberge JN, Murato M, Quattrociocchi-Longe T et al: Heparin-protamine complexes in the production of heparin rebound and other complications of extracorporeal bypass procedures, *Am J Clin Pathol* 87:210-217, 1987.

136. Morel DR, Costabella PM, Pittet JF: Adverse cardiopulmonary effects and increased plasma thromboxane concentrations following the neutralization of heparin with protamine in awake sheep are infusion rate-dependent [see comments], *Anesthesiology* 73:415-424, 1990.

137. Morel DR, Lowenstein E, Nguyenduy T et al: Acute pulmonary vasoconstriction and thromboxane release during protamine reversal of heparin anticoagulation in awake sheep. Evidence for the role of reactive oxygen metabolites following nonimmunological complement activation, *Circ Res* 62:905-915, 1988.

138. Morel DR, Zapol WM, Thomas SJ et al: C5a and thromboxane generation associated with pulmonary vaso- and bronchoconstriction during protamine reversal of heparin, *Anesthesiology* 66:597-604, 1987.

139. Nuttall GA, Murray MJ, Bowie EJ: Protamine-heparin-induced pulmonary hypertension in pigs: effects of treatment with a thromboxane receptor antagonist on hemodynamics and coagulation, *Anesthesiology* 74:138-145, 1991.

140. Cobel-Geard RJ, Hassouna HI: Interaction of protamine sulfate with thrombin, *Am J Hematol* 14:227-233, 1983.

141. Carr ME Jr, Carr SL: At high heparin concentrations, protamine concentrations which reverse heparin anticoagulant effects are insufficient to reverse heparin anti-platelet effects, *Thromb Res* 75:617-630, 1994.

142. Ammar T, Fisher CF: The effects of heparinase 1 and protamine on platelet reactivity, *Anesthesiology* 86:1382-1386, 1997.

143. Ellison N, Edmunds LH Jr, Colman RW: Platelet aggregation following heparin and protamine administration, *Anesthesiology* 48:65-68, 1978.

144. Cook JJ, Niewiarowski S, Yan Z et al: Platelet factor 4 efficiently reverses heparin anticoagulation in the rat without adverse effects of heparin-protamine complexes, *Circulation* 85:1102-1109, 1992.

145. Williams RD, D'Ambra MN, Maione TE et al: Recombinant platelet factor 4 reversal of heparin in human cardiopulmonary bypass blood, *J Thorac Cardiovasc Surg* 108:975-983, 1994.

146. Levy JH, Cormack JG, Morales A: Heparin neutralization by recombinant platelet factor 4 and protamine, *Anesth Analg* 81:35-37, 1995.

147. Linhardt RJ, Grant A, Cooney CL et al: Differential anticoagulant activity of heparin fragments prepared using microbial heparinase, *J Biol Chem* 1257:7310-7313, 1982.

148. Linhardt RJ, Fitzgerald GL, Cooney CL et al: Mode of action of heparin lyase on heparin, *Biochim Biophys Acta* 702:197-203, 1982.

149. Heres E VRD, Marquez J et al: Heparin reversal with heparinase I (Neutralase) in coronary artery bypass (CAB) patients, *Anesth Analg* 84:SCA32 (abstract), 1997.

150. Michelsen LG, Kikura M, Levy JH et al: Heparinase I (neutralase) reversal of systemic anticoagulation, *Anesthesiology* 85:339-346, 1996.

151. Gollub S: Heparin rebound in open heart surgery, *Surg Gynecol Obstet* 124:337-346, 1967.

152. Despotis GJ, Joist JH, Goodnough LT: Monitoring of hemostasis in cardiac surgical patients: impact of point-of-care testing on blood loss and transfusion outcomes, *Clin Chem* 43:1684-1696, 1997.

153. Kuitunen AH, Salmenpera MT, Heinonen J et al: Heparin rebound: a comparative study of protamine chloride and protamine sulfate in patients undergoing coronary artery bypass surgery, *J Cardiothorac Vasc Anesth* 5:221-226, 1991.

154. Khuri SF, Valeri CR, Loscalzo J et al: Heparin causes platelet dysfunction and induces fibrinolysis before cardiopulmonary bypass [see comments], *Ann Thorac Surg* 60:1008-1014, 1995.

155. Despotis GJ, Santoro SA, Spitznagel E et al: On-site prothrombin time, activated partial thromboplastin time, and platelet count. A comparison between whole blood and laboratory assays with coagulation factor analysis in patients presenting for cardiac surgery, *Anesthesiology* 80:338-351, 1994.

156. Despotis GJ, Santoro SA, Spitznagel E et al: Prospective evaluation and clinical utility of on-site monitoring of coagulation in patients undergoing cardiac operation, *J Thorac Cardiovasc Surg* 107:271-279, 1994.

157. Spiess BD, Tuman KJ, McCarthy RJ et al: Thromboelastography as an indicator of post-cardiopulmonary bypass coagulopathies, *J Clin Monit* 3:25-30, 1987.

158. Tuman KJ, Spiess BD, McCarthy RJ et al: Comparison of viscoelastic measures of coagulation after cardiopulmonary bypass, *Anesth Analg* 69:69-75, 1989.

159. Kang YG, Martin DJ, Marquez J et al: Intraoperative changes in blood coagulation and thrombelastographic monitoring in liver transplantation, *Anesth Analg* 64:888-896, 1985.

160. Kang Y: Thromboelastography in liver transplantation, *Semin Thromb Hemost* 21:34-44, 1995.

161. Kang Y: Transfusion based on clinical coagulation monitoring does reduce hemorrhage during liver transplantation [see comments], *Liver Transpl Surg* 3:655-659, 1997.

162. Shore-Lesserson L, Manspeizer HE, DePerio M et al: Thromboelastography-guided transfusion algorithm reduces transfusions in complex cardiac surgery, *Anesth Analg* 88:312-319, 1999.

163. Despotis GJ, Levine V, Filos KS et al: Evaluation of a new point-of-care test that measures PAF-mediated acceleration of coagulation in cardiac surgical patients, *Anesthesiology* 85:1311-1323, 1996.

164. Despotis GJ, Levine V, Saleem R et al: Use of point-of-care test in identification of patients who can benefit from desmopressin during cardiac surgery: a randomised controlled trial [see comments], *Lancet* 1354:106-110, 1999.

165. Khuri SF, Wolfe JA, Josa M et al: Hematologic changes during and after cardiopulmonary bypass and their relationship to the bleeding time and nonsurgical blood loss, *J Thorac Cardiovasc Surg* 104:94-107, 1992.

CHAPTER 13

Minimally Invasive Cardiac Surgery

Lawrence C. Siegel, M.D. ■ Jan Komtebedde, D.V.M.

OUTLINE

Cardiac surgery offers highly effective treatment methods for a variety of serious cardiovascular diseases. Minimally invasive and less invasive surgical techniques have gained broad acceptance in other surgical disciplines such as general surgery, gynecology, and orthopedics. A number of important cardiovascular diseases may be treated with catheter-based interventional methods such as coronary artery stent insertion. These advances underscore the desirability of less invasive surgical techniques for cardiac surgery. The goals of minimally invasive and less invasive cardiac surgery are to provide an efficacious and durable surgical result with less trauma than that of conventional surgical methods. Opportunities to reduce morbidity are of keen interest. To improve the patient's experience, surgeons wish to provide for a more rapid rehabilitation with less pain. Patients also seek approaches that are cosmetically more

desirable. Economic factors are important in the delivery of health care, spanning the resources used in the hospital and during rehabilitation, as well as the loss of productivity of a disabled patient.

Several approaches have been pursued in bringing minimally invasive and less invasive methods to cardiac surgery. Surgical incisions that are less traumatic than the median sternotomy have been introduced. These approaches parallel those of other surgical disciplines in which surgeons have found that technologic enhancements allow them to achieve desired surgical results without large and traumatic incisions. Progress in technology may also allow surgeons to perform procedures with methods that may be less disruptive to tissues. For example, balloon occlusion of the aorta during cardiopulmonary bypass (CPB) is of interest to some clinicians as an alternative to crushing the aorta with an external steel cross-clamp. Surgeons have also taken the opportunity to reconsider the value of CPB when operating on the surface of the heart. Avoidance of CPB when constructing coronary artery bypass grafts may provide a less traumatic and less invasive procedure.

New techniques and technologies bring changes in practice methods for anesthesiologists and provide new

Portions of this chapter adapted from *Advances in Anesthesia*, vol 16, Mosby, 1999; and *Seminars in Cardiothoracic and Vascular Anesthesia*, vol 3, WB Saunders, 1999. Heartport, EndoVent, DirectFlow, Quick-Draw, EndoReturn, EndoClamp, EndoPlege, StillSite, EndoDirect, PrecisionOp, and EndoCPB are registered trademarks and Port-Access, StraightShot, and FlexSite are trademarks of Heartport, Inc.

opportunities to provide sophisticated patient care in the perioperative period. A thorough understanding of this growing field will enable anesthesiologists to prepare appropriately now and in the future.

MINIMALLY INVASIVE CARDIAC SURGERY WITH CARDIOPULMONARY BYPASS
Aortic Valve Surgery

Advances in the field of minimally invasive cardiac surgery have been rapid as a result of new technology that has allowed surgeons to refine surgical techniques and perform a variety of increasingly complex procedures both thoracoscopically and under direct visualization through markedly smaller incisions. There has been considerable interest in minimally invasive approaches to aortic valve surgery and a number of choices for incisions and for cannulation methods have been pursued. Through cadaver evaluations, Reardon et al[1] noted that the anatomic relationship between valve structures and surface anatomy does not change when using different surgical approaches. The upper partial sternotomy approach with a partial or full transverse sternotomy was evaluated for aortic valve procedures. The partial upper sternotomy to the level of the fourth intercostal space gives excellent exposure of the aortic valve, and allows central cannulation and rapid conversion to full sternotomy. This sternal incision does not typically require sacrifice or mobilization of the internal mammary artery.

Cohn et al[2] described experience in 50 patients with three different minimally invasive aortic valve replacement methods: right parasternal incision, transverse sternotomy, and partial upper sternotomy. The upper partial sternotomy into the right third or fourth intercostal space spares the left half of the sternum and the left internal mammary artery. Central cannulation for CPB is easily accomplished because the aorta, the right atrium, and the right superior pulmonary vein are accessible. Femoro-femoral CPB is commonly used with the right parasternal approach to reduce the number of cannulae in the operative field. Axillary arterial and venous cannulation is feasible as well. The right internal mammary artery is mobilized and retracted laterally. Although central cannulation for CPB is feasible and coronary artery bypass graft (CABG) after previous aortic valve replacement is uncommon, a disadvantage of the transverse sternotomy is loss of both the right and left internal mammary artery. With all approaches, the importance of commissural stay sutures to elevate the aortic annulus into the incision is emphasized. Complex aortic valve procedures can be performed through these incisions. Homograft root replacement is easier through the upper partial sternotomy. Venting is

achieved through the aortic annulus or the right superior pulmonary vein and de-airing can be achieved through the ascending aorta or the dome of the left atrium. Ventricular pacing wires are typically placed before removal of the cross-clamp with the heart arrested and decompressed. The authors conclude that minimally invasive aortic valve operations reduce exposure of the patient to surgical trauma and blood use while achieving the same general quality operation as with the conventional operative approach. Early- and medium-term results show a reduction in pain, earlier return to full-time activity, and a reduction in cost and rehabilitation resources.

Retrograde cardioplegia delivery is widely practiced in aortic valve surgery for myocardial protection. Direct transatrial cannulation may fail during minimally invasive surgical approaches because of the unfavorable angle of introduction, the reduced ability to maneuver, and the decreased ability to palpate the position of the catheter in the coronary sinus. Relying solely on antegrade cardioplegia delivery not only increases the cross-clamp time resulting from interruptions in the surgical procedure, but also carries the risk of incomplete myocardial protection and ostial dissection. Kaur et al[3] noted the value of percutaneous coronary sinus cannulation both from the standpoint of improved ability to cannulate the coronary sinus during less invasive approaches and of reduced interference of catheters with the surgical field providing improved surgical exposure.

Mächler et al[4] prospectively evaluated 120 patients undergoing first-time isolated aortic valve replacement procedures with either a conventional approach ($n = 60$) or with a partial upper sternotomy approach ($n = 60$). Patient demographics were similar between both groups. Conventional cannulation was performed in both groups and venting was achieved via the right superior pulmonary vein or pulmonary artery. Cardioplegia delivery was delivered in an antegrade fashion only. Operative times, including CPB duration, cross-clamp time, and skin-to-skin times were similar. The right internal mammary artery was injured in two patients in the less invasive group. Duration of mechanical ventilation, chest tube drainage during the first 24 hours and next 24 hours, pericardial effusion greater than 1 cm, and incidence of supraventricular arrhythmias were significantly reduced in the patients with the less invasive procedure. Reoperation for bleeding was required in five hemisternotomy patients and three full sternotomy patients. Thirty-day mortality rate in the hemisternotomy group was 1.6%. Overall survival rates were 95% and 97% for the hemisternotomy and full-sternotomy groups respectively, with a mean follow-up of 294 days.

Byrne and colleagues[5] reported on 24 conventional and 21 upper partial sternotomy isolated aortic valve reoperations. Central cannulation was preferred; however, peripheral CPB was established before resternotomy whenever a patent left internal mammary artery graft to the left anterior descending coronary artery was present in either group. Venting was performed either via the aortic root or the right superior pulmonary vein. Percutaneous retrograde cardioplegia delivery and peripheral venous cannulation limit the need for right atrial dissection. There were no operative deaths or valve-related complications in either group. The amount of blood loss, transfusion requirements, and operative time were significantly less in the less invasive group. These benefits were achieved without compromising the efficacy of the operative procedure and without compromising myocardial protection.

An anterior mini-thoracotomy approach to aortic valve replacement (AVR) by using the right third intercostal space for access to the aorta has been described. This method does not typically require transection of the costal cartilage or ribs. Pericardial stay sutures are used to expose the aorta and commissural stay sutures are used to expose the aortic valve.[6] Aortic valve surgery can readily be accomplished by using catheters and cannulae specifically developed for a minimally invasive approach. A percutaneous pulmonary artery vent catheter and a percutaneous coronary sinus catheter are combined with a femoral venous drainage cannula and a thin-wall direct aortic cannula. CPB performed with these devices allows venting and retrograde cardioplegia delivery with minimal clutter of the surgical field. The surgeon is thereby able to achieve excellent exposure of the aortic annulus and optimal access through a variety of incisions.

The EndoCPB and EndoDirect Systems

A very broadly applicable method for minimally invasive cardiac surgery is minimal-access surgery performed on an arrested and decompressed heart by using endovascular-based CPB and cardioplegic arrest. Port-Access (Heartport, Inc., Redwood City, Calif.) minimally invasive cardiac surgery with the EndoCPB and EndoDirect systems (Heartport) provide a motionless, bloodless operative field, as in traditional, open-chest cardiac surgery with a median sternotomy. Consequently, a variety of cardiac procedures can be performed through the minimum appropriate incision, or access port, that is necessary to open, turn, and manipulate the heart. These conditions allow surgeons to perform intracardiac procedures such as valve surgery and atrial-septal defect repair, as well as permit surgical access for complete myocardial revascularization to all areas of the heart's surface.

The catheter-based EndoCPB and EndoDirect systems use an extracorporeal circuit to accomplish the same functions as a standard CPB system for open-chest cardiac surgery. Five cannulae and catheters are con-

nected to the extracorporeal circuit to drain and return blood and to deliver cardioplegia for cardiac arrest. Cannulae and catheter placement are guided by using transesophageal echocardiography (TEE), or fluoroscopic imaging, or both, and specific monitoring techniques are used to evaluate the functioning of all system components to ensure appropriate CPB and myocardial protection.

The anesthesiologist has an important role in Port-Access minimally invasive cardiac surgery. The anesthesiologist is typically responsible for percutaneously inserting and positioning the jugular catheters into the coronary sinus and pulmonary artery and for working collaboratively to monitor flows and pressures.

The external components of the endovascular CPB system include pumps for arterial blood flow, delivery of cardioplegia, pulmonary artery and aortic root venting, cardiotomy suction, and assisted venous drainage to augment return to the heart-lung machine; a venous reservoir; an oxygenator; a heat exchanger; and in-line monitors and safety devices. The endovascular components of the EndoDirect and EndoCPB Systems include two cannulae and three catheters that drain deoxygenated blood from the right atrium, return oxygenated blood to the arterial circulation, partition the arterial circulation by providing total occlusion or "clamping" of the ascending aorta, deliver crystalloid or blood cardioplegia into the coronary circulation, and vent the pulmonary artery and aortic root—all without the need for a median sternotomy. Figs. 13-1 and 13-2 schematically illustrate the placement of these catheters and cannulae.

Venous drainage is provided by the 22- or 25-Fr QuickDraw cannula (Heartport), which is introduced through a femoral vein. Typically, the 22-Fr cannula is placed percutaneously by using the Seldinger technique. The ultrathin wall of this cannula optimizes flow rates, and multiple side holes provide for increased venous drainage. Drainage may be augmented by 20% to 40% by using vacuum-assisted venous drainage or a centrifugal venous drainage pump placed between the venous cannula and the venous reservoir.

Arterial inflow is provided by using a CPB pump, and flow passes through the dual-armed, Y-shaped, DirectFlow cannula, which is placed in the ascending aorta, or through the 21- or 23-Fr EndoReturn Cannula (Heartport), which is introduced into a femoral artery. One arm of the cannula is connected to the arterial line of the CPB circuit to deliver oxygenated blood to the systemic vasculature. The other arm serves as a conduit for introducing, maintaining, and removing the EndoClamp aortic occlusion catheter (Heartport). This 10.5-Fr, triple-lumen, balloon-tipped catheter performs four functions. Inflation of the balloon at the catheter's tip occludes the ascending aorta to partition the aortic root and coronary arteries from the remainder of the arterial

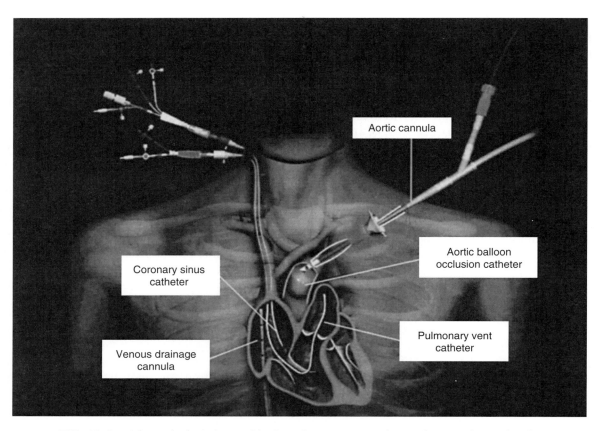

FIG. 13-1 Schematic depicting positioning of Port-Access endovascular cannulae and catheters in the heart. This system allows direct cannulation of the ascending aorta for arterial return. (Copyright Heartport. Reprinted with permission.)

circulation. In addition, the EndoClamp catheter delivers antegrade cardioplegia to the coronary arteries via the aortic root, vents blood from the aortic root, and permits measurement of aortic root pressure. When the surgical procedure requires an aortotomy, as in aortic valve surgery, aortic occlusion is typically achieved with an external steel cross-clamp and the EndoClamp catheter is not used. In this case, the ascending aorta may be cannulated with the single-arm StraightShot cannula (Heartport), which, like the DirectFlow cannula, includes an incising introducer for single-step incision and cannulation of the aorta.

The EndoPlege catheter (Heartport) is a triple-lumen catheter with a balloon near its tip to occlude the coronary sinus and permit coronary sinus pressure measurement and infusion of crystalloid or blood cardioplegia in a retrograde fashion into the coronary circulation. This 9-Fr preshaped catheter is positioned in the coronary sinus via an 11-Fr right internal jugular vein introducer sheath.

A pulmonary artery vent catheter (EndoVent catheter, Heartport) assists in draining and decompressing the heart. Multiple ventilation holes arranged around the circumference of the catheter's tip help to maintain the high flow rates necessary to ensure that the venting via the pulmonary artery is adequate. This 8.3-Fr catheter is introduced into the main pulmonary artery by using balloon-tip flotation through a 9-Fr percutaneous internal jugular vein introducer sheath. The radiopaque shafts of these catheters allow visualization with either TEE or fluoroscopy.

Patient Selection and Preoperative Evaluation

The evaluation and selection of candidates for Port-Access minimally invasive cardiac surgery are largely the same as for patients having open-chest cardiac surgery. Severe abnormalities of the chest wall may limit surgical exposure and contraindicate a minimally invasive surgical approach.

The vascular system should be evaluated preoperatively to determine whether the patient's vasculature permits introduction and placement of the catheters and cannulae. Peripheral arterial atherosclerosis does not contraindicate ascending aortic cannulation with the EndoDirect system; however, femoral artery cannulation with the EndoCPB system may be precluded. The

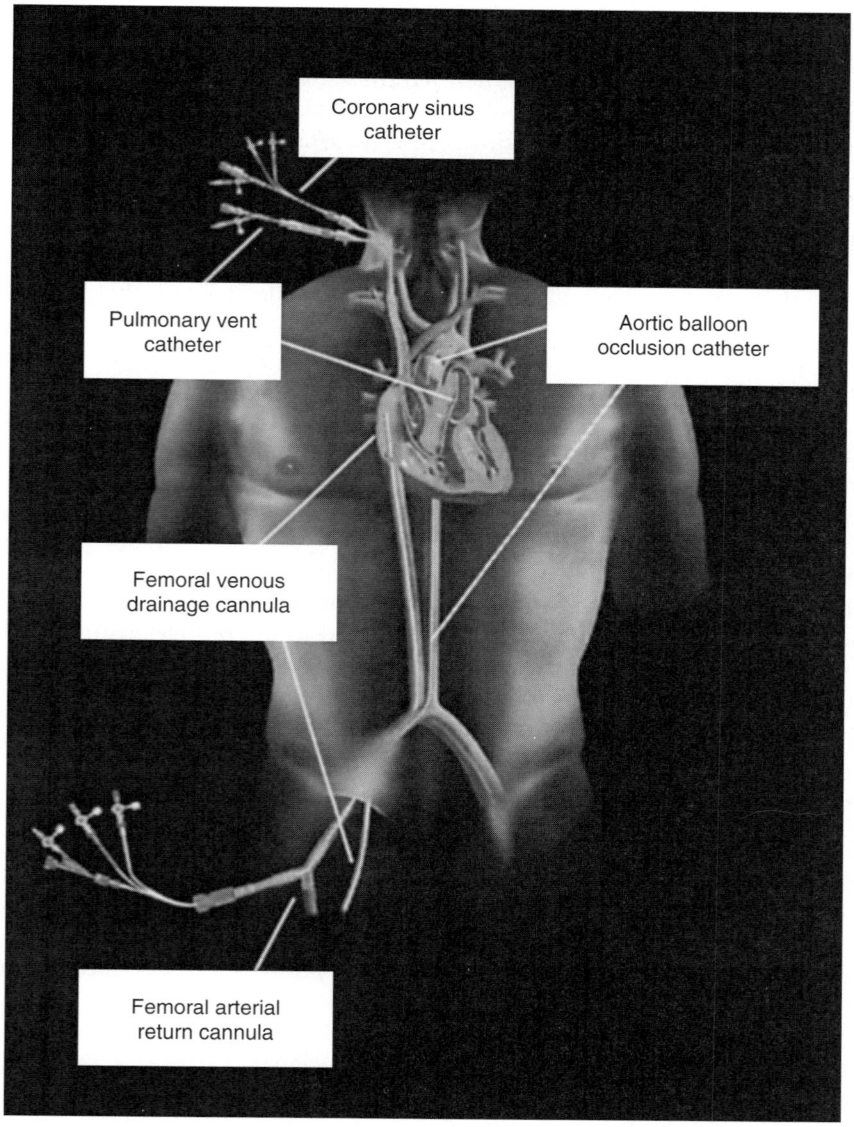

FIG. 13-2   Schematic depicting positioning of Port-Access endovascular cannulae and catheters in the heart. This system uses femoral arterial return.

(Copyright Heartport. Reprinted with permission.)

severity of aortic atherosclerosis merits consideration. Aneurysm of the ascending aorta may limit the ability to achieve appropriate balloon occlusion with the EndoClamp catheter. Severe aortic regurgitation may hinder effective antegrade delivery of cardioplegia.

Various tests are used preoperatively to evaluate the patient's cardiovascular anatomy, such as chest X-ray, aortography, iliofemoral arteriography, vascular magnetic resonance imaging methods, vascular ultrasound, and TEE. The referring cardiologist can facilitate the screening process by considering the patient a potential candidate for Port-Access surgery at the time of cardiac catheterization. An evaluation of aortic "runoff" is readily accomplished at that time.

Single-lung ventilation is often used to facilitate surgical exposure during Port-Access procedures; thus, the pulmonary function of patients with severe lung disease should be evaluated preoperatively. Tests may include chest X-ray, arterial blood gas analysis, and pulmonary function tests.

Intraoperative Management

Before Cardiopulmonary Bypass. Many clinicians prefer to insert a right radial arterial line and an intravenous (IV) line before induction of anesthesia. The anesthetic agents and techniques selected should be appropriate for the patient's condition and pathophysiology, as in conventional cardiac surgery. IV anesthetic medication is given in moderation to facilitate early postoperative emergence if desired. A double-lumen endobronchial tube or a bronchial blocker may be inserted for selective lung ventilation. Exposure of the aorta for cannulation with the DirectFlow cannula is facilitated with single-lung ventilation. The surgeon may also find that single-lung ventilation is helpful during dissection of the internal mammary artery in CABG procedures.

Following induction of anesthesia, a baseline TEE examination is conducted to survey the patient's anatomy before catheter insertion. Specific imaging information is obtained after a standard comprehensive examination. The diameter of the ascending aorta is measured and the presence and grade of aneurysm or atherosclerosis is evaluated. Complete examination of the thoracic aorta is desirable. The aortic valve is evaluated for insufficiency. The interatrial septum is examined for presence of an atrial septal defect or patent foramen ovale. With multiplane imaging, multiple views of the coronary sinus are obtained to determine the imaging strategy to be used during EndoPlege catheter placement. Similarly, views of the right ventricle, right ventricular outflow tract, pulmonary arteries, inferior vena cava, and superior vena cava are reviewed to facilitate the process of catheter and cannula placement. The anesthesiologist is responsible for inserting the EndoVent and EndoPlege catheters and provides valuable guidance in the placement of the other intravascular components.

Heparin is administered before the EndoPlege and EndoVent catheters are inserted in a dose sufficient to prevent thrombus formation (e.g., 100 U/kg). The remainder of a full dose of heparin (300 U/kg) is required before initiation of CPB and adequate activated clotting time is confirmed. By using TEE or fluoroscopy or both, the EndoPlege catheter is carefully advanced into the right atrium and the tip is placed in the coronary sinus. Positioning is also facilitated by observing the distal catheter tip pressure, which immediately indicates catheter advancement across the tricuspid valve into the right ventricle. The EndoVent catheter uses a flow-directed balloon to guide the tip across the tricuspid and pulmonic valves into the main pulmonary artery. Measurement of distal catheter pressure and imaging of the catheter with TEE, or fluoroscopy, or both allow appropriate catheter positioning.

The surgeon introduces the flexible QuickDraw cannula through a femoral vein and positions the cannula at the junction of the superior vena cava and right atrium for maximum drainage. A dilator and guidewire kit provided with the cannula facilitates placement. Final positioning is guided by TEE or fluoroscopy or both. Single-lung ventilation is used to facilitate exposure of the ascending aorta for placement of the DirectFlow cannula. Purse string sutures are placed via the main thoracic incision in the third or fourth intercostal space and the cannula is introduced through the first intercostal space. A spring-loaded blade within the tip of the DirectFlow incising introducer is used to make an incision in the aorta, and the tapered tip allows for easy single-step introduction of the cannula into the aorta.

The EndoClamp catheter is inserted through the Y-arm of the DirectFlow cannula and positioned for aortic occlusion. When femoral arterial return is planned by using the EndoReturn cannula, the surgeon performs a surgical cutdown of a femoral artery and introduces a guidewire into the artery. Imaging with TEE, fluoroscopy, or both ensures proper positioning of the wire in the descending thoracic aorta. The EndoReturn cannula is then advanced over the guidewire in the femoral artery and into position. The EndoClamp catheter is inserted coaxially into the EndoReturn cannula and advanced to the ascending aorta over a guidewire. The EndoClamp catheter is positioned appropriately in the ascending aorta by using TEE or fluoroscopy or both as a visual guide.

During Cardiopulmonary Bypass. A variety of specific monitoring techniques are used to evaluate venous drainage, arterial flow, venting, cardioplegia delivery, aortic occlusion, and regional perfusion to ensure that all catheters are maintained in the proper position and are functioning as desired. A coordinated team effort permits rapid adjustments to optimize system functioning. The anesthesiologist has an important role in gathering information and facilitating the appropriate interpretation, communication, and team response.

Venous drainage is evaluated by measuring centrifugal pump flow, inlet pressure of the centrifugal pump, right atrial pressure, pulmonary vent flow, right atrial pressure, TEE (to assess cardiac chamber size), and direct visualization or video-assisted thoracoscopy. Specific changes in flow and pressure can be traced to a variety of potential problems that may develop during CPB. Venous drainage inlet pressures more negative than −100 mm Hg could signal collapse of the right atrium around the QuickDraw catheter. In this situation, adjusting the pump's inertia to an inlet pressure less negative than −80 mm Hg typically improves venous drainage. A gradual loss of venous drainage without a progressively more negative inlet pressure may suggest hypovolemia and volume replacement may be necessary. The position of the QuickDraw catheter is monitored by using TEE imaging or fluoroscopy. For mitral valve procedures, surgical palpation is also possible through the right thoracic incision. Correct cannula positioning is essential to the proper conduct of endovascular CPB. Excessive flow through the EndoVent catheter may indicate that the QuickDraw cannula is placed in a less-than-optimal position. Arterial flow is monitored by measuring CPB pump flow and pressure as well as radial artery pressure. Typically, a vacuum relief valve is inserted into the pulmonary artery vent line and the EndoVent catheter is connected to a standard roller pump that aspirates blood from the pulmonary artery into the venous reservoir. The pressure relief valve vents air along with the blood as necessary to keep vacuum pressures from exceeding −80 mm Hg. A transit-time ultrasonic flowmeter and outlet pressures can be used to evaluate pulmonary artery venting. Venting of the aortic root is assessed by considering flow and aortic root pressures as well as by direct inspection.

Measurements of cardioplegia pump flow and pressure and of distal catheter pressures are used to evaluate antegrade or retrograde delivery of cardioplegia. TEE is used to image cardioplegia flow, and myocardial temperature and electrocardiogram (ECG) are observed for evidence of effective cardioplegia delivery. Resistance to delivery of antegrade cardioplegia by the EndoClamp catheter is evaluated continuously. Pump pressure should not exceed 350 mm Hg at a maximum flow rate of 250 to 300 ml/min. The aortic root pressure typically increases to between 60 and 90 mm Hg as the cardioplegia solution is infused into the catheter. Cardioplegia is delivered in a retrograde fashion via the EndoPlege catheter, and flow typically reaches 200 to 250 ml/min. The balloon at the catheter's tip is inflated before and during each infusion of cardioplegia and is typically deflated at the completion of each dose. During delivery of cardioplegic solution, the catheter's pressure-monitoring lumen is used to assess coronary sinus pressure. Kinks or partial occlusion of the cardioplegia lines or catheter malposition are usually indicated by excessive resistance or pressures in the cardioplegia circuit. Low pressure at the site of cardioplegia delivery may signal inadequate pump function, inadequate balloon occlusion, catheter malposition, or transducer problems. Pressures should be monitored in both the cardioplegia circuit and at the site of cardioplegia delivery.

The aortic root can be vented through the Endo-Clamp catheter. Aortic root pressure should be monitored during venting, and negative pressures should be avoided to keep air from being entrained into the aortic root as a result of a coronary arteriotomy or atriotomy. Adequate balloon catheter occlusion of the ascending aorta is evaluated by comparing simultaneous measurements of aortic root and radial artery pressures. Balloon pressure is also noted to verify static inflation. TEE and color flow Doppler aid in visualizing the balloon in the ascending aorta and in detecting any leakage around the balloon. Multiple monitoring techniques also verify proper positioning of the balloon in the ascending aorta and unimpeded fluid flow to the aortic arch vessels. Right radial artery pressure is monitored to detect any potential migration of the balloon that causes obstruction of the brachiocephalic artery. Some clinicians may choose to obtain and compare simultaneous measurements of left and right radial artery pressures. Transcranial Doppler monitoring of middle cerebral artery flow may also be useful. TEE is used to visualize the ascend-

ing aorta and the location of the balloon within the ascending aorta.

After Cardiopulmonary Bypass. Patients are weaned from CPB with the aid of TEE and pulmonary artery pressure measurements via the EndoVent catheter. TEE is used to evaluate ventricular and valvular function after separation from CPB. After removal of the catheters, a thermodilution pulmonary artery catheter is inserted when necessary for postoperative management. Before emergence, local anesthetics (e.g., bupivacaine with epinephrine) may be used for wound infiltration or intercostal nerve blocks. Emergence in the operating room is appropriate for some patients. Alternatively, the patient is transported to the intensive care unit (ICU) and then weaned from mechanical ventilation. The double-lumen endobronchial tube is exchanged for a single-lumen tube when postoperative mechanical ventilation is intended. Some clinicians prefer using a single-lumen endotracheal tube with a bronchial blocker to avoid the need to change the endobronchial tube at the end of surgery. Parenteral opioids or other analgesics such as ketorolac are typically administered in the immediate postoperative period for pain relief. Intercostal nerve blocks, intrathecal opiates, and epidural analgesia have also been used.

Investigational Experience

There have been reports of multiple laboratory investigations demonstrating the adequacy of endovascular CPB and the feasibility of Port-Access minimally invasive cardiac surgery by using the EndoCPB System. Schwartz et al[7] evaluated the effectiveness of endovascular CPB in achieving myocardial protection during aortic clamping. No differences were noted when comparing measures of left ventricular (LV) contractility in animals supported with endovascular CPB and those undergoing conventional CPB. Measurements included end-diastolic stroke work, preload recruitable stroke work, stroke work end-diastolic length relationship, maximal elastance, myocardial temperature, and ultrastructural biopsy. Ventricular performance was evaluated in Port-Access mitral valve replacement with endovascular CPB, demonstrating excellent recovery after CPB.[8] Preload recruitable stroke work, LV elastance, and preload recruitable work area were not significantly different 30 and 60 minutes after CPB as compared with baseline measurements before CPB. TEE demonstrated normal regional and global ventricular wall motion and normal prosthetic valve function.

Peters et al[9] evaluated the adequacy of endovascular CPB used to support 54 dogs during Port-Access cardiac surgical procedures. Cardioplegia delivery produced appropriate reductions in myocardial temperature. CPB time was 111 ± 27 minutes (mean ± standard deviation) and cardiac arrest time was 66 ± 21 minutes. Cardiac output was unchanged postoperatively versus preoperatively. Animal and human cadaver studies demonstrated the feasibility of Port-Access minimally invasive CABG in which the internal thoracic artery was used to bypass to various coronary arteries.[10-13] Additional studies demonstrated that Port-Access techniques can be used for mitral valve replacement and repair as well as other cardiac surgical procedures.[14] Laboratory experience demonstrated the feasibility of monitoring during endovascular CPB.[15]

Clinical Experience

CABG. Clinical reports have demonstrated broad applicability of Port-Access procedures with favorable outcomes. Galloway et al[16] reported the results of 1004 completed Port-Access procedures, including 555 completed CABG procedures and 299 completed mitral valve repairs and replacements from 121 centers performed from April 1, 1997, through January 1, 1998, and maintained in a registry of U.S. cases. Morbidity and mortality rates compared favorably with reported rates for conventional surgery. For Port-Access CABG, the mortality and myocardial infarction (MI) rates were 1.0% each and the stroke rate was 2.2%. The mortality rates for mitral valve repair and replacement were 1.5% and 3.3%, respectively. The incidence of new-onset postoperative atrial fibrillation was significantly lower in the Port-Access cases than has been reported in conventional cardiac surgery. More recent data from the Port-Access International Registry are shown in Table 13-1. In another report on the Port-Access International Registry, Shemin et al[17] noted increasing application in

multivessel CABG.[17] The application to multivessel CABG was reported by Groh et al,[18] who examined graft and target vessel usage in 228 consecutive patients from 21 sites. Multivessel CABG comprised 64% of cases with an average of 1.9 grafts per patient and left internal mammary artery (LIMA) to left anterior descending artery (LAD) used in 92% of cases. Saphenous vein grafts attached to the aorta were used in 79% of cases and all coronary beds were successfully grafted, suggesting that complete revascularization for all coronary beds can be accomplished with the Port-Access method by using a variety of venous and arterial conduits.

Port-Access methods use standard techniques for coronary artery revascularization on a motionless heart to afford the same level of myocardial protection through cardioplegic cardiac arrest and bypass as provided by traditional open-chest surgery. In a series of 32 Port-Access CABG procedures, Ribakove et al[19] reported 98% overall predischarge graft patency and 100% patency of left internal mammary-to-left anterior descending grafts. Reichenspurner et al[20] reported 100% angiographically documented graft patency in the first 10 Port-Access CABG patients from a series of 42 patients. Three-month follow-up angiography of 29 of these patients showed no evidence of stenosis in 27 patients. One patient had a new stenosis 2 cm distal to the LIMA graft site, which was not seen with a cardiac catheterization 5 months before surgery, and one patient had diffuse left anterior descending artery stenosis and sclerosis.[21] Barlow et al[22] reported that all 14 Port-Access patients were angina free and had no ischemia on exercise ECG at 12 weeks; coronary angiography was performed in the first 10 patients and disclosed 100% patency with no anastomotic narrowing. The patients in Barlow's series received single LIMA to LAD grafts. All the other reported series included up to three distal anastomoses. In the multicenter experience, Galloway noted a 1% incidence of MI in 583 patients and minimal need for primary procedure reoperations, providing evidence that the technique is reproducible with anastomotic accuracy.[16]

Several investigators have considered risk-adjusted mortality rates by considering preoperative patient characteristics and comorbid conditions. Shemin et al[23] analyzed data from 432 consecutive Port-Access CABG patients collected from 21 centers and used the New York State Department of Health multivariable risk-adjusted mortality rate model. The observed mortality rate with 30-day follow-up of 1.16% was not significantly different from the predicted in-hospital morality rate of 1.12%. Grossi et al[24] reported on 302 consecutive patients who underwent isolated Port-Access CABG and observed a 30-day mortality rate of 0.99% as compared with the predicted risk of death of 1.2% based on the Society of Thoracic Surgeons (STS) database risk-adjustment model. Groh et al[25] reported on their

OUTCOME (%)	CABG (n = 1676)
Death	1.6
Stroke	2.3
Myocardial infarction	0.8
New-onset atrial fibrillation	7.5
Reoperation for primary procedure	0.5
Reoperation for bleeding	3.6
Multisystem failure	0.4
Renal failure	1.0
Deep vein thrombosis	0.2

TABLE 13-1
Multicenter Morbidity and Mortality Rates Reported as Intention to Treat with Port-Access Coronaray Artery Bypass Graft (CABG)

experience with 229 consecutive Port-Access CABG cases from December of 1996 through July of 1998. Their observed mortality rate was 0.9%, compared with the predicted mortality rate of 1.3% based on the STS database risk-adjustment model (Table 13-2). Postoperative complications were compared with a matched cohort of conventional access patients. Complications of stroke and perioperative MI were not significantly different between the two groups. Reoperation for bleeding was more likely in the Port-Access group, while infections were more frequent in the sternotomy group. The length of hospital stay (LOS) postoperatively was significantly shorter for the Port-Access patients (4.3 days vs. 6.0 days), and transfusion therapy was significantly less frequent for the Port-Access patients (25.8% vs. 33.6%).

Analyzing the Port-Access International Registry, Siegel et al[26] found that the median duration of postoperative tracheal intubation following multivessel Port-Access CABG was 5 hours, the median duration of intensive care stay was 21 hours, and the median postoperative hospital stay was 4 days. These data were compared with results from the University Health System Consortium study of nonemergent, nonfatal, first-time CABG procedures performed at 40 academic hospitals in which the median duration of tracheal intubation was 15.2 hours, the median duration of intensive care stay was 31.5 hours, and the median postoperative hospital stay was 5 days. Chaney et al[27] noted reduced time to extubation and hospital discharge when comparing their initial Port-Access surgery experience with historic controls. Rogers et al[28] reported single center experience with the development and implementation of perioperative care protocols and a clinical pathway for Port-Access patients.

A retrospective analysis of 94 Port-Access CABG and 181 conventional CABG procedures performed during the same time period at a single institution was reported by Boova et al[29] The mean number of grafts was 2.7 in the Port-Access cohort and 3.5 in the conventional group. Significantly more of the Port-Access patients received total arterial revascularization than

did the conventional group (62% vs. 31%). Operating time was longer for the Port-Access procedures by approximately 85 minutes; however, perfusion time was equivalent and aortic clamp time was shorter. Duration of mechanical ventilation, ICU stay, and hospital stay were less for the Port-Access. Hospital complications including blood transfusion, incisional complications, reexploration, respiratory insufficiency, and atrial fibrillation were less for the Port-Access patients. Hospital charges for CABG without cardiac catheterization were not significantly different for the two surgical techniques.

Grossi et al[30] compared postoperative pain, stress response, and functional recovery in 14 Port-Access CABG and 15 standard sternotomy CABG patients. There were no differences between the two groups in gender or preoperative comorbid conditions, although the mean age was greater in the sternotomy group. Norepinephrine levels were significantly lower over the first 3 postoperative days in the Port-Access group as compared with the sternotomy group. Pulmonary function testing revealed significantly better forced expiratory volume in the Port-Access group than for sternotomy patients postoperatively (1.59 L/sec vs. 0.97 L/sec at 1 day and 2.20 L/sec vs. 1.49 L/sec at 3 days). Pain was significantly less over the first 4 weeks postoperatively in the Port-Access group as compared with the sternotomy group (Fig. 13-3). Patients in the Port-Access cohort also had significantly less muscle soreness, shortness of breath, fatigue, and poor appetite at 1, 2, 4, and 8 weeks postoperatively. Significantly more of the Port-Access patients than the sternotomy patients were able to walk one to two blocks at 1 week postoperatively, climb stairs at 1 and 2 weeks, perform light or moderate housework at 1 and 2 weeks, and engage in moderate recreational activities and perform heavy housework at 4 and 8 weeks postoperatively.

Valve Surgery. Mohr et al[31] updated their initial mitral valve surgery experience with a report of 2 years of experience in Leipzig with 129 Port-Access surgeries in which they commented on their learning curve. They

TABLE 13-2
Risk-Adjusted Mortality for Port-Access CABG

PUBLICATION	PATIENTS	CENTERS	PREDICTION MODEL	PREDICTED MORTALITY RATES (%)	OBSERVED MORTALITY RATES (%)
Shemin et al[23]	432	21	New York State	1.12	1.16
Grossi et al[24]	302	3	Society of Thoracic Surgeons	1.2	0.99
Groh et al[25]	229	1	Society of Thoracic Surgeons	1.3	0.9

FIG. 13-3 Grossi et al compared postoperative pain and functional recovery in 14 Port-Access coronary artery bypass graft (CABG) and 15 standard sternotomy CABG patients. Pain was significantly less over the first 4 weeks postoperatively in the Port-Access group compared with the sternotomy group. Patients in the Port-Access cohort also had significantly less muscle soreness, shortness of breath, fatigue, and poor appetite at 1, 2, 4, and 8 weeks postoperatively. Significantly more of the Port-Access patients than the sternotomy patients were able to walk one to two blocks at 1 week postoperatively, climb stairs at 1 and 2 weeks, perform light or moderate housework at 1 and 2 weeks, and engage in moderate recreational activities and perform heavy housework at 4 and 8 weeks postoperatively. (Adapted from Grossi EA, Zakow PK, Ribakove GH et al: *Eur J Cardiothorac Surg* 16[S2]:S39-S42, 1999.)

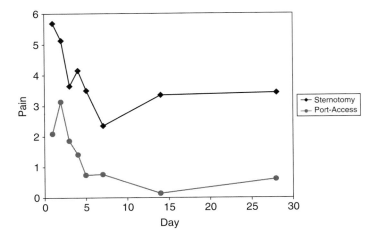

noted that the hospital mortality rate was 8% in the early 62 cases and 3% in the recent experience. Surgery, bypass, and clamp times improved during the experience, averaging 152 minutes, 107 minutes, and 48 minutes, respectively, in the most recent 67 patients.[32]

Grossi et al[33] prospectively gathered data on all patients undergoing Port-Access isolated valve surgery at their institution in New York and performed a case-match study with patients who had undergone isolated valve surgery with a conventional sternotomy approach during the prior year. In this study, the 109 Port-Access patients had significantly shorter LOS and received fewer transfusions than did the sternotomy group. In a series of 41 consecutive patients undergoing isolated mitral valve replacement or repair, Glower et al[34] demonstrated return to normal activity levels in 4 weeks after Port-Access mitral valve surgery as compared with 9 weeks by using open-chest methods (Fig. 13-4). In a retrospective comparison of 241 patients undergoing redo mitral operations, patients treated with minimally invasive Port-Access surgery had less transfusion therapy, less chest tube output, lower 30-day mortality rate, and earlier return to normal activity than patients treated with a standard median sternotomy or a right thoracotomy; however, these benefits came at the expense of longer procedure time.[35]

Glower et al[36] performed logistic regression analysis on valve surgery data from the Port-Access International Registry, a prospective, multicenter, longitudinal observational study of patients undergoing isolated aortic valve replacement, mitral repair, or mitral replacement by use of Port-Access techniques from 1997 to 1999. Aortic valve procedures were performed predominantly via partial sternotomy (40%) or right anterior thoracotomy (47%), and mitral valve surgery was performed by using a right anterior (87%) or lateral (10%) thoracotomy. Median length of the chest incision was 8 cm for aortic valve surgery and 6 cm for mitral valve surgery.

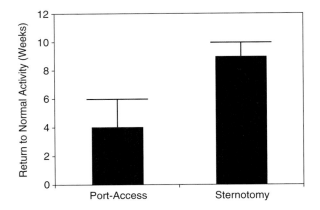

FIG. 13-4 Return to normal activity was significantly more rapid ($p = 0.01$) for patients who received Port-Access mitral valve surgery ($n = 21$) as compared with patients who had mitral valve surgery via sternotomy ($n = 20$). Values are expressed as mean and standard deviation. (Adapted from Glower DD, Landolfo K, Clements F et al: *Eur J Cardiothorac Surg* 14:S143-S147, 1999.)

Conversion to a full sternotomy occurred in 3.8% of cases. Endoaortic balloon occlusion was used in 93% of mitral repair, 90% of mitral valve replacement, and 2% of aortic valve replacements. The early mortality rate was 3.8% and onset of new atrial fibrillation occurred in 11% of patients (Tables 13-3 and 13-4). Most patients were discharged home without home care services (82% aortic valve replacement, 83% mitral valve repair, 74% mitral valve replacement) and rates of readmission within 30 days were low in all groups at 6.0% for aortic valve replacement, 8.4% for mitral valve repair, and 7.5% for mitral valve replacement. The authors examined potential independent predictors of mortality, stroke, and reoperation for bleeding by considering institutional case volume, age, previous cardiac operation,

TABLE 13-3
Preoperative Status of Patients Who Underwent Port-Access Isolated Aortic or Mitral Valve Surgery

PATIENT CHARACTERISTICS	AORTIC VALVE REPLACEMENT	MITRAL VALVE REPAIR	MITRAL VALVE REPLACEMENT
Age (yr, mean ± SD)	65 ± 15	57 ± 14	60 ± 14
Gender (% male)	63	66	39
Elective (%)	98	99	98
Reoperation (%)	12	8	23
Diabetes (%)	11.1	5.9	9.1
Renal failure (%)	3.0	2.3	4.3
Hypertension (%)	54	39	38
Pulmonary hypertension (%)	11	25	39
COPD (%)	8.0	6.5	15
Myocardial infarction (%)	8.0	8.2	6.0
NYHA class III-IV (%)	57	53	75

Adapted from Glower DD, Siegel LC, Frischmeyer KJ et al: *Ann Thorac Surg* 70:1054-1059, 2000.
COPD, Chronic obstructive pulmonary disease; *NYHA,* New York Heart Association.

TABLE 13-4
Perioperative Morbidity for Patients Who Underwent Port-Access Isolated Aortic or Mitral Valve Surgery

OUTCOME	AORTIC VALVE REPLACEMENT (n = 252)	MITRAL VALVE REPAIR (n = 491)	MITRAL VALVE REPLACEMENT (n = 568)
Death (%)	4.4	1.6	5.5
Stroke: unresolved (%)	2.4	2.6	2.8
Myocardial infarction (%)	0	0.4	0.2
Failed valve repair (%)	—	2.0	—
Paravalvular leak (%)	0	0.6	0.5
Reoperation for bleeding (%)	4.4	2.6	6.2
Renal failure (%)	2.8	2.1	3.3
Multisystem failure (%)	1.2	0.6	2.6
Deep vein thrombosis (%)	0	0	0.5
New-onset atrial fibrillation (%)	12.7	10.4	10.0
Pleural effusion (%)	4.0	4.5	4.0

Adapted from Glower DD, Siegel LC, Frischmeyer KJ et al: *Ann Thorac Surg* 70:1054-1059, 2000.

history of heart failure, and type of surgical procedure. Institutional Port-Access minimally invasive cardiac surgery case volume did not affect mortality, stroke, or reoperation for bleeding. The major predictors of mortality were previous cardiac operation, older age, and mitral valve replacement or aortic valve replacement as opposed to mitral valve repair. Older age was the only predictor of stroke. Older age, mitral valve replacement, and previous cardiac operation were independent pre-dictors of reoperation for bleeding. These results are consistent with previous reports of risk-prediction models including factors such as age. Similar patient outcomes from a variety of institutions suggest that Port-Access methods and technology can be mastered with an appropriate learning curve.

Atrial Fibrillation. Atrial fibrillation is the most common complication occurring after cardiac surgery. Supraventricular tachycardias (SVTs), including atrial fibrillation, have been detected in as many as 100% of patients after CABG surgery.[37] Clinically relevant postoperative atrial fibrillation, which may last for greater than 5 minutes or require an intervention for termination, has an incidence of 20% to 40%.[38] The most common episode of atrial fibrillation is a brief paroxysm, and the peak time-to-occurrence is on the second and third postoperative days with the possibility of episodes recurring or persisting for weeks.[38,39] The incidence of atrial fibrillation after cardiac surgery far exceeds its reported prevalence in the general population and in patients after major noncardiac surgery regardless of status of cardiac disease (Table 13-5).

The pathophysiology underlying the high incidence of atrial fibrillation after cardiac surgery is complex, and possible mechanisms include β-blocker withdrawal, CPB, inadequate atrial protection, and manipulation of the right atrium.[40] All of these factors may be interrelated or partially responsible. Clinical predictors of atrial fibrillation include age, male gender, concomitant valvular heart disease, history of atrial fibrillation, and history of congestive heart failure.[39,41] Surgical practices such as venting through the pulmonary vein, direct right atrial cannulation, use of an intraaortic balloon pump, and extended cross-clamp time are independent predictors of postoperative atrial fibrillation.[42]

There are important clinical consequences of postoperative atrial fibrillation.[43] Impaired systolic and diastolic function may cause congestive heart failure and hypotension. Postoperative atrial fibrillation increases the risk of stroke twofold to threefold, an excess comparable to patients with atrial fibrillation unrelated to surgery. Management of this risk is complicated by a reluctance to anticoagulate postoperative patients. Iatrogenic complications may result from attempts to avoid or treat postoperative atrial fibrillation. β-Adrenergic blockers, diltiazem, and sotalol may cause severe hypotension and impair hemodynamics. Cardioversion may cause bradycardia, tachycardia, and myocardial damage. Antiarrhythmic drugs can be proarrhythmic and cause life-threatening ventricular arrhythmia.

Atrial fibrillation increases duration of hospitalization and hospital costs (Table 13-6). Atrial fibrillation being the most frequent complication following CABG, its cumulative cost exceeds that of all other complications. Atrial fibrillation is identified as the primary factor for increasing the LOS, ahead of respiratory insufficiency, pneumonia, and wound infection.[44] After adjusting age, gender, and other potential correlates, atrial fibrillation is independently associated with an increased LOS of 4.9 days.[40] Various investigators reported an increase of LOS from 1 to 10 days with an overall average of 5 days.[38] Treatment with amiodarone for 7 days preoperatively and during hospitalization reduces the incidence of postoperative atrial fibrillation, LOS, and hospitalization costs.[45]

Several investigators have observed low frequencies of new-onset atrial fibrillation following Port-Access cardiac surgical procedures. Grossi et al[46] performed a multicenter case-matched comparison of Port-Access CABG ($n = 302$) with the STS database ($n = 9674$) and observed atrial fibrillation in 12.6% of Port-Access cases as compared with 17.9% in the sternotomy group ($p = 0.02$). Boova et al[29] compared 94 Port-Access CABG cases with 181 conventional CABG cases performed at the same institution and observed atrial fibrillation

TABLE 13-5
Reported Incidence of Atrial Fibrillation

POPULATION	n	INCIDENCE (%)	REFERENCE
CABG	211,622	17.2	STS database
CABG	570	33	Aranki et al, 1996[40]
CABG	2,458	26.7	Andrews et al, 1991[174]
All heart operations	3,983	34.6	Creswell et al, 1993[41]
CABG/valvular surgery	2,417	27	Mathew et al, 1996[42]
CABG	258	30.6	Chung et al, 1996[175]
General population		1.7	Kannel et al, 1982[176]
Noncardiac patients diagnosed		4.8 women	Furberg et al, 1994[177]
		6.2 men	
Atherosclerotic CAD		3.6	
Noncardiac surgery		5	Goldman et al, 1978[178]

CABG, Coronary artery bypass graft; *CAD*, coronary artery disease; *STS*, Society of Thoracic Surgeons.

in 9.6% of Port-Access cases and in 18.8% of conventional cases ($p < 0.05$). Groh et al[25] considered 229 consecutive Port-Access CABG cases at a single institution and compared these cases with a cohort of conventional access patients matched for morality risk. Atrial fibrillation was observed in 14.4% of Port-Access cases and 16.6% of conventional cases. The Port-Access International Registry, a prospective multicenter observational cohort study, reported new-onset atrial fibrillation in 7.5% of 1676 Port-Access CABG cases.[16,17] In smaller single-center series, investigators reported postoperative atrial fibrillation ranging in frequency from 3% to 7%.[19,20,28,47] Arom et al[48] found a significantly lower frequency ($p < 0.05$) of postoperative atrial fibrillation in Port-Access valve cases (8%, $n = 40$) as compared with valve procedures performed through a partial sternotomy (26%, $n = 66$). Glower et al[34] reviewed 41 consecutive mitral valve surgeries and noted atrial fibrillation in 29% of Port-Access cases and 50% of conventional cases. A low incidence of new-onset atrial fibrillation was reported by the Port-Access International Registry for mitral valve repair (10.4%, $n = 491$), mitral valve replacement (10.0%, $n = 568$), aortic valve replacement (12.7%, $n = 252$), and atrial septal defect repair (3.1%, $n = 223$).[16,36] Several investigators suggested that new methods be developed to combine minimally invasive mitral valve surgery with ablation therapy of the pulmonary veins to provide an effective treatment for atrial fibrillation.[49,50]

In summary, postoperative atrial fibrillation is common after cardiac surgery occurring in as many as one third of patients. The arrhythmias may cause hypotension, congestive heart failure, increased risk for stroke, or subjective discomfort and anxiety. Lengthened postoperative hospitalization and increased medical care costs are also associated with postoperative atrial fibrillation. A lower incidence of postoperative atrial fibrillation has been noted in a number of Port-Access cardiac surgical procedures. Additional investigation will facilitate an understanding of the pathophysiology of this important clinical observation.

Catheter and Cannula Insertion and Monitoring. There have been several clinical reports relating to the catheters and cannulae of the EndoCPB system regarding insertion and monitoring. Effective catheter insertion and monitoring techniques were demonstrated in the initial clinical series.[51] Plotkin et al[52] and Lewis et al[53] reported percutaneous cannulation of the coronary sinus by using TEE without fluoroscopy in a residency training program setting with cannulation time of 12.9 ± 3 minutes (mean $\pm$ standard deviation) and successful cannulation in 86% of cases. Yen et al[54] reported a multicenter experience with 58 patients in which cannulation of the coronary sinus was successful in 97% of cases and cannulation time was 5.2 ± 3.5 minutes (mean $\pm$ standard deviation). Ostrowski et al[55] noted an overall success rate of 76% for coronary sinus cannulation among 10 anesthesiologists in a teaching institution. They observed evidence of a reasonable learning curve by noting a statistically significant decrease in patient preparation time in the operating room when comparing the first and second 10 cases. Cardiac perforation during attempted coronary sinus cannulation has been reported.[56] Proper technique by using all available information coupled with a good understanding of cardiac anatomy and physiology is important for minimizing the likelihood of this complication.[57,58]

Applebaum et al[59] evaluated the utility of TEE in 36 patients during Port-Access surgical procedures. Retrograde cardioplegia was used in 21 procedures and percutaneous catheter placement was achieved in 95% of cases; one patient required catheter placement by direct surgical visualization. Percutaneous placement was thought to be hampered in this case by a prominent eustachian valve. TEE was also beneficial for imaging

---

TABLE 13-6

Postoperative Atrial Fibrillation Is Associated with a Longer Hospital Stay and Increased Medical Care Costs

STUDY	n	PATIENTS WITH ATRIAL FIBRILLATION (%)	INCREASE OF LOS (DAYS)	MEAN CHARGES INCREASE PER PATIENT ($)
Kowey et al[38]	157	28	3	21,504
Redle et al[163]	143	33	3.8	7,011
Creswell et al[41]	3,983	34.6	2.3 days in ICU plus 3.4 days in ward	—
Aranki et al[40]	570	33	4.9 (Adjusted LOS)	10,055

ICU, Intensive care unit; *LOS,* length of hospital stay.

venous cannulation and EndoClamp catheter placement.[59] In a subsequent report, the authors updated this experience by examining the role of TEE in 449 Port-Access procedures performed at a single institution from May of 1996 through July of 1998.[60] Schulze described the use of TEE in 51 Port-Access surgery cases and noted that TEE imaging was supplemented with intermittent fluoroscopy in 10% of the cases for positioning of the guidewire or EndoClamp catheter.[61] A detailed discussion of TEE imaging techniques in Port-Access surgical procedures is available.[62] In a comparison between aortic and femoral artery cannulation, Glower et al[63] demonstrated the elimination of Endo-Clamp migration with aortic cannulation and the groin and femoral arterial morbidity associated with femoral arterial cannulation. The 30-day mortality rate was 0% with aortic cannulation and 1% with femoral cannulation. The authors concluded that transthoracic direct aortic cannulation is technically easy in a wide variety of patients and expands the pool of patients eligible for minimally invasive cardiac surgery. Transcranial Doppler monitoring is useful to detect aortic balloon malposition.[64]

Robotics

Robotic technologies have been introduced to further facilitate minimally invasive surgery. Endoscopic visualization systems facilitated by a voice-activated camera control allow the general surgeon to perform laparoscopic procedures without the assistance of another surgeon. This technology has been applied to Port-Access minimally invasive mitral valve and atrial septal defect surgery.[65-67] Robotic systems offering "telepresence" facilitate suturing and tissue manipulation via small ports with video-assisted visualization. These systems consist of an interface device for manipulation by the surgeon, a controller, and robotic arms connected to instruments. The instrument tips are introduced into the body through small ports. The surgeon manipulates handles on the interface that are analogous to those of traditional surgical instruments. The surgeon's motions are replicated by the robotic arms, which manipulate the instrument tips. Signal processing allows for filtering of surgeon tremor and for scaling motion. For example, 3:1 scaling would allow the surgeon to have a movement of 3 cm at the interface device translated into a 1-cm movement by the robotic arm instrument tip. Initial clinical studies demonstrated the feasibility of using this technology.[68-70] Different robotic systems have been developed and the potential importance of various features such as the number of degrees of freedom, or the dimensions of the instruments is subject to investigation.[71] The role of robotic technology, the optimal clinical techniques for its application, and the associated clinical benefits are active areas of current clinical investigation.

Saphenous Vein Harvesting

Surgical techniques and technology have advanced to permit less invasive harvesting of saphenous veins for aortocoronary bypass grafts. Traditional methods include harvesting vein by using a single long incision. Bridging techniques are a series of small incisions used to access the vein. These bridging techniques are enhanced with improvements in lighting and retraction devices analogous to a laryngoscope. Endoscopic technologies allow for indirect visualization with a video camera and magnified video display. Balloon technologies facilitate dissection and visualization. Closed systems use carbon dioxide insufflation to create an operative tunnel. In open systems, the operative tunnel is maintained with a long and narrow U-shaped retractor. Endoscopic vein harvesting is associated with a significantly lower frequency of wound complications when compared with traditional vein harvesting (4% vs. 19%) in a prospective, randomized study of 112 patients.[72] Morris and colleagues compared 27 patients having endoscopic saphenous vein harvesting with 24 patients having traditional saphenous vein harvesting and noted less edema, less pain, and increased postoperative mobility in the patients who received the endoscopic procedure.[73]

CORONARY ARTERY SURGERY: OPCABG AND MIDCABG
History and Definitions

CABG without CPB was first reported during the mid to late 1960s and early 1970s.[74,75] Development of CPB and improvements in CPB equipment and technology made distal anastomoses less technically challenging and increased the surgeon's ability to access more distal coronary sites; thus, CABG without CPB was mostly abandoned. Myocardial revascularization without CPB regained popularity during the 1990s. This resurgence was based on the development and improvements of mechanical stabilization devices,[76-80] the recognition of adverse effects of CPB, and increased prevalence of comorbidities in an aging CABG patient population. Economic circumstances also played a role with the need to reduce the use of health care resources and with increased surgical and interventional competition. Controversy about CABG without CPB exists with the need to maintain the efficacy of the established standard of care for treatment of symptomatic coronary artery disease (CAD). These standards include low reintervention rates for failed primary procedure, complete revascularization, and long-term patency rates. The quality of outcome for conventional CABG has also been challenged,[70] both based on a review of the STS database, operative mortality rate and incidence of complication data, and a review of hospital discharge data from health insurance records.[71] Operative mortality rate increases with age from 1.1% at age 20 to 50 years to 7.2% at age 81 to 90 years. No complications are reported in only 65.4% of patients. Among patients 65 years old or more, 4.3% of them die in the hospital, only 81.9% are discharged within 14 days, 0.7% die in the first 2 months after discharge, and 9.9% are readmitted for cardiovascular, cerebrovascular, or respiratory complications.[81]

The terminology for less invasive CABG is evolving and is subject to confusion. MIDCABG typically refers to direct vision grafting of one or two anterior coronary vessels without CPB through a minithoracotomy. Minimally invasive direct coronary artery bypass grafting (MIDCABG) is sometimes combined with endoscopic mobilization of the internal mammary artery. Off pump coronary artery bypass grafting (OPCABG) typically refers to direct vision grafting of multiple coronary vessels without CPB via a median sternotomy.

Investigational Experience and Current Technology

The major challenges of CABG without CPB include accurate anastomosis suture placement, maintenance of acceptable hemodynamics, and avoidance of myocardial injury and hemostasis at the distal anastomosis site. Interruption of recipient artery flow may induce regional ischemia, arrhythmias, and hemodynamic deterioration. Retrograde blood flow in the arteriotomy may obscure the edges and hamper suturing. Displacement of the heart to expose posterior targets may interfere with normal pump function. Working space is limited and target vessel identification may be difficult. Although the adverse effects of CPB and cardiac arrest may be avoided, new problems are generated. These issues and potential solutions have been evaluated clinically and experimentally over the last decade.

Grafting of the posterior targets is still a major challenge because of hemodynamic deterioration. The hemodynamic consequences of exposing and stabilizing these targets is primarily related to deformation of the right ventricle.[82,83] Biventricular dysfunction in OPCABG patients[84] and impaired LV diastolic function may also occur.[85,86] Coronary flow itself does not appear to be mechanically obstructed during experimental cardiac displacement to expose posterior targets.[87] Hemodynamic deterioration is observed during mechanical stabilization of the LAD and caused by direct ventricular compression with reduced stroke volume.[88] The Trendelenburg position minimizes hemodyna-

mic deterioration.[82,87] Assisted circulation reduces the negative hemodynamic effects observed during CABG without CPB. Right heart bypass without an oxygenator improves stroke volume and mean arterial blood pressure.[83,89-91] Right heart bypass and left heart assist without an oxygenator permits OPCABG in patients with severely depressed LV function.[92-94]

Myocardial injury from global or regional ischemia may be reduced by pharmacologic or mechanical preconditioning. Ischemic preconditioning, defined as previous exposure to transient myocardial ischemia, is an endogenous adaptation of the heart providing protection to subsequent prolonged myocardial ischemia. This adaptive mechanism is created by mechanically occluding the coronary artery for a brief period during CABG surgery without CPB to protect the myocardium from potential ischemic injury during the surgical anastomosis. Evidence exists that mechanical ischemic preconditioning attenuates myocardial injury (endothelial dysfunction, apoptosis, and neutrophil accumulation) associated with temporary ischemia,[95-97] whereas other studies question its protective effect.[98,99] Pharmacologic preconditioning by using adenosine, isoflurane, and enflurane has also been reported.[100-102] Only minor changes in myocardial energy metabolism occur in OPCABG patients.[103]

Traction sutures and instruments provide an immobile coronary artery to perform the distal anastomosis.[104-107] The introduction of mechanical stabilizers attached to the operating table or a rib retractor in the mid 1990s has greatly facilitated local epicardial motion restraint.[76-79,82] Alternative approaches to create a motionless field without the use of stabilizers have also been investigated.[108-112] Pharmacologic agents slow or temporarily stop the heart to facilitate the anastomosis. Alternatively, the thoracic vagus nerve is directly or indirectly (intravascular) electrically stimulated to temporarily stop the heart.

Interruption of coronary flow is tolerated because of well-developed collateral circulation in many patients with CAD.[113] However, hemodynamic instability may occur as a result of ischemia or arrhythmia. Temporary shunts and distal perfusion systems are effective in reducing myocardial injury associated with temporary interruption of native coronary flow.[113-115] A variety of different methods are used to interrupt segmental coronary flow or provide coronary artery hemostasis.[116] Temporary shunts, intravascular or extravascular vessel occluders, and arteriotomy seals prevent blood from obscuring the arteriotomy edges.[113-115,117,118]

Technology for CABG without CPB principally consists of devices that provide a stable and bloodless anastomosis site. Three methods of stabilization are provided by current coronary artery stabilizers. A relatively motionless anastomosis site is achieved either by compressing the myocardium adjacent to the artery, immobilizing the myocardium with suction achieved with a remote vacuum source, or using a combination of limited compression of the myocardium and lifting of the coronary artery segment with elastic tapes. The coronary artery stabilizers are secured to a standard or special sternal (OPCABG) or a rib (MIDCABG) retractor. The coronary artery stabilizing component is connected to a rigid or articulating shaft that is attached to a base placed on a retractor. The impact of the different individual stabilizers systems on hemodynamics is unclear, especially when considering the impact of cardiac displacement. Compression systems currently on the market include the Access Ultima (Guidant, Inc., Santa Clara, Calif.) and the Precision-OP (Heartport, Fig. 13-5). Suction systems include the Octopus Stabilizer (Medtronic, Inc., Minneapolis, Fig. 13-6), the Vortex Stabilizer (Guidant), and Flexsite Stabilizer Systems (Heartport). The Cohn Cardiac Stabilizer (OPCAB Elite System, Genzyme, Inc., Fig. 13-7) represents a combination compression and lifting system. The elastic tapes used for immobilization with the Cohn Cardiac Stabilizer simultaneously provide proximal and distal vessel occlusion.

Devices used to provide a relatively bloodless anastomosis site consist of temporary intracoronary shunts, intravascular and extravascular vessel occluders, so-called "blower-mister" devices that displace blood by delivery of a combination of gas (CO_2) and liquid (saline), and standard suction devices. In addition to providing a relatively bloodless field, the blower-mister devices also open the arteriotomy to facilitate suture placement.

Patient Selection and Preoperative Evaluation

Indications for CABG without CPB are not well established and vary among clinicians. High-risk patients (older, multiple comorbidities, severely impaired LV function) have better outcomes if their CABG is performed off pump.[119-121] Current indications include favorable anatomy and high-risk patients. Most surgeons individualize the indication for each patient. Key issues are complete revascularization of all intended coronary arteries and durability of the anastomoses, the two principle advantages of surgery over percutaneous revascularization.[122] The difference between complete surgical revascularization and optimal revascularization is important. High-risk patients, for example, may benefit from incomplete surgical revascularization combined with percutaneous revascularization.[123] The durability of the anastomosis is largely based on vessel size, location, disease state, choice of conduit, and surgical technique.

Indications for MIDCABG are based on the location of the anastomosis and number of vessels that require revascularization. Patients requiring first-time or reoperative anterior vessel revascularization (proximal right coronary artery [RCA], LAD and diagonal, left main

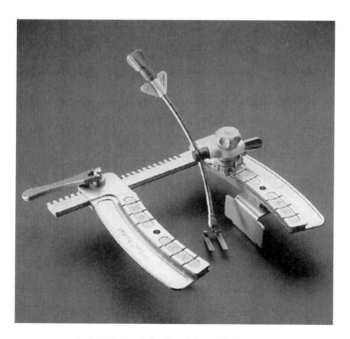

FIG. 13-5 The Precision-OP System.

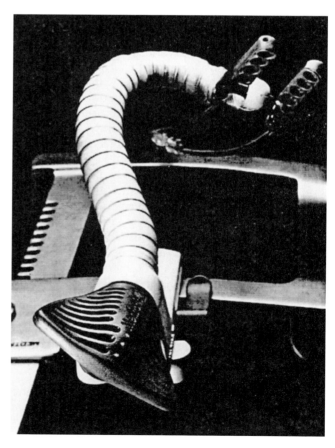

FIG. 13-6 The Octopus 2+ Tissue Stabilization System.

disease), with anastomoses at easily accessed locations, are good candidates for MIDCABG either as sole therapy or as a combination (so-called hybrid therapy) of surgical and percutaneous therapy.

Patients selected for OPCABG typically have multivessel surgical disease, in the presence or absence of comorbidities (heart failure, renal failure, respiratory failure, cerebrovascular disease). OPCABG has been performed in patients with a variety of medical problems, yielding acceptable morbidity rates.[124,125] Grafting circumflex and posterolateral branches is still a major challenge because of hemodynamic deterioration associated with surgical exposure. Arrhythmias and COPD may make OPCABG more challenging because of increased motion and decreased exposure, respectively.

Preoperative evaluation of patients specifically considered for CABG without CPB includes the number of distal anastomoses, suitability of distal targets, evaluation of hemodynamic and respiratory status, assessment of comorbidities, and determination of anesthetic and surgical risks. Calcification or vessel diameter of less than 1.5 mm at the anastomosis site, intramyocardial anastomosis site, and the need for endarterectomy are considered relative or absolute contraindications to OPCABG, emphasizing the need for evaluation of the diagnostic angiogram. It is important to identify cardiomegaly preoperatively because distal target exposure, especially of posterior vessels, is more likely to be associated with hemodynamic deterioration in patients with cardiomegaly. It is easier to convert an OPCABG case intraoperatively to conventional CABG than to convert MIDCABG. Comorbidities require increased attention, especially because patients who were not considered candidates for surgical revascularization, on the

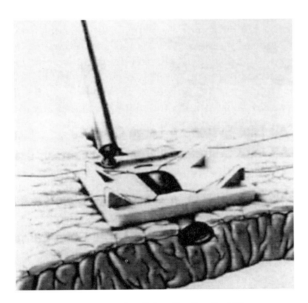

FIG. 13-7   The Cohn Cardiac Stabilizer.

basis of severe cardiac, renal, or respiratory dysfunction, are increasingly considered candidates for CABG without CPB.[119-121]

Surgical Technique

MIDCABG via a minithoracotomy was promoted in the early 1990s, and, although still practiced, the current indications for MIDCABG are limited. OPCABG via a median sternotomy became the more popular approach to CABG without CPB during the late 1990s. The ease and familiarity of internal mammary artery mobilization, target vessel identification and exposure, and increased ability to achieve complete revascularization are the main factors underlying the shift from MIDCABG to OPCABG. Industry continues to provide devices that enable this shift, but success or failure of CABG without CPB still depends on surgical technique.

General considerations regardless of the MIDCABG or OPCABG approach include having perfusion backup or on standby. The decision to have a primed or non-primed CPB circuit as backup depends on experience, the patient, and whether or not another patient requires CPB. The need for a cell saver is based on the number of grafts and the chosen surgical approach. External defibrillation and pacing pads are placed when access to the heart is limited.

During OPCABG, the grafts are harvested as in conventional CABG. Heparin is administered at the conclusion of internal mammary artery (IMA) harvesting. Chest tubes are occasionally placed while the retractor used for IMA harvesting is still in place. A standard pericardotomy is performed, including incisions for the IMA pedicle. The pericardiotomy may be extended posteriorly in a reverse T-fashion.

The decision to continue without CPB is made based on the hemodynamic response to temporary manual exposure of all distal targets and digital palpation of the intended anastomosis sites to determine the feasibility of OPCABG. The specific surgical revascularization strategy is determined at this time. This includes determination of the distal target order and the sequence of proximal and distal anastomoses. In general, the distal anastomoses are performed first. The goal is to establish adequate perfusion of the most critical vascular bed first to improve myocardial perfusion and performance during subsequent manipulations to revascularize other target areas. The LAD territory is often revascularized first because the IMA anastomosis provides immediate perfusion and requires minimal displacement.

Distal target exposure can be challenging during OPCABG, especially for exposure of the posterior targets. The objective is to place the target in a position that is comfortable for the surgeon while minimizing hemodynamic compromise. The physiologic tolerance to manipulation is unpredictable and depends on the degree

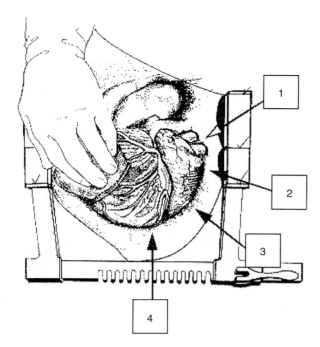

FIG. 13-8 Deep pericardial stay suture placement. The site of the pericardial stitches used to verticalize the heart. The first stitch (1) is located between the superior and the inferior left pulmonary veins close to the pericardial reflection (<1 cm from the vein bifurcation). The second stitch (2) is placed below the left inferior pulmonary vein. Once the first two stitches are anchored, a pericardial "ridge" is formed, which serves as a guide for implantation of the other stitches. The third stitch (3) is located between the second and the inferior vena cava, and the last stitch (4) is located close to the inferior vena cava.

of myocardial ischemia, global myocardial performance, and the degree and speed of manipulation. Several techniques have been described for exposing the various distal targets.[125-127] The most common technique is the use of multiple left-sided and inferior deep pericardial stay sutures, placed posterior to the phrenic nerve (Fig. 13-8). Tourniquet tubing is often applied over these sutures to avoid epicardial injury. During placement of these sutures, the surgeon not only displaces the heart, but also compresses the heart manually, resulting in temporary but severe hemodynamic compromise. Ventilation may need to be temporarily interrupted. Recovery is typically immediate once the heart is returned to its anatomic position. Additional surgical exposure techniques include placement of stay sutures in the acute margin of the heart. Release of right-sided pericardial stay sutures, opening of the right pleura, and incising the right pericardium while lifting the right sternal edge creates space for the right heart when the left posterolateral vessels are exposed. Laparotomy sponges or saline-filled gloves may also be placed under the heart. The operating table position is adjusted in both Trendelenburg and right tilt to provide increased access to the anastomosis area.

Regional stabilization is accomplished with the surgeon's device of choice. The use of pharmacologic agents such as adenosine or β-blockers to create a motionless anastomosis has largely been abandoned by most clinicians because of the improvements in stabilizing devices. Mechanical ischemic preconditioning, if performed, is conducted before the coronary arteriotomy. Analysis of the ECG, including ST-segment trend, is important during this evaluation of myocardial tolerance to ischemia. Occlusion is generally better tolerated with more severe coronary stenosis. The arteriotomy is made after external occlusion of the coronary artery proximal (and distal) to the anastomosis site. If a coronary occluder or shunt is used, external vessel occlusion is not required. Remaining blood flow from the arteriotomy is displaced with the blower-mister and suction devices. After completion of the distal anastomosis, strict avoidance of air embolization is of critical importance to avoid the detrimental effects of immediate hemodynamic compromise.

Proximal anastomoses are generally performed last, and, in contrast to CABG with CPB, more sequential grafts with fewer proximal anastomoses are performed. Before and during the period of partial aortic occlusion, blood pressure is typically lowered to reduce potential complications associated with the use of external aortic clamping. Conduit and anastomosis integrity are assessed by using a variety of methods, including direct observation, intraoperative angiography, Doppler-based flow assessment, TEE analysis with ultrasonic contrast agents,[128,129] and a modified Allen test.[130] Chest tubes and pacing wires are placed, hemostasis is achieved, and the chest is closed in routine fashion.

For MIDCABG, the typical surgical approach is through a left or right anterolateral minithoracotomy through the fourth or fifth interspace. Costal cartilages may be divided and resected and a limited pericardiotomy is performed. As with OPCABG, distal target suitability is assessed. The IMA is mobilized by using the exposure provided by specially designed rib retractors. Single-lung ventilation is used during IMA dissection. Heparin is administered after IMA mobilization. Pericardial stay sutures are placed to facilitate movement of the anastomosis site to the surface of the thoracotomy.

The management of the anastomosis area is similar to OPCABG. A stabilizing system is secured to the rib retractor and the anastomosis is performed. Anastomosis flow is assessed, pacing wires and a chest tube are placed, hemostasis is achieved, and regional intercostal anesthesia is provided with bupivacaine or cryoanalgesia before the incision is closed.

Alternative surgical approaches include a posterolateral thoracotomy approach for circumflex lesions during first-time operations or reoperations after sternotomy. A subxiphoid approach has been used for revascularization of posterior distal targets. A lower partial sternotomy has been described for multivessel revascularization. A hybrid approach using percutaneous transluminal coronary angioplasty and MIDCABG has also been reported. Endoscopic techniques in combination with MIDCABG are under evaluation as part of closed-chest CABG without CPB. Mechanical circulatory support overcomes the hemodynamic compromise associated with CABG without CPB.[91,92] Widespread acceptance of these latter techniques appears to be unlikely.

Intraoperative conversion from CABG without CPB to CABG with CPB may be required. The most common causes are hemodynamic compromise, unsuitable distal target, inability to expose obtuse marginal (OM) branches, regional myocardial ischemia, and cardiac tissue injury. When conversion is required, cardioplegic arrest may or may not be used, depending on the reason for conversion.

Intraoperative Management

A modified anesthetic approach is provided for MIDCABG[131-134] and OPCABG.[135] CABG without CPB requires enhanced attention and proactive care to achieve the goals of safe induction and maintenance of anesthesia, maximum myocardial protection, maintenance of adequate hemodynamics and end-organ perfusion, maintenance of normothermia, facilitation of surgical exposure and early emergence and ambulation. Maintenance of acceptable or desired hemodynamics is especially challenging with cardiac manipulation, displacement, compression, and temporary coronary occlusion. Deterioration of cardiac output is most severe during rapid exposure of posterolateral and posterior targets and during compression stabilization of anterior targets. Regional myocardial ischemia associated with coronary occlusion occurs during temporary occlusion of incompletely obstructed coronary vessels and may contribute to decreases in cardiac output, rhythm disturbances, myocardial stunning, infarction, or subclinical myocardial injury.

General patient management includes temperature homeostasis by manipulation of room temperature, low-flow inhalational anesthesia, heated airway humidification, warm IV solutions, and a warm air convection system or head cover. Normal pH and ventilation are maintained. Choice of anesthetic agents is directed by the goal of early extubation. For MIDCABG, tracheal intubation enabling single-lung ventilation is required. Equipment for temporary cardiac pacing and defibrillation should be available.

The degree of cardiac monitoring used for CABG without CPB is a dilemma. Additions to standard noninvasive monitoring techniques include continuous three-lead ECG ST-segment trend analysis, especially during coronary occlusion; continuous cardiac output and mixed venous oxygen saturation monitoring; left atrial pressure monitoring; and TEE evaluation of cardiac filling and regional wall motion. Use of pulmonary artery catheters varies among clinicians. There is a delayed time response of continuous cardiac output pulmonary artery catheters that must be considered during periods of abrupt hemodynamic change.[136] Nonpathologic ECG changes are caused by cardiac displacement. The transgastric short axis midpapillary muscle view is often used for volume and wall-motion analysis. This view may not detect many regional wall-motion abnormalities associated with intraoperative ischemia. Additional long-axis views and ultrasound contrast agents are also used to evaluate myocardial perfusion.[128,129,137] TEE interpretation and image acquisition during cardiac displacement is challenging.

Hemodynamic management is focused on end-organ perfusion by optimizing blood pressure and maintaining cardiac output. Elevations in pulmonary artery pressure, pulmonary artery occlusion pressure, and central venous pressure and decreases in cardiac output are commonly observed. External volume loading and internal volume loading by using the Trendelenburg position are frequently required to maintain acceptable end-organ perfusion. Standard pharmacologic agents are also used to manage blood pressure. Frequent adjustments of vasoactive and anesthetic agents are typical during CABG without CPB. Cardiac arrhythmias are managed with lidocaine, magnesium, and calcium antagonists to control SVT, and ischemia- and reperfusion-induced dysrhythmias. Blood pressure is typically reduced with a vasodilator before application of the partial occlusion clamp for proximal anastomosis.

The myocardium is protected with control of blood pressure, mechanical or pharmacologic ischemic preconditioning, use of calcium antagonists, β-blockers, and nitrates that reduce myocardial oxygen demand and dilate coronary and arterial grafts. Reduction of heart rate and contractility or pharmacologic cardiac arrest to facilitate suture placement is rarely practiced. Pacing may be required during right coronary occlusion, especially with right coronary dominance, because cardiac arrest may occur.

Anticoagulation is important but variable among clinicians during CABG without CPB. A target activated clotting time of greater than 300 to 400 seconds is most common. A platelet-independent increased procoagulant activity has been observed in OPCABG patients.

Strategies for postoperative pain management include intercostal nerve blocks for MIDCABG, epidural bupivacaine delivery, continuous bupivacaine infusion in the wound, patient-controlled analgesia pumps, and IV morphine or nonsteroidal antiinflammatory agents.[138]

Extubation is planned to occur in the operating room or in the immediate postoperative period.

Postoperative Care

As surgical techniques become less invasive, a corresponding less invasive perioperative care approach is also considered. Such efforts yield an accelerated in-hospital recovery and allow earlier discharge. This reduces the cost of cardiovascular care, estimated at $12 billion for 300,000 CABG procedures in the United States,[139] because a significant amount of the total cost is spent for postoperative (ICU) care. An integrated multidisciplinary recovery care pathway plays an important role in achieving these goals.

Most patients are candidates for a less intensive postoperative management plan, as described in several prospective studies.[140-143] This management plan begins preoperatively, with the selection of intraoperative anesthetic agents (low-dose narcotics, more inhalation anesthesia, minimal use of benzodiazepines), continues intraoperatively with maintaining normothermia, management of ventilation with the goal of early extubation, and aggressive pain management. Postoperative management also includes a review of indications for patient transfer from the operating room to ICU, patient management in the cardiac step-down unit, management of chest tubes and patient mobilization, and choice of recovery.

Clinical Experience

The resurgence of CABG without CPB was motivated by the drive toward improving the clinical results of conventional coronary artery revascularization by reducing the incidence and severity of perioperative complications while maintaining the efficacy of the standard of care method. There is an absence of randomized prospective clinical trial data that evaluate the outcome of CABG without CPB against the established outcome associated with conventional CABG surgery. Several controlled observational studies have compared specific outcome measures of CABG with and without CPB. It is important to recognize that the clinical results of CABG with CPB are not static. Advances in CPB, surgical technique, postoperative patient management, and a changing patient population are some of the factors affecting the changing outcome of CABG with CPB. The influence of complete versus incomplete revascularization on outcome and less than excellent outcomes with conventional CABG[80] are also important to consider when examining outcome data. Long-term anastomosis patency depends on several factors, including patient selection, conduit selection (arterial vs. venous), location of grafting, vessel size (<1.5 mm diameter), anastomosis stability, and surgical technique.

OPCABG. No randomized prospective triple vessel revascularization clinical trial data are available. Controlled observational studies report short-term and midterm outcomes, several with matched control groups. No long-term outcome data are available at this time. Short-term outcomes in general are comparable to those of conventional CABG with CPB. Specific outcome endpoints were found to be significantly different in a few well-controlled studies. The overall incidence of intraoperative complications such as cardiogenic shock, cardiac arrest, cardiac tissue injury, and coronary artery and aortic dissection is unknown.

The incidence of major adverse clinical events (MACE) from several studies[104,125,126,144-148] are reported in Table 13-7 . The MACE incidence of 30-day mortality rate, neurologic (cerebrovascular accident, transient ischemic attack, coma), cardiac (MI, use of intraaortic balloon pump, use of inotropic agents,

TABLE 13-7
Major Adverse Clinical Events Associated with OPCABG

AUTHOR	NO. OF PATIENTS	NO. OF GRAFTS/PATIENTS	MORTALITY (%)	CVA (%)	MI (%)	IABP (%)	AF (%)
Bergsland et al, 1998[144]	505	—	4.0	0.2	2.2	2.4	—
Calafiore et al, 1998[145]	280	1.8	0.2	0	0	—	—
Tasdemir et al, 1998[104]	2052	—	1.9	0.5	2.9	1.4	1.7
Cartier et al, 1999[146]	140	3.1	0.7	—	2.7	—	28
Baumgartner et al, 1999[125]	141	3.3	0	0.75	0	—	—
Hart et al, 1999[126]	374	1.96	0.26	0.26	—	0	12.8
Cartier et al, 2000[147]	300	2.92	1.3	1.6	4.0	0.8	30

AF, Atrial fibrillation; *CVA,* cerebrovascular accident; *IABP,* intraaortic balloon pump; *MI,* myocardial infarction; *OPCABG,* off-pump coronary artery bypass grafting.

new-onset atrial fibrillation, incidence of SVT), renal (dialysis), respiratory complications, and reoperation (failed primary procedure, bleeding, deep sternal infection) are similar to those of CABG with CPB. The incidence of MACE for high-risk patients is less for CABG without CPB compared with CABG with CPB.[121,144,149-151] Certain outcome measures are significantly decreased, including postoperative neuropsychologic and neuropsychiatric deficits,[152] subclinical myocardial injury,[147,153,154] use of inotropic drugs,[154] and a significant increase in creatinine. Perioperative blood loss, use of homologous blood products, ICU stay, duration of mechanical ventilation, postoperative LOS, 6-month readmission rate, and hospital cost are also significantly reduced.[147,154-159]

Patency rates are of crucial importance and could very well determine the future of OPCABG. Reported short-term patency rates are similar to those for CABG with CPB. One study reported overall patency rates of 98.9% and OM branch patency rates of 98.2%, a mean of 33 days postoperative.[146] The degree of revascularization is also important. Most studies report a lower number of grafts per OPCABG patient and a lower frequency of circumflex revascularization compared with CABG patients with CPB. In contrast, only a few studies demonstrate similar data to CABG with CPB.[135,136,144,146,160] Failure to revascularize diseased circumflex vessels is a significant risk factor for perioperative mortality, MI, and low-output syndrome.[104] Long-term and event-free survival rates for OPCABG are unknown.

MIDCABG Clinical Experience. The MIDCABG clinical experience started earlier, and longer-term outcome data are now available. However, surgical techniques and devices have changed significantly during this time. Caution must be exercised when interpreting midterm data for anticipated outcomes of current MIDCABG procedures. Outcomes of MIDCABG are difficult to compare with conventional CABG with CPB because of the underlying differences in surgical approach. Left IMA to LAD anastomosis via median sternotomy with CPB is associated with a low incidence of MACE.[161] Patency rates should be compared, although interpretation of patency rates for LIMA to LAD anastomosis may be problematic.[162] Consideration must be given to comorbidities. Another comparison for MIDCABG surgery is with an established database for CABG with CPB via a minithoracotomy.[17]

Table 13-8 lists outcomes associated with MIDCABG.[164-169] A prospective randomized study comparing MIDCABG and conventional CABG with CPB for isolated LAD stenosis reported significantly shorter duration of operation, decreased blood loss, shorter ventilatory time, and shorter LOS.[170] Morbidity and resource use significantly favored MIDCABG over conventional CABG with CPB.[171] Short-term results of MIDCABG for high-risk patients with respect to MACE are improved when compared with conventional CABG with CPB.[119-121,151]

Short-term patency rates have improved with new stabilization methods and range from the mid eighties to the high nineties.[166-169,172] Lower patency rates

---

TABLE 13-8
Adverse Clinical Events and Outcomes Associated with MIDCABG

AUTHOR	NO. OF PATIENTS	30 DAY MORTALITY RATE (%)	EARLY REINTERVENTION (%)	EARLY PATENCY RATE (%)	OUTCOME (%, TIME)
Mariani et al, 1997[165]	50	1.1	1.1*	—	—
Subramanian et al, 1997[166]	199	3.8	1.1*	89[†]	98,[§] 9M
				97[c]	93,[∥] 9M
Possati et al, 1998[167]	77	1.2	2.6*	82[†]	2 late death
				100[‡]	98.5,[¶] 18M
Calafiori et al, 1998[170]	434	1.1	6[†]	88.9[†]	91,[§] 13.5M
			2.1[‡]	96.3[‡]	
Allen et al, 1999[164]	93	—	—	87.5, 2Y	95, 2Y
Mack et al, 1999[171]	103	1.9	3.9	91	—
Diegeler et al, 1999[168]	271	—	3.1	91	—

MIDCABG, Minimally invasive direct coronary artery bypass grafting.
* Reoperation.
[†] Without mechanical stabilization.
[‡] With mechanical stabilization.
[§] Survival.
[∥] Event-free.
[¶] Angina-free.

may be explained by technical difficulties or difficulty with interpretation of immediate postoperative angiograms.[169] Early stenosis may improve in at least 25% of patients over 6 months.[168]

Midterm (1 year) and long-term (6-7 years) patency rates of the initial MIDCABG experience were poor.[76,173] A reference standard of care for long-term patency has been established with LIMA to LAD anastomosis with CPB. Improved methods of stabilization have increased midterm MIDCABG patency rates.[166,167]

Although still developing, both OPCABG and MIDCABG have become accepted revascularization procedures. The number of OPCABG procedures is likely to grow during the next few years as more surgeons become comfortable performing OPCABG. Continuous technology improvements and an ever-aging patient population continue to present increasing challenges to CABG with CPB. The growth of OPCABG depends on the emergence of long-term outcome data, in particular for patency rates. Future studies will also focus on objectively evaluating potential differences between OPCABG and CABG with CPB for MACE, with particular emphasis on neuropsychologic outcomes. Technologic advances, especially in the area of proximal and distal anastomoses and assisted circulation, are likely to have an impact as well. Because endoscopic CABG is technically very challenging, one particular challenge for minimally invasive multivessel CABG without CPB is to make the procedure less invasive without alienating the majority of surgeons by increasing the technical complexity.

CONCLUSION

Minimally invasive and less invasive cardiac surgery is a rapidly developing field that is now an important component of clinical practice. Substantial clinical experience has accumulated, demonstrating excellent clinical outcomes with Port-Access minimally invasive cardiac surgery. The anesthesiologist has a substantial role that includes placement of catheters and monitoring the conduct of CPB. Clinical experience continues to expand the indications for Port-Access minimally invasive cardiac surgery and to refine and enhance surgical procedures. Coronary artery surgery without the use of CPB has been adopted with enthusiasm when applied by using a median sternotomy. Further investigation will allow clinicians to refine the selection of minimally invasive surgical approaches for specific patients and clinical conditions. Technologic advancements are likely to continue to develop and will undoubtedly play a significant role in shaping this field. Anesthesiologists have a critical role to play both now and in the future.

KEY POINTS

1. Minimally invasive and less invasive cardiac surgical techniques and technologies have been developed to permit cardiac surgery through small incisions or access ports supported by CPB, or through a median sternotomy without the support of CPB.
2. Catheters and cannulae have been developed to enable surgeons to obtain appropriate myocardial protection, circulatory support, and operating conditions while operating through a small intercostal incision or access port.
3. TEE, fluoroscopy, or both are used to evaluate patient anatomy, including assessment of the aorta, to facilitate the placement of catheters and cannulae, and to monitor the conduct of CPB.
4. Clinical reports have demonstrated broad applicability of Port-Access procedures with favorable outcomes. Morbidity and mortality rates compare favorably with conventional surgery, including risk-adjustment models.
5. Clinical studies suggest that Port-Access surgery is associated with earlier postoperative extubation, shorter ICU and hospital stay, a low incidence of new-onset atrial fibrillation, and rapid functional recovery and return to normal activities.
6. The major challenges of CABG without CPB include accurate anastomosis suture placement, maintenance of acceptable hemodynamics, avoidance of myocardial injury, and hemostasis at the distal anastomosis site.
7. Technology for CABG without CPB principally consists of devices that provide a stable anastomosis site and devices that provide a relatively bloodless anastomosis site.
8. Specific indications for CABG without CPB are not well developed and vary among clinicians.
9. Randomized prospective clinical data that compare the outcome of CABG without CPB against the established outcome associated with CABG with CPB are absent. Short-term outcomes, however, are comparable.
10. Ongoing investigation and the introduction of new technologies, such as robotic telemanipulation, are part of this rapidly evolving field of minimally invasive cardiac surgery and offer the potential to further expand patient benefits and comfort.

KEY REFERENCES

Applebaum RM, Colvin SB, Galloway AC et al: The role of transesophageal echocardiography during Port-Access minimally invasive cardiac surgery: a new challenge for the echocardiographer, *Echocardiography* 16:595-602, 1999.

Arom K, Flavin T, Emery R et al: Safety and efficacy of off-pump coronary artery bypass grafting, *Ann Thorac Surg* 69:704-710, 2000.

Baumgartner FJ, Gheissari A, Capouya ER et al: Technical aspects of total revascularization in off-pump coronary bypass via sternotomy approach, *Ann Thorac Surg* 67:1653-1658, 1999.

Calafiore AM, Di Giammarco G, Teodori G et al: Midterm results after minimally invasive coronary surgery (LAST operation), *J Thorac Cardiovasc Surg* 115:763-771, 1998.

Cartier R, Brann S, Dagenais F et al: Systematic off-pump coronary artery revascularization in multivessel disease: experience of three hundred cases, *J Thorac Cardiovasc Surg* 119:221-229, 2000.

Galloway AC, Shemin RJ, Glower DD et al: First report of the Port-Access international registry, *Ann Thorac Surg* 67:51-58, 1999.

Glower DD, Landolfo K, Clements F et al: Mitral valve operation via port access versus median sternotomy, *Eur J Cardiothorac Surg* 14:S143-S147, 1998.

Glower DD, Siegel LC, Frischmeyer KJ et al: Predictors of outcome in a multicenter Port-Access valve registry, *Ann Thorac Surg* 70:1054-1059, 2000.

Groh MA, Sutherland SE, Burton HG et al: Port-Access coronary artery bypass grafting: technique and comparative results, *Ann Thorac Surg* 68:1506-1508, 1999.

Grossi EA, Groh MA, Lefrak EA et al: Results of a prospective multi-center study on port access coronary artery bypass, *Ann Thorac Surg* 68:1475-1477, 1999.

Grossi EA, Zakow PK, Ribakove GH et al: Comparison of post-operative pain, stress response, and quality of life in port access vs. standard sternotomy coronary bypass patients, *Euro J Cardiothorac Surg* 16(suppl 2):S39-42, 1999.

Nierich AP, Diephuis J, Jansen EWL et al: Embracing the heart: perioperative management of patients undergoing off-pump coronary artery bypass grafting using the Octopus tissue stabilizer, *J Cardiothorac Vasc Anesth* 13:123-129, 1999.

Pfister AJ, Zaki MS, Garcia JM et al: Coronary artery bypass without cardiopulmonary bypass, *Ann Thorac Surg* 54:1085-1091, 1992.

Siegel LC, St. Goar FG, Stevens JH et al: Monitoring considerations for Port-Access cardiac surgery, *Circulation* 96:562-568, 1997.

Tasdemir O, Vural KM, Karagoz H et al: Coronary artery bypass grafting on the beating heart without the use of extracorporeal circulation: review of 2052 cases, *J Thorac Cardiovasc Surg* 116:68-73, 1998.

References

1. Reardon MJ, Conklin LD, Philo R et al: The anatomical aspects of minimally invasive cardiac valve operations, *Ann Thorac Surg* 67:266-268, 1999.
2. Cohn LH, Adams DH, Couper GS et al: Minimally invasive aortic valve replacement, *Semin Thorac Cardiovasc Surg* 9:331-336, 1997.
3. Kaur S, Balaguer J, Vander Salm TJ: Improved myocardial protection in minimally invasive aortic valve surgery with the assistance of Port-Access technology, *J Thorac Cardiovasc Surg* 116:874-875, 1998.
4. Mächler HE, Bergmass P, Anelli-Monti M et al: Minimally invasive versus conventional aortic valve operations: a prospective study in 120 patients, *Ann Thorac Surg* 67:1001-1005, 1999.
5. Byrne JG, Aranki SF, Couper GS et al: Reoperative aortic valve replacement: partial upper hemi-sternotomy versus conventional full sternotomy, *J Thorac Cardiovasc Surg* 118:991-997, 1999.
6. Benetti FJ, Mariani MA, Rizzardi JL et al: Minimally invasive aortic valve replacement, *J Thorac Cardiovasc Surg* 113:806-807, 1997.
7. Schwartz DS, Ribakove GH, Grossi EA et al: Minimally invasive cardiopulmonary bypass, *J Thorac Cardiovasc Surg* 111:556-566, 1996.
8. Schwartz DS, Ribakove GH, Grossi EA et al: Minimally invasive mitral valve replacement: Port-Access technique, feasibility, and myocardial functional preservation, *J Thorac Cardiovasc Surg* 113:1022-1031, 1997.
9. Peters WS, Siegel LC, Stevens JH et al: Closed chest cardiopulmonary bypass and cardioplegia for less invasive cardiac surgery, *Ann Thorac Surg* 63:1748-1754, 1997.
10. Stevens JH, Burdon TA, Peters WS et al: Port-Access coronary artery bypass grafting: a proposed surgical method, *J Thorac Cardiovasc Surg* 111:567-573, 1996.
11. Peters WS, Burdon TA, Siegel LC et al: Port-Access bilateral internal mammary artery grafting for left main coronary artery disease: canine feasibility study, *J Card Surg* 12:1-7, 1997.
12. Fann JI, Peters WS, Burdon TA : Port-Access two-vessel coronary revascularization in the dog, *J Am Coll Cardiol* 2:466A, 1997.
13. Stevens JH, Burdon TA, Siegel LC : Port access coronary artery bypass with cardioplegic arrest: acute and chronic canine studies, *Ann Thorac Surg* 62:435-441, 1996.
14. Pompili MF, Stevens JH, Burdon TA et al: Port access mitral valve replacement in dogs, *J Thorac Cardiovasc Surg* 112:1268-1274, 1996.
15. Siegel LC, Peters WS, St. Goar FG et al: Anesthetic considerations for Port-Access cardiac surgery, *Anesth Analg* 82:SCA79, 1996.
16. Galloway AC, Shemin RJ, Glower DD et al: First report of the Port-Access international registry, *Ann Thorac Surg* 67:51-58, 1999.
17. Shemin RJ, Groh MA, Galloway AC et al: World's largest registry of minimally invasive CABG with endoCPB demonstrates excellent results with minimal morbidity and mortality, *J Am Coll Cardiol* 33S:567A, 1999.
18. Groh MA, Robinson NB, Galloway AC et al: Grafting strategies in minimally invasive CABG with endoCPB, *J Am Coll Cardiol* 33S:551A, 1999.
19. Ribakove GH, Miller JS, Anderson RV et al: Minimally invasive Port-Access coronary artery bypass grafting with early angiographic follow-up: initial clinical experience, *J Thorac Cardiovasc Surg* 115:1101-1110, 1998.

20. Reichenspurner H, Gulielmos V, Wunderlich J et al: Port-Access coronary artery bypass grafting with the use of cardiopulmonary bypass and cardioplegic arrest, *Ann Thorac Surg* 65: 413-419, 1998.

21. Reichenspurner H, Weltz A, Gulielmos V et al: Port-access cardiac surgery using endovascular cardiopulmonary bypass: theory, practice, and results, *J Card Surg* 13:275-280, 1998.

22. Barlow CW, Hildick-Smith D, Sayeed RA et al: Minimal access aortocoronary bypass surgery with endovascular balloon clamp: technical precision, operative times, complications, *J Am Coll Cardiol* 31: 28A, 1998.

23. Shemin RJ, Baker JW, Galloway AC et al: Risk adjusted mortality rate for minimally invasive port-access coronary artery bypass grafting is equivalent to conventional surgery: a multi-center study, *Circulation* 100: I-667, 1999 (abstract).

24. Grossi EA, Groh MA, Lefrak EA et al: Results of a prospective multi-center study on port access coronary bypass grafting, *Ann Thorac Surg* 68:1475-1477, 1999.

25. Groh MA, Sutherland SE, Burton HG et al: Port-access coronary artery bypass grafting: technique and comparative results, *Ann Thorac Surg* 68:1506-1508, 1999.

26. Siegel LC, Galloway AC, Shemin RJ et al: Port-Access minimally invasive multi-vessel CABG is associated with short post-operative duration of tracheal intubation, ICU stay and hospital stay, *Anesth Analg* 88:SCA 122, 1999 (abstract).

27. Chaney MA, Durazo-Arvizu RA, Fluder EM et al: Port-Access minimally invasive cardiac surgery increases surgical complexity, increases operating room time, and facilitates early postoperative hospital discharge, *Anesthesiology* 92:1637-1645, 2000.

28. Rogers JP, Novchich TM, Pearce GL et al: Port-Access cardiac surgery protocols and early outcomes, *Crit Care Nurs Clin North Am* 10:61-73, 1998.

29. Boova RA, Davis PK, Martella AT et al: Port access coronary artery bypass grafting: early clinical results and comparison with conventional CABG, *Chest* 118:226, 2000 (abstract).

30. Grossi EA, Zakow PK, Ribakove GH et al: Comparison of post-operative pain, stress response, and quality of life in port access vs. standard sternotomy coronary bypass patients, *Eur J Cardiothorac Surg* 16:S39-S42, 1999.

31. Mohr FW, Falk V, Diegler A et al: Minimally invasive Port-Access mitral valve surgery, *J Thorac Cardiovasc Surg* 115:567-576, 1998.

32. Mohr FW, Onnasch J, Falk V et al: The evolution of minimally invasive mitral valve surgery—2 years experience, *Eur J Cardiothorac Surg* 15:233-239, 1999.

33. Grossi EA, Galloway AC, Ribakove GH et al: Impact of minimally invasive approach on valvular heart surgery: a case controlled study, *J Am Coll Cardiol* 33S:554A, 1999.

34. Glower DD, Landolfo K, Clements F et al: Mitral valve operation via port access versus median sternotomy, *Eur J Cardiothorac Surg* 14:S143-S147, 1998.

35. Glower DD, Davis RD, Landolfo K et al: Comparison of minimally invasive port-access to sternotomy or thoracotomy for redo mitral operation, *Heart Surg Forum* 2:V5, 1999 (abstract).

36. Glower DD, Siegel LC, Frischmeyer KJ et al: Predictors of outcome in a multicenter Port-Access valve registry, *Ann Thorac Surg* 70:1054-1059, 2000.

37. White HD, Antman EM, Glynn MA et al: Efficacy and safety of timolol for prevention of supraventricular tachy-arrhythmias after coronary artery bypass surgery, *Circulation* 70:479-484, 1984.

38. Kowey PR, Dalessandro DA, Herbertson R et al: Effectiveness of digitalis with or without acebutolol in preventing atrial arrhythmias after coronary artery surgery, *Am J Cardiol* 79:1114-1117, 1997.

39. Ommen SR, Odell JA, Stanton MS: Atrial arrhythmias after cardiothoracic surgery, *N Engl J Med* 336:1429-1434, 1997.

40. Aranki SF, Shaw DP, Adams DH et al: Predictors of atrial fibrillation after coronary artery surgery. Current trends and impact on hospital resources, *Circulation* 94:390-397, 1996.

41. Creswell LL, Schuessler RB, Rosenbloom M et al: Hazard of postoperative atrial arrhythmias, *Ann Thorac Surg* 56:539-549, 1993.

42. Mathew JP, Parks R, Savino JS et al: Atrial fibrillation following coronary artery bypass graft surgery: predictors, outcomes and resource utilization, *JAMA* 276:300-306, 1996.

43. Olshansky B: Management of atrial fibrillation after coronary artery bypass graft, *Am J Cardiol* 78:27-34, 1996.

44. Lazar HL, Fitzgerald C, Gross S et al: Determinants of length of stay after coronary artery bypass graft surgery, *Circulation* 92: 20-24, 1995.

45. Daoud EG, Stickberger SA, Man KC et al: Preoperative amiodarone as prophylaxis against atrial fibrillation after heart surgery, *N Engl J Med* 337:1785-1791, 1997.

46. Grossi EA, Muhlbaier LH, Groh MA et al: Multicenter case-match comparison of port access CABG with STS database, *Cardiothoracic Techniques & Technologies Current Trends in Thoracic Surgery VI* Abstract 16, 2000.

47. Gulielmos V, Wagner F, Waetzig B et al: Clinical experience with minimally invasive coronary artery and mitral valve surgery with the advantage of cardiopulmonary bypass and cardioplegic arrest using the port-access technique, *World J Surg* 23:480-485, 1999.

48. Arom KV, Emery RW, Kshettry VR et al: Comparison between port-access and less invasive valve surgery, *Ann Thor Surg* 68: 1525-1528, 1999.

49. Melo J, Adragao P, Neves J et al: Endocardial and epicardial radiofrequency ablation in the treatment of atrial fibrillation with a new intra-operative device, *Eur J Cardiothorac Surg* 18: 182-186, 2000.

50. Holmes DS, Chintz LA, Pierce WJ et al: Rapid pulmonary vein isolation for atrial fibrillation during minimally invasive mitral valve surgery, *Circulation* 102:SII-484, 2000 (abstract).

51. Siegel LC, St. Goar FG, Stevens JH et al: Monitoring considerations for Port-Access cardiac surgery, *Circulation* 96:562-568, 1997.

52. Plotkin IM, Collard CD, Aranki SF et al: Percutaneous coronary sinus cannulation guided by transesophageal echocardiography, *Ann Thorac Surg* 66:2085-2087, 1998.

53. Lewis K, Smith B, Plotkin IM et al: Safety of percutaneous coronary sinus cannulation during minimally invasive cardiac surgery, *Anesth Analg* 90:SCA49, 2000 (abstract).

54. Yen ES, Brown GA, Carlson JL et al: Rapid cannulation of the coronary sinus during Port-Access cardiac surgery, *Anesthesiology* 89:A307, 1998.

55. Ostrowski JW, Cutler WM, Bhardwaj N et al: Experience improves anesthesia time in port-access cardiac surgery, *Anesth Analg* 88:SCA126, 1999 (abstract).

56. Abramson DC, Giannoti AG: Perforation of the right ventricle with a coronary sinus catheter during preparation for minimally invasive cardiac surgery, *Anesthesiology* 519-521, 1998.

57. Siegel LC: Coronary sinus catheterization for minimally invasive cardiac surgery, *Anesthesiology* 90:1232-1233, 1999.

58. Clements F, Wright S, deBruijn NP: Coronary sinus catheterization made easy for Port-Access minimally invasive cardiac surgery, *J Cardiothorac Vasc Anesth* 12:96-101, 1998.

59. Applebaum RM, Cutler WM, Bhardwaj N et al: Utility of transesophageal echocardiography during Port-Access minimally invasive cardiac surgery, *Am J Cardiol* 82:183-188, 1998.

60. Applebaum RM, Colvin SB, Galloway AC et al: The role of transesophageal echocardiography during Port-Access minimally invasive cardiac surgery: a new challenge for the echocardiographer, *Echocardiography* 16:595-602, 1999.

61. Schulze C, Wildhirt S, Boehm DH et al: Continuous transesophageal echocardiographic (TEE) monitoring during port-access cardiac surgery, *Heart Surg Forum* 2:54-59, 1999.

62. Coddens J, Deloof T, Hendrickx J et al: Transesophageal echocardiography for Port-Access surgery, *J Cardiothorac Vasc Anesth* 13:614-622, 1999.

63. Glower DD, Komtebedde J, Clements FM et al: Direct aortic cannulation for Port-Access mitral or coronary artery bypass grafting, *Ann Thorac Surg* 68:1878-1880, 1999.

64. Grocott HP, Stafford-Smith M, Glower DD et al: Endovascular aortic balloon clamp malposition during minimally invasive cardiac surgery: detection by transcranial Doppler monitoring, *Anesthesiology* 88:1396-1399, 1998.

65. Falk V, Walther T, Autschbach R et al: Robot-assisted minimally invasive solo mitral valve operation, *J Thorac Cardiovasc Surg* 115:470-471, 1998.

66. Reichenspurner H, Boehm DH, Zwissler B: 3D-Video-and robotic-assisted minimally-invasive ASD-closure using the Port-Access surgical method, *Heart Surg Forum* 1:104-106, 1998.

67. Reichenspurner H, Boehm DH, Gulbins H et al: Three-dimensional video and robot-assisted Port-Access mitral valve operation, *Ann Thorac Surg* 69:1176-1182, 2000.

68. Damiano RJ, Ehrman WJ, Ducko CT et al: Initial United States clinical trial of robotically assisted endoscopic coronary artery bypass grafting, *J Thoracic Cardiovasc Surg* 119:77-82, 2000.

69. Bohmer R, Reichenspurner H, Gulbins H et al: Early experience with robotic technology for coronary artery surgery, *Ann Thorac Surg* 68:1542-1546, 1999.

70. Falk V, Diegeler A, Walther T et al: Total endoscopic computer enhanced coronary artery bypass grafting, *Eur J Cardiothorac Surg* 17:38-45, 2000.

71. LaPietra A, Grossi E, Derivaux CC et al: Robotic-assisted instruments enhance minimally invasive mitral valve surgery, *Ann Thorac Surg* 70:835-838, 2000.

72. Allen KB, Griffith GL, Heimansohn DA et al: Endoscopic versus traditional saphenous vein harvesting: a prospective, randomized trial, *Ann Thorac Surg* 66:26-31, 1998.

73. Morris RJ, Butler MT, Samuels LE: Minimally invasive saphenous vein harvesting, *Ann Thorac Surg* 66:1026-1028, 1998.

74. Kolessov VL: Mammary artery-coronary artery anastomosis as a method of treatment for angina pectoris, *J Thorac Cardiovasc Surg* 54:535-544, 1967.

75. Ankeney JL: To use or not to use the pump oxygenator in coronary bypass operations, *Ann Thorac Surg* 19:108-109, 1975.

76. Calafiore AM, Di Giammarco G, Teodori G et al: Midterm results after minimally invasive coronary surgery (LAST operation), *J Thorac Cardiovasc Surg* 115:763-771, 1998.

77. Jansen EWL, Borst C, Lahpor JR: Coronary artery bypass grafting without cardiopulmonary bypass using the Octopus method: results in the first 100 patients, *J Thorac Cardiovasc Surg* 116:60-67, 1998.

78. Borst C, Jansen EWL, Tulleken CAF et al: Coronary artery bypss grafting without cardiopulmonary bypass and without interruption of native coronary flow using a novel anastomosis site restraining device ("Octopus"), *J Am Coll Cardiol* 27:1356-1364, 1996.

79. Shennib H, Lee AGL, Akin J: Safe and effective method of stabilization for coronary artery bypass grafting on the beating heart, *Ann Thorac Surg* 63:9889-9892, 1997.

80. Borst C, Gründeman PF: Minimally invasive coronary artery bypass grafting. An experimental perspective, *Circulation* 99:1400-1403, 1999.

81. Cowper PA, Peterson ED, DeLong ER et al: Impact of early discharge after coronary artery bypass graft surgery on rates of hospital readmission and death, *J Am Coll Cardiol* 30:908-913, 1997.

82. Gründeman PF, Borst C, van Herwaarden JA et al: Hemodynamic changes during displacement of the beating heart by the Utrecht Octopus method, *Ann Thorac Surg* 63:S88-S92, 1997.

83. Gründeman PF, Borst C, Verlaan CWF et al: Exposure of circumflex branches in the tilted, beating porcine heart: exposure of circumflex branches in the tilted, beating porcine heart: echocardiographic evidence of right ventricular deformation and the effect of right or left heart bypass, *J Thorac Cardiovasc Surg* 118:316-323, 1999.

84. Edgerton J, Mathison M, Horswell J et al: Hemodynamic changes in the displaced human heart during beating heart surgery, *The Society of Thoracic Surgery 36th Annual Meeting*, 134-135, 2000.

85. Isserles SA, Breen PH: Can changes in end-tidal PCO_2 measure changes in cardiac output? *Anesth Analg* 73:808-814, 1991.

86. Oh JK, Appleton CP, Hatle LK et al. The noninvasive assessment of left ventricular diastolic function with two-dimensional and doppler echocardiography, *J Am Soc Echocardiogr* 10:246-270, 1997.

87. Gründeman PF, Borst C, van Herwaarden JA, et al: Vertical displacement of the beating heart by the octopus tissue stabilizer: Influence on coronary flow, *Ann Thorac Surg* 65:1348-1352, 1998.

88. Burfeind, Jr., WR, Duhaylongsod, FG, Samuelson D et al: The effects of mechanical cardiac stabilization on left ventricular performance, *Eur J Cardiothorac Surg* 14:285-289, 1998.

89. Dekker AL, Geskes GG, Cramers AA et al: The enabler right heart support system for posterior and inferior wall access during beating heart surgery in sheep, *Heart Surg Forum ISMICS Meeting* Abstract 026, 1999.

90. Matheny R, Mack M, Robbins R et al: Right heart support facilitates cardiac manipulation in off-pump coronary bypass, *Evolving Techniques & Technology in Minimally Invasive Cardiac Surgery (V)* 82, 1999.

91. Mathison M, Buffolo E, Jatene A et al: Right heart circulatory support facilitates coronary artery bypass without cardiopulmonary bypass, *Cardiothoracic Techniques and Technologies, Current Trends in Thoracic Surgery (VI)* 25, 2000.

92. Esteves LL, Mack M, Sebatovics N et al: A-med system for right heart support facilitates posterior vessel revascularization without CPB (initial clinical experience), *Cardiothoracic Techniques and Technologies, Current Trends in Thoracic Surgery (VI)* 75, 2000.

93. Sweeney MS, Frazier OH: Device-supported myocardial revascularization: safe help for sick hearts, *Ann Thorac Surg* 54:1065-1070, 1992.

94. Mack M, Mullangi AJ, Edgerton J et al: Effects of mini-pump flow rate during right heart support for off-pump bypass, *Heart Surg Forum ISMICS* Abstract C93, 1999.

95. Thourani VH, Nakamura M, Durate IG et al: Ischemic preconditioning attenuates postischemic coronary artery endothelial dysfunction in a model of minimally invasive direct coronary artery bypass grafting, *J Thorac Cardiovasc Surg* 117:383-389. 1999.

96. Wang NP, Bufkin BL, Nakamura M et al: Ischemic preconditioning reduces neutrophil accumulation and myocardial apoptosis, *Ann Thorac Surg* 67:1689-1695, 1999.

97. Lucchetti V, Caputo M, Suleiman MS et al: Beating heart coronary revascularization without metabolic myocardial damage, *Eur J Cardiothorac Surg* 14:443-444, 1998.

98. Jahania MS, Lasley RD, Mentzer, Jr., RM: Ischemic preconditioning does not acutely improve load-insensitive parameters of contractility in *in vivo* stunned porcine myocardium, *J Thorac Cardiovasc Surg* 117:810-817, 1999.

99. Malkowski MJ, Kramer CM, Parvizi ST et al: Transient ischemia does not limit subsequent ischemic regional dysfunction in humans: a transesophageal echocardiographic study during minimally invasive coronary artery bypass surgery, *J Am Coll Cardiol* 31:1035-1039, 1998.

100. Uematsu M, Gaudette GR, Laurikka JO et al: Adenosine-enhanced ischemic preconditioning decreases infarct in the regional ischemic sheep heart, *Ann Thorac Surg* 66:382-387, 1998.
101. Belhomme D, Peynet J, Louzy M et al: Evidence for preconditioning by isoflurane in coronary artery bypass graft surgery, *Circulation* 100:SII 340-344, 1999.
102. de Peppo AP, Polisca P, Tomai F et al: Recovery of LV contractility in man is enhanced by preischemic administration of enflurane, *Ann Thorac Surg* 68:112-118, 1999.
103. Penttilä HJ, Lepojärvi MVK, Kaukoranta PK et al: Myocardial metabolism and hemodynamics during coronary surgery without cardiopulmonary bypass, *Ann Thorac Surg* 67:683-688, 1999.
104. Tasdemir O, Vural KM, Karagoz H et al: Coronary artery bypass grafting on the beating heart without the use of extracorporeal circulation: review of 2052 cases, *J Thorac Cardiovasc Surg* 116:68-73, 1998.
105. Buffolo E, Gerola LR: Coronary artery bypass grafting without cardiopulmonary bypass through sternotomy and minimally invasive procedure, *Int J Cardiol* 62:S89-S93, 1997.
106. Benetti FJ, Naselli G, Wood M, et al: Direct myocardial revascularization without extracorporeal circulation: experience in 700 patients, *Chest* 100:312-316, 1991.
107. Doty JR, Fonger JD, Salazar JD et al: Early experience with minimally invasive direct coronary artery bypass grafting with the internal thoracic artery, *J Thorac Cardiovasc Surg* 117:873-880, 1999.
108. Sakwa M, McCue MG, Shannon F et al: Pharmacologic electrical arrest with intermittent pacing facilitates off-pump bypass surgery, *Heart Surg Forum ISMICS Meeting* Abstract C18, 1999.
109. Bel A, Perrault LP, Faris B et al: Inhibition of the pacemaker current: a bradycardic therapy for off-pump coronary operations, *Ann Thorac Surg* 66:148-152, 1998.
110. McCue MG, Sakwa MP, Ayers G et al: Preservation of ventricular performance during pharmacologically induced electrical arrest for off-pump coronary bypass surgery, *Heart Surg Forum ISMICS Meeting* Abstract C104, 1999.
111. Ronson RS, Puskas JD, Velez DA et al: Controlled intermittent asystole for off-pump coronary surgery does not cause myocardial or neural injury, *Heart Surg Forum ISMICS Meeting* Abstract C37, 1999.
112. Robinson MC, Thielmeier KA, Hill BB: Transient ventricular asystole using adenosine during minimally invasive and open sternotomy coronary artery bypass grafting, *Ann Thorac Surg* 63:S30-S34, 1997.
113. van Aarnhem E, Nierich A, Jansen E: Ischemia in off-pump coronary artery bypass grafting: prevalence and effective management, *Cardiothoracic Techniques and Technologies, Current Trends in Thoracic Surgery (VI)* 99, 2000.
114. Dapunt OE, Raji MR, Jeschkeit S et al: Intracoronary shunt insertion prevents myocardial stunning in a juvenile porcine MID-CAB model absent of coronary artery disease, *Eur J Cardiothorac Surg* 15:173-179, 1999.
115. Guyton RA, Thourani VH, Puskas JD et al: Perfusion-assisted direct coronary artery bypass: selective graft perfusion in off-pump cases, *Ann Thorac Surg* 69:171-175, 2000.
116. Heijmen RH, Borst C, van Dalen R et al: Temporary luminal arteriotomy seal. II. Coronary artery bypass grafting on the beating heart, *Ann Thorac Surg* 66:471-476, 1998.
117. Perrault LP, Menasché P, Bidouard JP et al: Snaring of the target vessel in less invasive bypass operations does not cause endothelial dysfunction, *Ann Thorac Surg* 63:751-755, 1997.
118. Perrault LP, Nickner C, Desjardins N et al: Effects on coronary endothelial function of the Cohn stabilizer for minimally invasive coronary artery bypass surgery, *Cardiothoracic Techniques and Technologies, Current Trends in Thoracic Surgery (VI)* 100, 2000.
119. Pfister AJ, Zaki MS, Garcia JM et al: Coronary artery bypass without cardiopulmonary bypass, *Ann Thorac Surg* 54:1085-1091, 1992.
120. Magovern JA, Benckart DH, Landreneau RJ et al: Morbidity, cost, and six-month outcome of minimally invasive direct coronary artery bypass grafting, *Ann Thorac Surg* 66:1224-1229, 1998.
121. Del Rizzo DF, Boyd WD, Novich RJ et al: Safety and cost-effectiveness of MIDCABG in high-risk CABG patients, *Ann Thorac Surg* 66:1002-1007, 1998.
122. BARI Investigators: Comparison of coronary bypass surgery with angioplasty in patients with multivessel disease, *N Engl J Med* 335:217-225, 1996.
123. Angelini GD, Wilde P, Salerno TA et al: Integrated left small thoracotomy and angioplasty for multi-vessel coronary artery revascularisation, *Lancet* 347:757-758, 1996.
124. Buffolo E, Andrade JCS, Branco JNR et al: Coronary artery bypass grafting without cardiopulmonary bypass, *Ann Thorac Surg* 61:63-66, 1996.
125. Baumgartner FJ, Gheissari A, Capouya ER et al: Technical aspects of total revascularization in off-pump coronary bypass via sternotomy approach, *Ann Thorac Surg* 67:1653-1658, 1999.
126. Hart JC, Spooner T, Edgerton J et al: Off-pump multivessel coronary artery bypass utilizing the octopus® tissue stabilization system: initial experience in 374 patients from three separate centers, *Heart Surg Forum* 2:15-28, 1999.
127. Benetti FJ, Mariani MA: Off-pump coronary artery bypass surgery. In Szabo Z, editor, *Cardiovascular surgery surgical technology international* (VII). Hong Kong, 1999, Universal Medical Press, pp 219-226.
128. Erb JM, Shanewise JS, Michelsen LG et al: Changes in intraoperative regional wall motion assessment using contrast echocardiography during cardiac surgery, *J Cardiothoracic Vase Anesth* 12:214-217, 1998.
129. Kim WC, Balon KD, DuPont FW et al: Effect of contrast echocardiography in intraoperative regional wall motion assessment, *(Novice and expert echocardiographers)*, *Anesthesiology* 91:A134, 1999 (abstract).
130. Aronson S, Albertucci M: Assessing flow during minimally invasive coronary artery bypass. An Allen's test equivalent, *Ann Thorac Surg* 671:1173-1174, 1999.
131. Maslow AD, Park KW, Pawlowski J et al: Minimally invasive direct coronary artery bypass grafting (MID CABG). Changes in anesthetic management and surgical procedure, *J Cardiothorac Vasc Anesth* 13:417-423, 1999.
132. Wasnick JD, Hoffman WJ, Acuff T et al: Anesthetic management of coronary artery by pass via minithoracotomy with video assistance, *J Cardiothorac Vasc Anesth* 9:731-733, 1995.
133. Gayes JM, Emery RW, Nissen MD: Anesthetic considerations for patients undergoing minimally invasive coronary artery bypass surgery: mini-sternotomy and mini-thoracotomy approaches, *J Cardiothorac Vasc Anesth* 10:531-535, 1996.
134. Gayes JM, Emery RW: The MIDCAB experience: a current look at evolving surgical and anesthetic approaches, *J Cardiothorac Vasc Anesth* 11:625-628, 1997.
135. Nierich AP, Diephuis J, Jansen EWL et al: Embracing the heart: perioperative management of patients undergoing off-pump coronary artery bypass grafting using the octopus tissue stabilizer, *J Cardiothorac Vasc Anesth* 13:123-129, 1999.
136. Siegel LC, Hennessy MM, Pearl RG: Delayed time response of the continuous cardiac output pulmonary artery catheter, *Anesth Analg* 83:1173-1177, 1996.
137. Rouine-Rapp K, Lonescu P, Balea M et al: Detection of intraoperative segmental wall-motion abnormalities by transesophageal echocardiography. The incremental value of additional cross sections in the transverse and longitudinal planes, *Anesth Analg* 83:1141-1148, 1996.

138. Lin JC, Szwerc MF, Magovern JA: Non steroidal anti-inflammatory drug-based pain control for minimally invasive direct coronary artery bypass surgery, *Heart Surg Forum* 2:169-171, 1999.

139. ACC/AHA guidelines and indications for coronary artery bypass graft surgery: The report of the American College of Cardiology. American Heart Association task force on assessment of diagnostic and therapeutic cardiovascular procedures, *Circulation* 83: 1125, 1991.

140. Chong JL, Pillai R, Fisher A et al: Cardiac surgery: moving away from intensive care, *Br Heart J* 68:430-433, 1992.

141. Westaby S, Pillai R. Parry A et al: Does modern cardiac surgery require conventional intensive care? *Eur J Cardiothorac Surg* 7:313-318, 1993.

142. Jacobsohn E, De Brouwere R, Kenny S et al: ICU admission is not required after uncomplicated cardiac surgery, *Anesth Analg* 88: S-82, 1999.

143. Syslak P, De Brouwere R, Kenny S et al: Low-dose intrathecal morphine-bupivacaine for cardiac surgery does not delay extubation, *Can J Anaesth* 46:A3A, 1999.

144. Bergsland J, Schmid S, Yanulevich J et al: Coronary artery bypass grafting (CABG) without cardiopulmonary bypass (CPB): a strategy for improving results in surgical revascularization. *Heart Surg Forum* 1:107-110, 1998.

145. Calafiore AM, Giammarco GD, Teodori G et al: Recent advances in multivessel coronary grafting without cardiopulmonary bypass, *Heart Surg Forum* 1:20-25, 1998.

146. Cartier R, Blain R: Off-pump revascularization of the circumflex artery: technical aspect and short-term results, *Ann Thorac Surg* 68:94-99, 1999.

147. Cartier R, Brann S, Dagenais F et al: Systematic off-pump coronary artery revascularization in multivessel disease: experience of three hundred cases, *J Thorac Cardiovasc Surg* 119: 221-229, 2000.

148. Kshettry VR, Flavin TF, Emery RW et al: Does multi-vessel, off-pump coronary artery bypass (OPCABG) reduce postoperative morbidity? *The Society of Thoracic Surgeons 36th Annual Meeting*, 58, 2000.

149. Grosso MA, Anderson WA, McGrath LB et al: Salvage of high risk CABG patients utilizing an off-pump revascularization strategy, *West Thoracic Surgery Association 25th Annual Meeting*, 66-67, 1999.

150. Arom KV, Flavin TF, Emery RW et al: Is low EF safe for off-pump coronary bypass surgery? *Cardiothoracic Techniques and Technologies, Current Trends in Thoracic Surgery (VI) meeting* 45, 2000.

151. Pfister AJ, Stamou SC, Dullum MKC et al: Reoperative coronary artery bypass without cardiopulmonary bypass, *Cardiothoracic Techniques and Technologies, Current Trends in Thoracic Surgery (VI)* 65, 2000.

152. Murkin JM, Boyd D, Ganapathy S et al: OPCAB lowers incidences of neurobehavioural dysfunction vs conventional CABG, *Evolving Techniques & Technology in Minimally Invasive Cardiac Surgery (V)* 53, 1999.

153. Bonatti J, Hangler H, Hörmann C et al: Myocardial damage after minimally invasive coronary artery bypass grafting on the beating heart, *Ann Thorac Surg* 66:1093-1096, 1998.

154. Ascione R, Loyd CT, Gomes WJ et al: Beating versus arrested heart revascularization: evaluation of myocardial function in a prospective randomized study, *Eur J Cardiothorac Surg* 15: 685-690, 1999.

155. Ascione R, Lloyd CT, Underwood MJ et al: On-pump versus off-pump coronary revascularization: evaluation of renal function, *Ann Thorac Surg* 68:493-498, 1999.

156. Novitzky D, Fabri PJ, Perry RW et al: Total myocardial revascularization without cardiopulmonary bypass, *Evolving Techniques & Technology in Minimally Invasive Cardiac Surgery (V)* 44, 1999.

157. Puskas JD, Wright CE, Ronson RS et al: Clinical outcomes and angiographic patency in 125 consecutive off-pump coronary bypass patients, *Evolving Techniques & Technology in Minimally Invasive Cardiac Surgery (V)*, 1999.

158. Arom K, Flavin T, Emery R et al: Safety and efficacy of off-pump coronary artery bypass grafting, *Ann Thorac Surg* 69:704-710, 2000.

159. Novitzky D, Peniston RL, Lorenz BT et al: Differences between coronary artery bypass on and off cardiopulmonary bypass, *Cardiothoracic Techniques and Technologies, Current Trends in Thoracic Surgery VI:* 31, 2000.

160. D'Ancona G, Karamanoukian HL, Salerno TA et al: Flow measurement in coronary surgery, *Heart Surg Forum* 2:121-124, 1999.

161. Øvrum E, Tangen G, Åm Holen E: Facing the era of minimally invasive coronary grafting: current results of conventional bypass grafting for single-vessel disease, *Ann Thorac Surg* 64: 159-162, 1997.

162. Mack MJ, Osborne JA, Shennib H: Arterial graft patency in coronary artery bypass grafting: what do we really know? *Ann Thorac Surg* 66:1055-1059, 1998.

163. Redle JD, Khurana S, Marzan R et al: Prophylactic oral amiodarone compared with placebo for prevention of atrial fibrillation after coronary artery bypass surgery, *Am Heart J* 138: 144-150, 1999.

164. Allen KB, Matheny RG, Heimansohn DA et al: Minimally invasive direct coronary artery bypass grafting versus single vessel conventional coronary artery bypass, *J Am Coll Cardiol* 31S:70A, 1998 (abstract).

165. Mariani MA, Boonstra PW, Grandjean JG et al: Minimally invasive coronary artery bypass grafting without cardiopulmonary bypass, *Eur J Cardiothoracic Surg* 11:881-886, 1997.

166. Subramanian VA, McCabe JC, Geller CM: Minimally invasive direct coronary artery bypass grafting: two-year clinical experience, *Ann Thorac Surg* 64:1648-1655, 1997.

167. Possati G, Gaudino M, Alessandrini F et al: Systematic clinical and angiographic follow-up of patients undergoing minimally invasive coronary artery bypass, *J Thorac Cardiovasc Surg* 115: 785-790, 1998.

168. Diegeler A, Matin M, Kayser S et al: Angiographic results after minimally invasive coronary bypass grafting using the minimally invasive direct coronary bypass grafting (MIDCAB) approach, *Eur J Cardiothoracic Surg* 15:680-684, 1999.

169. Mack MJ, Magovern JA, Acuff TA et al: Results of graft patency by immediate angiography in minimally invasive coronary artery surgery, *Ann Thorac Surg* 68:383-390, 1999.

170. Gu YJ, Mariani MA, van Oeveren W et al: Reduction of the inflammatory response in patients undergoing minimally invasive coronary artery bypass grafting, *Ann Thorac Surg* 65:420-424, 1998.

171. Zenati M, Domit TM, Saul M et al: Resource utilization for minimally invasive direct and standard coronary artery bypass grafting, *Ann Thorac Surg* 63:S84-S87, 1997.

172. Cremer J, Mügge A, Wittwer T et al: Early angiographic results after revascularization by minimally invasive direct coronary artery bypass (MIDCAB), *Eur J Cardiothorac Surg* 15:383-387, 1999.

173. Gundry SR, Romano MA, Shattuck OH et al: Seven year follow-up of coronary artery bypasses performed with and without cardiopulmonary bypass, *J Thorac Cardiovasc Surg* 115: 1273-1278, 1998.

174. Andrews TC, Reimold SC, Berlin JA et al: Prevention of supraventricular arrhythmias after coronary artery bypass surgery, *Circulation* 84:S236-S244, 1991.

175. Chung MK, Asher CR, Dykstra D et al: Atrial fibrillation increases length of stay and cost after cardiac surgery in low risk patients targeted for early discharge, *J Am Coll Cardiol* 27:309A, 1996 (abstract).
176. Kannel WB, Abbott RD, Savage DD et al: Epidemiologic features of chronic atrial fibrillation: the Framingham study, *N Engl J Med* 306:1018-1022, 1982.
177. Furberg CD, Psaty BM, Manolio TA et al: Prevalence of atrial fibrillation elder subjects (The Cardiovascular Health Study), *Am J Cardiol* 74:236-241, 1994.
178. Goldman L: Supraventricular tachyarrhythmia in hospitalized adults after surgery: clinical correlates in patients over 40 years of age after major noncardiac surgery, *Chest* 73:450-454, 1978.

CHAPTER **14**

Thoracic Aortic Surgery

Christopher J. O'Connor, M.D.

OUTLINE

The surgical approach to disorders of the thoracic aorta began in the early 1950s when Debakey, Cooley, and colleagues reported the successful repair of aneurysms of the descending thoracic aorta (DTA).[1,2] In 1956 and 1957, they reported the first operative repair of aneurysms of both the ascending aorta and the aortic arch by using cardiopulmonary bypass (CPB).[3] These initial experiences paved the way for profound advancements in the surgical and anesthetic management of complex lesions of the entire thoracic aorta. Despite improvements in the perioperative management of patients undergo-ing thoracic aortic surgery, these surgeries remain the most demanding and technically challenging cardiovascular procedures encountered by the anesthesiologist. Safe intraoperative management of these cases requires not only a thorough comprehension of the physiology of CPB, but also a familiarity with the different techniques of cerebral protection, the physiology of one-lung ventilation, and the pathophysiologic events associated with cross-clamping of the DTA, the sentinel event that characterizes descending thoracic aortic surgery.

This chapter first describes the etiology, classification,

pathogenesis, and clinical presentation of thoracic aortic disease. The intraoperative anesthetic management of ascending and arch aortic disease as well as descending thoracic lesions are then reviewed separately, because the surgical and anesthetic approaches differ significantly for the two anatomic sites.

CLASSIFICATION

Thoracic aortic disease is classified according to the underlying pathologic condition, the presence or absence of dissection, and the location of the lesion. A simple classification scheme based on the underlying cause is shown in Box 14-1.

For aortic dissection, two classification schemes are widely used (Fig. 14-1). In the DeBakey classification, Type I dissections originate from an intimal tear in the ascending aorta and extend for variable lengths into the descending thoracic and abdominal aorta. Type II lesions are confined to the ascending aorta, and Type III dissections begin in the DTA and extend from the left subclavian artery either to the diaphragm (Type IIIa) or below it into the abdominal aorta (Type IIIb).[1] In contrast to this system, the Stanford classification described by Daily and colleagues designates any dissection that involves the ascending aorta as Type A, regardless of their extent, and all other dissections as Type B.[4] Because the Stanford classification is widely used in clinical practice, dissections are commonly termed either proximal or distal on the basis of their involvement of the ascending aorta.[4] This classification has practical significance since isolated acute distal dissections are initially treated medically, whereas proximal lesions are considered surgical emergencies.[1] Dissections less than 2 weeks old are

further classified as acute, whereas those beyond this period are considered chronic.

In contrast to aortic dissections, thoracoabdominal aortic aneurysms are classified by their extent of involvement of the distal thoracic and abdominal aorta (Fig. 14-2).[5] Preoperative identification of Crawford type I

BOX 14-1
Classification of Thoracic Aortic Disease

Aneurysm
    Congenital or developmental (i.e., Marfan's syndrome, Ehlers-Danlos syndrome)
    Degenerative
        Cystic medial degeneration
        Nonspecific (atherosclerotic)
    Traumatic
    Inflammatory
        Takayasu's arteritis, Behcet's syndrome, Kawasaki's disease
        Microvascular disorders (i.e., polyarteritis)
    Infectious (mycotic)
        Bacterial, fungal, spirochetal, viral
    Mechanical
        Poststenotic, associated with arteriovenous fistula
    Anastomotic (after arteriotomy)
Pseudoaneurysm
Dissection
    Type A (DeBakey Types I and II)
    Type B (DeBakey Type III)
Penetrating atherosclerotic ulcer
Intramural hematoma
Atherosclerotic disease

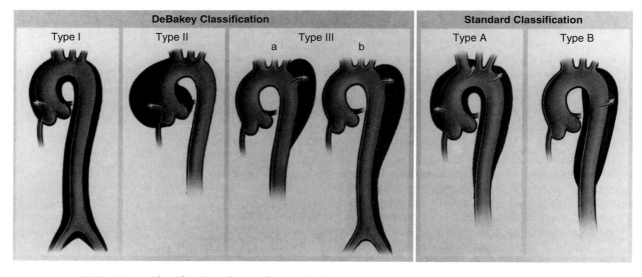

FIG. 14-1 Classification schemes for aortic dissection. See text for description. (From Kouchoukos NT, Dougenis D: *N Engl J Med* 336:1876-1887, 1997.)

and II thoracoabdominal aneurysms is essential because these lesions require the most extensive surgical resection and are associated with the highest incidence of postoperative paraplegia. Awareness of the anticipated complexity of a specific type of aneurysm resection permits appropriate anesthetic preparation.

Morphologically, aneurysms most often involve the entire circumference of the aorta and are termed *fusiform aneurysms*, but they may also enlarge asymmetrically to form saccular aneurysms.[6] Lesions of the thoracic aorta are also classified histopathologically according to the following underlying cellular pathologies: medial degenerative disease (loss of elastic fibers), medial necrosis (loss of smooth muscle), atherosclerosis (usually superimposed on medial degenerative disease), or inflammatory.[7]

ETIOLOGY
Aortic Aneurysms

Degenerative aneurysms associated with atherosclerosis most commonly involve the descending thoracic and thoracoabdominal aorta,[1] whereas the primary histopathologic cause of ascending aortic aneurysms is cystic medial degeneration. Pseudoaneurysms represent dilation of the aorta that involves a variable extent of the aortic media and adventitia, but not the entire aortic wall. Pseudoaneurysms typically occur following chest trauma, infectious processes, or surgical procedures that involve the ascending aorta (i.e., coronary bypass procedures, aortic surgery).[1]

A major factor postulated to contribute to the formation of aortic aneurysms is the abnormal production of elastase and other proteolytic enzymes that destroy the

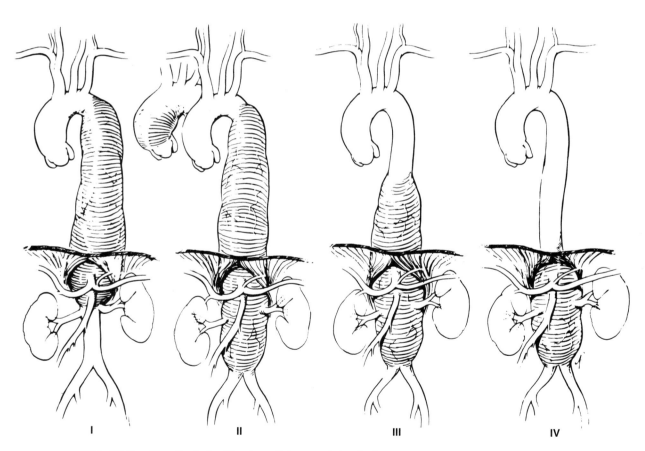

FIG. 14-2   Crawford classification of thoracoabdominal aortic aneurysms. Type I aneurysms extend from the proximal descending thoracic aorta (DTA) to the upper abdominal aorta but terminate before the renal arteries. Type II aneurysms extend more distally to the level of the aortic bifurcation. Type III lesions begin in the distal half of the DTA and extend to the aortic bifurcation. Type IV lesions extend from the twelfth intercostal space to the aortic bifurcation and do not include the intercostal arteries from T7 to T12.

(From Svensson LG, Crawford ES: *Curr Probl Surg* 29:922-1011, 1992.)

elastic fibers of the aortic wall and produce a nonelastic aorta that is prone to dilation, aneurysm formation, and possible rupture.[1,7] Other etiologic factors include deficiencies of collagen and elastin, and immune-mediated changes in the aortic wall.[7]

Aortic Dissection

Aortic dissection is a pathophysiologic process, distinct from degenerative aneurysm formation, that occurs when blood under pressure separates the aortic wall through a tear in the intima, cleaving the medial layer into two planes. The forward driving force of aortic blood flow extends the dissection in an antegrade direction along the aortic wall. Less commonly, dissection may occur in a retrograde direction. The blood-filled space between the dissected layers of the aortic wall becomes the *false lumen*, which may communicate with the *true lumen* through more distal reentry sites. The *intimal flap* is commonly visualized by echocardiography and represents the inner portion of the dissected aortic wall. The false lumen usually extends from the outer curve of the ascending aorta along the anterior portion of the arch and down the left side of the aorta, functionally involving more than 50% of the aortic circumference.[4] Although the majority of intimal tears occur in the ascending aorta, they may also be seen in the DTA or aortic arch.[8] The false lumen may compress the true lumen and may also obstruct the orifice of aortic branch vessels. This occurs in 30% of patients, by obstruction of the vessel orifice, compression of the artery, or shearing of the branch vessel from the true lumen.[4] Perfusion from the false lumen then maintains flow to these vessels.

Cystic medial degeneration is the most common pathophysiologic feature of aortic dissection. It is an essential component of many connective tissues disorders, most notably Marfan syndrome, which accounts for almost 10% of all aortic dissections.[9] Hypertension is also a critical risk factor for aortic dissection, possibly by facilitating the development of cystic medial degeneration. An association has also been observed between pregnancy and aortic dissection because 50% of all dissections in women younger than 40 years of age occur during the third trimester of pregnancy.[9] Other risk factors for aortic dissection include trauma, connective tissue disorders, iatrogenic dissection from surgery involving the aorta,[10] aortic coarctation, and bicuspid aortic valves.[1]

Variants of Aortic Dissection

There has been a recent appreciation of the importance of so-called variants of aortic dissection. The two most important of these pathologic variants are intramural hematoma (IMH) without a dissection flap and penetrating atherosclerotic aortic ulcer.[11] IMH has been attributed to rupture of the vaso vasorum, hemorrhage within an atherosclerotic plaque, or traumatic hematoma formation.[12] Importantly, these lesions may not be detected by conventional contrast angiography, so that transesophageal echocardiography (TEE) and contrast-enhanced computed tomography (CT) are the preferred initial diagnostic techniques. Penetrating atherosclerotic aortic ulcers have a similar clinical presentation to IMH and aortic dissection, presenting as chest or back pain in elderly, hypertensive patients.[11,13,14] These lesions are produced by atherosclerotic plaques that ulcerate through the elastic lamina into the media, precipitating either localized intramural hemorrhage, classic aneurysm formation, rupture through the adventitia that produces a pseudoaneurysm, or complete aortic rupture.[13,14]

Another variant of aortic dissection, described by Svensson et al,[15] is an aortic intimal tear without an IMH. This is a clinical entity that, although clinically similar to aortic dissection, may require aortography for accurate diagnosis since it may not be detected by noninvasive tests such as TEE, CT, or magnetic resonance imaging (MRI). Patients with any of these "acute aortic syndromes" should be treated as if they have acute aortic dissection, with involvement of the ascending aorta an indication for immediate surgical intervention, and medical therapy reserved for stable lesions of the DTA.[11,13,14,16] As noted by O'Gara and DeSanctis,[11] distinctions between these variants and classic aortic dissections are clinically artificial and should not delay an aggressive approach to surgical management.

Traumatic Lesions

Traumatic aortic injury characteristically results from high-speed deceleration injuries such as those observed after automobile accidents, blast injuries, or severe falls.[17] The abrupt deceleration of the body creates enormous shearing forces that act maximally on those areas of the aorta where a highly mobile segment joins a fixed one.[18,19] The most common location for aortic rupture is at the aortic isthmus just distal to the origin of the left subclavian artery where the relatively mobile thoracic aorta joins the fixed aortic arch. Traumatic aortic rupture is frequently a lethal event, although surgical intervention can limit the mortality rate, albeit with a potentially high incidence of paraplegia.[20]

CLINICAL PRESENTATION

Many patients with thoracic aortic aneurysms are asymptomatic at the time of presentation and the lesion is detected at the time of another medical evaluation.[1] However, when symptoms develop they are usually a result of aneurysm enlargement and compression of adjacent structures. Thoracic aneurysms may produce interscapular back pain or left-sided pleuritic pain, whereas thoracoabdominal aneurysm expansion is often associated with abdominal pain.[1] In contrast to pain, certain less common symptoms may indicate compression of structures that have significant implications for the anesthesiologist. These include hoarseness from stretching of the recurrent laryngeal nerve, stridor from tracheal or left mainstem bronchial compression, dysphagia and weight loss from esophageal compression, and dyspnea from left lung or left pulmonary artery compression.[1] Placement of left-sided double-lumen endobronchial tubes (DLTs) or TEE probes may be hazardous in the presence of airway or esophageal compression.

The symptoms of patients with acute aortic dissection typically include the sudden onset of severe pain in the chest, neck, or interscapular area.[1] The pain is classically described as a tearing sensation and is frequently accompanied by acute hypertension.[4] In addition, occlusion of aortic branch vessels by the dissection process can also produce signs or symptoms of myocardial ischemia, central nervous system (CNS) dysfunction, renal failure, visceral ischemia, paraplegia, or lower extremity claudication. Ninety percent of patients with untreated acute proximal aortic dissection die within 3 months. The diagnosis is more favorable for those with acute distal dissections, where the 1-year survival rate is 60%.[1,4] The most common causes of death in patients with acute dissection are rupture into the pericardium resulting in pericardial tamponade and exsanguination from rupture into the pleural space or mediastinum.[1,4]

SURGICAL INDICATIONS

Because the majority of patients with untreated thoracic or thoracoabdominal aortic aneurysms eventually die from aortic rupture, the timing of surgical intervention for patients with known aneurysms becomes critical. Unfortunately, the size-to-rupture correlation established for abdominal aortic aneurysms is not directly applicable to thoracic aortic lesions.[21] Moreover, the morbidity and mortality of thoracic aortic resection is significantly higher than for abdominal aortic surgery, especially for procedures involving the DTA. Elective resection is recommended for patients with chronic degenerative aneurysms of the ascending aorta when the aortic diameter is 5 to 5.5 cm,[21] since aneurysms greater than 5 to 6 cm have a faster growth rate and a greater subsequent risk of rupture than do smaller aneurysms.[1] Surgery is indicated for patients with Marfan syndrome when the aneurysm size is 5 to 5.5 cm or less, since most deaths from this disorder are related to complications from ascending aortic aneurysms and because rupture has been observed with aneurysms less than 5 cm.[1,4,21,22] Because of the greater risk of neurologic injury, elective resection for asymptomatic patients with aortic arch aneurysms is usually indicated only when the aneurysm exceeds 5.5 to 6 cm.[1] Similarly, because of the higher perioperative complication rate and the risk of spinal cord injury, resection of descending thoracic aortic aneurysms is advised when the aneurysm diameter exceeds 6.5 cm.[21]

In contrast to chronic processes, surgery is indicated for all acute proximal dissections and for acute distal dissections when there is persistent and intractable pain, evidence for impending rupture, branch vessel involvement with end-organ ischemia, or rapid expansion of the involved segment of aorta.[11]

INTRAOPERATIVE MANAGEMENT
Ascending Aortic Disease

Surgical Aspects. To protect the brain and the heart effectively during ascending aortic surgery, the anesthesiologist must understand the often complex surgical approach to these lesions.

Degenerative aneurysms or isolated dissections of the ascending aorta without associated aortic valvular disease are treated with Dacron graft replacement of the affected aortic segment by using standard methods of CPB.[1] If the lesion extends beyond the ascending aorta in the setting of aortic dissection, the disrupted layers of the distal aorta are sutured together before anastomosis to the graft.[1] If the aortic valve is normal but aortic regurgitation is present, then the aortic wall is approximated and the aortic valve resuspended. If aortic valve disease is also present (i.e., a bicuspid valve) or the patient has Marfan syndrome, then the ascending aorta and aortic valve are most commonly replaced with a composite valve graft containing a mechanical valve.[1,4,7] A critical aspect of composite valve graft insertion is attachment of the coronary ostia, which can be accomplished by using one of three techniques. In the Bentall repair, segments of the proximal graft are resected and the coronary ostia are directly attached to the prosthetic graft (Fig. 14-3). The button technique involves dissection of the coronary ostia as buttons of tissue that are then attached to the graft. This approach appears to decrease the rate of bleeding and false aneurysm formation at the coronary ostia-graft anastomosis site that has been observed with the Bentall procedure (as a result of tension of the anastomoses that pull free from the graft).[4] The Cabrol repair involves end-to-end attachment of the coronary ostia to a tube graft that is then attached in a side-to-side fashion to the aortic graft (Fig. 14-4).

By definition, aortic arch lesions extend from the origin of the innominate artery to the distal origin of the left subclavian artery. Resection of the aortic arch is a technically demanding procedure that requires either a period of deep hypothermic circulatory arrest (DHCA) or selective antegrade cerebral perfusion (ACP) with

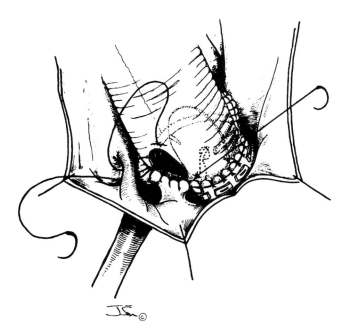

FIG. 14-3 The Bentall procedure. During aortic valve-conduit replacement of the ascending aorta, the coronary ostia are anastomosed directly to the graft.

(From Stowe CL, Baertlein MA, Wierman MD et al: *Ann Thorac Surg* 66:388-395, 1998.)

moderate systemic hypothermia to protect the brain during the period of arch reconstruction. For both approaches, CPB is achieved via cannulation of the femoral artery for retrograde aortic perfusion and of the right atrium (with or without the femoral vein) for venous drainage. A median sternotomy is performed, CPB is initiated, hypothermia is induced, and the heart is arrested. If DHCA is used, then the aorta is left unclamped and the arch is repaired with excision of the brachiocephalic vessels as a Carrel patch that is reinforced with Teflon pledgets and reattached to the aortic graft.[4] Once the anastomoses are completed, CPB is restarted, air and debris are flushed and aspirated from the graft, and the proximal graft is clamped to allow retrograde femoral perfusion of the arch vessels while the proximal aortic anastomsis is completed. Alternatively, the arterial cannula can be moved (or a side arm graft attached) to the aortic graft to provide antegrade flow to the cerebral vessels while the proximal anastomosis is performed. This may reduce the risk of cerebral air and debris embolization from retrograde femoral blood flow.[4]

Replacement of the entire arch or repair of the distal aortic arch is also technically difficult and is approached from either a left thoracotomy or median sternotomy, both by using CPB and DHCA. The elephant trunk procedure has simplified the ease and safety of extensive arch surgery and is commonly used for these complex lesions[4] (Fig. 14-5). This technique involves invaginating an aortic graft and inserting the proximal end into the proximal DTA. The distal anastomosis is then completed, after which the proximal graft sleeve is withdrawn and the arch vessels are reattached. The cerebral vessels are reperfused antegrade or retrograde by femoral artery perfusion as previously described, and the proximal anastomosis is finished with the graft clamped just below the innominate artery.

Early mortality rates after ascending aortic surgery range from 3% to 10%, with higher rates reported for aortic dissections and emergency procedures.[1] Five-year survival rates range from 60% to 80%. In contrast, early mortality rates for aortic arch surgery are nearly twice as high as for isolated ascending aortic procedures and the 5-year survival rate is only 50%.[1] The incidence of permanent neurologic deficits ranges from 3% to 10% in patients undergoing ascending and arch aortic surgery by using DHCA.[23-27] The incidence of transient delirium was 19% in a series of 200 patients after thoracic aortic surgery with DHCA.[27]

Anesthetic Issues. The anesthetic management of ascending aortic surgery is similar in many respects to routine cardiac surgery requiring CPB. However, there are notable differences because of the increased potential for cerebral ischemia and the effects of profound hypothermia and prolonged periods of CPB.

Monitors. The left radial or brachial artery is routinely chosen for invasive blood pressure monitoring because of the possible inclusion of the innominate artery within the cross-clamped segment of aorta. However, the right radial artery pressure is also frequently monitored to detect possible malperfusion of the innominate artery resulting from inadequate blood supply from the false lumen of a dissected aorta or obstruction by an intimal flap. In addition, it is important to monitor innominate artery pressure (and thus cerebral perfusion pressure) when selective ACP is used. Alternatively, the femoral artery may be used for systemic arterial blood pressure monitoring instead of the left radial artery, and is frequently monitored to assess the adequacy of distal perfusion during retrograde femoral CPB. In the presence of aortic dissection, the catheter is placed in the left femoral artery since the left side is supplied by the false lumen in 80% of patients with aortic dissection.[28] Communication between the two lumens by reentry sites theoretically allows an accurate measurement of distal pressure. The right femoral artery is then used for the aortic perfusion cannula, which ensures that retrograde aortic perfusion will more likely occur through the true, rather than the false, lumen. The choice of arterial monitoring sites is thus guided by several anatomic and surgical considerations and should be discussed in advance with the surgical team.

Pulmonary artery catheterization is typically indi-

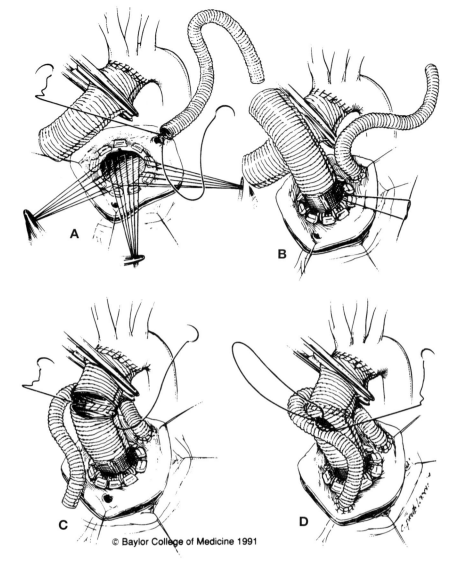

FIG. 14-4 The Cabrol procedure. In contrast to a Bentall repair, in this procedure the coronary ostia are anastomosed to the ends of a tube graft (**A** & **B**), which is then attached side to side to the aortic graft (**D**).

(From Svensson LG, Crawford ES: *Curr Probl Surg* 29:922-1011, 1992.)

© Baylor College of Medicine 1991

cated to precisely control systemic and intracardiac pressures in patients with significant aortic lesion and underlying hypertension who are undergoing prolonged periods of CPB. The pulmonary artery catheter is useful to guide fluid management and blood product replacement during complex aortic resections complicated by hypothermia and coagulation disturbances.

TEE is considered by many to be the initial diagnostic procedure of choice for suspected acute aortic dissection[29-33] and in some centers has replaced angiography as the most commonly performed diagnostic study in the evaluation of aortic dissection.[34] In addition to its role in the initial evaluation of aortic dissections, TEE is a valuable intraoperative monitor because of its ability to (1) confirm the diagnosis of aortic dissection, (2) identify the site of intimal tears and the extent of dissection, (3) evaluate the adequacy of ventricular filling and the quality of retrograde femoral

aortic and cerebral perfusion, (4) define the quality of surgical repair and the presence of residual reentry sites, (5) assess the adequacy of valvular and ventricular function,[32,35,36] and (6) evaluate the adequacy of left atrial and left ventricular (LV) decompression during distal circulatory support.[37]

Confirmation of the preoperative diagnosis and identification of the true and false lumens and the site of intimal tears are important components of the intraoperative TEE examination during aortic dissection repair. This information is probably most critical during surgery for ascending aortic lesions, where identification of the true lumen and possible intimal compression of coronary ostia, as well as assessment of the aortic valve, all provide the surgeon with important clinical information. In addition, evaluation of the aortic arch, the arch branch vessels, and the proximal DTA may be especially critical for emergency procedures where there is limited

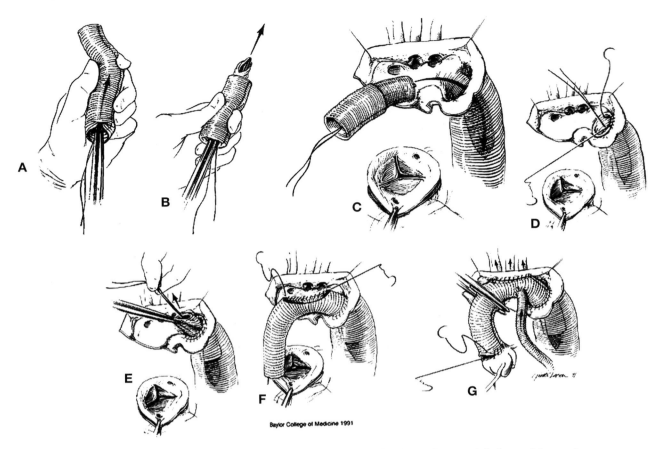

FIG. 14-5 The elephant trunk procedure. This procedure is used to repair lesions of the aortic arch and proximal descending thoracic aorta. As described in the text, this repair involves invagination of the proximal end of a graft and anastomosis of the distal end to the distal aortic arch (**A-D**). The invaginated portion of the graft is then pulled back, and the arch vessel and proximal anastomoses are completed (**E-G**).

(From Svensson LG, Crawford ES: *Curr Probl Surg* 29:922-1011, 1992.)

information available from hastily performed preoperative studies.

An important limitation of TEE in the assessment of the ascending aorta is the limited view of the distal ascending aorta because of interference by the air-filled trachea.[38] In addition, reverberation artifacts in the ascending aorta may mimic an intimal flap and are a common cause of false-positive findings that must be considered in any TEE evaluation of possible aortic dissection.[30,39,40] Recent evidence suggests that contrast echocardiography may eliminate the linear artifacts often encountered in the ascending aorta and allow for more precise identification of true aortic dissection.[41]

Differentiating between the true and false lumens may be difficult. Typically, color and pulsed Doppler evaluation demonstrate systolic forward flow with high velocities in the true lumen and low flow or flow reversal in the false lumen.[30] Two-dimensional analysis often shows spontaneous echo contrast in the false lumen

that results from stasis of blood (Fig. 14-6). In addition, the true lumen is typically smaller and tends to expand with systole and collapse during diastole. Entry sites can be located with color Doppler by detecting systolic flow from the true to the false lumen. Absent flow in the false lumen indicates no communication or a more distal communication between the two lumens, or occlusion of the false lumen by thrombus, a common finding.[30]

An important aspect of monitoring during ascending and arch aortic surgery is assessment of the CNS. Because of the risk of stroke and transient neurologic dysfunction, an aggressive approach toward intraoperative assessment of the adequacy of brain protection and cerebral perfusion is essential. Electroencephalography (EEG) is commonly used to measure cellular function and ensure electrical silence during procedures requiring DHCA. Although devices that record and display processed EEG data, such as the compressed spectral array or density-modulated spectral array systems, are less

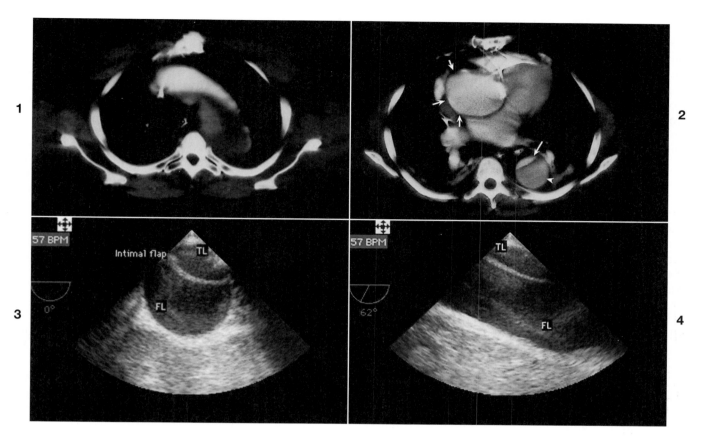

FIG. 14-6 Diagnostic images from a patient undergoing reoperation for a recurrent type I aortic dissection. **1,** A computed tomography (CT) scan demonstrates dye in the true lumen (outer, anterior portion) of the aorta. No dye is present in the false lumen. **2,** More distal CT scan images reveal aneurysmal dilation of the ascending aorta (*three arrows*) with a residual but only partial dissection flap that produces incomplete separation of the ascending aorta. The smaller true lumen and larger false lumen of the descending aorta are also apparent in this scan (*arrow* and *arrowhead,* respectively). **3,** A short-axis 0° transesophageal echocardiography (TEE) image of the proximal descending aorta demonstrates the true lumen (*TL*), an intimal flap, and the false lumen (*FL*). Spontaneous echo contrast is also evident in the false lumen. **4,** A long-axis TEE image at the same level of the descending aorta.

sensitive for the detection of cerebral ischemia than multichannel analogue EEG instruments, they are typically used because of their convenience and simplicity of data display.[42] Other potentially useful, although less commonly employed monitors, include (1) internal jugular vein oximetric catheters that measure jugular venous oxygen saturation (Sjo_2) and reflect the balance between cerebral oxygen delivery and cerebral oxygen consumption, (2) transcranial Doppler devices that measure middle cerebral artery blood flow and detect cerebral embolic events, (3) near-infrared spectroscopy that attempts to measure the adequacy of brain oxygen saturation,[43] and (4) somatosensory-evoked potentials (SSEPs).[44,45]

Anesthetic and Hemostasis Management. The choice of anesthetic for ascending aortic surgery is less important than is the control of hyperdynamic responses to intubation and surgical stimulation that may increase aortic shear forces and precipitate aortic dissection, aneurysm rupture, or myocardial ischemia. Commonly, moderate doses of short-acting opioids such as fentanyl or sufentanil provide satisfactory analgesia while allowing for a timely awakening in the intensive care unit. This will allow an early assessment of mental status and neurologic function to determine whether a new neurologic deficit has occurred. The use of barbiturates, volatile anesthetics, or both for cerebral protection will provide further hypnosis during the intraoperative period.

Ascending aortic surgery is frequently performed by using DHCA. The profound degree of hypothermia encountered and the prolonged period of CPB required for cooling, performance of the repair, and rewarming all produce alterations in hemostasis. Interestingly, although the hemostatic changes associated with CPB and moderate hypothermia have been extensively evaluated, there are little data on the hematologic consequences of DHCA. Available evidence suggests that hypothermia produces abnormalities in platelet function by activation of platelets and release of their granules. Hypothermia also reversibly impairs the enzymatic activity of clotting factors. These abnormalities promote abnormal clot formation,[46,47] and in conjunction with the disruption of vascular integrity from extensive aortic anastomoses, contribute to greater blood product requirements than are typically encountered for routine cardiac surgery. Blood product requirements range from 4 to 9 units of packed red blood cells (PRBCs), 4 to 10 units of fresh frozen plasma (FFP), and 2 to 4 units of platelets and cryoprecipitate.[4,48-50] Svensson et al[49] demonstrated, however, that 69% of 45 patients undergoing ascending and arch aortic surgery required no homologous blood transfusions when a blood conservation strategy of preoperative autologous blood donation was used, suggesting that ascending aortic surgery can be safely performed without homologous transfusions in select patients. The strongest predictors of in-hospital transfusion requirements were age and CPB time.

Aprotinin has been advocated because of its documented hemostatic effects to reduce the risk of hemorrhage associated with ascending aortic surgery. However, controversy has surrounded the use of aprotinin for procedures requiring DHCA since an early report from Sundt et al[51] suggested an increased incidence of intravascular coagulation and renal dysfunction in patients receiving aprotinin for thoracic aortic surgery with DHCA. Although inadequate heparinization was felt to be responsible for the diffuse thromboses reported by these authors, other more contemporary descriptions have suggested a higher incidence of renal dysfunction,[52,53] thrombosis,[54,55] and postoperative complications[50] in aprotinin-treated patients undergoing DHCA. In contrast to these unfavorable reports, several contemporary studies have noted significant reductions in transfusion requirements and no increased incidence of renal dysfunction in circulatory arrest patients treated with aprotinin.[56,57] Contemporary data also suggest that more aggressive heparinization during DHCA with aprotinin by using activated clotting time (ACT)-independent measures of anticoagulation may be associated with better platelet preservation and less hypercoagulability compared with monitoring and heparin dosing according to standard ACT measurements, where results may be spuriously prolonged by the effects of both aprotinin and hypothermia.[58]

In summary, the use of aprotinin for thoracic aortic procedures requiring DHCA is controversial, and existing data are inconclusive regarding both its potential deleterious effects and its beneficial effects. If aprotinin is used, the adequacy of heparin anticoagulation should be established by using satisfactory prolongation

(at least 500-600 seconds) of the kaolin, rather than celite-based ACT.[58] In addition, it may be prudent to use additional tests of heparin activity to ensure satisfactory anticoagulation. Despite these recommendations, some authors maintain that, until more extensive study of the risks and benefits of aprotinin during DHCA is done, aprotinin should not be used during procedures requiring circulatory arrest.

Cerebral Protection. Surgery of the ascending thoracic aorta and aortic arch presents a unique challenge to the operative team because cerebral perfusion cannot be achieved with standard CPB techniques when the arch vessels are temporarily isolated from the native aortic circulation. Techniques that allow for brain protection and cerebral perfusion during the period of aortic arch reconstruction are therefore required. These approaches include the use of DHCA, selective ACP, and DHCA in conjunction with retrograde cerebral perfusion (RCP) (Fig. 14-7). Hypothermia is the principal component of all of these methods of cerebral protection.

Hypothermic Circulatory Arrest. Borst et al first successfully used the technique of hypothermic circulatory arrest for aortic arch disease in 1964. Since that time, profound hypothermia has become an essential aspect of ascending aortic and aortic arch surgery and has permitted the safe repair of complex thoracic aortic lesions.

The CNS is entirely dependent on aerobic metabolism for energy production and any interruption in blood flow will lead to ischemic brain injury.[59] Hypothermia is highly effective in suppressing brain energy consumption via suppression of cerebral metabolism and provides far better protection against ischemic injury than do pharmacologic agents that similarly depress neuronal function.[59] The primary protective effect of hypothermia is via a temperature-induced reduction in intracellular enzymatic reactions and therefore cerebral metabolic rate. As metabolic rate is reduced, oxygen requirements and cerebral blood flow are also proportionately reduced. This relationship between cerebral metabolic rate and temperature has been classically described by the quotient, Q_{10}. The Q_{10} represents the ratio between the cerebral metabolic rate at two temperatures separated by $10°$, or the multiple by which metabolism decreases for each $10°$ decrease in temperature.[60] Although there is a wide range of reported values, most contemporary data suggest a value of 2.8 for humans.[60]

In addition to effects on metabolic rate, hypothermia also appears to protect neural tissue by preserving tissue pH and adenosine triphosphate stores, preventing the release of excitatory neurotransmitters, and delaying the onset of the ischemic cascade.[59] The use of DHCA also provides a bloodless operating field that is unobstructed by clamps or cannulas. In addition, it obviates the need for aortic cross-clamping and may lessen the risk of neurologic injury from clamp-induced cerebral embolization of aortic atheromatous debris.[61]

Following the institution of CPB, patients are cooled for at least 30 minutes until the esophageal temperature is 13° to 15° C and there is electrical silence on the EEG. Some institutions also measure internal SjO_2 as an additional measure of cerebral perfusion, targeting a saturation of greater than 95% to ensure adequate suppression of cerebral metabolism.[59] Packing of the head in ice is recommended for additional brain cooling and to prevent brain rewarming. Experimental data suggest that this maneuver may provide additional cerebral protection.[62,63] Once the repair is complete, the patient is placed in the Trendelenburg position and the graft is flushed free of air and debris by antegrade and retrograde perfusion. Rewarming is performed slowly to avoid cerebral hyperthermia, which may impair metabolic recovery in recently ischemic brain tissue and worsen neurologic outcome.[60] For these reasons, neither perfusate nor nasopharyngeal temperatures (nor other surrogate measures of cerebral temperature such as tympanic membrane temperature) should exceed 37° C.[59,60,64] After an adequate period of rewarming, the patient is weaned from CPB. Mild hypothermia is tolerated early in the postoperative period to protect the brain and hypotension is avoided to maintain cerebral perfusion pressure.[59]

There is significant controversy regarding the appropriate method of pH management during DHCA. Patients undergoing cardiac surgery with moderate hypothermia appear to have better neurobehavioral outcomes when an alpha-stat strategy is used, presumably because of reduced cerebral blood flow, which, in turn, limits the delivery of emboli to the cerebral circulation.[65-67] In contrast, the increased cerebral blood flow associated with pH-stat management may improve cerebral cooling and decrease the risk of cerebral anoxia during DHCA.[68] An improvement in neurobehavioral outcomes has been demonstrated experimentally[68-71] and in studies in infants undergoing

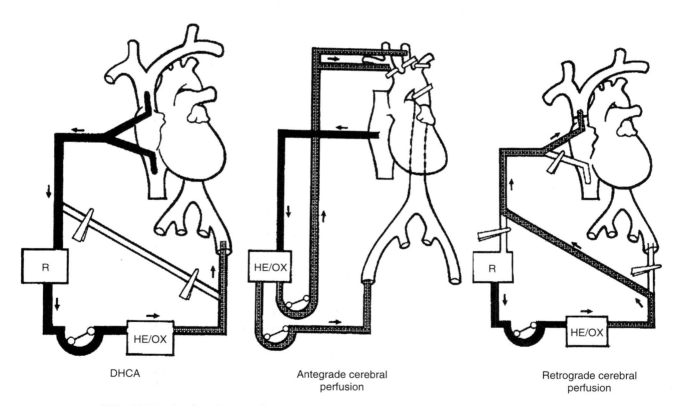

DHCA   Antegrade cerebral   Retrograde cerebral
              perfusion   perfusion

FIG. 14-7   Cardiopulmonary bypass circuits and perfusion systems for ascending and arch aortic surgery. The circuit for deep hypothermic circulatory arrest (*DHCA*) involves standard venous drainage and retrograde femoral artery perfusion. Separate cerebral perfusion catheters and a designated roller pump are used for antegrade cerebral perfusion with a different roller pump providing retrograde perfusion of the lower body. During retrograde cerebral perfusion, the femoral arterial inflow line and inferior vena cava are clamped after circulatory arrest is achieved, and blood is diverted retrograde across a bridge into the superior vena cava. *HE/OX*, Heat exchanger/oxygenator; *R*, reservoir.

(Adapted from Chanyi S: *J Cardiothorac Vasc Anesth* 10[1]:75-82, 1996.)

DHCA with pH-stat management,[72,73] supporting this approach in patients undergoing DHCA.

In addition to temperature and pH management, it is also essential to maintain hemodilution during DHCA because hypothermia-induced hemoconcentration and red blood cell sludging may reduce cerebral blood flow.[59] However, some experimental data suggest that extreme hemodilution during DHCA should be avoided because inadequate oxygen delivery may occur early during cooling and impair subsequent cerebral recovery.[74] Finally, intraoperative hyperglycemia should be aggressively treated because of substantial experimental and clinical evidence demonstrating cerebral intracellular acidosis and adverse neurologic outcome in patients who become hyperglycemic during or after periods of cerebral ischemia.[59,75-78]

Despite the utility of DHCA for complex thoracic aortic lesions, the absolute safe interval of circulatory arrest is unknown. Experimental data suggest an increased risk of cerebral injury when the period of DHCA exceeds 90 minutes.[79] Clinical data suggest an increased risk of stroke and early mortality when the arrest period exceeds 40 and 65 minutes, respectively.[80] Ergin et al[59] demonstrated a significant increase in the incidence of temporary neurologic dysfunction with arrest time exceeding 60 minutes, especially in elderly patients. From the same institution, Reich et al[81] established a higher incidence of memory and fine motor deficits in adults when arrest time exceeds 25 minutes. Finally, evidence from children undergoing congenital heart surgery with DHCA also shows a linear relationship between cognitive dysfunction and the duration of hypothermic arrest.[82] Low-flow CPB with moderate hypothermia or intermittent periods of low flow during DHCA may improve outcome and permit longer arrest intervals.[79,83,84]

In summary, these data suggest that a limited duration of DHCA is critical for the prevention of CNS complications during thoracic aortic surgery. Unfortunately, complex aortic repairs often require prolonged periods of circulatory arrest and thus other methods of cerebral perfusion and CNS protection have been investigated to increase the safe period of circulatory arrest.

Antegrade Cerebral Perfusion. Cerebral perfusion can be maintained during aortic arch procedures by using ACP via selective catheterization of the innominate and left common carotid arteries (Fig. 14-7). Typically, the innominate and left carotid arteries are preferentially perfused, although cannulation of the right common carotid artery, innominate artery, or bilateral common carotid arteries has been reported.[85] The femoral artery is used for retrograde perfusion and the induction of moderate systemic hypothermia. After cannulation of one or both of the cerebral vessels, the DTA is occluded either by placement of an external cross-clamp, or by insertion of an endoaortic intraluminal balloon that

effectively occludes the distal arch and proximal DTA. After proximal and distal aortic occlusion, separate pump heads are used to perfuse the brain with 500 to 700 ml/min of cold blood while the distal aorta is perfused at normal systemic flow rates.[61,86] Modifications of ACP include selective innominate perfusion alone with monitoring of cerebral function by EEG to ensure adequate collateral flow via the circle of Willis,[87] low-flow perfusion to the lower body by using a single arterial pump head, separate pumps and heat exchangers to allow differential cooling of the cerebral and systemic circulations, and the use of low-flow systemic perfusion at 22° C with an open distal aortic anastomosis.[61,88] The latter technique involves spillage of the retrograde systemic perfusate from the open distal anastomosis into the operative field, where it is returned to the venous reservoir via cardiotomy suction. The advantage of this technique is avoidance of aortic cross-clamping and the associated risks of aortic injury and embolization of atheromatous debris.[88]

ACP during aortic arch procedures has been associated with a 1% to 8% neurologic complication rate and mortality comparable to other series that use DHCA for these procedures.[85-89] Experimental evidence, however, clearly demonstrates preserved blood flow, superior brain protection, improved recovery of evoked potentials compared with RCP,[90] and improved neurologic outcome with ACP compared with DHCA, with or without RCP[62,63,91-93] (Fig. 14-8). The ability to deliver metabolic substrate to the brain, remove toxic ischemic metabolites and inflammatory mediators, and effectively maintain uniform cerebral hypothermia are the probable mechanisms by which ACP provides brain protection. The major disadvantage of ACP is the technical complexity of selectively cannulating and perfusing the cerebral vessels. The additional time required for isolation and cannulation of these vessels, together with the risk of carotid and innominate artery injury and potential dislodgement of atheromatous debris into the cerebral circulation, are significant disadvantages of this approach.[61] These concerns, along with cluttering of the operative field, limit the widespread acceptance of this approach and have led to increased use of the technique of RCP. A comparison of the advantages and disadvantages of ACP versus RCP is shown in Table 14-1.

Retrograde Cerebral Perfusion. Mills and Ochsner originally described the clinical use of RCP in 1980 as a treatment for massive cerebral air embolism occurring during CPB.[94] The theoretical advantages of RCP during aortic arch surgery include the maintenance of cerebral cooling, the removal of ischemic metabolites, the delivery of metabolic substrate to the brain, and the reduction of embolic events by the retrograde flushing of air and debris out of the cerebral arterial circulation.[95] An additional advantage is its technical simplicity, especially compared with ACP. Despite the more common

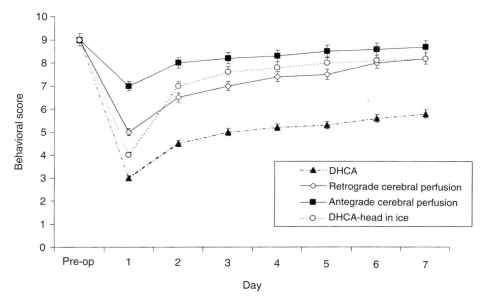

FIG. 14-8   Behavioral scores in pigs after aortic clamping by using different methods of cerebral perfusion and neuroprotection. On the first three postoperative days, scores were significantly higher when antegrade cerebral perfusion was used compared with the three methods. Scores were lowest with deep hypothermic circulatory arrest (*DHCA*) alone, even at 7 days. Packing the head in ice significantly improved behavioral scores and provided additional cerebral protection to DHCA.

(Adapted from Midulla PS, Gandsas A, Sadeghi AM et al: *J Card Surg* 9:560-575, 1994.)

TABLE 14-1
Advantages and Disadvantages of Retrograde and Antegrade Cerebral Perfusion

	ADVANTAGES	DISADVANTAGES
Retrograde cerebral perfusion	1. Maintains effective cerebral cooling 2. *May* minimize cerebral embolization 3. *May* provide substrate to brain 4. Simplicity of delivery system 5. Avoids manipulation of cerebral vessels 6. *Suggestive* favorable clinical data	1. May produce cerebral edema 2. Unreliable substrate delivery 3. Venous valves may hinder flow 4. Venovenous collaterals may divert cerebral flow 5. Retrograde drainage from arch vessels may obscure surgical field 6. More complex than DHCA alone
Antegrade cerebral perfusion	1. Clear experimental evidence of cerebral blood flow 2. Favorable neurologic outcomes in experimental studies 3. Effective and homogeneous cerebral cooling 4. Adequate cerebral substrate delivery 5. Can be used with moderate systemic hypothermia, avoiding DHCA	1. Complex set-up 2. Potentially cluttered operative field 3. Need to manipulate and clamp diseased vessels 4. Risk of cerebral embolization 5. Limited utility with fragile or severely diseased/dissected arch vessels

DHCA, Deep hypothermic circulatory arrest.

use of RCP, considerable controversy exists regarding the efficacy and potential detrimental effects of this approach.

Although there are multiple modifications of RCP, the basic approach involves standard bicaval venous and femoral arterial cannulation for the institution of DHCA. During the period of circulatory arrest, a clamp is placed on the arterial inflow line and blood is diverted via a bridge to the superior vena cava (SVC) catheter (Fig. 14-7). Blood at 8° to 14° C is then infused at rates of 100 to 500 ml/min to achieve a jugular venous pressure of 15 to 25 mm Hg.[96] After completion of the distal aortic and arch vessel anastomoses, the graft and the arch vessels are flushed clear of air and debris by RCP via the SVC cannula and retrograde femoral perfusion, and the proximal anastomosis is completed with antegrade or retrograde femoral perfusion.[61] Modifications of this technique include inferior vena cava (IVC) drainage to allow simultaneous RCP and retrograde aortic perfusion via the femoral artery with drainage from the IVC and the opened aorta; the addition of femoral venous or IVC drainage with or without systemic perfusion; total retrograde perfusion via the SVC, IVC, and coronary sinus; and clamping of the IVC to increase retrograde cerebral blood flow.[61]

Unfortunately, the evidence supporting a beneficial impact of RCP on postoperative neurologic function when it is used as an adjunct to DHCA for aortic procedures is sharply controversial. Concerns have emerged regarding competent venous valves that may prevent effective retrograde flow,[97] limited inflow because of venovenous shunting,[98] inadequate protection,[92] limited substrate supply and brain edema from high cerebral venous pressures,[99,100] and diminished perfusion because of diversion of retrograde flow from the SVC to the IVC.[101] Although extensive clinical data and some experimental evidence suggest that RCP may prolong the safe interval of circulatory arrest and produce favorable clinical outcomes when compared with DHCA alone,[24-26,62,93,102-105] Griepp et al[97] believe methodological problems with many clinical reports limit valid conclusions regarding the efficacy of RCP. Most studies have been neither prospective nor randomized; have included small numbers of patients, used historical controls, and applied a variety of other protective strategies and perfusion schemes that may have influenced the results; and have compared nonhomogeneous patient populations at different risk for neurologic injury. Griepp et al recommend that RCP be used with DHCA for only limited periods of time. This conservative viewpoint of the limited role of RCP is supported by evidence from a multicenter study in Japan of 228 patients undergoing aortic surgery with RCP where the risk of permanent neurologic injury increased abruptly when the retrograde perfusion time exceeded 60 minutes.[106] Despite this controversy, RCP is still extensively used by

many cardiac surgeons and holds promise as an additional method to provide cerebral protection during prolonged periods of circulatory arrest.

In summary, RCP is a commonly used technique for cerebral protection during aortic arch surgery that may improve neurologic outcome via prevention of brain injury from cerebral embolization and effective maintenance of cerebral cooling during periods of circulatory arrest. *Limiting* the duration of circulatory arrest rather than *extending* it with RCP may, however, be a more prudent approach to the surgical and perfusion management of aortic arch disease. Further study is required to clarify both the beneficial and potentially detrimental consequences of this technique and to compare neurologic outcome with randomized prospective analyses of RCP, ACP, and other neuroprotective strategies.

Other Cerebroprotective Adjuncts. The usefulness of pharmacologic agents for CNS protection during aortic surgery or during procedures requiring DHCA have not been evaluated in any prospective, randomized manner. Barbiturates, corticosteroids, or both are frequently administered for cerebral protection in many of the published studies on the surgical management of ascending aortic disease. Unfortunately, it is impossible to isolate the selective impact of these agents separate from the protective effects of other surgical and perfusion interventions. Barbiturates have been shown to exert a protective effect in experimental models of focal cerebral ischemia, but little data support a beneficial role for barbiturates during severe global cerebral ischemia.[107,108] Moreover, the putative incremental benefit provided by barbiturates (via reductions in cerebral metabolic rate) when used in conjunction with conditions of EEG isoelectricity, such as hypothermic circulatory arrest, is unproven and unlikely to be of significant additional value.

Shenkman et al[109] have reported a novel modification of RCP using the retrograde administration of pharmacologic agents. They administered small doses of etomidate (total 50 mg) or sodium pentothal (total 500 mg) into the SVC retrograde perfusate to abolish recurrent EEG activity. They also injected nitroprusside and nitroglycerin into the perfusate and were able to increase retrograde flow twofold to threefold.[109] This unique approach to the administration of cerebroprotective agents and vasodilators during circulatory arrest produced pharmacologic suppression of EEG activity and improved retrograde flow in the absence of systemic perfusion.

Recent evidence suggests that antagonism of the neurotoxic effects of the neurotransmitter glutamate may protect against focal and global cerebral ischemia.[108,110,111] Several agents appear to inhibit glutamate neurotransmission and antagonize the toxic effects of glutamate. These include the noncompetitive N-methyl-D-aspartate (NMDA) receptor antagonists

MK-801, GYKI-52466, and ketamine; the competitive NMDA receptor antagonist CGS-19755; the competitive NMDA receptor antagonist NBQX; and the anticonvulsant riluzole.[111,112] Sodium-channel blockade by local anesthetics may also reduce ischemic neuropathologic findings.[113] Given the experimental evidence that DHCA causes increased intracerebral glutamate levels,[114,115] agents that counter cerebral glutamate excitotoxicity may contribute additional neuroprotection during periods of circulatory arrest. Other anesthetic agents such as etomidate, propofol, and volatile anesthetics have also been shown to have neuroprotective effects in experimental models of cerebral ischemia.[116,117] Although no data support a beneficial neuroprotective role for glucocorticoids during cerebral ischemia, promising experimental and early clinical results have been obtained with the 21-aminosteroids.[110,118]

In summary, despite favorable experimental results with a wide variety of pharmacologic agents, there are little clinical data to support a beneficial role for any specific agent. Continued research into ways to modulate sodium channels and inhibit glutamate excitotoxicity may provide additional options for cerebroprotection during thoracic aortic surgery. Hypothermia remains the only proven neuroprotective intervention during periods of circulatory arrest. The additional protection provided by other pharmacologic interventions remains to be demonstrated.

Descending Thoracic Aortic Surgery

In contrast to ascending aortic surgery that more closely resembles standard cardiac surgical procedures requiring CPB, surgery of the DTA involves different yet equally significant changes in systemic hemodynamics, cardiopulmonary function, and spinal cord blood flow. Safe intraoperative management requires a clear understanding of the physiology of one-lung ventilation and the hemodynamic events that accompany cross-clamping of the DTA.

Monitors. Rapid and profound changes in arterial pressure are common during descending thoracic aortic surgery, and invasive arterial pressure monitoring is essential. Preoperatively, blood pressure should be assessed in each arm since clinically significant differences may be present as a result of atherosclerotic occlusive disease or aortic dissection involving the subclavian or innominate arteries.[119] In contrast to ascending aortic surgery, the right radial or brachial arteries should be used during descending aortic surgery to monitor proximal blood pressure because the aortic cross-clamp may be applied between the left subclavian and common carotid arteries, precluding use of left upper extremity arteries.

The use of a pulmonary artery catheter may be more important during procedures of the descending rather than ascending thoracic aorta because of the marked hemodynamic changes that accompany thoracic aortic cross-clamping, coupled with the large fluid and blood product requirements often necessary during extensive aortic repairs. Together with monitoring of ventricular end-diastolic volumes by TEE, pulmonary artery catheters facilitate the careful management of fluids and guide the titration of vasoactive medications. Accurate interpretation of data derived from pulmonary artery catheters can, however, be difficult during one-lung ventilation. If the tip of the catheter is in the left pulmonary artery when the left lung is collapsed, the measured pulmonary artery occlusion pressure (PAOP) will overestimate left atrial and left ventricular end-diastolic pressures (LVEDP) because of Starling resistor forces that produce venocompression. In addition, decreased left lung blood flow during one-lung ventilation may effectively "insulate" the thermistor at the tip of the catheter if it lies within the left pulmonary artery, potentially causing a spurious overestimation of the thermodilution cardiac output. Nonetheless, with attention to these issues, pulmonary artery catheters will continue to provide valuable information during and especially after descending thoracic aortic procedures.

Anesthetic Technique. Coronary artery disease and hypertension are common in patients undergoing surgery of the DTA. Consequently, intraoperative hemodynamic management is important to avoid myocardial ischemia and LV dysfunction. Both afterload and end-diastolic pressures increase significantly after clamping of the DTA, potentially causing myocardial oxygen supply/demand imbalance and the risk of myocardial ischemia or ventricular failure. Many approaches to the induction and maintenance of anesthesia can be used but all have a common feature of maintaining adequate myocardial and vital organ perfusion while avoiding hypertension and reducing ventricular stress. As with patients with ascending aortic disease, patients with descending thoracic aortic disease who are undergoing anesthesia may be safely induced by using a variety of anesthetic techniques, with the common goal of controlling unfavorable hyperdynamic responses that might produce an increase in aortic shear forces and jeopardize the integrity of the aortic wall. Anesthesia is often achieved with small doses of a hypnotic agent followed by the addition of moderate doses of fentanyl (10-20 mcg/kg) or sufentanil (2-5 mcg/kg). Intravenous β-blockers such as esmolol or metoprolol, and vasodilators, such as nitroglycerin (50-mcg boluses), are often necessary to consistently attenuate these potentially adverse responses. Since most patients are mechanically ventilated for up to 24 hours after surgery, high-dose opioid techniques (e.g., fentanyl 50 mcg/kg) are suitable alternatives, especially for individuals with underlying ventricular dysfunction. However, the use of high dosages of sedatives and opioids and the residual effects of long-acting muscle relaxants may prevent a prompt assessment of lower extremity neurologic function after descending thoracic aortic surgery. For patients with new neurologic deficits, this may delay the institution of potentially therapeutic interventions to correct spinal cord ischemia, such as cerebrospinal fluid (CSF) drainage and augmentation of perfusion pressure. Ultimately, a balance must be achieved between the competing goals of intraoperative cardiovascular stability and rapid recovery from general anesthesia.

One-Lung Ventilation. Exposure of the DTA is accomplished via a left-thoracotomy approach. Because aneurysm exposure is greatly facilitated by collapse of the left lung, DLTs are routinely used. Lung collapse and isolation improve exposure and protect the left lung from the trauma of surgical retraction. In addition, the dependent lung is protected from blood entering the left mainstem bronchus because of left lung intrapulmonary hemorrhage, especially during procedures requiring systemic heparinization or when the left lung is adherent to an inflammatory aneurysm.

Left-sided DLTs are typically recommended because of the potential for right upper lobe obstruction with right-sided DLTs. However, placement of left-sided DLTs may be technically difficult and hazardous in the presence of very large aneurysms because of compression of the left mainstem bronchus or distal trachea by the aneurysm.[120-124] Compression occurs because of the close anatomic relationship of the descending aorta to the tracheobronchial tree and pulmonary artery. Prolonged tracheobronchial compression by large thoracic aneurysms may also produce tracheomalacia, which may increase the risk of tracheobronchial disruption with DLT placement. To avoid these complications in patients with very large aneurysms or with respiratory symptoms suggesting airway compromise, left DLT placement is best accomplished by initially visualizing the anatomy of the distal trachea and left mainstem bronchus with a fiberoptic bronchoscope before left endobronchial intubation. Pulsatile compression of the airway contraindicates placement of a left-sided DLT or left mainstem bronchial blocker. Under these circumstances, it may be prudent to use a right-sided DLT instead.

In addition to endobronchial tubes, Univent tubes (Fuji Systems, Tokyo) have gained increasing popularity for lung isolation during thoracic surgery. These single-lumen endotracheal tubes have a hollow moveable bronchial blocker that can be positioned in the left mainstem bronchus, producing collapse of the left lung. A potential advantage of Univent tubes for DTA surgery is that they obviate the need to change from a DLT to a single-lumen tube at the end of the case. A possible disadvantage, however, is the high occlusion pressure of the blocker cuff and the higher transmural wall pressures it may produce. Theoretically, these higher pressures might increase the risk of aneurysm rupture when large aneurysms compress the left mainstem bronchus. For intubated patients who arrive at the operating room for emergent repair of acute aortic dissection or traumatic aortic rupture, it may be appropriate to use a Fogarty embolectomy catheter as a bronchial blocker rather than risk loss of the airway during placement of a DLT or Univent tube, which are technically more difficult to place, even in an elective situation.

A final important element of airway management during descending thoracic aortic procedures involves replacement of the DLT with a single-lumen endotracheal tube at the completion of the procedure. The combination of massive fluid and blood losses encountered during extensive aortic resections, the influence of Trendelenburg and right lateral decubitus positions on upper-body venous pressures, and the potential local effects of prolonged placement of TEE probes and DLTs on the oropharyngeal mucosa, may lead to impressive and potentially life-threatening upper airway edema and airway obstruction if the DLT is removed. Laryngoscopy and fiberoptic bronchoscopy may be extremely difficult in this situation and changing the DLT may be hazardous. If glottic visualization is difficult with the DLT in place, especially with a previously difficult intubation, the bronchial cuff should be deflated and the DLT withdrawn into the trachea. It can be left in place for 24 hours or until the edema has resolved, after which the tube may be safely changed.

Management of Hemostasis and Intraoperative Blood Loss. Intraoperative hemorrhage remains a major cause of morbidity after thoracic aortic surgery and may contribute to 23% of early deaths from acute aortic dissection.[125] Profound blood loss is secondary to multiple factors including surgical bleeding from vascular interruptions and opened vascular channels, dilutional thrombocytopenia, factor deficiencies, the effects of heparin and hypothermia, and disseminated intravascular coagulation from prolonged hypotension and hypoperfusion. Gertler et al[126] demonstrated a reduction in factor levels and an increase in D-dimer concentrations after supraceliac cross-clamping during thoracoabdominal aortic surgery. These changes suggest that visceral and lower-body ischemia may initiate a mild form of disseminated intravascular coagulation that may increase the risk of hemorrhage. Although there was no correlation between coagulation disturbances and the duration of aortic cross-clamping in this study, clamp times were short and bleeding complications were infrequent.[126] It is likely that with more prolonged clamp times and more extensive procedures hemostatic and hemorrhagic complications would increase accordingly.

The average intraoperative blood product requirements reported from two large series of patients undergoing thoracoabdominal aneurysm resection were 3 L of banked and autotransfused red cells, 6 units of FFP, 10 units of platelets, and 4 units of cryoprecipitate.[127,128] In high-risk procedures, however, transfusion requirements may exceed these values. Hemorrhage is most pronounced during thoracoabdominal aneurysm resection, during traumatic aneurysm repairs when systemic heparinization is used, and during acute aortic dissection repair.[129,130]

Initial blood product orders during these procedures should include type and cross-matching for 5 to 10 units each of PRBC, platelets, and FFP, with additional products obtained in advance of continued hemorrhage. When CPB is used, antifibrinolytic agents such as epsilon aminocaproic acid, tranexamic acid, or aprotinin may be useful, although no data from prospective, randomized trials are available regarding the efficacy of these agents for descending thoracic aortic surgery. If DHCA is used for extensive aneurysms of the DTA, the same issues as discussed for ascending aortic surgery regarding the safety of aprotinin must be considered. In addition to a pulmonary artery catheter and two large-bore (14-gauge) peripheral intravenous catheters, it is useful to insert a large (e.g., 9 French) introducer sheath in an internal jugular vein. A rapid infusion device, such as the Rapid Infusion System (Haemonetics Corp., Braintree, Mass.) or Level One blood-warming device (Level One Technologies Inc., Rockland, Mass.), is also useful to facilitate the rapid infusion of large volumes of warmed blood products. This will minimize the risk of hypovolemia and inadvertent hypothermia. In addition, blood scavenging devices are recommended to salvage blood lost into the operative field and are commonly used by most surgical teams, both intraoperatively and postoperatively. Other interventions, such as the use of platelet-rich plasma and acute hemodilution, have not been systematically evaluated during descending thoracic aortic surgery, although preoperative autologous blood donation has been advocated. Finally, intraoperative monitoring of coagulation function with frequent assessment of platelet counts, prothrombin and partial thromboplastin times, fibrinogen levels, and thromboelastography can help guide blood-component therapy.

Physiologic Effects of Cross-Clamping of the Descending Thoracic Aorta

Hemodynamic Changes. The pathophysiology of cross-clamping of the DTA is complex and incompletely defined, despite abundant experimental work examining both the mechanism and the magnitude of the hemodynamic changes associated with aortic cross-clamping (Fig. 14-9). In both animal and clinical studies, severe proximal hypertension is the most consistent and dramatic response to proximal aortic occlusion.[131-136] Although the cause of this response has been attributed to an increase in systemic vascular resistance and a sudden impedance to aortic outflow,[134,137] other factors may contribute to the observed hypertension. Increased plasma concentrations of catecholamines, renin, and angiotensin have been demonstrated after thoracic aortic occlusion and these may, in conjunction with other humoral factors released from ischemic tissues below the cross-clamp, increase vascular tone in vessels proximal to the cross-clamp.[134,138-140] Gelman and others have also noted a significant increase in blood volume in organs and tissues above the level of the cross-clamp due to diversion of blood from splanchnic venous capacitance beds (which collapse during thoracic aortic cross-clamping) to the central venous compartment.[134,141,142] This blood volume redistribution from the lower to upper body increases preload and may account for the increases in central venous pressure (CVP) and LV end-diastolic volumes observed after thoracic aortic occlusion.[133,143] It is theorized that proximal hypertension may be caused, in part, by changes in cardiac output from this preload-augmenting shift in blood volume via the Frank-Starling mechanism.[134,144]

Myocardial contractility may increase with thoracic aortic occlusion via an augmentation of endocardial blood flow, a physiologic process termed the *Anrep effect*.[134] Although this may explain the increase or absence of change in cardiac output observed in numerous animal models,[142,144-147] clinical studies of patients undergoing thoracic aortic cross-clamping have consistently demonstrated a reduction in cardiac output and global ventricular function after thoracic occlusion. Kouchoukos et al[131] assessed the hemodynamic effects of clamping the DTA in 8 patients and the subsequent response to placement of a Gott shunt. Mean arterial pressure (MAP), CVP, mean pulmonary artery pressure, and PAOP increased by 35%, 56%, 43%, and 90%, respectively, and cardiac output decreased by 29% (Table 14-2). All values returned to baseline after the shunt was opened, although cardiac output remained below baseline values. Roizen et al[143] provided more definite evidence of cross-clamp-induced ventricular dysfunction in a study of 12 patients undergoing aortic surgery involving infrarenal, suprarenal, and supraceliac cross-clamping. Using TEE analysis of LV dimensions and ejection fraction, they noted substantial increases in LV end-systolic and end-diastolic areas and decreased ejection fractions after supraceliac aortic clamping, despite the use of anesthetics and vasodilators to maintain preclamp hemodynamics (Table 14-3). In contrast, there were minimal hemodynamic changes with infrarenal clamping. Connelly et al[148] observed similar alterations of global LV systolic function, as shown by increases in end-systolic wall stress and decreased frac-

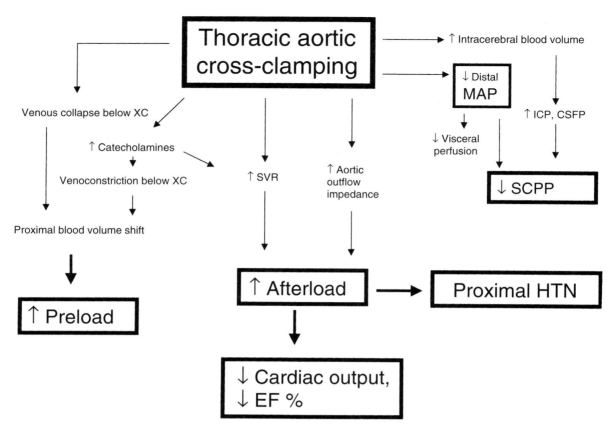

FIG. 14-9   Schematic diagram of the pathophysiologic events associated with cross-clamping of the descending thoracic aorta. See text for discussion. In animal models, cardiac output and EF % may *increase* with thoracic aortic cross-clamping. *CSFP,* Cerebrospinal fluid pressure; *EF,* ejection fraction; *HTN,* hypertension; *ICP,* intracranial pressure; *MAP,* mean arterial pressure; *SCPP,* spinal cord perfusion pressure; *SVR,* systemic vascular resistance.

(Adapted from Gelman S: *Anesthesiology* 82:1026-1060, 1995.)

tional area shortening in patients after thoracic aortic cross-clamping. Although myocardial ischemia may contribute to these decrements in cardiac output, it appears that the marked increase in afterload is primarily responsible for the global impairment in LV function.

Experimentally, coronary blood flow increases with thoracic aortic occlusion, presumably because of increased perfusion pressure or coronary blood flow autoregulation induced by increases in myocardial oxygen demand and consumption.[134,146,147] However, an increase in LVEDP may reduce the effective coronary perfusion pressure gradient. This is not uncommon in patients with underlying coronary artery disease and LV hypertrophy, which may produce an imbalance of myocardial oxygen supply and demand.[146] Although myocardial ischemia may contribute to a reduction in ejection fraction, inadequate control of proximal hypertension may also precipitate deterioration in ventricular function, especially in patients with impaired contractility who are intolerant of increases in afterload.

Arterial pressure distal to the level of the cross-clamp decreases considerably (to 20-40 mm Hg) and is strongly dependent on proximal aortic pressure.[134] Blood flow to vascular beds below the level of the cross-clamp is via collateral vessels and is dependent primarily on perfusion pressure rather than on cardiac output, suggesting that proximal aortic pressures should be maintained as high as possible to ensure distal perfusion.[134] TEE can be used to monitor the LV response to aortic clamping and to serve as a guide to the degree of proximal hypertension that can be safely tolerated.

Decrements in cardiac output after thoracic aortic cross-clamping may occur not only because of ischemia or altered loading conditions, but may also occur as an appropriate response to a decrease in total body oxygen consumption.[142] Evidence suggests that thoracic aortic clamping is accompanied by a 43% to 57% reduction in oxygen consumption caused by exclusion from the circulation of a substantial amount of metabolically active tissue below the level of the cross-clamp.[142] Thus, some

TABLE 14-2

Hemodynamic Response to Aortic Clamping and to Decompression with a Temporary Shunt in Eight Patients Undergoing DTA Repair

	BASELINE (PERIOD I)	AORTA CLAMPED (PERIOD II)	SHUNT OPENED (PERIOD III)
MAP (mm Hg)	90.3 ± 4.0	$122.1 \pm 4.1\dagger$	86.8 ± 4.4
MPAP (mm Hg)	21.3 ± 2.1	$30.5 \pm 3.1\dagger$	19.9 ± 1.7
CVP (mm Hg)	7.0 ± 0.5	$11.5 \pm 2.2\dagger$	7.8 ± 1.5
PAOP (mm Hg)	9.6 ± 1.9	$17.6 \pm 2.4\dagger$	10.4 ± 1.9
CI (L/min/m^2)	2.66 ± 0.34	$1.88 \pm 0.25*$	$2.18 \pm 0.24\dagger$
HR (bpm)	85.2 ± 7.6	89.8 ± 11.8	86.6 ± 4.5
SVI (mL/beat/m^2)	34.0 ± 6.4	23.0 ± 3.8	26.0 ± 3.0
LVSWI (g/m/m^2)	35.6 ± 4.9	31.8 ± 4.6	$25.8 \pm 2.4\dagger$

From Kouchoukos NT, Lell WA, Karp RB et al: *Surgery* 85:25-30, 1979.

CI, Cardiac index; *CVP*, central venous pressure; *DTA*, descending thoracic aorta; *HR*, heart rate; *LVSWI*, left ventricular stroke work index; *MAP*, mean arterial pressure; *MPAP*, mean pulmonary arterial pressure; *PAOP*, pulmonary artery occlusion pressure; *SVI*, stroke volume index. All values given are mean ± standard error.

$* p < 0.05$ (I v II).

$\dagger p < 0.05$ (I v III).

TABLE 14-3

Percent Change in Cardiovascular Variables on Initiation of Aortic Occlusion

	PERCENTAGE OF CHANGE AFTER OCCLUSION AT		
LEVEL OF AORTIC OCCLUSION	SUPRACELIAC	SUPRARENAL-INFRACELIAC	INFRARENAL
Mean arterial blood pressure	+ 54	+ 5*	+ 2*
Pulmonary capillary wedge pressure	+ 38	+ 10*	0*
End-diastolic area	+ 28	+ 2*	+ 9*
End-systolic area	+ 69	+ 10*	+ 11*
Ejection fraction	− 38	− 10*	− 8*
Patients with wall-motion abnormalities	+ 92	+ 33	0
New myocardial infarctions	+ 8	+ 0	0

From Roizen MF, Beaupre PN, Albert RA et al: *J Vasc Surg* 1:300-305, 1984.

* Statistically different ($p < 0.05$) from group undergoing supraceliac aortic occlusion.

fraction of the reduction in cardiac output may be in response to a decrease in oxygen consumption rather than from myocardial dysfunction.

Central Nervous System. Simple cross-clamping of the DTA leads to intracranial hypertension and increased cerebrospinal fluid pressure (CSFP).[134,149,150] The precise mechanism responsible for the rise in intracranial pressure (ICP) is unknown, although postulated mechanisms include proximal hypertension-induced engorgement of the intracranial space,[151] increased cerebral blood flow,[152] altered dural venous capacitance, and blood volume redistribution into cerebral venous capacitance beds.[134] The increased CSFP and decreased distal MAP reduce the spinal cord perfusion pressure (SCPP = distal MAP − CSFP). A more extensive discussion of spinal cord perfusion follows.

Metabolic Effects. Clamping of the DTA induces anaerobic metabolism and an increase in lactic acid production in tissues below the aortic cross-clamp. By reducing hepatic blood flow, simple aortic cross-clamping also reduces hepatic clearance of lactate and further contributes to metabolic acidosis.[153] Increased lactate levels with metabolic acidosis are observed with release of the cross-clamp and are more profound after prolonged cross-clamping without distal circulatory support. One study documented an average pH of 7.29 after thoracic aortic cross-clamp release.[129]

Renal Effects. Although the etiology of renal dysfunction after thoracic aortic surgery is multifactorial, renal hypoperfusion during the period of aortic cross-clamping and subsequent reperfusion injury after clamp release are important risk factors for the development of postoperative renal failure.[154,155] Renal hypoperfusion develops because of the 85% to 94% reduction in renal blood flow, glomerular filtration rate, and urine output during thoracic aortic cross-clamping.[134,156] In addition, blood flow within the kidney becomes abnormal, with a decrease in renal cortical blood flow and an associated decrease in glomerular filtration rate.[134] Alterations in renal hemodynamics caused by activation of the renin-angiotensin system and prostaglandin pathway may also produce tubular injury, with reperfusion-mediated oxygen free radical release producing further renal damage.[134,140]

Although it is common practice to administer mannitol, furosemide, or low-dose dopamine during these procedures in an attempt to improve renal blood flow, limit oxygen free radical injury, reduce intrarenal oxygen consumption, and maintain a diuresis, there are no data demonstrating a distinct outcome advantage with any of these agents. The obvious discrepancy between the favorable results of experimental studies on the use of diuretics and low-dose dopamine and the clinical studies of these agents is probably related to several factors. These factors include the small sample size of most clinical studies, differing degrees of renal ischemia observed during experimental and clinical situations, the influence of confounding clinical factors such as dye-induced renal injury and intraoperative embolic insults to the kidney, inadequate intravascular volume loading during surgery, and the low dose and suboptimal timing of intraoperative diuretics used.[134] Optimization of systemic hemodynamics and maintenance of cardiac output, along with surgical techniques to maintain renal blood flow, remain the most critical elements of intraoperative renal protection during descending thoracic aortic surgery.

In summary, clamping of the DTA produces a complex cascade of events including severe proximal arterial hypertension and distal hypotension; increased ventricular preload and reduced cardiac output; increased ICP; and decreased renal, visceral, and spinal cord blood flow.

Management of Thoracic Aortic Cross-Clamping. The management of the hemodynamic and metabolic consequences of thoracic aortic cross-clamping depends, in part, on the surgical technique used. With simple clamp and sew techniques, the hemodynamic changes are sudden and profound and require immediate intervention. The prevention of proximal hypertension must therefore begin *before* application of the cross-clamp, with vasodilators titrated to reduce the preclamp systolic blood pressure to approximately 90 mm Hg. This, in conjunction with gradual cross-clamp application by the surgeon, will attenuate the dramatic increase in blood pressure with thoracic aortic occlusion.

Pharmacologic Control of Proximal Hypertension. The control of clamp-induced hypertension associated with clamp and sew techniques can be achieved with a variety of pharmacologic agents. Typically, nitrovasodilators such as nitroprusside and nitroglycerin are used along with short-acting β-blockers such as esmolol or labetalol. In addition, isoflurane or other volatile anesthetics are often added to lower the dosage requirements for nitroprusside. Experimental data suggest that isoflurane can effectively control proximal hypertension with less neurologic injury than can nitroprusside,[157] although the high concentrations required and the relatively slow onset of isoflurane limit its usefulness as a single agent. Some evidence also indicates that nitroprusside, by altering the compliance of the spinal cord and by reducing proximal blood pressure, may increase the risk of paraplegia via an increase in CSFP and a reduction in distal arterial pressure, the combination of which will reduce SCPP.[134,158-163] For these reasons, avoidance of large doses of nitroprusside has been advocated.[134]

Intravenous calcium channel blockers, such as nicardipine, are appealing as antihypertensive agents because they have been shown to protect the spinal cord during experimental ischemia.[164] Similarly, fenoldopam is an effective antihypertensive agent that may have favorable effects on the kidney as a result of dopamine-1 (DA_1) receptor-mediated renal vasodilation.[165-167] Unfortunately, neither agent has been evaluated clinically during thoracic aortic surgery.

Nitroglycerin is a useful agent because coronary vasodilation and preload reduction accompany its antihypertensive effects. Unfortunately, nitroglycerin is a weak vasodilator and is often inadequate as a sole agent to control proximal hypertension. It may also have unfavorable effects on experimental spinal cord blood flow when used without CSF drainage.[168] One reasonable approach is a combination of nitroprusside and nitroglycerin, with a background of low concentrations of a volatile anesthetic. This combination allows for the rapid termination of pharmacologic vasodilation before aortic unclamping.

Distal Circulatory Support. The rationale behind distal perfusion is twofold: first, to attenuate proximal

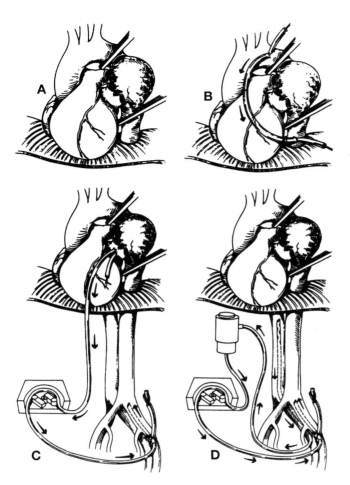

FIG. 14-10 Types of distal circulatory support. **A,** Simple cross-clamping of the descending thoracic aorta (DTA) without adjuncts for distal perfusion. **B,** A passive aorto-aortic shunt extending from the proximal DTA to the aorta below the level of the cross-clamp. **C,** Left atriofemoral bypass by using a centrigual pump to divert oxygenated blood from the left atrium to the femoral artery. **D,** Femoral artery to femoral vein cardiopulmonary bypass by using a pump oxygenator.

(From Ochsner J, Ancalmo N: *Chest Surg Clin N Am* 6:291, 1992.)

hypertension for cardiac and CNS protection, and second, to provide perfusion to vascular beds below the level of the aortic cross-clamp. Although their beneficial effects on outcome are controversial,[128,169] bypass and shunt techniques appear to reduce the incidence of renal failure and paraplegia after thoracic aortic surgery.[4,127,130,170-180] They also attenuate the metabolic acidosis and dramatic hypotension characteristic of the declamping syndrome that accompanies clamp release after simple clamp and sew procedures. Bypass techniques and aortic shunts control proximal hypertension by different mechanisms (Fig. 14-10): aortic shunts divert blood from the proximal to the distal aorta and thus reduce afterload, whereas bypass circuits con-

trol proximal blood pressure by reducing preload and cardiac output. Distal flow rates of 1.5 to 2.5 L/min and mean femoral artery pressures of 50 to 70 mm Hg are typical target flows and pressures during active pump bypass techniques.

Shunts. Shunts from the proximal to distal aorta are passive methods of distal perfusion that use a transparent heparin-coated conduit to perfuse the lower body (Fig. 14-10, *B*). Heparin coating of the bypass shunt precludes the need for systemic heparinization. The proximal end of the shunt is typically placed in the ascending aorta, although the proximal DTA, the aortic arch, and the left subclavian artery are acceptable though less common proximal cannulation sites. Verdant et al[177] reported a 0% incidence of paraplegia by using aortic shunts in 366 consecutive patients undergoing descending thoracic aortic surgery. They noted mean femoral artery pressures of 64 mm Hg and mean shunt flow rates of 2.5 L/min. Shunt flow, which is directly related to proximal pressure and inversely related to peripheral resistance, was highest with proximal cannulation in the ascending aorta and least with cannulation in the descending aorta. A flow probe is often used to ensure the adequacy of shunt flow and shunt function (e.g., low flow may represent shunt malposition or kinking). An interesting albeit complex alternative to standard shunts is use of a temporary axillofemoral bypass graft that is constructed before resection of the descending aorta.[181,182] The additional operative time and complexity of this approach are significant disadvantages that have limited its clinical use.

Atriofemoral bypass. Atriofemoral bypass is a popular form of distal perfusion and involves use of a centrifugal pump to divert oxygenated blood through heparinized circuits from the left atrium to the femoral artery (Fig. 14-10, *C*). In contrast to systems incorporating a reservoir, centrifugal pump bypass circuits require either no or minimal heparin to maintain an ACT of approximately 200 seconds. Experimental work suggests that shunt flows of 35 ml/kg/min improve ventricular function to near control values.[183] Clinically, bypass flow rates of 25 to 40 ml/kg/min appear sufficient to normalize proximal pressures and maintain adequate distal perfusion.[184-187] Careful monitoring of PAOPs and LV end-diastolic areas will detect hypovolemia if excess blood is pumped from the left atrium, and proximal hypotension will be evident if this occurs.[37]

Femoral venoarterial cardiopulmonary bypass. Femoral venoarterial partial CPB is an increasingly popular form of distal perfusion that uses a standard roller pump and oxygenator to circulate oxygenated blood from the femoral vein to the femoral artery (Fig. 14-10, *D*). In a manner similar to left heart bypass techniques, femoral CPB removes blood from the IVC and lowers preload and cardiac output and thus proximal systemic blood pressure. The main advantage of partial CPB over left heart bypass is the ability to provide supplementary oxygenation and full flow support without manipulating the heart or cluttering the operative field. The main disadvantage of femoral-femoral CPB is the requirement for full heparinization, which may have been responsible for the increased mortality observed during traumatic aortic rupture repairs.[130] Both bypass techniques provide the ability to regulate flow and actively warm the patient, distinct advantages compared with passive heparinized shunts.

Careful monitoring of preload during active distal bypass is essential to prevent excess removal of left atrial or femoral venous blood, which may produce hypovolemia and proximal hypotension. An adjustable clamp on the venous line controls gravity venous return. Clamp removal and collection of blood in the venous reservoir reduces venous return to the heart and cardiac output, and effectively decreases proximal aortic pressure. Conversely, clamping of the venous line increases IVC flow and proximal LV end-diastolic and aortic pressures. Control of venous return thus becomes critical to maintain stable hemodynamics because individual patients may demonstrate marked changes in proximal pressures with translocation of as little as 200 ml of blood into the central circulation. In addition, if technical factors such as suboptimal venous cannula positioning or small cannula size limit venous return, any increase in pump flow rates will only augment central venous return and potentially increase cardiac output and proximal aortic pressure, since blood will preferentially flow into the IVC rather than into the venous reservoir. Of course, increasing pump flows in the face of inadequate venous return will rapidly deplete the venous reservoir, necessitating either a reduction in pump flows or addition of fluid or blood to the venous reservoir. Because these technical problems with venous drainage will reduce the effectiveness of the bypass circuit to unload the left ventricle and control proximal blood pressure, it is *essential* that the anesthesiologist assess LV filling by using TEE and PAOPs and communicate with the perfusionist regarding the adequacy of venous drainage if LV filling seems excessive.

Ideally, pulmonary artery pressures (PAPs) and end-diastolic areas should be *reduced* by approximately 30% to 40% of preclamp values when distal inflows and venous return are adequate. Higher filling pressures and higher proximal aortic blood pressure suggest inadequate drainage and poor decompression of the proximal circulation. Careful attention to these aspects of distal perfusion will prevent unnecessary and potentially detrimental use of vasodilators to reduce proximal aortic pressures. Table 14-4 provides guidelines for hemody-

---

TABLE 14-4
Hemodynamic Management During Femoral Venoarterial Cardiopulmonary Bypass for Repair of the DTA

PROXIMAL AORTIC PRESSURE*	FEMORAL ARTERY PRESSURE†	PAOP/ LVEDA‡	DIAGNOSIS	INTERVENTION
Normal	Normal	Low	Optimal hemodynamics and proximal decompression	None
High	Low	Normal	Inadequate decompression vs. primary HTN	↑ VR to pump, ↑ pump flows, § vasodilators
Low	Low	Very low	Hypovolemia	↓ VR to pump, volume replacement
Low	Normal	Very low	Excess VR to pump, +/− hypovolemia	Clamp venous line and ↓ VR to pump, volume replacement if reservoir volumes low
Low	Low	High	Rule out LVF	Check CO/contractility, inotropes, ↑ VR to pump, ↑ pump flows

CO, Cardiac output; DTA, descending thoracic aorta; HTN, hypertension; LVEDA, left ventricular end-diastolic area by transesophageal echocardiography; LVF, left ventricular failure; PAOP, pulmonary artery occlusion pressure; VR, venous return (to pump).

* Increased pump flows must be accompanied by an increase in venous return to the pump, i.e., equilibrium between VR and arterial pump flow.

† Femoral pressures are considered "normal" if flows and pressures are adequate (i.e., 25 to 35 cc/kg/min and 40 to 60 mm Hg), and low if below these values. The highest distal flows compatible with normal proximal pressure and PAOPs should be maintained. Femoral pressures are presumed to reflect flow, although this agreement is not absolute.

‡ "Normal" values for PAOP/LVEDA are those at baseline. "Low" values (20%-30% decrease from preclamp values) are appropriate and reflect adequate decompression of the proximal circulation.

§ Proximal pressures are considered "normal" when at or slightly above baseline, i.e., prox. pressures are frequently maintained above the normal range to ensure distal perfusion. "High" proximal pressures are those well-above desired or baseline values.

namic management during distal perfusion when femoral-femoral CPB is used.

Physiologic Sequelae and Management of Thoracic Aortic Unclamping.

When distal perfusion is not used, thoracic aortic unclamping results in profound hemodynamic and metabolic changes that have been termed *declamping shock*[188] (Fig. 14-11). The severity of this syndrome will vary with the duration of aortic cross-clamping; the blood pressure and adequacy of ventricular preload before clamp release; and the continued influence of vasodilators, β-adrenergic antagonists, and anesthetic agents. The typical changes include a 70% to 80% decrease in vascular resistance and MAP, a decrease in CVP and PAOP, and increased PAPs.[140,147,189,190] In addition, there is an increase in end-tidal carbon dioxide, arterial carbon dioxide pressure, and plasma lactate levels, accompanied by a decline in arterial pH[129,175,191] (Fig. 14-11). Although preload decreases, cardiac output frequently increases, probably resulting from the marked decrease in vascular resistance. The observed increase in PAP is likely secondary to the effects on pulmonary vascular tone of lactate, hypercarbia, and vasoactive mediators released from ischemic tissues.[191] The main causes of hypotension with thoracic aortic unclamping include (1) central hypovolemia from pooling of blood in reperfused tissues below the level of the aortic cross-clamp (reactive hyperemia); (2) vasodilation and venodilation from the vascular effects of distal tissue hypoxia and vasoactive mediators released from previously underperfused tissues,[134,136] and (3) possible myocardial depression by circulating humoral substances.[134,188] Endogenous vasoactive mediators implicated in this complex hemodynamic response appear to be formed in ischemic and reperfused tissues below the level of the aortic cross-clamp. As delineated by Gelman, they include components of the renin-angiotensin and sympathetic nervous systems, oxygen free radicals, prostaglandins, endotoxins and cytokines, anaphylatoxins and components of the complement system, and activated platelets and neutrophils. Cohen et al[192] documented increases in intestinal permeability after supraceliac aortic cross-clamping in dogs. These alterations in gut mucosal integrity may allow translocation of endotoxin and intestinal bacteria into the portal circulation and may contribute to the vasodilation observed with aortic unclamping.

In summary, unclamping of the thoracic aorta is associated with a variety of pathophysiologic reactions that ultimately produce a severe reduction in preload and possibly cardiac output, an increase in pulmonary vascular resistance, metabolic and respiratory acidoses, and extreme hypotension.

Attenuation of declamping hypotension associated with simple clamp and sew techniques without distal

perfusion is most effectively achieved by aggressive volume administration before removal of the cross-clamp, discontinuation of vasodilators, β-adrenergic antagonists, and volatile anesthetics well in advance of cross-clamp release, increased minute ventilation, and

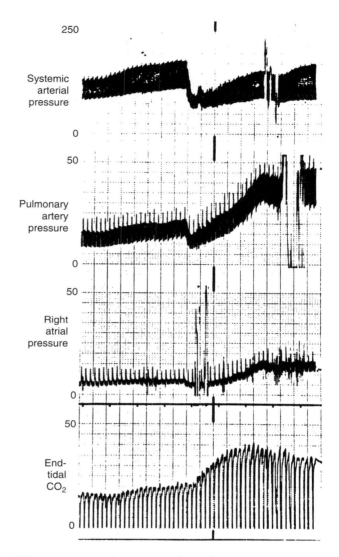

FIG. 14-11 Continuous recording of arterial, pulmonary artery, and right atrial pressures and end-tidal carbon dioxide *(CO₂)* before and after release of a supraceliac aortic cross-clamp. Pressures increase before the cross-clamp is released because vasodilators are discontinued and preload is augmented with volume administration. A dramatic increase in the arterial pressure is seen with release of the cross-clamp accompanied by an initial decrease in the pulmonary artery pressure. Vasopressors and volume administration then return the blood pressure to preclamp values. Pulmonary artery pressures and end-tidal CO_2 increase significantly because of the effects of lactic acid and other ischemic metabolites released from tissues below the level of the aortic cross-clamp.

(From Beattie C, Frank SM: Anesthesia for major vascular surgery. In Tinker T, Covino B, editors: *Principles and practice of anesthesiology*, St Louis, 1993, Mosby, pp 1931-1967.)

gradual release of the cross-clamp over 2 to 4 minutes. Gradual cross-clamp release may limit the impact of vasodepressant substances released from ischemic tissues and may also reduce the severity of renal and spinal cord reperfusion injury.[134] Some authors recommend the use of a sodium bicarbonate infusion during the period of simple aortic cross-clamping to minimize the metabolic acidosis observed with unclamping,[128,171,193] although the efficacy of this approach remains unproven. Despite these prophylactic maneuvers, hypotension is commonly observed and usually requires brief administration of vasopressors such as phenylephrine or norepinephrine. However, vasopressors should be administered cautiously and in small doses because even transient hypertension may precipitate bleeding from the aortic anastomosis. In addition, inappropriate vasopressor use may produce severe hypertension if reapplication of the aortic cross-clamp is required.

With appropriate volume loading and vasopressor administration, hypotension is usually transient and well tolerated. The PAPs eventually return to normal as the effects of lactic acidosis, hypercarbia, mediator release, prior volume loading, and previous vasopressor administration dissipate (Fig. 14-11).

Spinal Cord Perfusion and Postoperative Spinal Cord Injury. The most feared complication of thoracic aortic surgery is paraplegia from spinal cord ischemia. Unfortunately, it is not completely preventable, despite advances in the surgical approach to descending thoracic aortic surgery and a significant reduction in the incidence of this complication in recent years.[187,194-196] Although a number of techniques have been advocated for the prevention of neurologic injury, no prospective randomized studies have shown any single approach to be effective. It is likely that a multimodal approach that uses several agents and techniques will continue to be the most successful strategy to reduce the incidence of this complication.[197]

Incidence. The incidence of spinal cord injury ranges from less than 2% for children undergoing coarctation repair, where extensive collateral vessels maintain spinal cord blood flow, to 43% in patients after extensive thoracoabdominal aortic aneurysm resections.[198,199] Aneurysm rupture or acute dissection also substantially increases the risk of paraplegia since collateral blood flow to the spinal cord is either inadequately developed (rupture) or disrupted (dissection)[128,178,194,200] (Fig. 14-12). Approximately 50% of patients with immediate-onset paralysis never recover neurologic function.[134]

Spinal Cord Blood Supply. The complex and unpredictable anatomy of the spinal cord vasculature is an essential aspect of spinal cord injury after thoracic aortic surgery (Fig. 14-13). A pair of continuous posterior spinal arteries supplies the posterior one third of the spinal

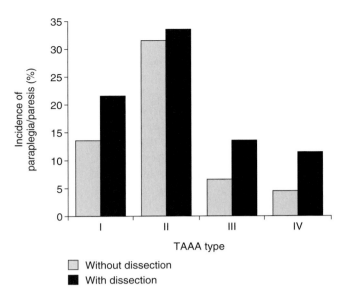

FIG. 14-12 The incidence of paraplegia/paresis is higher with more extensive aneurysms (Crawford Type I and II TAAA [thoracoabdominal aneurysms]), and is higher in the presence of aortic dissection.

(Data from Svensson LG, Crawford ES, Hess KR et al: *J Vasc Surg* 17:357-370, 1993.)

cord, and the anterior two thirds of the spinal cord are supplied by the discontinuous anterior spinal artery.[168,197] In fact, the anterior spinal artery is not a single, well-defined vessel but rather a network of interconnected vascular anastomoses.[201] It receives its blood supply from radicular branches of the left vertebral artery, the thyrocervical trunk, the intercostal arteries, and the lateral sacral artery. The major radicular supply to the anterior spinal artery in the thoracic and upper abdominal region is from three to five anterior radicular arteries, the largest of which is termed the *arteria radicularis magna*, the so-called artery of Adamkiewicz (Adam-káy-vich). In the majority of patients it originates from T_9 to L_3 and in 80% of cases has a left-sided origin.[168,201] It is this region of the spinal cord, where the collateral blood supply is minimal and dependent on the artery of Adamkiewicz, that is most susceptible to ischemia during aortic cross-clamping and after sacrifice of intercostal vessels. The combination of the variable origin of these feeding vessels and the segmental and discontinuous blood supply of the anterior portion of the spinal cord account for the variable incidence of paraplegia after thoracic aortic surgery.[197]

Etiology of Spinal Cord Injury. Two patterns of spinal cord injury are observed: immediate-onset paraplegia seen immediately on awakening from anesthesia, and delayed-onset paraplegia, an event that occurs in about 30% of cases of paraplegia and may be seen from 1 to 30 days postoperatively.[179,202] Delayed para-

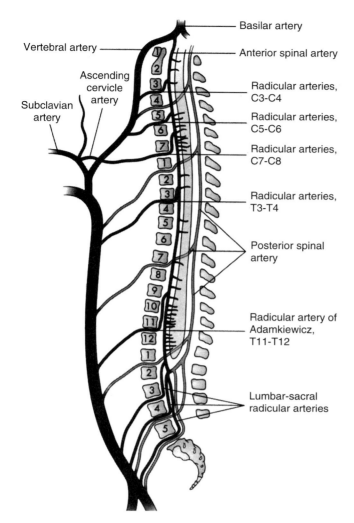

Basilar artery

Vertebral artery

Anterior spinal artery

Ascending cervicle artery

Radicular arteries, C3-C4

Subclavian artery

Radicular arteries, C5-C6

Radicular arteries, C7-C8

Radicular arteries, T3-T4

Posterior spinal artery

Radicular artery of Adamkiewicz, T11-T12

Lumbar-sacral radicular arteries

FIG. 14-13 The anatomy of the blood supply to the spinal cord.

(From Smith MS, Grichnik KP: Anesthetic considerations for lung transplantation and thoracic aortic surgery. In Reves JG, editor: *Atlas of anesthesia, cardiothoracic anesthesia*, vol 8, Philadelphia, 1999, Current Medicine.)

plegia is believed to be secondary to postoperative hypotension, spinal cord edema, reperfusion injury, or thromboembolic occlusion of reattached intercostal vessels.[127,200,203,204]

The risk of spinal cord injury is essentially determined by four major events occurring during and after thoracic aortic surgery[180] (Fig. 14-14): (1) reduction of spinal cord blood flow during the period of aortic cross-clamping; (2) permanent interruption of spinal cord blood flow from the loss of critical intercostal and lumbar arteries sacrificed during surgery or occluded by thromboembolic events postoperatively; (3) reperfusion injury; and (4) spinal cord hypoperfusion from postoperative hypotension. The prevention of spinal cord injury aims to minimize the impact of each of these pathologic events.

Substantial evidence suggests that the incidence of paraplegia is highly correlated with the duration of aortic cross-clamping.[127,172,178,205] The risk of spinal cord injury increases in a sigmoid fashion after 30 to 40 minutes of aortic cross-clamping without distal circulatory support, although the absolute safe ischemic interval may be as short as 18 minutes[158] (Fig. 14-15). In addition, the extent and location of the aneurysm influences the incidence of spinal cord injury because of the number of intercostal arteries involved and the prolonged duration of aortic cross-clamping required[179,194,200] (Fig. 14-12).

Intraoperative hypotension may also compromise SCPP by decreasing blood flow via collateral vessels. Experimental data suggest that nitroprusside, and possibly nitroglycerin, may increase the risk of paraplegia by decreasing proximal and distal aortic pressures and increasing CSFP, thus lowering SCPP.[159,160,168,206] Theoretically, blood is shunted away from high-resistance collateral vessels supplying the spinal cord to low-resistance proximal vascular beds. This risk, however, must be weighed against the danger of ventricular dysfunction, myocardial ischemia, and increased ICP resulting from uncontrolled proximal hypertension. In addition, severe proximal hypertension jeopardizes the integrity of fragile aortic walls above the cross-clamp.[200] For these reasons, lower proximal pressures must often be tolerated (or distal perfusion used) at the expense of potentially impaired spinal cord perfusion. A balance must therefore be achieved when using nitroprusside for blood pressure control during simple clamp and sew procedures. Not all data substantiate this increased risk,[207] however, and most operative teams continue to use nitroprusside as the primary antihypertensive agent because of its rapid onset, short duration of action, and proven efficacy. Ultimately, an approach that uses distal perfusion, modest proximal hypertension, alternative antihypertensive agents, and limited doses of nitroprusside may minimize this potential risk.

The failure to reimplant critical intercostal vessels is also cited as a cause of spinal cord injury.[179,180,203] Griepp et al[194] noted that the incidence of paraplegia was directly related to the number of intersegmental arteries sacrificed, and Svensson et al[208] and Safi et al[179] demonstrated a lower incidence of paraplegia when patent intercostal arteries from T_7 to L_1 were reimplanted. Others, however, advocate early ligation of all intercostals immediately after aortic occlusion to reduce the duration of aortic cross-clamping and to minimize backbleeding from the intercostal vessels into the aortic lumen.[169,196,205] Backbleeding appears to shunt blood away from the spinal cord, producing a steal phenomenon (i.e., reverse flow *out of* rather than *into* the intercostal arteries)[196] (Fig. 14-16). In fact, using SSEP guidance, Griepp et al[194] demonstrated that even when up to

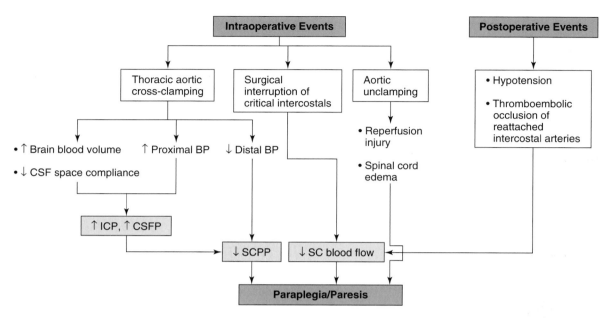

FIG. 14-14 The pathophysiology of spinal cord injury during descending thoracic aortic surgery. The etiology of paraplegia/paresis is multifactorial and related to several intraoperative and postoperative events. See text for detail. *BP,* Blood pressure; *CSF,* cerebrospinal fluid; *CSFP,* cerebrospinal fluid pressure; *ICP,* intracranial pressure; *SC,* spinal cord; *SCPP,* spinal cord perfusion pressure.

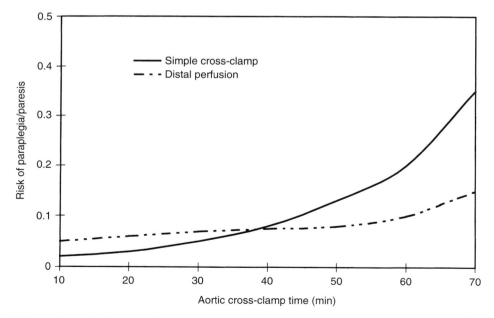

FIG. 14-15 The impact of aortic cross-clamp duration and distal perfusion on the incidence of paraplegia/paresis during repair of Type II thoracoabdominal aortic aneurysms. The risk of spinal cord injury increases in a sigmoid fashion after 40 minutes of aortic cross-clamping. This risk is reduced by the use of distal perfusion.

(Adapted from Svensson LG, Crawford ES, Hess KR et al: *Chest* 104:1248-1253, 1993.)

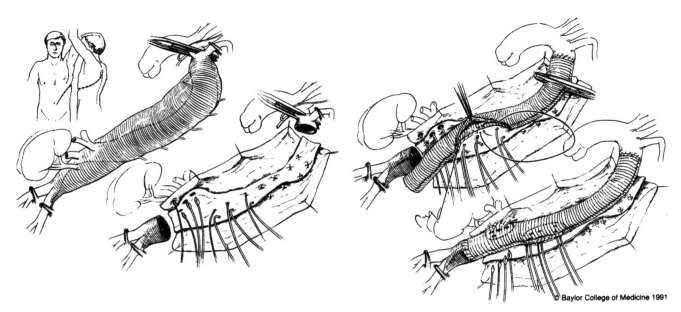

FIG. 14-16   Thoracoabdominal aortic aneurysm repair. Fogarty balloon catheters are placed in the intersegmental and visceral arteries to prevent backbleeding into the aortic lumen and embolization of air and debris into these vessels. This may prevent a ''steal'' phenomenon whereby blood flows *into* the aortic lumen and *away* from the spinal cord.

(From Svensson LG, Crawford ES: *Curr Probl Surg* 29:922-1011, 1992.)

10 pairs of intercostal arteries were ligated, no patients became paraplegic. Ultimately, the benefit of reimplanting intercostal arteries must be weighed against the additional period of cross-clamping required to reliably identify and reattach these vessels. Despite these contradictory findings, however, most authorities recommend reimplantation of all patent lower intercostal and lumbar arteries.*

Monitoring Spinal Cord Function. Evoked potential monitoring can detect subtle changes in spinal cord perfusion and is the primary method used to monitor spinal cord function during thoracic aortic surgery. Several authors have reported satisfactory results by using SSEPs to assess the adequacy of distal perfusion and to identify critical intercostal vessels[210-213] (Fig. 14-17). In a study involving a small number of patients, Cunningham et al[210] showed that loss of the SSEP signal for longer than 30 minutes resulted in a 71% incidence of paraplegia. Unfortunately, SSEPs monitor the more ischemia-resistant neurons of the dorsal columns, rather than the more ischemia-sensitive anterior horn cells.[180] In addition, the occurrence of motor deficits despite

unchanged or recovered SSEPs,[214] the technical difficulties associated with SSEP monitoring (effects of peripheral nerve ischemia, effect of anesthetics, etc.), and the inability of SSEPs to clearly detect ischemia of motor neurons in the anterior horn of the spinal cord have led to an interest in motor-evoked potentials (MEPs) and spinal cord-evoked potentials.[182,215-218] De Haan et al and Jacobs et al[219] used MEP to guide perfusion management and intercostal reimplantation during descending thoracic aortic surgery, and correctly predicted postoperative neurologic events with no false-negative findings (Fig. 14-18). These findings suggest that MEP may overcome some of the limitations of SSEP for the detection and management of spinal cord ischemia. However, if clamp and sew techniques are used without distal perfusion and without a selective approach to intercostal artery reattachment, evoked potential monitoring is likely to be of little value, since no active intervention can be used to reduce spinal cord ischemia. It is important to remember that evoked potential monitoring does not *prevent* spinal cord injury per se, but rather alerts the surgeons to spinal cord ischemia and the need for active intervention in the form of intercostal reattachment or increased distal perfusion.[220]

*References 172, 179, 180, 202, 204, 208, 209.

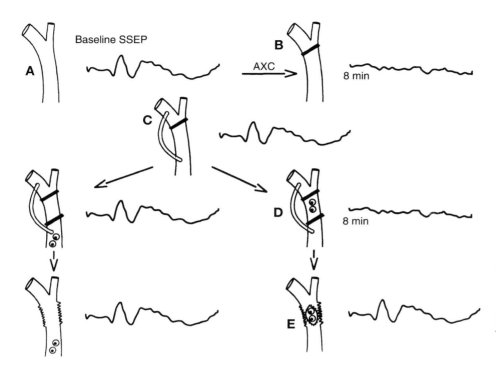

FIG. 14-17 Use of somatosensory evoked potentials *(SSEP)* during descending thoracic aortic cross-clamping *(AXC)*. The baseline SSEP recording (**A**) shows a decrease in amplitude and increase in latency after 8 minutes of AXC (**B**). When a shunt is placed from the proximal to distal aorta (**C**), critical intercostal arteries are perfused and the SSEP trace returns to baseline *(bottom left portion of figure)*. If the critical intercostal arteries arise from the segment of aorta that is cross-clamped (**D**), then shunting has little effect on spinal cord perfusion and the SSEP trace remains abnormal until the intercostal vessels are reattached and the aorta is unclamped (**E**).

(From Robertazzi RR, Cunningham, Jr, JN: *Semin Thorac Cardiovasc Surg* 10[1]:29-34, 1998.)

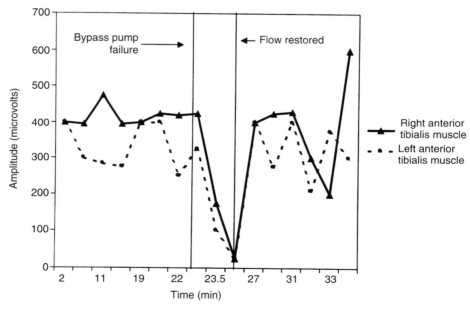

FIG. 14-18 Motor evoked potentials (MEP) in a patient undergoing repair of a type I thoraco-abdominal aortic aneurysm by using left atriofemoral bypass. During aortic cross-clamping, a technical failure of the bypass pump caused a decrease in the amplitude of the MEPs, indicative of spinal cord ischemia. These changes in the MEPs appeared within 2 minutes of the interruption of distal perfusion and returned to baseline immediately after restoration of normal bypass flows, emphasizing the utility of MEPs as a monitor of spinal cord ischemia.

(Adapted from de Haan P, Kalkman CJ, de Mol BA et al: *Semin Thorac Cardiovasc Surg* 10:45-49, 1998.)

Methods of Spinal Cord Protection. Although no one method of spinal cord protection has been proven to prevent spinal cord injury, a number of techniques and pharmacologic interventions have been attempted in an effort to preserve spinal cord function after thoracic aortic surgery (Box 14-2).

Distal circulatory support. Distal perfusion has become an essential adjuvant during thoracic aortic surgery, although some authors still report comparable results by using simple clamp and sew techniques without distal perfusion.[169,205,209,221] The impact of distal perfusion remains controversial because no randomized, prospective trials have been performed to investigate its independent influence on neurologic outcome. However, several studies have documented a reduction in the incidence of spinal cord injury when distal perfusion is used compared with historical control patients in whom no distal perfusion was used.* Distal perfusion appears to be most efficacious when used during extensive thoracoabdominal aortic aneurysm resections, since these procedures are technically complex and require prolonged cross-clamp times and thus are associated with the highest risk of neurologic injury. Svensson et al[127] demonstrated that atriofemoral bypass reduced the risk of spinal cord injury in 832 patients after thoracic aortic surgery when aortic cross-clamp times exceeded 40 minutes. Safi et al[178] noted a 38% incidence of neurologic deficits in 111 patients with type II thoracoabdominal aortic aneurysms by using a simple clamp technique compared with a 7% incidence when CSF drainage and distal perfusion were used. In addition, a meta-analysis

*References 127, 130, 173, 177, 178, 194.

of paraplegia after repair of traumatic aortic rupture revealed a paraplegia rate of 6% when distal perfusion was used compared with a 19% incidence with simple clamping alone.[130]

The optimal distal arterial pressures to maintain collateral blood flow to the spinal cord during distal circulatory support has yet to be ascertained. However, data from studies using SSEPs and MEPs to monitor spinal cord function suggest that pressures of 60 to 70 mm Hg maintain cord perfusion and intact evoked potentials[210,219] (Fig. 14-19), although pressures as low as 48 mm Hg were adequate in some patients. Distal flows should be regulated to achieve this pressure, although some centers additionally administer vasopressors into the distal circulation if increased flows fail to achieve these target pressures.

Unfortunately, perfusion techniques cannot completely prevent spinal cord ischemia since critical intercostal arteries are often included within the segment of aorta that is cross-clamped. Thus, there may be compromised blood flow to this segment of the spinal cord despite excellent distal perfusion. However, distal circulatory support may provide perfusion when there is inadequate collateral flow from above the level of the cross-clamp. In this way, it can prolong the safe period of aortic occlusion to allow for the repair of extensive aneurysms and the reattachment of important intercostal arteries.

Cerebrospinal fluid drainage. CSF drainage is a commonly used adjuvant during thoracic aortic surgery because a reduction in CSFP may theoretically produce an improvement in SCPP. Typically, a 19-gauge lumbar epidural catheter is placed preoperatively and 20 to 50 ml of CSF are removed immediately before aortic clamping. CSFP is then maintained below 10 mm Hg throughout the entire procedure by the intermittent removal of 10 to 15 ml of CSF.[220] Safi et al[178] and Acher et al[222] reported mean and maximum CSF drainage volumes of 80 to 100 ml and 220 to 250 ml, respectively. Safi et al[178] also maintain continuous CSF drainage for 3 postoperative days and reinsert the catheter if neurologic deficits become apparent after this period. Potential risks of CSF drainage include cerebral herniation and epidural hematoma formation. If postoperative paraplegia develops, MRI should be performed to exclude a traumatic epidural hematoma, although this event has yet to be reported despite the frequent intraoperative use of moderate doses of heparin.

In theory, CSF drainage improves SCPP by reducing CSFP (SCPP = distal MAP − CSFP). Unfortunately, the benefit of CSF drainage in reducing the incidence of spinal cord injury is controversial, with many studies reporting conflicting results.[223-230] Despite favorable experimental results, Crawford et al[231] failed to show a decrease in the incidence of paraplegia in a randomized prospective trial in 98 patients undergoing thoraco-

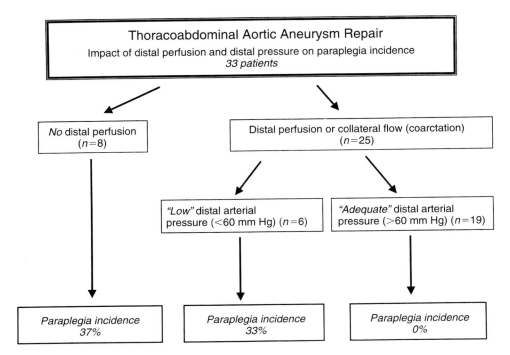

FIG. 14-19 The impact of distal perfusion and "adequate" perfusion pressure on the incidence of paraplegia in 33 patients undergoing thoracoabdominal aortic aneurysm repair. This study by Cunningham et al demonstrated that distal arterial pressures of less than or equal to 60 mm Hg during distal circulatory support resulted in a high paraplegia rate (33%) that was similar to the frequency observed when no distal perfusion was used. These data suggest that adequate distal pressures are necessary to ensure satisfactory collateral flow to the spinal cord during thoracic aortic surgery with distal perfusion.

(Modified from Cunningham JN, Laschinger JC, Spencer FC: *J Thorac Cardiovasc Surg* 94:275-285, 1987.)

abdominal aortic aneurysm repair. Murray et al[232] noted similar results in a retrospective clinical analysis of CSF drainage during descending thoracic aortic surgery. Critics of Crawford's study suggest that limiting the volume of CSF removed to 50 ml may have been inadequate to decrease CSFP and that, in some patients, large volumes of CSF may need to be removed to achieve a beneficial effect.[229,233-235] CSF drainage *alone* is of limited efficacy, however, since it decreases CSFP by only 8 to 10 mm Hg and is unlikely to increase SCPP to levels necessary to prevent ischemia.[151,229] CSF removal may be more effective when used in conjunction with distal perfusion or other adjuvants such as intravenous naloxone,[222,236] methylprednisolone,[163] or intrathecal papaverine.[199,237] Intrathecal papaverine may dilate the anterior spinal artery and increase spinal cord blood flow.[238] Svensson et al[199] demonstrated that CSF drainage and intrathecal papaverine reduced the incidence of neurologic injury and improved postoperative motor scores in 33 patients undergoing high-risk type I and II thoracoabdominal aortic aneurysm resection (Fig. 14-20). In addition to intraoperative use, case reports have suggested that large-volume CSF removal effectively and immediately reversed delayed-onset para-

plegia noted in the early postoperative period.[229,233] Finally, it must be noted that many centers performing large numbers of descending thoracic aortic procedures use intraoperative CSF drainage for spinal cord protection.

In summary, despite the controversial and inconclusive evidence regarding the efficacy of CSF drainage, it continues to be an important and likely efficacious component of a multimodal approach to spinal cord protection during thoracic aortic surgery.

Hypothermia. Hypothermic reduction of spinal cord metabolism has a clear protective effect on spinal cord function by prolonging the tolerable period of spinal cord ischemia.[209,239-242] Hypothermia may also exert its beneficial effect on the ischemic spinal cord by reducing intrathecal glutamate concentrations[243] and preventing secondary spinal cord damage from peroxidation of lipid membranes.[244] Clinical studies have documented the success of several different methods of hypothermia during thoracic aortic surgery including DHCA,[240,241,245,246] moderate systemic hypothermia,[178,194,196,247] regional aortic perfusion cooling,[248] and epidural cooling.[128,209,249]

Cambria and Davison et al[209] have reported a novel

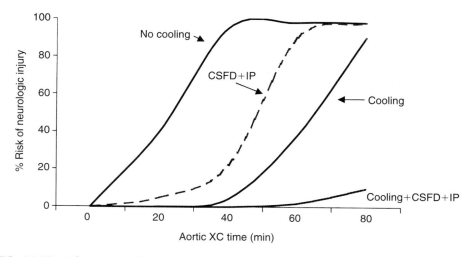

FIG. 14-20 The impact of cerebrospinal fluid drainage *(CSFD)*, intrathecal papaverine *(IP)*, and moderate systemic hypothermia on the risk of neurologic injury in patients undergoing high-risk thoracoabdominal aortic aneurysm surgery. These curves were created by extrapolation from data obtained in patients treated with CSFD+IP or no interventions (no cooling or control group). Moderate systemic hypothermia provided additional neurologic protection and the combination of CSFD, IP, and hypothermia was associated with the lowest theoretical risk of spinal cord injury.

(From Svensson LG, Hess KR, D'Agostino RS et al: *Ann Thorac Surg* 66:132-138, 1998.)

approach to regional epidural cooling that involves placement of an epidural catheter at the T_{10} to T_{12} level for the administration of cold normal saline (4° C). A 4 French intrathecal catheter with a thermistor tip for temperature monitoring is placed at the L_3-L_4 level. An iced saline infusion is started at a rate of 4 to 5 ml/min and adjusted to maintain a CSF temperature of 23° C before aortic cross-clamping. A significant advantage of this ingenious, albeit complex, system is the local cooling effect of the epidural solution without potentially detrimental systemic hypothermia (Fig. 14-21). The primary limitation is the significant rise in CSFP noted during the period of epidural cooling. However, the authors reported a low rate of neurologic deficits (2.9%) by using this technique in 70 patients undergoing thoracic and thoracoabdominal aneurysm repair. Moreover, they noted a significant reduction in the risk of spinal cord injury when compared with historical controls. This promising approach to spinal cord protection awaits further validation from other clinical studies.

In summary, hypothermia is an effective and established form of spinal cord protection during descending thoracic aortic surgery. Although DHCA and local epidural cooling are less common approaches that are successfully used at certain institutions, moderate systemic hypothermia (33° to 34° C) should be considered an *essential* aspect of spinal cord protection for *all* patients at risk for spinal cord injury undergoing descending thoracic aortic surgery.

Pharmacologic agents. A variety of pharmacologic agents have been used experimentally to reduce the de-

gree of spinal cord injury, although the clinical efficacy of these agents remains unproven (Box 14-3). Corticosteroids may decrease the incidence of experimental spinal cord injury by stabilizing cell membranes and reducing oxygen free-radical injury.[250] Opiate receptor antagonists such as naloxone and nalmefene block neuronal activity and reduce tissue metabolism and appear to be beneficial in limited clinical and experimental studies.[196,222,251] Although corticosteroids, barbiturates, and mannitol are commonly administered during thoracic aortic surgery, their efficacy has not been established. Calcium channel antagonists such as nimodipine have been used both experimentally[164,252] and clinically[197,253] with variable and inconsistent results. Experimental data suggest that NMDA receptor antagonists,[254] sodium channel blockade,[254] and glutamate antagonism with riluzole[255] may reduce the degree of ischemic neuronal injury during thoracic aortic occlusion. Systemic and intrathecal magnesium may similarly improve neurologic outcome via blockade of NMDA receptors.[239,256] In addition to intravenous medications, a number of agents including magnesium, papaverine, and tetracaine have been administered intrathecally for spinal cord protection.[197,256,257] Other agents investigated during experimental spinal cord ischemia include vasodilators such as adenosine and prostacyclin,[258] oxygen free radical scavengers such as allopurinol and superoxide dismutase, mannitol,[259] and perfluorocarbons.[197]

In summary, spinal cord injury during thoracic aortic surgery is a multifactorial event that is not com-

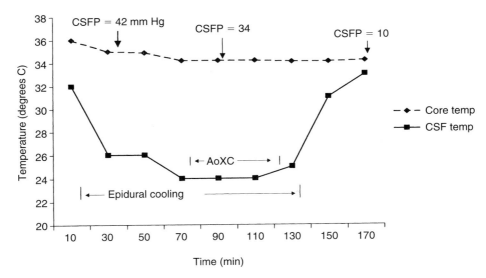

FIG. 14-21   Cerebrospinal fluid pressure *(CSFP)*, CSF temperature, and core temperature during thoracic aortic cross-clamping and epidural cooling in patients undergoing thoracic aortic surgery. Core temperature remains constant despite a significant decrease in CSF temperature during epidural cooling, and CSFP is significantly higher during epidural cooling than after active cooling has stopped. *AoXC,* Aortic cross-clamping.

(Adapted from Cambria RP, Davison JK: *Semin Thorac Cardiovasc Surg* 10:61-65, 1998.)

BOX 14-3
Pharmacologic Methods of Spinal Cord Protection During Descending Thoracic Aortic Surgery

Systemic
- Corticosteroids
- Barbiturates
- Naloxone
- Calcium channel antagonists
- O_2 free radical scavengers
- N-methyl-D-aspartate receptor antagonists
- Mannitol
- Magnesium
- Vasodilators (adenosine, papaverine, prostacyclin)
- Perfluorocarbons
- Colchicine

Intrathecal
- Papaverine
- Magnesium
- Tetracaine
- Perfluorocarbons

---

pletely preventable. However, a combination of measures, including limitation of the duration of aortic cross-clamping, the use of distal perfusion, maintenance of modest degrees of proximal hypertension and systemic or local hypothermia, CSF drainage, reimplanta-tion of critical intercostal arteries, and the use of certain pharmacologic agents may be the most promising and sensible approach to reduce the incidence of this dreaded complication.

ENDOVASCULAR STENT-GRAFT PLACEMENT FOR THE TREATMENT OF THORACIC AORTIC DISEASE

The significant morbidity and mortality associated with surgical repair of descending thoracic aortic lesions, along with the prohibitive risk associated with this procedure in patients with serious comorbid conditions, has prompted evaluation of nonsurgically placed endoluminal aortic stent-grafts. Originally described by Parodi et al[260] in 1991 for the treatment of abdominal aortic aneurysms in high-risk patients, stent-grafts are designed to stabilize aortic aneurysms by directing blood flow through the stent-graft and promoting subsequent thrombosis of the aneurysm around the stent-graft, thus excluding the fragile aortic wall from the systemic circulation and preventing aortic rupture.

The stent-graft device is a self-expanding endoprosthesis composed of interlocking self-expanding stents covered with a woven Dacron graft. They are compressed into a loading capsule and under fluoroscopic guidance, are advanced through a 27 French sheath positioned within the aneurysm.[261,262] Each device is custom-made for each patient according to measure-

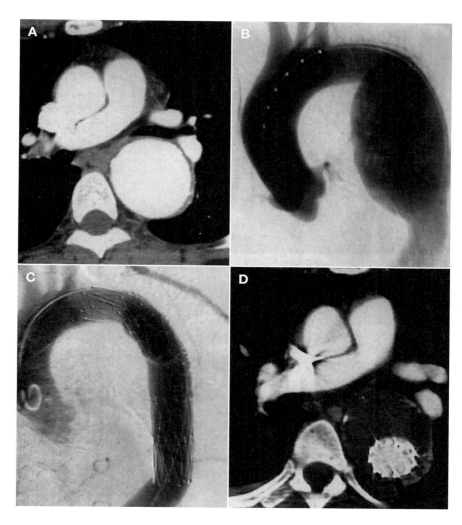

FIG. 14-22   The use of a stent-graft for the treatment of a descending thoracic aortic aneurysm. **A** and **B** show a large thoracic aortic aneurysm identified by computed tomography and angiography, respectively. After placement of the stent-graft, angiography reveals no flow outside the device (**C**), and computed tomography demonstrates successful thrombosis of the aneurysm and exclusion from the native circulation (**D**).

ments obtained from diagnostic imaging studies. After surgical exposure of the femoral or iliac artery, a wire is positioned in the thoracic aorta by using fluoroscopy and TEE (or in some centers, intravascular ultrasound). The sheath with the stent, a pusher, and, in some cases, a deflated latex balloon, is introduced until the device is positioned proximal to the aneurysm. Just before unloading of the stent-graft device, the MAP is lowered to 50 to 60 mm Hg with vasodilators and β-adrenergic blockers to reduce the risk of distal migration of the device by the force of arterial inflow.[263] If a balloon is used, it is inflated to expand the stent. The stent-graft is then deployed by holding the pusher firmly in place and quickly withdrawing the sheath, thereby allowing rapid expansion of the prosthesis.[263] Angiographic and echocardiographic images are obtained to confirm proper positioning of the device and to ensure that flow has been excluded from the aneurysm (Fig. 14-22). When stent-grafts are used to treat aortic dissections, these postprocedure imaging studies are also used to confirm that flow no longer exists in the false lumen. The sheath and guide are then removed and the incision is closed.

The average duration of the procedure in one series of aortic dissections was 1.6 hours.

These procedures are usually performed in the angiography suite, although they may also be performed in the operating room.[264] Most patients require general anesthesia since TEE is frequently used for monitoring the success of stent-graft placement. The use of thoracic epidural anesthesia as an adjunct to general anesthesia, as well as lumbar epidural anesthesia alone, have also been described, but appear to be less popular anesthetic techniques.[264] The major intraoperative concern is the satisfactory control of arterial blood pressure, especially when the stent-graft is deployed. This is most commonly achieved with nitroprusside, although nitroglycerin, epidural local anesthetics, and temporary asystole with adenosine have also been used successfully. Blood loss may be significant because of backbleeding from femoral sheath insertion sites, although recent data suggest transfusion is rarely needed.[261] Central venous access is recommended, but double-lumen tubes are not routinely inserted.[264] Preparations should be made, however, for possible emergent thoracotomy should procedural complications develop, such as branch vessel occlusion or aortic rupture.

The first reported series of patients managed with stent-grafts had isolated aneurysms of the DTA or penetrating ulcers associated with IMH,[265] although more recent investigations have described the successful use of stent-grafts for the treatment of both type A and type B acute aortic dissections. Nienaber et al[261] reported their results in 24 patients undergoing either stent-graft placement or conventional surgery, and noted no morbidity or mortality in the stent-graft group versus a 33% mortality in the operative group. The entry site was sealed and the false lumen thrombosed in all 12 stent-graft patients.[261] No patient in the stent-graft group required blood product transfusions and there were no postoperative complications. Dake et al[266] reported a 16% early mortality rate in a similar group of 19 patients with acute dissection involving the DTA treated with stent-grafts, and there were no cases of aortic rupture in any patients after 1 year. Complete and partial thrombosis of the false lumen was achieved in 79% and 21% of patients, respectively, and revascularization of branch vessels with relief of corresponding ischemic symptoms was noted in 76% of obstructed branches. The incidence of paraplegia was only 3%.

These data suggest that stent-grafts are a viable and increasingly common option for the treatment of both aortic aneurysmal disease as well as acute aortic dissection, and may represent reasonable alternative treatment modalities for high-risk patients with thoracic aortic disease. Unfortunately, these approaches are currently still evolving, are not available in all centers, and may not be applicable for some patients because of anatomic considerations, such as unfavorable aneurysm dimensions and prohibitive atherosclerotic disease of the femoral and iliac arteries. Nonetheless, these procedures will undoubtedly increase in frequency and will require that anesthesiologists apply similar principles of anesthetic management as used for open procedures, yet in an environment distant from the operating room.

MAJOR POSTOPERATIVE COMPLICATIONS
Cardiac

Cardiac complications, including myocardial infarction, low cardiac output syndrome, and arrhythmias, occur in 7% to 34%[23,26,27] and 10% to 15%[128,172,173,200] of patients after ascending and descending thoracic aortic surgery, respectively (Table 14-5). In 1509 patients undergoing thoracoabdominal aortic resections, cardiac complications occurred in 12% of patients, but accounted for 38% of all deaths.[200] Similarly, cardiac events were the leading cause of mortality in 227 patients undergoing aortic arch surgery.[23] Because ascending aortic surgery involves clamping of the ascending

TABLE 14-5
Complications after Thoracic Aortic Surgery

COMPLICATION	ASCENDING AORTIC SURGERY (%)	DESCENDING THORACIC AORTIC SURGERY (%)
Cardiac	10-34	10-38
Pulmonary	27-38	25-33
Renal failure	5-9	10-25
Hemorrhage	9-11	3-14
Stroke	3-10	2-3
Infection/sepsis	3-18	3-8
Aortointestinal fistulas	< 1	2-3
Gastrointestinal bleeding	—	2-3

From references 23, 26-27, 128, 172-173, and 200.

aorta and arrest of the heart, as well as occasional reimplantation of the coronary ostia, ischemic cardiac complications are not unexpected.

Pulmonary

Pulmonary complications are especially common after thoracic and thoracoabdominal aortic surgery because of the detrimental effects on pulmonary function of a rib-splitting thoracotomy incision and division of the diaphragm.[267] In addition, surgical trauma to the left lung and intrapulmonary hemorrhage also impair postoperative pulmonary function. Other commonly recognized risk factors for postoperative pulmonary complications include the presence of chronic obstructive pulmonary disease, advanced age, extent of the aneurysm, coexisting renal and cardiac complications, and the volume of blood products transfused.[267-269] After thoracic aortic surgery, the incidence varies between 24% and 33%, depending on the criteria used to define pulmonary complications.[128,200] Reported complications include respiratory insufficiency requiring prolonged ventilation, acute lung injury, pneumonia, pleural effusions, atelectasis, pneumothorax and chronic air leaks, and the need for tracheostomy. Judicious administration of fluids, aggressive pulmonary toilet, the use of bronchodilators, and adequate postoperative analgesia are important elements of postoperative pulmonary care. Although a thoracic epidural catheter is routinely used in stable postoperative patients after descending thoracic aortic procedures in many centers, no controlled studies have evaluated the impact of epidural analgesia on the incidence of pulmonary complications in this setting.

Renal Failure

The incidence of renal failure after thoracic and thoraco-abdominal aortic surgery ranges from 11% to 25% and is a lethal event in 50% of patients who develop this complication,[154] a rate that emphasizes the importance of identifying high-risk patients and developing preventative strategies. It occurs less often after ascending aortic surgery (5%-9%). In addition to the duration of aortic cross-clamping, other risk factors for renal failure after descending thoracic aortic surgery include advanced age, preoperative renal dysfunction, the use of simple cross-clamping without distal perfusion, the duration of renal ischemia, and the volume of red blood cell transfusion.[127,154,155,270] Preoperative renal insufficiency is the most consistently noted risk factor for postoperative renal failure and the need for dialysis, with a greater than tenfold increased risk noted in one study.[154] Unfortunately, there are no data to support the use of a specific pharmacologic agent or surgical technique that consistently reduces the incidence of this serious complication. Some evidence suggests that the use of distal circulatory support,[127,154] intraoperative diuretic administration,[134] and hypothermic renal perfusion[155] may reduce the degree of renal injury after thoracic aortic procedures.

Hemorrhage

Postoperative bleeding complications occur in 3% to 10% of patients after both ascending and descending thoracic aortic surgery. Although bleeding and coagulopathy are slightly less common after descending compared with ascending aortic surgery, hemostatic prob-

lems may contribute significantly to the occurrence of death.[271] In a series of 110 patients after thoracoabdominal aortic aneurysm resection, Gilling-Smith et al[271] reported that hemorrhage accounted for 39% of all deaths. This complication is typically a multifactorial event influenced by bleeding from multiple vascular anastomoses, hypothermic effects on the coagulation system, dilutional changes in coagulation factors and platelets secondary to massive transfusion, and alterations in hemostasis induced by CPB. Frequent monitoring of hemostatic parameters and aggressive therapy with FFP, platelet concentrates, and cryoprecipitate is recommended.

Central Nervous System Complications

Stroke occurs in 2% to 3%[127,128] of patients after descending thoracic aortic procedures. CNS complications after ascending aortic surgery were discussed previously.

CONCLUSIONS

The intraoperative management of thoracic aortic procedures will remain challenging and complex for the anesthesiologist as newer approaches to spinal cord protection, such as epidural cooling and DHCA, are adopted. Future developments in thoracic aortic surgery will continue to focus on surgical, perfusion, and pharmacologic techniques to reduce the incidence of renal, spinal cord, and CNS injury. The use of stent-grafts to treat aortic disease represents an exciting new alternative to surgery that may reduce the substantial morbidity currently encountered with standard operative approaches.

KEY POINTS

1. In addition to aortic aneurysms and aortic dissection, IMH and penetrating atherosclerotic ulcer are less well recognized but important etiological factors in thoracic aortic disease.

2. Existing data are inconclusive regarding both the beneficial and potentially deleterious effects of aprotinin when used during thoracic aortic surgery requiring circulatory arrest, and some authors maintain that aprotinin should not be used in this situation.

3. DHCA is an essential aspect of surgery of the ascending thoracic aorta and aortic arch, although the risk of neurologic injury increases with arrest times exceeding 40 minutes.

4. RCP may prolong the safe interval of circulatory arrest and possibly reduce the incidence of cerebral embolic injury, although the evidence supporting a beneficial impact on postoperative neurologic function is sharply controversial.

5. Clamping of the DTA produces a cascade of hemodynamic events that includes severe proximal arterial hypertension and distal hypotension; increased preload and reduced cardiac output; increased ICP; and decreased renal, visceral, and spinal cord blood flow.

6. The management of thoracic aortic clamping and unclamping is most effectively managed with distal circulatory support, which attenuates proximal hypertension, provides blood flow to vascular beds below the level of the aortic cross-clamp, and reduces the incidence of postoperative renal failure and paraplegia.

7. Spinal cord injury is due to cross-clamp-induced reductions in spinal cord blood flow, surgical interruption of critical intersegmental arteries, perioperative hypoperfusion, and postoperative thromboembolic events.

8. The critical elements of spinal cord protection during descending thoracic aortic surgery include limitation of the duration of aortic clamping, the use of distal perfusion, maintenance of regional or systemic hypothermia, CSF drainage, and reimplantation of critical intersegmental arteries.

9. Endovascular stent-grafts represent a nonsurgical approach to the treatment of thoracic aortic disease that may reduce the morbidity of standard operative repairs and provide an effective treatment option for high-risk patients.

KEY REFERENCES

Cambria RP, Davison JK: Regional hypothermia for prevention of spinal cord ischemic complications after thoracoabdominal aortic surgery: experience with epidural cooling, *Semin Thorac Cardiovasc Surg* 10:61-65, 1998.

Crawford ES, Svensson LG, Hess KR et al: A prospective randomized study of cerebrospinal fluid drainage to prevent paraplegia after high-risk surgery on the thoracoabdominal aorta, *J Vasc Surg* 13:36-46, 1990.

Ergin MA, Galla JD, Lansman SL et al: Hypothermic circulatory arrest in operations on the thoracic aorta, *J Thorac Cardiovasc Surg* 107:788-799, 1994.

Gelman S: The pathophysiology of aortic cross-clamping and unclamping, *Anesthesiology* 82:1026-1060, 1995.

Gharagozloo F, Neville, Jr, RF, Cox JL: Spinal cord protection during surgical procedures on the descending thoracic and thoracoabdominal aorta: a critical overview, *Semin Thorac Cardiovasc Surg* 10:73-86, 1998.

Griepp RB, Ergin MA, Galla JD et al: Looking for the artery of Adamkiewicz: a quest to minimize paraplegia after operations for aneurysms of the descending thoracic and thoracoabdominal aorta, *J Thorac Cardiovasc Surg* 112:1202-1215, 1996.

Griepp RB, Juvonen T, Griepp EB et al: Is retrograde cerebral perfusion an effective means of neural support during deep hypothermic circulatory arrest? *Ann Thorac Surg* 64: 913-916, 1997.

Kouchoukos NT, Daily BB, Rokkas CK et al: Hypothermic bypass and circulatory arrest for operations on the descending thoracic and thoracoabdominal aorta, *Ann Thorac Surg* 60:67-77, 1995.

Kouchoukos NT, Dougenis D: Surgery of the thoracic aorta, *N Engl J Med* 336:1876-1888, 1997.

Nienaber CA, Fattori R, Lund G et al: Nonsurgical reconstruction of thoracic aortic dissection by stent-graft placement, *N Engl J Med* 340:1539-1545, 1999.

Roizen MF, Beaupre PN, Albert RA et al: Monitoring with two-dimensional transesophageal echocardiography. Comparison of myocardial function in patients undergoing supraceliac, suprarenal-infraceliac, or infrarenal aortic occlusion, *J Vasc Surg* 1:300-305, 1984.

Svensson LG, Crawford ES, Hess KR et al: Deep hypothermia with circulatory arrest, *J Thorac Cardiovasc Surg* 106:19-31, 1993.

Svensson LG, Crawford ES, Hess KR et al: Variables predictive of outcome in 832 patients undergoing repairs of the descending thoracic aorta, *Chest* 104:1248-1253, 1993.

Svensson LG, Crawford ES, Hess KR et al: Experience with 1509 patients undergoing thoracoabdominal aortic operations, *J Vasc Surg* 17:357-370, 1993.

References

1. Kouchoukos NT, Dougenis D: Surgery of the thoracic aorta, *N Engl J Med* 336:1876-1888, 1997.
2. Debakey ME, Cooley DA: Successful resection of aneurysms of thoracic aorta and replacement by graft, *JAMA* 152:673-676, 1953.
3. Cooley DA, DeBakey ME: Resection of entire ascending aorta in fusiform aneurysm using cardiac bypass, *JAMA* 162:1158-1159, 1956.
4. Svensson LG, Crawford ES: Aortic dissection and aortic aneurysm surgery. Clinical observations, experimental investigations, and statistical analyses, Part II, *Curr Probl Surg* 29:922-1011, 1992.
5. Crawford ES: The diagnosis and management of aortic dissection, *JAMA* 264:2537-2541, 1990.
6. Beckman JA, O'Gara PT: Diseases of the aorta, *Adv Intern Med* 44:267-291, 1999.
7. Svensson LG, Crawford ES: Aortic dissection and aortic aneurysm surgery: clinical observations, experimental investigations, and statistical analyses, Part III, *Curr Probl Surg* 30:163, 1993.
8. Van Arsdell GS, David TE, Butany J: Autopsies in acute type A aortic dissection. Surgical implications, *Circulation* 98:II299-304, 1998.
9. Isselbacher EM, Eagle KA, Desanctis RW: Diseases of the aorta. In Braunwald E, editor: *Heart disease: a textbook of cardiovascular medicine*, vol 2, ed 5, Philadelphia, 1997, WB Saunders, pp 1546-1581.

10. O'Connor CJ, Najafi HN: Sudden death due to retrograde aortic dissection during repair of a descending thoracic aneurysm, *J Cardiothorac Vasc Anesth* 10(3):380-384, 1996.
11. O'Gara PT, DeSanctis RW: Acute aortic dissection and its variants: toward a common diagnostic and therapeutic approach, *Circulation* 92:1376-1378, 1995.
12. Bolognesi R, Manca C, Dimitri T et al: Aortic intramural hematoma: an increasingly recognized aortic disease, *Cardiology* 89: 178-183, 1998.
13. Vilacosta I, San Roman JA, Aragoncillo P et al: Penetrating atherosclerotic aortic ulcer: documentation by transesophageal echocardiography, *J Am Coll Cardiol* 32:83-89, 1998.
14. Coady MA, Rizzo JA, Hammond GL et al: Penetrating ulcer of the thoracic aorta: what is it? how do we recognize it? how do we manage it? *J Vasc Surg* 27:1006-1016, 1998.
15. Svensson LG, Labib SH, Eisenhauer AC et al: Intimal tear without hematoma. An important variant of aortic dissection that can elude current imaging techniques, *Circulation* 99:1331-1336, 1999.
16. Muluk SC, Kaufman JA, Torchiana DF et al: Diagnosis and treatment of thoracic aortic intramural hematoma, *J Vasc Surg* 24: 1022-1029, 1996.

17. O'Connor C: Chest trauma: the role of transesophageal echocardiography, *J Clin Anesth* 8(7):605-613, 1996.
18. Mattox KL: Traumatic rupture of the thoracic aorta, *Adv Card Surg* 10:271-283, 1998.
19. Shkrum MJ, McClafferty KJ, Green RN et al: Mechanisms of aortic injury in fatalities occurring in motor vehicle collisions, *J Forensic Sci* 44(1):44-56, 1999.
20. Attar S, Cardarelli MG, Downing SW et al: Traumatic aortic rupture: recent outcome with regard to neurologic deficit, *Ann Thorac Surg* 67(4):959-964, 1999.
21. Coady MA, Rizzo JA, Hammond GL et al: What is the appropriate size criterion for resection of thoracic aortic aneurysms? *J Thorac Cardiovasc Surg* 113:476-491, 1997.
22. Gott VL, Greene PS, Alejo DE et al: Replacement of the aortic root in patients with Marfan's syndrome, *N Engl J Med* 340(17):1307-1313, 1999.
23. Coselli JS, Büket S, Djukanovic B: Aortic arch operation: current treatment and results, *Ann Thorac Surg* 59:19-27, 1995.
24. Coselli JS, LeMaire SA: Experience with retrograde cerebral perfusion during proximal aortic surgery in 290 patients, *J Card Surg* 12:322-325, 1997.
25. Safi HJ, Letsou GV, Iliopoulos DC et al: Impact of retrograde cerebral perfusion on ascending aortic and arch aneurysm repair, *Ann Thorac Surg* 63:1601-1607, 1997.
26. Okita Y, Takamoto S, Ando M et al: Mortality and cerebral outcome in patients who underwent aortic arch operations using deep hypothermic circulatory arrest with retrograde cerebral perfusion: no relation of early death, stroke, and delirium to the duration of circulatory arrest, *J Thorac Cardiovasc Surg* 115:129-138, 1998.
27. Ergin MA, Galla JD, Lansman SL et al: Hypothermic circulatory arrest in operations on the thoracic aorta, *J Thorac Cardiovasc Surg* 107:788-799, 1994.
28. Svensson LG, Crawford ES: Aortic dissection and aortic aneurysm surgery: clinical observations, experimental investigations, and statistical analyses, Part I, *Curr Probl Surg* 29:817-911, 1992.
29. Cigarroa JE, Isselbacher EM, DeSanctis RW et al: Diagnostic imaging in the evaluation of suspected aortic dissection. Old standards and new directions, *N Engl J Med* 328:35-43, 1993.
30. Erbel R: Role of transesophageal echocardiography in dissection of the aorta and evaluation of degenerative aortic disease, *Cardiol Clin* 11:461-472, 1993.
31. Armstrong WF, Bach DS, Carey LM et al: Clinical and echocardiographic findings in patients with suspected acute aortic dissection, *Am Heart J* 136:1051-1060, 1998.
32. Armstrong WF, Bach DS, Carey L et al: Spectrum of acute dissection of the ascending aorta: a transesophageal echocardiographic study, *J Am Soc Echocardiogr* 9(5):646-656, 1996.
33. Bryan AJ, Barzilai B, Kouchoukos NT: Transesophageal echocardiography and adult cardiac operations, *Ann Thorac Surg* 59(3):773-779, 1995.
34. Torossov M, Singh A, Fein SA: Clinical presentation, diagnosis, and hospital outcome of patients with documented aortic dissection: the Albany Medical Center experience, 1986-1996, *Am Heart J* 137(1):154-161, 1999.
35. Yamada E, Matsumura M, Kimura S et al: Usefulness of transesophageal echocardiography in detecting changes in flow dynamics responsible for malperfusion phenomena observed during surgery of aortic dissection, *Am J Cardiol* 79(8):1149-1152, 1997.
36. Coletti G, Torracca L, La Canna G et al: Diagnosis and management of cerebral malperfusion phenomena during aortic dissection repair by transesophageal Doppler echocardiographic monitoring, *J Card Surg* 11(5):355-358, 1996.
37. Martin K, Schmitz S, Rank N et al: Hemodynamic monitoring during left atriofemoral bypass for resection of a postductal aortic isthmus stenosis: current role of intraoperative transesophageal echocardiography, *J Cardiothorac Vasc Anesth* 13(2):207-209, 1999.
38. Konstadt SN, Reich DL, Quintana C et al: The ascending aorta: how much does transesophageal echocardiography see? *Anesth Analg* 78(2):240-244, 1994.
39. Appelbe AF, Walker PG, Yeoh JK et al: Clinical significance and origin of artifacts in transesophageal echocardiography of the thoracic aorta, *J Am Coll Cardiol* 21(3):754-760, 1993.
40. Losi MA, Betocchi S, Briguori C et al: Determinants of aortic artifacts during transesophageal echocardiography of the ascending aorta, *Am Heart J* 137(5):968-973, 1999.
41. Kimura BJ, Phan JN, Housman LB: Utility of contrast echocardiography in the diagnosis of aortic dissection, *J Am Soc Echocardiogr* 12(2):155-159, 1999.
42. Frost EAM: Electroencephalography and evoked potential monitoring. In Saidman LJ, Smith NT, editors: *Monitoring in anesthesia,* ed 3, Boston, 1993, Butterworth-Heinemann, p 203.
43. Deeb M, Jenkins E, Bolling SF et al: Retrograde cerebral perfusion during hypothermic circulatory arrest reduces neurologic morbidity, *J Thorac Cardiovasc Surg* 109:259-268, 1995.
44. Guérit JM, Verheist R, Rubay J et al: The use of somatosensory evoked potentials to determine the optimal degree of hypothermia during circulatory arrest, *J Card Surg* 9:596-603, 1994.
45. Cheung AT, Bavaria JE, Weiss SJ et al: Neurophysiologic effects of retrograde cerebral perfusion used for aortic reconstruction, *J Cardiothorac Vasc Anesth* 12(3):252-259, 1998.
46. Westaby S: Coagulation disturbance in profound hypothermia: the influence of anti-fibrinolytic therapy, *Semin Thorac Cardiovasc Surg* 9(3):246-256, 1997.
47. Wilde JT: Hematological consequences of profound hypothermic circulatory arrest and aortic dissection, *J Card Surg* 12:201-206, 1997.
48. Eaton MP, Deeb GM: Aprotinin versus ε-aminocaproic acid for aortic surgery using deep hypothermic circulatory arrest, *J Cardiothorac Vasc Anesth* 12(5):548-552, 1998.
49. Svensson LG, Sun J, Nadolny E et al: Prospective evaluation of minimal blood use for ascending aorta and aortic arch operations, *Ann Thorac Surg* 59(6):1501-1508, 1995.
50. Parolari A, Antona C, Alamanni F et al: Aprotinin and deep hypothermic circulatory arrest: there are no benefits even when appropriate amounts of heparin are given, *Eur J Cardiothorac Surg* 11(1):149-156, 1997.
51. Sundt III, TM, Kouchoukos NT, Saffitz JE et al: Renal dysfunction and intravascular coagulation with aprotinin and hypothermic circulatory arrest, *Ann Thorac Surg* 55(6):1418-1424, 1993.
52. Goldstein DJ, DeRosa CM, Mongero LB et al: Safety and efficacy of aprotinin under conditions of deep hypothermia and circulatory arrest, *J Thorac Cardiovasc Surg* 110(6):1615-1621, 1995.
53. Regragui IA, Bryan AJ, Izzat MB et al: Aprotinin use with hypothermic circulatory arrest for aortic valve and thoracic aortic surgery: renal function and early survival, *J Heart Valve Dis* 4(6):674-677, 1995.
54. Westaby S, Forni A, Dunning J et al: Aprotinin and bleeding in profoundly hypothermic perfusion, *Eur J Cardiothorac Surg* 8(2):82-86, 1994.
55. Alvarez JM, Goldstein J, Mezzatesta J et al: Fatal intraoperative pulmonary thrombosis after graft replacement of an aneurysm of the arch and descending aorta in association with deep hypothermic circulatory arrest and aprotinin therapy, *J Thorac Cardiovasc Surg* 115(3):723-724, 1998.
56. Ehrlich M, Grabenwoger M, Cartes-Zumelzu F et al: Operations on the thoracic aorta and hypothermic circulatory arrest: is aprotinin safe? *J Thorac Cardiovasc Surg* 115(1):220-225, 1998.
57. Rooney SJ, Bonser RS: The management of bleeding following surgery requiring hypothermic circulatory arrest, *J Card Surg* 12(suppl 2):238-242, 1997.
58. Okita Y, Takamoto S, Ando M et al: Coagulation and fibrinolysis system in aortic surgery under deep hypothermic circulatory arrest with aprotinin: the importance of adequate heparinization, *Circulation* 96(9S):II376-381, 1997.

59. Ergin MA, Griepp EB, Lansman SL et al: Hypothermic circulatory arrest and other methods of cerebral protection during operations on the thoracic aorta, *J Card Surg* 9:525-537, 1994.

60. Mangano CM: Cardiac surgery and central nervous system injury: the importance of hypothermia during cardiopulmonary bypass. In Blanck TJJ, editor: *Neuroprotection*, Baltimore, 1997, Williams & Wilkins, p 197.

61. Chanyi S: Cerebral perfusion and hypothermic circulatory arrest, *J Cardiothorac Vasc Anesth* 10(1):75-82, 1996.

62. Midulla PS, Gandsas A, Sadeghi AM et al: Comparison of retrograde cerebral perfusion to antegrade cerebral perfusion and hypothermic circulatory arrest in a chronic porcine model, *J Card Surg* 9:560-575, 1994.

63. Crittenden MD, Roberts CS, Rosa L et al: Brain protection during circulatory arrest, *Ann Thorac Surg* 51(6):942-947, 1991.

64. Hindman BJ, Dexter F: Estimating brain temperature during hypothermia, *Anesthesiology* 82(2):329-330, 1995.

65. Murkin JM: The role of CPB management in neurobehavioral outcomes after cardiac surgery, *Ann Thorac Surg* 59:1308-1311, 1995.

66. Murkin JM, Martzke JS, Buchan AM et al: A randomized study of the influence of perfusion technique and pH management strategy in 316 patients undergoing coronary artery bypass surgery, II, Neurologic and cognitive outcomes, *J Thorac Cardiovasc Surg* 110(2):349-362, 1995.

67. Patel RL, Turtle MR, Chambers DJ et al: α-Stat acid-base regulation during cardiopulmonary bypass improves neuropsychologic outcome in patients undergoing coronary artery bypass grafting, *J Thorac Cardiovasc Surg* 111(6):1267-1279, 1996.

68. Kirshbom PM, Skaryak LR, DiBernardo LR et al: pH-stat cooling improves cerebral metabolic recovery after circulatory arrest in a piglet model of aortopulmonary collaterals, *J Thorac Cardiovasc Surg* 111:147-157, 1996.

69. Kurth CD, O'Rourke MM, O'Hara IB: Comparison of pH-stat and α-stat cardiopulmonary bypass on cerebral oxygenation and blood flow in relation to hypothermic circulatory arrest in piglets, *Anesthesiology* 89:110-118, 1998.

70. Aoki M, Nomura F, Stromski ME et al: Effects of pH on brain energetics after hypothermic circulatory arrest, *Ann Thorac Surg* 55:1093-1103, 1993.

71. Hiramatsu T, Miura T, Forbess JM et al: pH strategies and cerebral energetics before and after circulatory arrest, *J Thorac Cardiovasc Surg* 109:948-958, 1995.

72. Jonas RA, Bellinger DC, Rappaport LA et al: Relation of pH strategy and developmental outcome after hypothermic circulatory arrest, *J Thorac Cardiovasc Surg* 106(2):362-368, 1993.

73. du Plessis AJ, Jonas RA, Wypij D et al: Perioperative effects of α-stat versus pH-stat strategies for deep hypothermic cardiopulmonary bypass in infants, *J Thorac Cardiovasc Surg* 114(6): 991-1000, 1997.

74. Shin'oka T, Shum-Tim D, Jonas RA: Higher hematocrit improves cerebral outcome after deep hypothermic circulatory arrest, *J Thorac Cardiovasc Surg* 112(6):1610-1621, 1996.

75. Anderson RV, Siegman MG, Balaban RS et al: Hyperglycemia increases cerebral intracellular acidosis during circulatory arrest, *Ann Thorac Surg* 54(6):1126-1130, 1992.

76. Bruno A, Biller J, Adams, Jr, HP: Acute blood glucose level and outcome from ischemic stroke. Trial of ORG 10172 in Acute Stroke Treatment (TOAST) Investigators, *Neurology* 52(2): 280-284, 1999.

77. Ceriana P, Barzaghi N, Locatelli A et al: Aortic arch surgery: retrospective analysis of outcome and neuroprotective strategies, *J Cardiovasc Surg* 39(3):337-342, 1998.

78. Anderson RE, Tan WK, Martin HS et al: Effects of glucose and PaO_2 modulation on cortical intracellular acidosis, NADH redox state, and infarction in the ischemic penumbra, *Stroke* 30(1): 160-170, 1999.

79. Mezrow CK, Gandsas A, Sadeghi AM et al: Metabolic correlates of neurologic and behavioral injury after prolonged hypothermic circulatory arrest, *J Thorac Cardiovasc Surg* 109:959-975, 1995.

80. Svensson LG, Crawford ES, Hess KR et al: Deep hypothermia with circulatory arrest, *J Thorac Cardiovasc Surg* 106:19-31, 1993.

81. Reich DL, Uysal S, Sliwinski M et al: Neuropsychologic outcome after deep hypothermic circulatory arrest in adults, *J Thorac Cardiovasc Surg* 117:156-163, 1999.

82. Oates RK, Simpson JM, Turnbull JAB et al: The relationship between intelligence and duration of circulatory arrest with deep hypothermia, *J Thorac Cardiovasc Surg* 110:786-792, 1995.

83. Niwa H, Nara M, Kimura T et al: Prolongation of total permissible circulatory arrest duration by deep hypothermic intermittent circulatory arrest, *J Thorac Cardiovasc Surg* 116(1):163-170, 1998.

84. Bellinger DC, Jonas RA, Rappaport LA et al: Developmental and neurologic status of children after heart surgery with hypothermic circulatory arrest or low-flow cardiopulmonary bypass, *N Engl J Med* 332(9):549-555, 1995.

85. Testolin L, Roques X, Laborde MN et al: Moderately hypothermic cardiopulmonary bypass and selective cerebral perfusion in ascending aorta and aortic arch surgery. Preliminary experience in twenty-two patients, *Cardiovasc Surg* 6(4):398-405, 1998.

86. Veeragandham RS, Hamilton, Jr, IN, O'Connor CJ et al: Experience with antegrade bihemispheric cerebral perfusion in aortic arch operations, *Ann Thorac Surg* 66:493-499, 1998.

87. Wozniak G, Dapper F, Schindler E et al: An assessment of selective cerebral perfusion via the innominate artery in aortic arch replacement, *Thorac Cardiovasc Surg* 46:7-11, 1998.

88. Kazui T, Kimura N, Yamada O et al: Surgical outcome of aortic arch aneurysms using selective cerebral perfusion, *Ann Thorac Surg* 57(4):904-911, 1994.

89. Tabayashi K, Ohmi M, Togo T et al: Aortic arch aneurysm repair using selective cerebral perfusion, *Ann Thorac Surg* 57:1305-1310, 1994.

90. Sakurada T, Kazui T, Tanaka H et al: Comparative experimental study of cerebral protection during aortic arch reconstruction, *Ann Thorac Surg* 61:1348-1354, 1996.

91. Filgueiras CL, Ryner L, Ye J et al: Cerebral protection during moderate hypothermic circulatory arrest: histopathology and magnetic resonance spectroscopy of brain energetics and intracellular pH in pigs, *J Thorac Cardiovasc Surg* 112:1073-1080, 1996.

92. Ye J, Yang L, Del Bigio MR et al: Neuronal damage after hypothermic circulatory arrest and retrograde cerebral perfusion in the pig, *Ann Thorac Surg* 61:1316-1322, 1996.

93. Ye J, Ryner LN, Kozlowski P et al: Retrograde cerebral perfusion results in flow distribution abnormalities and neuronal damage. A magnetic resonance imaging and histopathological study in pigs, *Circulation* 98(19):II313-318, 1998.

94. Mills ML, Ochsner JL: Massive air emboli during cardiopulmonary bypass, *J Thorac Cardiovasc Surg* 80:708-717, 1980.

95. Coselli JS: Retrograde cerebral perfusion is an effective means of neural support during deep hypothermic circulatory arrest, *Ann Thorac Surg* 64:908-912, 1997.

96. Bavaria JE, Pochettino A: Retrograde cerebral perfusion (RCP) in aortic arch surgery: efficacy and possible mechanisms of brain protection, *Sem Thorac Cardiovasc Surg* 9(3):222-232, 1997.

97. Griepp RB, Juvonen T, Griepp EB et al: Is retrograde cerebral perfusion an effective means of neural support during deep hypothermic circulatory arrest? *Ann Thorac Surg* 64:913-916, 1997.

98. Loubser PG: Assessment of arteriovenous blood flow during retrograde cerebral perfusion, *J Cardiothorac Vasc Anesth* 13(2): 173-175, 1999.

99. Usui A, Oohara K, Liu T et al: Comparative experimental study between retrograde cerebral perfusion and circulatory arrest, *J Thorac Cardiovasc Surg* 107:1228-1236, 1994.

100. Yoshimura N, Okada M, Ota T: Pharmacologic intervention for ischemic brain edema after retrograde cerebral perfusion, *J Thorac Cardiovasc Surg* 109:1173-1181, 1995.

101. Boeckxstaens CJ, Flameng WJ: Retrograde cerebral perfusion does not perfuse the brain in nonhuman primates, *Ann Thorac Surg* 60:319-328, 1995.

102. Bavaria JE, Woo YJ, Hall A et al: Retrograde cerebral and distal aortic perfusion during ascending and thoracoabdominal aortic operations, *Ann Thorac Surg* 60:345-353, 1995.

103. Lin PJ, Chang CH, Tan PPC et al: Prolonged circulatory arrest in moderate hypothermia with retrograde cerebral perfusion. Is brain ischemic? *Circulation* 94(II):II169-172, 1996.

104. Stowe CL, Baertlein MA, Wierman MD et al: Surgical management of ascending and aortic arch disease: refined techniques with improved results, *Ann Thorac Surg* 66:388-395, 1998.

105. Pangano D, Boivin CM, Faroqui MH et al: Surgery of the thoracic aorta with hypothermic circulatory arrest: experience with retrograde perfusion via the superior vena cava and demonstration of cerebral perfusion, *Eur J Cardiothorac Surg* 10:833-839, 1996.

106. Usui A, Abe T, Murase M et al: Early clinical results of retrograde cerebral perfusion for aortic arch operations in Japan, *Ann Thorac Surg* 62:94-104, 1996.

107. Schmid-Elsaesser R, Schröder M, Zausinger S et al: EEG burst suppression is not necessary for maximum barbiturate protection in transient focal cerebral ischemia in the rat, *J Neurol Sci* 162:14-19, 1999.

108. Hemmings, Jr, HC: Neuroprotection by sodium channel blockade and inhibition of glutamate release. In Blanck TJJ, editor: *Neuroprotection*, Baltimore, 1997, Williams & Wilkins, p 23.

109. Shenkman Z, Elami A, Weiss YG et al: Cerebral protection using retrograde cerebral perfusion during hypothermic circulatory arrest, *Can J Anaesth* 44(10):1096-1101, 1997.

110. Hurn PD, Kirsch JR, Traystman RJ: Pharmacologic neuroprotection: fact or fantasy? In Blanck TJJ, editor: *Neuroprotection*, Baltimore, 1997, Williams & Wilkins, p 47.

111. Arias RL, Tasse RP, Bowlby MR: Neuroprotective interaction effects of NMDA and AMPA receptor antagonists in an in vitro model of cerebral ischemia, *Brain Res* 816:299-308, 1999.

112. Mantz J, Chéramy A, Thierry AM et al: Anesthetic properties of riluzole (54274 RP), a new inhibitor of glutamate neurotransmission, *Anesthesiology* 76:844, 1992.

113. Wang D, Wu X, Zhong Y et al: Effect of lidocaine on improving cerebral protection provided by retrograde cerebral perfusion: a neuropathologic study, *J Cardiothorac Vasc Anesth* 13(2):176-180, 1999.

114. Tseng EE, Brock MV, Kwon CC et al: Increased intracerebral excitatory amino acids and nitric oxide after hypothermic circulatory arrest, *Ann Thorac Surg* 67:371-376, 1999.

115. Tseng EE, Brock MV, Lange MS et al: Nitric oxide mediates neurologic injury after hypothermic circulatory arrest, *Ann Thorac Surg* 67:65-71, 1999.

116. Hoffman WE, Charbel FT, Edelman G et al: Thiopental and desflurane treatment for brain protection, *Neurosurgery* 43(5):1050-1053, 1998.

117. Miura Y, Grocott HP, Bart RD et al: Differential effects of anesthetic agents on outcome from near-complete but not incomplete global ischemia in the rat, *Anesthesiology* 89:391-400, 1998.

118. Kassell NF, Haley EC, Apperson-Hansen C et al: Randomized, double-blind, vehicle-controlled trial of tirilazad mesylate in patients with aneurysmal subarachnoid hemorrhage: a cooperative study in Europe, Australia, and New Zealand, *J Neurosurg* 84:221-230, 1996.

119. Frank SM, Norris E, Crawley H: Right and left arm blood pressure discrepancies in vascular surgery patients, *Anesthesiology* 73:A105, 1983.

120. Campos JH, Ajax TJ, Knutson RM et al: Case Conference 5-1990. A 76 year old man undergoing an emergency descending thoracic aortic aneurysm repair has multiple intraoperative and postoperative complications, *J Cardiothorac Anesth* 4:631-645, 1990.

121. Cohen JA, Denisco RA, Richards TS et al: Hazardous placement of a Robertshaw-type endobronchial tube, *Anesth Analg* 65:100-101, 1986.

122. Mora M, Chuma R, Kiichi Y et al: The anesthetic management of patient with a thoracic aortic aneurysm that caused compression of the left mainstem bronchus and the right pulmonary artery, *J Cardiothorac Vasc Anesth* 7:579-584, 1993.

123. Verdant A: Chronic traumatic aneurysm of the descending thoracic aorta with compression of the tracheobronchial tree, *Can J Surg* 27:278-279, 1984.

124. Gorman RB, Merritt WT, Greenspun H et al: Aneurysmal compression of the trachea and right mainstem bronchus complicating thoracoabdominal aneurysm repair, *Anesthesiology* 79:1424-1427, 1993.

125. Jex RK, Schaff HV, Piehler JM et al: Early and late results following repair of dissections of the descending thoracic aorta, *J Vasc Surg* 3:226-237, 1986.

126. Gertler JP, Cambria RP, Brewster DC et al: Coagulation changes during thoracoabdominal aneurysm repair, *J Vasc Surg* 24:936-945, 1996.

127. Svensson LG, Crawford ES, Hess KR et al: Variables predictive of outcome in 832 patients undergoing repairs of the descending thoracic aorta, *Chest* 104:1248-1253, 1993.

128. Cambria RP, Davison K, Zannetti S et al: Perspectives over a decade with the clamp-and-sew technique, *Ann Surg* 226:294-305, 1997.

129. Von Segesser LK, Killer I, Jenni R et al: Improved distal circulatory support for repair of descending thoracic aortic aneurysms, *Ann Thorac Surg* 56:1373-1380, 1993.

130. Von Oppell UO, Dunne TT, De Groot KM et al: Spinal cord protection in the absence of collateral circulation: meta-analysis of mortality and paraplegia, *J Cardiovasc Surg* 9:685-691, 1994.

131. Kouchoukos NT, Lell WA, Karp RB et al: Hemodynamic effects of aortic clamping and decompression with a temporary shunt for resection of the descending thoracic aorta, *Surgery* 85:25-30, 1979.

132. Gelman S, McDowell H, Varner PD et al: The reason for cardiac output reduction following aortic crossclamping, *Am J Surg* 155:578-586, 1988.

133. Gelman S, Khazalei MB, Orr R et al: Blood volume redistribution during cross-clamping of the descending aorta, *Anesth Analg* 78:219-224, 1994.

134. Gelman S: The pathophysiology of aortic cross-clamping and unclamping, *Anesthesiology* 82:1026-1060, 1995.

135. Mutch WAC, Thomson IR, Teskey J et al: Phlebotomy reverses the hemodynamic consequences of thoracic aortic cross-clamping, *Anesthesiology* 73:A630, 1990.

136. Normann NA, Taylor AA, Crawford ES et al: Catecholamine release during and after cross clamping of descending thoracic aorta, *J Surg Res* 34:97-103, 1983.

137. Silverstein PR, Caldera DL, Cullen DJ et al: Avoiding the hemodynamic consequences of aortic cross-clamping and unclamping, *Anesthesiology* 50:462-466, 1979.

138. Berkowitz HD, Shetty S: Renin release and renal cortical ischemia following aortic cross-clamping, *Arch Surg* 109:612-617, 1974.

139. Joob AW, Harman PK, Kaiser DL et al: The effect of renin-angiotensin system blockade on visceral blood flow during and after thoracic cross-clamping, *J Thorac Cardiovasc Surg* 91:411-418, 1986.

140. Symbas PN, Pfaender LM, Drucker MH et al: Cross-clamping of the descending aorta, *J Thorac Cardiovasc Surg* 85:300-305, 1983.

141. Barcroft H, Samaan A: The explanation of the increase in systemic flow caused by occluding the descending thoracic aorta, *Am J Physiol* 85:47-61, 1935.

142. Gregoretti S, Gelman S, Henderson T et al: Hemodynamics and oxygen uptake below and above aortic occlusion during cross-clamping of the thoracic aorta and sodium nitroprusside infusion, *J Thorac Cardiovasc Surg* 100:830-836, 1990.

143. Roizen MF, Beaupre PN, Albert RA et al: Monitoring with two-dimensional transesophageal echocardiography. Comparison of myocardial function in patients undergoing supraceliac, suprarenal-infraceliac, or infrarenal aortic occlusion, *J Vasc Surg* 1:300-305, 1984.

144. Stokland O, Miller MM, Ilebekk A et al: Mechanism of hemodynamic responses to occlusion of the descending thoracic aorta, *Am J Physiol* 238:H423-429, 1980.

145. Aakhus S, Aadahl P, Strømholm, T, Myhre HO et al: Increased left ventricular contractility during cross-clamping of the descending thoracic aorta, *J Cardiothorac Vasc Anesth* 9:497-502, 1995.

146. Brusoni B, Colombo A, Merlo L et al: Hemodynamic and metabolic changes induced by temporary clamping of thoracic aorta, *Eur Surg Res* 10:206-216, 1978.

147. Longo T, Marchetti G, Vercellio G: Coronary hemodynamic changes induced by aortic cross-clamping, *J Cardiovasc Surg* 10: 36-42, 1969.

148. Connelly GP, Arkoff H, McKenney PA et al: Left ventricular function during proximal aortic crossclamping and left atrial-femoral bypass, *Anesthesiology* 83:A56, 1995.

149. D'Ambra NM, Dewhirst W, Jacobs M et al: Cross-clamping the thoracic aorta: Effect on intracranial pressure, *Circulation* 78(Suppl III):198-202, 1988.

150. Hantler CB, Knight PR: Intracranial hypertension following cross-clamping of the thoracic aorta, *Anesthesiology*: 56(2): 146-147, 1982.

151. Kazama S, Masaki Y, Maruyama S et al: Effect of altering cerebrospinal fluid pressure on spinal cord blood flow, *Ann Thorac Surg* 58:112-115, 1994.

152. Saether OD, Juul RM, AadahlP et al: Cerebral haemodynamics during thoracic- and thoracoabdominal aortic aneurysm repair, *Eur J Vasc Endovasc Surg* 12:81-85, 1996.

153. O'Rourke K, Beattie C, Walman AT: Acidosis during high cross-clamp surgery, *Anesthesiology* 63:A266, 1985.

154. Safi HF, Harlin SA, Miller CC et al: Predictive factors for acute renal failure in thoracic and thoracoabdominal aortic aneurysm surgery, *J Vasc Surg* 24(3):338-345, 1996.

155. Kashyap VS, Cambria RP, Davison JK et al: Renal failure after thoracoabdominal aortic failure, *J Vasc Surg* 26:949-957, 1997.

156. Gelman S, Reves JG, Fowler K et al: Regional blood flow during cross-clamping of the thoracic aorta and infusion of sodium nitroprusside, *J Thorac Cardiovasc Surg* 85:287-291, 1983.

157. Godet G, Bertrand M, Coriat P et al: Comparison of isoflurane with sodium nitroprusside for controlling hypertension during thoracic aortic cross-clamping, *J Cardiothorac Anesth* 4:177-184, 1990.

158. Marini CP, Cunningham, Jr, JN: Issues surrounding spinal cord protection. In RB Karp editor: *Advances in cardiac surgery*, vol 4, St Louis, 1993, Mosby-Year Book, pp 89-107.

159. Simpson JI, Eide TR, Schiff GA et al: Isoflurane versus sodium nitroprusside for the control of proximal hypertension during thoracic aortic cross-clamping: effects on spinal cord ischemia, *J Cardiothorac Vasc Anesth* 9:491-496, 1995.

160. Cernaianu AC, Olah A, Cilley, Jr, JH et al: Effect of sodium nitroprusside on paraplegia during cross-clamping of the thoracic aorta, *Ann Thorac Surg* 56:1035-1038, 1993.

161. Marini CP, Grubbs PE, Toporoff B et al: Effect of sodium nitroprusside on spinal cord perfusion and paraplegia during aortic cross-clamping, *Ann Thorac Surg* 47:379-383, 1989.

162. Shine T, Nugent M: Sodium nitroprusside decreases spinal cord perfusion pressure during descending thoracic aortic cross-clamping in the dog, *J Cardiothorac Anesth* 4:185-193, 1990.

163. Woloszyn TT, Marini CP, Coons MS: Cerebrospinal fluid drainage and steroids provide better spinal cord protection during aortic cross-clamping than does either treatment alone, *Ann Thorac Surg* 49:78-83, 1990.

164. Schittek A, Bennink GBWE, Cooley DA et al: Spinal cord protection with intravenous nimodipine, *J Thorac Cardiovasc Surg* 104: 1100-1105, 1992.

165. Aronson S, Goldberg LI, Glock D et al: Effects of fenoldopam on renal blood flow and systemic hemodynamics during isoflurane anesthesia, *J Cardiothorac Vasc Anesth* 5(1):29-32, 1991.

166. Murphy MB, McCoy CE, Weber RR et al: Augmentation of renal blood flow and sodium excretion in hypertensive patients during blood pressure reduction by intravenous administration of the dopamine 1 agonist fenoldopam, *Circulation* 76(6): 1312-1318, 1987.

167. Brogden RN, Markham A: Fenoldopam. A review of its pharmacodynamic and pharmacokinetic properties and intravenous clinical potential in the management of hypertensive urgencies and emergencies, *Drugs* 54(4):634-646, 1997.

168. Marini CP, Levison J, Caliendo F et al: Control of proximal hypertension during aortic cross-clamping: its effects on cerebrospinal fluid dynamics and spinal cord perfusion pressure, *Semin Thorac Cardiovasc Surg* 10:51-56, 1998.

169. Cooley DA: Single-clamp repair of aneurysms of the descending thoracic aorta, *Semin Thorac Cardiovasc Surg* 10:87-90, 1998.

170. Najafi H: Descending aortic aneurysmectomy without adjuncts to avoid ischemia—1993 update, *Ann Thorac Surg* 55: 1042-1045, 1993.

171. Safi HJ, Bartoli S, Hess KR et al: Neurologic deficit in patients at high risk with thoracoabdominal aortic aneurysms: the role of cerebral spinal fluid drainage and distal aortic perfusion, *J Vasc Surg* 20:434-443, 1994.

172. Coselli JS: Thoracoabdominal aortic aneurysms: experience with 372 patients, *J Card Surg* 9:638-647, 1994.

173. Lawrie GM, Earle N, De Bakey ME: Evolution of surgical techniques for aneurysms of the descending thoracic aorta: twenty-nine years experience with 659 patients, *J Card Surg* 9:648-661, 1994.

174. Nicolosi AC, Almassi GH, Bousamra M et al: Mortality and neurologic morbidity after repair of traumatic aortic disruption, *Ann Thorac Surg* 61:875-878, 1996.

175. Biglioli P, Spirito R, Pompilio G et al: Descending thoracic aorta aneurysmectomy: left-left centrifugal pump versus simple clamping technique, *Cardiovasc Surg* 3:511-518, 1995.

176. Bavaria JE, Woo J, Hall RA et al: Retrograde cerebral and distal aortic perfusion during ascending and thoracoabdominal aortic operations, *Ann Thorac Surg* 60:345-353, 1995.

177. Verdant A, Cossette R, Pagé A et al: Aneurysms of the descending thoracic aorta: three hundred sixty-six consecutive cases resected without paraplegia, *J Vasc Surg* 21:385-391, 1995.

178. Safi HJ, Winnerkvist A, Miller III, CC et al: Effect of extended cross-clamp time during thoracoabdominal aortic aneurysm repair, *Ann Thorac Surg* 66:1204-1209, 1998.

179. Safi HJ, Miller III, CC, Carr C et al: Importance of intercostal artery reattachment during thoracoabdominal aortic aneurysm repair, *J Vasc Surg* 27:58-68, 1998.

180. Svensson LG: Management of segmental intercostal and lumbar arteries during descending and thoracoabdominal aneurysms repairs, *Semin Thorac Cardiovasc Surg* 10:45-49, 1998.

181. Comerota AJ, White JV: Reducing morbidity of thoracoabdominal aneurysm repair by preliminary axillofemoral bypass, *Am J Surg* 170:218-222, 1995.

182. Stühmeier KD, Grabitz K, Mainzer B et al: Use of the electrospinogram for predicting harmful spinal cord ischemia during repair of thoracic or thoracoabdominal aortic aneurysms, *Anesthesiology* 79:1170-1176, 1993.

183. Mandelbaum I, Webb MK: Left ventricular function during cross-clamping of the descending thoracic aorta, *JAMA* 186: 229-231, 1963.

184. Ataka K, Okada M, Yoshimura N et al: Surgical treatment for aneurysms of the descending aorta using temporary perfusion by a centrifugal pump: clinical analysis of 33 cases, *Artif Organs* 17:901-905, 1993.

185. Sander-Jensen K, Krogager G, Pettersson G: Left atrial-aortic/femoral bypass with a centrifugal pump without systemic heparin during surgery on the descending aorta, *Artif Organs,* 19: 774-776, 1995.

186. Borst HG, Jurmann M, Bühner B et al: Risk of replacement of descending aorta with a standardized left heart bypass technique, *J Thorac Cardiovasc Surg* 107:126-133, 1994.

187. Safi HJ, Campbell MP, Ferreira ML et al: Spinal cord protection in descending thoracic and thoracoabdominal aortic aneurysm repair, *Semin Thorac Cardiovasc Surg* 10:41-44, 1998.

188. Brant B, Armstrong R, Vetto RM: Vasodepressor factor in declamp shock production, *Surgery* 67:650, 1970.

189. Roberts AJ, Nora JD, Hughes WA et al: Cardiac and renal responses to cross-clamping of the descending thoracic aorta, *J Thorac Cardiovasc Surg* 86:732-741, 1983.

190. Livesay JJ, Cooley DA, Ventemiglia RA et al: Surgical experience in descending thoracic aneurysmectomy with and without adjuncts to avoid ischemia, *Ann Thorac Surg* 39:37-46, 1985.

191. Beattie C, Frank SM: Anesthesia for major vascular surgery. In Rogers M, Tinker T, Covino B, editors: *Principles and practice of anesthesiology,* St Louis, 1993, Mosby, pp 1931-1967.

192. Cohen JR, Sardari F, Paul J et al: Increased intestinal permeability: implications for thoracoabdominal aneurysm repair, *Ann Vasc Surg* 6:433-437, 1992.

193. Van Norman G, Pavlin E, Pavlin J: Hemodynamic and metabolic changes after thoracic aortic unclamping, *Anesthesiology* 71:A59, 1989.

194. Griepp RB, Ergin MA, Galla JD et al: Looking for the artery of Adamkiewicz: a quest to minimize paraplegia after operations for aneurysms of the descending thoracic and thoracoabdominal aorta, *J Thorac Cardiovasc Surg* 112:1202-1215, 1996.

195. Griepp RB, Ergin MA, Galla JD et al: Minimizing spinal cord injury during repair of descending thoracic and thoracoabdominal aneurysms: the Mount Sinai approach, *Semin Thorac Cardiovasc Surg* 10:25-28, 1998.

196. Acher CW, Wynn MM: Multifactoral nature of spinal cord circulation, *Semin Thorac Cardiovasc Surg* 10(1):7-10, 1998.

197. Gharagozloo F, Neville, Jr, RF, Cox JL: Spinal cord protection during surgical procedures on the descending thoracic and thoracoabdominal aorta: a critical overview, *Semin Thorac Cardiovasc Surg* 10:73-86, 1998.

198. Safi HJ, Miller III, CC, Reardon MJ et al: Operation for acute and chronic aortic dissection: recent outcome with regard to neurologic deficit and early death, *Ann Thorac Surg* 66:402-411, 1998.

199. Svensson LG, Hess KR, D'Agostino RS et al: Reduction of neurologic injury after high-risk thoracoabdominal aortic operation, *Ann Thorac Surg* 66:132-138, 1998.

200. Svensson LG, Crawford ES, Hess KR et al: Experience with 1509 patients undergoing thoracoabdominal aortic operations, *J Vasc Surg* 17:357-370, 1993.

201. Heinemann MK, Brassek F, Herzog T et al: The role of spinal angiography in operations on the thoracic aorta: myth or reality? *Ann Thorac Surg* 65:346-351, 1998.

202. Kouchoukos NT, Rokkas CK: Descending thoracic and thoracoabdominal aortic surgery for aneurysm or dissection: how do we minimize the risk of spinal cord injury? *Semin Thorac Cardiovasc Surg* 5:47-54, 1993.

203. Svensson LG: Intraoperative identification of spinal cord blood supply during repairs of descending aorta and thoracoabdominal aorta. *J Thorac Cardiovasc Surg* 112:1455-1461, 1996.

204. de Haan P, Kalkman CJ, de Mol BA et al: Efficacy of transcranial motor-evoked myogenic potentials to detect spinal cord ischemia during operations for thoracoabdominal aneurysms, *J Thorac Cardiovasc Surg* 113:87-101, 1997.

205. Biglioli P, Spirito R, Porqueddu M et al: Quick, simple clamping technique in descending thoracic aortic aneurysm repair, *Ann Thorac Surg* 67(4):1038-1043, 1999.

206. Ryan T, Mannion D, O'Brien W et al: Spinal cord perfusion pressure in dogs after control of proximal aortic hypertension during thoracic aortic cross-clamping with esmolol or sodium nitroprusside, *Anesthesiology* 78:317-325, 1993.

207. Clark FJS, Mutch WAC, Sutton IR et al: Treatment of proximal aortic hypertension after thoracic cross-clamping in dogs: phlebotomy versus sodium nitroprusside/isoflurane, *Anesthesiology* 77:357-364, 1992.

208. Svensson LG, Hess KR, Coselli JS et al: Influence of segmental arteries, extent, and atriofemoral bypass on postoperative paraplegia after thoracoabdominal aortic operations, *J Vasc Surg* 20(2):255-262, 1994.

209. Cambria RP, Davison JK: Regional hypothermia for prevention of spinal cord ischemic complications after thoracoabdominal aortic surgery: experience with epidural cooling, *Semin Thorac Cardiovasc Surg* 10:61-65, 1998.

210. Cunningham JN, Laschinger JC, Spencer FC: Monitoring of somatosensory evoked potentials during surgical procedures on the thoracoabdominal aorta, Part IV, *J Thorac Cardiovasc Surg* 94:275-285, 1987.

211. Schepens MAAM, Boezeman EHJF, Hamerlijnck RPHM et al: Somatosensory evoked potentials during exclusion and reperfusion of critical aortic segments in thoracoabdominal aortic aneurysm surgery, *J Card Surg* 9:692-702, 1994.

212. Guerit JM, Verhelst R, Rubay J et al: Multilevel somatosensory evoked potentials (SEPs) for spinal cord monitoring in descending thoracic and thoraco-abdominal aortic surgery, *Eur J Cardiothorac Surg* 10:93-103, 1996.

213. Galla JD, Ergin MA, Sadeghi AM et al: A new technique using somatosensory evoked potential guidance during descending and thoracoabdominal aortic repairs, *J Card Surg* 9:662-672, 1994.

214. Crawford ES, Mizrahi EM, Hess KR: The impact of distal aortic perfusion and somatosensory evoked potential monitoring on prevention of paraplegia after aortic aneurysm operation, *J Thorac Cardiovasc Surg* 95:357-367, 1988.

215. Yamamoto N, Takano H, Kitagawa H et al: Monitoring for spinal cord ischemia by use of the evoked spinal cord potentials during aortic aneurysm surgery, *J Vasc Surg* 20:826-833, 1994.

216. Matsui Y, Goh K, Shiiya N et al: Clinical application of evoked spinal cord potentials elicited by direct stimulation of the cord during temporary occlusion of the thoracic aorta, *J Thorac Cardiovasc Surg* 107:1519-1527, 1994.

217. Mongan PD, Peterson RE, Williams D: Spinal evoked potentials are predictive of neurologic function in a porcine model of aortic occlusion, *Anesth Analg* 78:257-266, 1994.

218. Shiiya N, Yasuda K, Matsui Y et al: Spinal cord protection during thoracoabdominal aortic aneurysm repair: results of selective reconstruction of the critical segmental arteries guided by evoked spinal cord potential monitoring, *J Vasc Surg* 21: 970-975, 1995.

219. Jacobs MJHM, Meylaerts SA, de Haan P et al: Strategies to prevent neurologic deficit based on motor-evoked potentials in type I and II thoracoabdominal aortic aneurysm repair, *J Vasc Surg* 29(1):48-57, 1999.

220. Robertazzi RR, Cunningham, Jr, JN: Intraoperative adjuncts of spinal cord protection, *Semin Thorac Cardiovasc Surg* 10(1):29-34, 1998.

221. Grabitz K, Sandmann W, Stuhmeier K et al: The risk of ischemic spinal cord injury in patients undergoing graft replacement for thoracoabdominal aortic aneurysms, *J Vasc Surg* 23(2):230-240, 1996.

222. Acher CW, Wynn MM, Hoch JR et al: Combined use of cerebral spinal fluid drainage and naloxone reduces the risk of paraplegia in thoracoabdominal aneurysm repair, *J Vasc Surg* 19:236-248, 1994.

223. McCullough JL, Hollier LH, Nugent M: Paraplegia after thoracic aortic occlusion: influence of cerebrospinal fluid drainage, *J Vasc Surg* 7:153-160, 1988.

224. Bower TC, Murray MJ, Gloviczki P: Effects of thoracic aortic occlusion and cerebrospinal fluid drainage on regional spinal cord blood flow in dogs: correlation with neurologic outcome, *J Vasc Surg* 9:135-144, 1988.

225. Dasmahapatra HK, Coles JG, Wilson GJ: Relationship between cerebrospinal fluid dynamics and reversible spinal cord ischemia during experimental thoracic aortic occlusion, *J Thorac Cardiovasc Surg* 95:920-923, 1988.

226. Kaplan DK, Atsumi N, D'Ambra MN et al: Distal circulatory support for thoracic aortic operations: effects on intracranial pressure, *Ann Thorac Surg* 59:448-452, 1995.

227. Wadouh F, Lindemann EM, Arndt CF et al: The arteria radicularis magna anterior as a decisive factor influencing spinal cord damage during aortic occlusion, *J Thorac Cardiovasc Surg* 88:1-10, 1984.

228. Elmore JR, Glovickzi P, Harper M: Failure of motor evoked potentials to predict neurologic outcome in experimental thoracic aortic occlusion, *J Vasc Surg* 14:131-139, 1991.

229. Wisselink W, Becker MO, Nguyen JH et al: Protecting the ischemic spinal cord during aortic clamping: the influence of selective hypothermia and spinal cord perfusion pressure, *J Vasc Surg* 19:788-796, 1994.

230. Nugent M: Pro: cerebrospinal fluid drainage prevents paraplegia, *J Cardiothorac Vasc Surg* 6:366-368, 1992.

231. Crawford ES, Svensson LG, Hess KR et al: A prospective randomized study of cerebrospinal fluid drainage to prevent paraplegia after high-risk surgery on the thoracoabdominal aorta, *J Vasc Surg* 13:36-46, 1990.

232. Murray MJ, Bower TC, Oliver WC et al: Effects of cerebrospinal fluid drainage in patients undergoing thoracic and thoracoabdominal aortic surgery, *J Cardiothorac Vasc Anesth* 7:266-272, 1993.

233. Hill AB, Kalman PG, Johnston KW et al: Reversal of delayed-onset paraplegia after thoracic aortic surgery with cerebrospinal fluid drainage, *J Vasc Surg* 20:315-317, 1994.

234. Schoenwald P, Gottlieb A, Lewis B et al: Cerebrospinal fluid pressure (CSFP) during aortic cross-clamp (XC) as a predictor of neurologic outcome during thoracoabdominal aneurysm repair, *Anesthesiology* 77:A71, 1992.

235. Hollier LH, Money SR, Naslund TC et al: Risk of spinal cord dysfunction in patients undergoing thoracoabdominal aortic placement, *Am J Surg* 164:210-213, 1992.

236. Acher CW, Wynn MM, Archibald J: Naloxone and spinal fluid drainage as adjuncts in the surgical treatment of thoracoabdominal and thoracic aneurysms, *Surgery* 108:755-762, 1990.

237. Sun J, Hirsch D, Svensson G: Spinal cord protection by papaverine and intrathecal cooling during aortic crossclamping, *J Cardiovasc Surg* 39(6):839-842, 1998.

238. Svensson LG, Von Ritter CM, Grieneveld HT: Cross-clamping of the thoracic aorta, *Ann Surg* 204:38-47, 1986.

239. Vacanti FX, Ames AA: Mild hypothermia and Mg ++ protect against irreversible damage during CNS ischemia, *Stroke* 15:695-698, 1983.

240. Kouchoukos NT, Daily BB, Rokkas CK et al: Hypothermic bypass and circulatory arrest for operations on the descending thoracic and thoracoabdominal aorta, *Ann Thorac Surg* 60:67-77, 1995.

241. Rokkas CK, Kouchoukos NT: Profound hypothermia for spinal cord protection in operations on the descending thoracic and thoracoabdominal aorta, *Semin Thorac Cardiovasc Surg* 10(1):57-60, 1998.

242. Kakinohana M, Taira Y, Marsala M: The effect of graded post-ischemic spinal cord hypothermia on neurological outcome and histopathology after transient spinal ischemia in rat, *Anesthesiology* 90(3):789-798, 1999.

243. Wakamatsu H, Matsumoto M, Nakakimura K et al: The effects of moderate hypothermia and intrathecal tetracaine on glutamate concentrations of intrathecal dialysate and neurologic and histopathologic outcome in transient spinal cord ischemia in rabbits, *Anesth Analg* 88(1):56-62, 1999.

244. Tuzgen S, Kaynar MY, Guner A et al: The effect of epidural cooling on lipid peroxidation after experimental spinal cord injury, *Spinal Cord* 36(9):654-657, 1998.

245. Kieffer E, Koskas F, Walden R et al: Hypothermic circulatory arrest for thoracic aneurysmectomy through left-sided thoracotomy, *J Vasc Surg* 19:457-464, 1994.

246. Grabenwöger M, Ehrlich M, Simon P et al: Thoracoabdominal aneurysm repair: spinal cord protection using profound hypothermia and circulatory arrest, *J Card Surg* 9:679-684, 1994.

247. Frank SM, Parker SD, Rock P et al: Moderate hypothermia, with partial bypass and segmental sequential repair for thoracoabdominal aortic aneurysm, *J Vasc Surg* 19:687-697, 1994.

248. Fehrenbacher JW, McCready RA, Hormuth DA et al: One-stage segmental resection of extensive thoracoabdominal aneurysms with left-sided heart bypass, *J Vasc Surg* 18:366-371, 1993.

249. Tabayashi K, Niibori K, Konno H et al: Protection from post-ischemic spinal cord injury by perfusion cooling of the epidural space, *Ann Thorac Surg* 56:494-498, 1993.

250. Laschinger JC, Cunningham JN, Cooper MM: Prevention of ischemic spinal cord injury following aortic cross-clamping: use of corticosteroids, *Ann Thorac Surg* 38:500-507, 1984.

251. Yum SW, Faden AI: Comparison of the neuroprotective effects of the N-methyl-D-aspartate antagonist MK-801 and the opiate-receptor antagonist nalmefene in experimental spinal cord ischemia, *Arch Neurol* 47:277-281, 1990.

252. Rhee RY, Gloviczki P, Cambria RA et al: The effects of nimodipine on ischemic injury of the spinal cord during thoracic aortic cross-clamping, *Int Angiol* 15:153-161, 1996.

253. Westaby S, Katsumata T, Vaccari G: Arch and descending aortic aneurysms: influence of perfusion technique on neurological outcome, *Eur J Cardiothorac Surg* 15:180-185, 1999.

254. Follis FM, Blisard KS, Varvitsiotis PS et al: Selective protection of gray and white matter during spinal cord ischemic injury, *Ann Thorac Surg* 67(5):1362-1369, 1999.

255. Lang-Lazdunski L, Heurteaux C, Vaillant N et al: Riluzole prevents ischemic spinal cord injury caused by aortic crossclamping, *J Thorac Cardiovasc Surg* 117(5):881-889, 1999.

256. Simpson JI, Eide TR, Schiff GA et al: Intrathecal magnesium sulfate protects the spinal cord from ischemic injury during thoracic aortic cross-clamping, *Anesthesiology* 81:1493-1499, 1994.

257. Breckwoldt WL, Genco CM, Connolly RJ: Spinal cord protection during aortic occlusion: efficacy of intrathecal tetracaine, *Ann Thorac Surg* 51:959-963, 1991.

258. Attar A, Tuna H, Sargon MF et al: Early protective effects of Iloprost after experimental spinal cord injury, *Neurol Res* 20:353-359, 1998.

259. Mutch WAC, Thiessen DB, Girling LG et al: Neuroanesthesia adjunct therapy (mannitol and hyperventilation) is as effective as cerebrospinal fluid drainage for prevention of paraplegia after descending thoracic aortic cross-clamping in the dog, *Anesth Analg* 81:800-805, 1995.

260. Parodi JC, Palmaz JC, Barone HD: Transfemoral intraluminal graft implantation for abdominal aortic aneurysms, *Ann Vasc Surg* 5(6):491-499, 1991.

261. Nienaber CA, Fattori R, Lund G et al: Nonsurgical reconstruction of thoracic aortic dissection by stent-graft placement, *N Engl J Med* 340:1539-1545, 1999.

262. Mitchell RS, Miller DC, Dake MD: Stent-graft repair of thoracic aortic aneurysms, *Semin Vasc Surg* 10(4):257-271, 1997.

263. Dake MD, Miller DC, Semba CP et al: Transluminal placement of endovascular stent-grafts for the treatment of descending thoracic aortic aneurysms, *N Engl J Med* 331(26):1729-1734, 1994.

264. Baker AB, Lloyd G, Fraser TA et al: Retrospective review of 100 cases of endoluminal aortic stent-graft surgery from an anaesthetic perspective, *Anaesth Intens Care* 25:378-384, 1997.

265. Dake MD, Miller DC, Mitchell RS et al: The "first generation" of endovascular stent-grafts for patients with aneurysms of the descending thoracic aorta, *J Thorac Cardiovasc Surg* 116(5):689-703, 1998.

266. Dake MD, Kato N, Mitchell RS et al: Endovascular stent-graft placement for the treatment of acute aortic dissection, *N Engl J Med* 340:1546-1552, 1999.

267. Engle J, Safi HJ, Miller III, CC et al: The impact of diaphragm management on prolonged ventilator support after thoracoabdominal aortic repair, *J Vasc Surg* 29(1):150-156, 1999.

268. Svensson LG, Hess KR, Coselli JS et al: A prospective study of respiratory failure after high-risk surgery on the thoracoabdominal aorta, *J Vasc Surg* 14(3):271-282, 1991.

269. Money SR, Rice K, Crockett D et al: Risk of respiratory failure after repair of thoracoabdominal aortic aneurysms, *Am J Surg* 168(2):152-155, 1994.

270. Godet G, Fleron MH, Vicaut E et al: Risk factors for acute postoperative renal failure in thoracic or thoracoabdominal aortic surgery: a prospective study, *Anesth Analg* 85(6):1227-1232, 1997.

271. Gilling-Smith GL, Worswick L, Knight PF et al: Surgical repair of thoracoabdominal aortic aneurysm: 10 years' experience, *Br J Surg* 82(5):624-629, 1995.

CHAPTER 15

Cardiac Transplantation

Ivan S. Salgo, M.D. ■ Rebecca Barnett, M.D.

OUTLINE

One of the great medical achievements of the latter twentieth century has been the advent of organ transplantation. At one time, heart transplantation was reserved for newspaper headlines, but now it is commonly performed at many major medical centers. Approximately 2500 heart transplants are performed each year in the United States, and heart transplantation has a 10-year survival rate approaching 50%.[1]

The most common indications for transplantation include idiopathic dilated cardiomyopathy and ischemic heart disease, each of which accounts for nearly half of the transplant population in any given year.[2]

Alternatives to cardiac allotransplantation include xenotransplantation, cardiomyoplasty, left ventricular volume reduction surgery, and long-term mechanical circulatory support. Immunosuppression, graft vasculopathy, and the potential transfer of animal infection to humans are current limitations to xenotransplantation. Cardiomyoplasty (use of a latissimus dorsi muscle pedicle around the heart to assist the cardiac pumping) has not had optimal survival rates.[2] The Batista operation and other forms of ventricular volume reduction surgery are more common in countries with a minimum or lack of donor hearts. Active research in ventricular

remodeling surgery may eventually increase this application, as will advances in gene therapy research to restore or regrow healthy myocytes. Permanent implantable systems are emerging, including axial flow devices and devices that are wrapped around the heart.

Immunosuppression is central to the successful outcome of cardiac transplantation and remains one of the great medical challenges of the early twenty-first century.[3] The technical issues of implantation are dwarfed by the complexities of immunosuppression and transplant rejection. Although a straightforward heart transplant is a routine operation, complexities in coexisting organ disease require expertise by the anesthesiologist in managing patients through surgery. A rigorous understanding of the management of right and left ventricular dysfunction is fundamental to successful outcome.[4-6]

Heart transplantation remains the only means to life for those with end-stage heart disease. There are, unfortunately, insufficient donor hearts to accommodate the urgent need for many patients in congestive heart failure.[7] Advancements in ventricular assist device (VAD) technology have increased survival and increased the number of patients awaiting cardiac transplantation. Hearts are typically matched to recipient size and ABO blood group.

The logistics of actual resource coordination is complicated by the relatively short allowable ischemic time of the donor heart (approximately 4 to 6 hours).[8] The donor is frequently in another city. Rigorous communication between the attending anesthesiologist and surgeon is critical for coordinating the surgical procedure and minimizing ischemic time of the donor heart.

The cardiac condition of patients awaiting cardiac transplantation varies in severity, from well compensated with intravenous medications or VADs, to severe cardiac decompensation. The most critical patients have congestive heart failure, renal insufficiency, and pulmonary edema. Modern practice involves selecting patients who are optimally compensated by medical or surgical therapy before they receive their transplant so that they can tolerate the concomitant physiologic insult of surgery and immunosuppression.

TREATMENT OF CHRONIC HEART FAILURE

Congestive heart failure represents a major health problem affecting more than 2 million Americans, with 500,000 new cases diagnosed each year.[9]

The failing heart is characterized by decreased force of contractility, impaired relaxation, and decreased response to β-adrenergic stimulation (Figs. 15-1 and 15-2). Heart failure involves a complex interplay between cardiac mechanics and neurohumoral regulation.[10-12] Etiologic factors for heart failure include coronary artery disease, hypertension, valvular lesions, and primary cardiomyopathies (e.g., viral or postpartum). There are less understood risk factors for women who develop heart failure.[13] The decreased capacity for ejection of blood leads to an imbalance between oxygen delivery and tissue consumption and an inability to regulate fluid homeostasis.

Therapy includes reducing systemic vascular resistance, increasing cardiac contractility, and reducing total body sodium and fluid. Common drugs used to support the failing heart include inotropic agents, diuretics, angiotensin-converting enzyme inhibitors (ACEIs), nitrates, calcium channel blockers, and, more recently, β-blockers.[14] Although digitalis has been used in selected cases of heart failure, its use is declining with the advent of newer therapies.[9,15] ACEIs have been shown repeatedly to prolong survival.[9]

A decreased risk of sudden death and reinfarction is observed in patients with heart failure who tolerate β-blockade.[16] Carvedilol is a β-blocker and vasodilator that provides substantial improvement in left ventricular ejection fraction for both idiopathic dilated and ischemic cardiomyopathy.[17] The physiologic benefits of β-blockers include a slower heart rate, fewer arrhythmias, a myocyte protective effect from the toxic effects of catecholamines, upregulated β-receptor density, restored receptor coupling to the postreceptor pathway, and improved myocardial contractility.[18] Support with mechanical VADs improves myocyte contractile properties and increases β-adrenergic responsiveness. Newer drugs for treating congestive heart failure facilitate more effective management. Common errors in the management of congestive heart failure include prescribing digitalis for diastolic dysfunction and prescribing high-dose negative inotropic agents such as β-blockers.[9] Other problems include insufficient monitoring of electrolyte levels with the use of diuretics and combinations of β-blockers and calcium blockers that produce bradycardia.

The spectrum of medical therapy must be weighed

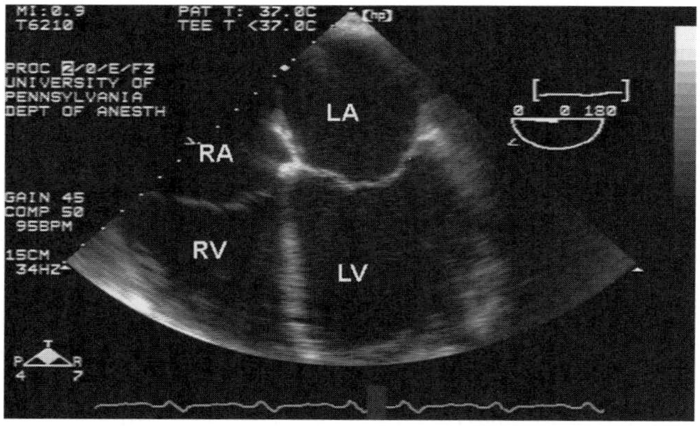

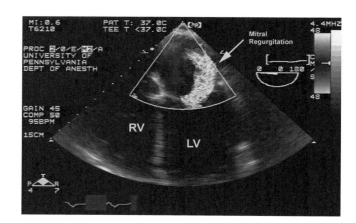

FIG. 15-1 Echocardiographic view of dilated cardiomyopathy. Midesophageal four-chamber view of left and right atria and ventricles. *LA*, Left atrium; *LV*, left ventricle; *RA*, right atrium; *RV*, right ventricle.

FIG. 15-2 Echocardiographic view of mitral regurgitation. Dilation of the left ventricle can increase the size of the mitral annulus. This affects leaflet coaptation and patients with dilated cardiomyopathy can frequently have severe mitral regurgitation. This figure demonstrates Doppler mapping of a large jet. *LV*, Left ventricle; *RV*, right ventricle.

against the common side effects. The following questions are considered preoperatively. Is the patient well optimized with the regimen? Does the patient have signs or symptoms of left and right heart failure such as pulmonary edema, hepatic congestion, renal insufficiency, and peripheral edema? If the patient is not optimized, what effect will the anesthetic and surgery have on physiologic function?

PATIENT SELECTION

Common indications for cardiac transplantation include congestive heart failure refractory to maximum medical therapy, intractable angina pectoris with inoperable coronary artery disease, and malignant ventricular arrhythmias unaffected by pharmacologic or surgical intervention. The most common causes are ischemic heart disease or viral myocarditis, but many cases are idiopathic in origin.[3,19] Exclusion criteria are conditions that complicate postoperative recovery or long-term survival with a transplanted heart.[20] These criteria can include severe fixed pulmonary hypertension, debilitating stroke, severe peripheral vascular disease, the presence of human immunodeficiency virus (HIV) antibody, sepsis, and active malignancy. Carefully selected patients with malignancy in remission have been treated successfully.[21] Hepatic and renal failure are only relative contraindications in this era of combined organ transplantation. The presence of coexisting disease and the patient's social situation are evaluated by a hospital's heart transplant committee, comprising surgeons, cardiologists, anesthesiologists, nurses, and social workers. Heart transplantation requires both psychologic and physical preparation. The recipient patient requires a strong social support network of friends and family to help with the postoperative recovery and long-term medical compliance. Patients who are unable to discontinue the use of recreational drugs, alcohol, or tobacco are poor candidates.

Heart transplant allocation is managed by the United Network For Organ Sharing (UNOS). UNOS is a private, not-for-profit organization that contracts with the U.S. Department of Health and Human Services to administer the national Organ Procurement and Transplantation Network and the U.S. Scientific Registry on Organ Transplantation.[22] Patients are classified according to the list in Table 15-1.

VENTRICULAR ASSIST DEVICE THERAPY

Patients awaiting heart transplantation face two major dilemmas. Many patients sustain reversible end-organ ischemia and total body fluid overload because of cardiogenic shock. Others wait for protracted periods before an organ becomes available, provided their native heart sustains life. Patients in the initial phases of shock experience pulmonary edema, hepatic congestion, and renal insufficiency. The increased preoperative morbidity of these patients worsens their survival, even if a heart became available within days. Use of mechanical support in patients with end-stage heart disease may improve the outcome of heart transplantation. The hemodynamic benefits of mechanical assistance convert high-risk, terminally ill patients into reconditioned heart-transplant recipients.[1,23] The routine clinical use of mechanical assist overcomes many problems, if only to increase the population of those waiting for too few donor hearts.

VADs include extracorporeal membrane oxygenation (ECMO), univentricular and biventricular extracorporeal nonpulsatile devices, extracorporeal and implantable pulsatile devices, and the complete artificial heart.

VADs are useful in two types of patients. The first consists of patients who require ventricular assistance to allow the heart to rest and recover its function by unloading the ventricle, diminishing myocardial work, and maximizing perfusion. Mechanical unloading attenuates development of myocardial histologic abnormalities, including normalization of fiber orientation and regression of myocyte hypertrophy.[1,24] Left ventricular assist device (LVAD) support can reveal functional plasticity even in the most severely failing human hearts, supporting the concept that mechanical circulatory support improves myocardial function. Contraction magnitude, rates of shortening and relengthening, and β-adrenergic responsiveness are increased. Hence, LVAD support promotes favorable ventricular remodeling.[25]

The second indication for VAD implantation is irreversible heart disease from myocardial infarction, acute myocarditis, or end-stage heart disease. These patients are not expected to recover adequate cardiac function and require mechanical support as a bridge to transplantation.[26] Less than 5% of these patients recover without cardiac transplantation.[10,27-29]

TABLE 15-1 UNOS Policy 3.7, Heart Transplant Status Listing	
IA	VAD <1 mo, artificial heart, ECMO, IABP, VAD complication, intubation, use of a single high-dose inotropic agent
IB	VAD >30 days, IV drugs
II	Not status I but suitable
VII	Temporarily unsuitable

ECMO, Extracorporeal membrane oxygenation; *IABP*, intraaortic balloon pump; *IV*, intravenous; *VAD*, ventricular assist device.

TABLE 15-2
Ventricular Assist Device (VAD) Characteristics

	THORATEC VAD	ABIOMED BVS 5000	TCI HEARTMATE NOVACOR N100
Pump drive	Pneumatic	Pneumatic	Pneumatic or electric
Patient size	Small-large	BSA > 1.3	BSA > 1.5
Pump placement	"Paracorporeal"	Extracorporeal	LVAD
Ventricular support	LVAD, RVAD, BiVAD	LVAD, RVAD, BiVAD	LVAD
Cannulation	Ventricular and atrial	Atrial	Ventricular
Anticoagulation	IV or oral	IV	Heartmate: minimal
			Novacor: IV or oral
Mobilization	Yes	No	
Transfer from ICU	Yes	No	
Duration	Short-long	Short	Long

BiVAD, Biventricular assist device; *BSA*, body surface area; *ICU*, intensive care unit; *IV*, intravenous; *LVAD*, left ventricular assist device; *RVAD*, right ventricular assist device; *TCI*, thermo cardiosystems.

The first cardiopulmonary bypass device was used clinically in 1953.[2] By the third quarter of the twentieth century, only perioperative mechanical assist pumps requiring *full anticoagulation* were available. These were used for periods of days as ECMO or mechanical assist devices. The profound bleeding complications and eventual infection precluded long-term (i.e., weeks, months, or years) support. Research focus shifted to developing artificial hearts as human heart transplantation became common and organ shortage became real.

The two fundamental design goals for long-term mechanical assist devices are the prevention of both thromboembolism and infection. Engineering of the design has focused on developing "blood-friendly" surfaces that generate pulsatile flow. Some of these devices are fully implantable (HeartMate, Thermo Cardiosystems, Woburn, Mass.; Novacor, Baxter Healthcare, Oakland, Calif.) and others are external (Thoratec VAS, Thoratec Laboratories, Pleasanton, Calif.) (Table 15-2).

The more recent implantable devices have smaller portable consoles that allow patients to be active and participate in work activities. Electrical devices are smaller than externally powered pneumatic devices. In 1994 the U.S. Food and Drug Administration approved VADs as a bridge to transplantation. The Thermo Cardiosystems HeartMate 1205 VE device (Thermo Cardiosystems) and the Novacor N100 left ventricular assist system (Baxter Healthcare) are implanted through a median sternotomy. The inflow cannula is inserted into the left ventricular apex and an outflow conduit is connected to a cannula in the ascending aorta. (The device's pumping chamber is placed within the abdominal wall.)

Typical pulsatile VAD is operated in either a fixed-rate mode or, more often, an automatic mode that more closely resembles normal physiologic conditions. In automatic mode, the device ejects when the pump becomes 90% full or when it senses a decreased filling rate. As activity increases, the pump fills faster and the rate automatically increases. This results in an increase in pump output. The heart frequently does not override the device and eject blood. Hence the aortic valve does not open and total body cardiac output is provided entirely from the VAD. These devices require an "air vent" tunneled through the skin that allows the diaphragm to move inside the pumping chamber. (There is air on one side of the diaphragm and blood on the other.)

Abiomed

The Abiomed (Danvers, Mass.) BVS 5000 is a two-chambered extracorporeal device that is useful for short-term management of heart failure over a period of days to 2 weeks[30,31] (Figs. 15-3 and 15-4). Patients with failed heart transplantation, myocarditis, or ventricular failure after cardiopulmonary bypass are typical recipients. This device is not intended as a long-term bridge to transplantation. These patients undergo intrinsic myocardial recovery and are weaned from the device or are reimplanted with a long-term device. The device is implanted with conventional surgical techniques. It is a widely available emergency device in cardiac surgical centers that may or may not have a mechanical assist program. Patients with this device remain intubated in an intensive care unit (ICU). Meticulous anticoagula-

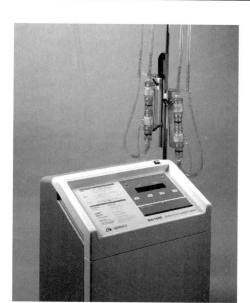

FIG. 15-3 Abiomed BVS 5000 console and pumping chambers.

(Courtesy Abiomed, Danvers, Mass.)

tion with heparin is required to prevent stroke or pulmonary embolus.

HeartMate

The Thermo Cardiosystems HeartMate contains a sintered titanium surface that encourages cellular deposition and formation of an autologous tissue lining.[2] Tissue valves within the device provide unidirectional flow, obviating the need for full anticoagulation. The LVAD receives blood from the apex of the left ventricle and returns blood to the ascending aorta (Fig. 15-5). Its pumping chamber consists of a diaphragm that is pneumatically compressed; the rate of compression is determined by a flow sensor that determines the amount of blood entering the VAD device. The pneumatic drive console is portable and contains electronics that regulate LVAD flow and detect problems. A battery-sustained, electrically driven HeartMate with a smaller console is used both as a bridge to transplantation and as a permanent alternative in patients who are unable to receive a donor heart (Fig. 15-6).

Novacor

The Novacor LVAD contains a smooth blood-contacting surface. Blood is propelled by a pusher plate acting on a polyurethane sac.[2] As with the HeartMate, blood is received from the left ventricular apex and returned via the aortic root. The device is operated through a console

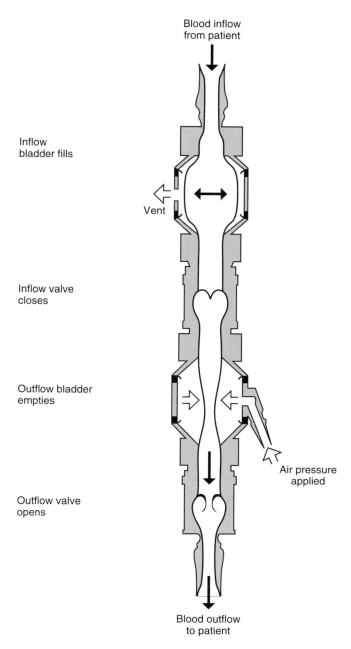

FIG. 15-4 Abiomed BVS 5000 pumping chambers schematic. Blood enters the top of the chamber and is pneumatically ejected. Note the presence of an artificial valve.

(Courtesy Abiomed, Danvers, Mass.)

unit or by a small wearable vest for portable modus. The level of anticoagulation required is similar to that required for mechanical heart valves.

Thoratec

Right ventricular (RV) failure, hypovolemia, and venodilatation decrease LVAD flow. Appropriate initial treatment consists of volume repletion while assessing right heart function. Central venous pressure is evaluated with central venous catheter placement or physical exam. Hepatic congestion and elevated filling of the external jugular vein indicate increased central venous pressure. The Thoratec VAD system consists of an externally positioned, pneumatically driven, diaphragm

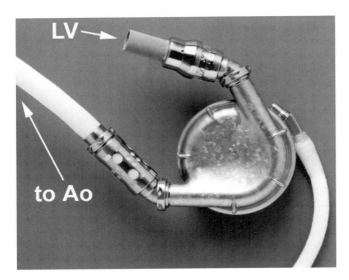

FIG. 15-5 Thermo Cardiosystems HeartMate. This pumping chamber is implanted within the abdomen. The inflow (from left ventricle *[LV]*) and outflow (to aorta *[Ao]*) are shown.

(Courtesy Thermo Cardiosystems, Woburn, Mass.)

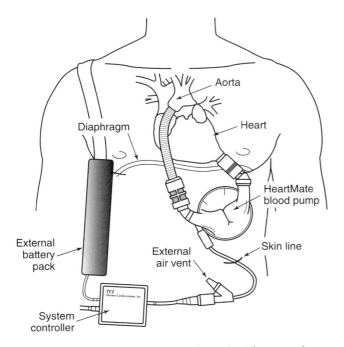

FIG. 15-6 Electric HeartMate schematic. The cannula arrangement is shown. Note the air vent and controller.

(Courtesy Thermo Cardiosystems, Woburn, Mass.)

pump that is used for right circulation, left circulation, or both (Figs. 15-7 and 15-8). This device is useful as a bridge to transplantation in patients with severe biventricular failure.

COMPLICATIONS OF VENTRICULAR ASSIST DEVICE THERAPY

Bleeding, right-sided heart failure, air embolism, and multisystem organ failure are frequent causes of early morbidity after left VAD placement. Later complications include infection, thromboembolism, and device failure.

Aprotinin is commonly used at the time of implant to reduce postoperative bleeding.[32] Right heart failure resolves with lowering left ventricular end diastolic pressure and treatment of pulmonary hypertension. RV failure is probably the single most difficult issue in managing these patients.

Thromboembolic events are relatively rare with textured devices. Patients do not typically receive full-dose heparin or warfarin therapy; rather, they receive aspirin or dipyridamole. Transcranial Doppler reveals a 34% to 67% incidence of microemboli, although neurologic outcome is generally good.[1] Although most patients do well, complications of VADs are nosocomial and device-related infections from immobilization, prolonged tracheal intubation, poor nutritional status, and the need for multiple intravascular and urinary catheters.[33] The most common infections are those related to the drive exit site and are manageable with local wound care and antibiotics. Surgical debridement is sometimes necessary.

ECHOCARDIOGRAPHIC DETERMINANTS OF PROPER VENTRICULAR ASSIST DEVICE FUNCTION

Transesophageal echocardiography (TEE) is essential for managing proper functioning of mechanical assist devices. TEE provides assessment of the existing pathology and identifies problems that occur with VAD dysfunction after separation from cardiopulmonary bypass. Certain structural cardiac abnormalities interfere with blood flow within the heart (Figs. 15-9 and 15-10). The left atrium and ventricle are a conduit for blood flow with a Thermo Cardiosystems or Thoratec left VAD. Functionally, this device does not require pumping action of the native left heart, but the presence of mitral stenosis interferes with passive flow. Table 15-3 summarizes cardiac pathology that interferes with the function of LVADs.

Aortic insufficiency permits regurgitation of blood from the aortic root to the left ventricle. A "backward" shunt is created by the aortic insufficiency and LVAD. A 5-L/min LVAD flow with 2 L/min regurgitation provides only 3 L/min flow to the aortic arch distally. This is easily corrected by the surgeon who sutures the native aortic valve closed. An atrial septal defect (ASD) or ventricular septal defect (VSD) also creates shunting with LVAD use. These septal defects, furthermore, interfere with oxygenation. Thrombus predisposes the patient to stroke. Left ventricular apical akinesis is often associated with a mural thrombus. The apical cannula is positioned so that flow is not obstructed when imaged with TEE (Fig. 15-11). The right atrial cannula (RVAD inflow)

position is also assessed with echocardiography (Fig. 15-12).

The standard cardiopulmonary bypass and permanent VAD cannulae present before separation from bypass obscure the TEE views. Epicardial echocardiography is useful during these cases for detecting problems with VAD function. A patient who requires both right and left ventricular device placement with pulmonic regurgitation will shunt RVAD flow into the right ventricle and away from the lungs. This causes RV dilation and

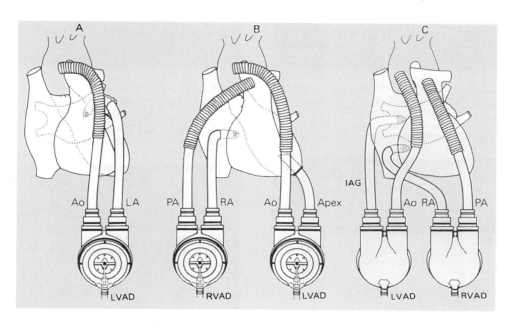

FIG. 15-7   Thoratec VAS system. Right ventricular assist device *(RVAD)* and left ventricular assist device *(LVAD)* arrangements are shown. The pumping chambers are external to the body. *Ao,* Aorta; *IAG,* intra-atrial graft (cannula to left atrium); *LA,* left atrium; *PA,* pulmonary artery; *RA,* right atrium.

(Courtesy Thoratec.)

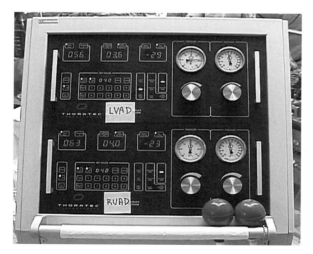

FIG. 15-8   Thoratec console. Drive console for a patient with biventricular assist device support. The dials indicate pneumatic pressure (ejection) and suction (filling). *LVAD,* Left ventricular assist device; *RVAD,* right ventricular assist device.

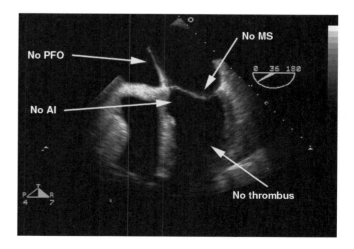

FIG. 15-9   Echocardiogram demonstrating key points to be excluded in patients using ventricular assist devices. *AI,* Aortic insufficiency; *MS,* mitral stenosis; *PFO,* patient foramen ovale.

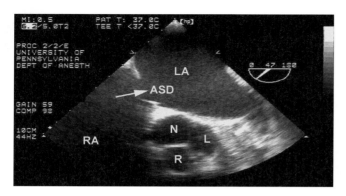

FIG. 15-10   Atrial septal defect *(ASD)*. *L,* Left coronary cusp of the aortic valve; *LA,* left atrium; *N,* noncoronary; *R,* right coronary; *RA,* right atrium.

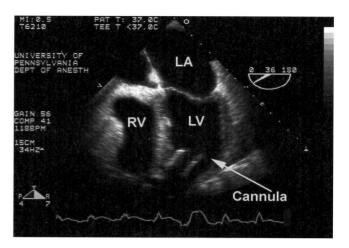

FIG. 15-11   Apical position of left ventricular assist device cannula. It is important that if the cannula is tilted, it is not obstructed from left ventricular blood flow. *LA,* Left atrium; *LV,* left ventricle; *RV,* right ventricle.

TABLE 15-3
Coexisting Cardiac Pathology that Interferes with Left Ventricular Assist Device Placement

Mitral stenosis
Aortic insufficiency
Atrial septal defect
Ventricular septal defect
Pulmonic insufficiency (BiVAD placement)
Thrombus

These pathologies should be screened in the prebypass exam.
BiVAD, Biventricular assist device.

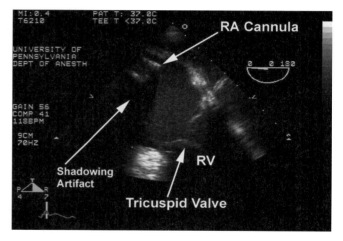

FIG. 15-12   Thoratec right ventricular assist device inflow cannula in the right atrium. Note how the presence of the cannula can create "shadow" artifacts. *RA,* Right atrium; *RV,* right ventricle.

elevated central venous pressure. TEE is essential for assessing pulmonic regurgitations, but if TEE cannot image the valve appropriately, epicardial imaging is used. Figs. 15-13 and 15-14 demonstrate pulmonic insufficiency as imaged by an epicardial linear phased array probe. The presence of retained intracardiac air is also evaluated with TEE. Significant collections of air require venting of the left heart or aorta to minimize cerebral embolization of the air.

VENTRICULAR VOLUME REDUCTION SURGERY

Palliative procedures for heart failure that have been developed in response to the shortage of donor hearts include partial left ventriculectomy and endoventricular patch plasty.[34-37] The Batista procedure entails resecting portions of (possibly viable) left ventricular myocar-

dium and repairing mitral regurgitation (invariably present with dilated cardiomyopathy) (see Fig. 15-2). The left ventricular end-diastolic diameter is thus reduced (Figs. 15-15 and 15-16). The mitral valve repair usually consists of an edge-to-edge mitral leaflet suture known as an *Alfieri repair.*[38-40] This suture creates a double mitral orifice that is imaged by TEE as a "figure of eight." These procedures alter ventricular mechanics to reduce wall stress and stroke volume.[34] Although some patients improve according to their New York Heart Association functional status, others sustain significant morbidity and mortality. The preoperative indicators for predicting postoperative outcome are poorly understood. Echocardiography is used to measure ventricular dilation and

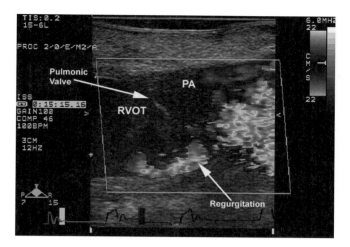

FIG. 15-13 Epicardial echocardiography demonstrating pulmonic insufficiency (see Fig. 15-14). This created backflow into the right ventricle. Right ventricular assist device flows were significantly higher in this patient than were left ventricular assist device flows because of shunt. A linear 6- to 15-MHz probe was used to generate the image. Note that the image is not wedge (or "pie") shaped. *PA*, Pulmonary artery; *RVOT*, right ventricular outflow tract.

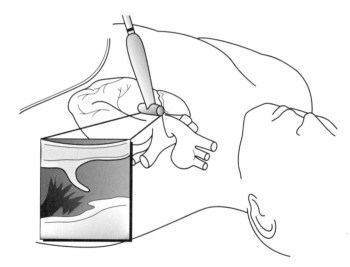

FIG. 15-14 Epicardial echocardiography probe positioning. The schematic demonstrates color Doppler imaging of the pulmonic valve.

(Courtesy Agilent Technologies).

to guide the extent of ventricular resection for providing a specific end-diastolic dimension. The Alfieri repair is assessed for residual regurgitation or acquired stenosis.

Endoventricular patch plasty uses a similar concept but with resection of a myocardial scar.[41] *Dyskinetic* ventricular segments are resected to reduce ventricular work that is lost to the dyskinetic area instead of to LV outflow ejection. The scar is opened and a patch of artificial material is sewn to the mechanical border

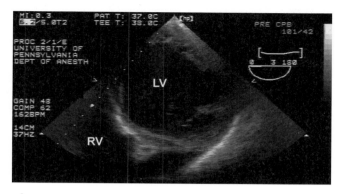

FIG. 15-15 Transesophageal echocardiogram of the left ventricle *(LV)* in short axis. This patient was scheduled for a "Batista" procedure. Note the ventricular diameter. *RV*, Right ventricle.

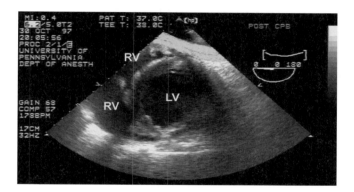

FIG. 15-16 Transesophageal echocardiography of the left ventricle *(LV)* in short axis: after reduction. The LV is smaller in diameter than in Fig. 15-15. The right ventricle *(RV)* is large and encloses a large circumference of the LV septal wall.

zone, thus reducing the global size of the ventricle (Fig. 15-17). Preoperative evaluation includes viability studies (e.g., stress echocardiography or positron emission tomography) to determine noninfarcted segments for coronary artery revascularization. This procedure has also been used for *akinetic* segments with some success[42-44] and as a treatment for refractory ventricular tachycardia.[45]

These procedures are possibly the most challenging to manage of all cardiac surgical maneuvers (i.e., transplantation or VAD placement) because the ventricular function is not dramatically improved after bypass. Anesthetic management is similar to other procedures discussed in this chapter.[46] TEE is important for determining ventricular size and valvular function. Most centers perform endoventricular patch plasty with the availability of VAD backup. Before the advent of portable vented

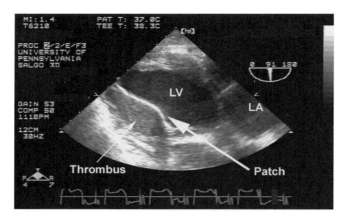

FIG. 15-17   Endoventricular patch plasty. The patch is seen in this long axis view of the left ventricle *(LV)*. *LA,* Left atrium.

electric VADs for out-of-hospital use, only heart transplant candidates received VADs.

PREOPERATIVE ASSESSMENT FOR HEART TRANSPLANTATION

Patients considered for transplantation undergo a rigorous medical evaluation before they are accepted onto a transplant list. Most of the medical information is readily available when the anesthesiologist is informed of the transplant. Laboratory evaluation includes viral and protozoal titers for HIV, cytomegalovirus (CMV), Epstein-Barr virus (EBV), hepatitis B surface antigen, hepatitis B core antigen, hepatitis C surface antigen, herpes simplex viruses (HSV) 1 and 2, varicella-zoster virus (VZV) (shingles, chicken pox), and toxoplasmosis. The dates of cardiac imaging studies such as echocardiography or radionuclide ventriculography are considered. Older studies are discounted because of congestive heart failure progression. All patients require cardiac catheterization to measure pulmonary artery (PA) pressure. Pulmonary function testing is indicated for patients with known pulmonary disease or cigarette abuse. Patients with a history of numerous blood transfusions (e.g., as part of a VAD operation) require a panel-reactive antibody (PRA) screen to determine the degree of alloimmunization. A significant PRA makes donor selection more difficult in finding a better human leukocyte antigen (HLA) match (see the section on immune function following). Complete dental examination is performed to determine the presence of infection. Women undergo screening mammograms and gynecologic evaluation. Men undergo a serum prostate-specific antigen test as a screen for carcinoma.

Heart transplantation is by definition an emergent procedure since donor availability is not an elective circumstance. Patients have mild chronic renal or hepatic dysfunction as a consequence of their compensated state. Patients are either called from home for their transplant or, more commonly, are hospitalized for days to months on a heart failure service. Inotropic agents such as milrinone or dobutamine are frequently infused during their hospitalization. These patients have extreme psychologic pressure and commonly form a support network among family and friends of other heart failure victims. Patients with an O blood group antigen may have a protracted waiting period and see other "healthier" patients receive a transplant before them.

The goal before transplantation is stabilization of other organ function, so that most patients are reasonably well compensated physiologically. Inotropic agents or VAD therapy improves perfusion to other organ systems in preparation for transplantation. Less optimal circumstances include the patient who has been on the transplant list for an extended period and is failing inotropic therapy. These patients commonly present for VAD insertion without the benefit of a previous anesthetic preconsultation. There are many psychologic issues for both the patient and family. The anesthesiologist plays a very important role during the preanesthetic interview to build a rapport that helps soothe the energized atmosphere surrounding this event. This approach minimizes the need for anxiolytic premedication. Collection of history includes data about prior anesthetics, particularly for cardiac operations and allergies.[47] Examination of the airway is particularly important. Anesthetic induction balances a slow, careful induction, avoiding hypotension, with securing the airway and avoiding aspiration. Fasting is not always feasible because the availability of a donor heart is unpredictable. Premedication includes a histamine (H_2) antagonist and a propulsive agent (e.g., ranitidine and metoclopramide, respectively). Sedative premedication is given to patients that are monitored for oxygen saturation, consciousness, and blood pressure. Poor venous access resulting from multiple cardiac procedures such as coronary artery bypass graft or VAD placement is common. Frequently, the only existing venous access will be a peripherally inserted central catheter (PICC) for dobutamine or milrinone infusion. Communication with the surgical team ensures that blood chemistries, complete blood count, coagulation profile, chest X-ray, and consents are current.

PREPARATION FOR ANESTHETIC INDUCTION

On notification of a heart transplant, the anesthesiologist coordinates the patient's transport to the operating room, placement of monitoring devices, and time of induction. Constant communication with other team members (surgeons, nurses, and perfusionists) is essential. Difficulty in obtaining arterial and venous access is anticipated to avoid delays in starting the induction. Timing is critical because of the inherent risk of increased donor ischemic time. *Heart failure after bypass should not be the result of a protracted ischemic time from delayed induction.*

Monitoring

Monitoring for heart transplantation is similar to elective cardiac surgery, with minor changes. Pulse oximetry, noninvasive blood pressure measurement, and electrographic monitoring are initiated before attempting vascular access. Because of the stressful nature of the situation, the patient benefits from small, titrated doses of a benzodiazepine and a compassionate rapport with the anesthesiologist. An intraarterial catheter is placed for blood gas analysis and continuous monitoring of blood pressure. A PA catheter allows measurement of *cardiac output, pulmonary vascular resistance (PVR) and pressure,* and *central venous pressure,* providing an estimate of RV filling and function. Continuous monitoring of mixed venous oxygen saturation (Svo_2) by a more expensive PA catheter is controversial because of the additional cost and lack of definitive data showing improved outcome.[48] Nonetheless, alterations in cardiac output, hemoglobin concentration, and arterial oxygenation are reflected instantaneously by changes in Svo_2. Successful therapeutic intervention during hemodynamic decompensation is also recognized promptly by an increase in Svo_2. An abnormally high Svo_2 in the functioning donor heart may indicate a left-to-right intracardiac shunt. A similar defect in the recipient's native heart is inconsequential after a new heart is implanted. The PA catheter is placed in the left internal jugular vein to allow intracardiac biopsy after transplant from the right internal jugular vein. Prior cardiac surgery with intrathoracic adhesions can make insertion of a central catheter from the left side problematic. Many patients have an implantable cardioverter-defibrillator (ICD) or PICC. These devices occupy intravascular space and predispose the patient to thrombus formation. The neck vessels are imaged with an ultrasound device to locate the vein, avoid the artery, and determine the absence of thrombus.[49] Multiple attempts to acquire vascular access require valuable time that may increase donor heart ischemic time. A long (80-cm) sterile sleeve for the introducer allows the withdrawal of the PA catheter from the recipient heart before explantation.

The failing heart results in a delayed upstroke of the arterial waveform and reduced systolic and mean arterial pressures. Electrocardiogram (ECG) analysis reveals ventricular premature contractions, particularly during the prebypass surgical dissection. PA catheter insertion may be difficult in patients with a dilated right ventricle or severe tricuspid regurgitation. Rhythm disturbances are common during PA catheter insertion and may be refractory to electrical or chemical cardioversion. For this reason, PA catheter insertion can be delayed until the chest is open and the heart is exposed. Emergent institution of cardiopulmonary bypass is performed if refractory ventricular fibrillation ensues.

Invasive hemodynamic monitoring may reveal a low Svo_2 (<50%) or a decreased cardiac index (<1.8 L/min/m^2). Calculation of *PVR* is important for predicting difficulty in separation from cardiopulmonary bypass. Patients with an elevated PVR (>2.5 Wood units) are at increased risk for RV failure. A comparison of PVR is made between the pretransplant cardiac catheterization values and the intraoperative values. Patients with poor ventricular function may require inotropic support *before* induction of anesthesia. Dobutamine or milrinone are used for patients with pulmonary hypertension and a systolic arterial blood pressure greater than 130 mm Hg. Patients with cardiogenic shock benefit from a norepinephrine infusion. Vasoactive infusions are titrated while waiting for the harvest team to arrive with the donor organ.

Induction of Anesthesia

The recipient patient is prepared for induction of anesthesia with approval by the procurement team. Health of the donor heart is assessed by ECG, echocardiography, and occasionally cardiac catheterization. The donor is matched for size, ABO compatibility, and infectious agents.[8] Malignancies in the donor (except glioblastoma multiforme) are a contraindication to transplantation.

The general anesthetic considerations of airway anatomy and fasting status are imposed on the potential for hemodynamic perturbations. The preinduction administration of inotropic agents or pressors optimizes circulation and minimizes transit time of subsequently administered anesthetic agents. It is more difficult to treat hypotension in the setting of a low cardiac output because of the delayed circulation time. Dantrolene, with its theoretic negative inotropic action, has been used with caution in patients undergoing heart transplantation with a history of malignant hyperthermia syndromes.[50]

Induction is performed in the presence of the cardiac surgeon, scrub nurse, and perfusionist in anticipation of cardiovascular collapse. Discretion dictates the choice of anesthetic induction agent.[51,52] Barbiturates depress cardiac output and blood pressure. Most common techniques use a high-dose narcotic induction with administration of muscle relaxant to minimize chest wall rigidity.[53] Alternatively, a modified rapid sequence induction with etomidate is used for patients with delayed gastric emptying (who have received H_2 blockade and a gastric motility agent). Etomidate causes minimal change in hemodynamics but does not generally blunt the hypertensive response to laryngoscopy. Myoclonus is attenuated by concomitant administration of a short-acting benzodiazepine. The dose of etomidate is supplemented before laryngoscopy with narcotic (e.g., 5-10 mcg/kg of fentanyl, depending on prevailing hemodynamics). Many newer paralytic agents lack significant hemodynamic side effects. Succinylcholine is used with caution in patients with renal insufficiency and hyperkalemia.

Gastric suctioning is performed after intubation unless one of the older transplant protocols is used with oral administration of azathioprine before admission to the operating room. Indiscriminate gastric suction in such cases will remove this medication. Narcotic agents supplement the anesthesia for incision while amnesia is achieved with benzodiazepine or scopolamine. Addition of a low dose of potent inhalational agent is worthwhile unless the patient is in cardiogenic shock.

Induction should take in the presence of the surgeon, scrub nurse, and perfusionist in preparation for cardiovascular collapse, should it occur. Transcutaneous defibrillator pads are placed on patients with prior sternotomy. The surgeon is unable to gain prompt access to the heart with epicardial paddles because of adhesions. Aprotinin, ε-aminocaproic acid, or tranexamic acid attenuate postoperative bleeding in patients with prior chest surgery. These infusions are begun before incision for optimum effect. High-dose methylprednisolone is administered during cardiopulmonary bypass immediately before the donor heart is reperfused.

TRANSESOPHAGEAL ECHOCARDIOGRAPHY DURING CARDIAC TRANSPLANTATION

TEE provides an accurate anatomic and physiologic assessment of the beating heart. The *classic survey for routine cardiac surgery* includes evaluation of ventricular and valvular function, allowing optimal management during *the prebypass state* in titrating inotropic support. Uncommon findings such as vegetations or metastatic tumor (both pathologic, not echocardiographic diagnoses) can indicate otherwise unrecognized problems such as systemic infection or cancer. TEE is used to guide PA catheter insertion in patients with cardiomegaly or severe tricuspid regurgitation if this was not possible before induction. Newer technologies such as three-dimensional echocardiography can be used to assess the global shape of the ventricle.[54,55]

Atrial anatomy is different in the transplanted heart because of features of the anastomosis. Newer techniques of right circulatory anastomoses include a bicaval suture technique to avoid sizing issues between the right atrium of the donor and recipient. Each atrial anastomosis provides the patient with two "subchambers," one atrium from the recipient and one from the donor (Fig. 15-18). The long-axis four-chamber view is sometimes termed *six-chamber view*.[56] The atria ap-

pear slightly different in each recipient because suture lines vary from patient to patient. This interatrial anastomosis can be mistaken for a mass.

Significant size mismatch between donor and recipient is a prelude to difficulties and requires close communication between the surgeon and echocardiographer. Kinking or obstruction of the right or left ventricular outflow tracts may be observed, and torsion of the atrial anastomosis can lead to ventricular inflow problems detected by elevated Doppler inflow velocities. Mild mitral regurgitation is relatively common and insignificant. Mild regurgitation is caused by preexisting pathology or mild distortion of the annulus.[56,57] Although mild or even moderate tricuspid regurgitation is common, it may be a sign of RV pressure overload from pulmonary hypertension. Concomitant findings in the early postoperative setting include RV dilation and an elevated central venous pressure. Preoperative pulmonary hypertension may normalize with a new left ventricle and allow RV remodeling despite the pressure overload immediately after transplantation.

SEPARATION FROM CARDIOPULMONARY BYPASS

Two crucial issues determine the ease of separation from cardiopulmonary bypass: *the ability of the heart to recover from its ischemic state* (4-6 hours) and *the absence of pulmonary hypertension.* The denervated heart benefits from a chronotropic agent and a pulmonary vasodilator. The classic agent of choice is isoproterenol. Preoperative pacing ICD is not helpful because the myocardial electrode leads are severed during removal of the native heart. Epicardial leads are placed for electrical pacing.

Global and regional ventricular function are assessed by TEE as the heart begins to eject. The donor heart

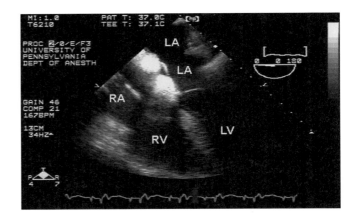

FIG. 15-18 Transesophageal echocardiography of a transplanted heart. The elongated atria are shown. The visualized anatomy varies from patient to patient depending on suture lines. *LA,* Left atrium; *LV,* left ventricle; *RA,* right atrium; *RV,* right ventricle.

with left ventricular hypertrophy requires elevated filling pressures. The patient is weaned with concurrent hyperventilation to facilitate dilation of the pulmonary vasculature in patients with reversible pulmonary hypertension. The donor heart is not accustomed to increased RV afterload. Every effort should be made to minimize this acute exposure to elevated PA pressure to avoid RV dysfunction. Other factors such as donor ischemic time and brain death can contribute to RV dysfunction.[58] Hemodynamic information is obtained by inserting the PA catheter as intracardiac flow is restored. A steep "step-down" between RV and PA systolic pressures suggests the presence of a right ventricular outflow tract (RVOT) anastomotic stricture.

RV failure is diagnosed by right heart dilation observed in the operative field, an elevated central venous pressure, and RV dilation on TEE with moderate or severe tricuspid regurgitation. Pharmacologic therapy is used to increase RV inotropy. Milrinone, a phosphodiesterase fraction III inhibitor, causes pulmonary vasodilatation and increases myocardial performance synergistically with β-adrenergic agonists such as isoproterenol or epinephrine. Systemic vasodilatation caused by milrinone or isoproterenol is problematic. Systemic vasoconstrictors such as phenylephrine or vasopressin are slowly titrated to counteract these effects. Patients with

infection are prone to developing a systemic inflammatory response syndrome to bypass.[59,60] A left atrial infusion catheter minimizes the pulmonary effects of vasoconstrictors but the morbidity associated with these catheters does not justify this approach. Inhaled nitric oxide is useful in the management of RV failure by dilating the pulmonary vasculature without inducing systemic vasodilation.[61-67]

TEE is used to examine the donor heart systematically after cardiopulmonary bypass.[68] Disorders such as ASD or bicuspid aortic valve should have been noted by echocardiography at the donor site or by the surgeon before implantation.

POSTOPERATIVE INTENSIVE CARE

Management of the cardiac transplant patient in the ICU is best organized by an organ systems approach (Fig. 15-19). Routine management includes appropriate mechanical ventilation, monitoring of urine output, and treating coagulation deficiencies with the appropriate blood products.[69] Management of hemodynamic physiology is different than for routine cardiac surgery.

A common problem among transplant recipients is RV dysfunction in the immediate postoperative period. Common causes of RV failure include pulmonary hy-

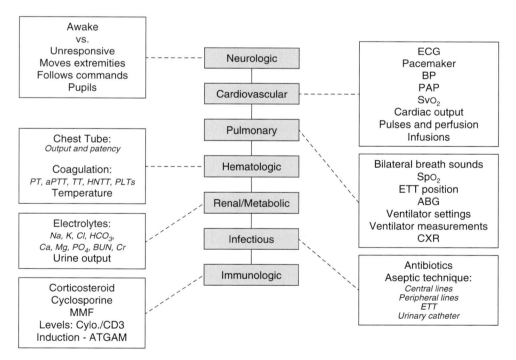

FIG. 15-19 Organ systems approach to intensive care unit care of the patient for cardiac transplant. *ABG*, Arterial blood gases; *aPTT*, activated partial thromboplastin time; *ATGAM*, antithymocyte immunoglobulin; *BP*, blood pressure; *BUN*, blood urea nitrogen; *CD3*, T-cell marker; *CXR*, chest X-ray; *cylo*, serum cyclosporine level; *ECG*, electrocardiogram; *ETT*, endotracheal tube; *HNTT*, heparin-neutralized thrombin time; *MMF*, mycophenolate mofetil; *PAP*, pulmonary artery pressure; *PLTs*, platelets; *PT*, prothrombin time; *Spo$_2$*, peripheral oxygen saturation; *Svo$_2$*, mixed venous oxygen saturation; *TT*, thrombin time.

pertension, long ischemic time, and rejection. The donor heart compensates for the elevated PVR, which requires approximately 3 or 4 weeks to decline.[56] RV overload is manifested by apicalization of the ventricle with septal flattening. Careful monitoring and aggressive management of PVR is essential. *Pulmonary arterial pressures may actually be low despite elevated PVR when cardiac output is low.* RV failure is typically manifested by elevated central venous pressure and peripheral edema. Milrinone, dobutamine, prostaglandin E_1, and inhaled nitric oxide are used to treat pulmonary hypertension.[61,62,64,65] The urge to treat hypotension by the administration of fluids must be tempered in the setting of RV overload. Overzealous fluid administration creates a downward spiral of RV distention, ischemia, RV failure, and greater distention that may require reopening the chest for cardiac arrest. Isoproterenol is the optimal inotropic agent for this situation because of its ability to induce pulmonary vasodilatation, increase contractility, and cause mild tachycardia (95-110 beats/min). Prophylactic use of isoproterenol before the onset of RV failure is common practice in patients with elevated PVR. A declining cardiac output must prompt the associated calculation of systemic vascular resistance and PVR to determine therapy. Venodilation is common during rewarming, necessitating the administration of intravenous fluid (or packed red blood cells if anemic) as the initial therapy. Both packed red blood cells and platelets should be leukocyte depleted or filtered to prevent alloimmunization of the recipient. The ICU central venous pressure and PA pressure are compared with intraoperative values obtained after successful weaning from cardiopulmonary bypass. A poor response to fluid administration indicates the need for an increase in inotropic support and hyperventilation. Postoperative surgical bleeding and tamponade should be considered.[70] TEE is useful in differentiating the cause of hypotension in terms of volume status, tamponade, or biventricular function.

A normally functioning donor heart facilitates rapid weaning of the patient from mechanical ventilation. Patients are typically extubated during the first postoperative day. Immunosuppression therapy is provided early in the ICU course. Cyclosporine is administered intravenously while patients are intubated but is converted to microemulsified cyclosporine (Neoral) to establish steady-state serum levels.[71] Daily trough monitoring of cyclosporine is mandatory for assuring adequate immunosuppression. Urine output and serum creatinine levels are closely monitored because cyclosporine causes renal vasoconstriction. Patients with transient renal dysfunction and patients with greater risk for rejection (high PRA screen) are treated with antithymocyte immunoglobulin (ATGAM). Assays for $CD4^+$ lymphocyte counts tailor daily ATGAM dosing.

Complications of heart transplantation include heart failure, renal failure, and infection. Patients with poor outcome have protracted duration of stays in the ICU. These patients may present for noncardiac surgery for placement of feeding tube, tracheostomy, or reparative plastic surgery for incisional wound. ICU care of the cardiac transplant patient requires close communication between the intensivist, cardiac surgeon, transplant cardiologist, and ICU nursing staff. Preoperative demographics, morbidity, and indices of organ failure during the first 24 hours after surgery are not predictive of hospital mortality. After 28 days in the ICU, the indices of organ failure predictive of hospital mortality include infusions of dopamine or norepinephrine, diminished Glasgow Coma Scale score, elevated bilirubin, elevated arterial partial pressure of carbon dioxide, decreased serum albumin, and advanced age. Preoperative health status and early organ failure are not predictive of late hospital mortality.[72] Complex issues involving hemodynamic, pulmonary, renal, infectious, and immunotherapy status requires multidisciplinary collaboration.

IMMUNE FUNCTION

The most difficult aspect of transplant management is preventing rejection. Improved donor and recipient selection criteria, better preservative solutions, and faster personnel transport have contributed to improved outcome in transplantation. However, human transplantation is not possible without recipient immunosuppression. Organ rejection or undesirable secondary effects of immunosuppression provide challenges for appropriate management. Anesthesiologists must understand immunosuppression therapy rationale for patients undergoing transplantation or during their care in either the immediate or long-term posttransplant setting. Cardiac, renal, hepatic, and pancreatic dysfunction have potential origins from the complex drugs used to allow tolerance of a "foreign" heart.

The basis of rejection involves lymphocyte recognition of foreign donor protein on cardiac cells associated with the major histocompatibility complex (MHC).[73] In humans, the MHC is sometimes denoted as human leukocyte antigen (HLA). A minor histocompatibility complex also exists that can stimulate rejection. Class I HLA (types -A,-B,-C) antigens of MHC are expressed in almost all donor cells, and antigen specificity is mediated by the T-cell receptor. During development, random arrangements of gene sequences in developing T cells in the thymus generate a vast library of "foreign" and "self" binding sites.[74] T-cell lines that recognize "self" are destroyed to prevent autoimmunity. Antigen recognition is amplified by costimulatory ligands from antigen-presenting cells.[75]

The T cell responds by secreting interleukin-2 (IL-2), a substance that induces proliferation of more T cells. In the absence of antigen-presenting cells, a programmed

CD4$^+$ T cell becomes unresponsive to antigen and undergoes apoptosis (programmed cell death). Activated CD4$^+$ T cells upregulate the activity of monocytes, macrophages, antibody-producing B cells, and cytotoxic CD8$^+$ T cells. Therefore, the CD4$^+$ T cell is central to the rejection response.

Antigen-presenting cells (e.g., macrophages) process "foreign" protein and are carried to their cell surface with MHC molecules. Clonal lines of CD4$^+$ T cells that are stimulated to respond are amplified by IL-2. Other cytokines (IL 1-6,9,10; interferons; and tumor necrosis factor α and β) are also involved. Donor and recipient may be HLA matched but this is not routine practice unless the recipient is known to be highly sensitized (as judged by a PRA screen).

Rejection

The introduction of cyclosporine has increased survival after heart transplantation to 63% at 5 years and 43% at 10 years.[56,76] There are generally three forms of rejection: hyperacute, acute, and chronic. **Hyperacute rejection** represents a reaction by preformed antibodies. This reaction can occur when the arterial clamps are removed and the recipient's blood begins to perfuse the myocardium. Preformed antibodies activate complement, leading to formation of microthrombi.[77] Thrombosis ensues and the donor heart becomes necrotic. This is the primary rejection mechanism for xenotransplant (non-human) organ rejection. Cross matching individuals for ABO compatibility nearly eliminates this form of rejection.

Acute rejection is the most problematic aspect of perioperative transplantation and occurs within days to weeks (Table 15-4). IL-2 stimulates T cells and γ-interferon activates macrophages to react against donor tissue through a complex series of lymphokine pathways and immune cell activation. Interstitial edema oc-

curs from endovascular damage and capillary leak because the donor heart's endothelium is regarded as foreign tissue.[78] Echocardiography is used to determine changes in ventricular compliance that are characteristic of rejection. Both systolic and diastolic function are affected.[78] Myocardial edema creates changes in the cyclic variation of ultrasound backscatter, which prompts new areas of research.[79] Difficulties with specificity affect integrated backscatter studies. Tissue Doppler is also used to assess myocardial function.[80] Acute rejection is clinically manifested as heart failure and is the form of rejection that is targeted for therapy in the perioperative setting. Myocardial biopsy is used to determine the efficacy of immunotherapy.

Chronic rejection is one of the most poorly understood problems in the long-term management of heart transplant patients. This form of rejection is manifested by small-vessel arteriosclerotic disease and affects several transplanted organs, including heart, kidney, and liver. Cardiac graft vasculopathy is immune mediated and affects both intramyocardial and epicardial coronary arteries.[81] Intimal proliferation of smooth muscle leads to luminal narrowing and eventual ischemia.[82] Noninvasive testing such as exercise electrocardiography, thallium scintigraphy, exercise radionuclide ventriculography, or ambulatory electrocardiography are not sufficiently sensitive or specific to be reliable screening tests of mild disease.[81] Coronary angiography is specific for the diagnosis of chronic rejection but underestimates the presence of disease. Intracoronary ultrasound is used for evaluating intimal thickening,[81,83] and dobutamine stress echocardiography is a useful screening tool for detecting small-vessel arteriosclerosis.[84] Unfortunately, neither percutaneous transluminal coronary angioplasty (PTCA) nor surgical coronary artery bypass grafting is useful for treating this disorder because of the diffuse nature of the atherosclerosis.[81] Retransplantation is problematic as a result of subsequent surgical complications and is not generally associated with positive outcome. This is mitigated by the shortage of donor organs.

Xenotransplantation is the transplantation of organs from different species. The major problem with xenotransplantation is the presence of preformed antibodies that induce hyperacute rejection. Although primates (baboons) have been used for experimental cardiac transplantation, there is less social and ethical conflict in using specially bred porcine donors.[85] The other major obstacle is coinfection by animal agents such as retroviruses.[86,87]

Immunosuppressive Agents

The immune system depends on *upregulating cytokine pathways, cell surface receptors,* and *activating nucleotide pathways.* Immune therapy targets these aspects of im-

TABLE 15-4
Biopsy Classification of Stages of Rejection

0	None
1 A	**Focal** aggregates of lymphocytes
1 B	**Diffuse** but sparse aggregate of lymphocytes
2	One focus of **myocyte damage**
3 A	**Multifocal** areas of myocyte damage
3 B	**Borderline** severe rejection
4	Diffuse mixed infiltrates with vasculitis, hemorrhage, and **necrosis**

Griffith BP: Heart transplantation. In Edmunds LH, editor: *Cardiac surgery in the adult,* New York, 1997, McGraw-Hill, pp 1385-1407.

TABLE 15-5
Drugs that Elevate or Diminish Cyclosporine Serum Levels

ELEVATE	DIMINISH
Fluconazole	Phenobarbital
Itraconazole	Phenytoin
Ketoconazole	Carbamazepine
Diltiazem	Nafcillin
Verapamil	Octreotide
Nicardipine	Isoniazid
Erythromycin	
Clarithromycin	

mune function. Common agents used to prevent rejection include **corticosteroids**, **calcineurin inhibitors**, **nucleic acid pathway inhibitors** (a form of chemotherapy), and **antilymphocyte antibodies**. Biologic therapies such as genetically engineering human murine chimeric antibodies are emerging. These include antibodies against other immune targets (e.g., anti–T-cell receptor, anti–IL-2, etc.). Significant side effects of immunosuppression include infection, nephrotoxicity, hypertension, and hyperlipidemia. The prevalence of malignant disease is increased in patients who have undergone long-term immunosuppression.[87]

Corticosteroids are part of the mainstay of therapy but untoward side effects limit total dose and chronic exposure. Corticosteroids act both on nuclear factors (nuclear factor kappa B) and affect gene promoter sites responsible for IL-2 synthesis. Common side effects include hyperglycemia, weight gain, osteopenia, avascular necrosis, acne, poor wound healing, skin atrophy, gastrointestinal bleeding, protein catabolism, fat redistribution, cataract formation, glaucoma, and mood swings. Synergistic combinations of other drugs are used to supplement glucocorticoids. Agents such as oral prednisone or intravenous methylprednisolone are preferred over hydrocortisone because they have less mineralocorticoid activity (and hence less sodium retention).

One of the most important contributions to modern transplant immunology is the development of **calcineurin inhibitors: cyclosporine or tacrolimus**. Both cyclosporine and tacrolimus bind cytoplasmic receptors (cyclophylin and FK-binding protein 12, respectively[75]). The resulting complexes inactivate calcineurin and IL-2 synthesis. Plasma levels of cyclosporine are sampled daily during the initial postoperative period to achieve a therapeutic, minimally toxic steady state. Cytochrome-P450 is an important human metabolic pathway for cyclosporine. Several drugs that interact with P-450 increase or decrease plasma cyclosporine levels[74] (Table 15-5).

Oral preparations of cyclosporine include an older oil suspension and a newer microemulsion known as "Neoral" (Novartis, Hanover, NJ). Trough monitoring of cyclosporine blood levels minimizes toxicity and ensures adequate immunosuppression. There is a lower incidence of rejection in patients receiving Neoral because of more predictable blood levels. Long-term monitoring of calcineurin inhibitor effect is performed with myocardial biopsies and serum creatinine levels. Dosage is adjusted in patients with renal insufficiency. Cyclosporine can cause intense renal vasoconstriction and worsen renal function. The other major side effects of cyclosporin include hypertension and hirsutism. Less common reactions include seizure and cholestasis. Tacrolimus, a more potent IL-2 inhibitor than cyclosporine, is frequently used in liver transplantation because it is more water soluble and less dependent on bile salt absorption.[75,88]

Purine antimetabolites (cytotoxic agents) are the third leg in the triad of current transplant immunosuppression. **Azathioprine** (6-mercaptopurine, Immuran) inhibits rapidly dividing cells of the immune system by its systemic conversion to 6-thioguanine and incorporation into DNA. Azathioprine reduces the amount of other immunosuppressive agents. Side effects include bone marrow suppression, hair loss, pancreatitis, nausea, and, rarely, hepatic dysfunction. A newer agent, **mycophenolate mofetil** (MMF, CellCept, Syntex, Palo Alto) inhibits inosine monophosphate dehydrogenase and guanosine monophosphate guanylic acid. These are part of the de novo purine pathway and are more specific to T cells. Several studies have shown MMF to be superior to azathioprine for maintenance and rescue therapy.[75]

Patients at increased risk for acute rejection (i.e., presensitized by prior pregnancy or multiple blood transfusions) are treated with "induction" therapy of either **polyclonal** antilymphocyte antibody (antithymocyte or antilymphocyte) or **monoclonal anti-CD3$^+$ antibodies**. The ATGAM is an (equine) polyclonal antibody that binds to several T-cell receptors. This interaction damages and clears the T-cell population and is commonly used for induction and therapy. It may also be used in place of cyclosporine in the perioperative setting for patients with severe renal dysfunction. A newer hybridoma-engineered technologic product is OKT3. This is a murine monoclonal antibody against T cells and is quite potent.[75] It induces complement-mediated lysis of T cells. The polyclonal agent is directed against many cell receptors, whereas the monoclonal is directed against CD3$^+$ T cells. These drugs can cause serum sickness, thrombocytopenia, and granulocytopenia. Repeated use predisposes patients to infection or malignancy.

Immunosuppressive agents can induce profound immunosuppression. When associated with EBV, immunosuppression is associated with posttransplant lym-

TABLE 15-6
Common Opportunistic Infections and Selected Drug Therapy

INFECTIOUS AGENT	TYPE	COMMON PHARMACOTHERAPY
HSV 1 and 2	Viral	Acyclovir, valacyclovir, famciclovir (ganciclovir alone with CMV)
VZV	Viral	
CMV	Viral	Ganciclovir, foscarnet
HHV-6	Viral	
Candida spp. (most)	Fungal	Fluconazole amphotericin B
Torulopsis glabrata	Fungal	Amphotericin b
Aspergillus (invasive)	Fungal	
Cryptococcus neoformans	Fungal	Flucytosine + amphotericin B
Pneumocystis carinii	Parasitic	Trimethoprim/sulfamethoxazole
Toxoplasma gondii	Parasitic	Pyrimethamine

CMV, Cytomegalovirus; *HHV*, human herpesvirus; *HSV*, herpes simplex virus; *VZV*, varicella-zoster virus.

phoproliferative disorder (PTLD), a B-cell lymphoma. It is generally associated with an initially "EBV naïve" (i.e., negative) recipient. Primary EBV infection and OKT3 use are risk factors for developing PTLD. The clinical presentation ranges from a self-limited mononucleosis-like syndrome to nodal or extranodal disease.[89] Reduced immunosuppression is the mainstay of therapy. The efficacy of acyclovir, ganciclovir, interferon-α, or anti–B-cell antibodies in the treatment of PTLD is unclear.[89] Older age, tumor monoclonality, and longer interval after transplantation are associated with worse outcome.[89,90] More than 90% of the world's population is EBV+.[91] The problem with EBV-negative recipients is the difficulty in finding donors without EBV. Other forms of cancer, such as lip and skin, also occur in the transplant population.

Infection

No discussion of immunotherapy is complete without an infection survey. Patients or donors with HIV are excluded from transplant consideration. Hepatitis C–positive donors have been used in emergent circumstances. Table 15-6 lists common infectious agents and therapies. The herpesviruses CMV, HSV, EBV, VZV, and human herpesvirus-6 (HHV-6) are the most significant pathogens after transplantation.[89] An important feature of all herpesviruses is latency: Once infected, the viral genome remains in the infected cells of the host for life. Seropositivity or the detection of antibodies to the virus, is indicative of latency. Immunosuppression can activate a latent herpesvirus. Fungal and bacterial infection are also problematic. Patients transplanted in a septic state, such as those with VAD infection, are at increased risk for septic complications.

Routine prophylaxis for most patients includes acyclovir (or similar agent) and trimethoprim/sulfameth-

oxazole. The situations mentioned earlier require therapy modification according to seropositivity.

ANESTHESIA FOR PREVIOUS TRANSPLANT

Overall survival for patients with a previous transplant is greater than 45% at 10 years.[76] In the transplant era 1995 to 1998, the number of patients surviving 3 years was approximately 74%. Many of these patients require another anesthetic for surgery that may or may not be related to their transplant.

Most patients return to New York Heart Association Class 1 functional capacity after cardiac transplantation. Preoperative preparation includes reevaluation of cardiac function.[92,93] Repeated biopsy for routine transplant management may cause injury to the tricuspid valve and severe tricuspid regurgitation, necessitating valve replacement.

Echocardiography is useful in the presurgical evaluation. Portions of detached leaflets should not be interpreted as vegetations.[56] Systolic function remains normal in the majority of patients, but a significant proportion develop diastolic dysfunction, manifested by exercise intolerance.[56] Mild rejection is not always evident with two-dimensional echocardiography. Abnormalities in isovolumic relaxation time correspond to varying degrees of rejection.[56] Increased peak inflow velocity and mitral deceleration are indicators of restrictive filling. Rejection produces an inflammatory infiltrate that causes edema.

A history of good exercise tolerance and the absence of cardiac failure symptoms comprise sufficient preoperative evaluation for minor procedures. Major procedures with considerable fluid shifting or hemodynamic challenges require a more extensive cardiac evaluation.

Patients should also be evaluated for evidence of acute or chronic rejection. The presence of rejection increases perioperative morbidity and the incidence of asymptomatic arrhythmias.

The gold standard for determining the presence of acute rejection is endomyocardial biopsy. Because this is an invasive procedure, new efforts are directed to developing a noninvasive method to detect rejection, including magnetic resonance (MR) imaging with MR spectroscopy, changes in atrial electrophysiology, and serial dobutamine stress echocardiography. Chronic rejection is manifested as ischemic heart disease. Extensive disease places these patients at risk for significant morbidity. Meticulous attention is required to maintain hemodynamic variables at preoperative levels.

All patients receive immunosuppression, and preoperative evaluation includes serum sampling to determine adequate levels. Daily perioperative measurement is necessary because shifts and other drugs may alter serum levels. Complications related to immunosuppression should be considered, including opportunistic infections. Side effects are related to specific immunosuppressive agents; for example, cyclosporine is both nephrotoxic and neurotoxic, as is tacrolimus. Cyclosporine is associated with increased risk of cholelithiasis, increasing the incidence of cholecystectomy in these patients.[94,95]

Choice of anesthetic technique depends on the type of surgery and condition of the patient.[96,97] Regional and general anesthesia can be used for patients with previous heart transplant. Cardiovascular monitoring is dependent on the nature of planned surgery. The ECG may have a double P wave, reflecting atrial activity in the native atrial cuff and the transplanted atrium. Cardiac output of the transplanted heart is preload dependent, indicating a low threshold for central venous monitoring in cases where significant fluid shifts are expected perioperatively.

Pharmacology of the transplanted heart is of particular interest to the anesthesiologist. The transplanted heart is considered to be completely denervated and does not respond acutely to exercise or hypotension with an increase in heart rate. Sympathetic reinnervation occurs over years.[98,99] Changes in cardiac output rely on changes in stroke volume, the classic Frank-Starling mechanism. The heart remains sensitive to circulating catecholamines because receptor density does not change, but will eventually respond to increases in circulating levels. Resting heart rate is usually faster than normal, representing a lack of vagal tone, but it does respond to isoproterenol, epinephrine, and norepinephrine. It was believed that neostigmine had no effect on the heart rate until recent work suggested otherwise.[100,101] Anticholinesterase agents decrease heart rate in a dose-dependent fashion, but this phenomenon is more apparent in more distant rather than recent transplants.

In summary, patients with previous heart transplant who present for surgery do not usually require invasive monitoring for minor procedures. Invasive hemodynamic monitoring is extremely useful if large fluid shifts are anticipated because these patients are very preload dependent.[102,103] Epidural or spinal anesthesia is used cautiously, with the knowledge that these patients cannot mount the usual response to vasodilation and hypotension. Patients with prior heart transplant have undergone successful pregnancies.[104,105] Ephedrine, isoproterenol, or both should be readily available to treat bradycardia since atropine has no effect on the denervated heart. It is useful to have the capability to pace transcutaneously. Finally, intraoperative echocardiography plays a significant role in managing the volume status of these patients.

KEY POINTS

1. Each year, 500,000 cases of heart failure are diagnosed.
2. Medical therapies for heart failure includes inotropic agents (milrinone or dobutamine), ACEIs, nitrates, calcium channel blockade, and β-blockade.
3. Once thought to be a contraindication in heart failure, β-blockade is useful in selected patients.
4. VADs are more commonly used to compensate heart failure patients in shock for weeks to months before transplant.
5. Coagulation therapy for VAD depends on the type of device and its blood-exposed surfaces. Stroke is a major complication of VAD therapy.
6. Preoperative evaluation of transplant candidates not only includes assessment of cardiac systolic function but also of renal and hepatic function.
7. Line placement is difficult in cardiac transplant patients. Adequate time should always be allowed for difficulties with placement of central and arterial lines.
8. Preoperative sedation is carefully titrated to avoid loss of consciousness or hypotension.
9. Induction is coordinated with the surgeon who is physically present in the operating room.
10. Anesthetic induction balances the risk of aspiration of gastric contents with hemodynamic changes on induction.

11. Inotropic therapy is started *before* induction to maintain hemodynamic stability immediately *after* induction.
12. TEE allows assessment of function before bypass and can diagnose the following complications associated with cardiac transplantation: atrial torsion, RV outflow obstruction, and decreased right or left ventricular systolic function after bypass.
13. RV dysfunction from elevated PVR is the most common cause of perioperative heart failure.
14. PA pressure can be *low* in right heart failure, even with elevated PVR. This is due to decreased ejection. Elevations in central venous pressure are a marker of RV failure.
15. Patients with prior heart transplant need an assessment of acute and chronic rejection before proceeding with surgery.

Key References

Coodley E: Newer drug therapy for congestive heart failure, *Arch Intern Med* 159:1177-1183, 1999.

Denton MD, Magee CC, Sayegh MH: Immunosuppressive strategies in transplantation, *Lancet* 353:1083-1091, 1999.

Hunt SA: Current status of cardiac transplantation, *JAMA* 280:1692-1698, 1998.

Hunt SA, Frazier OH: Mechanical circulatory support and cardiac transplantation, *Circulation* 97:2079-2090, 1998.

Schrier RW, Abraham WT: Hormones and hemodynamics in heart failure, *N Engl J Med* 341:577-585, 1999.

Shanewise JS, Cheung AT, Aronson S et al: ASE/SCA guidelines for performing a comprehensive intraoperative multiplane transesophageal echocardiography examination: recommendations of the American Society of Echocardiography Council for Intraoperative Echocardiography and the Society of Cardiovascular Anesthesiologists Task Force for Certification in Perioperative Transesophageal Echocardiography, *Anesth Analg* 89:870-884, 1999.

Steudel W, Hurford WE, Zapol WM: Inhaled nitric oxide: basic biology and clinical applications, *Anesthesiology* 91:1090-1121, 1999.

References

1. Goldstein DJ, Oz MC, Rose EA: Implantable left ventricular assist devices, *N Engl J Med* 339:1522-1533, 1998.
2. Hunt SA, Frazier OH: Mechanical circulatory support and cardiac transplantation, *Circulation* 97:2079-2090, 1998.
3. Hunt SA: Current status of cardiac transplantation, *JAMA* 280:1692-1698, 1998.
4. Firestone L: Heart transplantation, *Int Anesthesiol Clin* 29:41-58, 1991.
5. Hussain A: Anaesthesia for heart transplantation, *Br J Hosp Med* 54:466-468, 1995.
6. Sharpe MD: Anaesthesia and the transplanted patient, *Can J Anaesth* 43:R89-R98, 1996.
7. Kottke TE, Pesch DG, Frye RL et al: The potential contribution of cardiac replacement to the control of cardiovascular diseases. A population-based estimate, *Arch Surg* 125:1148-1151, 1990.
8. Fleischer KJ, Baumgartner WA: Heart transplantation. In Edmunds LH, editor: *Cardiac surgery in the adult*, New York, 1997, McGraw-Hill, pp 1409-1449.
9. Coodley E: Newer drug therapy for congestive heart failure, *Arch Intern Med* 159:1177-1183, 1999.
10. Mann DL: Mechanisms and models in heart failure: a combinatorial approach, *Circulation* 100:999-1008, 1999.
11. Pepper GS, Lee RW: Sympathetic activation in heart failure and its treatment with β-blockade, *Arch Intern Med* 159:225-234, 1999.
12. Schrier RW, Abraham WT: Hormones and hemodynamics in heart failure, *N Engl J Med* 341:577-585, 1999.
13. Petrie MC, Dawson NF, Murdoch DR et al: Failure of women's hearts, *Circulation* 99:2334-2341, 1999.
14. Pamboukian SV, Carere RG, Webb JG et al: The use of milrinone in pre-transplant assessment of patients with congestive heart failure and pulmonary hypertension, *J Heart Lung Transplant* 18:367-371, 1999.
15. Hauptman PJ, Kelly RA: Digitalis, *Circulation* 99:1265-1270, 1999.
16. Crilley JG, Dark JH, Hall JA: Reversal of severe pulmonary hypertension with β blockade in a patient with end stage left ventricular failure, *Heart* 80:620-622, 1998.
17. Metra M, Nardi M, Giubbini R et al: Effects of short- and long-term carvedilol administration on rest and exercise hemodynamic variables, exercise capacity and clinical conditions in patients with idiopathic dilated cardiomyopathy, *J Am Coll Cardiol* 24:1678-1687, 1994.
18. Quaife RA, Gilbert EM, Christian PE et al: Effects of carvedilol on systolic and diastolic left ventricular performance in idiopathic dilated cardiomyopathy or ischemic cardiomyopathy, *Am J Cardiol* 78:779-784, 1996.
19. Costanzo MR, Augustine S, Bourge R et al: Selection and treatment of candidates for heart transplantation. A statement for health professionals from the Committee on Heart Failure and Cardiac Transplantation of the Council on Clinical Cardiology, American Heart Association, *Circulation* 92:3593-3612, 1995.
20. Torre-Amione G, Kapadia S, Short D III et al: Evolving concepts regarding selection of patients for cardiac transplantation. Assessing risks and benefits, *Chest* 109:223-232, 1996.
21. Goldstein DJ, Seldomridge JA, Addonizio L et al: Orthotopic heart transplantation in patients with treated malignancies, *Am J Cardiol* 75:968-971, 1995.
22. United Network for Organ Sharing. http://www.unos.org/, 2000.
23. Gronda EG, Barbieri P, Frigerio M et al: Prognostic indices in heart transplant candidates after the first hospitalization triggered by the need for intravenous pharmacologic circulatory support, *J Heart Lung Transplant* 18:654-663, 1999.
24. Levin HR, Oz MC, Chen JM et al: Reversal of chronic ventricular dilation in patients with end-stage cardiomyopathy by prolonged mechanical unloading, *Circulation* 91:2717-2720, 1995.

25. Dipla K, Mattiello JA, Jeevanandam V et al: Myocyte recovery after mechanical circulatory support in humans with end-stage heart failure, *Circulation* 97:2316-2322, 1998.

26. Scherr K, Jensen L, Koshal A: Mechanical circulatory support as a bridge to cardiac transplantation: toward the 21st century, *Am J Crit Care* 8:324-337, 1999.

27. McCarthy PM, James KB, Savage RM et al: Implantable left ventricular assist device. Approaching an alternative for end-stage heart failure. Implantable LVAD Study Group, *Circulation* 90:II83-II86, 1994.

28. Mann DL, Willerson JT: Left ventricular assist devices and the failing heart: a bridge to recovery, a permanent assist device, or a bridge too far? *Circulation* 98:2367-2369, 1998.

29. Jaski BE, Lingle RJ, Kim J et al: Comparison of functional capacity in patients with end-stage heart failure following implantation of a left ventricular assist device versus heart transplantation: results of the experience with left ventricular assist device with exercise trial, *J Heart Lung Transplant* 18:1031-1040, 1999.

30. Jett GK: ABIOMED BVS 5000: experience and potential advantages, *Ann Thorac Surg* 61:301-304, 1996.

31. Marelli D, Laks H, Amsel B et al: Temporary mechanical support with the BVS 5000 assist device during treatment of acute myocarditis, *J Card Surg* 12:55-59, 1997.

32. Goldstein DJ, Seldomridge JA, Chen JM et al: Use of aprotinin in LVAD recipients reduces blood loss, blood use, and perioperative mortality, *Ann Thorac Surg* 59:1063-1067, 1995.

33. Herrmann M, Weyand M, Greshake B et al: Left ventricular assist device infection is associated with increased mortality but is not a contraindication to transplantation, *Circulation* 95:814-817, 1997.

34. Batista R: Partial left ventriculectomy—the Batista procedure, *Eur J Cardiothorac Surg* 15 (suppl 1):S12-S19, 1999.

35. Dor V, Di Donato M: Ventricular remodeling in coronary artery disease, *Curr Opin Cardiol* 12:533-537, 1997.

36. Dor V: Left ventricular aneurysms: the endoventricular circular patch plasty, *Semin Thorac Cardiovasc Surg* 9:123-130, 1997.

37. Dor V, Sabatier M, Montiglio F et al: Endoventricular patch reconstruction in large ischemic wall-motion abnormalities, *J Card Surg* 14:46-52, 1999.

38. Fucci C, Sandrelli L, Pardini A et al: Improved results with mitral valve repair using new surgical techniques, *Eur J Cardiothorac Surg* 9:621-626, 1995.

39. Maisano F, Torracca L, Oppizzi M et al: The edge-to-edge technique: a simplified method to correct mitral insufficiency, *Eur J Cardiothorac Surg* 13:240-245, 1998.

40. Maisano F, Redaelli A, Pennati G et al: The hemodynamic effects of double-orifice valve repair for mitral regurgitation: a 3D computational model, *Eur J Cardiothorac Surg* 15:419-425, 1999.

41. Fantini F, Barletta G, Toso A et al: Effects of reconstructive surgery for left ventricular anterior aneurysm on ventriculoarterial coupling [published erratum appears in *Heart* 81(4):452, 1999], *Heart* 81:171-176, 1999.

42. Dor V: Reconstructive left ventricular surgery for post-ischemic akinetic dilatation, *Semin Thorac Cardiovasc Surg* 9:139-145, 1997.

43. Dor V, Sabatier M, Di Donato M et al: Efficacy of endoventricular patch plasty in large postinfarction akinetic scar and severe left ventricular dysfunction: comparison with a series of large dyskinetic scars, *J Thorac Cardiovasc Surg* 116:50-59, 1998.

44. Di Donato M, Sabatier M, Dor V et al: Akinetic versus dyskinetic postinfarction scar: relation to surgical outcome in patients undergoing endoventricular circular patch plasty repair, *J Am Coll Cardiol* 29:1569-1575, 1997.

45. Dor V: The treatment of refractory ischemic ventricular tachycardia by endoventricular patch plasty reconstruction of the left ventricle, *Semin Thorac Cardiovasc Surg* 9:146-155, 1997.

46. Aronson SL, Hensley FA Jr: Case 1—1998. Anesthetic considerations for the patient undergoing partial left ventriculectomy (Batista procedure), *J Cardiothorac Vasc Anesth* 12:101-110, 1998.

47. Johnson RF, Lobato EB, Eckard JB: Perioperative management of a patient with latex allergy undergoing heart transplantation, *Anesth Analg* 87:304-305, 1998.

48. Gattinoni L, Brazzi L, Pelosi P et al: A trial of goal-oriented hemodynamic therapy in critically ill patients. SvO2 Collaborative Group, *N Engl J Med* 333:1025-1032, 1995.

49. Troianos CA, Savino JS: Internal jugular vein cannulation guided by echocardiography, *Anesthesiology* 74:787-789, 1991.

50. Koehntop DE, Beebe DS, Belani KG: The safety of dantrolene in a patient with a severe cardiomyopathy requiring a heart transplant, *Anesth Analg* 85:229-230, 1997.

51. Jayamaha JE, Dowdle JR: Acceleration of ventricular tachycardia following propofol in a patient with heterotopic cardiac transplant. Cardioversion of ventricular tachycardia in the native heart, *Anaesthesia* 48:889-891, 1993.

52. Myles PS, Hall JL, Berry CB et al: Primary pulmonary hypertension: prolonged cardiac arrest and successful resuscitation following induction of anesthesia for heart-lung transplantation, *J Cardiothorac Vasc Anesth* 8:678-681, 1994.

53. Berberich JJ, Fabian JA: A retrospective analysis of fentanyl and sufentanil for cardiac transplantation, *J Cardiothorac Anesth* 1:200-204, 1987.

54. Shiota T, McCarthy PM, White RD et al: Initial clinical experience of real-time three-dimensional echocardiography in patients with ischemic and idiopathic dilated cardiomyopathy, *Am J Cardiol* 84:1068-1073, 1999.

55. Salgo IS: Three-dimensional echocardiography, *J Cardiothorac Vasc Anesth* 11:506-516, 1997.

56. St John Sutton MG, Plappert T, Wiegers SE: *Doppler echocardiography in the transplanted heart, echocardiography in adult cardiac surgery*, Izzat MB, Sanderson JE, St John Sutton MG, editors, Oxford, 1999, Isis Medical Media, pp 301-316.

57. Chatel D, Paquin S, Oroudji M et al: Systolic anterior motion of the anterior mitral leaflet after heart transplantation, *Anesthesiology* 91:1535-1537, 1999.

58. Bittner HB, Chen EP, Biswas SS et al: Right ventricular dysfunction after cardiac transplantation: primarily related to status of donor heart, *Ann Thorac Surg* 68:1605-1611, 1999.

59. Johnson MR: Low systemic vascular resistance after cardiopulmonary bypass: are we any closer to understanding the enigma? *Crit Care Med* 27:1048-1050, 1999.

60. Argenziano M, Choudhri AF, Oz MC et al: A prospective randomized trial of arginine vasopressin in the treatment of vasodilatory shock after left ventricular assist device placement, *Circulation* 96:II-90, 1997.

61. Chiche JD, Dhainaut JF: Inhaled nitric oxide for right ventricular dysfunction in chronic obstructive pulmonary disease patients: fall or rise of an idea? *Crit Care Med* 27:2299-2301, 1999.

62. Hare JM, Shernan SK, Body SC et al: Influence of inhaled nitric oxide on systemic flow and ventricular filling pressure in patients receiving mechanical circulatory assistance [published erratum appears in *Circulation* 96(3):1065, 1997], *Circulation* 95:2250-2253, 1997.

63. Loh E, Stamler JS, Hare JM et al: Cardiovascular effects of inhaled nitric oxide in patients with left ventricular dysfunction, *Circulation* 90:2780-2785, 1994.

64. Stamler JS, Loh E, Roddy MA et al: Nitric oxide regulates basal systemic and pulmonary vascular resistance in healthy humans, *Circulation* 89:2035-2040, 1994.

65. Steudel W, Hurford WE, Zapol WM: Inhaled nitric oxide: basic biology and clinical applications, *Anesthesiology* 91:1090-1121, 1999.

66. Carrier M, Blaise G, Belisle S et al: Nitric oxide inhalation in the treatment of primary graft failure following heart transplantation, *J Heart Lung Transplant* 18:664-667, 1999.

67. Rajek A, Pernerstorfer T, Kastner J et al: Inhaled nitric oxide reduces pulmonary vascular resistance more than prostaglandin E(1) during heart transplantation, *Anesth Analg* 90:523-530, 2000.

68. Shanewise JS, Cheung AT, Aronson S et al: ASE/SCA guidelines for performing a comprehensive intraoperative multiplane transesophageal echocardiography examination: recommendations of the American Society of Echocardiography Council for Intraoperative Echocardiography and the Society of Cardiovascular Anesthesiologists Task Force for Certification in Perioperative Transesophageal Echocardiography, *Anesth Analg* 89:870-884, 1999.

69. Mair P, Balogh D: Anaesthetic and intensive care considerations for patients undergoing heart or lung transplantation, *Acta Anaesthesiol Scand Suppl* 111:78-79, 1997.

70. D'Cruz IA, Overton DH, Pai GM: Pericardial complications of cardiac surgery: emphasis on the diagnostic role of echocardiography, *J Card Surg* 7:257-268, 1992.

71. Cantarovich M, Elstein E, de Varennes B et al: Clinical benefit of neoral dose monitoring with cyclosporine 2-hr post-dose levels compared with trough levels in stable heart transplant patients, *Transplantation* 68:1839-1842, 1999.

72. Ryan TA, Rady MY, Bashour CA et al: Predictors of outcome in cardiac surgical patients with prolonged intensive care stay, *Chest* 112:1035-1042, 1997.

73. Harlan DM, Kirk AD: The future of organ and tissue transplantation: can T-cell costimulatory pathway modifiers revolutionize the prevention of graft rejection? *JAMA* 282:1076-1082, 1999.

74. Khanna A, Rosenbloom AJ, Bonham CA et al: *Principles of immunosuppression, textbook of critical care*, ed 4, Grenvik A, Ayres SM, Holbrook PR et al, editors, Philadelphia, 2000, WB Saunders, pp 1925-1938.

75. Denton MD, Magee CC, Sayegh MH: Immunosuppressive strategies in transplantation, *Lancet* 353:1083-1091, 1999.

76. Hosenpud JD, Bennett LE, Keck BM et al: The Registry of the International Society for Heart and Lung Transplantation: fourteenth official report—1997, *J Heart Lung Transplant* 16:691-712, 1997.

77. VanBuskirk AM, Pidwell DJ, Adams PW et al: Transplantation immunology, *JAMA* 278:1993-1999, 1997.

78. Barry WH: Mechanisms of immune-mediated myocyte injury, *Circulation* 89:2421-2432, 1994.

79. Lieback E, Meyer R, Nawroci M et al: Non-invasive diagnosis of cardiac rejection through echocardiographic tissue characterization, *Ann Thorac Surg* 57:1164-1170, 1994.

80. Mankad S, Murali S, Kormos RL et al: Evaluation of the potential role of color-coded tissue Doppler echocardiography in the detection of allograft rejection in heart transplant recipients, *Am Heart J* 138:721-730, 1999.

81. Weis M, von Scheidt W: Cardiac allograft vasculopathy: a review, *Circulation* 96:2069-2077, 1997.

82. Sayegh MH, Turka LA: The role of T-cell costimulatory activation pathways in transplant rejection, *N Engl J Med* 338:1813-1821, 1998.

83. Allen-Auerbach M, Schoder H, Johnson J et al: Relationship between coronary function by positron emission tomography and temporal changes in morphology by intravascular ultrasound (IVUS) in transplant recipients, *J Heart Lung Transplant* 18:211-219, 1999.

84. Akosah KO, Mohanty PK: Role of dobutamine stress echocardiography in heart transplant patients, *Chest* 113:809-815, 1998.

85. Martin RD, Bailey LL, Jacobsen WK et al: Anesthesia for neonatal orthotopic cardiac xenograft, *J Cardiothorac Anesth* 1:132-135, 1987.

86. Weiss RA: Xenotransplantation, *BMJ* 317:931-934, 1998.

87. Dorling A, Riesbeck K, Warrens A et al: Clinical xenotransplantation of solid organs, *Lancet* 349:867-871, 1997.

88. Kelly PA, Burckart GJ, Venkataramanan R: Tacrolimus: a new immunosuppressive agent, *Am J Health Syst Pharm* 52:1521-1535, 1995.

89. Singh N: Infections in solid-organ transplant recipients, *Am J Infect Control* 25:409-417, 1997.

90. Nagele H, Bahlo M, Klapdor R et al: Fluctuations of tumor markers in heart failure patients pre and post heart transplantation, *Anticancer Res* 19:2531-2534, 1999.

91. Haque T, Crawford DH: The role of adoptive immunotherapy in the prevention and treatment of lymphoproliferative disease following transplantation, *Br J Haematol* 106:309-316, 1999.

92. Schwaiblmair M, von Scheidt W, Uberfuhr P et al: Lung function and cardiopulmonary exercise performance after heart transplantation: influence of cardiac allograft vasculopathy, *Chest* 116:332-339, 1999.

93. Hauptman PJ, Gass A, Goldman ME: The role of echocardiography in heart transplantation, *J Am Soc Echocardiogr* 6:496-509, 1993.

94. Joshi GP, Hein HA, Ramsay MA et al: Hemodynamic response to anesthesia and pneumoperitoneum in orthotopic cardiac transplant recipients, *Anesthesiology* 85:929-933, 1996.

95. Levecque JP, Benhamou D, Zetlaoui P et al: Laparoscopic cholecystectomy in a patient with a transplanted heart, *Anesthesiology* 86:1425-1427, 1997.

96. Cheng DC, Ong DD: Anaesthesia for non-cardiac surgery in heart-transplanted patients, *Can J Anaesth* 40:981-986, 1993.

97. Boscoe M: Anesthesia for patients with transplanted lungs and heart and lungs, *Int Anesthesiol Clin* 33:21-44, 1995.

98. Estorch M, Camprecios M, Flotats A et al: Sympathetic reinnervation of cardiac allografts evaluated by 123I-MIBG imaging, *J Nucl Med* 40:911-916, 1999.

99. Steinfaith M, Schmitz W, Scholz H et al: β-adrenergic receptor number in surgically denervated, transplanted human hearts, *Anesthesiology* 76:863-864, 1992.

100. Beebe DS, Shumway SJ, Maddock R: Sinus arrest after intravenous neostigmine in two heart transplant recipients. *Anesth Analg* 78:779-782, 1994.

101. Backman SB, Ralley FE, Fox GS: Neostigmine produces bradycardia in a heart transplant patient, *Anesthesiology* 78:777-779, 1993.

102. Shenaq SA, Schultz S, Noon GP et al: Case 3—1993. Combined abdominal aortic aneurysm resection and cholecystectomy following prior heart transplantation, *J Cardiothorac Vasc Anesth* 7:610-614, 1993.

103. Kanter SF, Samuels SI: Anesthesia for major operations on patients who have transplanted hearts, a review of 29 cases, *Anesthesiology* 46:65-68, 1977.

104. Kim KM, Sukhani R, Slogoff S et al: Central hemodynamic changes associated with pregnancy in a long-term cardiac transplant recipient, *Am J Obstet Gynecol* 174:1651-1653, 1996.

105. Camann WR, Goldman GA, Johnson MD et al: Cesarean delivery in a patient with a transplanted heart, *Anesthesiology* 71:618-620, 1989.

CHAPTER 16

Cardiothoracic Intensive Care

J.G.T. Augoustides, M.D. ■ C. William Hanson III, M.D.

OUTLINE

Cardiothoracic intensive care begins during the transport of the patient to the cardiothoracic intensive care unit (CTICU). The vulnerable period of transport proceeds under the direct supervision of the anesthesiologist when the patient's clinical condition is stable. The electrocardiogram (ECG), blood pressure, and systemic oxygen saturation are continuously monitored during transport. Temporary cardiac pacing continues the intraoperative pacing mode or is set at a ventricular rate below the patient's intrinsic rate (usually 50 to 60 beats/min). The operative in-

struments remain sterile and available for possible emergent sternotomy until the patient leaves the operating room in a stable condition. On arrival to the CTICU, a full report regarding relevant history and intraoperative details is provided to the CTICU team. Hemodynamic monitoring, mechanical ventilation, initial laboratory tests, and initial patient orders are instituted.

The patient's course in the CTICU typically follows one of three tracks:

1. The **fast-track** patient (discharged within days from the CTICU)

2. The **short-term** patient (develops complications and is discharged from the CTICU within days to weeks)
3. The **long-term** patient (discharge delayed over weeks to months)

THE FAST-TRACK CARDIOTHORACIC PATIENT

Postoperative cardiothoracic care is a focal point of intensive cost reduction in the managed care era. Postoperative cardiothoracic care contributes significantly to the overall cost of cardiac surgery.[1] Fast-track care aims to improve postoperative cost-efficiency and patient outcome by minimizing the postoperative length of stay. Delayed patient movement from the CTICU inhibits opportunities for increasing surgical case load and may lead to case cancellations for lack of CTICU beds. These factors contribute to suboptimal use of operating room resources and personnel. Postoperative cost reduction focuses on fast-track patient care within the CTICU or fast-track patient care in alternative facilities. These fast-track options are discussed in the following sections.

Fast-Track Postoperative Care within the CTICU

Fast-track CTICU care begins with appropriate patient selection. The CTICU team determines the fast-track selection criteria.[2] The ideal patient has discrete cardiothoracic pathologic findings and no additional major organ system insufficiency. Comorbid conditions do not necessarily disqualify a patient, especially if the deficit is static (e.g., a residual hemiplegia). Although fast tracking began with patients undergoing primary coronary revascularization, this approach has been extended to CTICU patients undergoing valve replacement, lung resection, and heart and lung transplantation. Teamwork is essential to the success and safety of this approach.[2] Patient-care protocols standardize patient care and allow individual disciplines to function congruently. CTICU data collection and analysis evaluate the success of fast-track protocol implementation. Evidence-based feedback serves as ongoing quality and safety assessment within the CTICU. Fast-track CTICU care requires a systems approach to protocol implementation. Figs. 16-1 and 16-2 show examples of a fast-track CTICU physician orders and a patient care pathway.

Respiratory. The weaning of mechanical ventilation, arterial blood gas sampling, weaning parameters, timing of tracheal extubation, and subsequent weaning of fractional inspired oxygen concentration are all standardized. The patient begins the fast-track pathway on arrival to the CTICU. The fast-track process requires physician consultation only in problem cases. Expedited

tracheal extubation is usually achieved within 6 hours of CTICU admission.[3] The patient should be alert and cooperative, normothermic, hemodynamically stable, not bleeding significantly, and have adequate respiratory mechanics. A fast-track ventilator weaning protocol is shown in Fig. 16-3.

Cardiothoracic. The weaning of hemodynamic infusions, the withdrawal of invasive monitoring, the removal of pericardial and pleural drains, and the use of temporary pacing wires are standardized.

Hematologic. The criteria and practice of blood component transfusion and anticoagulation are standardized. Antithrombolytic drug selection and dosing are also standardized. These agents possess proven efficacy and enhance cost savings.[4,5]

Renal and Metabolic. Electrolyte repletion (especially potassium and magnesium), glucose homeostasis with an insulin infusion or sliding-scale insulin coverage, and Foley catheter management are standardized.

Hepatic and Gastrointestinal. The commencement and advancement of intake per os is encouraged and standardized.

Protocol-driven patient management is tailored to the particular patient population. The pathway for primary myocardial revascularization is therefore distinct from the primary valve replacement pathway. Common areas have uniform management for consistency and ease of implementation in the CTICU. Protocol-driven care represents efficient consensus-based management for the cardiothoracic patient with an uncomplicated postoperative course. Cardiothoracic clinical pathways vary from institution to institution, reflecting regional preference. The CTICU team must be intimately involved with protocol design. Protocol implementation is designed to succeed in a particular CTICU. The CTICU fast-track pathway interfaces with overall perioperative management to achieve total perioperative fast tracking. Cardiothoracic patient flow must be safe and efficient from the operating room through the CTICU and surgical floor to home.

Advances in cardiothoracic surgery and anesthesia have enhanced the success of fast-track patient care. The expanding role of advanced cardiothoracic surgery relates significantly to CTICU fast-track care. The percentage of cardiothoracic patients suitable for fast-track care increases where these advanced techniques are implemented. Minimally invasive and off-pump cardiac surgery allows shorter operative times, smaller incisions, and avoidance of cardiopulmonary bypass (CPB), thus shortening the CTICU stay. Cardiothoracic anesthetic techniques have evolved in tandem with cardiothoracic surgery to facilitate fast-track CTICU care. The fast-track

Text continued on p. 467

DATE	TIME	ORDERS NOTED BY NURSE	PLEASE LIST ALL DRUG ALLERGIES AND SENSITIVITIES WHEN WRITING ADMISSION ORDERS. PLEASE CHECK DRUG ALLERGIES AND SENSITIVITIES BEFORE WRITING MEDICATION ORDERS.			
			TREATMENT ORDERS	DATE	TIME	STUDY ORDERS
			SICU ADMISSION ORDERS (Page 1 of 3)			
			1. Admit to SICU			
			2. Operation:			
			3. Surgeon:			
			4. Allergies:			
			5. Vital Signs per protocol:			
			6. Daily weight @ 5:00 am, I&O q1h; 1200 cc fluid restriction			
			7. NPO until extubation, then ice chips/clear liquids, advance to Low-Cholesterol/Low-Fat/NAS as tolerated			
			8. Nasogastric tube to 60 cm suction; irrigate q4h with 30 cc normal saline, D/C upon extubation			
			9. Foley catheter to straight drainage; D/C foley by 0900 POD #1			
			10. Chest tube to 20 cm H_2O per protocol; autotransfusion per protocol			
			Maintain monitor lines heparinized saline per protocol			
			Rewarming unit to patient; remove when T36.5°C			
			11. Soft restraints as needed			
			12. Continuous pulse oximetry per protocol			
			13. OR dressing remains intact ×24 hrs then change per protocol			
			14. PACEMAKER ORDERS:			
			Mode: _____ Rate: _____ M.A.: _____	Sensitivity: _____ A.V. delay: _____		
			15. Bedrest until post-op day 1 then dangle legs; advance to OOB as tolerated			
			16. Initial vent settings:			
			Mode: _____ Respiratory Rate: _____ Tidal Volume (10-15 cc/kg): _____ FiO_2: _____ %			
			PEEP: _____ Pressure Support: _____			
			17. Weaning parameters for FiO_2 using pulse oximetry (refer to weaning protocol)			
			18. Incentive Spirometry q2-4h and prn post extubation			
			19. Medications:			
			☐ Meperidine (Demerol) 25 mg IV prn shivering, repeat ×1 in 15 min if needed. Notify MD if shivering			
			persists. (NB: Discontinue if patient on MAO inhibitors)			
			☐ Nitroprusside (Nipride) 100 mg/250 cc D5W to maintain MAP _____ to _____ mmHg			
			☐ NTG 100 mg/250 cc D5W to maintain MAP _____ to _____ mmHg			
			MD Signature _____			Beeper # _____
			Name (printed) _____			

FIG. 16-1   Sample fast-track CTICU physician orders.

Continued

DATE	TIME	ORDERS NOTED BY NURSE	PLEASE LIST ALL DRUG ALLERGIES AND SENSITIVITIES WHEN WRITING ADMISSION ORDERS. PLEASE CHECK DRUG ALLERGIES AND SENSITIVITIES BEFORE WRITING MEDICATION ORDERS.			
			TREATMENT ORDERS	DATE	TIME	STUDY ORDERS
			SICU ADMISSION ORDERS (Page 2 of 3)			
			19. Medications (continued):			
			☐ Once extubated, begin metoprolol 25 mg po q6h (If SBP <100, give 12.5 mg for that dose.			
			If SBP <90, hold dose)			
			☐ (**In Diabetic Patient**) Insulin Sliding Scale: Regular Humulin Insulin sq q4h			
			Glucose <200 _____ units (suggested 0 units)			
			Glucose 201-250 _____ units (suggested 3 units)			
			Glucose 251-300 _____ units (suggested 6 units)			
			Glucose 301-350 _____ units (suggested 9 units)			
			Glucose 351-400 _____ units (suggested 12 units)			
			Glucose >400 _____ units (Notify House Officer)			
			☐ KCl 10-20 mEq IV q1h prn to maintain K+ 4.0-4.5			
			☐ Magnesium <2.0 give 1 g Magnesium Sulfate in 50 mg D5W over 1 hr until POD 1			
			☐ Aspirin 325 mg QD, begin 6 hrs post-op via NG tube or pr. If receiving blood products, give 12 hrs			
			post-op. Once taking po, use enteric coated.			
			☐ Maalox 30 cc q4h per NGT if drainage Heme + or pH <4.5			
			☐ Sucralfate (Carafate) 1 g q6h prn per NGT if drainage Heme + or pH <4.5 or Hx of ulcers			
			☐ Cefazolin (Ancef) 500 mg IV q8h × 72h (Delete if penicillin allergic)			
			PRN Medications			
			☐ Acetaminophen 650 mg q3-4h prn temp >38.5°C or pain			
			☐ Morphine _____ mg IV q _____ hrs			
			☐ Midazolam _____ mg IV q _____ hrs if intubated			
			☐ Oxycodone/Acetaminophen (Percocet) 1-2 po q3-4h prn pain postextubation			
			Other medications:			
			MD Signature _____			Beeper # _____
			Name (printed) _____			

FIG. 16-1, cont'd   Sample fast-track CTICU physician orders.

Continued

DATE	TIME	ORDERS NOTED BY NURSE	PLEASE LIST ALL DRUG ALLERGIES AND SENSITIVITIES WHEN WRITING ADMISSION ORDERS. PLEASE CHECK DRUG ALLERGIES AND SENSITIVITIES BEFORE WRITING MEDICATION ORDERS.			
			TREATMENT ORDERS	DATE	TIME	STUDY ORDERS
			SICU ADMISSION ORDERS (Page 3 of 3)			
			20. Lab data:			
			Chest X-ray (portable), ordered upon arrival in SICU and QD as long as chest tube in place			
			EKG 12 lead STAT upon arrival and post-op day 1			
			21. Admission Blood Work:			
			ABG, K, Na, Mg, Cl, CO_2, Glucose, Ca, Hgb/Hct, PT/PTT			
			22. A.M. Lab (**to lab no later than 1 am**)			
			Send routine panel 7, Mg, CBC			
			23. Notify House Officer:			
			MAP or mm/Hg			
			CVP or mm/Hg			
			PAD/PAW or mm/Hg			
			HR or BPM			
			Urine output ≤30 cc/hr ×2h			
			Temp ≥38.5°C			
			MD Signature _____			Beeper # _____
			Name (printed) _____			

FIG. 16-1, cont'd   Sample fast-track CTICU physician orders.

	Office Visit	Before Procedure	Day of Surgery (Before Surgery)	Day of Surgery (Intensive Care Unit)
TESTS		• Blood tests • Urine test • Chest X-ray (if ordered) • Electrocardiogram (if ordered)		• Blood tests • Chest X-ray • Electrocardiogram
TREATMENTS				• Deep breathing exercises after breathing tube removed • Incentive spirometry
LINES AND TUBES				• Breathing tube until able to breathe on your own, then oxygen • Special equipment to monitor blood pressure and heart function • Pacemaker wires • IV fluids • Catheter tube for urine • Chest tubes for drainage
MEDICATIONS			• Medications as instructed by your surgeon or anesthesiologist	• IV antibiotics • IV pain medications • IV heart medications (if needed) • Aspirin
DIET			• Nothing to eat or drink after 12M day of surgery	• Ice chips after breathing tube removed • Fluids restricted
ACTIVITY			• No restrictions unless told otherwise • Bring only essential belongings to the hospital. Valuables should be given to your family to take home.	• Turn side to side in bed with nurse's help
TEACHING	• Your doctor will discuss the surgical procedure with you, explaining the benefits and risks • Sign the consent forms for the procedure and for blood transfusion	• The anesthesiologist will discuss anesthesia with you, explaining the benefits and risks.	• Incentive spirometry (deep breathing exercises) • Pain control methods and pain scale • Ask any unanswered questions • Family should wait in waiting area until surgery is complete.	• After surgery, family can wait in ICU waiting area.

FIG. 16-2   Fast-track CTICU patient care pathway.
Continued

Post-Operative Day 1 SICU	Post-Op Day 2	Post-Op Day 3	Post-Op Day 4	Post-Op Day 5 or 6 Discharge to Home
——→ ——→ ——→	——→ ——→ ——→		• Blood tests	
• Weight on transfer • Deep breathing exercises • Incentive spirometry • Dressing removed from wounds today	• Daily weight ——→ • Dressing change to chest and legs (incisions open to air if dry)	——→ ——→ ——→	——→ ——→	——→ • Staples removed today; Steri-strips (paper strips) applied
• Some monitoring equipment removed • Telemetry (heart rhythm monitor) • Urine catheter removed • Chest tubes may be removed today or tomorrow • IV capped • Oxygen	——→ • Oxygen removed when oxygen level in blood is sufficient	——→ ——→	• Pacemaker wires removed	• Heart monitor removed • IV removed
• Heart medications (if necessary) • IV antibiotics • Aspirin • Pain medicine switched to pills • Medications for bowels	——→ ——→ ——→ • Pain pills • Medications for bowels as needed	——→ ——→ ——→ ——→	——→ ——→ ——→ ——→	——→
• Liquids advanced to regular diet as tolerated • Fluids restricted	• Regular - no added salt, low cholesterol diet		——→	——→
• Out of bed twice today • Walk 50 feet with assistance twice today • Physical therapy evaluation	• Out of bed three times with meals • Walk 75 feet with assistance three times today • Begin to bathe yourself with assistance from nurse	• Out of bed at least three times/day • Walk to bathroom with assistance • Walk in hall 100 feet four times today with help	• Out of bed for meals • Walk to bathroom • Walk in hall 150 feet four times/day with help	• May shower today with assistance • Walk four times/day • Climb one flight of stairs
	• Review "Moving Right Along" booklet • Activity progression • Sternal precautions • Start discharge instructions: signs/symptoms of infection	• Attend Phase I Cardiac rehab class: - Cardiac risk factors - Benefits of exercise - Pulse taking - Energy conservation techniques - Instruction in home program • Attend discharge class	——→	——→ • Review copy of discharge instructions/ when to call doctor • Receive prescriptions • Receive information about follow-up visits to doctor(s)

FIG. 16-2, cont'd   Fast-track CTICU patient care pathway.

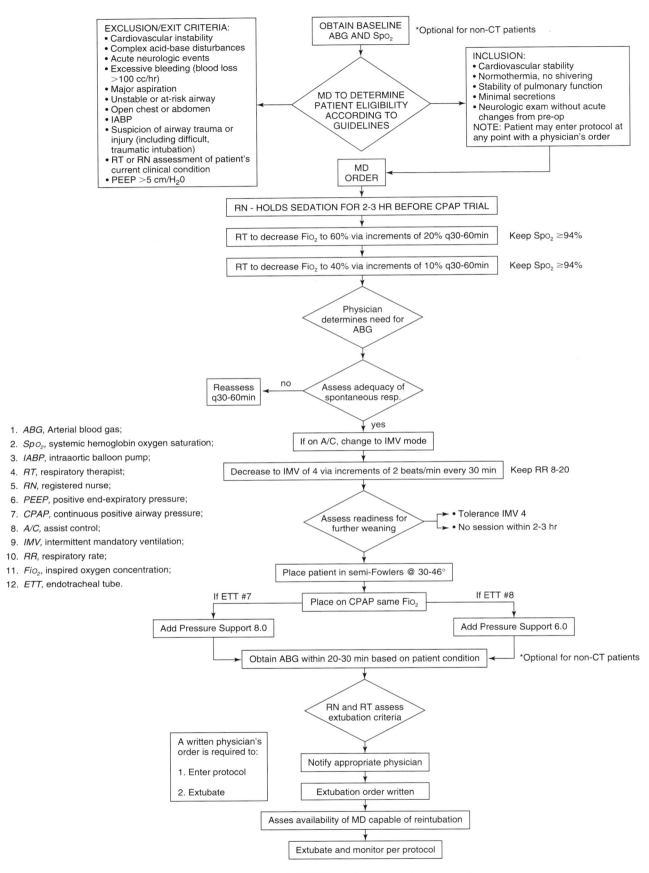

FIG. 16-3   Fast-track CTICU ventilator weaning protocol.

anesthetic technique achieves smooth and rapid emergence without sacrificing intraoperative goals such as hemodynamic stability and neurohumoral stress reduction. Amnesia is provided by administering short-acting benzodiazepines, volatile anesthetics, and propofol infusions at 25 to 75 mcg/kg/min.[6] Analgesia is provided by administering reduced intravenous fentanyl at 12.5 to 37.5 mcg/kg.[7] Opioid-sparing drugs such as ketorolac and trazodone augment postoperative analgesia as part of a multimodal approach to postoperative pain management. Neuromuscular blockade is tailored for early postoperative extubation. The choice of paralytic agent depends on cost, length of surgical procedure, and the degree of renal or hepatic failure.[8] At the Hospital of the University of Pennsylvania the primary long-acting neuromuscular blocker is pancuronium.

Further opioid reduction may be achieved with remifentanil, α_2-agonists, and central neuraxial blockade. Remifentanil is an ultrashort-acting opioid. Although remifentanil facilitates expedited tracheal extubation, postoperative opioid supplementation is indicated.[9] α_2-Agonists such as clonidine and dexmedetomidine reduce the surgical neurohumoral stress response and facilitate CTICU fast-track care.[10] Intrathecal or epidural local anesthetics with or without opioids may also expedite tracheal extubation.[11] This approach is currently limited by the risk of spinal hematoma with concomitant heparinization and a paucity of data to demonstrate superiority over a balanced reduced opioid technique. In cardiothoracic surgery without cardiopulmonary bypass (CPB), epidural analgesia can be considered to expedite tracheal extubation and reduce total postoperative opioid dosage.

Fast-Track Postoperative Care outside the CTICU

Postoperative cost reduction may dictate patient recovery in alternative facilities such as a cardiac surgery recovery area (CSRA) located within the operating room environment. The CSRA as described by Westaby et al[12] was staffed by cardiac recovery nurses who were supervised by anesthesiologists and surgeons. The driving force for this innovation was a shortage of CTICU beds. Westaby et al demonstrated a reduced length of stay with equivalent patient outcome. Their patient population was young and had shorter aortic cross-clamp and surgery times. These patient criteria must be considered before adopting this model in another institution. The choice and organization of the postoperative cardiothoracic care facility depends on institutional preference. The fast-track approach seeks to optimize postoperative cardiothoracic care for appropriate patients within the institutional model selected.

Fast-track care enhances patient flow from the CTICU or CSRA via telemetry beds to discharge from the hospital. The rate-limiting step for CTICU discharge may be the availability of telemetry beds. A discharge holding area can accept patients from telemetry, allowing patient transfer from the CTICU or CSRA and preventing unnecessary CTICU days. This broader perioperative perspective will continue to affect postoperative cardiothoracic management. These alternatives within and without the conventional model must be tested for patient safety as reflected by mortality and morbidity rates.

Patient outcome analysis is essential to demonstrate the patient safety of fast-track postoperative cardiac care. Johnson et al[13] evaluated respiratory outcome after expedited tracheal extubation. The fast-track group, as compared with a control group, had similar postextubation parameters except for a radiographic atelectasis score that was worse in the control group. This may reflect the earlier return of spontaneous ventilation, an effective cough, and earlier mobility in the fast-track group. Cheng et al[14] demonstrated that fast-track care has equivalent rates of myocardial ischemia or infarction, bleeding, stroke, and overall mortality. Their fast-track group had less intrapulmonary shunting, a faster return to cognitive baseline, and a lower major complication rate. This may reflect, in part, different patient populations. Hall et al[15] demonstrated that low-dose or high-dose propofol sedation did not change the incidence of myocardial ischemia as detected by Holter ST-segment monitoring in a randomized controlled clinical trial.

The economic impact of fast-track postoperative patient care has been extensively evaluated. Expedited CTICU tracheal extubation provides savings as high as 25%.[14] Reduced costs using fast-track CTICU care have been demonstrated in many recent studies.[10,16] Fast-track CTICU care is safe and cost-effective. It is now firmly established in the CTICU and continues to evolve as new anesthetic and surgical techniques enter the clinical arena. These advances, coupled with the economic demands of managed care, will shape the future of fast-track CTICU care.

THE SHORT-TERM CARDIOTHORACIC PATIENT

The complications of the CTICU short-term patient are examined according to a systems approach in the following section. The relevant diagnostic modalities and appropriate management are also reviewed.

New Neurologic Deficit

The neurologic lesion may be central or peripheral. Recovery from structural neural damage is highly variable. A full diagnostic evaluation is the platform for rational management, as summarized in Table 16-1.

Delirium. Delirium is described as a clouded consciousness and disorientation with respect to person,

TABLE 16-1
New Neurologic Deficit in the Cardiothoracic Intensive Care Unit

NEUROLOGICAL ENTITY	ETIOLOGY	DIAGNOSTIC EVALUATION	CLINICAL MANAGEMENT

Delirium	Hypoxia
	Hypercarbia
	Infection
	Metabolic drugs
	Drug withdrawal
	ICU psychosis
		Arterial blood gas
		Serum glucose
		Serum sodium
		Serum calcium
		Renal function
		Liver function
		Body fluid culture
			Ventilation
			Oxygenation
			Correct metabolic milieu
			Appropriate antibiotics
			Rehydration and sedation
			    for drug withdrawal
			    and ICU psychosis

Cerebrovascular accident	Macroemboli Microemboli	Serial physical exams Neuroimaging Echocardiogram Carotid Doppler	Anticoagulation for embolic event Rehabilitation
Paraplegia	Epidural Hematoma Anterior spinal artery syndrome	Serial physical exam Neuroimaging	Laminectomy for hematoma Spinal drainage Rehabilitation
Periphral nerve lesions	Compression traction	Serial physical exam Electromyography	Rehabilitation

ICU, Intensive care unit.

place, or time. Because delirium is often a symptom, reversible organic causes are explored and corrected. "ICU psychosis" is a diagnosis made after exclusion of organic causes. This phenomenon may be due to disturbance of the sleep-wake cycle in the CTICU, and it is treated with haloperidol and judicious nocturnal sedation.

Cerebrovascular Accident. Central structural lesions are typically embolic in origin. Macroemboli are atherosclerotic debris released during intraoperative aortic manipulation. Gaseous microemboli during CPB have been reduced by membrane oxygenators and arterial line filters.[17,18] The embolic lesion may be focal (e.g., internal capsule) or diffuse (e.g., multiple small cerebral infarcts). The final neurologic deficit depends on the site, extent, and reversibility of neural damage.

Paraplegia. New postoperative paraplegia in the setting of an epidural catheter or lumbar spinal drain is an epidural hematoma until proven otherwise. Emergency laminectomy is indicated if neuroimaging demonstrates epidural hematoma. The anterior spinal artery syndrome typically follows spinal devascularization during thoracic aortic surgery. Sparing of touch and proprioception is typical. Cerebrospinal fluid drainage may improve spinal perfusion and allow neurologic recovery.

Peripheral Nerve Lesions. Brachial plexopathy after median sternotomy has a frequency of 2% to 25%.[19] Most lesions are subclinical and resolve within 6 to 8 weeks.[20] About 50% of ulnar nerve injuries resolve in 6 months, but 25% persist beyond 2 years.[21] A comprehensive baseline assessment, including electromyogram testing, facilitates detection and monitors recovery.

Respiratory Failure

Progressive hypoxemia or hypercarbia mandates the mechanical support of oxygenation or ventilation. A diagnostic evaluation strategy determines cause and severity before prompt appropriate management is instituted. This clinical approach is summarized in Table 16-2.

Respiratory Drive. Inadequate respiratory drive is caused by pharmacologic inhibition or ischemic insult to the medullary respiratory control center. Pharmacologic inhibition is reversed by the appropriate antagonist and by allowing adequate time for drug clearance. An ischemic medullary lesion is usually irreversible; prolonged dependence on mechanical ventilation is typical.

Respiratory Muscle Strength. Inadequate cough is usually a marker of respiratory muscle weakness. Resid-

TABLE 16-2
Respiratory Failure in the Cardiothoracic Intensive Care Unit

RESPIRATORY ENTITY	ETIOLOGY	DIAGNOSTIC EVALUATION	CLINICAL MANAGEMENT
Inadequate respiratory drive	Pharmacologic Ischemic	Neurologic exam Rule out other etiologies	Ventilatory support Antagonists Time
Inadequate muscle strength	Neuromuscular blockade Diaphragmatic dysfunction Postoperative pain	Pharmacologic reversal Fluoroscopy	Ventilatory support Physiotherapy Brochoscopy Pain management
Alveolar infiltration	*Transudate:* Ventricular failure *Exudate:* Aspiration; ARDS; infection	Ventricular evaluation Chest x-ray Body fluid culture	Ventilatory support Diuresis Antibiotics V/Q matching maneuvers
Pleural collection	Gas Fluid	Physical exam Chest x-ray	Ventilatory support Drainage

ARDS, Adult respiratory distress syndrome; *V/Q,* ventilation/perfusion.

ual neuromuscular blockade is pharmacologically reversed. Diaphragmatic dysfunction may follow intraoperative phrenic nerve injury. Postoperative pain also inhibits respiratory excursion and postoperative cough. Consequent aspiration and inadequate clearance of epithelial mucus result in progressive atelectasis and ventilation/perfusion (V/Q) mismatch. Aggressive chest physiotherapy and incentive spirometry are treatments for postoperative atelectasis. Intermittent bronchoscopic lavage is used to remove large mucous plugs. Concomitant bronchospasm and respiratory infection must be aggressively managed.

Alveolar Infiltration. Alveolar infiltration is either transudative or exudative. The transudate of left ventricular (LV) failure resolves with diuresis and support of ventricular function. Exudative alveolar etiologic factors include aspiration, infection, and the adult respiratory distress syndrome (ARDS). Inadequate cough or swallowing causes aspiration. The main central risk factor is impairment of consciousness from any cause. The main peripheral risk factor is swallowing dysfunction. The natural history depends on the amount and type of aspirated material. Methylene blue in nasoenteric feeds is a useful marker for aspiration. A speech and swallowing evaluation allows for appropriate nutritional planning.

The immunocompromised transplant patient is at risk for opportunistic viral, bacterial, and fungal infections. These patients may not manifest infection with a fever or leukocytosis. Bronchoscopy or open lung biopsy may be required for diagnostic and culture

samples. Lung rejection may resemble alveolar infection. The balance between immunosuppression and antibiotic therapy often requires expert consultation with infectious disease specialists and pulmonologists.

ARDS is an asymmetric alveolar process that may accompany the multiorgan-failure syndrome. Mechanical ventilation with small tidal volumes and limited peak pressures reduces barotrauma and improves survival.[22] Pressure-cycled ventilation and inverse inspiratory-to-expiratory ratio ventilation limit peak inspiratory pressure. Sedation lowers oxygen consumption and allows the patient to tolerate this mode of ventilation. Ventilation trials customize mechanical ventilation for each patient on the basis of serial blood gases and overall clinical status of the patient.

Ventilation-perfusion matching in ARDS improves oxygenation. Hypoxic pulmonary vasoconstriction (HPV) diverts blood from nonventilated to ventilated pulmonary segments. Ventilation (V) is thus coupled with perfusion (Q) and gas exchange is optimized. Intravenous administration of a vasoconstrictor such as phenylephrine augments this HPV-mediated V/Q coupling.[23] Inhaled nitric oxide (NO) is a selective pulmonary vasodilator with a role in ARDS.[24] NO vasodilates capillaries in ventilated pulmonary segments and couples V with Q. Intravenous phenylephrine administered simultaneously with inhaled NO in ARDS synergistically augments O_2 transfer in the lung.[23] NO vasodilates capillaries in the ventilated lung units while phenylephrine-enhanced HPV shunts perfusion away from hypoxic lung units.

Gravity also determines V/Q matching.[25] The prone

position improves oxygenation in ARDS by improving V/Q matching.[26] The prone position preserves functional residual capacity and minimizes airway closure.[27] Greater diaphragmatic excursion in the prone position augments the regional V/Q.[28] The risks associated with the prone position are unintentional tracheal extubation, pressure necrosis of dependent body parts, and retinal infarction.[29] Careful nursing care minimizes the risks of the prone position while improving oxygenation in ARDS.

Pleural Collection. Tension pneumothorax mandates immediate needle thoracostomy. The needle thoracostomy is then revised to a regular tube thoracostomy when the patient is stable. Drainage of a pleural effusion reverses regional atelectasis and improves respiratory mechanics.

Cardiac Failure

The etiologic factors for cardiac failure are considered anatomically as conductive, pericardial, myocardial, or valvular. The electrocardiogram (ECG) and echocardiogram facilitate the analysis of myocardial rhythm and function. The diagnostic and management approaches for cardiac failure are summarized in Table 16-3.

Conductive Disease. Hemodynamically unstable tachycardias are managed by urgent electrical cardioversion or defibrillation. Pharmacologic cardioversion or rate control is used to manage a hemodynamically stable tachycardia. Serum pH, potassium, and mag-

nesium are corrected. Pharmacologic rate control of postoperative atrial fibrillation (AF) is achieved with digoxin, esmolol,[30] and diltiazem. Esmolol has minimal bronchoconstricting effects in patients with chronic obstructive pulmonary disease.[31] Procainamide is effective for conversion of AF to sinus rhythm, but is also associated with hypotension and impaired ventricular function. Procainamide administration is titrated to clinical effect and serum levels of procainamide and N-acetylprocainamide that depend on renal and hepatic function. Amiodarone is used to manage AF both for rate control and cardioversion.[32] It appears safe for use in patients with depressed ventricular function. Intravenous administration is devoid of the chronic adverse effects such as photosensitivity, corneal deposits, lung fibrosis, and thyroid disease.

If AF persists for 48 hours, the risk of atrial thromboembolism is addressed with anticoagulation or electrical cardioversion. The choice depends on the presence of preoperative AF, patient lifestyle, and another indication for long-term anticoagulation.

Ventricular tachycardia is treated with lidocaine. Lidocaine-resistant ventricular tachyarrhythmias may respond to procainamide, amiodarone, or bretylium. The causes of the ventricular arrhythmia are sought while the serum pH, potassium, and magnesium are normalized. Ventricular ischemia and inappropriate pacing should be excluded.

A hemodynamically significant bradycardia is managed by temporary pacing. An adequate cardiac rhythm that persists postoperatively may require permanent pacing. Heart block typically occurs after extensive dis-

TABLE 16-3
Cardiac Failure in the Cardiothoracic Intensive Care Unit

CARDIAC ENTITY	ETIOLOGY	DIAGNOSTIC EVALUATION	CLINICAL MANAGEMENT
Conductive disease	Acidosis	ECG	Cardioversion
	Potassium and magnesium	Arterial blood sample	Defibrillation
	Ischemia	Electrolytes	Drugs
	Surgical edema and dissection	Echocardiography	Pacemaker
Pericardial disease	Bleeding	Clinical exam	Pericardial drainage
	Surgical dissection	Invasive monitoring	Medical support of ventricular function
		Echocardiography	
Myocardial and	Ischemia	ECG	Volume expansion
valvular disease	Failed surgery	Echocardiography	Inotropes
	Hypertension	Invasive monitoring	Pressors
			Surgery
			Mechanical assistance

ECG, Electrocardiogram.

section around the conductive system. An adequate rhythm may return when the postoperative edema has resolved.

Pericardial Disease. Pericardial tamponade typically presents with hypotension and equalization of intracardiac pressures. Echocardiography demonstrates a pericardial collection with diastolic chamber collapse and greater than 50% respiratory variation in chamber filling pressures. The decision for mediastinal exploration is clinical: the unstable patient returns to the operating room for pericardial evacuation. The markedly unstable patient may require sternotomy in the CTICU to acutely relieve the tamponade.

Pericardiectomy increases ventricular volume loading. Ventricular failure may result from the increased ventricular preload. Pharmacologic ventricular support allows the ventricle to adapt to the new loading conditions.

Myocardial Disease and Valvular Disease. Right ventricular (RV) failure is caused by ischemia, tricuspid regurgitation (TR), or high pulmonary vascular resistance (PVR). RV ischemia occurs from inadequate RV protection during CPB, right coronary graft insufficiency, atherosclerotic emboli, and air. Air typically embolizes to the right coronary artery because the right coronary ostium is anterior in the aortic root and air migrates anteriorly in the supine patient.

TR protects the right ventricle from volume and pressure overload by providing a "pop off" for RV ejection. Surgical correction of TR may cause postoperative RV failure if the right ventricle cannot tolerate the increase in afterload. Severe TR in the heart-transplant population may develop postoperatively after RV endomyocardial biopsy.

High PVR is typically secondary to pulmonary emboli, mitral valve disease, or LV failure. High PVR places considerable strain on the transplanted heart right ventricle that previously experienced normal PVR. Temporary postoperative support is indicated until the donor right ventricle adapts to this higher PVR. The management of RV failure includes providing pharmacologic support of RV function and proceeding with prompt surgery when indicated. Pharmacologic therapy of right ventricle support lowers PVR and augments RV contractility, as outlined in Table 16-4. NO effectively lowers PVR for the donor ventricle.[33] NO weaning should be gradual because rebound PVR may occur.[34]

LV failure is caused by ischemia, mitral regurgitation (MR), and LV outflow tract (LVOT) obstruction. LV ischemia is caused by inadequate LV protection during CPB, coronary graft insufficiency,[35] atherosclerotic emboli, and air. ECG and echocardiography identify specific cor-

TABLE 16-4
Management of Pulmonary Hypertension in the Cardiothoracic Intensive Care Unit

INTERVENTION	RATIONALE	ACTION	USE
Metabolic	Ensure Hyperoxia Hypocarbia Alkalosis Normothermia	Decrease pulmonary vascular resistance and unload right ventricle	Initial strategy titrated to clinical effect and serial arterial blood gases
Epinephrine	Classic inotrope with direct cAMP increase	Enhances right ventricular contractility but increases pulmonary vascular resistance	Dosage titrated to clinical effect and increase in pulmonary vascular resistance
Milrinone	Inodilator and phosphodiesterase inhibitor with indirect cAMP increase	Enhances right ventricular contractility and decreases pulmonary vascular resistance	Useful agent (especially with epinephrine) titrated to clinical effect but limited by systemic hypotension
Prostaglandins E_1 and I_2	Relatively selective pulmonary vasodilator	Decreases pulmonary vascular resistance and unloads right ventricle	Useful agent titrated to clinical effect but limited by systemic hypotension
Inhaled nitric oxide	True selective pulmonary vasodilator	Decreases pulmonary vascular resistance and unloads right ventricle	Useful agent titrated to clinical effect with inotropes and prostaglandins

cAMP, Cyclic adenosine monophosphate.

onary graft insufficiency by localizing LV ischemia. Nitroglycerin, nicardipine, or milrinone infusion minimize coronary graft spasm.[36,37] Intraaortic balloon counterpulsation via the femoral artery reduces LV afterload and augments diastolic coronary perfusion.

Acute severe MR from ischemia or failed mitral surgery may require emergent mitral valve repair or replacement. Dynamic MR is caused by LVOT obstruction resulting from systolic anterior motion of the mitral valve. Dynamic LVOT obstruction may occur after aortic valve replacement in patients with severe LV hypertrophy (LVH) from aortic stenosis. Enhanced intravascular volume, an atrial rhythm, a slower rate, and high systemic vascular resistance (SVR) are used to manage LVOT obstruction. Atrial contraction normally contributes 15% to 20% of LV filling. The atrial contribution approaches 40% in patients with LVH. A higher mean arterial pressure (MAP) is required to perfuse the hypertrophied subendocardium. Hypovolemia, loss of sinus rhythm, and low SVR all contribute to LVOT obstruction. LVOT obstruction lowers MAP and produces subendocardial ischemia and MR. LV filling and SVR are increased to reduce LVOT obstruction and improve subendocardial perfusion, thus aborting this cycle.

The heart-transplant patient may experience LV failure in the CTICU as a result of acute rejection. This is uncommon because of rigorous donor and recipient testing. Chronic rejection is more common and is manifested by small-vessel coronary artery disease.

The management of ventricular failure requires pharmacologic support and prompt surgery when indicated. If the ventricle does not respond despite aggressive medical management, a ventricular assist device (VAD) may be indicated. VAD placement reduces the complications of ventricular failure such as liver and renal dysfunction. A temporary VAD is indicated for ventricular failure that is expected to resolve within days to weeks. Ventricular recovery is determined at the bedside by hemodynamics and echocardiography as the VAD flows are slowly weaned. The VAD is explanted when ventricular function is sustained with weaning. A long-term VAD is indicated for mechanical support as a bridge to heart transplantation. Concomitant anticoagulation is indicated. The long-term VAD is explanted during heart transplantation.

Low cardiac output in a patient with a VAD is due to inadequate filling or inadequate ejection of blood. Inadequate filling is due to hypovolemia or a blocked inflow cannula. In the case of an isolated left VAD, RV function is linked to the filling of the LV. NO provides successful application in this setting since it unloads the RV, thus improving RV ejection.[38] Inadequate LV ejection is due to high SVR, pulmonic regurgitation, or aortic regurgitation. The CTICU staff must be appropriately trained in VAD management. Chest compression is contraindicated during cardiac arrest in a patient with a VAD.

Renal Failure

Postoperative renal failure may be prerenal, renal, or postrenal. CTICU management determines the cause where possible and maintains fluid and electrolyte homeostasis.

Prerenal Failure. Inadequate glomerular flow results from LV failure or inadequate intravascular volume. Urine osmolality is elevated and the fractional excretion of sodium is typically less than 1%. Adequate therapeutic response is urine production of greater than 1 cc/kg/hr. Dopamine infusion of 2 to 4 mcg/kg/min dilates the renal arteries and is thus protective by augmenting glomerular flow and diuresis. Renal-dose dopamine increases renal vascular resistance in certain patients.[39] In a pneumonectomy or lung transplant patient, deliberate intravascular dehydration is used to minimize postoperative lung edema[40] because the mortality of postpneumonectomy pulmonary edema is as high as 25%.[41]

Renal Failure. The glomerulus, tubule, or interstitium of the kidney may be the cause of renal failure. Dilute urine and epithelial casts reflect renal tubular damage. Common renal toxins that CTICU patients are exposed to include intravenous contrast dye, CPB, antibiotics (vancomycin, gentamicin), cyclosporine, and sepsis.

Postrenal Failure. Postrenal failure is rare in the CTICU. An obstructed Foley catheter must be excluded initially.

Although diuresis maintains urine output, it has not been definitively linked to patient outcome. Dialysis is indicated with volume or metabolic (pH, potassium, urea) overload. Continuous venovenous hemodialysis allows exact volume and metabolic adjustment. The patient may become dialysis dependent and require a renal transplant.

Fluid and Electrolyte Management

Hypernatremia. Acute hypernatremia is manifested by delirium, seizures, and coma. Hypovolemic hypernatremia from either a renal or gastrointestinal cause is treated with volume expansion. The fluid loss may be renal or gastrointestinal. Diabetes insipidus may be central or nephrogenic. The central type responds to vasopressin. Hypervolemic hypernatremia is due to mineralocorticoid excess, whether exogenous or endogenous. Rapid correction of hypernatremia causes neural edema with seizures and coma. Slow correction is appropriate and based on the calculated water deficit.[42]

Hyponatremia. Hyponatremia is manifested by delirium, seizures, and coma. Pseudohyponatremia exhibits a normal serum osmolality associated with hyperlipidemia and hyperproteinemia. A low serum osmolality implies excess water or excessive sodium loss. The syndrome of inappropriate antidiuretic hormone secretion (SIADH) is caused by disease processes in the brain or chest. SIADH is managed with water restriction and treatment of the underlying cause. Excessive sodium loss occurs by renal or extrarenal routes that include skin and the gastrointestinal and respiratory tracts. Hyponatremia is corrected slowly to avoid quadriplegia from central pontine myelinolysis.[43] Hypervolemic hyponatremia is treated with diuresis and dialysis.

Hyperkalemia. Hyperkalemia may cause ventricular fibrillation or asystole. Spurious hyperkalemia is associated with hemolysis, thrombocytosis, and leukocytosis. Hyperkalemia is due to intracellular potassium release or inadequate renal potassium clearance. Intracellular release occurs with acidosis, succinylcholine administration, insulin deficiency, and β-blockade. Intravenous calcium administration stabilizes cardiac membranes. Redistribution is achieved with sodium bicarbonate and a bolus of regular insulin with dextrose. Potassium-binding resins, diuresis, and dialysis eliminate potassium.

Hypokalemia. Hypokalemia is manifested by ECG changes, neuromuscular weakness, and ileus.[44] Hypokalemia enhances digitalis toxicity. Excessive intracellular redistribution occurs with alkalosis and insulin therapy. Renal potassium wasting occurs with iatrogenic diuresis and mineralocorticoid excess. Extrarenal losses include the gastrointestinal tract. Emergent potassium replacement for arrhythmias is at an intravenous administration rate of 1 mEq per 3 to 5 minutes until clinical resolution of the arrhythmia. Intravenous repletion for less urgent hypokalemia is a rate of 10 mEq per hour. Gradual repletion of potassium occurs via the gastrointestinal route.

Hypercalcemia. Hypercalcemia is manifested by delirium, renal calculi, and gastrointestinal disturbance. Excess parathyroid hormone stimulates bone resorption and inhibits renal calcium excretion. It occurs with solid malignancies such as lung cancer. Forced saline diuresis with furosemide augments calcium elimination. Second-line agents include plicamycin (an osteoclast toxin) and diphosphonates (bone resorption inhibitors) such as etidronate and pamidronate.

Hypocalcemia. Hypocalcemia reduces ventricular function and vascular tone. The citrate contained in packed red blood cells and fresh frozen plasma (FFP) binds calcium. Massive transfusion causes dilutional hypocalcemia in addition to calcium binding, leading to severe hypocalcemia. Hypocalcemia is treated with intravenous calcium chloride in increments of 100 to

200 mg. Larger doses (1 g) are used if the patient is hypotensive.

Hypomagnesemia. Hypomagnesemia is a significant problem in the CTICU.[45] It is caused by renal wasting of magnesium, acidosis, severe potassium deficiency, and drugs (diuretics, aminoglycosides, amphotericin B, cyclosporine, and digoxin). Nonrenal mechanisms include gastrointestinal losses, skin losses, poor intake, redistribution (insulin, sepsis, and catecholamines), and dilution. Arrhythmias caused by hypomagnesemia resolve with 1 to 2 g IV magnesium sulfate over 5 minutes. An infusion of 1 to 2 g for several hours provides further repletion.

Gastrointestinal Complications

Table 16-5 summarizes the major gastrointestinal presentations in the CTICU.

Upper Gastrointestinal Bleeding. A decreasing hematocrit, "coffee grounds" emesis, or bright red blood per os or nasogastric tube suggest significant upper gastrointestinal bleeding that may occur despite stress ulcer prophylaxis. Upper endoscopy is used to localize the bleeding and cauterize the source. Medical management is supportive.

Lower Gastrointestinal Bleeding. Colonoscopy is reserved for significant bleeding. Massive colonic bleeding may necessitate radiographic embolization and, rarely, colectomy.

Gastrointestinal Perforation. Partial perforation refers to mucosal transgression by local bacteria. Bacterial translocation across the protective intestinal mucosa contributes to the multiorgan-failure syndrome.[46,47] Complete perforation produces a local abdominal syndrome that presents atypically in the immunosuppressed patient. Prompt exploratory laparotomy is the appropriate management. Thromboembolic intestinal ischemia presents with metabolic acidosis.

Intestinal Obstruction. Mechanical intestinal obstruction is characterized by symptoms and signs of hyperperistalsis. Laparotomy is indicated for progressive severe mechanical obstruction. Sigmoid volvulus is hydrostatically reduced. Acute colonic pseudoobstruction is manifested by marked dilation of the colon in the absence of mechanical obstruction. Ninety-five percent of patients with this condition have had recent surgery or serious infection.[48] Perforation or ischemia is possible when the cecal diameter exceeds 12 cm. The risk of cecal perforation is 3% when the cecal diameter exceeds 12 cm.[49] Colonoscopic decompression is indicated for cecal diameter greater than 12 cm on abdominal radio-

TABLE 16-5
Gastrointestinal Presentations in the Cardiothoracic Intensive Care Unit

GASTROINTESTINAL ENTITY	SELECTED ETIOLOGIES	DIAGNOSTIC EVALUATION	CLINICAL MANAGEMENT
Bleeding	Stress ulceration Varices Ischemia Anticoagulation	Serial hematocrit Abdominal x-ray Lavage Endoscopy	Drugs Transfusion Endoscopic intervention Embolization surgery
Perforation	Ischemia	Abominal exam Abdominal x-ray Computed tomography	Antibiotics Circulatory support Surgery
Obstruction	Adhesions Ileus Volvulus	Abdominal exam Abdominal x-ray	Intravenous hydration Drugs Endoscopy Surgery
Hypermotility	*Clostridium difficile*	Stool analysis and culture	Antibiotics
Jaundice	Drugs TPN Acalculous Cholecystitis	Liver function tests Ultrasound Nuclear scans Endoscopy	Drug modification Endoscopy Surgery

TPN, Total parenteral nutrition.

graph or worsening clinical status. The 70% success rate is enhanced with colon drainage.[50] Colonic decompression after intravenous neostigmine was demonstrated in a double-blind controlled trial.[51] Atropine reversed any associated bradycardia.

Intestinal Hypermotility. Diarrhea is typically toxic, osmotic, or infectious. *Clostridium difficile* responds to oral metronidazole. Osmotic diarrhea from enteral feeding responds to dietary adjustments. Infection is more likely in the immunosuppressed patient or in a CTICU outbreak.

Jaundice. Prehepatic jaundice or unconjugated hyperbilirubinemia follows hemolysis or hematoma reabsorption. Hepatic jaundice or mixed hyperbilirubinemia occurs from hepatotoxic drugs, RV failure, and sepsis. Fatty liver from excess glucose in total parenteral nutrition (TPN) causes a high-serum alkaline phosphatase, perhaps on the basis of biliary canalicular distortion.[52] Cholestasis from TPN resolves with enteral feeding. The implanted drive lines for a VAD may cause duodenal compression and consequent cholestasis. Acalculous cholecystitis occurs with the absence of duodenal lipid because of TPN. Right upper quadrant pain is absent in 30% of cases.[53] Liver function tests are neither sensitive nor specific markers of this entity.[54] Ultrasound findings of biliary sludge, gallbladder dilation, and thickening are nonspecific.[54] Cholecystectomy

or cholecystostomy may be indicated. Vitamin K is fat-soluble and requires bile salts for absorption. Because it supports hepatic synthesis of factors II, V, VII, and IX, cholestasis induces a coagulopathy that is corrected by parenteral vitamin K administration. Hepatic encephalopathy varies from subclinical delirium to frank coma. Lactulose improves mental status by augmenting intestinal transit, thus minimizing absorption of proteins and colonic bacterial toxins.

Nutrition

If the patient tolerates intake per os, the diet is advanced as tolerated to the goal diet. Nasoenteral feeding is preferred because it has less infectious risk and is cheaper than TPN. The nasoenteral tube is positioned distal to the pylorus to minimize aspiration. The enteral regimen depends on the patient's age and weight, caloric requirement, and disease processes. TPN is typically administered via a central intravenous catheter over a 24-hour period. TPN is ordered the day before and mixed under sterile conditions to minimize infectious risk. The formulation depends on the patient's age and weight, caloric requirement, and disease processes. The components are fat, protein, carbohydrate, trace minerals, vitamins, and electrolytes. The electrolyte formulation is tailored to the daily serum electrolytes. High-acetate formulation is used to treat metabolic acidosis. Serum glucose is managed with an insulin sliding scale or insulin in the TPN based on the most recent 24-hour insulin requirements.

Hematologic Complications

The infectious risks, immunosuppressive properties, and practice parameters of red cell transfusion have been reviewed.[55,56] Red cell transfusion for immunosuppressed patients should be free of cytomegalovirus and leukocytes. Leukocyte depletion prevents graft-versus-host disease.

Normal coagulation provides a delicate balance between clot formation and clot breakdown (fibrinolysis). Clot formation requires interaction between functional platelets and functional coagulation proteins. Thrombocytopenia is caused by decreased production, dilution, or consumption. Progressive thrombocytopenia should prompt a drug review for heparin and histamine blockers. If necessary, heparin administration may be continued with a platelet count above $50,000/mm^3$. Thrombocytopenia with sepsis is due to bone marrow suppression or platelet consumption. Management includes appropriate antibiotics and platelet transfusion. The indications for platelet transfusion include active hemorrhage despite a platelet count of greater than $50,000/mm^3$ and less than $20,000/mm^3$ platelets in patients at risk for bleeding. CPB, renal failure, hepatic failure, and preoperative aspirin also induce a qualitative disturbance in platelet function.[57] Dialysis and desmopressin acetate promote recovery of platelet function with renal failure. Postoperative residual blockade of the IIa/IIIb platelet receptor is managed with platelet transfusion. There is currently no clinical antagonist.

The prothrombin time (PT) and partial thromboplastin time (PTT) remain normal despite coagulation factor levels of only 20% to 30% of normal. Bleeding occurs with factor concentrations below 20% to 30%. Factor deficiency is due to decreased hepatic production or hemodilution. Liver disease, cholestasis, and preoperative warfarin (Coumadin) administration decrease hepatic production. Hemodilution occurs with CPB and non-FFP transfusion. Bedside PT/PTT monitors help guide FFP therapy more accurately. Residual heparin after CPB is neutralized with additional protamine. Residual fibrinolysis is treated with an antifibrinolytic.

Infectious Disease in the CTICU

The CTICU is colonized with antibiotic-resistant bacteria. Handwashing and patient isolation are important for limiting bacterial colonization.

Catheter-Based Infections. Vascular catheters present in all patients are a potential site for infection. Many patients have multiple catheters including arterial, central venous, and pulmonary artery catheters. The femoral site is the most common site for infection.[58] Catheter-based infection (CBI) prevention includes sterile catheter insertion, local care of the entry site, and prompt catheter removal. Bacterial seeding occurs along the soft tissue tract or along the catheter. The site of indwelling vascular catheters is changed if the entry site appears infected or the patient is septic without an identifiable source.[59] The catheter tip is cultured after removal. If the source of sepsis is identified in a location distant from the catheter, the catheter may be changed over a wire and the tip cultured. For chronic sepsis, the catheter is changed over a wire every 7 days and the catheter tip is cultured each time. The site of central line placement is chosen ipsilateral to a coexisting pleural drain in anticipation of an unintentional pneumothorax.

Antibiotic selection for a CBI is initially empiric and broad-spectrum against Gram-positive bacteria and Gram-negative bacteria. Subsequent antibiotic selection is based on culture and sensitivity data. The CBI resolves within 7 to 10 days of appropriate antibiotics and catheter management.

Respiratory Tract Infections. Upper respiratory tract colonization often precedes nosocomial pneumonia.[60] The indigenous flora are eliminated by perioperative antibiotics, and portals such as endotracheal and nasogastric tubes provide colonization. Bacterial and fungal sinusitis result from sinus blockage by nasal tubes. Cultures and Gram stain guide antibiotic selection. Fungal sinusitis (especially mucormycosis) is a serious infection in diabetic and immunosuppressed patients. Systemic amphotericin B is indicated for fungemia. Lower respiratory tract infections range from bronchitis to pneumonia. The pathogenesis is usually aspiration from the upper respiratory tract or the gastrointestinal tract. Gastric colonization occurs with pharmacologic achlorhydria, enteral feeding, and advanced age. Gram-negative bacteria predominate and include *Escherichia coli, Enterobacter, Klebsiella, Proteus,* and *Pseudomonas aeruginosa.* Gram-positive bacteria cultured from lower respiratory tract infections include staphylococcal and streptococcal species, and fungi include *Candida* and *Aspergillus.* Nosocomial pneumonia presents with fever, cough, purulent sputum, and new or changing pulmonary infiltrates on chest radiograph. The emphasis on new or changing pulmonary infiltrates stems from the frequency of pulmonary infiltrates in the CTICU. These frequent infiltrates result from many different noninfectious processes such as ventricular failure, postoperative atelectasis, ARDS, aspiration, and lung rejection.[61] Correlating the dynamic radiographic trend with the clinical picture and course of the patient is the best diagnostic method for CTICU pneumonia. Sputum sampling includes nasotracheal suctioning and bronchoscopy. Blood culture isolates the infectious agent with bacteremia. Antibiotic selection is on a case-by-case basis. The variables considered in antibiotic selection include the putative infectious agent based on the clinical picture, prior antibiotic selection, culture and antibiotic sensitivity profiles, CTICU bacterial patterns, and antibiotic usage. Patient allergies and the degree of renal and hepatic function are also relevant.

Urinary Tract Infections. The Foley catheter is almost always associated with urinary tract infections (UTIs).[62] Foley catheters should be promptly discontinued when no longer required. Gram-negative bacteria predominate. Fungi such as *Candida albicans* are common in the diabetic or immunosuppressed patient. These organisms reach the bladder at the time of catheterization or via the urinary catheter. A UTI is defined as greater than 100,000 colony-forming units per cubic centimeter of urine. Antibiotic sensitivity profiles guide therapy. The clinical features of a UTI vary from sepsis, to the fever and flank tenderness of pyelonephritis, to the dysuria and frequency of a cystitis. Asymptomatic bacteriuria or candiduria resolves with removal of the Foley catheter. Antibiotic selection for nosocomial bacterial UTI includes broad-spectrum penicillins, cotrimoxazole, or a quinolone for 7 days. An aminoglycoside such as gentamicin is added in the event of associated bacteremia. Persistent candiduria resolves with continuous bladder irrigation with amphotericin B.[63] Alternative therapy includes systemic amphotericin B and fluconazole for 7 days.

Soft Tissue Infections. Cardiothoracic surgery is classified as a clean surgical wound. Surgeries that involve the respiratory tract are classified as clean contaminated with a higher wound-infection rate. The bacterial organisms found in wound infections are usually staphylococcal and streptococcal species. The incubation period is 4 to 6 days. A wound swab sent for Gram stain and culture guides antibiotic selection. Severe cases mandate intravenous antibiotics and surgical debridement. Infections that extend to the sternum necessitate sternal rewiring, sternal debridement, and possible soft tissue flapping.

Sepsis. The source of sepsis is not always known. Septic physiology is characterized by low SVR and high cardiac output. The mortality from sepsis is approximately 25% to 50%.[64] Management includes appropriate antibiotic coverage and circulatory support with pressors or inotropic agents. Phenylephrine and norepinephrine augment SVR. Vasopressin augments SVR but does not increase PVR because of the lack of vasopressin receptors in the lung.

BOX 16-1
Management of Thyroid Storm

STEP 1: Propylthiouracil blockade
STEP 2: Iodine blockade
STEP 3: Hydrocortisone supplementation
STEP 4: β-Blockade with esmolol
STEP 5: Supportive care for hyperthermia, dehydration, and hypoglycemia or hyperglycemia

---

The low SVR in sepsis occurs with NO overproduction by endothelial NO synthase. NO synthase inhibitors improve SVR but do not affect outcome. Mortality is not affected by the novel choice of a particular pressor or inotropic agent, because the reduction in SVR is only a marker of the severity of sepsis and not the cause of mortality.[65]

Endocrine Considerations in the CTICU

Diabetes. Hyperglycemia during neurologic injury is associated with a worse neurologic outcome and predisposes patients to surgical wound infections.[66] Hyperglycemia occurs with TPN, catecholamine administration, pain, and the stress response to surgery.[67] Postoperative euglycemia is accomplished with a perioperative insulin infusion, which is started preoperatively in diabetic patients. The rate of insulin administration is titrated by serial blood glucose determinations. Blood glucose levels are determined at least every 2 hours in the immediate postoperative period, particularly if an epinephrine infusion is used. Diabetic ketoacidosis is managed with vigorous intravascular volume expansion and an insulin infusion titrated to frequent blood glucose determinations. Electrolyte repletion is guided by serial serum electrolyte determinations and intravenous bicarbonate is administered for a pH of less than 7.20. Dextrose-containing solutions are used when the blood glucose approaches the 200- to 250-mg/dl range to allow the continued infusion of insulin and to prevent reexacerbation of this problem. A precipitating factor such as infection is sought and managed appropriately.

Thyroid Disease. Inadequately controlled hyperthyroidism may present in the CTICU as postoperative thyroid storm.[68] The diagnosis is clinical and thyroid tests are confirmatory. The mortality rate from thyroid storm is 20%.[69] Box 16-1 summarizes its management.

Patients with mild-to-moderate hypothyroidism typically have an uncomplicated postoperative course. The hypothyroid patient with a complicated CTICU stay (e.g., respiratory insufficiency, poor mental status) should have thyroid function testing and appropriate replacement with thyroid hormone.

Adrenal Insufficiency. The CTICU patient who has taken steroids within the previous year has underlying adrenal insufficiency. The patient may first present with catecholamine-resistant shock in the CTICU. Perioperative steroid replacement is necessary treatment for the surgical stress response.

THE LONG-TERM PATIENT

The long-term patient remains in the CTICU for a variety of reasons. A patient with a long-term left-ventricular assist device remains in the CTICU until a more appropriate facility becomes available. Options include transfer to a special unit for VAD patients, which is present in major institutions. The patient may be discharged home, in selected cases, with regular outpatient follow-up.

Respiratory failure and dependency on mechanical ventilation is the most common reason for long-term CTICU stay. Slow weaning from mandatory ventilation involves the gradual decrease in the rate of the synchronized intermittent mechanical ventilation ventilator mode or the gradual decrease of the pressure support in a continuous positive airway pressure ventilator mode. Failure to wean may occur because of hypercapnia due to excess CO_2 production from hypertonic dextrose,[70] hypoventilation from metabolic alkalosis, or pulmonary infection. Acetazolamide alkalizes the urine and neutralizes the metabolic alkalosis. Prolonged failure to wean necessitates transfer to the medical ICU for further weaning trials or to a facility for chronic ventilator-dependent patients.

A third reason for long-term CTICU stay is the neurologically disabled patient who requires transfer to a nursing home. This patient is typically transferred to the surgical floor and the appropriate arrangements are made for the nursing home transfer. Because the nursing home arrangements may require a few weeks, it is advisable to contact a social worker early in the clinical course.

The long-term patient with continued systemic illness is managed according to the clinical approaches that were outlined earlier. Clinical improvement allows eventual discharge from the CTICU, whereas significant clinical deterioration prompts discussion with the family as to the level of appropriate intervention.

WITHDRAWAL OF CARE

It is not universally appropriate to aggressively manage every patient in the CTICU. It is always appropriate to relieve suffering but the decision for cessation of aggressive and invasive management is made at certain times. Care is withdrawn in stages with consultation between the family and surgeon. Care withdrawal begins with a decision not to proceed with cardiopulmonary resuscitation in the event of a cardiac arrest. It progresses to not allowing significant changes in patient management even as the patient's clinical status deteriorates. It then progresses to the withdrawal of significant interventional therapies such as dialysis or mechanical ventilation. Generally, a universal agreement on the prognosis is made before such withdrawal decisions are made.

KEY POINTS

1. The transport of the CTICU patient must be organized and safe. Continuous hemodynamic monitoring and trained personnel accompany the patient during transport.

2. The length of stay in the CTICU defines the CTICU patients as fast-track, short-term, and long-term patients.

3. The fast-track patient is appropriately selected and undergoes expedited tracheal extubation by a protocol-driven withdrawal of support.

4. Postoperative delirium mandates a search for and treatment of an underlying organic cause. A new postoperative paraplegia is an epidural hematoma until proven otherwise.

5. Respiratory failure mandates aggressive support of oxygenation or ventilation. The cause is addressed in an organized fashion.

6. A hemodynamically unstable tachyarrhythmia merits prompt cardioversion or defibrillation.

7. The management of heart failure includes improving perfusion, determining the cause, and reoperating when indicated.

8. Inhaled NO is a selective pulmonary vasodilator but is not the initial management of pulmonary hypertension.

9. Closed-chest cardiopulmonary resuscitation is contraindicated with the presence of a ventricular assist device.

10. Renal failure is prerenal, renal, or postrenal. Dialysis is reserved for severe volume and metabolic overload.

11. Stress ulceration prophylaxis is essential. Neostigmine may be helpful in acute colonic pseudoobstruction. *Clostridium difficile* is treated with oral metronidazole.

12. Vitamin K is administered intravenously in patients with cholestasis. Acalculous cholecystitis causes fever and abdominal pain.

13. Mixed coagulopathies are common in the CTICU.
14. Enteral feeding is safer and less expensive than parenteral nutrition.

15. The Foley catheter should be discontinued as soon as possible because it is frequently associated with nosocomial UTI.
16. Failure to wean is caused by excess CO_2 production, metabolic alkalosis, or infection.

KEY REFERENCES

The Acute Respiratory Distress Syndrome Network: Ventilation with lower tidal volumes as compared with traditional tidal volumes for acute lung injury and the acute respiratory distress syndrome, *N Engl J Med* 342:1301, 2000.

Aranda M, Pearl RG: The pharmacology and physiology of nitric oxide-understanding its use in anesthesia and critical care medicine, *Anesthesiol Clin North Am* 16:236, 1998.

Balser JR: The rational intravenous use of amiodarone in the perioperative period, *Anesthesiology* 86:974, 1999.

Cheng DCH: Fast track cardiac surgery pathways: early extubation, process of care, and cost-containment, *Anesthesiology* 88:1429, 1998.

Cheng DCH, Karski J, Peniston C et al: Early tracheal extubation after coronary artery bypass graft surgery reduces cost and improves resource use, *Anesthesiology* 85:1300, 1996.

Clark RE, Brillman J, Davis DA et al: Microemboli during coronary artery bypass grafting. Genesis and effect on outcome, *J Thorac Cardiovasc Surg* 109:249, 1995.

Doering EB, Hanson CW, Reily DJ et al: Improvement in oxygenation by phenylephrine and nitric oxide in patients with adult respiratory distress syndrome, *Anesthesiology* 87:18, 1997.

Eyer S, Brummit C, Crosseley K et al: Catheter-related sepsis: prospective, randomized study of three methods of long-term catheter maintenance, *Crit Care Med* 18:1073, 1990.

Liu JJ, Doolan LA, Xie B et al: Direct vasodilator effect of milrinone, an inotropic drug, on arterial bypass graft, *J Thorac Cardiovasc Surg* 113:108, 1997.

Ponec RJ, Saunders MD, Kimmey MB: Neostigmine for the treatment of acute colonic pseudo-obstruction, *N Engl J Med* 341:137, 1999.

Task force on blood component therapy: Practice guidelines for blood component therapy, *Anesthesiology* 84:732, 1996.

Zeldin RA, Normadin D, Landtwing BS et al: Postpneumonectomy pulmonary edema, *J Thorac Cardiovasc Surg* 87:359, 1984.

References

1. Prakash O, Johnson B, Meij S et al: Criteria for early extubation after intracardiac surgery in adults, *Anesth Analg* 56:703, 1977.
2. Cheng DCH: Fast track cardiac surgery pathways: early extubation, process of care, and cost-containment, *Anesthesiology* 88:1429, 1998.
3. Higgins TL: Pro: early endotracheal extubation is preferable to delayed extubation in patients following coronary artery bypass surgery, *J Cardiothorac Vasc Anesth* 6:488, 1992.
4. Laupacis A, Fergusson D: Drugs to minimize perioperative blood loss in cardiac surgery; meta-analyses using perioperative blood transfusion as the outcome, *Anesth Analg* 85:1258, 1997.
5. Cheng DCH: Fast-track cardiac surgery: economic implications in postoperative care, *J Cardiothorac Vasc Anesth* 12:72, 1998.
6. Bell J, Sartain J, Wilkinson GAL et al: Propofol and fentanyl anesthesia for patients with low cardiac output state undergoing cardiac surgery: comparison with high-dose fentanyl anesthesia, *Br J Anaesth* 73:162, 1994.
7. Mora CT, Dudek C, Epstein RH et al: Cardiac anesthesia techniques: fentanyl alone or in combination with enflurane or propofol, *Anesth Analg* 61:972, 1982.
8. Demonaco HJ, Shah AS: Economic considerations in the use of neuromuscular drugs, *J Clin Anesth* 6:383, 1994.
9. Royston D: Remifentanil in cardiac surgery, *Eur J Anaesthiol* 10:S77, 1995.
10. Jalonen J, Hynynen M, Kuitunen A et al: Dexmedetomidine as an anesthetic adjunct in coronary artery bypass grafting, *Anesthesiology* 86:331, 1997.
11. Chaney MA: Intrathecal and epidural anesthesia and analgesia for cardiac surgery, *Anesth Analg* 84:1211, 1997.
12. Westaby S, Pillai R, Parry A et al: Does modern cardiac surgery require conventional intensive care? *Eur J Cardiothor Surg* 7:313, 1993.
13. Johnson D, Thomson D, Myck T et al: Respiratory outcomes with early extubation after coronary artery bypass surgery, *J Cardiothorac Vasc Anesth* 11: 474, 1997.
14. Cheng DCH, Karski J, Peniston C et al: Early tracheal extubation after coronary artery bypass graft surgery reduces cost and improves resource use, *Anesthesiology* 85:1300, 1996.
15. Hall RI, Maclaren C, Smith MS et al: Light versus heavy sedation after cardiac surgery: myocardial ischemia and the stress response, *Anesth Analg* 85:971, 1997.
16. Chong JL, Pillai R, Fisher A et al: Cardiac surgery: moving away from intensive care, *Br Heart J* 68: 430, 1992.
17. Pusgley W, Klinger L, Paschalis C et al: The impact of microemboli during cardiopulmonary bypass on neuropsychological functioning, *Stroke* 25:1393, 1994.
18. Clark RE, Brillman J, Davis DA et al: Microemboli during coronary artery bypass grafting. Genesis and effect on outcome, *J Thorac Cardiovasc Surg* 109:249, 1995.
19. Stoelting RK: Brachial plexus injury after median sternotomy: an unexpected liability for anesthesiologists, *J Cardiothorac Vasc Anesth* 8:2, 1994.
20. Lederman RJ, Breuer AC, Hanson MR et al: Peripheral nervous system complications of coronary bypass graft surgery, *Ann Neurol* 12:297, 1982.

21. Alvine FG, Schurrer ME: Postoperative ulnar nerve palsy, *J Bone Joint Surg Am* 69A:255, 1987.
22. The Acute Respiratory Distress Syndrome Network: Ventilation with lower tidal volumes as compared with traditional tidal volumes for acute lung injury and the acute respiratory distress syndrome, *N Engl J Med* 342:1301, 2000.
23. Doering EB, Hanson CW, Reily DJ et al: Improvement in oxygenation by phenylephrine and nitric oxide in patients with adult respiratory distress syndrome, *Anesthesiology* 87:18, 1997.
24. Aranda M, Pearl RG: The pharmacology and physiology of nitric oxide-understanding its use in anesthesia and critical care medicine, *Anesthesiol Clin North Am* 16:236, 1998.
25. West JB: Regional differences in gas exchange in the lung of erect man, *J Appl Physiol* 17: 893, 1962.
26. Lamm WJE, Graham MM, Albert RK: Mechanism by which the prone position improves oxygenation in acute lung injury, *Am J Respir Crit Care Med* 150:184, 1994.
27. Rehder K, Knopp TJ, Sessler AD: Regional intrapulmonary gas ventilation in awake and anesthetised-paralysed prone man, *J Appl Physiol* 45:528, 1978.
28. Beck KC, Vetterman J, Rehder K: Gas exchange in dogs in the prone and supine position, *J Appl Physiol* 72:2292, 1992.
29. Givner I, Jaffe N: Occlusion of the central retinal artery following anesthesia, *Arch Ophthalmol* 43:197, 1950.
30. Morganroth J, Horowitz LN, Anderson J et al: Comparative efficacy and tolerance of esmolol to propanolol for control of supraventricular arrhythmia, *Am J Cardiol* 56:33F, 1985.
31. Steck J, Sheppard D, Byrd RC et al: Pulmonary effects of esmolol-an ultra-short acting β-adrenergic blocking agent, *Clin Res* 33:472A, 1985.
32. Balser JR: The rational intravenous use of amiodarone in the perioperative period, *Anesthesiology* 86:974,1999.
33. Girard C, Lehot JJ, Pannetier JC et al: Inhaled nitric oxide for right ventricular failure after heart transplantation, *J Cardiothorac Vasc Anesth* 7:181, 1993.
34. Miller OI, Tang SF,Keech A et al: Rebound pulmonary hypertension on withdrawal from inhaled nitric oxide, *Lancet* 346:51, 1995.
35. Buxton AE, Goldberg S Harken A et al: Coronary-artery spasm immediately after myocardial revascularization: recognition and management, *N Engl J Med* 304:1249, 1981.
36. Cooper GJ, Wilkinson GA, Angelini G: Overcoming perioperative spasm of the internal mammary artery; which is the best vasodilator? *J Thorac Cardiovasc Surg* 104: 465, 1992.
37. Liu JJ, Doolan LA, Xie B et al: Direct vasodilator effect of milrinone, an inotropic drug, on arterial bypass graft, *J Thorac Cardiovasc Surg* 113:108, 1997.
38. Macdonald PS, Keogh A, Mundy J et al: Adjunctive use of inhaled nitric oxide during implantation of a left ventricular assist device, *J Heart Lung Transpl* 17:312, 1998.
39. Garwood S, Hines R, Harris S: Does dopamine exacerbate renal ischemia? *Anesth Analg* 88(4S):SCA 9, 1999.
40. Zeldin RA, Normadin D, Landtwing BS et al: Postpneumonectomy pulmonary edema, *J Thorac Cardiovasc Surg* 87:359, 1984.
41. Verheijen-Breemhar L, Bogaard JM, Van Den Berg B et al: Postpneumonectomy pulmonary edema, *Thorax* 43:323, 1988.
42. Torres N: Electrolyte abnormalities: sodium. In Faust RJ, editor: *Anesthesiology review*, ed 2, New York, 1994, Churchill Livingstone, p 34.
43. Sterns RH: The management of hyponatremic emergencies, *Crit Care Clin* 7:127, 1991.
44. Stoelting RK, Dierdorf SF, McCammon RL: Water and electrolyte disturbances. In *Anesthesia and co-existing disease*, New York, 1988, Churchill Livingstone, p 445.
45. Salem M, Munoz R, Brodsky MA: Hypomagnesemia in critical illness. A common and clinically important problem, *Crit Care Clin* 7:225, 1991.
46. Wilmore DW, Smith RJ, O'Dweyer ST et al: The gut: a central organ after surgical stress, *Surgery* 104: 917, 1988.
47. Cerra FB: Metabolic manifestations of multiple systems organ failure, *Crit Care Clin* 5:119, 1989.
48. Vanek VW, Al-salti M: Acute pseudo-obstruction of the colon (Ogilvie's syndrome): an analysis of 400 cases, *Dis Colon Rectum* 29:203, 1986.
49. Rex DK: Colonoscopy and acute colonic pseudo-obstruction, *Gastrointest Endosc Clin N Am* 7: 499, 1997.
50. Harig JM, Fumo DE, Loo FD et al: Treatment of acute nontoxic megacolon during colonoscopy: tube placement versus simple decompression, *Gastrointest Endosc* 34:23, 1988.
51. Ponec RJ, Saunders MD, Kimmey MB: Neostigmine for the treatment of acute colonic pseudo-obstruction, *N Engl J Med* 341:137, 1999.
52. Baker AL, Rosenberg IH: Hepatic complications of total parenteral nutrition, *Am J Med* 82:489, 1987.
53. Orlando R, Gleason E, Drezner AD: Acute acalculous cholecystitis in the critically ill patient, *Am J Surg* 145:472, 1983.
54. Savino JA, Scalea TM, Del Guercio LRM: Factors encouraging laparotomy in acalculous cholecystitis, *Crit Care Med* 13:377, 1985.
55. Vamvakas E, Moore SB: Perioperative blood transfusion and colorectal cancer recurrence: a qualitative statistical overview and meta-analysis, *Transfusion* 33:754, 1993.
56. Task force on blood component therapy: Practice guidelines for blood component therapy, *Anesthesiology* 84:732, 1996.
57. Taggart DP, Siddiqui A, Wheatley DJ: Low-dose preoperative aspirin therapy, postoperative blood loss and transfusion requirements, *Ann Thorac Surg* 50:425, 1990.
58. Kemp L, Burge J, Choban P et al: The effect of catheter types and site on infection rates in total parenteral nutrition patients, *JPEN J Parenter Enteral Nutr* 18:71, 1994.
59. Eyer S, Brummitt C, Crosseley K et al: Catheter-related sepsis: prospective, randomized study of three methods of long-term catheter maintenance, *Crit Care Med* 18:1073, 1990.
60. Neiderman MS: Microbial flora of the respiratory tract: normal inhabitants and abnormal colonization. In Bone RC, editor: *Pulmonary and critical care medicine*, St Louis, 1993, Mosby.
61. Andrews CP, Coalson JJ, Smith JD et al: Diagnosis of nosocomial bacterial pneumonia in acute, diffuse lung injury, *Chest* 80:254, 1981.
62. Platt R, Polk BF, Murdock B et al: Mortality associated with nosocomial urinary tract infection, *N Engl J Med* 307:637, 1982.
63. Wise GJ, Kozinn PJ, Goldberg P: Amphotericin B as a urologic irritant in management of noninvasive bacteriuria, *J Urol* 128:82, 1982.
64. Pinner RW, Teutsch SM, Simonsen L et al: Trends in infectious diseases mortality in the United States, *JAMA* 275:189, 1996.
65. Groeneveld ABJ, Bronsveld W, Thijs LG: Hemodynamic determinants of mortality in human septic shock, *Surgery* 99:140, 1986.
66. Wallace LK, Starr NJ, Leventhal MJ et al: Hyperglycemia on ICU admission after CABG is associated with increased risk of mediastinitis or wound infection, *Anesthesiology* 85:A286, 1996.
67. Werb MR, Zinman B, Teasdale SJ et al: Hormonal and metabolic responses during coronary artery bypass surgery: role of infused glucose, *J Clin Endocrinol Metab* 69:1010, 1989.
68. Gregg-Smith SJ: Thyroid storm following chest trauma, *Injury* 24:422, 1993.
69. Burch HB, Wartofsky L: Life-threatening thyrotoxicosis. Thyroid storm, *Endocrinol Metab Clin North Am* 22:262, 1993.
70. Amene PC, Sladen RJ, Feeley TW et al: Hyperrcapnea during total parenteral nutrition with hypertonic dextrose, *Crit Care Med* 15: 171, 1988.

PART IV

Noncardiac Surgical Settings

CHAPTER 17

Vascular Surgery

Christopher J. O'Connor, M.D. ■ Kenneth J. Tuman, M.D.

OUTLINE

The perioperative management of vascular surgical procedures is demanding because of the high-risk profile of the patient population undergoing surgery and the potentially deleterious surgical and hemodynamic events encountered during the intraoperative period. The surgery itself poses an intrinsic ischemic risk to the end organ supplied by the operative vascular bed because of the risk of embolism or thrombosis of the grafted or revascularized arterial segment. The unfavorable hemodynamic and cerebrovascular events seen during surgery further increase the risk of significant postoperative complications, including renal insufficiency, central nervous system dysfunction, and respiratory insufficiency. A balance must therefore be attained between reducing the ischemic threat to the tissues or organs supplied by the diseased vessels, and maintaining adequate myocardial, cerebral, and renal blood flow and oxygen delivery to effectively reduce operative morbidity.

The important contribution of postoperative cardiac events to overall mortality after vascular surgery mandates that cardiac protection be an essential component of the perioperative management of vascular surgical patients. It also demands cautious intraoperative control of myocardial oxygen supply and demand to minimize the occurrence of myocardial ischemia and ventricular dysfunction in at-risk individuals. Contemporary data also suggest that effective control of postoperative pain with epidural analgesia can reduce the incidence of thrombotic events after certain vascular procedures and control some of the adverse hemodynamic and metabolic responses elicited by painful stimuli. The management of these patients and procedures therefore requires a global perioperative perspective and a multifaceted approach to intraoperative anesthesia and postoperative analgesia (Fig. 17-1).

This chapter reviews current issues pertaining to the anesthetic management of vascular surgical procedures and discusses the choice of anesthetic, pertinent surgical aspects of each procedure, important intraoperative hemodynamic and hemostatic events that influence outcome and require intervention, and important features of postoperative care. These features include successful analgesic techniques and relevant complications. Topics are discussed as they pertain to individual vascular procedures, so that all aspects of a specific procedure of interest to the reader can be identified and reviewed in a simple and clinically useful manner.

FIG. 17-1 A paradigm for the management of perioperative stress in patients undergoing major vascular surgery. The global management of these high-risk patients includes the perioperative administration of agents that reduce anxiety and pain (opioid and nonopioid agents, sedatives, and neuraxial analgesics), modulate sympathetic activity (α_2-agonists, β-blockers, epidural local anesthetics, and inhalation anesthetics), and inhibit postoperative hypercoagulable states (anticoagulants and platelet inhibitors). A multimodal approach is thus recommended to reduce perioperative stress and minimize the risk of adverse cardiopulmonary events. *PCA*, Patient-controlled analgesia.

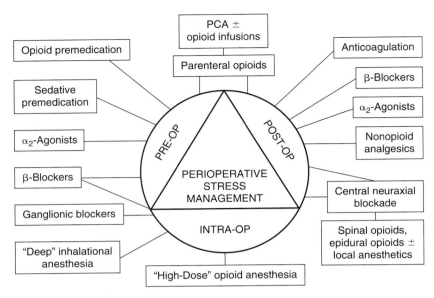

COEXISTING DISEASE IN PATIENTS UNDERGOING VASCULAR SURGERY

Patients requiring major vascular surgery often have atherosclerotic involvement of multiple areas of the vascular system, including the coronary, renal, and cerebral vessels.[1] The involvement of these important organ systems is variable and frequently asymptomatic. Each patient who is to undergo major vascular surgery therefore requires careful assessment, beginning with a thorough history and physical examination. Coexistent coronary artery disease (CAD) remains a major cause of morbidity and mortality after vascular surgery, and assessment of the severity of CAD is an important aspect of preoperative evaluation.[2] Although a fraction of patients with peripheral vascular disease are not limited by lower extremity claudication, can tolerate an acceptable level of exercise, and have no important cardiac risk factors, the majority require further cardiac evaluation preoperatively[3] (Fig. 17-2). The decision to proceed with preoperative testing to assess cardiac risk should be based on the presence of clinical markers (major, intermediate, or minor predictors), functional capacity, and the surgical procedure–specific cardiac risk (stratified as high, intermediate, and low risk). For example, carotid endarterectomy (CEA) is typically considered an intermediate-risk procedure, and specific preoperative cardiac testing is generally not indicated in this setting in the absence of major clinical predictors of increased cardiac risk (unstable coronary syndromes such as recent myocardial infarction [MI] with evidence of important ischemic risk and unstable or severe angina, decompensated congestive heart failure [CHF], significant arrhythmias, or severe valvular disease). The specific methodology of this type of preoperative evaluation and subsequent interventions are discussed elsewhere in Chapter 1.

Patients with peripheral vascular disease also commonly have comorbid conditions that can increase perioperative risk. Chronic hypertension is very common in patients with peripheral vascular disease. When long-standing, chronic hypertension can have deleterious effects on myocardial and renal function. When end-organ dysfunction is present, perioperative risk is probably increased. When end-organ damage is not present, chronic preoperative hypertension may or may not affect outcome.[4] Although adequate preoperative blood pressure control should logically be associated with decreased incidence of cardiac and neurologic morbidity, there are at present no conclusive prospective data to confirm that delaying vascular surgery to achieve a certain level of preoperative blood pressure actually reduces morbidity and no data to define how long a period of control might be required to realize such a potential benefit. What is known is that poorly controlled hypertensive patients frequently have labile intraoperative blood pressure and are also more likely to have both postoperative hypotension and hypertension.[5] Retrospective data indicate that hypertensive patients whose blood pressure is pharmacologically controlled before surgery have a lower incidence of postoperative hypertension than do patients with poorly controlled blood pressure ($\geq$170/95 mm Hg).[6] Given the known alterations in the cerebral blood flow autoregulatory curve of patients with chronic hypertension, blood pressure reductions should be undertaken gradually, and complete normalization of blood pressure is probably not required and may even have detrimental neurologic effects in the presence of extracranial or in-

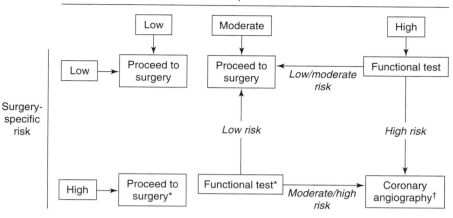

FIG. 17-2   A simplified approach to preoperative cardiac risk assessment that involves evaluation of both patient-specific and surgery-specific risk factors. *Depending on functional capacity. †Only if the patient is a candidate for coronary artery bypass surgery or percutaneous transluminal coronary angioplasty.

tracranial cerebral vascular disease. Evidence that blood pressure need not be greatly reduced but that it is important to stabilize it, is suggested by data demonstrating that hypertensive patients with blood pressures not exceeding 170/90 mm Hg on antihypertensive therapy did not have neurologic outcomes significantly different from normotensive patients; however, patients with blood pressures greater than 170/95 mm Hg had a greater incidence of transient neurologic deficits after CEA.[6] Another common preoperative condition in patients with peripheral vascular disease is diabetes mellitus, which is also associated with a greater incidence of CAD, ischemic cardiomyopathy, autonomic neuropathy, and nephropathy. These factors further aggravate the risk of cardiovascular instability and cardiac morbidity, and increase the risk of perioperative renal insufficiency, especially when such patients have been exposed to radiocontrast dye in the immediate perioperative period.

Cardiac complications are the most common cause of morbidity and mortality in patients undergoing major vascular surgery.[2] Perioperative myocardial ischemia occurs with similar frequency in the presence of abnormal hemodynamics as in the absence of hemodynamic aberrancy. Nonetheless, there is strong association between myocardial ischemia and tachycardia, and perioperative β-adrenergic blockade can reduce the incidence of myocardial ischemia and cardiac events in such high-risk patients (Table 17-1), probably via a number of mechanisms.[7,8] α_2-Agonists such as clonidine and dexmedetomidine can also reduce the incidence of tachycardia and myocardial ischemia.[9,10] In addition to demand ischemia, increased coronary vasomotor tone can result in supply ischemia despite normal systemic hemodynamics, necessitating therapy with coronary vasodilating drugs such as nitroglycerin or cal-

cium channel blockers. However, prophylactic use of nitrates or calcium channel blockers has not been demonstrated to be effective in preventing perioperative ischemia.[11-13]

The critical level of anemia that results in inadequate myocardial oxygen delivery is dependent on all of the other factors that determine the balance of myocardial oxygen supply and demand. In general, because of the

TABLE 17-1
Predictors of Death Among Patients Undergoing Noncardiac Surgery from the McSPI Database (*n* = 2000)*

PREDICTOR	HAZARD RATIO (95% CI)	P VALUE
Univariate Models		
Atenolol	0.4 (0.2-0.9)	0.03
Diabetes mellitus	3.1 (1.4-6.8)	0.01
Ischemia on Holter monitoring on postoperative days 0-2	2.3 (1.0-5.3)	0.04
Multivariate Models		
Diabetes mellitus	2.8 (1.4-6.2)	0.01
Atenolol	0.5 (0.2-1.1)	0.06

Adapted from Mangano DT, Layug EL, Wallace A et al: *N Engl J Med* 335:1713-1720, 1996.
CI, Confidence interval.
*A hazard ratio of less than 1 indicates a protective effect of the predictor and a lower risk of death, whereas a hazard ratio greater than 1 indicates a detrimental effect and a greater risk of death.

frequent coexistence of ischemic heart disease in patients requiring peripheral vascular surgery, most clinicians apply a perioperative threshold for transfusion that is at a higher hemoglobin level than for healthier patients. Although a specific transfusion trigger cannot be generally defined, at least one study has demonstrated an increased incidence of myocardial ischemia and cardiac events in patients with lower hematocrits (<28%) after major vascular surgery.[14]

LOWER EXTREMITY REVASCULARIZATION
Anesthetic Choice

Numerous anesthetic options are available for lower extremity vascular surgery, including general anesthesia (GA), GA combined with spinal or epidurally administered local anesthetics or opioids, and intraoperative neuraxial blockade alone. Epidural anesthesia and analgesia are also frequently continued into the postoperative period. This discussion focuses on outcome data from clinical trials that compare neuraxial blockade with GA (Table 17-2).

Reiz et al[15] were among the first investigators to report outcome data with different anesthetic and analgesic regimens in high-risk patients undergoing emergency major vascular surgery in the face of recent MI. There was a lower incidence of myocardial ischemia and ventricular dysfunction and a lower myocardial reinfarction rate when patients were randomized to receive epidural anesthesia and analgesia.[15] Subsequently, Yeager et al[16] demonstrated that high-risk patients had fewer cardiovascular, infectious, and overall complications when

they received epidural anesthesia and analgesia compared with a GA group that received 60 mcg/kg fentanyl. A subset of patients in the latter study underwent major vascular surgery and that subset also demonstrated similar beneficial effects of epidural anesthesia and analgesia. The conclusions of the study are constrained by the heterogeneity of the study population, the small sample size, and the comparison of two widely different GA techniques. Tuman et al[17] validated the findings of Yeager et al of decreased cardiac complications with epidural anesthesia and analgesia, and reported additional benefits of reduced hypercoagulability and reduced thromboembolic complications in patients undergoing lower extremity revascularization. The incidence of pulmonary complications was also lower in the epidural analgesia group. A major limitation of this study was the comparison of significantly different postoperative pain control methods (continuous epidural analgesia vs. standard intermittent parenteral medication), raising the question of whether inferior pain control alone was responsible for the worse outcomes in the absence of epidural analgesia.

Subsequently, Baron et al[18] reported no difference in cardiac, pulmonary, or other operative morbidity when comparing GA with epidural-supplemented GA for abdominal aortic reconstructive surgery. The study population, surgical stress, and intraoperative management were homogeneous, but postoperative care and analgesia were not protocol directed. The authors did not report on postoperative lower extremity vascular patency and concluded that the study did not exclude the possibility that postoperative epidural analgesia could favorably influence postoperative outcome. The Periop-

TABLE 17-2
Summary of Outcome Studies Comparing General with Regional or Regional Supplemented Anesthesia

STUDIES	PROTOCOL CHARACTERISTICS			IMPROVED OUTCOMES		
	POSTOP NEURAXIAL ANALGESIA	TIGHT HEMO-DYNAMIC CONTROL	ROUTINE PAC AND ICU STAY	CARDIAC COMPLICATIONS	VASCULAR OCCLUSION OR REOPERATION	PULMONARY COMPLICATIONS
Yeager et al	Yes	No	No	Yes	NR	Yes
Tuman et al	Yes	No	No	Yes	Yes	Yes
Christopherson et al	Yes	Yes	No	No	Yes	No
Berlauk et al	No	Yes	Yes	Yes	Yes	NR
Baron et al	No	No	No	No	No	Possible*
Bode et al	No	Yes	Yes	No	NR	No
Pierce et al	No	Yes	Yes	No	No	No

The tendency of epidural anesthesia and analgesia and intensive medical management to be associated with similar outcomes is suggested.
ICU, Intensive care unit; *NR*, not reported; *PAC*, pulmonary artery catheterization.
*Decreased duration of mechanical ventilation with epidural compared with general anesthesia.

erative Ischemia Randomized Anesthesia Trial (PIRAT) study group contributed information that has clarified some of the controversies surrounding the effects of epidural anesthetic techniques on outcome.[19-21] Christopherson et al[19] found no difference in myocardial ischemia, major cardiac morbidity, or operative mortality between epidural anesthesia/analgesia and GA with patient-controlled analgesia (PCA) in patients undergoing lower extremity vascular surgery. This study was, however, inadequately powered to detect some of these outcomes that were the result of the early termination of enrollment because of an increased rate of reoperation for vascular graft failure in patients randomized to GA and postoperative PCA.[19] Data from the same group of patients demonstrated that preoperative plasminogen activator inhibitor-1 (PAI-1) levels were higher in individuals who developed thrombotic complications, whereas PAI-1 levels were unchanged in patients receiving epidural anesthesia and analgesia.[20] The investigators postulated that epidural anesthesia and analgesia may decrease the risk of arterial thrombotic complications in patients undergoing lower extremity revascularization by preventing the postoperative inhibition of fibrinolysis.

Breslow et al[21] investigated catecholamine and cortisol levels in patients undergoing lower extremity revascularization and found increased catecholamine levels at skin closure and into the postoperative period in patients not receiving epidural anesthesia and analgesia. Increased plasma catecholamine levels have been associated with a hypercoagulable state,[22] and attenuation of elevated blood catecholamine levels has therefore been suggested as an additional mechanism for the role played by epidural anesthesia/analgesia in the reduction of thrombotic complications.

The largest randomized trial of regional versus GA in peripheral vascular surgery compared spinal, epidural, and GA in 423 patients, and concluded that the choice of anesthesia does not affect cardiac morbidity and overall mortality in patients undergoing infrainguinal arterial revascularization.[23] Important aspects of this study included the systematic use of a pulmonary artery catheter in all patients and an absence in the study protocol of a specific provision for the use of postoperative epidural analgesia in patients randomly assigned to receive epidural anesthesia. Power calculations demonstrated that very large numbers of patients (>24,000) would be needed to achieve sufficient statistical power to demonstrate significant differences in outcome (on the basis of the low mortality rates) between anesthetic techniques. Although the identification of a lack of cardiovascular outcome difference related to the choice of intraoperative anesthetic, the study design precluded evaluation of the impact of continued neuraxial analgesia on outcome. Lower extremity vascular graft patency (30 day) and limb salvage rates in the latter study population

were compared and no difference in these outcomes, or length of hospital stay, were found between general, epidural, or spinal anesthesia.[24] As with other outcomes in the study of Bode et al,[23] the effect that epidural analgesia may have had on graft occlusion cannot be determined because epidural analgesia was not systematically applied.[23,24]

The inconsistent findings among several studies evaluating the impact of anesthetic technique on outcome after lower extremity revascularization deserves further analysis. The inability of the PIRAT study to show any significant difference in cardiac outcomes between anesthetic groups is probably related to the conservative vital-sign limits imposed by the study protocol as well as to the exclusion of similar patients undergoing more stressful operative procedures, such as aortic surgery.[19] These limitations create a more homogeneous study population, but likely make it more difficult to demonstrate differences in anesthetic technique. The very low overall incidence of complications reported by Bode et al also makes it difficult to detect differences related to anesthetic management. These excellent outcomes may be due to rapid medical interventions made possible by careful, continuous monitoring in the intensive care unit (ICU) for 48 to 72 hours after surgery in every patient.[23] It is possible that substantial physiologic parallels exist between the beneficial effects of epidural analgesia and the physiologic and pharmacologic interventions directed by intense monitoring. The results of Berlauk et al,[25] which indicated similar reductions in morbidity and graft complications via intensive optimization of systemic blood flow parameters, tend to support this hypothesis (see Table 17-2). The finding by Garnett et al of a burst of ischemia on the discontinuation of epidural analgesia is consistent with the concept that continuous epidural analgesia is associated with beneficial physiologic effects.[26] Finally, it may be that tightly controlled physiologic determinants of blood flow have effects similar to postoperative neuraxial blockade, and that when medical practices aimed at maintaining physiologic homeostasis are rigorously applied, the choice of anesthetic technique alone has only a small impact on postoperative outcome.

Some studies involving the continuous application of epidural anesthesia and analgesia after lower extremity revascularization suggest beneficial effects on thrombotic events such as vascular graft occlusion; these effects may be mediated via the attenuation of hypercoagulability or other mechanisms, such as reduced vasoconstriction and improved blood flow in the affected limb.[17,19] It has long been known that blood flow through femoral arterial grafts is better maintained under epidural anesthesia during and after surgery than with GA.[27] As previously noted, the failure of at least one randomized trial to identify any difference in graft occlusion rates among surgical anesthesia techniques is

---

BOX 17-1
Recommendations Regarding Anticoagulation and Neuraxial Anesthesia for Vascular Surgery

- The intraoperative use of unfractionated heparin for vascular surgery patients in whom neuraxial anesthetic techniques are used is acceptable with the following caveats:
  - Neuraxial anesthesia is avoided in the presence of other coagulopathies.
  - Heparin administration should be delayed for 1 hour after needle placement.
  - The catheter should be removed 1 hour before any subsequent heparin use, or 2 to 4 hours after the last heparin dose.
  - Careful postoperative neurologic monitoring should be performed to allow early detection of a new or persistent motor blockade; the use of low concentrations of local anesthetics to permit the early and accurate diagnosis of a spinal hematoma should be considered.
  - Traumatic needle placement with the appearance of blood in the needle or catheter *may* increase the risk of a spinal hematoma, although insufficient data exist to support cancellation of surgery. Clinical judgment should guide the decision to proceed with surgery, and frequent postoperative neurologic monitoring is recommended.
- If systemic anticoagulation with unfractionated heparin is begun with an epidural catheter in place, catheter removal should be delayed for 2 to 4 hours after discontinuation of anticoagulation and assessment of coagulation parameters.

- The concurrent use of other medications such as aspirin, NSAIDs, oral anticoagulants, and low-molecular-weight heparin (LMWH) may increase the risk of spinal hematoma in patients receiving standard heparin therapy.
- Subcutaneous, or minidose, heparin is not a contraindication to neuraxial techniques.
- Use of LMWH:
  - Needle placement for neuraxial anesthesia in patients treated with LMWH preoperatively should be performed at least 10 to 12 hours after the LMWH dose (24 hours after when higher dosages are used, e.g., enoxaparin 1 mg/kg twice daily), and is contraindicated when the dose is administered 2 hours before surgery.
  - Postoperative LMWH therapy can be safely used as long as continuous catheters are removed 2 hours before the start of LMWH therapy, or at least 10 to 12 hours after a dose of LMWH.
  - If LMWH therapy is begun with an indwelling neuraxial catheter *already in place*, extreme vigilance of the patient's neurologic status is *mandatory* because of possible increased risk of spinal hematoma. This decision should be made with care, and dilute local anesthetics are recommended to allow for the accurate and timely evaluation of neurologic function. Alternate forms of thromboprophylaxis or a delay in LMWH administration until catheter removal should be considered for catheter use beyond 24 hours.

Adapted from *Consensus Statements on Neuraxial Anesthesia and Anticoagulation*, American Society of Regional Anesthesia Consensus Conference, May 1998.
NSAIDs, Nonsteroidal antiinflammatory drugs.

---

probably not only related to the failure to evaluate postoperative neuraxial analgesia, but also to the very low overall frequency of graft occlusion observed at the study center.[24] The impact of surgical management on outcome has important implications for the decision process of whether to use neuraxial analgesia or other techniques on a specific patient. Indeed, a large number of surgical and patient variables (such as underlying vascular anatomy, type of material used for vascular conduits, reconstructive techniques, and distal extent of revascularization) influence outcome after peripheral vascular reconstruction.

Despite the potential for certain advantages over GA (e.g., reduced propensity toward postoperative hypercoagulability), regional anesthesia (RA) for lower extremity revascularization has limitations and disadvantages. Besides the usual adverse effects of central neuraxial blockade that can occur in any patient (e.g., excessive sympathetic blockade, ventilatory compromise secondary to excessive motor blockade of respiratory muscles, or the effects of neuraxial opioids), a special concern in patients undergoing lower extremity revascularization is

the risk of epidural hematoma. Anticoagulation with heparin is commonly used before vascular clamping and may be continued into the postoperative period. Based on reports of large series of patients, placement of epidural catheters before subsequent systemic heparinization appears to be safe.[28-32] Most practitioners advocate that epidural catheters not be removed postoperatively until a finite interval after heparin dosing, with a longer interval necessary if fractionated heparin (low-molecular-weight heparin or heparinoids) is used postoperatively.[33] Anecdotal reports suggest that RA is probably contraindicated when vascular thrombolytic therapy is used in these patients.[34] Recommendations for the use of neuraxial anesthesia when perioperative heparinization is anticipated are presented in Box 17-1.

CAROTID ENDARTERECTOMY
Preoperative Considerations

Current indications for CEA are based on prospective randomized trials of symptomatic and asymptomatic patients with carotid artery disease.[35,36] It is well accepted that symptomatic patients (previous transient ischemic attack, reversible ischemic neurologic deficit, or mild stroke within 6 months) with at least 70% carotid artery stenosis (CAS) are candidates for CEA. In addition, treatment of 60% or more asymptomatic CAS with aspirin and CEA reduces the 5-year risk of fatal and nonfatal strokes compared with aspirin alone.[36]

Preoperative conditions other than angiographic anatomy have not consistently been identified as predictive of adverse outcome in CEA patients. A multicenter review of nearly 700 CEA procedures found that only angiographic characteristics (ipsilateral carotid occlusion, stenosis near the carotid siphon, or intraluminal thrombosis) and age greater than 75 years were predictive of perioperative complications.[37] Another multivariate analysis was unable to identify any predictive association between age, gender, indication for surgery, bilaterality of CAS, hypertension, or smoking and adverse outcome after CEA.[38] In contrast, a larger multicenter study ($n = 1160$) identified several clinical predictors of adverse outcome (cerebrovascular accident, MI, or death) after CEA, including age greater than 75 years, symptom status (ipsilateral symptoms vs. asymptomatic or nonipsilateral symptoms), severe hypertension (diastolic blood pressure >110 mm Hg), CEA before coronary artery bypass graft surgery, history of angina, evidence of internal carotid artery thrombus, and internal CAS near the carotid siphon.[39] The presence of at least two factors was associated with a twofold increase in adverse events.

Patients with internal CAS often have associated impairment of cerebrovascular reactivity (CVR) and reduced ability to further dilate intracerebral arterioles in response to declines in cerebral perfusion pressure. The use of transcranial Doppler (TCD) to assess changes in middle cerebral artery blood flow velocity as a marker of CVR has been recommended for prediction of cerebral ischemic risk and to identify asymptomatic patients with CAS who are at greatest risk of stroke.[40] Patients with impaired CVR to carbon dioxide (CO_2), as demonstrated by preoperative TCD, have not been shown to have an increased risk of cerebral ischemia during CEA, as assessed by somatosensory-evoked potential recording (SEP).[41] Patients with residual cerebral ischemia after obstructive carotid artery lesions are removed or bypassed may have impaired CVR with an increased risk of stroke,[42] and hypotension should be meticulously avoided in such patients.

Intraoperative Considerations

The major intraoperative goals of management for patients undergoing CEA are modulation of the risks for myocardial and cerebral ischemia that are amenable to intervention. The essential elements of anesthetic management include maintenance of adequate cerebral

---

BOX 17-2
Intraoperative Monitors of Cerebral Perfusion

- Neurologic assessment of awake patient
- Assessment of cerebral blood flow
  - Stump pressures
  - Xe^{133} washout
  - Transcranial Doppler (middle cerebral artery flow)
- Cerebral electrical activity
  - EEG ± computer processing
  - Somatosensory-evoked potentials
- Cerebral oxygenation
  - Jugular venous oxygen saturation
  - Near-infrared spectroscopy (cerebral oximetry)

EEG, Electroencephalography; *Xe,* xenon.

---

perfusion, continual adjustment of important cardiovascular parameters, and appropriate monitoring of neurologic function to facilitate prompt intervention that may help reduce the risk of adverse postoperative neurologic or cardiovascular events.

Cerebral Monitoring. Many methods are available for intraoperative neurologic monitoring, although no single method is infallible, in large part because of the heterogeneity of the causes of cerebral ischemia, the complex sequelae of cellular events, and the variable location of ischemic insults (i.e., lacunar vs. cortical). The ideal method of monitoring cerebral perfusion during CEA remains controversial (Box 17-2). Available techniques include xenon blood flow, TCD ultrasonography, cerebral oximetry, SEPs, electroencephalography (EEG), and continual awake clinical neurologic evaluation during RA. The latter two methods are the most commonly used and are probably more accurate monitors of the adequacy of cerebral perfusion than carotid stump pressure alone.[43] Although reduced carotid stump pressure is generally associated with a greater risk of ischemic EEG changes, it is generally considered to be neither sufficiently sensitive nor specific enough to serve as a guide to selective carotid shunting,[44] and it is difficult to define a critical pressure that does not result in an unacceptably high number of false-positive or false-negative results (Fig. 17-3). Kwaan et al[45] determined that 25% of patients who had no neurologic changes during awake CEA had stump pressures less than 25 mm Hg and nearly a third of patients with carotid cross-clamp-induced neurologic changes had stump pressures greater than 50 mm Hg, underscoring the limited usefulness of stump pressure measurements to guide shunt placement.

Neurologic testing during CEA in the awake patient with RA is generally accepted as a sensitive monitor of

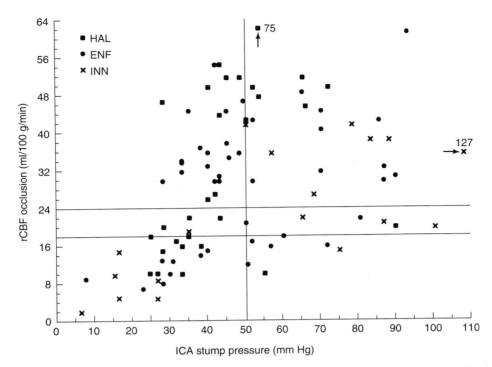

FIG. 17-3 The poor correlation between stump pressures and radiolabeled xenon-determined cerebral blood flow is clearly demonstrated by using three different anesthetics in this study of a large number of patients undergoing carotid endarterectomy. It is apparent that stump pressures below the critical value of 50 mm Hg are frequently associated with adequate cerebral blood flow, whereas stump pressures considered safe (i.e., >50 mm Hg) may be seen with low cerebral blood flow. *Enf,* Enflurane; *Hal,* halothane; *ICA,* internal carotid artery; *Inn,* Innovar; *rCBF,* regional cerebral blood flow.

(From McKay RD, Sundt TM, Michenfelder JD et al: *Anesthesiology* 45[4]:390-399, 1976.)

cerebral function and can reveal clinically significant cerebral ischemia even when sensitive EEG monitoring remains unchanged.[46] This may occur when the ischemic insult is located within deeper brain structures and when preexisting electrophysiologic abnormalities make it difficult to identify superimposed new abnormalities.[47] While processed EEG data are more "user friendly," sensitivity is reduced compared with multichannel analog EEG. For example, density spectral array analysis simplifies interpretation of EEG data, but it may not reliably detect mild analog EEG changes consistent with cerebral ischemia.[48] Compressed spectral array analyses of EEG data, especially declines in the spectral edge frequency, are also less sensitive than raw EEG data as a marker for ischemia.[49] One observational, noninterventional study collected EEG data during CEA without shunting and documented that 80% of immediate strokes after awakening from GA for CEA were associated with severe intraoperative EEG changes.[50] However, no data define how severe the intraoperative EEG changes must be or how long they must be present to accurately predict stroke after CEA, nor are there prospective data to define whether the EEG is decisively better than alternative methods of assessing the adequacy of cerebral perfusion.

TCD ultrasonography applied across the relatively thin temporal bone allows continuous measurement of blood flow velocity in the middle cerebral artery distribution and may be helpful in differentiating between intraoperative hemodynamic versus embolic neurologic events. Failure to obtain interpretable TCD signals occurs in 15% to 20% of cases because of temporal hyperostosis or other technical difficulties. Unfortunately, values for blood flow velocity or pulsatility index that correlate with critical cerebral blood flow reduction have not been identified. Patients with minimal changes in blood flow velocity during carotid clamping (with shunting) have been shown to have stroke rates similar to (or even slightly greater than) when flow velocity is unchanged and shunts are not used.[51] TCD-detected embolization occurs in more than 90% of patients during CEA[52] (Fig. 17-4). Emboli having TCD characteristics of air (occurring at shunt opening and during restoration of flow) are generally not associated with

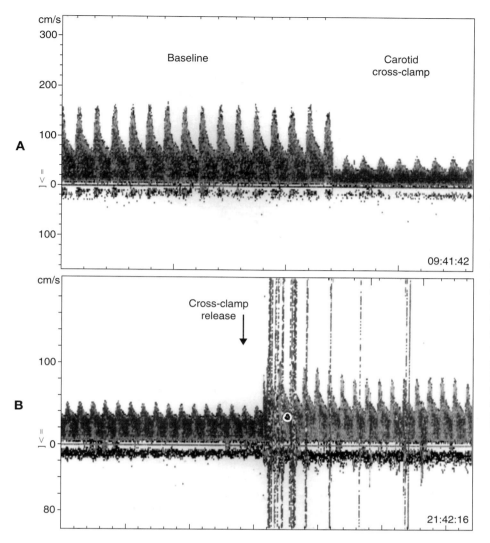

FIG. 17-4   **A,** Transcranial Doppler (TCD) tracing of middle cerebral artery blood flow velocity before and after clamping of the internal carotid artery during a carotid endarterectomy. Although the velocities decreased with clamping, they only decreased by 30% of the preclamp mean value, and thus represent competent collateral flow. In contrast, TCD velocities would have completely disappeared with inadequate collateral flow. **B,** Microemboli in the middle cerebral artery after carotid clamp release and restoration of cerebral blood flow. Embolic events appear as sharp spikes on the TCD recording and are common with reperfusion.

(From Davis DA: Intraoperative transcranial Doppler monitoring in carotid endarterectomy. In Bailes JE, Spetzler RF, editors: *Microsurgical carotid endarterectomy,* Philadelphia, 1996, Lippincott-Raven, pp 89-105, Figures 6,9.)

adverse clinical outcome. However, particulate emboli (>10) detected by TCD during carotid dissection correlate with significant deterioration in cognitive function after CEA,[52] postoperative ischemic events, and new ischemic lesions on magnetic resonance images of the brain.[53] More careful surgical dissection of the artery and more meticulous attention to backbleeding and flushing to avoid embolization may be guided by acoustic evidence for embolism, although it is unknown if such an approach alters outcome. TCD monitoring may also indicate which patients should have aggressive hemodynamic interventions or be anticoagulated, because cerebral embolic events and decreased cerebral blood flow velocity can be differentiated.

Near-infrared spectroscopy (NIRS) can also be used to assess changes in cerebral blood flow by measuring regional cerebral oxygenation. NIRS assesses oxygenation of arterial, capillary, and venous hemoglobin, and predominantly estimates venous oxygenation (the largest of the three cerebral vascular compartments). Ca-

rotid artery clamping results in a variable decrease in cerebrovascular hemoglobin oxygen saturation in the majority of patients undergoing CEA.[54] Declines in regional cerebral oxygenation correlate variably with decreases in evoked potential amplitude during CEA.[55-58] Specific regional cerebral saturation threshold values defining critical cerebral ischemia have not been definitively established, and the specific role of this monitor compared with other methods for cerebral ischemia detection remains to be defined.

Cerebral and Myocardial Ischemia. Hyperventilation has been proposed to redistribute blood flow from normal areas of the brain with preserved CO_2 reactivity to ischemic areas in which CO_2 reactivity has been lost, but controlled studies have not identified any benefit attributable to this "inverse steal" phenomenon.[59] Available data do not support reduction of arterial carbon dioxide pressure (Pa_{CO_2}) as a routine intervention to reduce cerebral injury, and maintaining normocapnia seems to be the most reasonable approach during CEA in most situations.

Cerebral ischemia during carotid clamping can be reduced with the use of a carotid shunt, although to optimize benefit the shunt should be functional within 2 to 4 minutes without dissection or embolization. Even functioning shunts do not guarantee adequacy of cerebral perfusion, and there are markedly variable flow rates for different types of shunts. For example, the flow through a long Inahara-Pruitt shunt is about half that through a Javid shunt under similar conditions.[60] Of course, hypotension and low cardiac output compound such flow discrepancies and may be associated with decreased cerebral perfusion despite shunt patency.

Most practitioners advocate maintenance of blood pressure close to the preoperative level, whereas some recommend a blood pressure of 10% to 20% above normal. The rationale for maintaining normal or mildly increased systemic blood pressure during CEA is based on three concerns: (1) the normally occurring reduction in cerebral perfusion pressure in boundary zones between principle vascular territories, (2) the increased vulnerability of these areas to declines in blood pressure if intracranial occlusive disease or cerebral infarction are present, and (3) alteration of normal autoregulation in the presence of volatile anesthetics or chronic hypertension. Definite neurologic benefits of intraoperative "hypertension" have not been documented, although concern has been raised about potential myocardial risks. Smith et al[61] showed that transesophageal echocardiography (TEE)-diagnosed myocardial ischemia (identified as new wall-motion abnormalities) occur frequently during CEA when phenylephrine is administered to support blood pressure when moderately deep levels of inhaled anesthesia are used. These changes may be related to changes in ventricular loading conditions when a pure α_1-agonist is administered in the presence of a volatile anesthetic with negative inotropic effects, resulting in altered regional wall motion and overdiagnosis of ischemia. Mutch et al[62] found no evidence for Holter-monitored ischemia when phenylephrine was infused to support mean arterial pressure (MAP) at $110 \pm 10\%$ of ward values during carotid artery clamping. However, Holter-diagnosed myocardial ischemia that is prolonged and that occurs during carotid artery clamping or within 2 hours following declamping is highly predictive of adverse cardiac complications.[63]

During CEA, myocardial ischemia can occur in close association with marked fluctuations in blood pressure that are partially related to carotid baroreceptor deactivation (during clamping) and reactivation (after declamping).[63] While intraoperative carotid sinus infiltration with local anesthetic has been recommended to reduce such hemodynamic fluctuations, this approach is associated with a greater frequency of intraoperative and postoperative hypertension.[64,65] The extent of surgical or pharmacologic denervation of the carotid sinus during CEA is likely an important determinant of postclamp hemodynamic responses. Perioperative hypertension has a multifactorial etiology, is dependent on the adequacy of preoperative blood pressure control and the presence of peripheral vascular disease, and may be impacted significantly by the choice of anesthesia.[66] Hemodynamic instability with episodes of tachycardia and hypertension on awakening and tracheal extubation after CEA are also associated with myocardial ischemia.[62]

Minimally Invasive Carotid Artery Revascularization. Minimally invasive techniques for management of carotid artery stenosis present significant challenges for the anesthesiologist. Percutaneous interventions for carotid angioplasty and stenting may be performed either via the femoral artery approach, or (less commonly) via direct puncture of the common carotid artery. Sedation is usually sufficient for groin cannulation, with the patient awake during carotid balloon inflation. Anticholinergic agents (atropine or glycopyrrolate) are administered to attenuate the baroreceptor response during balloon dilation or stent deployment. GA with short-acting agents is more commonly performed when direct carotid artery puncture is used, and prompt awakening at the end of the procedure is desirable to facilitate early neurologic evaluation. Particular vigilance in monitoring hemodynamic and neurologic status is required during these procedures, especially during balloon inflations and after sheath removal for the cervical approach. Control of hypertension is particularly important because it increases the risk of hematoma formation, a potentially catastrophic event, especially if residual anticoagulation is present. Maintenance of adequate perfusion pressure is particularly important to facilitate collateral blood flow during balloon dilation. Although CEA is currently the "gold standard" therapy for carotid artery stenosis, experience with endovascular techniques suggests complication rates comparable to CEA, with carotid patency even after 6-year follow-up.[67]

Choice of Anesthesia for CEA. Debate over the choice of RA versus GA persists because of differing conclusions regarding the risks and benefits of each from various studies. The main advantage of RA is the ability to predict cerebral ischemia after carotid artery clamping, although various retrospective analyses have not been able to identify a clear difference in stroke or mortality rate between GA and RA.[68,69] Uncontrolled retrospective studies have suggested that RA is associated with a lower frequency of carotid artery shunting,[68,70] a lower incidence of postoperative hemodynamic instability,[66,70,71] and a shorter postoperative hospital stay.[68,72]

However, other retrospective analyses have found no difference in cardiovascular outcome or hospital stay after CEA regardless of anesthetic technique.[69] Interestingly, one prospective investigation found RA for CEA to be associated with a high incidence of tachycardia,[73] which may be related to elevated levels of epinephrine and norepinephrine (Fig. 17-5). A retrospective review of GA versus RA for CEA found a greater incidence of ventricular arrhythmias with GA but other adverse cardiac and neurologic events occurred with similar frequency between the two techniques.[74] Another retrospective analysis of more than 1000 CEA (two thirds with cervical block) could not identify any difference in cardiac complication rates between GA and RA.[75] The latter retrospective study did, however, report a lower stroke rate after CEA with RA (1.3%) compared with GA (3.2%).[75] Most studies evaluating the influence of choice of anesthesia on the incidence of MI after CEA are not prospective and have screened for MI on the basis of clinical symptoms only, so that the question of whether there are differences in true rates of adverse cardiac outcome remains unresolved. No carefully controlled randomized trial has been conducted to identify whether any definite cardiac or neurologic outcome difference exists between RA and GA for CEA.

Opponents of RA for CEA are often concerned about its finite "failure rate" (defined as the need for conversion to GA), which occurs in about 1% to 2% of cases.[68] This may be reduced by supplemental infiltration with local anesthetic by the surgeon. A major factor for success of RA for CEA is gentle handling of tissues by the surgeon, as well as appropriate and frequent patient communication during the procedure. The success of RA is also improved with infiltration of local anesthetic at the ramus and lower border of the mandible. Even with these qualifiers, RA is not ideal for patients with an expected long operative time or difficult vascular anatomy, especially when there is a more cephalad carotid bifurcation or a high carotid plaque that requires vigorous submandibular retraction. In addition, unsatisfactory conditions may become manifest with RA in patients with short necks, where surgical exposure may be difficult. Intraoperative mandibular nerve block can relieve discomfort associated with forceful or prolonged retraction on the mandible. Patients who become uncomfortable or restless may require airway intervention under physically awkward conditions, and the clinician must be ready to deal with this circumstance whenever

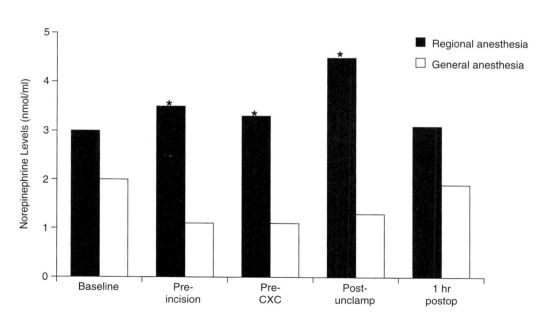

FIG. 17-5 A comparison of plasma norepinephrine levels at several time points during carotid endarterectomy in patients receiving either general anesthesia or regional anesthesia with a cervical plexus block. Norepinephrine levels were significantly (p <0.01) higher in the regional anesthesia group at the three designated time intervals (*).

(From Takolander R, Bergqvist D, Hulthen UL et al: *Eur J Vasc Surg* 4:265-270, 1990.)

TABLE 17-3
Comparison of Regional and General Anesthesia for CEA

TECHNIQUE	ADVANTAGES	DISADVANTAGES
Regional	• Less intraoperative hypotension	• More intraoperative hypertension, higher catecholamine levels
	• Technically simple block	• Potential unfamiliarity for operative team
	• Tracheal intubation not required	• Awkward airway control if GA required
	• Sensitive neurologic monitor	• Sedation may obscure neurologic monitoring or falsely suggest ischemia
	• Avoids postoperative somnolence seen with GA	• Patient discomfort if ischemia develops, or if procedure is lengthy
	• Provides postoperative analgesia	• Sedation-induced $\uparrow$ $Paco_2$, $\downarrow$ Pao_2 may increase cerebral ischemia
		• Need to convert to GA
General	• Reliable airway control	• Intubation/airway device required
	• Secure control of $Paco_2$, Pao_2	• More intraoperative hemodynamic changes
	• Possible neuroprotective effects of anesthetics	• Delayed emergence vs. new neurologic event

CEA, Carotid endarterectomy; *GA,* general anesthesia; *Paco₂,* arterial carbon dioxide pressure; *Pao₂,* arterial oxygen pressure.

embarking on RA for CEA. RA and GA are both acceptable options for CEA, and the decision to use one or the other technique should depend on the combined desires and experience of the anesthesiologist and surgeon, as well as patient preference. For RA techniques, a prospective, randomized comparison of deep versus superficial cervical plexus block for CEA found no differences in patient satisfaction or intraoperative conditions, although deep cervical plexus block resulted in a later onset of postoperative discomfort and a lower likelihood of requiring analgesia in the first 24 hours after CEA.[76] Table 17-3 summarizes the advantages and disadvantages of RA versus GA for CEA.

Most anesthetic agents commonly used for induction or maintenance of GA decrease cerebral metabolism, although it is likely that any neuroprotective influence of anesthetics is more related to complex biochemical effects on ischemic brain tissue than simply a reduction of cerebral metabolism. While isoflurane has been associated with fewer EEG changes during carotid clamping[77] and with a lower critical regional cerebral blood flow[78] when compared with older volatile agents such as halothane or enflurane, retrospective comparison of these three anesthetics could not identify any difference either in neurologic outcome[77] or in cardiac outcome after CEA.[79]

Hemodynamic stability during GA for CEA can be enhanced with moderate amounts of opioids such as fentanyl or its derivatives, although care must be exercised to avoid doses that compromise rapid emergence at the end of the procedure. The ultrashort duration of the new synthetic opioid remifentanil may be use-

ful for CEA because its pharmacokinetic profile allows effective modification of intraoperative hyperdynamic responses while permitting a rapid emergence from anesthesia. Judicious administration of β-adrenergic blockers is also useful to minimize increases in heart rate and blood pressure during stressful intraoperative periods, and perioperative β-blockade may have beneficial effects on cardiac outcome.[7,8] α_2-Receptor agonists are also useful to attenuate adverse hemodynamic responses during CEA.[9,10]

Postoperative Considerations

Although the efficacy of CEA for the prevention of stroke has been demonstrated for specific subsets of both symptomatic as well as asymptomatic patients, perioperative stroke remains an important and often devastating complication. Acute postoperative neurologic events usually occur early in the postoperative course,[80] which allows timely identification of patients who require overnight ICU admission. As with other surgical procedures, fast-track recovery without routine ICU admission and with early home discharge is being applied to patients after CEA. The feasibility and safety of fast-tracking protocols has been examined, and the majority of patients do not require ICU admission and may be safely discharged home 1 to 2 days after CEA.[81]

Stroke after CEA has many causes, with more than half of surgical etiology (ischemia during carotid clamping, postoperative thrombosis, and embolism), and the remainder because of other factors such as reperfusion

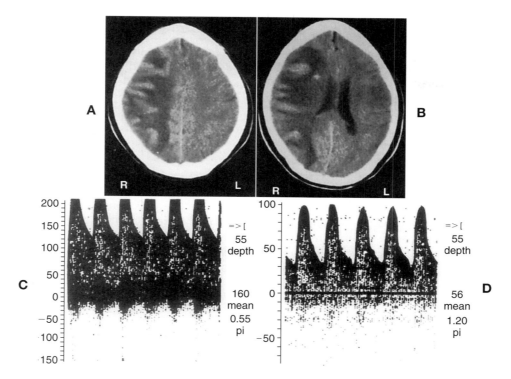

FIG. 17-6 Hyperfusion syndrome after carotid endarterectomy (CEA). **A,** Noncontrast head computed tomography scan on postoperative day 5 reveals diffuse edema in the right frontal and parietal lobes. **B,** Midline shift from right-sided edema and a small hyperdense lesion in the right frontal lobe, representing a small cerebral hemorrhage, are evident in this scan. **C,** Transcranial Doppler recordings from a different patient with the hyperperfusion syndrome noted one day following CEA. The mean velocity of 160 cm/sec was an increase of 400% over preoperative values and was accompanied by a severe unilateral headache. **D,** By postoperative day two, the mean velocity (56 cm/sec) had returned to normal and the symptoms had resolved. *Pi,* Pulsating index.

(**A** and **B** from Breen JC, Caplan LR, DeWitt LD et al: *Neurology* 46:175-181, 1996; **C** and **D** from Powers AD, Smith RR: *Neurosurgery* 26:56-60, 1990.)

injury, intracranial hemorrhage, or other postoperative events. Embolization is the most common cause of intraoperative strokes and is invariably associated with surgical events. It is estimated that only approximately 20% of intraoperative strokes are due to hemodynamic events (related to carotid clamping, intracranial occlusive disease, and shunt problems). Nonetheless, hemodynamically mediated strokes may follow a critical reduction in boundary zone perfusion secondary to intracranial occlusive disease, or may occur in areas around old cerebral infarcts, where apparently innocuous reductions in cerebral perfusion pressure may result in adverse outcome. After CEA, strokes tend to be related to embolization or thrombosis, although intracerebral hemorrhage may also occur. Early thrombosis may be related to intimal injury or flap formation, as well as to enhanced platelet activation or deposition at the operative site. Neurologic events occurring during CEA are not necessarily predictive of postoperative complications, which may explain the variable findings of studies ex-

amining the effects of intraoperative interventions on overall stroke incidence.

Another neurologic complication manifesting after CEA is the hyperperfusion syndrome. This syndrome consists of an abrupt increase in blood flow with loss of autoregulation in surgically reperfused brain tissue. Patients with severe hypertension after CEA are at increased risk of developing this syndrome, which may present with a spectrum of findings including headache, signs of transient cerebral ischemia, seizures, brain edema, and even intracerebral hemorrhage[82] (Fig. 17-6). Middle cerebral artery blood flow has been shown to be pressure dependent in patients with post-CEA hyperperfusion (consistent with defective autoregulation) and systemic blood pressure should, therefore, be controlled meticulously in the immediate period after CEA, especially when there was a large preoperative pressure gradient across a severe CAS.[83]

Postoperative blood pressure lability is common after CEA, and hypertension is seen in approximately

70% of patients.[84] Before CEA, carotid sinus baroreceptors may reset secondary to proximal arterial occlusion. After CEA, the reset baroreceptor may sense sudden increases in blood pressure, triggering subsequent baroreceptor-mediated hypotension. However, hypotension is less common than hypertension. As noted earlier, although anesthetizing the carotid sinus nerve can improve hemodynamic stability during CEA, this practice, as well as surgical denervation of the carotid sinus, compounds the risk of postoperative hypertension, especially in patients with significant preoperative hypertension.

Transient dysfunction of adjacent cranial nerves and their branches may occur despite gentle dissection and retraction during CEA. Injury to the superior laryngeal nerve can occur, which primarily results in mild relaxation of the ipsilateral vocal cord manifested by early fatigability of the voice and impairment of high-pitched phonation. Recurrent laryngeal nerve (RLN) dysfunction after CEA may result in paralysis of the ipsilateral vocal cord in the paramedian position, hoarseness, and impairment of the cough mechanism. If RLN injury occurs and contralateral CEA is planned, consideration should be given to postponing the subsequent operation until satisfactory RLN function returns, or at least precautions for postoperative airway management should be planned if surgery cannot be delayed. Although bilateral CEA is known to result in carotid body dysfunction and increases in resting Pa_{CO_2}, carotid body function can be abnormal even after unilateral CEA, with impaired ventilatory response to mild hypoxemia. Supplementary oxygen is therefore indicated in the immediate recovery period after CEA.

Upper airway obstruction after CEA is a rare but potentially fatal complication that occurs not only because of hematoma formation, but also more commonly because of glottic edema secondary to venous and lymphatic congestion. This diffuse type of neck edema (lateral and retropharyngeal) may be associated with markedly edematous supraglottic mucosal folds. Although such edema has also been postulated to be the effect of tissue trauma with increased capillary permeability induced by local vasoactive mediator release, steroid administration immediately before CEA does not reduce edema formation.[85] The presence of supraglottic edema after CEA may make intubation and mask ventilation extremely difficult. Opening of the neck wound at the bedside for evacuation of the hematoma is not uniformly effective in this situation, may induce significant hypertension that may aggravate further bleeding, and is best reserved for patients with impending respiratory arrest. The most prudent approach to this problem may be to return the patient to the operating room for controlled surgical exploration. Local anesthetic infiltration for evacuation of the hematoma is preferred over GA, because the latter approach may induce airway obstruc-

tion and difficulty in intubation. O'Sullivan et al[86] described six patients who developed wound hematomas after CEA, four of whom had respiratory distress. All six patients developed immediate airway obstruction on induction of anesthesia and all were difficult to intubate. Airway landmarks during laryngoscopy were described as "unrecognizable." Kunkel et al[87] reported a series of 15 patients who underwent surgical exploration for postoperative neck hematomas after CEA, only three of whom had respiratory distress. Six of seven patients developed airway obstruction with induction of anesthesia and were difficult to intubate; two sustained perioperative MIs, one developed respiratory failure, and one patient died. Of the remaining eight patients who received local anesthesia rather than GA, none sustained a complication. These reports emphasize the potential for upper airway obstruction with the induction of GA, despite the absence of respiratory distress preoperatively. Awake intubation is thus *strongly* advised if respiratory distress develops or surgical exploration is required to evacuate a neck hematoma after CEA. If severe bleeding develops within the first hour after surgery, then glottic edema and the risk of airway obstruction may be less pronounced than when neck swelling has been prolonged. Fig. 17-7 presents an approach to the postoperative management of patients with neck swelling and wound hematomas after CEA.

Phrenic nerve paresis is common after cervical plexus block. While this normally has little clinical consequence (except for a mildly increased Pa_{CO_2}), it is a potentially more serious problem in patients with severe pulmonary disease or who have preexisting contralateral diaphragmatic dysfunction.

ABDOMINAL AORTIC SURGERY
Epidemiology and Pathogenesis

Aneurysms of the infrarenal abdominal aorta are commonly defined by the presence of permanent dilation of the abdominal aorta at least 1.5 to 2 times the normal diameter of the abdominal aorta. They are typically fusiform in shape with a uniform increase in aortic size. The mechanism of aneurysm formation is likely multifactorial, although atherosclerosis is considered the most common pathologic factor. Thickening of the infrarenal aortic intima by the atherosclerotic process may limit the diffusion of oxygen and other nutrients across the intimal layer into the aortic media, leading to ischemic injury of the media and subsequent weakening of the aortic wall.[88] These changes, in concert with increased wall stress from hypertension, lead to medial degeneration, aneurysmal dilation of the aortic wall, and increases in wall tension that lead to further propagation of the aneurysmal process.[88] In addition to the classic theory of atherosclerosis, genetic factors are also important. Abdominal ultrasound screening has revealed

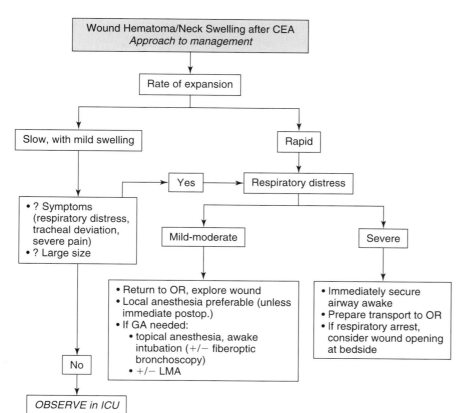

FIG. 17-7   A suggested approach to the management of wound hematomas accompanied by neck swelling after carotid endarterectomy *(CEA)*. Mild swelling with minimal symptoms may be managed conservatively with observation in an intensive care unit *(ICU)*. The presence of respiratory symptoms, or a rapid increase in neck diameter, requires immediate reexploration in the operating room *(OR)* and securing of the airway while the patient is awake. Neck swelling immediately (<1 hour) after surgery may produce less glottic edema because of the short duration of bleeding, but cautious assessment of the airway is still advised before proceeding with general anesthesia *(GA)* for reexploration. Opening of the wound at the bedside is probably only appropriate for acute respiratory arrest. *LMA,* Laryngeal mask airway.

that approximately 28% of patients with an infrarenal aortic aneurysm have a first-degree relative with a similar aneurysm.[88] Other proposed mechanisms of aneurysm formation include excessive activity of proteolytic enzymes such as collagenase and elastase, hemodynamic factors including aneurysm-induced increased wall tension that leads to further aneurysm expansion (according to the law of Laplace), and inflammatory changes because of cytokine activity and macrophage activation.[89] Other less common etiologic factors include infectious processes, trauma, congenital abnormalities, and vasculitis.[89]

Surgical Indications

The primary indication for surgical repair of abdominal aortic aneurysms is to prevent rupture, which is an important and preventable cause of mortality in men over 55 years of age.[89] In addition, lower extremity ischemic symptoms (claudication) resulting from aortoocclusive disease often require aortic bifurcation grafts to bypass stenotic or aneurysmal iliac vessels. Compared with aneurysmal disease of the abdominal aorta, patients with aortoiliac occlusive disease are younger and have a lower operative mortality, although their risk of postoperative cardiac complications is similar. The rate of growth of individual aneurysms and the risk of rupture are somewhat unpredictable, although rupture appears to be closely related to the diameter of the aneurysm.[90,91] Some data, in fact, suggest that aneurysm diameter is the *only* factor that has a significant impact on the frequency of rupture.[90] The accelerated growth rate observed with large aneurysms (>5 cm) increases the annual risk of rupture to 10% to 15% for aneurysms greater than 6 cm in size, compared with a risk of rupture of less than 5% for aneurysms less than 6 cm in diameter.[90] Aneurysms less than 4 cm rarely rupture and are not repaired unless there is a secondary indication for surgery.[89] Repair of aneurysms between 4 and 5 cm is controversial because of the low risk of rupture, although it is recommended for the young or low-risk patient because of the unpredictability of aneurysm rupture and because most patients will eventually come to surgery for resection.[92] In contrast to size factors, all symptomatic aneurysms and all saccular aneurysms should be repaired. The prohibitive risk of aneurysm rupture for very large aneurysms—over 20% per year for lesions greater than 7 cm—mandates operative repair even for patients with significant comorbid conditions.[89-92]

Surgical Approach

A midline abdominal incision and transperitoneal approach to the abdominal aorta is the standard operative procedure for repair of infrarenal aortic aneurysms. Although controversial, some data suggest that the retroperitoneal approach, where an incision is made in the left retroperitoneal space, avoids intestinal evisceration and thereby decreases fluid requirements, lowers the rate of pulmonary complications, reduces the risk of postoperative ileus, is less painful, and allows an earlier resumption of oral intake. These benefits ultimately reduce the duration of ICU stays and the overall duration of hospitalization.[93-95] Other investigators have not confirmed these findings,[96,97] and because of the perceived technical difficulties of this approach, many surgeons are reluctant to adopt this technique. Instead, it is reserved for patients with significant pulmonary disease or specific anatomic problems (e.g., previous surgery) that militate against use of the classic midline abdominal incision.[93]

The need to reduce the significant incidence of cardiopulmonary complications after conventional transperitoneal or retroperitoneal approaches has led to the development of less invasive transfemoral endovascular stent-graft techniques for the repair of abdominal aortic aneurysms. First described by Parodi and colleagues,[98] the endovascular stent-graft consists of an introducer sheath and a delivery system that contains a graft with self-expanding fixation devices at each end. The sheath is placed in the femoral artery and positioned within the aneurysm sac by using fluoroscopy. Once properly positioned, the delivery system is removed and a completion angiogram is performed to confirm the position and function of the graft and to establish the absence of an incomplete seal (which causes perianastomotic reflux of blood into the aneurysm sac).[99] The goal is complete exclusion of the aneurysm sac from the circulation, thereby "defunctionalizing" it and reducing the subsequent risk of rupture. The procedure is performed by a team of vascular surgeons and interventional radiologists, either in the operating room, or in a catheterization laboratory with full operative capabilities. Although initial reports described the use of GA, more contemporary experience has demonstrated the successful use of local anesthesia and intravenous sedation with propofol and midazolam.[100] Epidural anesthesia has also been successfully used and appears to reduce the length of hospitalization when compared with GA.[101] Monitoring for these procedures typically includes radial arterial and central venous catheters. Operative times range from 2 to 3 hours and blood loss averages 300 to 800 ml; the majority of patients are discharged within 48 to 72 hours of surgery.[94,100,102] Available data suggest shorter hospital and ICU stays and a lower incidence of pulmonary complications and overall operative morbidity compared with conventional open procedures.[94,103-105] Unfortunately, mortality rates and hospital costs are comparable to open procedures and local or vascular complications may occur in a disturbingly high percentage of patients.[94-102] It appears that the cost savings accrued from a reduced

hospital stay are offset by the increased cost of supplies and radiology resources. Ultimately, the lower pulmonary and cardiac morbidity associated with this technique offers an attractive option to conventional open procedures for the high-risk patient with substantial pulmonary or cardiac disease. It is to be hoped that mortality will decrease as additional clinical experience is gained and new devices are developed.

As a further alternative to transabdominal aortic surgery, minimally invasive laparoscopic aneurysm resection has been reported with equivalent mortality rates but with less ventilator support, shorter ICU stays, and a lower frequency of ileus compared with open procedures.[106] This technically demanding approach offers yet another potentially safer alternative to conventional transabdominal aortic surgery for the high-risk patient.

Intraoperative Management

Monitors and Vascular Access. The choice of monitoring for abdominal aortic surgery is controversial, and depends in large part on the preoperative renal and cardiopulmonary function of each patient. Invasive arterial blood pressure monitoring is considered essential because of the rapid and frequent fluctuations in blood pressure and because of the need to assess hemoglobin levels and changes in acid-base variables. The radial artery is typically chosen as the preferred site, although the brachial artery can be safely cannulated without fear of complications.

In contrast to invasive arterial blood pressure monitoring, the need for pulmonary artery catheterization for infrarenal aortic surgery remains controversial. Initial data suggested that use of a pulmonary artery catheter in conjunction with preoperative "hemodynamic optimization" resulted in more favorable outcomes compared with cases managed with central venous catheters and no preoperative preparation.[25] Berlauk et al[25] demonstrated reduced cardiac morbidity, fewer adverse intraoperative hemodynamic events, improved early graft patency, and fewer deaths in a series of patients undergoing infrainguinal bypass procedures randomized to this optimization strategy. More contemporary evidence, however, has failed to show that the use of pulmonary artery catheters to guide preoperative hemodynamic optimization confers any significant advantage in terms of reduced cardiopulmonary complications in patients undergoing aortic procedures.[107-111] It would appear that low-risk patients without significant left ventricular dysfunction, renal insufficiency, or severe obstructive lung disease can be safely managed in the perioperative period with central venous catheters alone.[111,112] The additional information regarding cardiac function obtained from a pulmonary artery catheter, including mixed venous oxygen saturation (Sv_{O_2}) and cardiac output measurement, may be especially useful for patients with impaired ventricular function, renal dysfunction, and severe lung disease in whom central venous pressure monitoring alone may be inadequate. TEE may also provide additional, more sensitive information regarding ventricular function and the presence of myocardial ischemia, and may prove to be a more reliable intraoperative monitor during aortic surgery.[113,114] Studies that examine myocardial ischemia during aortic surgery by using intraoperative TEE have demonstrated a 28% to 38% incidence of new segmental wall-motion abnormalities.[115-116] These echocardiographic changes have not, however, consistently predicted the occurrence of postoperative cardiac complications,[115-118] and this may reflect the influence of nonischemic causes of wall-motion changes, such as changes in preload and afterload, which are common during major aortic surgery. Catoire et al[119] noted a significant increase in segmental wall scores after infrarenal aortic clamping, again suggesting the possible influence of loading conditions on the incidence of new wall-motion changes. Wall-motion abnormalities are less frequent during infrarenal compared with supraceliac aortic cross-clamping,[120] and this may reflect the more modest increases in afterload observed with infrarenal aortic cross-clamping. The complexity of the hemodynamic and coronary vascular response to thoracic aortic clamping, however, precludes exclusion of myocardial ischemia as a possible mechanism of these changes distinct from the effects of altered loading conditions (see Chapter 14).

Because of the potential for sudden and severe hemorrhage, the placement of two large-bore (e.g., 14-gauge) intravenous catheters is recommended. If a central venous catheter is chosen for hemodynamic monitoring, a 12-French multilumen catheter can provide additional large-bore venous access to facilitate rapid transfusion. It is useful to use pressurized rapid infusion devices such as Level One blood warmers (Level One Technologies, Rockland, Mass.) that allow rapid administration of warmed fluid and blood products. The average operative blood loss for infrarenal aortic procedures is about 900 ml* and mean red blood cell transfusion rates are approximately 1 unit of homologous blood and 2 to 3 units of autotransfused blood.[121] Some data suggest a lower blood loss with retroperitoneal procedures compared with conventional transperitoneal approaches.[93] Serious bleeding occurs in approximately 5% of patients undergoing elective abdominal aortic surgery and in this instance blood loss can vary from 3 to 6 L.[122] In about 50% of patients, this bleeding is from the aortic anastomosis or from clamp-induced aortic injury, and in the remainder bleeding arises from major veins such as the inferior vena cava and renal veins.[122] Because of the risk of hemorrhage, blood should be immediately available

*References 93, 94, 97, 107, 109, 111.

and ordered in advance of ongoing losses. When major hemorrhage occurs, dilutional hemostatic changes from inadequate replacement of platelets and fresh frozen plasma, along with hypothermic alterations in hemostasis, ionized hypocalcemia, and low-grade consumptive coagulopathy, further exacerbate bleeding. Evaluation of platelet counts, thromboelastography, and serial hematocrit values allow a reasonable estimation of the need for factor and platelet transfusions.

Anesthetic Choice. The type of anesthetic used for abdominal aortic surgery varies and depends primarily on the dose of opioid used and whether or not adjuvant epidural anesthesia is used. Although some institutions use a high-dose opioid technique similar to that used for patients undergoing cardiac surgery, a common approach is the use of modest doses of fentanyl (5-10 mcg/kg), a barbiturate or etomidate for anesthetic induction, and a volatile anesthetic supplemented with additional opioids for the maintenance of anesthesia. This approach avoids the obligatory period of prolonged intubation and mechanical ventilatory support associated with high-dose opioids. Because of the high-risk cardiac profile of patients undergoing abdominal aortic surgery, short-acting β-adrenergic blockers such as esmolol may be necessary to control the hyperdynamic response to intubation. Similarly, vasoactive infusions such as nitroglycerin, nitroprusside, and phenylephrine should be readily available to promptly treat intraoperative fluctuations in blood pressure.

The use of epidural anesthesia and analgesia as an adjunct to GA for aortic surgery gained popularity with investigations performed in the late 1980s. Suggested benefits of epidural anesthesia and analgesia include a reduction of the neuroendocrine stress response to surgery, reduced opioid requirements, earlier mobilization, attenuation of hypercoagulability, decreased myocardial oxygen demand and intraoperative ischemia, improved postoperative analgesia, favorable changes in postoperative pulmonary function, and a reduction in cardiac morbidity. Yeager et al[16] were the first to demonstrate that compared with GA alone, the addition of epidural anesthesia for abdominal aortic surgery reduced postoperative cardiac morbidity by improving analgesia and reducing the systemic stress response. Other investigators have also demonstrated modest reductions in postoperative epinephrine and norepinephrine levels in patients receiving epidural analgesia[123-125] although Norman and Fink failed to show any demonstrable change in the cortisol, catecholamine, or cytokine response to surgical stress during aortic surgery with epidural anesthesia.[126] By using TEE, Saada et al[127] and Dodds et al[128] were unable to demonstrate any effect of thoracic epidural anesthesia on the incidence of segmental wall-motion abnormalities during abdominal aortic aneurysm resection compared with GA alone.

In addition, Baron et al[18] were unable to discern a difference in postoperative complications with thoracic epidural anesthesia in more than 100 patients undergoing aortic surgery by using combined thoracic epidural and GA compared with GA alone, although disparities in the quality of postoperative analgesia between groups may have influenced their unfavorable results. Other investigators have reported contrary results, including a reduction in the duration of ICU stay, a decrease in the incidence of postoperative cardiac complications, reduced intraoperative wall-motion abnormalities, and a decrease in the frequency of respiratory failure and need for postoperative mechanical ventilatory support with adjuvant epidural anesthesia and analgesia.[16,129-133] These encouraging findings, along with the widespread belief that epidural analgesia is superior to analgesia provided by conventional parenteral opioids, have led to the common use of epidural analgesia both during and after major abdominal aortic surgery,[134] and many clinicians believe that epidural analgesia facilitates early extubation by reducing pain and improving pulmonary function. Epidural anesthesia has also been used as the sole anesthetic for infrarenal aortic surgery via the retroperitoneal approach[135] with a low complication rate and an extremely low incidence of postoperative respiratory failure. Despite the frequent use of low-dose intraoperative heparin, the incidence of epidural hematoma appears to be reassuringly low.[136]

The favorable results encountered with adjunct epidural analgesia and anesthesia are tempered by potentially deleterious reductions in arterial blood pressure; cardiac filling pressures; and cerebral, renal, and coronary perfusion pressures when epidural local anesthetics are used intraoperatively. The degree of hypotension is magnified if fluid and blood replacement is inadequate and vasopressors are not judicially administered. Indeed, Baron et al[18] noted a substantial increase in vasopressor requirements in patients receiving thoracic epidural anesthesia during abdominal aortic surgery. The combination of significant blood and fluid losses, together with vasodilation induced by mediators released from ischemic tissues below the level of the aortic cross-clamp, may produce profound hypotension at aortic unclamping in the presence of an epidural anesthetic-induced sympathectomy. For these reasons, some clinicians advocate the intraoperative administration, through a low thoracic or high lumbar epidural catheter, of dilute local anesthetic/opioid solutions (e.g., 0.1% bupivacaine/fentanyl [5-10 mcg/ml]) rather than higher concentrations of local anesthetics. Moreover, the primary use of epidural anesthesia and analgesia after major blood loss has occurred but before the patient awakens from GA may reduce the incidence of hypotension. If systemic blood pressure remains adequate throughout the procedure, however,

supplemental local anesthetics can be administered as the operative procedure is completed. Alternatively, epidural opioids alone can be used before incision and throughout surgery for neuraxial analgesia. These techniques provide stable hemodynamics while simultaneously ensuring satisfactory analgesia, which facilitates tracheal extubation soon after the completion of the procedure.

Mesenteric Traction Syndrome. An important element of hemodynamic management during abdominal aortic surgery is recognition of the hypotension encountered during traction on the mesentery and eventration of the bowel during aneurysm exposure, the so-called "mesenteric traction syndrome." This is typically observed soon after opening of the peritoneum and is characterized by facial flushing, decreased systemic vascular resistance (SVR), reduced MAP, increased heart rate, and increased cardiac index.[137-140] These hemodynamic changes frequently require treatment with a vasopressor such as phenylephrine, and appear to be associated with increases in plasma concentrations of 6-keto-prostaglandin $F_{1\alpha}$ (6-K-PGF$_{1\alpha}$), the stable metabolite of prostacyclin, and also thromboxane B_2.[139,140] They usually peak within 10 minutes after the start of abdominal exploration and resolve over 30 minutes. Prostacyclin appears to originate from the intestinal mucosa and/or the intestinal mesentery, since the hemodynamic and humoral changes are not seen in patients undergoing a retroperitoneal compared with a transabdominal approach to exposure of the aneurysm.[141] In addition, the phenomenon is temporally related to bowel eventration and aneurysm exposure.[139] The increases in 6-K-PGF$_{1\alpha}$ and the associated hemodynamic and cutaneous responses are completely prevented by pretreatment with the cyclooxygenase inhibitors ibuprofen and aspirin[139,140] (Fig. 17-8). Seltzer et al[138] demonstrated that plasma from nonibuprofen-treated patients was able to dilate cat mesenteric artery preparations, compared with an absent vascular response to plasma from treated patients. It is essential that this phenomenon be recognized because it is often associated with dramatic reductions in MAP that may compromise coronary perfusion. It may be more profound in hypovolemic patients or when concomitant epidural anesthesia is used, and typically requires brief treatment with a vasopressor rather than fluids. Awareness of this syndrome and its occurrence during the very early stages of the procedure facilitates prompt treatment and the avoidance of potentially dangerous decreases in blood pressure.

Pathophysiologic Events Associated with Infrarenal Aortic Cross-Clamping. The hemodynamic consequences of infrarenal aortic cross-clamping are less substantial than aortic occlusion at the level of the de-

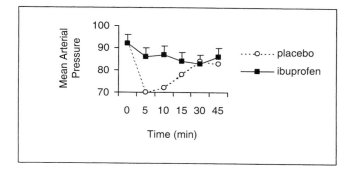

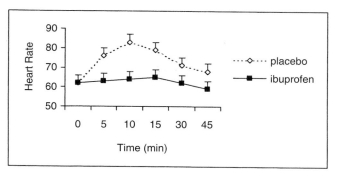

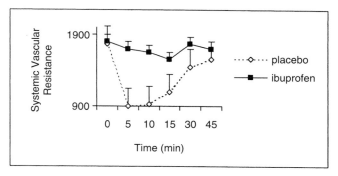

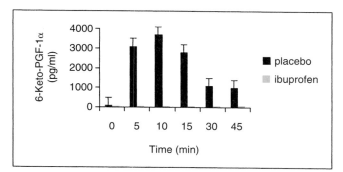

FIG. 17-8 The impact of ibuprofen pretreatment on the severity of hemodynamic changes and 6-keto-prostaglandin-1α (6-keto-PGF-1α) levels with abdominal exploration during infrarenal aortic surgery (placebo group [$n = 13$] and patients pretreated with ibuprofen [$n = 14$]). The horizontal axis represents time after exploration of the abdomen, with time zero preceding exploration. Hemodynamic changes at 5 and 10 minutes and 6-keto-PGF-1α levels at all time intervals were statistically different between groups. This study demonstrates the pathophysiologic role of prostacyclin in the mesenteric traction syndrome and the protective effect of pretreatment with the prostanoid inhibitor ibuprofen.

(From Hudson JC, Wurm WH, O'Donnell TF et al: *Anesthesiology* 72:443-449, 1990.)

scending thoracic aorta. An extensive discussion of the pathophysiology of aortic cross-clamping is presented in Chapter 14, but the essential clinical aspects of infrarenal cross-clamping are reviewed in the following discussion.

The hemodynamic changes induced by infrarenal aortic occlusion have been extensively investigated in both experimental and human studies. Unfortunately, interpretation of these investigations is limited by differences between animal and human cardiovascular responses; variations in baseline cardiac function of study subjects; and the ubiquitous use of volatile anesthetics, intravenous vasodilators, and β-adrenergic antagonists to control blood pressure after the application of the aortic cross-clamp. Thus the reported changes in vascular resistance and systemic blood pressure during human infrarenal aortic cross-clamping probably underestimate the true severity of clamping-induced events. In addition, variations in volume loading, baseline ventricular filling pressures, level of sympathetic tone,

and underlying cardiac function also influence the reported hemodynamic responses to aortic clamping. Nonetheless, the majority of clinical investigations reveal a consistent increase in SVR and MAP and a decrease in cardiac output, stroke volume, and ejection fraction.[113,142-147] There is little change in heart rate. Alterations in cardiac filling pressures are inconsistent, with some investigations suggesting no change or a modest increase in preload. In a well-conducted investigation that used radionuclide angiography and TEE to examine ventricular performance in 20 patients during infrarenal aortic cross-clamping, significant increases in MAP, meridional end-systolic wall stress, end-diastolic and end-systolic volumes, and reductions in ejection fraction were demonstrated (Table 17-4). There were significant changes in a reverse direction with release of the cross-clamp. In contrast to these findings, some investigations have observed a decrease in pulmonary artery occlusion pressure with infrarenal aortic occlusion,[142-145] while others have noted that increases in

TABLE 17-4

Hemodynamic Variables before and after Infrarenal Aortic Cross-Clamping and Unclamping

VARIABLE	PRECLAMP	AORTIC CLAMPING*	AORTIC UNCLAMPING†
Ejection fraction (%)	56	48	58
End-diastolic volume (ml)	171	225	187
End-systolic volume (ml)	85	127	94
Systolic blood pressure (mm Hg)	127	142	106
Mean arterial pressure (mm Hg)	82	91	69
LV end-systolic wall stress (10^3 dyne/cm^2)	53	67	46

Data from Harpole DH, Clements FM, Quill T et al: *Ann Surg* 209:356-362, 1989.
*Significant increase from all baseline values.
†Significant decrease from all aortic clamp values.

ventricular filling pressures are limited only to patients with underlying CAD.[143]

Despite the significant changes in cardiac function encountered with infrarenal aortic occlusion, the alterations are of modest clinical significance. They are easily treated with minor adjustments in anesthetic depth and vasodilator use and appear to be safely tolerated, even in patients with underlying ventricular dysfunction.[113] Some investigators have demonstrated myocardial ischemia in patients with underlying CAD after infrarenal aortic clamping[148] (Fig. 17-9), but others have failed to observe an increase in the incidence of intraoperative myocardial ischemia or postoperative myocardial infarction in these patients.[113,120,128]

The pathophysiologic mechanisms underlying the cardiovascular response to infrarenal aortic cross-clamping appear to be primarily related to an increase in afterload resulting from an impedance to aortic blood flow, which is manifested by an increase in systemic arterial pressure and SVR. Alterations in cardiac filling pressures depend, in part, on blood volume redistribution from distal venous capacitance beds to the proximal vasculature. This proximal redistribution effect has been well demonstrated during thoracic aortic cross-clamping (see Chapter 14), but is probably less frequent during infrarenal aortic cross-clamping because of variability in splanchnic venous tone and the preferential redistribution of blood from lower body venous capacitance beds to splanchnic vascular beds, rather than to the heart.[146] If blood volume redistribution does occur and if myocardial contractility is insufficient to accommodate these increases in preload and afterload, then ventricular function may deteriorate and filling pressures increase significantly.[146] It is also theorized that proximal arterial hypertension may be caused,

in part, by changes in cardiac output from this preload augmenting shift in blood volume. This mechanism may play a more significant role in the arterial hypertension observed with thoracic rather than with infrarenal aortic cross-clamping. In addition to these changes in aortic impedance and cardiac output, neurohumoral activation and sympathetic activation may produce increases in catecholamine, renin, and angiotensin levels that may contribute to increased vascular resistance.[146] These substances may, in conjunction with other humoral factors released from ischemic tissues below the cross-clamp, increase vascular tone in vessels proximal to the cross-clamp.

Unclamping of the infrarenal abdominal aorta is associated with hemodynamic changes that are directionally opposite to those observed with aortic clamping. Typically, modest reductions in SVR, end-diastolic and end-systolic volumes, and MAP are seen, accompanied by significant increases in cardiac output and ejection fraction.[113,142,149,150] The primary reasons for declamping hypotension include hypovolemia-induced reductions in stroke volume from pooling of blood in reperfused tissues below the level of the aortic cross-clamp, hypoxia-mediated distal arterial vasodilation, and the vasodilatory effects of ischemic metabolites and humoral mediators released from previously ischemic tissues (including endotoxin, endothelin,[151] cytokines [tumor necrosis factor, interleukin-1, interleukin-6], prostaglandins, oxygen-free radicals, and activated complement factors).[146,152-155]

A metabolic acidosis, as evidenced by increases in venous lactate levels and base deficits, is commonly observed after cross-clamp release and is presumably due to the washout of lactate and other metabolic byproducts from previously ischemic tissues below the

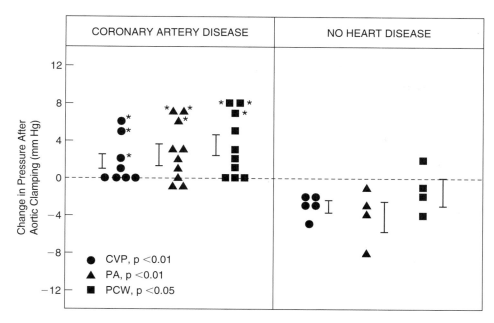

FIG. 17-9 Comparison of changes in central venous pressure *(CVP)*, pulmonary artery *(PA)* pressure, and pulmonary capillary wedge *(PCW)* pressure in patients with and without coronary artery disease during infrarenal aortic cross-clamping. Values with asterisks refer to patients who develop myocardial ischemia during infrarenal aortic cross-clamping. Significance values refer to the comparison between patients with and without heart disease.

(From Attia RR, Murphy JD, Snider M et al: *Circulation* 53:961-965, 1976.)

level of the cross-clamp.[147,156,157] Significant decreases in Sv_{O_2}[142,145] are also seen with unclamping and reflect increased oxygen extraction in ischemic tissues of the lower torso. The severity of the metabolic acidosis appears related to the duration of aortic clamping and the degree of clamp-induced increases in SVR.[156] Finally, dramatic increases in pulmonary artery pressure and pulmonary vascular resistance occur immediately after unclamping and probably represent the pulmonary vasoconstricting effects of CO_2 and ischemic metabolites, and to a lesser extent the impact of prior fluid loading and vasopressor use.[145,158]

Some data suggest that the changes induced by infrarenal aortic clamping and unclamping are less severe in patients undergoing surgery for aortoocclusive disease compared with patients having surgery for aneurysmal disease. Presumably, the presence of extensive collateral vessels allows continued perfusion of the lower extremities during the period of aortic occlusion. Thus less severe changes in SVR and blood pressure are encountered with aortic clamping and unclamping.[159-162] Other investigators, however, have failed to confirm this observation.[113,156]

In summary, infrarenal aortic cross-clamping produces modest increases in vascular resistance, arterial blood pressure, left ventricular wall stress, and, infre-

quently, ventricular filling pressures, whereas unclamping induces directionally opposite events accompanied by increases in venous lactate levels, pulmonary vascular resistance, and pulmonary artery pressures, and reductions in pH and mixed venous oxygen tensions.

Management of Infrarenal Aortic Clamping and Unclamping. The management of infrarenal aortic cross-clamping primarily involves control of the increase in SVR and arterial blood pressure. This is typically achieved with an increase in volatile anesthetic concentration, infusion of nitroglycerin or nitroprusside infusion, use of epidural local anesthetics, or the administration of β-adrenergic-receptor blocking agents such as esmolol or labetalol. Some investigators have achieved satisfactory blood pressure control and maintenance of cardiac output during the period of aortic clamping by using the phosphodiesterase inhibitor amrinone.[163] Intravenous calcium channel blockers such as nicardipine and the dopaminergic receptor agonist fenoldopam are alternative agents that may be potentially useful to maintain stable hemodynamics during the period of aortic clamping, although no clinical data from patients undergoing aortic surgery are available to confirm their usefulness as rapid-acting and safe antihypertensive agents.

It is essential to adequately replace fluid and blood losses during the period of infrarenal aortic cross-clamping. Hypotension accompanied by low ventricular filling pressures and diminished anesthetic and vasodilator requirements suggest considerable hypovolemia that, if not adequately replaced, will result in profound hypotension with release of the aortic cross-clamp. Declamping hypotension is most reliably attenuated by a combination of rapid volume infusion immediately before cross-clamp release,[147,149,150] discontinuation of vasodilators, temporary interruption of opioid infusions and volatile anesthetics in advance of clamp release, and the brief administration of vasopressors to counteract the well-recognized reduction in vascular resistance. Gradual cross-clamp release may attenuate the decrease in vascular resistance, but blood pressure almost always declines temporarily. With adequate restoration of intravascular volume, replacement of salvaged blood, and judicious vasopressor administration, blood pressure promptly returns to baseline levels. As discussed earlier, a transient increase in $Paco_2$ and lactate levels, accompanied by a decrease in pH and Svo_2, is commonly observed, but rarely requires treatment unless severe or protracted. Sodium bicarbonate administration before clamp release is advocated by some practitioners, but is neither routinely necessary nor consistently effective. With sequential unclamping of a single iliac or femoral artery during surgery for aortoocclusive disease, these hemodynamic changes are less dramatic than during aneurysm surgery, and reflect reperfusion of a smaller vascular bed (i.e., one extremity) and the effects of collateral vessels supplying infrarenal vascular beds during the period of aortic clamping.[161]

Renal Protection during Aortic Clamping. Substantial clinical data suggest that infrarenal aortic cross-clamping during abdominal aortic aneurysm surgery consistently reduces renal blood flow and glomerular filtration rate. In addition, these unfavorable changes in renal function may persist for several months after surgery.[164-169] These effects on renal function are not necessarily related to reductions in cardiac output or hypovolemia but instead appear secondary to primary alterations in renal vascular resistance. Gamulin et al[167] demonstrated a 75% increase in renal vascular resistance and a 38% decrease in renal blood flow after infrarenal aortic cross-clamping, despite an increase in cardiac output. In some instances, these reductions in renal blood flow have been correlated with a significant decrease in postoperative creatinine clearance.[169] The etiology of reduced renal blood flow is unclear, although it has long been recognized that embolization of ulcerated atheroma and/or mural thrombi occur in up to 77% of patients during infrarenal aortic reconstruction, probably during the dissection and clamping

phases.[170] In addition, renal vasoconstriction from alterations in renin-angiotensin levels, increases in sympathetic tone and concentrations of the potent endogenous vasoconstrictor endothelin,[171] and reductions in intrarenal vasodilatory prostaglandins probably also play a role in the observed deterioration in renal function after infrarenal aortic cross-clamping.[146,166] Methods to prevent these unfavorable changes in renal function during aortic surgery have included the use of low-dose dopamine,[172-173] angiotensin-converting enzyme inhibitors,[164] the dopamine receptor agonist dopexamine,[174] epidural anesthesia,[175] nifedipine,[171] furosemide,[176] and mannitol.[166,176-178] Although some of these experimental and human investigations have demonstrated increased urine output and favorable changes in renal blood flow, creatinine clearance, and glomerular filtration rate with these pharmacologic interventions, no clinically significant reduction in the incidence of postoperative renal failure has been realized. Despite the continued absence of supportive clinical data regarding the protective effect of any specific pharmacologic agent, it is common clinical practice to administer low-dose dopamine (1-3 mcg/kg/min), mannitol (0.2-0.5 g/kg), or furosemide (10-40 mg) alone or in combination before and during the period of infrarenal aortic cross-clamping.[93,128,146,179,180] Until further information becomes available regarding pharmacologic renal protection during aortic surgery, the intraoperative use of these agents seems acceptable in an attempt to improve renal blood flow and preserve tubular integrity. However, the most important and established elements of perioperative renal protection remain the preservation of intravascular volume and cardiac output, renal perfusion pressure, and oxygen delivery to the kidney.[146]

Complications. Operative mortality rates for abdominal aortic aneurysm surgery vary from 3% to 8% for elective repair and up to 68% for emergency repair of ruptured aneurysms[122,181-185] (Table 17-5). Cardiac events, including MI, CHF, and arrhythmias, are the most frequent complications after elective infrarenal aortic surgery and were the primary cause of death in two large, multicenter evaluations[122,185] (Table 17-6). An analysis of 72 articles encompassing 37,654 patients undergoing elective abdominal aortic aneurysm repair observed a 10% to 12% cardiac complication rate and a 5% to 10% risk of pulmonary complications.[183] Other important complications include hemorrhage, renal failure, and intestinal and limb ischemia.[186]

A variety of reports have delineated the risk factors for postoperative morbidity and mortality. These include advanced age, low preoperative ejection fraction, history of MI or CHF, severity of intraoperative blood loss, additional intraoperative procedures performed (especially renal revascularization), and opera-

TABLE 17-5

Complications after Elective Infrarenal Abdominal Aortic Aneurysm Repair

COMPLICATION	INCIDENCE (%)
Cardiac	10-5
Myocardial infarction	2-5
CHF	5-9
Arrhythmia	10
Pulmonary	3-8
Renal failure	5-10
Hemorrhage	1-8
Limb ischemia	3-5
Intestinal ischemia	2-3
Central nervous system	0.6-1

Data from Blankensteijn et al,[183] Johnston,[185] Diehl et al,[184] Martin et al,[188] Jarvinen et al.[186]
CHF, Congestive heart failure.

TABLE 17-6

Major Causes of Death after Elective Infrarenal Abdominal Aortic Surgery (*n* = 3786)

CAUSE OF DEATH	INCIDENCE (%)
Cardiac	40
Hemorrhage	20
Pulmonary	13
Renal	4
Ischemic extremity	6
Ischemic gut	5

Data from Galland RB: *Br J Surg* 85:633-636, 1998.

tive time.[182,184,187,188] Some data also suggest that because of a higher prevalence of diabetes and CAD, patients undergoing infrainguinal procedures have a higher risk of cardiac complications than do patients undergoing aortic procedures.[118]

RUPTURED ABDOMINAL AORTIC ANEURYSMS

In contrast to elective repair of abdominal aortic aneurysms, surgery for rupture of the abdominal aorta is a major vascular emergency that is associated with a high mortality rate. The anesthetic management of aortic rupture is especially challenging because patients are fre-

quently unstable on arrival in the operating room. The critical condition of these patients and the demanding nature of these procedures are highlighted by the observation that one fifth of patients undergoing emergency surgery for ruptured abdominal aortic aneurysms sustain an intraoperative cardiac arrest.[189]

Patients typically have sudden onset of acute, severe abdominal pain, often accompanied by syncope.[190] Because rupture frequently begins in the retroperitoneal space, severe low back or flank pain is a common initial symptom. Hypotension is seen in almost 40% of patients at initial evaluation[189] and probably accelerates the diagnosis of aortic rupture, since these patients tend to be operated on more promptly.[191] A pulsatile midepigastric mass accompanied by abdominal pain dictates the need for immediate surgery, although the classic triad of abdominal or back pain, a pulsatile mass, and shock is only present in 50% of cases.[191]

The duration of fluid resuscitation for hypotensive patients with known or suspected aortic rupture before surgery is controversial. Several studies have shown that a longer period of resuscitation before surgery improves survival, since this may reverse hypotension and restore vital organ and tissue perfusion.[192-194] This is consistent with data showing higher mortality in patients with preoperative hypotension.[189] However, data from a prospective evaluation of 598 patients with penetrating torso injuries indicate that aggressive fluid administration in hypotensive patients before corrective surgery can be associated with reduced survival and increased morbidity.[195] Presumably, fluids given before surgical control of intraabdominal bleeding may lead to disruption of an established thrombus and cause a fatal secondary hemorrhage.[195] In addition, aggressive fluid administration may lead to unfavorable dilutional changes in platelet and coagulation factor levels. Furthermore, most surgeons believe that immediate surgery with rapid control of bleeding by aortic cross-clamping is critical for survival and a favorable outcome. However, it is reasonable to proceed with judicious fluid administration while rapid diagnostic tests are performed and the patient is prepared for expeditious transport to the operating room.

When patients arrive in the operating room, they are often hypotensive, hypothermic, and potentially moribund. Some may even be receiving active resuscitation with chest compressions. Basic monitors including electrocardiography, noninvasive blood pressure, and pulse oximetry should be immediately applied. Intraarterial catheters for invasive blood pressure monitoring may be placed *only* if time and stable hemodynamics permit. At this time, priority should be given to the immediate placement of several large-bore (e.g., 14-gauge) intravenous catheters (if not already in place), because rapid fluid and blood product administration is critically important to successful intraoperative management. Central venous and pulmonary artery catheters, although helpful to guide further fluid therapy, are of secondary importance at the initial resuscitative stage, and can be placed later after anesthetic induction and after aortic clamping has reduced the immediate hemorrhage. Blood warmers and pneumatic devices that facilitate rapid transfusion are especially helpful to prevent hypothermia and correct hypovolemia. If time permits, 5 to 10 units of type-specific blood should be obtained, although unstable patients requiring immediate laparotomy may require transfusion with uncross-matched type O-negative blood because of the prohibitive time required for complete blood typing. Box 17-3 summarizes the items necessary for the appropriate intraoperative management of these patients.

Before the induction of anesthesia and while basic monitors are applied, fluid and blood replacement should continue, preferably with the assistance of additional personnel. Because intraabdominal hemorrhage may be constrained by the effects of localized thrombus formation, increased abdominal muscle tone, continued hypotension, and containment of the bleeding within the retroperitoneum,[191] the induction of anesthesia and abdominal exploration may induce precipitous and profound hypotension. Consequently, the abdomen is prepped and draped in preparation for surgical incision and before the induction of anesthesia. The choice of induction agents is largely determined by the hemodynamic status of the patient on arrival in the operating room. A moribund patient, if not already intubated, may only require a rapid-acting muscle relaxant and an amnestic agent such as scopolamine, whereas a more alert and stable patient may undergo a rapid sequence induction with reduced doses of ketamine, eto-

midate, or a combination of fentanyl and midazolam. Additional opioids, benzodiazepines, and volatile anesthetics can be added as hemodynamic stability is attained. Vasopressors such as dopamine, phenylephrine, epinephrine, or norepinephrine may be required at this time and throughout the operative period to maintain perfusion pressure while volume resuscitation is ongoing.

After incision, the aorta is manually compressed and a vascular clamp applied to either the infrarenal aorta or the supraceliac aorta at the level of the diaphragmatic hiatus (Fig. 17-10). In the latter situation, the clamp is usually repositioned to the level of the infrarenal aorta once bleeding has been controlled. Data suggest that use of intraoperative autotransfusion and rapid insertion of a simple aortic tube graft, rather than a more complex bifurcation graft, reduces operative time and improves survival.[196] It is essential for the surgeons, in their desire to rapidly control the rupture and expose the neck of the aneurysm, to avoid injury to the inferior vena cava, the renal veins, or the inferior mesenteric veins. Because of the difficulty of controlling venous hemorrhage, injury

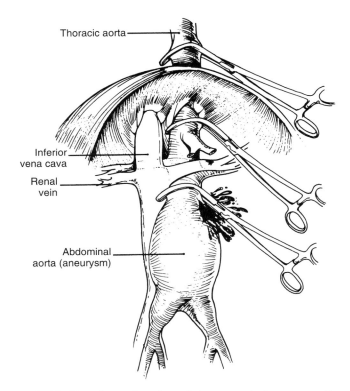

FIG. 17-10 Cross-clamping of the aorta during surgery for abdominal aortic aneurysm rupture. Once the abdomen is opened, the thoracic aorta may be clamped above the diaphragm, at a supraceliac location, or, preferably, at the level of the infrarenal aorta.

(From Haimovici H: Abdominal aortic aneurysms. In *Vascular emergencies*, New York, 1982, Appleton-Century-Crofts, pp 331-352, Figure 20.6.)

BOX 17-3
Intraoperative Preparation for Ruptured Abdominal Aortic Aneurysm Surgery

- Additional personnel
- Fluid/blood warmers
- Rapid infusion devices
- Large-bore central venous and peripheral intravenous catheters
- Pulmonary artery catheter
- Bladder catheter, temperature probe
- Forced-air upper-body warming units
- Drugs
  - Ketamine, etomidate, scopolamine, opioids, muscle relaxants
- Vasoactive infusions
  - Phenylephrine, norepinephrine, epinephrine, dopamine
  - Nitroglycerin, nitroprusside

to venous structures is a major surgical complication that significantly increases the mortality of ruptured aortic aneurysm repair.[189,196]

Thirty-day mortality from ruptured abdominal aortic aneurysms ranges from 48% to 60%, and nearly one fourth of patients die in the operating room.[189,193,197,198] Perioperative variables predictive of death include hypotension on admission (systolic blood pressure <90 mm Hg), preoperative loss of consciousness, hemoglobin level less than 10 g/dl, baseline creatinine level greater than 1.5 mg/dl, preoperative or intraoperative cardiac arrest, extent of intraoperative blood loss, and postoperative renal failure.[189,198] Halpern et al[189] established a mortality rate of 100% in hypotensive patients undergoing surgery for ruptured abdominal aortic aneurysms who had a hemoglobin level less than 10 g/dl and a history of loss of consciousness. These data highlight the importance of prompt restoration of blood volume and expeditious surgical control of aortic bleeding. Unfortunately, rupture of an abdominal aortic aneurysm remains a highly lethal event and little change in mortality has been observed over time, despite improvements in the perioperative management of these patients.

KEY POINTS

1. There is a high prevalence of CAD in patients undergoing major vascular surgery, and cardiac complications continue to be the primary cause of postoperative morbidity and mortality.

2. Epidural anesthesia and analgesia reduce hypercoagulability and thromboembolic complications after lower extremity revascularization, although their impact on the risk of postoperative cardiac events remain unresolved.

3. The main advantage of RA for CEA is the ability to accurately predict cerebral ischemia after carotid artery clamping; its impact on cardiovascular outcome is less clearly defined.

4. Upper airway obstruction after CEA is primarily due to glottic edema from venous and lymphatic obstruction, and immediate reexploration in the operating room by using local anesthesia is recommended because of the risk of complete airway obstruction with induction of GA.

5. Combined epidural and GA for abdominal aortic aneurysm surgery *may* reduce the incidence of postoperative cardiopulmonary complications, but may also aggravate intraoperative hypovolemia and hypotension.

6. The mesenteric traction syndrome is due to prostacyclin release from the intestinal mucosa and mesentery and is a common cause of vasodilation and hypotension during abdominal aortic aneurysm exposure.

7. Infrarenal aortic cross-clamping produces clinically modest increases in vascular tone, arterial blood pressure, left ventricular wall stress, and infrequently, ventricular filling pressures, whereas unclamping induces directionally opposite events accompanied by increases in venous lactate levels, pulmonary vascular resistance, and pulmonary artery pressures, and reductions in pH and mixed venous oxygen tensions.

8. Infrarenal aortic cross-clamping consistently reduces renal blood flow and glomerular filtration rate, and appears to be related to clamp-induced thromboembolic events and neurohumorally mediated increases in renal vascular resistance.

9. Despite the widespread use of low-dose dopamine and diuretics during infrarenal aortic surgery, no definitive impact of their use on the incidence of postoperative renal failure has been demonstrated, and the most important and established elements of renal protection remain the preservation of intravascular volume and cardiac output, renal perfusion pressure, and oxygen delivery to the kidney.

10. Surgery for ruptured abdominal aortic aneurysms is associated with a 50% to 60% mortality rate, and nearly one fourth of patients will experience a cardiac arrest during the intraoperative period.

KEY REFERENCES

ACC/AHA Task Force on Practice Guidelines: ACC/AHA guidelines for perioperative cardiovascular evaluation for noncardiac surgery, *Circulation* 93:1280-1317, 1996.

Allen BT, Anderson CB, Rubin BG et al: Influence of anesthetic technique on perioperative complications after carotid endarterectomy, *J Vasc Surg* 19:834-843, 1994.

Bickell WH, Wall MJ, Pepe PE et al: Immediate versus delayed fluid resuscitation for hypotensive patients with penetrating torso injuries, *N Engl J Med* 331:1105-1109, 1994.

Biller J, Feinberg WM, Castaldo JE et al: Guidelines for carotid endarterectomy: a statement for healthcare professionals from a special writing group of the stroke council, American Heart Association, *Circulation* 97:501-509, 1998.

Bode RH, Lewis KP, Zarich SW et al: Cardiac outcome after peripheral vascular surgery: comparison of general and regional anesthesia, *Anesthesiology* 84:3-13, 1996.

Cucchiara RF, Sundt TM, Michenfelder JD: Myocardial infarction in carotid endarterectomy patients anesthetized with halothane, enflurane, or isoflurane, *Anesthesiology* 69:783-784, 1988.

Gelman S: The pathophysiology of aortic cross-clamping and unclamping, *Anesthesiology* 82:1026-1060, 1995.

Harpole DH, Clements FM, Quill T et al: Right and left ventricular performance during and after abdominal aortic aneurysm repair, *Ann Surg* 209:356-362, 1989.

Hudson JC, Wurm H, O'Donnell, Jr, F et al: Ibuprofen pretreatment inhibits prostacyclin release during abdominal exploration in aortic surgery, *Anesthesiology* 72:443-449, 1990.

Johnston KW: Multicenter prospective study of nonruptured abdominal aortic aneurysm. Part II. Variables predicting morbidity and mortality, *J Vasc Surg* 9:437-447, 1989.

Mangano DT, Layug EL, Wallace A et al: Effects of atenolol on mortality and cardiovascular morbidity after noncardiac surgery. Multicenter Study of Perioperative Ischemia Research Group, *N Engl J Med* 335:1713-1720, 1996.

McCrory DC, Goldstein LB, Samsa GP et al: Predicting complications of carotid endarterectomy, *Stroke* 24:1285-1291, 1993.

Tuman KJ, McCarthy RJ, March RJ et al: Effects of epidural anesthesia and analgesia on coagulation and outcome after major vascular surgery, *Anesth Analg* 73:696-704, 1991.

References

1. Hertzer NR, Beven EG, Young JR et al: Coronary artery disease in peripheral vascular patients. A classification of 1000 coronary angiograms and results of surgical management, *Ann Surg* 199:223-233, 1984.

2. Fleisher L, Eagle K, Shaffer T et al: Perioperative and long-term mortality rates after major vascular surgery: the relationship to preoperative testing on the medicare population, *Anesth Analg* 89:849-955, 1999.

3. ACC/AHA Task Force on Practice Guidelines: ACC/AHA guidelines for perioperative cardiovascular evaluation for noncardiac surgery, *Circulation* 93:1280-1317, 1996.

4. Colombo J, O'Connor CJ, Tuman K: Perioperative hypertension and outcome, *Anesthesiol Clin North Am* 17:581-591, 1999.

5. Bove EL, Fry WJ, Gross WS et al: Hypotension and hypertension as consequence of baroreceptor dysfunction after carotid endarterectomy, *Surgery* 85:633-637, 1979.

6. Asiddao CB, Donegan JH, Witesell RC et al: Factors associated with perioperative complications during carotid endarterectomy, *Anesth Analg* 61:631-637, 1982.

7. Mangano DT, Layug EL, Wallace A et al: Effects of atenolol on mortality and cardiovascular morbidity after noncardiac surgery. Multicenter Study of Perioperative Ischemia Research Group, *N Engl J Med* 335:1713-1720, 1996.

8. Wallace A, Layug B, Tateo I et al: Prophylactic atenolol reduces postoperative myocardial ischemia, *Anesthesiology* 88:7-17, 1998.

9. Ellis JE, Drijvers G, Pedlow S et al: Premedication with oral and transdermal clonidine provides safe and efficacious postoperative sympatholysis, *Anesth Analg* 79:1133-1140, 1994.

10. Stuhmeier KD, Mainzer B, Cierpka J et al: Small, oral dose of clonidine reduces the incidence of intraoperative myocardial ischemia in patients having vascular surgery, *Anesthesiology* 85:706-712, 1996.

11. Dodds TM, Stone JG, Coromilas J et al: Prophylactic nitroglycerin infusion during noncardiac surgery does not reduce perioperative ischemia, *Anesth Analg* 76:705-713, 1993.

12. Chung F, Houston PL, Cheng DCH et al: Calcium channel blockade does not offer adequate protection from perioperative myocardial ischemia, *Anesthesiology* 69:343-347, 1988.

13. Slogoff S, Keats AS: Does chronic treatment with calcium entry blocking drugs reduce perioperative myocardial ischemia? *Anesthesiology* 68:676-680, 1988.

14. Nelson AH, Fleisher LA, Rosenbaum SH: Relationship between postoperative anemia and cardiac morbidity in high-risk vascular patients in the intensive care unit, *Crit Care Med* 21:860-866, 1993.

15. Reiz S, Balfors E, Sorenson MB et al: Coronary hemodynamic effects of general anesthesia and surgery: modification by epidural analgesia in patients with ischemic heart disease, *Reg Anesth* 7:8-20, 1982.

16. Yeager MP, Glass DD, Neff RK et al: Epidural anesthesia and analgesia in high risk surgical patients, *Anesthesiology* 66:729-735, 1987.

17. Tuman KJ, McCarthy RJ, March RJ et al: Effects of epidural anesthesia and analgesia on coagulation and outcome after major vascular surgery, *Anesth Analg* 73:696-704, 1991.

18. Baron JF, Bertrand M, Barre E et al: Combined epidural and general anesthesia versus general anesthesia for abdominal aortic surgery, *Anesthesiology* 75:611-618, 1991.

19. Christopherson R, Beattie C, Frank SM et al: Perioperative morbidity in patients randomized to epidural or general anesthesia for lower extremity vascular surgery, *Anesthesiology* 79:422-434, 1993.

20. Rosenfeld BA, Beattie C, Christopherson R et al: The effects of different anesthetic regimens on fibrinolysis and the development of postoperative arterial thrombosis, *Anesthesiology* 79:435-443, 1993.

21. Breslow MJ, Parker SD, Frank SM et al: Determinant of catecholamine and cortisol responses to lower extremity revascularization, *Anesthesiology* 79:1202-1209, 1993.

22. Rosenfeld BA, Faraday N, Campbell D et al: Hemostatic effects of stress hormone infusion, *Anesthesiology* 81:1116-1209, 1994.

23. Bode RH, Lewis KP, Zarich SW et al: Cardiac outcome after peripheral vascular surgery: comparison of general and regional anesthesia, *Anesthesiology* 84:3-13, 1996.

24. Pierce ET, Pomposelli, Jr, FB, Stanley GD et al: Anesthesia type does not influence early graft patency or limb salvage rate of lower extremity artery bypass, *J Vasc Surg* 25:226-232, 1997.

25. Berlauk J, Abrams JH, Gilmour IJ et al: Preoperative optimization of cardiovascular hemodynamics improves outcome in peripheral vascular surgery, *Ann Surg* 214:289-297, 1991.

26. Garnett RL, Macintyre A, Lindsay P et al: Perioperative ischaemia in aortic surgery: combined epidural/general anesthesia and epidural analgesia vs general anaesthesia and i.v. analgesia, *Can J Anaesth* 43:769-777, 1996.

27. Cousins MJ, Wright CJ: Graft, muscle, skin blood flow after epidural block in vascular surgical procedures, *Surg Gynecol Obstet* 133:59-64, 1971.

28. Baron HC, LaRaja RD, Rossi G et al: Continuous epidural analgesia in the heparinized vascular surgical patient: a retrospective review of 912 patients, *J Vasc Surg* 6:144-146, 1987.

29. Turnbull KW: Con: neuraxial block is useful in patients undergoing heparinization for surgery, *J Cardiothorac Vasc Anesth* 10: 961-962, 1996.

30. Rao TLK, El-Etr AA: Anticoagulation following placement of epidural and subarachnoid catheters: an evaluation of neurologic sequelae, *Anesthesiology* 55:618-620, 1981.

31. Odoom JA, Sih IL: Epidural analgesia and anticoagulant therapy: experience with one thousand cases of continuous epidurals, *Anaesthesia* 38:254-259, 1983.

32. Ellison N, Jobes DR, Schwartz AJ: Implications of anticoagulant therapy, *Int Anesthesiol Clin* 20:121-135, 1982.

33. Horlocker TT, Heit JA: Low molecular weight heparin: biochemistry, pharmacology, perioperative prophylaxis regimens, and guidelines for regional anesthetic management, *Anesth Analg* 85:874-875, 1997.

34. Onishchuk JL, Carlsson C: Epidural hematoma associated with epidural anesthesia: complications of anticoagulant therapy, *Anesthesiology* 77:1221-1223, 1992.

35. Moore WS, Barnett HJM, Beebe HG et al: Guidelines for carotid endarterectomy. A multidisciplinary consensus statement from the Ad Hoc committee, American Heart Association, *Circulation* 91:566-579, 1995.

36. Executive Committee for the Asymptomatic Carotid Atherosclerosis Study: Endarterectomy for asymptomatic carotid stenosis, *JAMA* 273:1421-1428, 1995.

37. Goldstein LB, McCrory DC, Landsman PB et al: Multicenter review of preoperative risk factors for carotid endarterectomy in patients with ipsilateral symptoms, *Stroke* 25:1116-1121, 1994.

38. Davies AH, Hayward JK, Currie I et al: Risk prediction of outcome following carotid endarterectomy, *Cardiovasc Surg* 4:338-339, 1996.

39. McCrory DC, Goldstein LB, Samsa GP et al: Predicting complications of carotid endarterectomy, *Stroke* 24:1285-1291, 1993.

40. Gur AY, Bova I, Bornstein NM: Is impaired cerebral vasomotor reactivity a predictive factor of stroke in asymptomatic patients? *Stroke* 27:2188-2190, 1996.

41. Thiel A, Zickmann B, Stertmann WA et al: Cerebrovascular carbon dioxide reactivity in carotid artery disease, *Anesthesiology* 82:655-661, 1995.

42. Yonas H, Smith HA, Durham, SR et al: Increased stroke risk predicted by compromised cerebral blood flow reactivity, *J Neurosurg* 79:483-489, 1993.

43. Whitley D, Cherry KJ: Predictive value of carotid artery stump pressures during carotid endarterectomy, *Neurosurg Clin N Am* 7:723-732, 1996.

44. Harada RN, Comerota AJ, Good GM et al: Stump pressure, electroencephalographic changes, and the contralateral carotid artery: another look at selective shunting, *Am J Surg* 170: 148-153, 1995.

45. Kwaan JH, Peterson GJ, Connolly JE: Stump pressure: an unreliable guide for shunting during carotid endarterectomy, *Arch Surg* 115:1083-1086, 1980.

46. Pruitt J: 1009 consecutive carotid endarterectomies using local anesthesia, EEG, and selective shunting with Pruitt-Inahara carotid shunt, *Contemp Surg* 23:49-53, 1983.

47. Silbert BS, Kluger R, Cronin KD et al: The processed electroencephalogram may not detect neurologic ischemia during carotid endarterectomy, *Anesthesiology* 70:356-358, 1989.

48. Kearse LA, Martin D, McPeck K et al: Computer-derived density spectral array in detection of mild analog electroencephalographic ischemic pattern changes during carotid endarterectomy, *J Neurosurg* 78:884-890, 1993.

49. Hanowell LH, Soriano S, Bennett HL: EEG power changes are more sensitive than spectral edge frequency variation for detection of cerebral ischemia during carotid artery surgery: a prospective assessment of processed EEG monitoring, *J Cardiothorac Vasc Anesth* 6:292-294, 1992.

50. Redekop G, Ferguson G: Correlation of contralateral stenosis and intraoperative electroencephalogram change with risk of stroke during carotid endarterectomy, *Neurosurgery* 30:191-194, 1992.

51. Halsey JH: Risks and benefits of shunting in carotid endarterectomy. The International Transcranial Doppler Collaborators, *Stroke* 23:1583-1587, 1992.

52. Gaunt ME, Martin PJ, Smith JL et al: Clinical relevance of intraoperative embolization detected by transcranial Doppler ultrasonography during carotid endarterectomy: a prospective study of 100 patients, *Br J Surg* 81:1435-1439, 1994.

53. Ackerstaff RGA, Jansen C, Moll FL et al: The significance of microemboli detection by means of transcranial Doppler ultrasonography monitoring in carotid endarterectomy, *J Vasc Surg* 21:963-969, 1995.

54. Samra SK, Dorje P, Zelenock GB et al: Cerebral oximetry in patients undergoing carotid endarterectomy under regional anesthesia, *Stroke* 27:49-55, 1996.

55. Cho H, Nemoto EM, Yonas H et al: Cerebral monitoring by means of oximetry and somatosensory evoked potentials during carotid endarterectomy, *J Neurosurg* 89:533-8, 1998.

56. Kuroda S, Houkin K, Abe H et al: Near-infrared monitoring of cerebral oxygenation state during carotid endarterectomy, *Surg Neurol* 45:450-458, 1996.

57. Duffy CM, Manninen PH, Chan A et al: Comparison of cerebral oximeter and evoked potential monitoring in carotid endarterectomy, *Can J Anaesth* 44:1077-1081, 1997.

58. Beese U, Langer H, Lang W et al: Comparison of near-infrared spectroscopy and somatosensory evoked potentials for the detection of cerebral ischemia during carotid endarterectomy, *Stroke* 29:2032-2037, 1998.

59. Michenfeder JD, Milde JH: Failure of prolonged hypocapnia, hypothermia, or hypertension to favorably alter acute stroke in primates, *Stroke* 8:87-91, 1977.

60. Grossi EA, Giangola G, Parish MA et al: Differences of flow rates in carotid shunts: consequences in cerebral perfusion, *Ann Vasc Surg* 19:206-216, 1994.

61. Smith JS, Roizen MF, Cahalan MK et al: Does anesthetic technique make a difference? Augmentation of systolic blood pressure during carotid endarterectomy: effects of phenylephrine versus light anesthesia and of isoflurane versus halothane on the incidence of myocardial ischemia, *Anesthesiology* 69:846-853, 1988.

62. Mutch WAC, White IWC, Donen N et al: Haemodynamic instability and myocardial ischaemia during carotid endarterectomy: a comparison of propofol and isoflurane, *Can J Anaesth* 42: 577-587, 1995.

63. Landesberg G, Erel J, Anner H et al: Perioperative myocardial ischemia in carotid endarterectomy under cervical plexus block and prophylactic nitroglycerin infusion, *J Cardiothorac Vasc Anesth* 7:259-265, 1993.

64. Gottlieb A, Satariano-Hayden P, Schoenwald P et al: The effects of carotid sinus nerve blockade on hemodynamic stability after carotid endarterectomy, *J Cardiothorac Vasc Anesth* 11:67-71, 1997.

65. Elliott BM, Collins GJ, Youkey JR et al: Intraoperative local anesthetic injection of the carotid sinus nerve, *Am J Surg* 152: 695-699, 1986.

66. Corson JD, Chang BB, Leopold PW et al: Perioperative hypertension in patients undergoing carotid endarterectomy: shorter duration under regional block anesthesia, *Circulation* 75(suppl I): 1-4, 1986.

67. Kachel R: Results of balloon angioplasty in the carotid arteries, *J Endovasc Surg* 3:22-30, 1996.

68. Allen BT, Anderson CB, Rubin BG et al: Influence of anesthetic technique on perioperative complications after carotid endarterectomy, *J Vasc Surg* 19:834-843, 1994.

69. Palmer MA: Comparison of regional and general anesthesia for carotid endarterectomy, *Am J Surg* 157:329-330, 1989.

70. Forssell C, Takolander R, Bergquist D et al: Local versus general anaesthesia in carotid surgery: a prospective randomized study, *Eur J Vasc Surg* 3:503-505, 1989.

71. Corson JD, Chang BB, Shah DM et al: The influence of anesthetic choice on carotid endarterectomy outcome, *Arch Surg* 122:807-812, 1987.

72. Muskett A, McGreevy J, Miller M: Detailed comparison of regional and general anesthesia for carotid endarterectomy, *Am J Surg* 152:691-694, 1986.

73. Davies MJ, Murrell GC, Cronin KD et al: Carotid endarterectomy under cervical plexus block: a prospective clinical audit, *Anaesth Intensive Care* 18:219-223, 1990.

74. Ombrellaro MP, Freeman MB, Stevens SL et al: Effect of anesthetic technique on cardiac morbidity following carotid artery surgery, *Am J Surg* 171:387-390, 1996.

75. Fiorani P, Sbarigia E, Speziale F et al: General anaesthesia versus cervical block and perioperative complications in carotid artery surgery, *Eur J Vasc Endovasc Surg* 13:37-42, 1997.

76. Stoneham MD, Doyle A, Knighton J et al: Prospective, randomized comparison of deep or superficial cervical plexus block for carotid endarterectomy, *Anesthesiology* 89:907-912, 1998.

77. Michenfelder JD, Sundt TM, Fode N et al: Isoflurane when compared to enflurane and halothane decreases the frequency of cerebral ischemia during carotid endarterectomy, *Anesthesiology* 67:336-340, 1987.

78. Messick JM, Casement B, Sharbrough FW et al: Correlation of regional cerebral blood flow (rCBF) with EEG changes during isoflurane anesthesia for carotid endarterectomy: critical rCBF, *Anesthesiology* 66:344-349, 1987.

79. Cucchiara RF, Sundt TM, Michenfelder JD: Myocardial infarction in carotid endarterectomy patients anesthetized with halothane, enflurane, or isoflurane, *Anesthesiology* 69:783-784, 1988.

80. Geary KJ, Ouriel K, Geary JE et al: Neurologic events following carotid endarterectomy: prediction of outcome, *Ann Vasc Surg* 7:76-82, 1993.

81. Kaufman JL, Frank D, Rhee SE et al: Feasibility and safety of 1-day postoperative hospitalization for carotid endarterectomy, *Arch Surg* 131:751-755, 1996.

82. Breen JC, Caplan LR, DeWitt LD et al: Brain edema after carotid surgery, *Neurology* 46:175-181, 1996.

83. Jorgensen LG, Schroeder TV: Defective cerebrovascular autoregulation after carotid endarterectomy, *Eur J Vasc Surg* 7:370-379, 1993.

84. Biller J, Feinberg WM, Castaldo JE et al: Guidelines for carotid endarterectomy: a statement for healthcare professionals from a special writing group of the stroke council, American Heart Association, *Circulation* 97:501-509, 1998.

85. Hughes R, McGuire G, Montanera W et al: Upper airway edema after carotid endarterectomy: the effect of steroid administration, *Anesth Analg* 84:475-478, 1997.

86. O'Sullivan JC, Wells DG, Wells GR: Difficult airway management with neck swelling after carotid endarterectomy, *Anaesth Intensive Care* 14:460-464, 1986.

87. Kunkel JM, Gomez ER, Spebar MJ et al: Wound hematomas after carotid endarterectomy, *Am J Surg* 148:844-877, 1984.

88. Isselbacher EM, Eagle KA, Desanctis RW: Diseases of the aorta. In Braunwald E, editor: *Heart disease: a textbook of cardiovascular medicine*, vol 2, ed 5, Philadelphia, 1997, WB Saunders, pp 1546-1581.

89. Sternbergh III WC, Gonze MD, Garrard CL et al: Abdominal and thoracoabdominal aortic aneurysm, *Surg Clin North Am* 78:827-843, 1998.

90. Perko MJ, Schroeder TV, Olsen PS et al: Natural history of abdominal aortic aneurysm: a survey of 63 patients treated nonoperatively, *Ann Vasc Surg* 7:113-116, 1993.

91. Vardulaki KA, Prevost TC, Walker NM et al: Growth rates and risk of rupture of abdominal aortic aneurysms, *Br J Surg* 85:1674-1680, 1998.

92. Hollier LH, Taylor LM, Ochsner J: Recommended indications for operative treatment of abdominal aortic aneurysms. Report of a subcommittee of the Joint Council of the Society for Vascular Surgery and the North American Chapter of the International Society for Cardiovascular Surgery, *J Vasc Surg* 15:1046-1056, 1992.

93. Darling III RC, Shah DM, Chang BB et al: Current status of the use of retroperitoneal approach for reconstructions of the aorta and its branches, *Ann Surg* 224:501-508, 1996.

94. Quiñones-Baldrich WJ, Garner C, Caswell D et al: Endovascular, transperitoneal, and retroperitoneal abdominal aortic aneurysm repair: results and costs, *J Vasc Surg* 30:59-67, 1999.

95. Sicard GA, Freeman MB, VanderWoude JC et al: Comparison between the transabdominal and retroperitoneal approach for reconstruction of the infrarenal abdominal aorta, *J Vasc Surg* 5:19-27, 1987.

96. Cambria RP, Brewster DC, Abbott WM et al: Transperitoneal versus retroperitoneal approach for aortic reconstruction: a randomized prospective study, *J Vasc Surg* 11:314-325, 1990.

97. Sieunarine K, Lawrence-Brown MMD, Goodman MA: Comparison of transperitoneal and retroperitoneal approaches for infrarenal aortic surgery: early and late results, *Cardiovasc Surg* 5:71-76, 1997.

98. Parodi JC, Palmaz JC, Barone HD: Transfemoral intraluminal graft implantation for abdominal aortic aneurysms, *Ann Vasc Surg* 5:491-499, 1991.

99. Moore WS, Vescera CL: Repair of abdominal aortic aneurysm by transfemoral endovascular graft placement, *Ann Surg* 220:331-341, 1994.

100. Henretta JP, Hodgson KJ, Mattos MA et al: Feasibility of endovascular repair of abdominal aortic aneurysms with local anesthesia with intravenous sedation, *J Vasc Surg* 29:793-798, 1999.

101. Cao P, Zannetti S, Parlani G et al: Epidural anesthesia reduces length of hospitalization after endoluminal abdominal aortic aneurysm repair, *J Vasc Surg* 30:651-657, 1999.

102. White GH, May J, McGahan T et al: Historic control comparison of outcome for matched groups of patients undergoing endoluminal versus open repair of abdominal aortic aneurysms, *J Vasc Surg* 23:201-212, 1996.

103. Blum U, Voshage G, Lammer J et al: Endoluminal stent-grafts for infrarenal abdominal aortic aneurysms, *N Engl J Med* 336:13-20, 1997.

104. Treharne GD, Thompson MM, Whiteley MS et al: Physiological comparison of open and endovascular aneurysm repair, *Br J Surg* 86:760-764, 1999.

105. Boyle JR, Thompson JP, Thompson MM et al: Improved respiratory function and analgesia control after endovascular AAA repair, *J Endovasc Surg* 4:62-85, 1997.

106. Edoga JK, James KV, Resnikoff M et al: Laparoscopic aortic aneurysm resection, *J Endovasc Surg* 5:335-344, 1998.

107. Valentine RJ, Duke ML, Inman MH et al: Effectiveness of pulmonary artery catheters in aortic surgery: a randomized trial, *J Vasc Surg* 27:203-212, 1998.

108. Ziegler DW, Wright JG, Choban PS et al: A prospective randomized trial of preoperative "optimization" of cardiac function in patients undergoing elective peripheral vascular surgery, *Surgery* 122:584-592, 1997.

109. Bender JS, Smith-Meek MA, Jones CE: Routine pulmonary artery catheterization does not reduce morbidity and mortality of elective vascular surgery, *Ann Surg* 226:229-237, 1997.

110. Isaacson IJ, Lowdon JD, Berry AJ et al: The value of pulmonary artery and central venous monitoring in patients undergoing abdominal aortic reconstructive surgery: a comparative study of two selected, randomized groups, *J Vasc Surg* 12:754-760, 1990.

111. Adams, Jr, JG, Clifford EJ, Henry RS et al: Selective monitoring in abdominal aortic surgery, *Am Surg* 59:559-563, 1993.

112. Joyce WP, Provan JL, Ameli FM et al: The role of central haemodynamic monitoring in abdominal aortic surgery: A prospective randomized study, *Eur J Vasc Surg* 4:633-636, 1990.

113. Harpole DH, Clements FM, Quill T et al: Right and left ventricular performance during and after abdominal aortic aneurysm repair, *Ann Surg* 209:356-362, 1989.

114. Gillepsie DL, Connelly GP, Arkoff HM et al: Left ventricular dysfunction during infrarenal abdominal aortic aneurysm repair, *Am J Surg* 168:144-147, 1994.

115. Smith JS, Cahalan MK, Benefiel DJ et al: Intraoperative detection of myocardial ischemia in high-risk patients: electrocardiography versus two-dimensional transesophageal echocardiography, *Circulation* 72:1015-1021, 1985.

116. Gewertz BL, Kremser PC, Zarins CK et al: Transesophageal echocardiographic monitoring of myocardial ischemia during vascular surgery, *J Vasc Surg* 5:607-613, 1987.

117. London MJ, Tubau JF, Wong MG et al: The "Natural History" of segmental wall motion abnormalities in patients undergoing noncardiac surgery, *Anesthesiology* 73:644-655, 1990.

118. Krupski WC, Layug EL, Reilly LM et al: Comparison of cardiac morbidity rates between aortic and infrainguinal operations: two year follow-up, *J Vasc Surg* 18:609-617, 1993.

119. Catoire P, Saada M, Liu N et al: Effect of preoperative normovolemic hemodilution on left ventricular segmental wall motion during abdominal aortic surgery, *Anesth Analg* 75:654-659, 1992.

120. Roizen MF, Beaupre PN, Alpert RA: Monitoring with two dimensional transesophageal echocardiography: comparison of myocardial function in patients undergoing supraceliac supraceliac-infraceliac or infrarenal aortic occlusion, *J Vasc Surg* 1:300-305, 1984.

121. Kelley-Patteson C, Ammar AD, Kelley H: Should the cell saver autotransfusion device be used routinely in all infrarenal abdominal aortic bypass operations? *J Vasc Surg* 18:261-265, 1993.

122. Galland RB: Mortality following elective infrarenal aortic reconstruction: a joint vascular research group study, *Br J Surg* 85:633-636, 1998.

123. Gold MS, DeCrosta D, Rizzuto C et al: The effect of lumbar epidural and general anesthesia on plasma catecholamines and hemodynamics during abdominal aortic aneurysm repair, *Anesth Analg* 78:225-230, 1994.

124. Breslow MJ, Jordan DA, Christopherson R et al: Epidural morphine decreases postoperative hypertension by attenuating sympathetic nervous system hyperactivity, *JAMA* 261:3577-3581, 1989.

125. Smeets HJ, Kievit J, Dulfer FT et al: Endocrine-metabolic response to abdominal aortic surgery: a randomized trial of general anesthesia versus general plus epidural anesthesia, *World J Surg* 17:601-607, 1993.

126. Norman JG, Fink GW: The effects of epidural anesthesia on the neuroendocrine response to major surgical stress: a randomized prospective trial, *Am Surg* 63:75-80, 1997.

127. Saada M, Catoire P, Bonnet F et al: Effect of thoracic epidural anesthesia combined with general anesthesia on segmental wall motion assessed by transesophageal echocardiography, *Anesth Analg* 75:329-335, 1992.

128. Dodds TM, Burns AK, DeRoo DB et al: Effects of anesthetic technique on myocardial wall motion abnormalities during abdominal aortic surgery, *J Cardiothorac Vasc Anesth* 11:129-136, 1997.

129. Major CP, Greer MS, Russell WL: Postoperative pulmonary complications and morbidity after abdominal aneurysmectomy: a comparison of postoperative epidural versus parental opioid analgesia, *Am Surg* 62:45-51, 1996.

130. Her Ch, Kizelshteyn G, Walker V et al: Combined epidural and general anesthesia for abdominal aortic surgery, *J Cardiothorac Anesth* 4:552-557, 1990.

131. Katz S, Reiten P, Kohl R: The use of epidural anesthesia and analgesia in aortic surgery, *Am Surg* 58:470-473, 1992.

132. Pecoraro JP, Dardik H, Mauro A et al: Epidural anesthesia as an adjunct to retroperitoneal aortic surgery, *Am J Surg* 160:187-191, 1990.

133. Gormezano G: Effect of thoracic epidural anesthesia combined with general anesthesia on segmental wall motion assessed by transesophageal echocardiography, *Anesth Analg* 75:329-347, 1992.

134. Stone WM, Larson JS, Young M et al: Early extubation after abdominal aortic reconstruction, *J Cardiothorac Vasc Anesth* 12:174-176, 1998.

135. Rosenbaum GJ, Arroyo PJ, Sivina M: Retroperitoneal approach used exclusively with epidural anesthesia for infrarenal aortic disease, *Am J Surg* 168:136-139, 1994.

136. Cunningham FO, Egan JM, Inahara T: Continuous epidural anesthesia in abdominal vascular surgery. A review of 100 consecutive cases, *Am J Surg* 139:624-627, 1980.

137. Seltzer JL, RItter DE, Starsnic MA et al: The hemodynamic response to traction on the abdominal mesentery, *Anesthesiology* 63:96-99, 1985.

138. Seltzer JL, Goldberg ME, Larijani GE: Prostacyclin mediation of vasodilation following mesenteric traction, *Anesthesiology* 68:514-518, 1988.

139. Hudson JC, Wurm H, O'Donnell, Jr, F et al: Ibuprofen pretreatment inhibits prostacyclin release during abdominal exploration in aortic surgery, *Anesthesiology* 72:443-449, 1990.

140. Gottlieb A, Skrinska VA, O'Hara P et al: The role of prostacyclin in the mesenteric traction syndrome during anesthesia for abdominal aortic reconstructive surgery, *Ann Surg* 209:363-367, 1989.

141. Hudson JC, Wurm WH, O'Donnell TF et al: Hemodynamics and prostacyclin release in the early phases of aortic surgery: comparison of transabdominal and retroperitoneal approaches, *J Vasc Surg* 7:190-198, 1988.

142. Galt SW, Bech FR, McDaniel MD et al: The effect of ibuprofen on cardiac performance during abdominal aortic cross-clamping, *J Vasc Surg* 13:876-884, 1991.

143. Gooding JM, Archie JP, McDowell H: Hemodynamic response to infrarenal aortic cross-clamping in patients with and without coronary artery disease, *Crit Care Med* 8:382-385, 1980.

144. Schuetz W, Radermacher P, Goertz A et al: Cardiac function in patients with treated hypertension during aortic aneurysm repair, *J Cardiothorac Vasc Anesth* 12:33-37, 1998.

145. Vandermeer TJ, Maini BS, Hendershott TH et al: Evaluation of right ventricular function during aortic operations, *Arch Surg* 128:582-585, 1993.

146. Gelman S: The pathophysiology of aortic cross-clamping and unclamping, *Anesthesiology* 82:1026-1060, 1995.

147. Falk JL, Rackow EC, Blumenberg R et al: Hemodynamic and metabolic effects of abdominal aortic crossclamping, *Am J Surg* 142:174-177, 1981.

148. Attia RR, Murphy JD, Snider M et al: Myocardial ischemia due to infrarenal aortic cross-clamping during aortic surgery in patients with severe coronary artery disease, *Circulation* 53:961-965, 1976.

149. Bush HL, LoGerfo FW, Weisel RD et al: Assessment of myocardial performance and optimal volume loading during elective abdominal aortic aneurysm resection, *Arch Surg* 112:1301-1306, 1977.

150. Reiz S, Peter T, Rais O: Hemodynamic and cardiometabolic effects of infrarenal aortic and common iliac artery declamping in man – an approach to optimal volume loading, *Acta Anaesthesiol Scand* 23:579-586, 1979.

151. Fukuda S, Taga K, Tanaka T et al: Relationship between tissue ischemia and venous endothelin-1 during abdominal aortic aneurysm surgery, *J Cardiothorac Vasc Anesth* 9:510-514, 1995.

152. Holmberg A, Bergqvsit D, Westman B et al: Cytokine and fibrinogen response in patients undergoing open abdominal aortic aneurysm surgery, *Eur J Vasc Endovasc Surg* 17:294-300, 1999.

153. Holzheimer RG, Gross J, Schein M: Pro- and anti-flammatory cytokine-response in abdominal aortic aneurysm repair: a clinical model of ischemia-reperfusion, *Shock* 11:305-310, 1999.

154. Swartbol P, Norgren L, Albrechtsson U et al: Biological responses differ considerably between endovascular and conventional aortic aneurysm surgery, *Eur J Vasc Endovasc Surg* 12:18-25, 1996.

155. Baigrie RJ, Lamont PM, Whiting S et al: Portal endotoxin and cytokine responses during abdominal aortic surgery, *Am J Surg* 166:248-251, 1993.

156. Whalley DG, Salevsky FC, Ryckman JV: Haemodynamic and metabolic consequences of aortic occlusion during abdominal aortic surgery, *Br J Anaesth* 70:96-98, 1993.

157. Perry MO: The hemodynamics of temporary abdominal aortic occlusion, *Ann Surg* 168:193-200, 1968.

158. Ueda N, Dohi S, Akamatsu S et al: Pulmonary arterial and right ventricular responses to prophylactic albumin administration before aortic unclamping during abdominal aortic aneurysmectomy, *Anesth Analg* 87:1020-1026, 1998.

159. Dunn E, Prager RL, Fry W et al: The effect of abdominal aortic cross-clamping on myocardial function, *J Surg Res* 22:463-468, 1977.

160. Johnston WE, Balestrieri FJ, Plonk G et al: The influence of periaortic collateral vessels on the intraoperative hemodynamic effects of acute aortic occlusion in patients with aorto-occlusive disease or abdominal aortic aneurysm, *Anesthesiology* 66:386-389, 1987.

161. Powelson JA, Maini BS, Bishop RL et al: Continuous monitoring of mixed venous oxygen saturation during aortic operations, *Crit Care Med* 20:332-336, 1992.

162. Cunningham AJ, O'Toole DP, McDonald N et al: The influence of collateral vascularisation on haemodynamic performance during abdominal aortic surgery, *Can J Anaesth* 36:44-50, 1989.

163. Dentz ME, Lubarsky DA, Smith LR et al: A comparison of amrinone with sodium nitroprusside for control of hemodynamics during infrarenal abdominal aortic surgery, *J Cardiothorac Vasc Anesth* 9:486-490, 1995.

164. Licker M, Bednarkiewicz M, Neidhart P et al: Preoperative inhibition of angiotensin-converting enzyme improves systemic and renal haemodynamic changes during aortic abdominal surgery, *Br J Anaesth* 76:632-639, 1996.

165. Colson P, Capdevilla X, Cuchet D et al: Does choice of the anesthetic influence renal function during infrarenal aortic surgery? *Anesth Analg* 74:481-485, 1992.

166. Paul MD, Mazer CD, Byrick RJ et al: Influence of mannitol and dopamine on renal function during elective infrarenal aortic clamping in man, *Am J Nephrol* 6:427-434, 1986.

167. Gamulin Z, Forster A, Morel D et al: Effects of infrarenal aortic cross-clamping on renal hemodynamics in humans, *Anesthesiology* 61:394-399, 1984.

168. Awad RW, Barham WJ, Taylor DN et al: The effect of infrarenal aortic reconstruction on glomerular filtration rate and effective renal plasma flow, *Eur J Vasc Surg* 6:362-367, 1992.

169. Welch M, Knight DG, Carr HMH et al: Influence of renal artery blood flow on renal function during aortic surgery, *Surgery* 115:46-51, 1994.

170. Thurlbeck WM, Castleman B: Atheromatous emboli to the kidneys after aortic surgery, *N Engl J Med* 257:442-447, 1957.

171. Antonucci F, Calo L, Rizzolo M et al: Nifedipine can preserve renal function in patients undergoing aortic surgery with infrarenal crossclamping, *Nephron* 74:668-673, 1996.

172. Schwartz LB, Bissell MG, Murphy M et al: Renal effects of dopamine in vascular surgical patients, *J Vasc Surg* 8:367-374, 1988.

173. Baldwin L, Henderson A, Hickman P: Effect of postoperative low-dose dopamine on renal function after elective major vascular surgery, *Ann Int Med* 120:744-747, 1994.

174. Welch M, Newstead CG, Smyth JV et al: Evaluation of dopexamine hydrochloride as a renoprotective agent during aortic surgery, *Ann Vasc Surg* 9:488-492, 1995.

175. Brinkman A, Seeling W, Wolf CE et al: Ibuprofen does not impair renal function in patients undergoing infrarenal aortic surgery with epidural anaesthesia, *Intensive Care Med* 24:322-328, 1998.

176. Hanley MJ, Davidson K: Prior mannitol and furosemide infusion in a model of ischemic acute renal failure, *Am J Physiol* 241:F556-564, 1981.

177. Abbott WM, Austen WG: The reversal of renal cortical ischemia during aortic occlusion by mannitol, *J Surg Res* 16:482-489, 1974.

178. Nicholson ML, Baker DM, Hopkinson BR et al: Randomized controlled trial of the effect of mannitol on renal reperfusion injury during aortic aneurysm surgery, *Br J Surg* 83:1230-1233, 1996.

179. McCoy D, Hargaden K, Kilfeather S et al: Neuroendocrine and haemodynamic responses to abdominal aortic cross clamp and release during high-dose opiate-oxygen-isoflurane anaesthesia, *Eur J Vasc Surg* 7:648-653, 1993.

180. Knos GB, Berry AJ, Isaacson IJ et al: Intraoperative urinary output and postoperative blood urea nitrogen and creatinine levels in patients undergoing aortic reconstructive surgery, *J Clin Anesth* 1:181-185, 1989.

181. Lawrence PF, Gazak C, Bhirangi L et al: The epidemiology of surgically repaired aneurysms in the United States, *J Vasc Surg* 30:632-640, 1999.

182. Huber TS, Harward TRS, Flynn TC et al: Operative mortality rates after elective infrarenal aortic reconstructions, *J Vasc Surg* 22:287-294, 1995.

183. Blankensteijn JD, Lindenburg FP, Van Der Graaf Y et al: Influence of study design on reported mortality and morbidity rates after abdominal aortic aneurysm repair, *Br J Surg* 85:1624-1630, 1998.

184. Diehl JT, Cali RF, Hertzer NR et al: Complications of abdominal aortic reconstruction. An analysis of perioperative risk factors in 557 patients, *Ann Surg* 197:49-56, 1983.

185. Johnston KW: Multicenter prospective study of nonruptured abdominal aortic aneurysm. Part II. Variables predicting morbidity and mortality, *J Vasc Surg* 9:437-447, 1989.

186. Jarvinen O, Laurikka J, Sisto T et al: Intestinal ischemia following surgery for aorto-iliac disease, *VASA* 25:148-155, 1996.

187. Calligaro KD, Azurin DJ, Dougherty MJ et al: Pulmonary risk factors of elective abdominal aortic surgery, *J Vasc Surg* 18:914-921, 1993.

188. Martin LF, Atnip RG, Holmes PA et al: Prediction of postoperative complications after elective aortic surgery using stepwise logistic regression analysis, *Am Surg* 60:163-168, 1994.

189. Halpern VJ, Kline RG, D'Angelo AJ et al: Factors that affect the survival rate of patients with ruptured abdominal aortic aneurysms, *J Vasc Surg* 26:939-948, 1997.

190. Eldrup-Jorgensen J, Hawkins RE, Bredenberg CE: Abdominal vascular catastrophes, *Surg Clin North Am* 77:1305-1320, 1997.

191. Brimacombe J, Berry A: A review of anaesthesia for ruptured abdominal aortic aneurysm with special emphasis on preclamping fluid resuscitation, *Anaesth Intensive Care* 21:311-323, 1993.

192. Katz SG, Kohl RD: Ruptured abdominal aortic aneurysms. A community experience, *Arch Surg* 129:285-290, 1994.

193. Farooq MM, Freischlag JA, Seabrook GR et al: Effect of the duration of symptoms, transport time, and length of emergency room stay on morbidity and mortality in patients with ruptured abdominal aortic aneurysms, *Surgery* 119:9-14, 1996.

194. Martin RS, Edwards, Jr, WH, Jenkins JM et al: Ruptured abdominal aortic aneurysms: a 25-year experience and analysis of recent cases, *Am Surg* 54:539-543, 1988.

195. Bickell WH, Wall MJ, Pepe PE et al: Immediate versus delayed fluid resuscitation for hypotensive patients with penetrating torso injuries, *N Engl J Med* 331:1105-1109, 1994.

196. Marty-Ané CH, Alric P, Picot MC et al: Ruptured abdominal aortic aneurysm: influence of intraoperative management on surgical outcome, *J Vasc Surg* 22:780-786, 1995.

197. Johnston KW: Ruptured abdominal aortic aneurysm: six-year follow-up results of a multicenter prospective study, *J Vasc Surg* 19:888-900, 1994.

198. Sasaki S, Sakuma M, Samejima M et al: Ruptured abdominal aortic aneurysms: analysis of factors influencing surgical results in 184 patients, *J Cardiovasc Surg* 40:401-405, 1999.

CHAPTER 18

Trauma

Victor C. Baum, M.D.

OUTLINE

Patients with traumatic cardiac injury are often cared for by noncardiac anesthesiologists. Patients who sustain cardiac injury and require emergent or urgent surgery often require noncardiac surgery, and so are not strictly within the purview of cardiac anesthesiologists. Many cardiac injuries can be repaired emergently without the use of cardiopulmonary bypass. In addition, there can be sequelae of cardiac injury, which persist for some time. This chapter addresses the patient with cardiac trauma who requires repair of either cardiac or noncardiac injuries. Injuries to major extracardiac, intrathoracic vascular structures are discussed in greater detail in Chapter 14. Issues specific to children are not covered.

EPIDEMIOLOGY AND PROGNOSIS

Cardiac trauma is classically separated into blunt and penetrating trauma. There is, in fact, adequate overlap in clinical injuries, to make this division somewhat artificial and of limited use. The true incidence of cardiac trauma is not currently known, which is somewhat surprising. An incidence varying between 16% and 76% in cases of blunt trauma is often quoted.[1,2] Using clinical criteria, more recent studies estimate the incidence of

cardiac injury following blunt trauma at approximately 13%.[3-7] The incidence of blunt cardiac injuries actually requiring treatment is probably much less, and is reported as 2.6% to 4.5%.[8]

Why the widely varying estimates? There are several readily apparent reasons for these discrepancies. Patient populations are identified from the emergency room, intensive care unit, or at autopsy. Different populations not only have different incidences of organ injury, but also different degrees of severity of organ injury and subsequent cardiac sequelae. There is no currently accepted "gold standard" to diagnose cardiac injury, particularly subtle blunt injury. There is not always a differentiation of abnormalities found on a diagnostic test versus clinically important injury,[3,9] and different studies do not agree on what constitutes "clinically important." Even when a specified laboratory test is used to diagnose cardiac injury, a commonly accepted threshold criterion may be lacking. For example, the minimum level of the cardiac isoenzyme of creatine kinase (CK-MB) used to make a diagnosis of cardiac injury has been variously defined as any, 2% of total CK, or 4% of total CK. Even criteria for that staid old diagnostic test, the electrocardiogram (ECG), are nonconsistent. Some studies accept sinus tachycardia alone as a diagnostic finding.[8] This lack of widely accepted diagnostic criteria makes the development of screening and treatment paradigms problematic. Again, this is particularly true for blunt cardiac injury (commonly referred to as *BCI*– and previously known as *cardiac contusion*).

The distribution of penetrating trauma has changed over the years. In the United States the incidence of stabbings is decreasing in "favor" of gunshot wounds that carry increased morbidity and mortality.[10] Unfortunately, this epidemiologic shift is also being found in other countries.[11]

Penetrating cardiac injury is accompanied by relatively high mortality, varying from 5% to 30%. Mortality remains at approximately 30% for gunshot wounds and 10% for stabbings, even if the patient arrives alive to the emergency room, although there is a range in reported series. A nonsinus rhythm on arrival in the emergency room or a cardiac arrest in the emergency room significantly decreases projected survival of patients with penetrating cardiac trauma.[10,12,13] The effect of tamponade on survival is unclear.[10,11,14,15]

Cardiac injury frequently does not occur in isolation, and may be encountered in patients requiring emergency repair of other traumatic injury. Patients with identified cardiac injury may have unsuspected noncardiac injury. Blunt trauma causing cardiac injury includes an average of 2.3 to 3.4 organ systems injured per patient.[5,16,17] The more critically ill the patient, the more likely he or she is to have cardiac injury. Approximately 44% of patients with penetrating cardiac trauma also have major noncardiac injury, and the leading cause of death in these patients in the past has been unsuspected noncardiac trauma.[18] Presumably, with increased diagnostic ability such as the availability of computed tomography scans to the trauma patient, the incidence of overlooked noncardiac trauma has decreased.

From the opposite perspective, cardiac injuries are the most frequently overlooked injuries in patients with fatal trauma.[19] Again, the increased availability of diagnostic tools such as echocardiography to the trauma patient has presumably decreased this incidence.

Risk factors and appropriate triage and observation of hemodynamically stable patients with cardiac injury remain issues of intense discussion, speculation, and research. Sequelae of cardiac injury may not become apparent for days to weeks, and may have anesthetic implications. Delayed sequelae include intracardiac shunts and fistulae, valve lesions, ventricular aneurysm, retained foreign body, postpericardiotomy syndrome, hemopericardium, constrictive pericarditis, and coronary thrombosis. It has also been suggested that some survivors of penetrating cardiac trauma have psychologic sequelae and complain of long-term symptoms and disability in the absence of demonstrable cardiac impairment.[20]

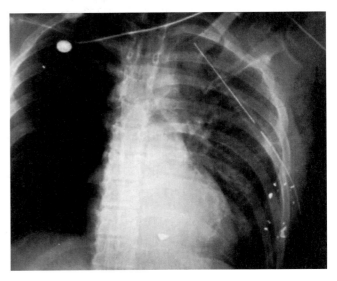

FIG. 18-1 While driving her car, this young woman was shot by a deranged sniper. She was treated for a hemopneumothorax. After penetrating the left ventricle, a large bullet fragment lodged in the interventricular septum. The left ventricular myocardium sealed the cardiac entrance wound.

(From Baum VC, Drinkwater DC: *Semin Anesthesiol* 3:210, 1989.)

Penetrating Cardiac Trauma

The most common sources of penetrating cardiac trauma are knives, ice picks, gunshot wounds, and rib or sternal fractures. Gunshot wounds tend to be large and cause blood loss and hypovolemia. Other penetrating cardiac injury is associated with hemopericardium 80% to 90% of the time. Thus, on occasion, there may be significant intracardiac injury in the absence of a hemopericardium.[21] The muscular left ventricular free wall, and to a lesser degree the right ventricular free wall, may seal off after penetration by a foreign object (Fig. 18-1). Atrial tears spontaneously seal infrequently.

The anterior right ventricle is the most commonly injured cardiac structure. Sites of injury are shown in Fig. 18-2. Multiple-chamber injury carries high mortality.[10] The ability of penetrating missiles to deflect off tissue planes and bony surfaces is well known, and cardiac injury may not be apparent from inspection of the surface entry site.

Blunt Cardiac Trauma

Blunt cardiac trauma (BCT) produces an array of cardiac injuries that can involve the myocardium, the cardiac

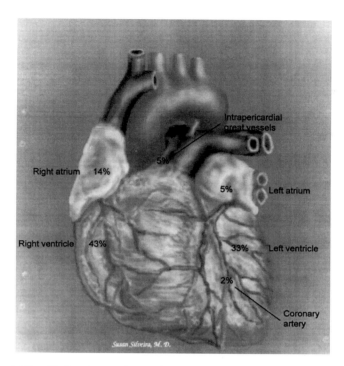

FIG. 18-2 Approximate location of penetrating cardiac trauma.

(From Baum VC: *J Cardiothorac Vasc Anesth* 14:73, 2000.)

valves, the coronary vessels, and the pericardium. The most common sequela is myocardial contusion, which is also the most problematic in terms of diagnosis and treatment. The ready availability of transesophageal echocardiography (TEE) in the emergency room may alter the historical distribution of injury because the right ventricle can be more fully evaluated.[22,23]

Although onset can be delayed, complications of blunt cardiac trauma are usually apparent within 12 hours of hospital admission.[6] Complications in otherwise asymptomatic patients admitted to monitored hospital beds are exceedingly rare.[24] Abnormal myocardial function as a result of blunt trauma resolves by several weeks after injury, as shown by a variety of imaging techniques.[22]

The mechanism of cardiac dysfunction following blunt trauma remains unclear. Although some studies implicate ischemia from disrupted coronary flow,[25-27] other animal studies exclude ischemia as a cause of myocardial dysfunction in the absence of gross coronary artery disruption.[28-31] Certainly, left ventricular dysfunction can be the consequence of right ventricular dysfunction within the constraints of the closed pericardium.[32] The most common complication of blunt cardiac injury is arrhythmias.[8] It is suggested that contusion causes reentrant arrhythmias around electrically silent zones.[33] A variety of animal studies implicate con-

comitant hypovolemia in worsening the prognosis of BCT.[34] This mirrors clinical experience.[17] Blunt injury can be associated with valve injury in up to 9% of cases (aortic > mitral > tricuspid), but these series have significant selection bias, so that the true incidence is almost certainly lower.

DIAGNOSIS

Readily accepted, reliable, and widely available diagnostic criteria for the diagnosis of clinically significant BCT remain elusive. The history and physical examination are often inadequate. The injury may have been unwitnessed and thoracic injury unappreciated. Preexisting cardiac disease confounds diagnostic tests such as the ECG. Pulsus paradoxus from hemopericardium may not be detected if only an automated blood pressure cuff is used. The neck needs to be examined for jugular venous distension, particularly when there is systemic hypotension, and for an inspiratory *increase* in distension (Kussmaul's sign). Muffled heart sounds or a pericardial friction rub is difficult to hear in a noisy emergency room. In addition to the general difficulties of making a diagnosis of traumatic cardiac injury by history and physical examination, it is particularly difficult in the elderly patient if cardiac injury is superimposed on a substrate of preexisting chronic cardiac disease. Treatment of preexisting disease, such as with β-adrenergic antagonists, may complicate matters by blunting the heart's ability to respond appropriately to injury.

A variety of diagnostic tests are available to diagnose or confirm the diagnosis of cardiac trauma. These tests are discussed in detail in the following sections, and the relative advantages and disadvantages of them are summarized in Table 18-1.

Chest Radiography

Widely available and relatively easily interpreted, chest radiographs have the limitation that cardiac injury is only inferred, and cardiac injury, even significant cardiac injury, can be radiologically silent early after injury. Anteroposterior and lateral radiographs can confirm the intracardiac location of radiopaque foreign bodies such as bullet fragments. The likelihood of cardiac injury is greater if there is evidence of additional major thoracic injury, such as hemothorax, first-rib fracture, or intrathoracic free air from bronchial or esophageal rupture. The pericardium is poorly compliant and will not stretch acutely, even with a hemodynamically significant hemopericardium. The cardiac silhouette is often normal with acute valve insufficiency. The mediastinum can be widened with aortic disruption; however, mediastinal widening is a nonspecific finding. Mediastinal bleeding following blunt trauma is due to nonaortic

TABLE 18-1
Advantages and Disadvantages of Diagnostic Tests for Cardiac Trauma

TEST	ADVANTAGES	DISADVANTAGES
Chest radiography	1. Identifies radiopaque foreign body 2. Readily available equipment and expertise 3. Inexpensive	1. Cardiac injury is only inferable, not directly shown 2. Cardiac silhouette acutely normal, even with hemodynamically significant hemopericardium or cardiac injury
Electrocardiography	1. Readily available equipment and expertise 2. Inexpensive	1. Findings may be due to hemodynamically insignificant acute trauma or may be due to preexisting abnormality 2. Abnormalities may not develop for 12-24 hr after injury 3. Findings nonspecific and can be found with noncardiac shock, hypovolemia, or hypotension
Echocardiography	1. Precisely defines myocardial, valvular, and pericardial disorders and their severity 2. TEE allows better examination of the right ventricle 3. TEE allows simultaneous evaluation of descending aorta	1. Expertise may not be immediately available
Cardiac enzymes	1. Troponins T and I are cardiac specific	1. Delay to process sample in laboratory 2. CK-MB not completely cardiac specific, especially with major noncardiac injury 3. Correlation of blood level with severity of cardiac injury unclear
Radionuclide scans		1. Poor correlation with hemodynamic instability or death 2. Specialized equipment and expertise may not be immediately available 3. Expensive

CK-MB, Cardiac isoenzyme of creatine kinase; *TEE,* transesophageal echocardiography.

injury in up to 80% of patients. In addition, approximately 5% of patients with an aortic tear have no mediastinal widening on chest radiographs.

Electrocardiography

As with the chest radiograph, the ECG is readily available and relatively easy to interpret. ECG findings are, however, nonspecific and may be associated with clinically unimportant cardiac injury.[35] The ECG can be affected by preexisting cardiac conditions.[36] ECG findings may develop 12 to 24 hours after injury.

A wide variety of ECG abnormalities are found in up to 30% of patients with significant blunt cardiac injury. These abnormalities include ischemic changes, bundle-branch or fascicular block, atrial or ventricular extrasystoles, atrioventricular block, and prolonged QT interval. ECG changes may mimic those of an acute myocardial infarction. In this context, QT prolongation with ST changes suggest myocardial injury. Electrical alternans, alternating height of the R wave with each beat, suggests pericardial injury.

Unfortunately, there is poor correlation between abnormalities of the ECG and abnormalities of cardiac function or the degree of cardiac injury as indicated by other modalities.[37] In addition, hypovolemia, hypotension, or shock of any cause can produce many of these same electrocardiographic findings.

The importance of the ECG in evaluating cardiac trauma patients has undergone a role reversal in recent years. After early enthusiasm, its importance was downgraded because of the limitations delineated earlier. However, it is now viewed as the most important emergency room screening test by a recent consensus panel[38] and others.[39] The ECG on admission to the emergency room correlates with the development of cardiac complications with a sensitivity of 96%, but with lower specificity (47%) as discussed earlier.[3,24] Almost all arrhythmias resolve spontaneously and do not degenerate into hemodynamically unstable rhythms. The uncommon late rhythm abnormalities that develop after a normal admission ECG only rarely require treatment.[5,24] A hemodynamically stable patient with a normal admission ECG is not likely to have blunt cardiac injury that requires treatment. Neither further diagnostic evaluation nor admission to a monitored hospital bed is warranted.[9,38,40] Patients with an abnormal admission ECG are admitted to a monitored bed.[38]

Echocardiography

Echocardiography provides evidence of blunt cardiac injury by imaging hemopericardium, valvular or vascular disruption, anterior myocardial dysfunction, or sequelae of penetrating injury. Echocardiographic evidence of myocardial injury includes decreased regional wall motion and end-systolic wall thickness, regionally increased end-diastolic wall thickness, focal increases in intensity, and focal echolucency consistent with an intramural hematoma.[30,41]

Emergency department physicians performed a limited echocardiographic examination in a nonrandomized retrospective review of patients with penetrating trauma for the sole purpose of determining the presence or absence of hemopericardium. Survival in the echocardiogram group was 100% versus 57% in the nonechocardiogram group, the time to diagnosis was shortened by 30 minutes, and there were no false-negative studies.[42] This study was limited because it was retrospective and nonrandomized. Very critically ill patients, for example, may have been excluded. Thourani et al[13] reported that surgeon-performed cardiac ultrasound successfully identified all cases of hemopericardium.

About 25% of patients with an abnormal echocardiogram develop cardiac problems requiring treatment in contrast to only 1% to 3% of patients with normal echocardiograms (sensitivity of 99%).[43,44] Echocardiography is very useful in delineating the cause of cardiac dysfunction: hemopericardium versus right ventricular contusion, for example.[44]

The earliest echocardiographic studies used the transthoracic approach. More recent studies demonstrate increased utility with TEE without increasing complications. Transthoracic images were suboptimal in 62% of patients in one study of cardiac trauma. TEE was successfully performed in 131 of 134 patients but was not performed in 3 patients with coexisting laryngeal or cervical spine trauma.[45] TEE is particularly good for imaging the right ventricle (because of the near field artifact seen with the transthoracic approach),[23] diagnosing traumatic injury to the interatrial septum,[46] and evaluating trauma patients for aortic disruption. It is equally sensitive as angiography for the diagnosis of major aortic injury, and is somewhat more sensitive for

demonstrating minor injury.[47] TEE is not as useful for imaging the aortic arch and its main branches. A negative TEE study result does not exclude significant intrathoracic vascular injury in this region.

Increased use of echocardiography probably decreases the incidence of unsuspected late complications of cardiac injury.[48,49] A consensus panel (of trauma surgeons), however, recommended use of echocardiography only for patients with hemodynamic instability.[38]

Cardiac Enzymes

Direct injury to the myocardium is probably best reflected by the liberation of myocardial enzymes or other proteins into the blood. CK-MB is more sensitive than ECG for indicating cardiac contusion. CK-MB is not elevated in patients with an abnormal ECG but with a normal echocardiogram.[50] Only 40% of patients with elevated CK-MB have an abnormal echocardiogram.[22] Although ECG abnormalities are more common in patients with elevated CK-MB,[51] CK-MB is neither sensitive nor specific for identifying patients who develop significant arrhythmias.[52] A markedly elevated CK-MB ($\geq$200 U/L) is nearly 100% specific (i.e., all patients with CK-MB $\geq$200 U/L develop cardiac complications) but identifies only 38% of patients who develop cardiac complications.[3]

CK-MB lacks cardiac specificity in the setting of major trauma because of extensive traumatic injury to noncardiac muscle. For this reason, determination of CK-MB levels has been replaced by measurement of other, more specific cardiac enzymes.[53-55] Serum troponin-T is used for the diagnosis of traumatic and ischemic cardiac injury,[54,55] with the ability to do qualitative bedside testing.[55] In one prospective study of patients with blunt injury there was significant overlap of troponin-T levels in the contusion and noncontusion groups (0.04-2.2 versus 0.04-4.08 μg/L), and there was no correlation of troponin-T level and left ventricular ejection fraction.[54] This series, however, did not include patients with cardiogenic shock, which is often apparent by other methods.

Serial measures of another myocardium-specific enzyme, troponin-I, has also been proposed as a specific marker of blunt cardiac injury. Troponin-I elevation mirrored cardiac injury in an animal study, with greater injury causing a more prolonged release of the enzyme.[56] A cutoff of 3.5 ng/ml in a clinical study provided no overlap of the cardiac injury and no injury groups (as defined by echocardiography).[53] Unfortunately, this study followed serial measures over 3 days and did not report the time to peak troponin-I. This test is of limited clinical utility if the time to peak troponin-I is delayed. Currently, neither CK-MB nor troponin levels are thought to be predictive of cardiac complications from BCI.[57]

Radionuclide Imaging

Radionuclide imaging techniques are less useful than other currently available techniques for a variety of reasons. Thallium imaging of hypoperfused myocardium is insensitive, and injured myocardium may be acutely hyperemic. Technetium imaging is also relatively insensitive.[58] First-pass or gated scans have been used to evaluate cardiac function after injury,[4,35,37,58,59] but the results of radionuclide scans do not correlate with myocardial injury, hemodynamic stability, or death.[8] One study reported improved specificity compared with CK-MB levels,[60] but with pronounced shortcomings. Evaluation of wall motion is difficult with an intraventricular conduction delay. Inferences of clinical severity are difficult to make. Most abnormal scans either normalize or markedly improve within several weeks. Finally, this technique is expensive and requires specialized equipment and expertise. Radionuclide imaging is of limited additional value with the availability of echocardiography.[38]

In an effort to synthesize the large amount of confusing and sometimes conflicting data concerning the variety of diagnostic tests available, Maenza et al[8] performed a metaanalysis of 2210 patients in 25 prospective studies of blunt trauma (their paper has the apt subtitle *"ending myocardial confusion"*). Abnormal ECG or abnormal CK-MB in the emergency room, but not radionuclide scans, correlated with clinically significant injury or complications that required treatment. Although abnormal echocardiograms also correlated with serious injury, the data were skewed by a single study. The most common complication was arrhythmias. There were inadequate additional complications to allow valid statistical analysis if arrhythmias were excluded. The conclusions were similar if an additional 2471 patients reported in 16 retrospective studies were included in the analysis.

SPECIFIC INJURIES
Cardiac Contusion

Myocardial abnormalities associated with blunt injury spans a spectrum from epicardial petichiae to transmural injury. Patients with myocardial contusion have precordial pain, angina unresponsive to nitrates, or arrhythmias. Traumatic myocardial injury is histologically similar to infarction, with healing by scarring. The only significant difference is a graded transition from infarcted tissue to normal tissue, and a sharp demarcation with traumatic injury. Extensive necrosis can cause generalized cardiomegaly with heart failure or late myocardial rupture. Focal injury can cause late true or false aneurysms. *Cardiac concussion* and *commotio cordis* are old terms used to describe cardiac injury without histologic changes. Although prolonged hypovolemia is capable of inducing myocardial hibernation, there is currently no information ascribing functional deficits from traumatic injury to current concepts of cellular level myocardial dysfunction.

The anterior right ventricle is particularly susceptible to blunt injury. Excessive "delta-down," and an excessive inspiratory decrease in systemic arterial blood pressure during positive-pressure ventilation are consistent with right ventricular contusion.

Posttrauma aneurysms are generally better tolerated than postinfarction aneurysms of a similar size. Trauma patients tend to be younger and have normal coronaries and healthier unaffected myocardium than do patients with ischemia-related aneurysms. Posttrauma aneurysms serve as a nidus for thrombus formation and arrhythmogenesis. Emboli and arrhythmias can occur late after injury. Other late sequelae of aneurysms include suppurative pericarditis, postpericardiotomy syndrome, and constrictive pericarditis.

Tricuspid and Mitral Insufficiency

An otherwise normal heart generally tolerates acute tricuspid insufficiency, which may not become clinically apparent for months or years. Tricuspid insufficiency can negatively impact cardiac output in the setting of significant myocardial injury.[61] In contrast, the patient with acute traumatic mitral insufficiency is usually quite ill. This is partly due to the increased energy needed to disrupt the posterior mitral valve, increasing the likelihood of associated myocardial injury.

Acute mitral insufficiency has different symptoms from chronic mitral insufficiency. Large v (or c) waves may be may be present on pulmonary artery occlusion (wedge) pressure tracings. Typical systolic murmurs of mitral insufficiency may be absent in the hypovolemic patient until intravascular volume is restored. Acute mitral insufficiency can cause pulmonary hypertension and pulmonary edema. This is reflected on the chest radiograph as pulmonary edema and Kerley B lines. The cardiac silhouette may be normal early after injury. Cardiomegaly develops later with dilation of the left ventricle, left atrium, right atrium, and superior vena cava. Similarly, the ECG is normal or has only nonspecific ST-T wave changes early after injury. Left ventricular hypertrophy (mitral insufficiency), incomplete right bundle-branch block, or minimal right ventricular hypertrophy (tricuspid insufficiency) develop as late sequelae.

Aortic Insufficiency

Acute aortic insufficiency is poorly tolerated and is worse than acute mitral insufficiency because of the deleterious effect on left ventricular wall tension (proportional to systolic pressure and ventricular radius). The volume-overloaded ventricle of aortic insufficiency must eject its entire stroke volume into the higher pressure aorta, as opposed to the situation in mitral insufficiency, in which wall tension is decreased by ejecting volume into the lower pressure left atrium. Left ventricular wall stress is markedly elevated with acute valve insufficiency because left ventricular hypertrophy takes time to develop and to lower wall tension. Pulmonary edema and pulmonary hypertension rapidly ensue. The initial chest radiograph may be normal. Rapid equilibration of left ventricular and aortic pressures in mid-diastole soften the first heart sound, in contrast to the normal sound heard in chronic aortic insufficiency.

Ventricular Septal Defect

Unlike the typical perimembranous location of the common congenital ventricular septal defect (VSD), the traumatic VSD occurs anywhere along the entire ventricular septum, but is usually within the muscular septum (Fig. 18-3). The murmur is maximal at the lower left sternal border or the apex, depending on the location of the VSD. The chest radiograph acutely shows increased pulmonary blood flow without cardiomegaly. The ECG is normal early after injury. If a pulmonary artery catheter has been placed, the diagnosis can be confirmed by measuring oxygen saturation in both the right atrium and the pulmonary artery and demonstrating a greater

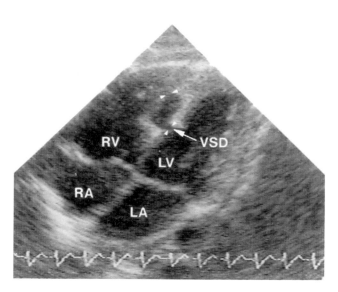

FIG. 18-3 Transthoracic echocardiogram of a traumatic ventricular septal defect *(VSD)* in a 5-year-old child. The *arrowheads* identify the entry points into the right and left ventricles. The midmuscular position and serpiginous pathway through the interventricular septum differentiate it from the typical perimembranous congenital VSD. *LA,* Left atrium; *LV,* left ventricle; *RA,* right atrium; *RV,* right ventricle.

(From Bromberg BI, Mazziotti MV, Canter CE et al: *J Pediatr* 128: 540, 1996.)

oxygen saturation in the pulmonary artery. Posttraumatic VSD is more common after penetrating injury, but the diagnosis is often delayed.

Atrial Septal Defect

The atrial septum is protected from penetrating trauma by the sternum. Traumatic atrial septal defects are therefore less common than traumatic VSDs. Easily overlooked on physical examination, atrial septal defects are readily apparent with echocardiography. The right ventricle and pulmonary artery eventually dilate from chronic volume overload.

Cardiac Rupture

Autopsy series, with their built-in selection bias, indicate cardiac rupture as the most common finding after cardiac trauma.[62] The diagnosis of cardiac rupture can be obscured or delayed in the setting of major noncardiac trauma and in the absence of newer imaging techniques in the emergency room. An older series of atrial tears demonstrated a delay of greater than 1 hour in making the diagnosis in 16 of 24 cases, despite hypotension and either elevated central venous pressure or distended neck veins in all 24 patients.[63]

Rupture of cardiac structures, in order of decreasing incidence, is right ventricle, left ventricle, right atrium, left atrium, interventricular septum, interatrial septum and aortic valve, mitral valve and tricuspid valve, and pulmonary valve.[62] It is important to note that these data are from an autopsy series and clinical studies may yield different results.

Rupture of a ventricle is often rapidly fatal in the field. One study demonstrated only 29 of 59 patients with ventricular rupture had vital signs present during admission to the emergency room.[64] Another series reported a 76% overall mortality, with a 52% mortality among patients who arrived at the emergency room with vital signs.[16] Survival after a stab wound is better than survival after a gunshot wound.[65] Survival is associated with less than 5 minutes of cardiopulmonary resuscitation in the field and with a return of organized electrical activity.[65] The patient who is alive during admission to the emergency room most likely has an atrial tear or coronary laceration as the bleeding source rather than ventricular rupture.

Pericardial Injury

A torn or disrupted pericardium predisposes the patient to the risk of herniation and potential strangulation of the left atrial appendage. In extreme cases, the entire heart may herniate through the defect. Pericardial lacerations may spontaneously seal by clot or overlying fat.

Hemopericardium

Pericardial tamponade is the most common finding in patients arriving at the hospital after penetrating cardiac injury.[13] The classic findings of tamponade from hemopericardium may be absent with concomitant hypovolemia. The classic Beck's triad (of distended neck veins, muffled heart sounds, and hypotension) is found in only 10% of trauma patients with tamponade,[15] and Kussmaul's pulses (an abnormal inspiratory increase in jugular venous distension) may only become apparent with anesthetic-mediated hypotension. Tamponade may compress coronary vessels in patients whose coronary flow is already diminished from hypotension and whose myocardial demands are increased due to tachycardia.

The pericardium is poorly compliant. Tamponade physiology can be acutely relieved by removal of only 40 to 50 ml of blood from the pericardial space. Poor pericardial distensibility causes the cardiac silhouette to appear normal on the chest radiograph despite hemodynamically significant collections of pericardial fluid. Intrapericardial blood may clot yielding increased chance of false-positive and false-negative needle pericardiocenteses. The incidence of false-negative aspirations is as high as 23%. A successful pericardiocentesis, however, temporarily relieves the tamponade and stabilizes the patient.[66] The availability of echocardiography for diagnosis and needle guidance decreases the concerns about needle pericardiocentesis for diagnosis, and improves the reliability of the procedure as a therapeutic technique. One large American trauma center reported that their surgeon-performed cardiac ultrasound correctly identified all cases of traumatic hemopericardium. This resulted in 100% survival for these patients and virtually eliminated the need for diagnostic and therapeutic needle pericardiocenteses in the emergency room.[13]

Coronary Artery Injury

Both blunt and penetrating trauma can cause disruption of coronary vessels. Coronary arteries are injured in about 2% of patients with penetrating trauma. Coronary artery dissection has also been reported after blunt injury. Coronary artery injury causes hemopericardium and tamponade, and leads to myocardial ischemia and possible fistula formation. The prognosis for patients with traumatic coronary thrombosis is better than that for patients with nontraumatic myocardial infarctions. This is probably because of the generally better condition, younger population, and lack of additional coronary artery involvement in trauma patients.

Great Vessel Injury

Approximately 5% of penetrating cardiac injuries affect the intrapericardial great vessels. The most common aortic injury after blunt trauma is disruption, which most commonly (90%-95%) occurs just distal to the left subclavian artery, where the aorta is anchored by the ligamentum arteriosus to the pulmonary artery. Tears in the ascending aorta are noted in 5% of surgical patients but in 25% of autopsy patients. Tears in the ascending aorta are located immediately above the aortic annulus at the typical location for spontaneous aortic dissections. The sinuses of Valsalva, the coronary arteries, and the aortic valve are rarely involved with tears of the ascending aorta, in contrast to nontraumatic dissection of the ascending aorta. Aortic tears are particularly uncommon in children. Hemodynamic instability is unlikely due to the isolated nature of these aortic dissections and, if present, suggests an additional site of injury.

Traumatic injury can cause hemorrhage, false aneurysms, arteriovenous fistulae, or thrombosis, which occurs from partial disruption of the vascular wall by the blast effect from gunshot wounds. Systemic arterial bleeding into the pleural space is not tamponaded by the lung, even during positive-pressure ventilation. Arterial, venous, or capillary bleeding into the pericardial space can cause tamponade, as can arterial bleeding into the mediastinum that is in close proximity to the pericardium. Disruption of the pulmonary veins from traumatic injury to the pulmonary hilum can cause fatal air embolism.

Fistulae

Fistula formation is usually a sequela of penetrating trauma, but can also be caused by blunt trauma. Fistulae are arteriovenous or arteriocameral (to a chamber of the heart). The left anterior descending coronary artery and its first diagonal branch are most commonly involved. Internal mammary right ventricular fistulae and a fistulous connection of the aorta and pulmonary artery can also occur.[67] Arteriocameral fistulae occur in decreasing incidence involving the right atrium and right ventricle, left ventricle, and left atrium. The two types of fistulae are distinguished by their murmur. The murmur of an arteriocameral fistula is continuous and louder during diastole, whereas the murmur of an arteriovenous fistula is louder during systole. Fistulae can potentially cause coronary steal and create an endocarditis risk.

Retained Foreign Body

The myocardium, particularly the thick left ventricle, can spontaneously seal itself after the entry of a foreign body (see Fig. 18-1). A retained foreign object is of particular danger on the left side of the heart because of the risk of systemic embolization. It is often medically unnecessary to remove foreign bodies, despite the significant long-term psychologic burden.[20]

SURGERY

Penetrating trauma is more likely to cause injury requiring emergency surgery than is blunt trauma because of the greater likelihood of injury to mediastinal and abdominal organs. This is true even if surface entry wounds appear innocuous. The approach for managing hemodynamically unstable traumatic cardiac injury is institutionally specific. Most clinicians advocate exploration in the operating room, rather than in the emergency room, because of the immediate availability of the full range of equipment, instruments, and expertise. While emergency room thoracotomy is life saving on rare occasions, it should not be considered routine. Thoracotomy in the emergency room is associated with poor survival: 14% overall, 8% in patients who arrive without vital signs, and only 2% in patients who lack vital signs in the field or on emergency room admission.[68] The sole survivor in this series (representing the 2%) was neurologically devastated. Other surgical series present similar results: Survival is best for patients not in shock, but is near zero for patients without vital signs in the field.[69] Lateral thoracotomy provides poor exposure to the anterior heart, which is more likely to be injured, provides more difficult access for cannulation should cardiopulmonary bypass be required, and does not allow for extension to a laparotomy incision for repair of multiple abdominal injuries.

Other clinicians, however, support the use of the lateral thoracotomy in the emergency room. Arsenio et al[10] reviewed their results of lateral thoracotomies for penetrating cardiac trauma at a large U.S. urban trauma center. Emergency thoracotomy was associated with a higher mortality rate than was operating room thoracotomy (86% vs. 27%), reflecting the high acuity of these patients. The need for cardiopulmonary bypass for definitive repair was identified as a significant incremental mortality risk for patients who had a thoracotomy in the emergency room. The clinical suspicion of tamponade did not affect mortality. Although these authors argue forcefully for emergency department thoracotomy, their data are solely descriptive and do not support the conclusion that emergency room thoracotomy improves outcome. Emergency thoracotomy is indicated for pulmonary vein disruption with entrainment of air and air embolism. The hilum is clamped and the left ventricle and ascending aorta de-aired.

The threat of tamponade takes precedence when prioritizing the surgical approach. A small vertical subxiphoid incision performed with local anesthesia relieves tamponade from a hemothorax and improves blood pressure to allow for transfer to the operating room for definitive treatment. A vertical subxiphoid incision can be extended for median sternotomy. This midline incision can also be extended caudad for abdominal exploration. The need for emergent operative repair of cardiac or great vessel injury is weighed against the consequences of delaying treatment for additional noncardiac injuries, such as an epidural hematoma. Traumatic tears of the ascending aorta are emergently repaired simultaneously with other emergent surgery (e.g., craniotomy or laparotomy). Aortic cross-clamping during repair of a traumatic dissection of the descending aorta has significant physiologic consequences, particularly in the setting of additional myocardial injury. Bypassing the clamped section of the aorta with either a Gott shunt or partial bypass with a centrifugal (Biomedicus) pump lessens the impact of aortic cross-clamping on the left ventricle.

Most causes of traumatic hemopericardium can be repaired without cardiopulmonary bypass and systemic heparinization. Most cardiac lacerations can be repaired with a single deep mattress suture without cardiopulmonary bypass, and larger, stellate injuries can be transiently controlled with brief inflow occlusion that allows visualization during repair.[18] Emergency cardiopulmonary bypass is always anticipated and occasionally required. The groins are prepped for every patient who sustains cardiac trauma in case femoral bypass is required. Disruption of a proximal coronary artery requires repair with coronary artery bypass grafting. Posterior disruptions of the atria or ventricles and disruption of the intrapericardial inferior vena cava require repair with cardiopulmonary bypass. Surgical repair can often be delayed for valve disruption, fistulae, or VSDs until the patient is hemodynamically stable.

INTRAOPERATIVE MANAGEMENT AND ANESTHESIA

Optimal fluid management of the cardiac trauma patient is complicated by acute or ongoing blood loss and myocardial injury, which limits the heart's ability to accommodate (iatrogenic) hypervolemia.[17] Intravenous fluid administered shortly after injury is required to augment cardiac filling during hypovolemia,[5] but patients with myocardial injury can rapidly decompensate with overzealous fluid administration. Concurrent hypovolemia can worsen cardiac injury,[34] and intravascular fluid alone may not adequately restore cardiac function in the presence of significant cardiac injury.[32]

Trauma patients can have suspected or unsuspected injuries that cause disruption of major vessels draining to the superior or the inferior vena cava. Large-bore intravenous catheters placed in both an upper and a lower extremity minimize unsuspected extravasation of fluids from the vascular space. An autotransfusion apparatus should be available because blood loss from cardiac disruption or associated lesions can be massive.

There are no current recommendations for placement of vascular pressure-monitoring catheters, either central venous or pulmonary arterial. The decision regarding monitors is a balance between the benefit of the added information versus the potential risks and time required to place these catheters. A large-bore central venous catheter, used initially for volume resuscitation, can later be used for monitoring or for inserting a pulmonary artery catheter. Preoperative echocardiography can now serve to identify patients who would particularly benefit from central venous or pulmonary arterial pressure measurement.

Intraoperative morbidity of the cardiac trauma patient requiring emergency surgery varies between 0%[4] and 58%.[39] Unfortunately, relatively little has been written about specific anesthetic management or implications. Most data on intraoperative morbidity and mortality are in surgical trauma literature.* Many studies combine emergent surgery with surgery several weeks after injury. Discussion regarding specific anesthetic techniques is lacking or ambiguous, including anesthesia-related morbidity. One example is a critical review of patients with cardiac contusion requiring emergent noncardiac surgery that reported no intraoperative morbidity despite the occurrence of anesthesia-related morbidity upon later review.[71]

A large series of patients with blunt chest trauma requiring emergent surgery demonstrated a significantly higher mortality rate in patients with cardiac injury (5% vs. 57%), but the authors attributed the findings to noncardiac causes.[59] Flancbaum et al[39] reported no intraoperative mortality in a series of severely injured patients during emergent noncardiac surgery; however, 11 of 19 required perioperative inotropic support, 90% had an abnormal admission ECG, and 9 of 19 were in shock on admission. Intraoperative hypotension and arrhythmias are common,[5,59,72] with varying frequency and severity among reports. Eisenach,[72] for example, reported a low incidence of intraoperative arrhythmias requiring therapy (3/43) among patients with blunt cardiac injury requiring surgery, but a significant incidence of hypotension (10/43).[72] Hemodynamic instability is particularly common during induction of general anesthesia.[71]

Studies critically evaluating specific induction techniques are lacking. Techniques that cause minimal vasodilatory and myocardial depressant effects are preferable for hemodynamic stability. The availability of intraoperative echocardiography provides valuable feedback regarding the effects of various anesthetic techniques on volume and contractility.

General anesthesia with positive pressure ventilation impairs venous return and inhibits the patient's ability to mount a hemodynamic response to incipient tamponade, potentially precipitating cardiac decompensation with hemopericardium. Patients with significant tamponade can have difficulty lying flat. Ketamine and intravascular fluid are traditionally recommended for

this situation. Ketamine maintains cardiac inotropy and venous tone to maximize preload. Ketamine's sympathomimetic actions are indirect and require endogenous catecholamines. Ketamine's direct myocardial depressant effects predominate in patients with chronic heart failure whose endogenous catecholamines are depleted, and in patients receiving β-blockers. Spontaneous ventilation is maintained when possible. Calhoon et al[16] provided anecdotal information on the care of patients with cardiac rupture and tamponade (and, by extension, traumatic tamponade in general). This group relieved tamponade by means of a small subxiphoid window under local anesthesia, as described earlier. The only death in their series involved a patient with suspected tamponade, taken directly to the operating room without the benefit of the subxiphoid incision to relieve the tamponade before induction of general anesthesia.

No anesthesia-related intraoperative complications in cardiac trauma patients have been reported for surgery performed longer than 1 month after injury.[72] This is consistent with a variety of radionuclide and echocardiographic studies that demonstrate return of normal cardiac function after 1 month.[22,37]

Patients with cardiac injury generally have a good prognosis if their injury is not associated with other major noncardiac injuries. Low perioperative hemodynamic mortality or major morbidity is particularly associated with patients who arrive at the hospital with stable hemodynamics and a normal ECG. Such patients undergo general anesthesia with low risk and complications are easily managed.

PATIENTS WITH UNDERLYING HEART DISEASE AND NONCARDIAC TRAUMA

Exclusion of cardiac injury in patients with preexisting, chronic heart disease who have multiorgan trauma may be difficult. Diagnostic test results are often unclear. Electrocardiographic abnormalities (arrhythmias, ischemic changes, or nonspecific ST-T changes) can be preexisting or indicative of acute cardiac injury. Cardiomegaly (chest radiograph), contractile dysfunction, or valve insufficiency (echocardiography) can also be preexisting or indicative of acute cardiac injury. A good history from the patient, family, or primary physician is paramount for elucidating the acute versus chronic nature of cardiac abnormalities.

Intraoperative management of the noncardiac trauma patient is affected by preexisting heart disease. Chronic cardiovascular medications alter the stress response. Heart rate does not increase in response to hypovolemia in the patient taking β-blockers. Medications with a long half-life exhibit their effects hours after injury. Fluid management is challenging for patients with significant blood loss and poor underlying cardiac function. Chronic cardiac abnormalities are often less significant than similar acute changes caused by traumatic

---

*References 3-5, 22, 39, 40, 44, 50, 52, 70.

injury, as discussed earlier. Patients suffering acute cardiac injury are presumed to benefit from invasive arterial and pulmonary arterial pressure monitoring, despite the lack of outcome data. Intraoperative TEE evaluates baseline cardiac function, volume status, and hemodynamic changes.

KEY POINTS

1. The incidence of cardiac injury with blunt thoracic trauma is between 16% and 76%. However, the incidence of blunt cardiac injuries actually requiring treatment is only 2.6% to 4.5%.
2. Cardiac injuries caused by penetrating injury can also occur with blunt trauma.
3. All diagnostic tests have limitations. Transthoracic and transesophogeal echocardiography can rapidly detect many life-threatening injuries.
4. The benefit of thoracotomy performed in the emergency department is minimal at best for patients without vital signs in the field.
5. Blunt cardiac injury with myocardial dysfunction can occur simultaneously with massive blood loss requiring rapid fluid replacement. The shift from compensated to uncompensated cardiac function after myocardial injury can be rapid if fluid is aggressively replaced.
6. Repair of cardiac injury can often be delayed, and penetrating injury can often be managed without cardiopulmonary bypass.
7. If unassociated with other major noncardiac injuries, patients with cardiac injury generally have a good prognosis with low perioperative hemodynamic mortality or major morbidity. Patients undergo general anesthesia with minimal risk and complications are easily managed.

KEY REFERENCES

Eisenach JC, Nugent M, Miller FA et al: Echocardiographic evaluation of patients with blunt chest injury: correlation with perioperative hypotension, *Anesthesiology* 64:364-366, 1986.

Frazee RC, Mucha, Jr, P, Farnell MB et al: Objective evaluation of blunt cardiac trauma, *J Trauma* 26:510-519, 1986.

Lorenz HP, Steinmetz B, Lieberman J et al: Emergency thoracotomy: survival correlates with physiologic status, *J Trauma* 32:780-785, 1992.

Maenza RL, Seaberg D, D'Amico F: A meta-analysis of blunt cardiac trauma: ending myocardial confusion, *Am J Emerg Med* 14:237-241, 1996.

Pasquale M, Fabian TC: Practice management guidelines for trauma from the Eastern Association for the Surgery of Trauma, *J Trauma* 44:941-956, 1998.

Shears LL, Hill RC, Timberlake GA et al: Myocardial performance after contusion with concurrent hypovolemia, *Ann Thorac Surg* 55:834-837, 1993.

Thourani VH, Feliciano DV, Cooper WA et al: Penetrating cardiac trauma at an urban trauma center: a 22-year perspective, *Am Surg* 65:811-816, 1999.

References

1. Leinoff HD: Direct nonpenetrating injuries to the heart, *Ann Intern Med* 14:653-666, 1940.
2. Sigler LH: Traumatic injury to the heart: incidence of its occurrence in 42 cases of severe accidental bodily injury, *Am Heart J* 30:459-478, 1945.
3. Healey MA, Brown R, Fleiszer D: Blunt cardiac injury: is this diagnosis necessary? *J Trauma* 137-146, 1990.
4. Fabian TC, Mangiante EC, Patterson CR et al: Myocardial contusion in blunt trauma: clinical characteristics, means of diagnosis, and implications for patient management, *J Trauma* 28:50-57, 1988.
5. Snow N, Richardson JD, Flint, Jr, LM: Myocardial contusion: implications for patients with multiple traumatic injuries, *Surgery* 92:744-749, 1982.
6. Baxter BT, Moore EE, Moore FA et al: A plea for sensible management of myocardial contusion, *Am J Surg* 158:557-561, 1989.
7. Torres-Mirabal P, Gruenberg JC, Brown RS et al: Spectrum of myocardial contusion, *Am Surg* 48:383-392, 1982.
8. Maenza RL, Seaberg D, D'Amico F: A meta-analysis of blunt cardiac trauma: ending myocardial confusion, *Am J Emerg Med* 14:237-241, 1996.
9. Gunnar WP, Martin M, Smith RF et al: The utility of cardiac evaluation in the hemodynamically stable patient with suspected myocardial contusion, *Am Surg* 57:373-377, 1991.
10. Asensio JA, Berne JD, Demetriades D et al: One hundred five penetrating cardiac injuries: a 2-year prospective evaluation, *J Trauma* 44:1073-1082, 1998.
11. Campbell NC, Thomson SR, Muckart DJ et al: Review of 1198 cases of penetrating cardiac trauma, *Br J Surg* 84:1737-1740, 1997.
12. Marshall WG, Bell JL, Kouchoukos NT: Penetrating cardiac trauma, *J Trauma* 24:147-149, 1984.
13. Thourani VH, Feliciano DV, Cooper WA et al: Penetrating cardiac trauma at an urban trauma center: a 22-year perspective, *Am Surg* 65:811-816, 1999.
14. Moreno C, Moore EE, Majure JA et al: Pericardial tamponade: a critical determinant for survival following penetrating cardiac wounds, *J Trauma* 26:821-825, 1986.

15. Demetriades D, van der Veen BW: Penetrating injuries of the heart: experience over two years in South Africa, *J Trauma* 23:1034-1041, 1983.

16. Calhoon JH, Hoffmann TH, Trinkle JK et al: Management of blunt rupture of the heart, *J Trauma* 26:495-502, 1986.

17. Jones JW, Hewitt RL, Drapanas T: Cardiac contusion: a capricious syndrome, *Ann Surg* 181:567-574, 1975.

18. Trinkle JK: Penetrating heart wounds: difficulty in evaluating clinical series, *Ann Thorac Surg* 38:181-182, 1984.

19. Liedtke AJ, DeMuth WEJ: Nonpenetrating cardiac injuries: a collective review, *Am Heart J* 86:687-697, 1973.

20. Abbott JA, Cousineau M, Cheitlin M: Late sequelae of penetrating cardiac wounds, *J Thorac Cardiovasc Surg* 75:510-518, 1978.

21. Pasteuning WH, Wonnink-de Jonge WF, Van Berge Henegouwen DP et al: Acquired ventricular septal defect and mitral insufficiency without pericardial effusion after stab wound to the chest, *J Am Soc Echocardiogr* 11:483-486, 1998.

22. Frazee RC, Mucha P, Jr., Farnell MB et al: Objective evaluation of blunt cardiac trauma, *J Trauma* 26:510-519, 1986.

23. Weiss RL, Brier JA, O'Connor W et al: The usefulness of transesophageal echocardiography in diagnosing cardiac contusions, *Chest* 109:73-77, 1996.

24. Wisner DH, Reed WH, Riddick RS: Suspected myocardial contusion. Triage and indications for monitoring, *Ann Surg* 212:82-86, 1990.

25. O'Connor C: Chest trauma: the role of transesophageal echocardiography, *J Clin Anesth* 8:605-613, 1996.

26. Liedtke AJ, Allen RP, Nellis SH: Effects of blunt cardiac trauma on coronary vasomotion, perfusion, myocardial mechanics, and metabolism, *J Trauma* 20:777-785, 1980.

27. Baxter BT, Moore EE, Synhorst DP et al: Graded experimental myocardial contusion: impact on cardiac rhythm, coronary artery flow, ventricular function, and myocardial contusion, *J Trauma* 28:1411-1417, 1988.

28. Doty DB, Anderson AE, Rose EF et al: Cardiac trauma: clinical and experimental correlations of myocardial contusion, *Ann Surg* 180:452-460, 1974.

29. Utley JR, Doty DB, Collins JC et al: Cardiac output, coronary flow, ventricular fibrillation and survival following varying degrees of myocardial contusion, *J Surg Res* 20:539-543, 1976.

30. Pandian NG, Skorton DJ, Doty DB et al: Immediate diagnosis of acute myocardial contusion by two-dimensional echocardiography: studies in a canine model of blunt chest trauma, *J Am Coll Cardiol* 2:488-496, 1983.

31. Pu Q, Mazoit X, Cao LS et al: Effect of lignocaine in myocardial contusion: an experiment on rabbit isolated heart, *Br J Pharmacol* 118:1072-1078, 1996.

32. Diebel LN, Tagett MG, Wilson RF: Right ventricular response after myocardial contusion and hemorrhagic shock, *Surgery* 114:788-793, 1993.

33. Robert E, de La Coussaye J, Aya AG et al: Mechanisms of ventricular arrhythmias induced by myocardial contusion: a high-resolution mapping study in left ventricular rabbit heart, *Anesthesiology* 92:1132-1143, 2000.

34. Shears LL, Hill RC, Timberlake GA et al: Myocardial performance after contusion with concurrent hypovolemia, *Ann Thorac Surg* 55:834-837, 1993.

35. McLean RF, Devitt JH, McLellan BA et al: Significance of myocardial contusion following blunt chest trauma, *J Trauma* 33:240-243, 1992.

36. Berk BA: ECG findings in nonpenetrating chest trauma: a review, *J Emerg Med* 5:209-215, 1987.

37. Harley JP, Mena I, Narahara KA et al: Traumatic myocardial dysfunction, *J Thorac Cardiovasc Surg* 87:386-393, 1984.

38. Pasquale M, Fabian TC: Practice management guidelines for trauma from the Eastern Association for the Surgery of Trauma, *J Trauma* 44:941-956, 1998.

39. Flancbaum L, Wright J, Siegel JH: Emergency surgery in patients with posttraumatic myocardial contusion, *J Trauma* 26:795-803, 1986.

40. Norton MJ, Stanford GG, Weigelt JA: Early detection of myocardial contusion and its complications in patients with blunt trauma, *Am J Surg* 160:577-581, 1990.

41. Skorton DJ, Collins SM, Nichols J et al: Quantitative texture analysis in two-dimensional echocardiography: application to the diagnosis of experimental myocardial contusion, *Circulation* 68:217-223, 1983.

42. Plummer D, Brunette D, Asinger R et al: Emergency department echocardiography improves outcome in penetrating cardiac injury, *Ann Emerg Med* 21:709-712, 1992.

43. Reif J, Justice JL, Olsen WR et al: Selective monitoring of patients with suspected blunt cardiac injury, *Ann Thorac Surg* 50:530-533, 1990.

44. Karalis DG, Victor MF, Davis GA et al: The role of echocardiography in blunt chest trauma: a transthoracic and transesophageal echocardiographic study, *J Trauma* 36:53-58, 1994.

45. Mollod M, Felner JM: Transesophageal echocardiography in the evaluation of cardiothoracic trauma, *Am Heart J* 132:841-849, 1995.

46. Kennedy NJ, Ireland MA, McConaghy PM: Transesophageal echocardiographic examination of a patient with venacaval and pericardial tears after blunt chest trauma, *Br J Anaesth* 75:495-497, 1995.

47. Goarin J, Cluzel P, Gosgnach M et al: Evaluation of transesophageal echocardiography for diagnosis of traumatic aortic injury, *Anesthesiology* 93:1373-1377, 2000.

48. Clements F: The role of transesophageal echocardiography in patients with cardiac trauma, *Anesth Analg* 77:1089-1090, 1993.

49. Porembka DT, Johnson DJI, Holt BD et al: Penetrating cardiac trauma: a perioperative role for transesophageal echocardiography, *Anesth Analg* 77:1275-1277, 1993.

50. Hiatt JR, Yeatman LA, Child JS: The value of echocardiography in blunt chest trauma, *J Trauma* 28:914-922, 1988.

51. Kettunen P: Cardiac damage after blunt chest trauma, diagnosed using CK-MB enzyme and electrocardiogram, *Int J Cardiol* 6:355-374, 1984.

52. Fabian TC, Cicala RS, Croce MA: A prospective evaluation of myocardial contusion: correlation of significant arrhythmias and cardiac output with CPK-MB measurements, *J Trauma* 31:653-659, 1991.

53. Adams JE III, Davila-Roman VG, Bessey PQ et al: Improved detection of cardiac contusion, *Am Heart J* 131:308-312, 1996.

54. Ferjani M, Droc G, Dreux S et al: Circulating cardiac troponin T in myocardial contusion, *Chest* 111:427-433, 1997.

55. Helm M, Hauke J, Lampl L: Diagnostic value of troponin T as a biochemical marker of myocardial contusion, *Anesthesiology* 89(Abstract):A467, 1998.

56. Okubo N, Hombrouck C, Fornes P et al: Cardiac troponin I and myocardial contusion in the rabbit, *Anesthesiology* 93:811-817, 2000.

57. Mattox KL, Flint LM, Carrico CJ et al: Blunt cardiac injury, *J Trauma* 33:649-650, 1992.

58. Fenner JE, Knopp R, Lee B: The use of gated radionuclide angiography in the diagnosis of cardiac contusion, *Ann Emerg Med* 13:688-694, 1984.

59. Devitt JH, McLean RF, McLellan BA: Perioperative cardio-vascular complications associated with blunt thoracic trauma, *Can J Anaesth* 40:197-200, 1993.

60. Sutherland GR, Driedger AA, Holliday RL et al: Frequency of myocardial injury after blunt chest trauma as evaluated by radionuclide angiography, *Am J Cardiol* 52:1099-1103, 1983.

61. Kantor G, Devitt JH: Blunt cardiac injury and intraoperative hypoxaemia, *Can J Anaesth* 40:515-517, 1993.

62. Parmley LF, Manion WC, Mattingly TW: Nonpenetrating traumatic injury of the heart, *Circulation* 18:371-396, 1958.

63. Patton AS, Guyton SW, Lawson DW et al: Treatment of severe atrial injuries, *Am J Surg* 141:465-471, 1981.

64. Fulda G, Brathwaite CE, Rodriguez A et al: Blunt traumatic rupture of the heart and pericardium: a ten-year experience (1979-1989), *J Trauma* 31:167-172, 1991.

65. Ivatury RR, Rohman M, Steichen FM et al: Penetrating cardiac injuries: twenty-year experience, *Am Surg* 53:310-317, 1987.

66. Trinkle JK, Toon RS, Franz JL et al: Affairs of the wounded heart: penetrating cardiac wounds, *J Trauma* 19:467-472, 1979.

67. Blackwell RA, Symbas PN: Delayed traumatic aorto-pulmonary artery fistula, *J Trauma* 44:212-213, 1998.

68. Millham FH, Grindlinger GA: Survival determinants in patients undergoing emergency room thoracotomy for penetrating chest injury, *J Trauma* 34:332-336, 1993.

69. Lorenz HP, Steinmetz B, Lieberman J et al: Emergency thoracotomy: survival correlates with physiologic status, *J Trauma* 32:780-785, 1992.

70. Kron IL, Cox PM: Cardiac injury after chest trauma, *Crit Care Med* 11:524-526, 1993.

71. Baum V: Anesthetic complications during emergency noncardiac surgery in patients with documented cardiac contusions, *J Cardiothorac Vasc Anesth* 5:57-60, 1991.

72. Eisenach JC, Nugent M, Miller FA et al: Echocardiographic evaluation of patients with blunt chest injury: correlation with perioperative hypotension, *Anesthesiology* 64:364-366, 1986.

CHAPTER 19
Neurosurgery

W. Andrew Kofke, M.D.

OUTLINE

Neural function is essential to human existence. Thus loss of any neural element in the course of a critical illness represents a major loss to a given individual. Neurons or supporting elements may be lost in a small, virtually unnoticeable manner or by widespread selective neuronal loss or tissue infarction. Because neural function is the essence of acceptable survival from criti-

cal illness, it is crucial for perioperative management of the cardiac patient to consider neural viability and the impact and interactions of cardiac diseases and therapy on the nervous system.

There are numerous clinical scenarios wherein a surgical patient with cardiac problems may have symptoms of a neurologic illness. In a general sense, these scenarios often involve cerebral ischemia, trauma, or neuroexcitation. The potential progression to brain death usually includes a period of decreased cerebral perfusion pressure (CPP), usually because of elevated intracranial pressure (ICP). Cerebral blood flow (CBF) is sufficiently compromised to produce permanent neuronal loss and whole brain death. A variety of distinct, yet interrelated, biochemical pathways play a major role in this process, which ultimately leads to neuronal death.

The patient with cardiac disease is subject to a variety of cardiovascular perturbations because of normal and disordered neurocardiac interactions and the cardiovascular effects of neurosurgical therapies. This chapter reviews many of these issues as they relate to specific neurologic problems and neurosurgical procedures.

INTRACRANIAL HYPERTENSION
Pathophysiology Relevant to the Cardiovascular System

The brain, spinal cord, cerebrospinal fluid (CSF), and blood are encased in the protecting but noncompliant skull and vertebral canal, constituting a nearly incompressible system (Fig. 19-1). In a totally incompressible system, pressure would rise linearly with increased volume. The capacitance of the system is thought to be provided by the intervertebral spaces. Once this capacitance is exhausted, the ICP increases dramatically with increased intracranial volume.

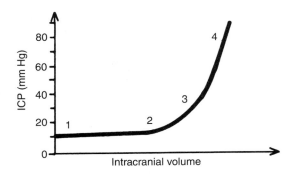

FIG. 19-1 Intracranial compliance: an idealized depiction of the intracranial volume-pressure relationship. During initial spatial compensation (between points *1* and *2*), intracranial pressure (*ICP*) increases slightly. At point *2*, compliance is reduced, and further volume additions elicit progressive ICP elevation. When ICP is already high (point *3*), even small increases in the intracranial volume will result in marked intracranial hypertension (between points *3* and *4*). In this circumstance, anesthetic agents and techniques altering cerebral blood volume will markedly change ICP.

(From Shapiro HM: Neurosurgical anesthesia and introcranial hypertension. In Miller RD, editor: *Anesthesia*, New York, 1981, Churchill Livingston.)

Based on the following relation:

$$CBF = (MAP-ICP)/CVR$$

where

$$MAP = mean\ arterial\ pressure$$
$$CVR = cerebral\ vascular\ resistance,$$

the concern is raised, mathematically, that increasing ICP is associated with decrements in CBF. However, the effect of increasing ICP on CBF is not straightforward. MAP may increase with ICP elevations,[1] and CVR compensates for decreasing CPP (increasing cerebral blood volume [CBV]) to maintain CBF until maximal vasodilatation occurs.[2,3] Maximal changes in CVR occur at CPP less than or equal to 50 mm Hg, with considerable individual heterogeneity. Thus, increasing ICP initially is often associated with vasodilation or increasing MAP to maintain CBF.

Normal ICP is less than 10 mm Hg. Patients with ICP greater than 20 mm Hg typically are treated with drugs that lower ICP.[4] However, this is an epidemiologically derived response. Patients with ICP greater than 20 mm Hg because of trauma generally have a poor outcome.[4] Simply elevating ICP to greater than 20 mm Hg in experimental animals is not necessarily associated with decrements in CBF or permanent sequelae, provided the aforementioned compensatory mechanisms occur.[5]

Increasing ICP because of mass lesions or obstruction of CSF outflow can exhaust compensatory mechanisms, leading to compromise of CBF. The initial decrease in the distal runoff of the cerebral circulation is followed by the interruption of the normally continuous (systole and diastole) cerebral perfusion. Ultimately, cerebral perfusion becomes discontinuous (systolic perfusion only)[6] (Fig. 19-2). Further compromise of CPP leads to anaerobic metabolism, exacerbation of edema, and ultimately intracranial circulatory arrest.[6] Early recognition of increasing ICP is important to determine whether a potentially lethal sequence of events is starting.

Contributors
Brain. The brain normally comprises about 80% of the intracranial contents. Edema increases ICP by increasing brain volume. Cerebral edema is either cytotoxic or vasogenic, depending on whether the cause is cellular or vascular.[7] Heterogeneously distributed ICP leads to ICP gradients and the potential for a variety of herniation syndromes.

Cerebrospinal Fluid. CSF is produced in the choroid plexus and absorbed in the arachnoid villi. Equilibrium normally exists between production and absorption. Disruption of this equilibrium leads to an excess of fluid in all or part of the CSF system, causing increased ICP with hydrocephalus. Hydrocephalus is categorized as communicating or noncommunicating, depending on whether the CSF circulation between the site of CSF production and absorption is intact. Decreased absorption or increased production results in a communicating hydrocephalus. Noncommunicating hydrocephalus is characterized by an interruption in CSF flow such that CSF cannot circulate to the convexity of the brain to be absorbed. CSF accumulates in the ventricles, producing distension.[8]

Blood. CBV is an important component of ICP, due in part to the wide variation of CBV that occurs with normal physiologic homeostasis and the effects of drugs and disordered physiology. ICP increases dramatically when CBV increases because of increased CBF and intracranial compliance is abnormal. Unlike ICP elevation resulting from increased CSF volume, edema, or a tumor, in which decreased CBF is expected, this variety of ICP increase is produced by increased CBF, making the clinical significance of the ICP elevation unclear. Increased CBV may also be caused by venous outflow obstruction. This leads to brain engorgement and CBV-mediated increased ICP without increased CBF.[9]

Masses. The fourth cause of increased ICP is pathologic masses in the form of hematoma or neoplasia. The faster the onset of the mass effect, the more acute the rise in ICP. Compensatory mechanisms in intracranial compliance can allow large, slow-growing masses to arise in the brain without elevated ICP. Similar size masses, arising acutely, are associated with symptomatic increases in ICP.

Two Types of Intracranial Hypertension. There are two types of intracranial hypertension, categorized according to whether CBF is hyperemic or oligemic (Fig. 19-3). Increased CBF is not associated with increased ICP when normal capacitive mechanisms compensate for the CBV-mediated increased intracranial volume. Disordered intracranial compliance allows small increases in intracranial volume to produce significant increases in ICP.[2,3]

An important issue to consider is the traditional concern that elevated ICP jeopardizes cerebral perfusion. The concern about elevated ICP may not be appropriate when the cause of the elevated ICP is intracranial hyperemia with associated increased CBV. The issue is unclear because of the lack of definitive studies. Some studies have allowed reasonable inferences about the significance of hyperemic intracranial hypertension.

Although abrupt noxious stimuli briefly increase ICP in the setting of decreased intracranial compliance, recent studies have revealed associated hyperemia, strongly suggesting that brief hyperemic intracranial hypertension is not a dangerous situation.[10] Hyperemia is a concern for three primary reasons. First, elevated ICP resulting from hyperemia in one portion of the brain might increase ICP to compromise CBF in other areas of the brain in which CBF is marginal. Second, increased pressure in one area of the brain may produce gradients, which might lead to a herniation syndrome. Third, there

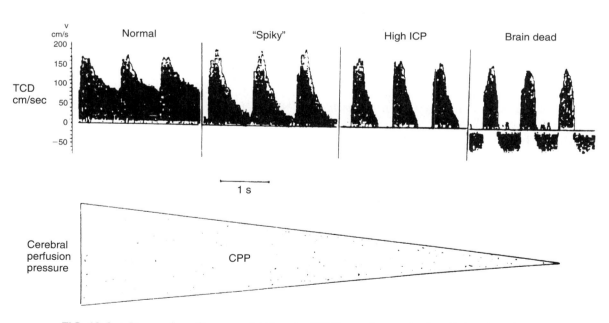

FIG. 19-2 Progression of transcranial Doppler (*TCD*) waveforms after head injury from intact cerebral blood flow and normal-appearing TCD waveform to intracranial hypertension sufficient to induce intracerebral circulatory arrest. Schematic of decreasing cerebral perfusion pressure (*CPP*) indicated in the lower panel. *ICP*, Intracranial pressure.

(From Hassler W, Steinmetz H, Gawlowski J: *J Neurosurg* 68:745, 1988.)

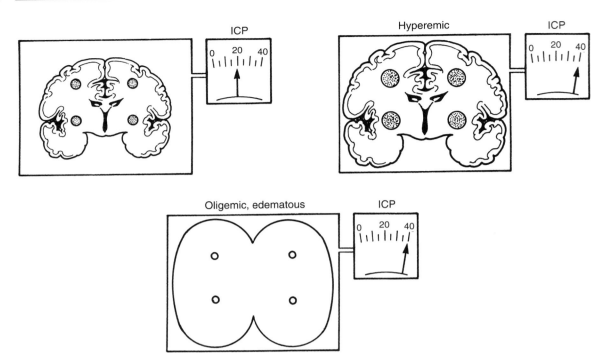

FIG. 19-3 Two types of intracranial hypertension. From a baseline condition, intracranial pressure (*ICP*) can increase in two ways. One is via an increase in cerebral blood volume associated with reflex vasodilation resulting from moderate blood pressure decreases or resulting from hyperemia. The second mechanism of intracranial hypertension is via malignant brain edema or other expanding masses encroaching on the vascular bed to produce intracranial ischemia.

(From Kofke WA, Yonas H, Wechsler L: Neurologic intensive care. In Albin M, editor: *Textbook of neuroanesthesia*, New York, 1997, McGraw-Hill.)

is theoretic concern that inappropriate hyperemia may predispose the brain to worsened edema or hemorrhage, as occurs with hyperperfusion syndromes. Thus hyperemic intracranial hypertension has a theoretic potential to be deleterious but this has yet to be demonstrated. For brief periods, as may occur during intubation or other limited noxious stimuli, it is suggested (but not proven) that hyperemic intracranial hypertension may not be problematic.[11]

In contrast, oligemic intracranial hypertension is associated with compromised cerebral perfusion and is clearly deleterious.[6] This is supported by the high mortality observed in head trauma patients in whom ICP rises because of brain edema with decrements in CBF.[4,12] Transcranial Doppler and CBF studies on these patients demonstrate low CBF and discontinuous perfusion during the cardiac cycle[4,12] (see Fig. 19-2). Jugular venous bulb data indicate markedly increased O_2 extraction, suggesting loss of reserve and increased likelihood of anaerobic metabolism.[12] Noxious stimuli further increase the ICP, leading to hyperemic intracranial hypertension in addition to oligemic intracranial hypertension. The hyperemic rise in ICP presumably further

reduces regional CBF in compromised areas with brain edema and may contribute to vasogenic edema.

Treatment

The general goals for treating intracranial hypertension are to promote adequate oxygen and nutrient supply by maintaining adequate CPP, oxygenation, and glucose supply (without hyperglycemia). The clinical strategy is to diagnose and treat the underlying cause, avoid exacerbating factors, and reduce ICP. Underlying causes include masses (tumors and hematomas), hydrocephalus, cerebral edema, and cerebrovascular dilation.

Therapy of intracranial hypertension is primarily directed at removing the cause if possible. If the cause cannot be removed, therapy is aimed at controlling ICP, in anticipation that the primary cause of the intracranial hypertension will resolve. Controlling ICP is then a supportive maneuver, intended to preserve viable neuronal tissue until the cause of the high ICP resolves. Therapeutic maneuvers generally involve one of five categories of therapy: (1) decrease CBV, (2) decrease CSF volume, (3) resect dead or injured brain tissue, (4) resect nonneural masses or hematomas, and (5) remove the calvarium to permit unopposed outward brain swelling.

CBV decreases with hyperventilation, CBF-decreasing drugs, mannitol, or hypothermia. CBF-decreasing (and therefore CBV-decreasing) drugs that decrease ICP include barbiturates,[13-15] benzodiazepines,[16] etomidate,[17,18] and propofol.[15,19] These drugs are central nervous system depressants with varying degrees of negative inotropic effects and vasodilation, causing hypotension and respiratory depression. Blood pressure may require pharmacologic support. Intubation and mechanical ventilation are mandatory. Lidocaine can also be used to decrease ICP by decreasing CBF and cerebral metabolic rate (CMR), with a less pronounced decrement in neurologic function.[20,21]

Hyperventilation decreases ICP by reducing CBF and CBV.[22-26] CBF may return to baseline within hours in a normal brain.[22,26] It is unclear why sustained decreases in ICP are achieved with hyperventilation. Hyperventilation is accomplished in the intubated patient by increasing tidal volume or rate.

Hyperventilation has several effects on cardiac function. Hypocapnic alkalosis interferes with myocardial O_2 supply in humans with coronary artery disease (CAD) by causing coronary vasoconstriction[27] and increased O_2 affinity of blood.[27] Respiratory alkalosis also produces prolongation of A-V conduction time on anesthetized animals, along with increased sympathetic influence of cardiac activity.[28] A recent study in anesthetized humans undergoing coronary artery bypass graft surgery indicated no decrement in myocardial blood flow with hyperventilation with a concomitant increase in systemic vascular resistance. Moreover, there was no change in myocardial oxygen or glucose use with hyperventilation.[29] An in vitro study by Onishi et al[30] demonstrated decreased oxygen cost of contractility with alkalosis. Despite these relatively benign cardiovascular effects of hyperventilation, there are numerous reports of coronary spasm in unanesthetized hyperventilating humans,[31-33] suggesting cautious use of hyperventilation in patients with CAD. Hyperventilation decreases venous return and induces a functional hypovolemic condition with its attendant sequelae for cardiovascular function.

Mannitol has a variety of relevant potential effects on the heart. Mannitol has been used in cardioplegia for many years. Perfused directly into the heart,[34-36] its protective effects arise from high local concentrations. Given systemically, mannitol has positive inotropic effects[37,38] and is a coronary vasodilator.[37,38] Notably, mannitol increases coronary blood flow in humans with CAD.[38] Myocardial perfusion and function improves when mannitol is administered to dogs during occlusion of a coronary artery.[39-42] Increased serum os-

molality decreases the extent of myocardial necrosis with a decrement in cell swelling and increased tissue perfusion.[41-43] The protective mechanisms of mannitol include free radical scavenging[41,44,45] and decreased cellular and tissue edema.[41,46] Despite these observed protective effects, more recent reports indicate potential harm caused by mannitol. Mannitol and other causes of increasing serum osmolality exacerbated ST changes on epicardial electrocardiogram (ECG) in one dog study.[47] Another study showed that intravenous infusion of mannitol before coronary occlusion does not decrease the extent of myocardial necrosis or increase myocardial blood flow 4 hours after occlusion.[48] Mannitol infusion before and during myocardial ischemia in a baboon model had no effect on ST segment changes or on the extent of myocardial necrosis.[49] Mannitol did not attenuate reperfusion-induced arrhythmias in a rat model.[50] **Overall the data suggest that mannitol has a potential to improve myocardial perfusion but without assurance. Use of mannitol for neurologic indications in the presence of CAD is not contraindicated.**

Mannitol has traditionally been used to induce a relative hypovolemic condition. However, the recently determined importance of maintaining CPP requires replacement of mannitol-induced urine losses with a balanced crystalloid, usually normal saline, or colloid. Mannitol has the potential to cause rapid intravascular volume changes that may have an adverse impact on overall cardiovascular function.

Blood Pressure Effects: Plateau Waves

Lundberg, in a pioneering 1960 study,[51] monitored ICP in hundreds of patients, identifying three characteristic pressure waves, one of which is the plateau wave. Plateau waves are associated with increased CBV[2] (Fig. 19-4), occur when the ICP abruptly increases to systemic blood pressure levels for 15 to 30 minutes, and are occasionally accompanied by neurologic deterioration. Rosner's analysis[3] of the data convincingly indicates that intracranial blood volume dysautoregulation is responsible for plateau waves. Rosner induced mild head trauma in cats and subsequently monitored the animals after the insult. He observed that mild decrements in blood pressure (mean of 70-80 mm Hg) preceded the development of plateau waves (Fig. 19-5). CBV in normally autoregulating brain tissue increases with decreasing blood pressure. However, the increase in CBV is nonlinear. There is an exponential increase in CBV as perfusion pressure decreases to 80 mm Hg and lower[3] (Fig. 19-6). Small decreases in the normotensive range of blood pressure produce exponential increases in CBV in a setting of abnormal intracranial compliance, with the ICP at the elbow of the ICP-intracranial volume curve. A small decrease in blood pressure introduces an

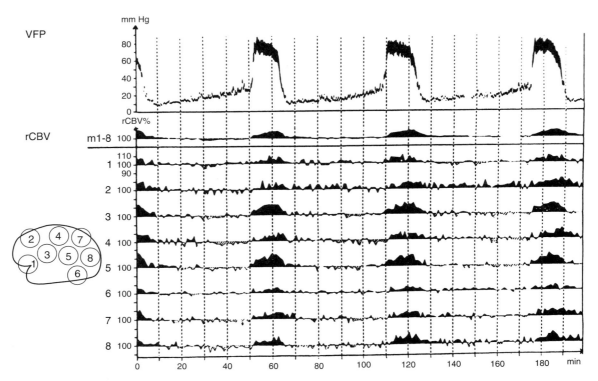

FIG. 19-4 Simultaneous recordings of regional cerebral blood volume (*rCBV*) and ventricular fluid pressure (*VFP*) during three consecutive plateau waves. The rCBF was measured in eight regions over the left hemisphere. The mean changes in the eight regions are shown in the uppermost curve of the rCBF diagram. Note that the rCBV and VFP curves show a very similar course during the three waves.

(From Risberg J, Lundberg N, Ingvar DH: *J Neurosurg* 31:303, 1969.)

FIG. 19-5 In an animal head trauma model, a trivial-appearing and transient decrease in systemic arterial blood pressure in the setting of borderline cerebral perfusion pressure (CPP) precipitates sufficient cerebral vasodilatations to markedly increase the intracranial pressure. Restoration of CPP is associated with abolition of the plateau wave.

(From Rosner MJ, Becker DP: *J Neurosurg* 50:312, 1984.)

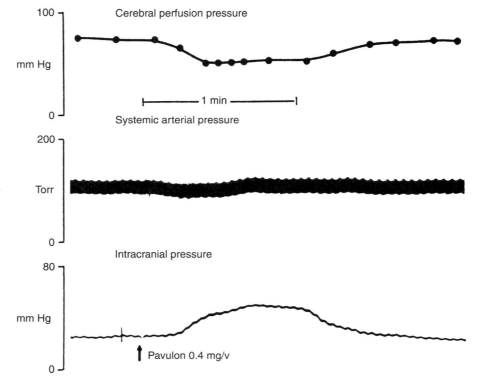

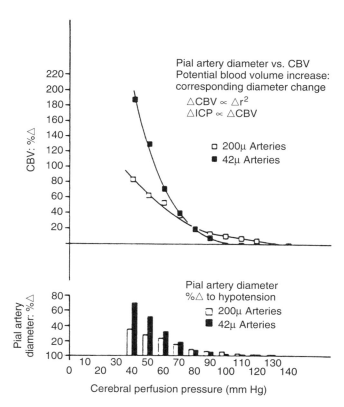

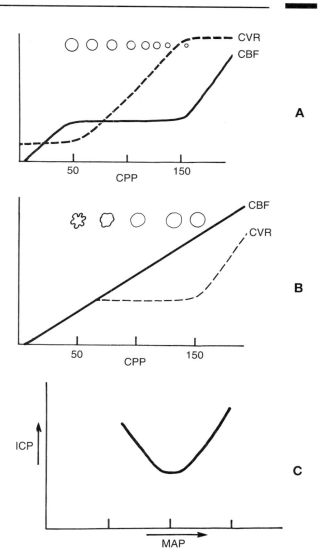

FIG. 19-6 Vasodilatation occurs at a logarithmic rate as cerebral perfusion pressure (CPP) is reduced. Intracranial pressure (*ICP*) increases at a proportional rate within each pressure range with the most rapid increase occurring below a CPP of 80 mm Hg. *CBV,* Cerebral blood volume; *r,* radius.

(From Rosner MJ, Becker DP: *J Neurosurg* 50:312, 1984.)

FIG. 19-7 Cerebral perfusion pressure (*CPP*) versus cerebral blood flow (*CBF*) and cerebrovascular resistance (*CVR*). **A,** Blood flow is normally maintained constant through changes in CVR, depicted as changes in vascular diameter (and therefore cerebral blood volume [*CBV*]) in the figure. CBV varies inversely with CPP. **B,** With vasoparalysis resulting from injury, CVR does not change with CPP variations, such that CBF and CBV vary directly with CPP. **C,** In the situation of decreased intracranial compliance, both of these factors in **A** and **B** may interact to increase intracranial pressure (*ICP*). Normally autoregulating tissue as in **A** will predispose to CBV-mediated ICP elevation with decreasing blood pressure, whereas vasoparalyzed tissue (**B**) will predispose to CBV-mediated ICP elevations with increasing blood pressure, leading to the notion of an ICP optimum (probably about 80-100 mm Hg) with varying CPP. *MAP,* Mean arterial pressure.

(From Kofke WA, Yonas H, Wechsler L: Neurologic intensive care. In Albin M, editor: *Textbook of neuroanesthesia,* New York, 1997, McGraw-Hill.)

exponential CBV change on an exponential ICP relation such that ICP increases significantly and abruptly. Plateau waves spontaneously resolve with a hypertensive response or with hyperventilation that opposes the increase in CBV. A plateau wave can only arise with concurrent heterogeneous autoregulation in which a portion of the brain with normally reactive vasculature is associated with other brain areas that have a mass effect and elevated ICP. To prevent and treat plateau waves it is important to maintain MAP in the 80 to 100 mm Hg range in patients with high ICP.

Conversely, hypertension can also increase ICP. Changes in blood pressure have no effect on ICP in normal brain within the normal autoregulatory range. In the presence of brain injury and the associated vasoparalysis, blood pressure increases mechanically produce cerebral vasodistension, increasing ICP[52] (Figs. 19-7 and 19-8). It thus appears that both increasing and decreasing blood pressure can increase ICP, suggesting the presence of a CPP optimum for ICP, probably in the 80 to 100 mm Hg range. Experimental confirmation of this CPP optimum is lacking.

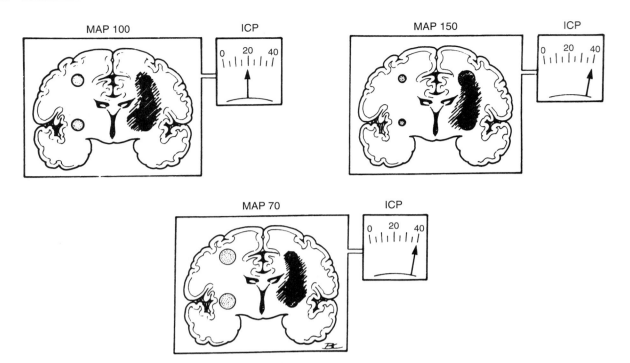

FIG. 19-8 In the setting of heterogeneous autoregulation in the brain, conditions may predispose to cerebral blood volume-mediated increases in intracranial pressure (*ICP*) with both increases or decreases in blood pressure. *MAP,* Mean arterial pressure.

(From Kofke WA, Yonas H, Wechsler L: Neurologic intensive care. In Albin M, editor: *Textbook of neuroanesthesia,* New York, 1997, McGraw-Hill.)

Positive End-Expiratory Pressure

Positive end-expiratory pressure (PEEP) can increase ICP by two mechanisms. PEEP impedes venous return, increasing cerebral venous pressure and ICP. PEEP also decreases blood pressure with a reflex increase of CBV, thereby increasing ICP (Fig. 19-9). The latter is probably the predominant mechanism.

Shapiro et al[53] demonstrated increased ICP with application of PEEP in head-injured humans with intracranial hypertension (Fig. 19-10). The most profound decreases in CPP with concomitant ICP increments occurred in patients with PEEP-induced decrements in MAP. Rosner[3] also concluded that decreases in blood pressure increase CBV and ICP. Aidinis et al[54] used a feline model to confirm these observations in a more controlled setting. They examined the role of pulmonary compliance, finding that PEEP had less impact on increasing ICP if pulmonary compliance was decreased by oleic acid injections. ICP is less likely to be affected in situations where PEEP is needed, that is, decreased pulmonary compliance. This coincides with the observation that the hemodynamic effects of PEEP are less apparent with less compliant lungs,[55,56] minimizing hypotensive-mediated increases in CBV.

The cerebral venous pressure must be equal to or greater than ICP for PEEP to increase cerebral venous

Low PEEP $\rightarrow$ $\downarrow$CO $\rightarrow$ $\downarrow$BP $\rightarrow$ $\uparrow$CBV $\rightarrow$ $\uparrow$ICP

High PEEP $\rightarrow$ $\uparrow$CVP $\rightarrow$ $\uparrow P_{SS} >$ ICP $\rightarrow$ $\uparrow$ICP

FIG. 19-9 Two mechanisms of positive end-expiratory pressure (*PEEP*)-mediated increases in intracranial pressure (*ICP*). Addition of PEEP decreases cardiac output (*CO*) and blood pressure (*BP*), leading to a reflex increase in cerebral blood volume (*CBV*). If cerebral perfusion pressure is marginal with heterogeneous autoregulation, this can lead to further increases in ICP. Conversely, to increase sagittal sinus pressure (*P_{SS}*) to an extent sufficient to further increase ICP, which is already elevated, PEEP levels at or greater than the ICP must be applied. *CVP,* Central venous pressure.

(From Kofke WA, Yonas H, Wechsler L: Neurologic intensive care. In Albin M, editor: *Textbook of neuroanesthesia,* New York, 1997, McGraw-Hill.)

pressure to levels that increase ICP. Higher ICP requires higher PEEP to cause a direct hydraulic effect on ICP. Huseby et al[57] used a canine model to demonstrate that increased PEEP is necessary to affect ICP as the baseline ICP progressively increases (Fig. 19-11). These investigators, however, prevented PEEP-induced decrements in blood pressure, thus avoiding any reflex increases in CBV. They suggested a hydraulic model to better conceptualize this phenomenon (Fig. 19-12). For example,

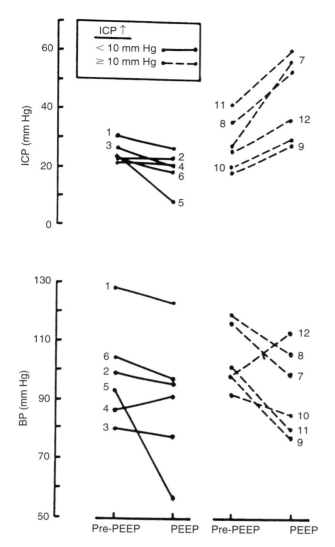

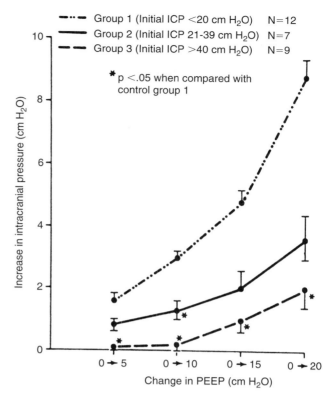

FIG. 19-10 Intracranial pressure (*ICP*) and arterial blood pressure (*BP*) before and with the application of positive end-expiratory pressure (*PEEP*, 4-8 cm H_2O) in severely head-injured patients. The patients are arbitrarily divided into two groups: those with an ICP increase equal to or above 10 mm Hg, and those with ICP gains below 10 mm Hg. Note that PEEP-induced blood pressure decreases appear to be more marked in patients sustaining larger ICP increases.

(From Shapiro HM, Marshall LF: *J Trauma* 18:254, 1978.)

FIG. 19-11 Increases in intracranial pressure (*ICP*) with positive end-expiratory pressure (*PEEP*) in dogs. Values are mean ± standard error of the mean. *Group 1* included 12 animals with initial ICP less than 20 cm H_2O; *group 2* included 7 animals with initial ICP of 21 to 39 cm H_2O; *group 3* included 9 animals with initial ICP greater than 40 cm H_2O. Blood pressure was maintained constant in all animals. Note that with blood pressure maintained constant the most significant increases in PEEP occur in the animals with the lowest starting PEEP level.

(From Huseby JS, Luce JM, Cary JM et al: *J Neurosurg* 55:704, 1981.)

if all of a 10-cm H_2O PEEP application was transmitted to the cerebral vasculature (unlikely given the decreased pulmonary compliance associated with the need for such PEEP), ICP will only be affected if it is less than or equal to 10 cm H_2O (7.7 mm Hg), increasing to a level no higher than the applied PEEP. This presupposes no PEEP-induced arterial pressure decrement. Thus the higher the ICP, the less likely it is that PEEP will sufficiently increase cerebral venous pressure to further increase ICP.

The rational approach to the use of PEEP in the patient with intracranial hypertension is to use PEEP if required, but to avoid any PEEP-induced decrements in blood pressure.

Systemic Hypertension

Significant increases in blood pressure occur in patients with intracranial hypertension. The sympathetic discharge associated with intracranial hypertension or associated traumatic injuries produces substantial increases in blood pressure. Similarly, concomitant medical or surgical problems can produce hypotension as can side effects of therapy or the sequelae of brain death. ICP is also influenced by antihypertensive therapy. Vasodilators such as nitroprusside,[58-60] nitroglycerin,[61,62] and nifedipine[63] can increase ICP. Conversely, nonvasodi-

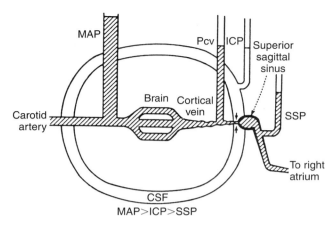

FIG. 19-12 Schematic illustration of the intracranial space during raised intracranial pressure (*ICP*). The *arrows* indicate the position of the hypothesized Starling resistor. Here, the mean arterial pressure (*MAP*) is greater than ICP, which is greater than sagittal sinus pressure (*SSP*). Cortical vein pressure (*Pcv*) cannot fall below ICP, and thus flow is dependent on MAP-ICP, and independent of small changes in SSP. *CSF*, Cerebrospinal fluid.

(From Huseby JS, Luce JM, Cary JM et al: *J Neurosurg* 55:704, 1981.)

lator (sympatholytic) antihypertensive drugs such as trimethophan, or β-adrenergic blocking drugs such as esmolol or labetalol,[64] generally have little or no effect on ICP. **These observations suggest that the rise in ICP because of vasodilators is caused by increased CBF with attendant increase in CBV.** The increase in ICP thus does not necessarily cause ischemia, although herniation and hyperperfusion syndromes may occur. There has been a report of neurologic deterioration with nitroprusside use despite no change in blood pressure.[60] Another consideration in the use of vasodilators is the propensity to reflexly increase plasma catecholamines.[65] Such increases in plasma catecholamines may be deleterious to the marginally perfused injured brain.[66-68]

Vasodilators. Vasodilators such as nitroprusside and hydralazine are frequently used in patients with severe arterial hypertension. Although nitroprusside has minimal CBF effect with induced hypotension,[69] data are not available on its CBF-CBV effects for treatment of hypertension in humans. Nitroprusside was reported to increase ICP and blood flow in a baboon model of intracranial hypertension.[70] Vasodilator-induced increases in ICP[71] suggest an element of cerebral hyperemia. This is supported by reports of cerebral dysautoregulation induced by nitroprusside.[72] The extent of this ICP elevation and hyperemia[69,73] appear to decrease as blood pressure is lowered. This is supported by observations during neurosurgery of the development of cerebral

swelling during nitroprusside administration.[74] Nitroprusside use for induced hypotension during neurosurgery causes the brain to be flaccid with no hyperemia evident. **Thus cerebral vasodilators appear to produce a cerebral dysoutaregulation/hyperperfusion syndrome, the extent of which is blood-pressure dependent.** Use of vasodilators has not been associated with exacerbation of cerebral edema or hemorrhage.

Angiotensin-Converting Enzyme Inhibitors. Angiotensin-converting enzyme (ACE) inhibitors reportedly do not increase ICP with normal pressure hydrocephalus,[75] but their effects when ICP is elevated are unknown. Because ACE inhibitors are not cerebral vasodilators,[76,77] they are unlikely to significantly increase ICP on a hyperemic basis. ACE inhibitors may possess brain-protective properties, as demonstrated in one animal study.[78]

β-Blockers. β-Blockers have no significant impact on ICP.[79,80] They may also produce a brain-protective side effect as suggested by animal studies with brain ischemia and sympatholytic treatment.[81]

Diuretics. Diuretics cause hypovolemia and a consequent decrease in blood pressure that may exacerbate ICP, as discussed under plateau waves. Furosemide may exert a primary effect of decreasing ICP distinct from its osmolar or volume effects.[81]

Coronary Artery Disease

Patients with CAD who develop intracranial hypertension experience exacerbation of myocardial ischemia. Previously described intracranial processes can lead to alterations in blood pressure, inotropic state, and heart rate that are detrimental to the myocardial oxygen supply-demand relationship. Accordingly, it may be necessary to implement or increase antiischemic therapy in patients with preexisting atherosclerotic coronary disease.

Nitroglycerin. Nitroglycerin dilates conductance vessels in the brain and tends to increase CBF.[82] Neurologic deterioration with nitroglycerin therapy is due to increases in ICP, presumably hyperemic in nature.[62,70,83]

Calcium Channel Blockers. Verapamil and diltiazem can increase ICP probably by a hyperemic mechanism[84] and do not cross the blood-brain barrier (BBB) to a substantial extent. These drugs are not brain-protective, unlike nimodipine and nicardipine, which are both brain-protective calcium channel blocking drugs.[85-91] In a group of head trauma patients[92] and in a group of postcardiopulmonary resuscitation patients,[93] nimodipine did not produce a statistically significant effect on ICP, whereas diltiazem and nicardipine had a mild ICP-increasing effect (nicardipine > diltiazem).[62]

β-Adrenergic Blockers. Ordinary doses of β-adrenergic blockers do not have significant effects on ICP[94,95] and are preferred for the treatment of CAD if there are no other contraindications.

Hypotension

The choice of fluids to maintain blood pressure is very important. The general principle is that hypo-osmolar fluids such as lactated Ringer's are avoided. Fluids that are isoosmolar or, preferably, slightly hyperosmolar such as normal saline are preferred. Use of albumin remains controversial. Recent evidence suggests that colloid infusion has a beneficial impact on brain edema.[96]

Vasopressors. Vasopressors used in the normal auto regulatory range have no impact on CBF or cerebral metabolic rate provided that the BBB is intact. If the BBB is disrupted, these drugs cross it and exhibit an excitatory effect on brain function. β-Adrenergic agonists increase CBF and increase metabolic rate in the presence of a disrupted BBB.[97-99] In one series of animal studies, catecholamine infusion exacerbated ischemic damage, whereas sympatholytic therapy was protective.[78,100,101]

Cardiomyopathy

Patients with preexisting cardiomyopathy may experience exacerbation of their symptoms resulting from alterations in preload, afterload, or contractility caused by the high ICP disease process or by therapy.

β-Agonists. β-Agonists have little impact on the brain. However, in the presence of a disrupted BBB, they cross into the brain and exert a stimulatory effect as noted earlier.[97-99]

Phosphodiesterase Inhibitors. Data are limited on cerebrovascular effects of milrinone and amrinone. There is some evidence that indicates a cerebral vasodilatory effect,[102,103] but no reports of their effect on ICP. Their cerebral vasodilatory properties would suggest a hyperemic increase in ICP.

Afterload-Reducing Agents. Afterload-reducing agents such as ACE inhibitors and vasodilators have cerebral effects as described previously.

Arrhythmias

A variety of cardiac arrhythmias can occur consequent to cerebral insults.[104-106] Tachyarrhythmias and bradyarrhythmias, ventricular ectopy, and supraventricular tachycardia are common arrhythmias associated with intracranial hypertension. Tachyarrhythmias are due to a hyperadrenergic state, whereas bradyarrhythmias are related to excessive vagal tone.[107,108]

Arrhythmia Therapy. β-Blockers and calcium channel blockers used to treat tachyarrhythmias were described earlier in the context of intracranial hypertension. While atropine may contribute to sedation,[109] there is no information on the cerebrovascular or ICP effects of atropine. Lidocaine decreases cerebral metabolic rate and CBF[110] and decreases ICP.[111,112] Lidocaine is neuroexcitatory at high dosages[113] and possesses some brain-protective side effects.[114]

CEREBROVASCULAR DISEASES AND PROCEDURES
Cerebral Ischemic Syndromes

Pathophysiology. Stroke is the third leading cause of death in the United States. For every patient who dies of a stroke there are about 13 survivors who survive with the effects of their loss of neural tissue.[115] The 2-year incidence of stroke is 10 per 1000 and the incidence because of atherothrombotic brain infarction is 4.4 per 1000.[115] Risk factors for atherothrombotic stroke include hypertension, left ventricular hypertrophy, cigarette use, elevated lipids, obesity, and polycythemia.[115]

Data from animal models of ischemia provide insight into the pathogenesis of neuronal death with cerebral ischemia. The primary event is energy failure. Consciousness is lost within 7 seconds after total cessation of brain flow in normal subjects, with cessation of electroencephalogram activity occurring within 10 seconds.[116] Brain adenosine 5-triphosphate is depleted to less than 20% of baseline in canine models within 5 minutes of no blood flow.[117] Recirculation after ischemic periods as long as 60 minutes is associated with return of brain high-energy phosphates to greater than 90% of baseline in animal models.[118-121] However, restoration of energy metabolism does not correlate with functional recovery,[121,122] suggesting other causes of neurologic deficit after cerebral ischemia. Most of the ischemia-susceptible neurons are innervated by glutamatergic fibers, indicating a relationship between glutamate-mediated synaptic transmission and postischemic neuronal death.

Pathologic studies indicate a heterogeneous susceptibility among neurons to ischemia-mediated death. Selectively vulnerable neurons and a hierarchy of vulnerability has been identified. Neurons die hours to days after the ischemic insult, implying delayed neuronal death with the potential for reversible pathophysiologic processes.[123-127] Postinsult deficits occur despite normalization of energy metabolism.

Cerebral infarction is due to one of three mechanisms of vascular insufficiency: (1) cerebral arterial hypotension (hemodynamic infarct), (2) embolism, and (3) thrombosis. *Cerebral arterial hypotension* occurs with systemic hypotension with CPP less than 60 mm Hg. Focal intracranial stenosis or stenoses cause cerebral arterial hypotension in normotensive patients who sustain intracranial hypotension. One notable example is the hypertensive patient undergoing antihypertensive therapy who develops cerebral ischemia as blood pressure is normalized. Another example is the patient with inadequate cerebrovascular reserve (e.g., carotid stenosis, edema) who becomes anemic or hypoxemic. *Cerebral embolism* arises from clots originating in the left chamber of the heart, aorta, or carotid artery, or from venous thromboembolism with right-to-left passage through the heart. *Thrombotic stroke* occurs when a thrombosis develops in a previously patent stenotic artery due to atherosclerosis and a low flow state. Nonlaminar flow predisposes to coagulation and results in thrombotic occlusion of the artery with ischemia to distal tissues.[128]

Therapy. Stroke has recently been identified as a medical emergency. Efforts to increase public awareness of signs and symptoms of stroke expedite entry of stroke patients into the emergency medical system, providing urgent institution of diagnostic and therapeutic procedures.

The primary concern of the anesthesiologist in stroke therapy is maintenance of normal physiologic homeostasis. Notable in this regard is blood pressure management. Hypertension associated with stroke should not be treated aggressively unless there is clinical concern that other systemic morbidity is being caused by the hypertension.

Reperfusion therapy is being used in many medical centers. There have been numerous anecdotes and clinical trials of this approach to the management of acute stroke in both the anterior and posterior intracranial circulations.[129-133] Outcome improves with earlier initiation of treatment. A recent meta-analysis of thrombolytic therapy for stroke indicated that the procedure is an effective technique.[129] A multi-institutional study of tissue plasminogen activator for acute ischemic stroke indicated a protective effect in terms of neurologic disability but not mortality, with an increased incidence of hemorrhage (6.4% vs. 0.6%).[134] A major concern with thrombolytic therapy is that it may produce hemorrhagic transformation of a bland ischemic stroke, leading to intracerebral hematoma and greater disability or death. The incidence of postthrombolysis hematoma appears to be related to the depth of ischemia before reperfusion.[135] Overall, thrombolytic therapy appears to be safe and efficacious, but the outcome is dependent on the elapsed time between onset of ischemia and institution of therapy. It is of utmost importance that stroke victims undergo transportation and evaluation in the most urgent manner. Treatment must be instituted within 3 hours of the onset of symptoms and, preferably, within 2 hours of symptom onset. Anecdotes suggest that complete recovery is possible when recanalization occurs promptly, as may occur with in-hospital strokes.[136]

These studies present important issues in the cardiovascular management of such patients. Hypertension should be tolerated while the artery is still occluded insofar as permanent cardiovascular injury is not produced. Blood pressure should be acutely normalized when the artery is opened to minimize the likelihood of postthrombolysis hemorrhagic conversion. Unfortunately, this management approach has not been validated and the appropriate target pressure or the most appropriate antihypertensive drugs have not been identified. Extrapolation from animal studies suggests the use of sympatholytic or calcium-blocking drugs such as labetalol, esmolol, or nicardipine.

Neurosurgery is indicated on an urgent basis in a few subsets of stroke patients. Procedures that may be used include urgent revascularization, strokectomy, decompressive craniectomy, cerebellar resection, and external ventricular drain placement. *Revascularization*, that is, carotid endarterectomy or extracranial-intracranial bypass, is occasionally performed when the onset time is brief, such as with an in-hospital stroke, and endovascular reperfusion techniques are not feasible.[137] Revascularization may also be indicated when the patient has progressive stroke in the presence of known ulcerating intraarterial plaque or when there are fluctuating symptoms of hemodynamic origin, where systemic perfusion-augmenting therapy is not appropriate. *Decompressive craniectomy* is somewhat controversial. It is used for malignant intracranial hypertension and involves resection of the skull and dura to allow unopposed outward brain swelling without intracranial hypertension after a large stroke. There is laboratory support for this procedure with encouraging anecdotal evidence in humans for its use.[138-142] *Strokectomy* is performed for malignant brain edema after ischemic stroke as a life-saving alternative to temporal lobe resection.[143] Cerebellar *decompression* can be life-saving when the deterioration is detected and decompression occurs in a timely manner.[139,140] *Ventriculostomy* is performed if ICP is increasing and ICP-reducing therapy is titrated by ICP measurements. A ventriculostomy drain is also used to remove CSF if ICP is high or hydrocephalus occurs after cerebellar infarction. All of these procedures require appropriate anesthetic management with the implicit impact on cardiovascular function.

Blood Pressure Management. Ischemic stroke produces a central ischemic core around which there is an ischemic penumbra, where flow is perfusion-pressure dependent via collateral vessels. This dependence of flow on blood pressure is supported by clinical observations in stroke patients,[142] emphasizing the hazard of decreasing blood pressure in a stroke patient without a strong indication. There are a variety of theoretic and demonstrated pros and cons to antihypertensive therapy with stroke. These complex considerations were reviewed in detail by Powers,[144] who concluded that data are indefinite regarding antihypertensive therapy in stroke. He suggests that blood pressure reduction is accompanied by a significant risk of extending ischemic damage. Blood pressure should only be reduced when there is a risk of hypertensive encephalopathy or cardiovascular compromise because of hypertension (e.g., myocardial ischemia, or low-output state with preexisting ventricular dysfunction).[139,143] If blood pressure reduction is contemplated, agents used should be short-acting, readily reversible, and not prone to increase ICP.[139] Sympatholytic drugs are preferred because they confer neuronal preservation.[78,100,101] Nicardipine is a primary consideration because of its brain-protective side effects.[86,89-91]

Ischemic stroke may be associated with ECG changes, myocardial ischemic injury,[145-148] and a significantly increased incidence of cardiac arrhythmias, particularly ventricular ectopy.[149,150] ECG changes indicate a poorer prognosis,[151] with 11% of patients with ECG changes developing elevations in cardiac isoenzymes[152] and an associated doubling of mortality rate.[139] These adverse cardiac outcomes are probably related to stroke-induced elevations of blood catecholamines,[153,154] emphasizing the fact that these ECG changes in stroke patients are not artifact. Any stroke patient who has ECG changes should have creatine phosphokinase (CPK) isoenzymes determined and continuous monitoring for cardiac arrhythmias.

Management of hypotension is somewhat enigmatic. Decreases in blood pressure are likely to worsen the outcome from a cerebral ischemic process. Decreases in blood pressure should be aggressively treated according to the cause of the hypotension.

Intracerebral Hemorrhage

Pathophysiology. Intracerebral hemorrhages (ICHs) are categorized pathologically on the basis of size as petechial, small, large, and massive. An ICH is considered massive when it is greater than 3 cm in the cerebrum, 2 cm in the cerebellum, and 1 cm in the brainstem.

The primary risk factor for developing an ICH is hypertension,[155,156] present in 72% to 81% of patients with ICHs.[157,158] Left ventricular hypertrophy is common in patients with ICH,[155,159,160] and their admission blood pressures are significantly higher

compared with patients who have other types of stroke.[161] Other conditions that predispose patients to ICH include blood dyscrasias, vascular malformations, and tumors, accounting for about 25% of ICHs.[162] Some authors suggest that hypertension accounts for only half of ICHs,[163,164] not three quarters as earlier reported.[157,158] Amyloid angiopathy accounts for most lobar hemorrhages.[165]

Therapy. The management of ICH is controversial. Some authors recommend an aggressive operative approach, whereas others prefer a nonsurgical approach.[166] It is recommended that patients who are alert with small ICH be treated medically, but those with larger or expanding ICHs undergo angiography to rule out a vascular abnormality such as arteriovenous malformation or aneurysm. Radiographic imaging is used to guide surgical removal of the ICH.[166] There are a variety of pros and cons to the surgical approach. Large hematomas can be associated with local tissue damage. Conversely, small hematomas limited to dissection through white matter planes locally resorb without injuring vital brain tissue. Performing surgery may cause brain tissue injury that would otherwise not have occurred. Decompressing ICH large enough to produce high ICP decreases ICP and prevents secondary brain damage from compromised CPP and herniation. The decision regarding surgery is based on a judgment about whether the mass effect of the hematoma is compromising blood flow to still-viable brain tissue.[166] This assessment is further complicated by the introduction of noncraniotomy methods of clot removal such as percutaneous aspiration with or without stereotactic guidance, local fibrinolysis, and endoscopic evacuation.[166]

Blood Pressure Management. Blood pressure management in the patient with ICH is controversial and enigmatic, particularly if the ICH is due to hypertension. It seems logical to control blood pressure if the ICH is due to hypertension. Drugs used to control blood pressure may increase ICP while decreasing blood pressure, possibly compromising CPP.[167] If hematoma compresses the brain tissue from which the bleed arose and there is a fibrin clot on the bleeding source, it seems unlikely that the high blood pressure being recorded peripherally is actually relevant to the cerebral microcirculation. In addition, an ICH seldom enlarges. The most appropriate course of treatment is to treat blood pressure when it is very high, for example, greater than about 180 to 200 mm Hg systolic or 130 to 140 mm Hg mean pressure. Any blood pressure reduction must be accompanied by careful neurologic assessment and discontinuation of antihypertensive therapy if deterioration occurs in temporal association with blood pressure reduction.

Subarachnoid Hemorrhage

Pathophysiology

Ictus. The initial bleed is associated with a transient increase in ICP to systemic levels. This has two predominant effects. The first is to produce a decrement in level of conscious, with unconsciousness occurring in 45% of patients. Usually the loss of consciousness is brief but it can last for days. The second effect of the high ICP is to stop the egress of blood from the arterial rupture to promote hemostatic clot formation.[168,169]

A complex series of events can occur subsequent to the bleed. These events include rebleeding, hydrocephalus, and vasospasm that produce a delayed neurologic deficit. Extracranial complications also contribute to postbleed morbidity and contribute to neurologic problems.

Rebleed. The probability of rebleeding is about 4% the first day after the bleed and 1.5% per day thereafter. The overall incidence of rebleeding is 19% the first 2 weeks, 64% by the end of the first month, and 78% by the end of 8 weeks after the initial bleed.[170-174] Predisposing factors for rebleeding include female gender, admission within the first day after subarachnoid hemorrhage (SAH; implying that survival outside the hospital for longer periods selects more stable patients), poor neurologic grade, poor general medical condition, and systolic blood pressure greater than 170 mm Hg.[170] A rebleed is associated with a mortality rate of 48% to 78%.[170,175]

Hydrocephalus. On the basis of temporal considerations, hydrocephalus is divided into three categories: acute, subacute, and delayed.[176-178] The ventricular dilation is caused by the effects of fresh blood in the CSF, which can fill the ventricles, block the aqueduct of Sylvius, fill and obstruct the fourth ventricle, fill the subarachnoid cisterns, or block the arachnoid villi. This results in obstruction of CSF circulation or reabsorption, leading to hydrocephalus, increased ICP, and a depressed level of consciousness.

Intraventricular hemorrhage in association with SAH produces a substantially worse outcome if hydrocephalus develops.[179,180] Hydrocephalus is the result of the CSF egress from the ventricles and absorption in the choroid plexus. The likelihood of hydrocephalus correlates with the amount of blood evident on computed tomography (CT) scan.[177] The overall mortality rate of patients with hydrocephalus after SAH is 64%.[180] Mortality rate remains high even after ventricular drainage.[180] Most patients admitted with hydrocephalus have a poorer neurologic grade. Morbidity is related to herniation and decrements in CBF that may already be compromised. Hydrocephalus can occur at any time after SAH, occurring acutely in 20% of patients,[178] and subacutely or chronically in 15% to 20% of patients.[170] Permanent CSF diversion is required in 5% to 10% of patients after SAH.[170]

Vasospasm. Post-SAH vasospasm occurs 3 to 21 days after SAH, more commonly within 4 to 14 days after SAH. The peak incidence is between days 6 and 8 after SAH with duration of up to 2 weeks.[181,182] The actual incidence of post-SAH vasospasm varies between 15% and 76%. The true incidence is probably in the 30% to 40% range.[170,183-193] Delayed cerebral ischemia because of delayed vascular narrowing remains one of the most frightening and devastating causes of stroke in a patient making a good recovery after SAH and surgery. Thirty percent of patients developing vasospasm sustain an ischemic deficit due to the vasospasm,[194] and 7% to 17% develop permanent neurologic deficit or death.[181,183,195] Cardiovascular issues are of paramount importance when vasospasm develops.

The pathogenesis of vasospasm correlates clinically with the amount of blood in the basal cisterns adhering to basal cerebral arteries.[177-182,196-200] These observations are supported by the in vivo and in vitro application of blood to cerebral arteries, producing contraction of the vessels.[201-203] The many components of blood have been studied for their potential to produce vasospasm.[201] Although many of these components cause spasm, no single spasmogen has been identified as the sole culpable substance. Many chemicals in the blood also cause spasm of cerebral arteries in the experimental situation.[201] Other potential contributors to vasospasm include mechanical wall disruption, inflammation, and free radicals.[201]

The cerebral vasculature maintains the appropriate vascular tone through the interplay of numerous factors. Important in this homeostasis is the balance between endothelin and nitric oxide. Endothelin is a potent vasoconstrictor and nitric oxide is a short-lived potent vasodilator. Oxyhemoglobin binds nitric oxide. Thus, with degradation of the erythrocytes in the CSF, the basal cerebral arteries are exposed to oxyhemoglobin, which binds nitric oxide, resulting in spasm.[201,204] Intracarotid nitric oxide infused into the vasospastic artery of a monkey relieves the spasm.[205]

Serum catecholamine levels increase dramatically after SAH, peaking at the same time as the peak incidence of vasospasm after SAH, with symptom development corresponding to serum catecholamine levels.[206-214] This has important implications with respect to cardiac function. Hypothalamic injury with excess catecholamine release is an important factor in the genesis of post-SAH spasm.[208] Several lines of evidence further support this hypothesis:

1. The cerebral vasculature is innervated with adrenergic nerves. Adrenergic receptors in the cerebral vessels decrease in quantity after SAH.[215,216] Denervation hypersensitivity may be occurring such that the increase in humoral catecholamines with SAH produces spasm in hyperreacting vessels.

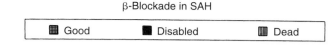

β-Blockade in SAH

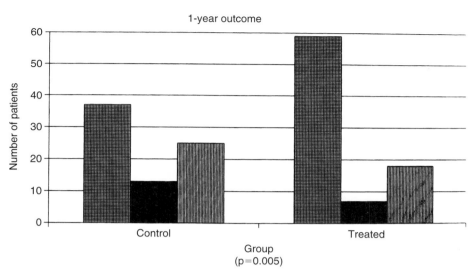

FIG. 19-13 Subarachnoid hemorrhage patients were randomly treated with propranolol or placebo. Neurologic outcome was better in patients undergoing β-blockade. *SAH,* Subarachnoid hemorrhage.

(Data from Neil-Dwyer et al. From Kofke WA, Yonas H, Wechsler L: Neurologic intensive care. In Albin M, editor: *Textbook of neuroanesthesia,* New York, 1997, McGraw-Hill.)

2. Treatment of SAH in humans with β- and α-adrenergic antagonists is associated with an improvement in neurologic outcome[217] (Fig. 19-13) and electrocardiographic abnormalities.[153]

3. Catecholamine release after SAH produces electrocardiographic abnormalities* with ventricular wall-motion abnormalities[222-224] and myocardial injury.[146,225-227]

4. Selective destruction of hindbrain adrenergic nuclei with cephalad projections prevents the development of vasospasm.[228-230] Vasopressin has an important role in vasospasm. Vasospasm cannot be produced in vasopressin-deficient rats.[231]

This hyperadrenergic state has important negative consequences for the patient with preexisting cardiovascular disease.

Seizures. Three percent to five percent of patients develop seizures during the acute phase after SAH.[232] Moreover, 13% to 15% develop epilepsy as a chronic complication of their SAH, with the incidence increasing to 30% when the SAH arises from a middle cerebral artery aneurysm, presumably because of proximity to the temporal lobe. The incidence increases from 5% in patients without neurologic deficit to 41% in patients with neurologic deficits.[233] Seizures cause tachycardia and hypertension, which may produce ischemia or cardiac decompensation in patients with ischemic or valvular heart disease.

Extracranial Complications. A variety of extracranial complications arise as a direct consequence of the SAH.

These include abnormalities in cardiovascular, pulmonary, endocrine, and electrolyte homeostasis, and arise from the post-SAH hyperadrenergic state or dysfunctional hypothalamus.

Systemic hypertension is very common after SAH[234] and is most likely related to elevated catecholamines and renin secondary to hypothalamic disturbance.[105,107] Other causes include intracranial hypertension, preexisting essential hypertension, seizures, vomiting, pain, bladder distension, agitation, or vasospasm. Hypertension, in addition to predisposing the patient to rebleeding, is associated with a higher incidence of vasospasm and death.[235]

Cardiac arrhythmias are observed in nearly all patients after SAH[105,106] and electrocardiographic changes suggestive of myocardial ischemia occur in 50% to 80% of patients after SAH.* The arrhythmias are severe or life threatening in 20% of patients.[105,106] A diverse array of ECG changes appear to indicate myocardial ischemia. It is likely that these changes represent more than simple artifact. Ventricular wall-motion abnormalities consistent with myocardial ischemia are observed after SAH, particularly with worsened neurologic grade.[222-224] CPK isoenzyme elevations indicating myocardial infarction,[225,226] and postmortem examination of myocardial necrosis have been associated with SAH.[236]

Neurogenic pulmonary edema is a rare complication of SAH, having been ascribed to the brief period of severe intracranial hypertension associated with the initial bleed or the postbleed surge in catechol-

*References 104-106, 153, 207, 210, 218-221.

*References 104-106, 153, 207, 218-220.

amines.[237-250] The post-SAH increase in blood-borne vasogenic substances leads to increased permeability of the pulmonary vasculature such that pulmonary edema occurs at lower hydrostatic pressures than normal.[237]

Abnormalities of fluid and sodium homeostasis occur in about 33% of patients.[239] Both hypovolemia and hyponatremia are commonly observed. The clinical presentation appears similar to the syndrome of inappropriate antidiuretic hormone secretion. Patients in the past were treated with fluid restriction.[241,243] In retrospect, this treatment would aggravate the more recently discovered SAH-associated hypovolemia and increased blood viscosity, both undesirable after SAH. More recent studies indicate that both fluid and sodium are lost after SAH,[239,245,247,249,251] indicating that the hyponatremia is not an isolated issue of dilution of sodium because of excessive water retention. Declines in blood volume are observed by using tracer techniques.[238,250,252] The kidney is unable to retain sodium,[252,253] consistent with observed increases in atrial natriuretic factor,[253,254] and constituting the so-called "cerebral salt-wasting" syndrome.[234,244,248,253] Atrial natriuretic factor levels in plasma peak 3 days after SAH and then decline within 7 days after the SAH.

Hypokalemia occurs frequently after SAH and is most likely due to vomiting, elevated circulating catecholamines, corticosteroids, renin, or diuretic use.[220]

Fever is a common concomitant condition with SAH,[255-257] which also affects cardiac function. The etiology of fever is unclear, but it can be an indicator of developing vasospasm.[257] Unfortunately, SAH patients commonly undergo instrumentation of the vasculature, bladder, brain, or trachea, all of which may independently lead to infection with accompanying fever. These patients also have other potential causes of fever, including deep vein thrombosis, biliary stasis, and multiple pyrogenic drug administrations. The presence of fever in this patient group is more serious because fever seriously exacerbates the consequences of cerebral ischemia.[258]

Therapy
Aneurysm Clipping. Intracranial surgery and clipping of the aneurysm is generally the most appropriate therapy. Left unclipped, the incidence of rebleeding is high.[259-261] The only reasons for not clipping an aneurysm are medical instability, technical difficulty, or patient or family refusal. Other techniques may be used in situations where definitive surgery is not feasible. These techniques include proximal arterial ligation or endovascular occlusion by using interventional neuroradiologic techniques. The timing of surgery has been the source of controversy. For a period of time the consensus was that surgery should be delayed until after the risk of vasospasm had subsided and acute edema had resolved to improve operating conditions. Studies

also indicated that operative morbidity and mortality rates were good when surgery was delayed.[262] Delaying surgery, however, increases the risk of rebleed during a phase of the disease wherein hypertension is induced or occurs spontaneously, and other medical complications of the SAH increase the likelihood of rebleed. Although the operative statistics may be good when surgery is delayed, the overall outcome of surgery appears to be better if surgery is performed in the first few days after SAH and before the onset of vasospasm.[263-274] A large epidemiologic study on the timing of aneurysm surgery, involving 3521 patients, supports early surgery for improving outcome, especially for grades I to IV patients.[275,276]

Calcium Channel Blockers. Nimodipine, an enterally administered calcium channel blocker, is the only clinically efficacious drug in prospective randomized trials for the treatment of vasospasm. Nimopidine prevents or reduces ischemic deficits by 40% to 70%.[277-283] On the basis of these data, it is generally recommended that all SAH patients receive nimodipine 30 to 60 mg enterally every 4 to 6 hours for 2 to 3 weeks after SAH. Its use is associated with hypotension, which opposes beneficial therapeutic effects. Treatment includes fluid administration, especially if hypovolemia is suspected, administering the same daily dose over smaller intervals, or reducing the overall dose.

Nicardipine is a calcium channel blocker that is administered intravenously. Its use is associated with a lower than expected incidence of angiographic narrowing,[284] a lower incidence of vasospasm, and a lower incidence of the use of hypertensive hypervolemic therapy drugs.[285] Final neurologic outcomes were similar for both treated and control groups in one controlled study.[285]

Hypervolemic, Hypertensive, Hemodilution (HHH) Therapy. Hypovolemia with contraction of circulating blood volume occurs after SAH.[244,252] This decrease in circulating blood volume is an important factor (or perhaps epiphenomenon) in the development of delayed ischemic deficits after SAH.[238,248,252] The onset of vasospasm sufficient to attenuate cerebrovascular reserve creates a situation in which CBF becomes a function of CPP.[244,286-288] Viscosity becomes an important factor in determination of CBF as luminal size decreases. These observations have led to the use of HHH therapy to prevent and actively treat delayed cerebral ischemia resulting from vasospasm, and it is consistently applied to patients after SAH. HHH therapy increases rCBF and ameliorates ischemic deficits because of post-SAH vasospasm.[289-294]

Hypervolemia is instituted with infusion of 5% albumin 75 to 125 ml/hr plus 250- to 500-ml infusions to maintain central venous pressure (CVP) or pulmonary capillary wedge pressure (PCWP) about 10 to 14 mm Hg. Notably, the PCWP often does not correlate with CVP.[167,295] Titrating fluid infusions by the

CVP alone may lead to elevated left ventricular pressure, pulmonary edema, or pleural effusion. Ventricular wall-motion abnormalities or electrocardiographic changes suggestive of ischemia predispose patients to myocardial diastolic dysfunction.* For these reasons, pulmonary artery catheterization is recommended for any SAH patient undergoing HHH therapy.

The physiologic basis for increased blood volume producing increased rCBF is obscure. Infusion of red-blood-cell-free solutions decreases hematocrit, which lowers blood viscosity.[296] Hemodilution increases rCBF as a result of decreased viscosity. Optimal hematocrit in animal studies is 33%; that is, O_2-carrying capacity is not compromised until hematocrit decreases below this level.[296] This concept is applied to clinical care for determining the endpoint for hemodilution therapy.[297] Phlebotomy is performed only after maximal hypervolemia therapy leaves the hematocrit above desired levels.

Increasing preload usually increases blood pressure. Patients tend to spontaneously increase their blood pressure as vasospasm worsens. Induced hypertensive therapy is indicated when increased preload and spontaneously increased blood pressure do not prevent delayed cerebral ischemia. Such therapy increases rCBF[292] and ameliorates ischemic deficits.[298] Hypertensive therapy is instituted with a titrated infusion of an intravenous vasopressor. The endpoint is reversal of neurologic deficits that may require a systolic blood pressure as high as 240 mm Hg. The blood pressure endpoint is attenuated if the heart is unable to tolerate the increased afterload. Increased afterload decreases cardiac output. Therapy is altered for decreases in cardiac output that compromise splanchnic flow, as indicated by decreasing urinary output or increasing lactate, increases in PCWP that threaten pulmonary edema, or ischemic changes on ECG. Therapy should include an inotrope or be abandoned in favor of another approach (e.g., cerebral angioplasty). The specific hypertensive drug chosen varies among investigators and physicians but includes phenylephrine, dopamine, dobutamine, and norepinephrine.[299] Although catecholamine-based vasopressors occasionally reverse neurologic deficits, their cerebrovascular and metabolic effects are unclear. Darby et al[300] demonstrated heterogenous rCBF throughout the brain with intravenous dopamine infusion by using stable xenon CT CBF. Many areas of the brain sustained significant decreases in rCBF. The areas of the brain with low baseline flow (presumably vasospastic areas) tended to increase rCBF with dopamine infusion (Fig. 19-14). When catecholamines cross the BBB, which is disrupted with vasospasm,[301-303] they produce hypermetabolism and hyperemia.[304] Con-

versely, catecholamines have no significant effect on CBF when administered with an intact BBB.[305] Despite numerous anecdotes of symptomatic improvement with vasopressor therapy, there is a theoretic basis for concern regarding catecholamine therapy on overall outcome.

Institution of HHH therapy often results in bradycardia. Urine output increases sufficiently to prevent the desired increase in preload. Atropine (1 mg intramuscularly [IM] q3-4 h) or vasopressin (5 U IM to keep urine output less than 200 ml/hr) may be required.[298]

Patients undergoing HHH therapy require intensive care with invasive hemodynamic monitoring, including central venous or pulmonary artery monitoring and intraarterial catheter placement for arterial blood gases and blood pressure monitoring. These monitors are associated with a risk of septicemia, which may cause decreased blood pressure and decreased rCBF.[306] The overzealous administration of fluids in the setting of decreased pulmonary vascular permeability and myocardial diastolic dysfunction predisposes patients to pulmonary edema and pleural effusion. Patients develop an increased risk of pneumonia if these complications result in prolonged tracheal intubation and mechanical ventilation. These pulmonary complications may also cause hypoxemia, predisposing the patient to stroke in the setting of decreased cerebrovascular reserve. The incidence of systemic complications associated with HHH therapy includes 7% to 17% pulmonary edema, 2% myocardial infarction, 3% to 35% dilutional hyponatremia, and 3% coagulopathy.[297,307-309] Other iatrogenic complications secondary to the intensive care required for HHH include urinary tract infection, pneumothorax, carotid artery puncture, agitation-induced rebleed, and barotrauma.

Interventional Neuroradiology Techniques. Transluminal angioplasty effectively reverses angiographic evidence of vasospasm of proximal accessible vessels in 75% of patients refractory to conventional treatment with HHH therapy.[310] Intraarterial papaverine is infused if vasospasm is present in distal vessels, producing a favorable reversal of vasospasm.[310,311] However, papaverine can transiently produce neurologic deterioration during infusion, according to the vascular territory infused. Neurologic deterioration includes seizure (personal observation), hemiparesis, pupillary changes, unconsciousness, increased ICP, or cardiovascular collapse.[311-315] Earlier use of angioplasty or papaverine therapy is advocated because of the morbidity associated with HHH therapy and the increasing experience with these procedures.

Occlusion of the aneurysm with coils to induce an intraaneurysmal clot is used in unstable patients or patients with severe neurologic dysfunction. This treatment is particularly helpful if the patient develops vasospasm, despite the need for HHH therapy. The coils protect the aneurysm lumen from the high pressures

*References 104, 218, 219, 225, 226, 236.

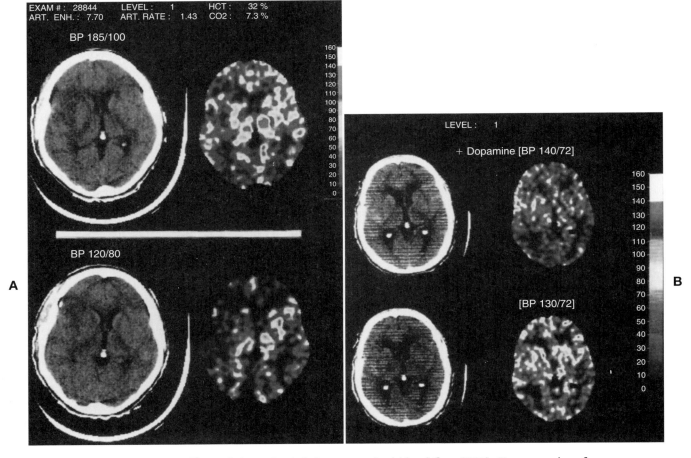

EXAM # : 28844   LEVEL : 1   HCT : 32 %
ART. ENH. : 7.70   ART. RATE : 1.43   CO2 : 7.3 %

BP 185/100

BP 120/80

A

+ Dopamine [BP 140/72]

[BP 130/72]

B

FIG. 19-14 Effects of dopamine infusion on cerebral blood flow (CBF). Two examples of disparate effects of dopamine infusion of CBF in subarachnoid hemorrhage patients with vasospasm. CBF scale is indicated on the right in ml/100 g/min. Computed tomography images are indicated in the left figures and CBF maps in the right figures. Blood pressures before and after dopamine infusion are indicated. **A,** Dopamine infusion is associated with a general increase in CBF, whereas in **B,** it is associated with a decrease in CBF.

(From Kofke WA, Yonas H, Wechsler L: Neurologic intensive care. In Albin M, editor: *Textbook of neuroanesthesia*, New York, 1997, McGraw-Hill.)

associated with HHH therapy, thus reducing the risk of rebleeding.[316,317]

Blood Pressure Management. SAH is accompanied by a hyperadrenergic state.* This is one contributing factor to hypertension associated with SAH. There is a concern that hypertension predisposes patients to rebleed early after SAH with an unclipped aneurysm. There are ample data in animal studies to indicate that catecholamines are deleterious neurologically.[78,100,101,319] Sympatholytic drugs are used to treat hypertension in the absence of medical contraindications. They include β-adrenergic blocking drugs, trimethaphan, clonidine, methyldopa, and ACE inhibitors. Nicardipine and nimodipine are advantageous in

this setting because of limited data suggesting brain-protective effects.

If surgery is performed early, before vasospasm, blood pressure is treated immediately postoperatively when it exceeds 160 mm Hg. Because the likelihood of vasospasm increases with time postbleed (about 5-15 days), blood pressure is not treated unless hypertension is deleterious to the heart, lungs, or kidneys (240 mm Hg systolic pressure or 150 mm Hg MAP). Many patients spontaneously develop blood pressure in this range.

There is not a consensus regarding the most appropriate pressor to use for hypertensive therapy. Increasing cardiac output theoretically increases CBF, supporting the use of dobutamine and dopamine, but the physiologic basis for this is not clear. An alternative approach is to primarily use vasoconstrictor drugs such as phenyl-

*References 104, 105, 153, 210, 218-220, 246, 318.

ephrine or norepinephrine, because rCBF in vasospastic areas varies primarily as a function of perfusion pressure. Each drug that is a neurotransmitter or neurotransmitter analog has unique effects on the cerebral vasculature independent of blood pressure or cardiac output effects, which vary according to permeability of the BBB. Darby et al[300] demonstrated highly disparate rCBF effects within the brain of individual subjects with SAH and between subjects with SAH. Further work is needed to properly decide the most appropriate drug to use and to ascertain whether outcome is actually improved with catecholamine infusion with SAH.

Head Trauma

Pathophysiology. Head trauma results in abnormalities of brain anatomy, perfusion, metabolism, and function. The initial impact of closed head trauma results in mechanical disruption of the integrity of cellular and supporting tissue membranes.[320-322] Numerous secondary phenomena follow the initial event that worsen the patient's condition.[323-327] As a consequence of the trauma, blood and edema fluid accumulate as normal compartmentation is disrupted. Consequent to vascular disruption and the accumulating edema, secondary ischemia then assumes primary pathophysiologic importance. As ischemia develops, a variety of adverse biochemical processes occur because of the mechanical disruption. These processes are secondarily exacerbated by ischemia and with a positive feedback cycle, the sequelae of ischemia worsen. These biochemical events include release of free radicals[328] with lipid peroxidation, excitatory amino acid release,[329,330] inflammatory mediators,[331] metabolic acidosis,[332,333] and others that worsen the neurologic outcome. Microcirculatory disturbances occur related to edema, BBB disruption, and abnormalities in substances that regulate blood flow. It is thought that areas of vasospasm are related to the presence of free blood in the CSF or locally near parenchymal blood vessels.[334]

CBF goes through several phases over time after a closed head injury.[323,335-339] Initially CBF is depressed, subsequently becoming hyperemic. CBF returns to normal with resolution of membrane abnormalities or progresses to zero with infarction as hyperemia exacerbates the edema.

The intracranial volume of blood and brain tissue increases with edema and hemorrhage. ICP rises.[327,338,340] Regional and/or global ICP increases progressively as edema worsens, resulting in lower CBF (oligemic form of intracranial hypertension) that clearly leads to permanent brain damage. Patients with head injury also exhibit cerebral dysautoregulation with altered intracranial compliance that results in hyperemia and manifests as high ICP (hyperemic intracranial hypertension). Hyperemic intracranial hypertension is exacerbated by in-

creased blood pressure (producing distension of injured vasculature), fever, cerebral stimulants, cerebral vasodilators, and noxious or painful stimuli. Hyperemic intracranial hypertension does not have the same dire significance as oligemic intracranial hypertension with respect to whole brain function because of elevated CBF. Intracranial hypertension at high levels may produce regional exacerbation of the brain damage, ultimately sustained in edematous brain areas with tenuous perfusion. The pathophysiology of hyperperfusion exacerbates the neurologic damage.

Mechanical effects of brain injury have a major impact on the ultimate outcome. Categories of structural abnormalities include penetrating injury, hematoma effects, contusion, and white matter shear. The specific effects of such anatomic disruption depend to a great extent on the anatomic location. Isolated cortical or white matter lesions tend to produce focal deficits. Injuries to the midbrain and hindbrain or diffuse and bilateral injuries to the cerebral hemispheres produce global effects on the level of consciousness. Penetrating injury produces irreversible structural abnormalities, whereas the effects of contusion and hematoma produce abnormalities that may resolve with resolution of the lesion. White matter shear occurs as a result of inertia between brain tissue, thereby disrupting neural circuitry.[341,342] These lesions are associated with petechial lesions on CT scan, but are not always evident. The diagnosis then depends on the clinical scenario with less clinical improvement than expected based on initial imaging studies.

Therapy. Therapy for head trauma entails good medical management to maintain nutritive perfusion, procedures to facilitate monitoring, and procedures to decompress the brain. Medical management encompasses optimal oxygenation, ventilation, temperature, perfusion pressure, and glycemia. Monitoring procedures include invasive monitoring to ascertain ICP, including insertion of devices such as subdural bolts, camino monitors, and ventriculostomy catheters. Decompressive procedures include resection of edematous or injured tissues, removal of foreign bodies, repair of depressed skull fractures, drainage of hematomas, and craniectomy.

Blood Pressure Management. Blood pressure issues are similar to those discussed earlier in the context of high ICP. MAP is maintained at 80 to 100 mm Hg to avoid plateau waves.

Pituitary Tumors

Pathophysiology. Pituitary tumors usually arise as discrete nodules in the anterior part of the gland. Tumors less than 1 cm in diameter are microadenomas, and larger tumors are adenomas. Medical problems arise when the tumor enlarges to produce a significant mass effect, or more commonly, when the neoplastic tissue secretes pituitary hormones free of normal homeostatic auto feedback control.

Therapy. Many smaller pituitary tumors are treated pharmacologically or with radiation. Surgery becomes the principal therapy if noninvasive therapy is not effective or there are immediate concerns regarding mass effect. A transsphenoidal approach is used if the tumor is small enough and positioned appropriately to allow safe removal. If the tumor has significant suprasellar extension, then a frontal craniotomy is performed.

Issues in Management of Cardiovascular Problems. Perioperatively, careful observation for the development of diabetes insipidus (DI) is indicated. Left undetected, DI leads to life-threatening hypernatremia and hypovolemic shock. Prompt therapy is required as soon as the diagnosis is made.

Awake patients complain of severe thirst.[343] Profound diuresis may be the first sign in the noncommunicative patient, often in excess of 1 L per hour. Patients also develop progressive hypernatremia that may exceed 170 mEq/L with hypovolemia. Other signs of hypernatremia include restlessness, irritability, ataxia, increased muscle tone, hyperreflexia, seizures, and intracranial hemorrhage.[344]

DI is diagnosed by hyperosmolar serum (mOsm >285), a urine specific gravity close to 1.000, and urine osmolarity less than 200 mOsm with little or variable sodium in the urine.[345] Incomplete DI exhibits intermediate values of urine and serum electrolytes.[345,346]

Serial plasma sodium concentrations are determined every 6 hours in the appropriate setting in which DI is considered. The frequency is increased if sodium is elevated or rising. If the patient is diuresing 1 L/hr, hourly sodium levels are required until the sodium becomes elevated, whereupon urine osmolarity and specific gravity are obtained with simultaneous serum sodium and osmolarity to establish the diagnosis unequivocally.

Patients are at high risk to develop temporary or permanent DI after pituitary surgery.[299,347,348] Fifty percent develop transient DI lasting 3 to 5 days, 33% develop permanent DI, and 33% develop a triphasic courses. The initially substantial diuresis lasts 12 to 24 hours. As ADH previously synthesized is released, the DI will appear to resolve with a risk of iatrogenic hyponatremia secondary to treatment of the initial DI. This phase recedes as fully established DI appears, which may or may not be permanent.[349]

Other causes of perioperative polyuria are considered, notably mannitol, excessive fluids, or hyperglycemia. These conditions differ from DI in that the urine specific gravity and osmolarity are higher than observed with DI.

Once the diagnosis of DI is made, therapy is initiated with either DDAVP (desmopressin) or vasopressin. DDAVP is administered 1 to 4 μg every 12 to 24 hours via intravenous, subcutaneous, or intramuscular routes. The specific dosage interval is determined by the resumption of polyuria. Vasopressin 5 to 10 units IM is given every 4 to 6 hours or as dictated by the occurrence of polyuria. Some authors recommend a more titratable continuous infusion of low-dose vasopressin to avoid overtreatment. Therapeutic effects last only 3 hours after cessation of infusion.[350,351]

Other perioperative concerns with pituitary surgery are related to loss of adrenocortical function. Prophylactic use of stress steroid coverage with hydrocortisone 100 mg is indicated every 8 hours.

Pituitary surgery for acromegaly requires consideration of the sequelae of prolonged growth hormone secretion. These include airway abnormalities, hypertension, cardiomegaly, glucose intolerance, and fluid balance abnormalities. A recent retrospective review indicated that such problems, although present in patients with acromegaly, do not pose significant difficulty with perioperative management.[352] Airway difficulties are a known risk for patients with acromegaly. If not fully awake at the end of surgery, these patients must be fully awake after anesthesia before extubation is performed. Hypertension predisposes these patients to blood pressure lability, although a recent retrospective review suggested that this is not a major intraoperative problem.[352] Preoperative evaluation of cardiovascular function is indicated to determine any ventricular dysfunction that makes fluid management more challenging in these patients.

Tumors and Tumor Surgery

Pathophysiology. The incidence of primary brain tumors is estimated to be 15 per 100,000 and of secondary brain tumors 46 per 100,000. The presenting symptoms are understood by using principles of physics and physiology. Tumors become symptomatic from high ICP or from local effects causing a neurologic deficit. A tumor leads to decreased consciousness by uncal transtentorial herniation, direct infiltration of the reticular activating system, hydrocephalus, seizures with a postictal condition, and intratumor bleeding.[353] Peritumor vasogenic edema exacerbates the effects of a tumor mass and is common with brain tumors.[354]

Patients exhibit personality or behavioral changes, headaches, papilledema, and vomiting as ICP increases. Twenty percent to fifty percent of patients with brain tumors develop seizures.[354]

Intracranial tumors require resection when they become symptomatic or are thought to be malignant. Therapy to reduce ICP or other mass effects is often used preoperatively, including steroids for vasogenic edema and mannitol or furosemide to reduce ICP.

Perioperatively, the major neurologic concerns are new hematoma, brain edema, hydrocephalus, and retractor-mediated deficits. Postoperative neurologic deterioration can be caused by any of these problems, mandating urgent CT scan to elucidate the cause and need for neurosurgical intervention. Hematomas most often occur within the first 6 hours after surgery and are usually on the operative site.[355,356] Posterior fossa hematoma is most notable, leading to abrupt and severe neurologic deterioration. Urgent therapy is required because patients have the greatest chance for recovery if decompression occurs quickly. They die from brainstem ischemia if hematoma evacuation is prolonged.[357] This justifies the occasional practice of performing a decompressive opening of the surgical wound in the neuro intensive care unit (NICU).

Blood Pressure Management. Postoperative hypertension is common after tumor resection, predisposing patients to postoperative hematoma. Control of blood pressure is very important for avoiding this complication. Hypertension is treated after other causes of postoperative hypertension are considered, such as hypercarbia, bladder distension, shivering, and pain. Vasodilator drugs such as nitroprusside or hydralazine are used if ICP is low after extensive tumor decompression. If there is concern that the ICP remains elevated or may become elevated, vasodilators are avoided when possible. Treatment for hypertension commonly uses labetalol, nifedipine, or nicardipine.

Brain Death
Pathophysiology
Definition. A person with irreversible cessation of all functions of the entire brain, including the brain stem, is dead.[358-360] Conceptually this definition is straightforward. The diagnosis of brain death must be cautiously approached by virtue of the beating heart and known situations that can imitate brain death. Numerous guidelines for determining brain death have been published.[361-363] No single set of specific diagnostic criteria is universally accepted or enacted by federal or international legislation.[363] Many authoritative groups use their own criteria.

Most brain death criteria share the following specific requirements: (1) establish irremediable structural damage; (2) exclude reversible causes of unresponsiveness; (3) demonstrate unresponsiveness and absence of brainstem function with a clinical examination; (4) verify with laboratory studies; and (5) retest over time to confirm an unchanging condition.

Patient History. An irremediable cause of brain death is established that accounts for the irreversible cessation of all brain function without resorting to angiography. The patient's history provides essential information that determines the appropriate tests for confirming the diagnosis. The history also reveals circumstances (e.g., drug use, anesthetic administration) or medical history (e.g., endocrine abnormalities or severe lung disease) that provide information to properly perform brain death certification.

Issues in Management of Cardiovascular Problems. Once brain death is confirmed, therapy is directed toward preservation and enhancement of donor organs. This issue has been nicely reviewed by Powner et al.[364] Previous treatment priorities are reversed or reconsidered in light of this new overall treatment goal. For example, the hyperosmolarity of the intravascular fluid used to treat the brain edema is no longer appropriate and may be undesirable during preparation for organ removal. New physiologic changes occur after brain death that must be anticipated, prevented, or treated. Patient care following brain death is not static and often presents major challenges.

The primary treatment goal during preparation for organ procurement is to maintain optimal intravascular volume and the delivery of oxygen and nutrients to the donor organs. Appropriate fluid supplementation and monitoring techniques are coordinated with members of the transplantation team. Issues include which artery to cannulate, desirability or need for pulmonary artery catheterization, arrhythmia management (atropine is ineffective), and type of fluid to administer.

Experimental and clinical evidence indicates that donor organs are harmed during hormonal changes after head injury and during the evolution of brain death.[365-367] Damage to these organs may cause them to fail in the donor patient. A higher incidence of early nonimmunologically mediated primary organ failure in the recipient follows. Current estimates indicate that 4% to 10% of transplanted hearts, for example, fail in the recipient soon after implantation for unexplained reasons.[368]

Abnormalities in cardiac biopsy specimens from human donors are reported.[369] These abnormalities correlate with an increased need for inotropic support and increased mortality rate among recipients. A myocytolytic cardiac lesion is also reported[370] in patients suffering a variety of intracranial insults, although the relationship of brain death to myocardial performance was not discussed. Serial liver biopsies after brain death in humans show histologic changes characteristic of central venous congestion in a majority of specimens. Changes consisting of fibrosis, cholangitis, piecemeal necrosis, and fatty metamorphosis were minimal at the time of brain death, but are prominent days later.[371]

Novitsky et al[372] studied hemodynamic events in the baboon after sudden cerebral herniation and brain death caused by abrupt inflation of a subdural balloon. Initial increases in ICP were associated with systemic hypertension, sinus bradycardia, and atrioventricular dissociation. Additional rises in ICP precipitated elevated left atrial pressure, PCWP, systemic vascular resistance, and further increases in systemic blood pressure. Aortic blood flow decreased and pulmonary edema developed, presumably because of the high systemic vascular resistance. Supraventricular and ventricular arrhythmias were also observed during this hypertensive phase. Histologic changes in the heart were noted, consisting of myocardial fiber disorganization and contraction bands.[373]

Novitsky et al hypothesized that catecholamine release from the injured brain and an accentuated discharge of the sympathetic nervous system causes severe vasoconstriction, ischemia, and histologic lesions in various organs, especially the heart.[374] Myocardial lesions are eliminated or reduced by pretreatment with a calcium channel blocker[375] or β-receptor blocker[372] and after cardiac sympathectomy[376] in a small number of animals. Similar in vivo and in vitro cardiac dysfunction was demonstrated in an ischemic brain death model in pigs[377] and dogs,[378] but data in humans are lacking.

Many clinical scenarios are consistent with Novitsky et al observed general pattern of hemodynamic change observed during brain death. The patient's cardiovascular system is often stable after acute resuscitation from the primary brain injury. As deterioration of the patient's neurologic condition ensues despite therapeutic measures, a period of remarkable arterial hypertension develops that lasts for 1 or 2 hours. Tachycardia and arrhythmias occur but are usually not life threatening.[379] Cerebral herniation likely occurs during the hypertensive period, and brain death is diagnosed shortly thereafter. Neurologic function present during the hypertensive period erodes as the patient's blood pressure falls. Profound hypotension may occur precipitously, and be refractory to fluid infusion, inotropic support, and α-adrenergic receptor stimulation.[379-382] This hypotension is caused by loss of sympathetic discharge from the brain, leading to arterial vasodilation and relative hypovolemia.[380,383] Other theories include reduced endogenous catecholamine production[380,384] and the stress-induced release of endorphins, for which naloxone administration has been suggested.[385] Although episodic elevations in blood pressure and heart rate may subsequently occur because of a spinal cord nociceptive reflex,[386] the brain-dead patient often remains hypotensive.

Treatment during brain death development is challenging. Vasoactive drugs that produce general or regional vasoconstriction are avoided, including norepinephrine, high-dose dopamine, and phenylephrine. Dopamine infusion at dosages of 10 μg/kg/min do not harm the human donor heart,[368] but dosages exceeding 15 μg/kg/min harmed the liver in a brain-dead dog preparation.[387] Dopamine may or may not be harmful to the donor pancreas[388,389] or kidney[390] in the human. Iwai et al[391] reported that a combination of intravenous vasopressin (Pitressin) at 1 to 2 units/hr and epinephrine are most helpful in treating hypotension and avoiding cardiac arrest.

Hypotension resolves over time, and pressor support is often reduced. This cycle of low perfusion followed by normal perfusion, with or without medicinal support, implies that a subsequent reperfusion type of injury occurs in organs.[392] Agents that reduce formation of free radicals and free radical scavengers have been proposed to minimize organ damage.[392,393]

Several animal and human studies demonstrate changes in circulating hormones and endocrine gland function. Novitzky et al[394] found low levels of triiodothyronine, thyroxine, cortisol, and insulin in a baboon model of brain death. Similar changes in circulating thyroid hormone levels were documented in brain-dead humans,[395-397] although insulin and cortisol levels were low, normal, or increased. The proposed benefits of hormonal therapy have been reviewed,[398] and are considered controversial.

These experimental data and clinical observations provide options in patient care that are considered experimental because they are untested and directed toward donor organ care in a patient who is not yet brain dead. Careful invasive vascular monitoring, titrated β-adrenergic receptor blockade, intravascular volume expansion or restriction, calcium channel blockers, agents that scavenge or reduce the production of free radicals, and intracellular buffers of acidosis, all remain possible untested techniques for use in cases of anticipated brain death and organ donation.

KEY POINTS

1. The brain, spinal cord, CSF, and blood are encased in the protecting but noncompliant skull and cerebral canal, constituting a nearly incompressible system.
2. There are two types of intracranial hypertension, categorized according to CBF as hyperemic or oligemic.
3. Low blood pressure can increase ICP, causing plateau waves via normal autoregulatory vasodilation.
4. Systemic hypertension can increase ICP through distension and hydrostatic edema in vasoparalyzed tissue.
5. PEEP increases ICP primarily through decreased systemic blood pressure.
6. Vasodilators should be avoided in patients with intracranial hypertension.

7. Sympatholytic drugs are preferable when there is a risk of cerebral ischemia or intracranial hypertension.

8. Intracranial processes can be associated with significant cardiac problems.

KEY REFERENCES

Cushing H: Concerning a definite regulatory mechanism of the vaso-motor centre which controls blood pressure during cerebral compression, *Johns Hopkins Hospital Bulletin* 126: 290, 1901.

Drummond JC, Patel PM, Cole DJ et al: The effect of the reduction of colloid oncotic pressure, with and without reduction of osmolality, on post-traumatic cerebral edema, *Anesthesiology* 88:993, 1998.

Huseby JS, Luce JM, Cary JM et al: Effects of positive end expiratory pressure on intracranial pressure in dogs with intracranial hypertension, *J Neurosurg* 55:704, 1981.

Lundberg N: Continuous recording and control of ventricular fluid pressure in neurosurgical practice, *Acta Psychiatr Scand* 36(suppl 149):1, 1960.

Marion DW, Segal R, Thompson ME: Subarachnoid hemorrhage and the heart, *Neurosurgery* 18:101, 1986.

Michenfelder JD: The 27th Rovenstine Lecture: neuroanesthesia and the achievement of professional respect, *Anesthesiology* 70:695, 1989.

Miller JD, Becker DP, Ward JD et al: Significance of intracranial hypertension in severe head injury, *J Neurosurg* 47:503, 1977.

Myers MG, Norris JW, Hachinski VC et al: Cardiac sequelae of acute stroke, *Stroke* 13:838, 1982.

Neil-Dwyer G, Walter P, Cruickshank JM: Beta-blockade benefits patients following a subarachnoid hemorrhage, *Eur J Clin Pharmacol* 28(suppl A):25, 1985.

Olesen J: The effect of intracarotid epinephrine, norepinephrine, and angiotensin on the regional CBF in man, *Neurology* 22:978, 1972.

Powers WJ: Acute hypertension after stroke: the scientific basis for treatment decisions, *Neurology* 43:461, 1993.

Raichle ME, Plum F: Hyperventilation and CBF, *Stroke* 3:566, 1972.

Rosner MJ, Becker DP: Origin and evolution of plateau waves. Experimental observations and a theoretical model, *J Neurosurg* 50:312, 1984.

Van Aken H, Puchstein C, Schweppe M-L et al: Effect of labetalol on intracranial pressure in dogs with and without intracranial hypertension, *Acta Anaesthesiol Scand* 26:615, 1982.

Werner C, Hoffman WE, Thomas C et al: Ganglionic blockade improves neurologic outcome from incomplete ischemia in rats: partial reversal by exogenous catecholamines, *Anesthesiology* 73:923, 1990.

References

1. Cushing H: Concerning a definite regulatory mechanism of the vaso-motor centre which controls blood pressure during cerebral compression, *Johns Hopkins Hospital Bulletin* 126: 290, 1901.

2. Risberg J, Lundberg N, Ingvar DH: Regional cerebral blood volume during acute rises in the intracranial pressure (plateau waves), *J Neurosurg* 31:303, 1969.

3. Rosner MJ, Becker DP: Origin and evolution of plateau waves. Experimental observations and a theoretical model, *J Neurosurg* 50:312, 1984.

4. Miller JD, Becker DP, Ward JD et al: Significance of intracranial hypertension in severe head injury, *J Neurosurg* 47:503, 1977.

5. Giulioni M, Ursino M, Alvisi C: Correlations among intracranial pulsatility, intracranial hemodynamics, and transcranial Doppler wave form: literature review and hypothesis for future studies, *Neurosurgery* 22:807, 1988.

6. Hassler W, Steinmetz H, Gawlowski J: Transcranial Doppler ultrasonography in raised intracranial pressure and in intracranial circulatory arrest, *J Neurosurg* 68:745, 1988.

7. Klatzo I: Evolution of brain edema concepts, *Acta Neurochir Suppl (Wien)*, 60:3-6, 1994.

8. von Haken MS, Aschoff AA: Acute obstructive hydrocephalus. In Hacke W, Hanley DF, Einhaupl KM et al, editors: *Neurocritical care*, New York, 1994, Springer-Verlag, p 869.

9. Bederson JB, Wiestler OD, Brustle O et al: Intracranial venous hypertension and the effects of venous outflow obstruction in a rat model of arteriovenous fistula, *Neurosurgery* 29:341-350, 1991.

10. Kofke WA, Dong ML, Bloom M et al: Transcranial Doppler ultrasonography with induction of anesthesia for neurosurgery, *J Neurosurg Anesthesiol* 6:89, 1994.

11. Michenfelder JD: The 27th rovenstine lecture: neuroanesthesia and the achievement of professional respect, *Anesthesiology* 70: 695, 1989.

12. Jaggi JL, Obrist WD, Gennarelli TA et al: Relationship of early CBF and metabolism to outcome in acute head injury, *J Neurosurg* 72:176, 1990.

13. Pierce EC, Lambertsen CJ, Deutsch S: Cerebral circulation and metabolism during thiopental anesthesia and hyperventilation in man, *J Clin Invest* 41:1664-1671, 1962.

14. Marshall LF, Shapiro HM, Rauscher A et al: Pentobarbital therapy for intracranial hypertension in metabolic coma. Reye's syndrome, *Crit Care Med* 6:1-5, 1978.

15. Hartung HJ: Intracranial pressure after propofol and thiopental administration in patients with severe head trauma, *Anaesthetist* 36:285-287, 1987.

16. Larsen R, Hilfiker O, Radle J et al: The effects of midazolam on the general circulation, the CBF and cerebral oxygen consumption in man, *Anaesthetist* 30:18-21, 1981.

17. Renou AM, Vernhiet J, Macrez P et al: CBF and metabolism during etomidate anaesthesia in man, *Br J Anaesth* 50: 1047-1051, 1978.

18. Prior JGL, Hinds CJ, Williams J et al: The use of etomidate in the management of severe head injury, *Int Care Med* 9:313-320, 1983.

19. Vandesteene A, Trempont V, Engelman E et al: Effect of propofol on CBF and metabolism in man, *Anaesthesia* 43(suppl):42-43, 1988.

20. Sakabe T, Maekawa T, Ishikawa T et al: The effects of lidocaine on canine metabolism and circulation related to the electroencephalogram, *Anesthesiology* 40:433-441, 1974.

21. Yano M, Nishiyama H, Yokota H et al: Effect of lidocaine on ICP response to endotracheal suctioning, *Anesthesiology* 64:651-653, 1986.

22. Raichle ME, Posner JB, Plum F: CBF during and after hyperventilation, *Arch Neuro* 23:3, 1970.

23. Lassen NA: Control of cerebral circulation in health and disease, *Circ Res* 34:749, 1974.

24. Shapiro HM: Intracranial hypertension: therapeutic and anesthetic considerations, *Anesthesiology* 43:445, 1975.

25. Shenkin HA, Bouzarth WF: Clinical methods of reducing intracranial pressure, *N Engl J Med* 282:1465, 1970.

26. Raichle ME, Plum F: Hyperventilation and CBF, *Stroke* 3:566, 1972.

27. Neill WA, Hattenhauer M: Impairment of myocardial O_2 supply due to hyperventilation, *Circulation* 52:854-858, 1975.

28. Samuelsson RG, Nagy G: Effects of respiratory alkalosis and acidosis on myocardial excitation, *Acta Physiol Scand* 97:158-165, 1976.

29. Kazmaier S, Weyland A, Buhre W et al: Effects of respiratory alkalosis and acidosis on myocardial blood flow and metabolism in patients with coronary artery disease, *Anesthesiology* 89:831-837, 1998.

30. Onishi K, Sekioka K, Ishisu R et al: Decrease in oxygen cost of contractility during hypocapnic alkalosis in canine hearts, *Am J Physiol* 270:H1905-1913, 1996.

31. Minoda K, Yasue H, Kugiyama K et al: Comparison of the distribution of myocardial blood flow between exercise-induced and hyperventilation-induced attacks of coronary spasm: a study with thallium-201 myocardial scintigraphy, *Am Heart J* 127:1474-1480, 1994.

32. Fujii H, Yasue H, Okumura K et al: Hyperventilation-induced simultaneous multivessel coronary spasm in patients with variant angina: an echocardiographic and arteriographic study, *J Am Coll Cardiol* 12:1184-1192, 1988.

33. Rasmussen K, Juul S, Bagger JP et al: Usefulness of ST deviation induced by prolonged hyperventilation as a predictor of cardiac death in angina pectoris, *Am J Cardiol* 59:763-768, 1987.

34. Roberts LA, Hughes MJ: Chronotropic response of spontaneously beating rabbit atria to hyperosmotic media, *Am J Physiol* 233:H228-233, 1977.

35. Wilson GJ, Axford-Gatley RA, Bush BG et al: European versus North American cardioplegia: comparison of Bretschneider's and Roe's cardioplegic solutions in a canine model of cardiopulmonary bypass, *Thorac Cardiovasc Surg* 38:10-14, 1990.

36. Dunphy G, Richter HW, Azodi M et al: The effects of mannitol, albumin, and cardioplegia enhancers on 24-h rat heart preservation, *Am J Physiol* 276:H1591-1598, 1999.

37. Hutton I, Marynick SP, Fixler DE et al: Changes in regional coronary blood flow with hypertonic mannitol in conscious dogs, *Cardiovasc Res* 9:47-55, 1975.

38. Willerson JT, Curry GC, Atkins JM et al: Influence of hypertonic mannitol on ventricular performance and coronary blood flow in patients, *Circulation* 51:1095-1100, 1975.

39. Hutton I, Curry GC, Templeton GH et al: Influence of hypertonic mannitol on regional myocardial blood flow and ventricular performance in awake, intact dogs with prolonged coronary artery occlusion, *Cardiovasc Res* 9:409-419, 1975.

40. Willerson JT, Watson JT, Hutton I et al: The influence of hypertonic mannitol on regional myocardial blood flow during acute and chronic myocardial ischemia in anesthetized and awake intact dogs, *J Clin Invest* 55:892-902, 1975.

41. Magovern, Jr, GJ, Bolling SF, Casale AS et al: The mechanism of mannitol in reducing ischemic injury: hyperosmolarity or hydroxyl scavenger? *Circulation* 70:I91-95, 1984.

42. Justicz AG, Farnsworth WV, Soberman MS et al: Reduction of myocardial infarct size by poloxamer 188 and mannitol in a canine model, *Am Heart J* 122:671-680, 1991.

43. Powell, Jr, WJ, DiBona DR, Flores J et al: The protective effect of hyperosmotic mannitol in myocardial ischemia and necrosis, *Circulation* 54:603-615, 1976.

44. Gardner TJ, Stewart JR, Casale AS et al: Reduction of myocardial ischemic injury with oxygen-derived free radical scavengers, *Surgery* 94:423-427, 1983.

45. Gauduel Y, Duvelleroy MA: Role of oxygen radicals in cardiac injury due to reoxygenation, *J Mol Cell Cardiol* 16:459-470, 1984.

46. Pine MB, Brooks WW, Nosta JJ et al: Hydrostatic forces limit swelling of rat ventricular myocardium, *Am J Physiol* 241:H740-747, 1981.

47. Kahles H, Hellige G, Hunnemann DH et al: Different effects of interventions suppressing free fatty acid metabolism on myocardial ischemia, *Clin Cardiol* 7:341-348, 1984.

48. Carlson RE, Aisen AM, Buda A: Effect of reduction in myocardial edema on myocardial blood flow and ventricular function after coronary reperfusion, *Am J Physiol* 262:H641-648, 1992.

49. Harada RN, Limm W, Piette LH et al: Failure of mannitol to reduce myocardial infarct size in the baboon, *Cardiovasc Res* 26:893-896, 1992.

50. Woodward B, Zakaria MN: Effect of some free radical scavengers on reperfusion induced arrhythmias in the isolated rat heart, *J Mol Cell Cardiol* 17:485-493, 1985.

51. Lundberg N: Continuous recording and control of ventricular fluid pressure in neurosurgical practice, *Acta Psychiatr Scand* 36(suppl 149):1, 1960.

52. Matakas F, Von Waechter R, Knupling R et al: Increase in cerebral perfusion pressure by arterial hypertension in brain swelling. A mathematical model of the volume-pressure relationship, *J Neurosurg* 42:282,1975.

53. Shapiro HM, Marshall LF: Intracranial pressure responses to PEEP in head-injured patients, *J Trauma* 18:254, 1978.

54. Gupta AK, Gupta S, Swart M et al: Comparison of brain tissue oxygen with jugular venous oxygen saturation during hyperventilation in head-injured patients, *J Neurosurg Anesth* 9:399, 1997 (abstract).

55. Aidinis SJ, Lafferty J, Shapiro HM: Intracranial responses to PEEP, *Anesthesiology* 45:275-286, 1976.

56. Harken AH, Brennan MF, Smith B et al: The hemodynamic response to positive end-expiratory ventilation in hypovolemic patients, *Surgery* 76:786-793, 1974.

57. Huseby JS, Luce JM, Cary JM et al: Effects of positive end expiratory pressure on intracranial pressure in dogs with intracranial hypertension, *J Neurosurg* 55:704, 1981.

58. Griswold WR, Roznik V, Mendoza SA: Nitroprusside induced intracranial hypertension, *JAMA* 246:2679, 1981.

59. Overgaard J, Skinhoj E: A paradoxical cerebral hemodynamic effect of hydralazine, *Stroke* 6:402, 1975.

60. Marsh ML, Shapiro HM, Smith RW et al: Changes in neurologic status and intracranial pressure associated with sodium nitroprusside administration, *Anesthesiology* 51:336, 1979.

61. Dohi S, Matsumoto M, Takahashi K: The effects of nitroglycerin on cerebrospinal fluid pressure in awake and anesthetized humans, *Anesthesiology* 54:511, 1981.

62. Hirayama T, Katayama Y, Kano T et al: Control of systemic hypertension with diltiazem, a calcium-antagonist, in patients with a mildly elevated intracranial pressure: a comparative study, *Neurol Res* 16:97-99, 1994.

63. Hayashi M, Kobashi H, Kawano H et al: Treatment of systemic hypertension and intracranial hypertension and intracranial hypertension in cases of brain hemorrhage, *Stroke* 19:314, 1988.

64. Van Aken H, Puchstein C, Schweppe M-L et al: Effect of labetalol on intracranial pressure in dogs with and without intracranial hypertension, *Acta Anaesth Scand* 26:615, 1982.
65. Stanek B, Zimpfer M, Fitzal S et al: Plasma catecholamines, plasma renin activity and haemodynamics during sodium nitroprusside-induced hypotension and additional beta-blockage with bunitrolol, *Eur J Clin Pharmacol* 19:317, 1981.
66. Werner C, Hoffman WE, Thomas C et al: Ganglionic blockade improves neurologic outcome from incomplete ischemia in rats: partial reversal by exogenous catecholamines, *Anesthesiology* 73:923, 1990.
67. Neil-Dwyer G, Walter P, Cruickshank JM: Beta-blockade benefits patients following a subarachnoid hemorrhage, *Eur J Clin Pharmacol* 28(A:suppl):25, 1985.
68. Hoffman WE, Kochs E, Werner C et al: Dexmedetomidine improves neurologic outcome from incomplete ischemia in the rat. Reversal by the alpha 2-adrenergic antagonist atipamezole, *Anesthesiology* 75(A:2):328, 1991.
69. Henriks C, Harmsen A, Christensen P et al: Controlled hypotension with sodium nitroprusside: effects on cerebral blood flow and cerebral venous blood gases in patients operated for cerebral aneurysms, *Acta Anaesth Scand* 27:62-67,1983.
70. Hartmann A, Buttinger C, Rommel T et al: Alteration of intracranial pressure, cerebral blood flow, autoregulation and carbon dioxide-reactivity by hypotensive agents in baboons with intracranial hypertension, *Neurochirurgia* 32:37-43, 1989.
71. Cottrell JE, Patel KP, Ransahoff JR et al: Intracranial pressure changes induced by sodium nitroprusside in patients with intracranial mass lesions, *J Neurosurg* 48:329, 1978.
72. Weiss MH, Spence J, Apuzzo ML et al: Influence of nitroprusside on cerebral pressure autoregulation, *Neurosurgery* 4:56-59 1979.
73. Candia GJ, Heros RC, Lavyne MH et al: Effect of intravenous sodium nitroprusside on cerebral blood flow and intracranial pressure, *Neurosurgery* 3:50-53, 1978.
74. Theard MA, Cheng MA, Crowder CM et al: Control of blood pressure during intracranial procedures: comparison between nicardipine and nitroprusside, *J Neurosurg Anesth* 9:388, 1997.
75. Schmidt JF, Andersen AR, Paulson OB et al: Angiotensin converting enzyme inhibition, CBF autoregulation, and ICP in patients with normal-pressure hydrocephalus, *Acta Neurochir (Wien)* 106:9-12, 1990.
76. Cutler NR, Sramek JJ, Luna A et al: Effect of the ACE inhibitor ceronapril on cerebral blood flow in hypertensive patients, *Ann Pharmacother* 30:578-582, 1996.
77. Demolis P, Chalon S, Annane D et al: Effects of an angiotensin converting enzyme inhibitor, ramipril, on intracranial circulation in healthy volunteers, *Br J Clin Pharmacol* 34:224-230, 1992.
78. Hoffman WE, Kochs E, Werner C et al: Dexmedetomidine improves neurologic outcome from incomplete ischemia in the rat. Reversal by the alpha 2-adrenergic antagonist atipamezole, *Anesthesiology* 75:328, 1991.
79. Qureshi AI, Wilson DA, Hanley DF et al: Pharmacologic reduction of mean arterial pressure does not adversely affect regional cerebral blood flow and intracranial pressure in experimental intracerebral hemorrhage, *Crit Care Med* 27:965-971, 1999.
80. Orlowski JP, Shiesley D, Vidt DG et al: Labetalol to control blood pressure after cerebrovascular surgery, *Crit Care Med* 16:765-768, 1988.
81. Cottrell JE, Marlin AE: Furosemide and human head injury, *Journal of Trauma* 21:805-806, 1981.
82. Dahl A, Russell D, Nyberg-Hansen R: Effect of nitro-glycerin on cerebral circulation measured by transcranial Doppler and SPECT, *Stroke* 20:1773-1736, 1989.
83. Ohar JM, Fowler AA, Selhorst JB et al: Intravenous nitro-glycerin-induced intracranial hypertension, *Crit Care Med* 13:867-868, 1985.
84. Bedford RF, Dacey R, Winn H et al: Adverse impact of a calcium entry-blocker (verapamil) on intracranial pressure in patients with brain tumors, *J Neurosurg* 59:800-802, 1983.
85. Kakarieka A, Schakel EH, Fritze J: Clinical experiences with nimodipine in cerebral ischemia, *J Neural Transm Suppl* 43:13, 1994.
86. Rosenbaum D, Zabramski J, Frey J et al: Early treatment of ischemic stroke with a calcium antagonist, *Stroke* 22:437, 1991.
87. Anonymous: A multicenter trial of the efficacy of nimodipine on outcome after severe head injury. The European Study Group on Nimodipine in Severe Head Injury, *J Neurosurg* 80:797, 1994.
88. Pickard JD, Murray GD, Illingworth R et al: Effect of oral nimodipine on cerebral infarction and outcome after subarachnoid haemorrhage: British aneurysm nimodipine trial, *BMJ* 298:636, 1989.
89. Kucharczyk J, Chew W, Derugin N et al: Nicardipine reduces ischemic brain injury. Magnetic resonance imaging/spectroscopy study in cats, *Stroke* 20:268, 1989.
90. Alps BJ, Calder C, Hass WK et al: Comparative protective effects of nicardipine, flunarizine, lidoflazine and nimodipine against ischaemic injury in the hippocampus of the Mongolian gerbil, *Br J Pharmacol* 93:877, 1988.
91. Grotta J, Spydell J, Pettigrew C et al: The effect of nicardipine on neuronal function following ischemia, *Stroke* 17:213, 1986.
92. Bailey I, Bell A, Gray J et al: A trial of the effect of nimodipine on outcome after head injury, *Acta Neurochir (Wien)* 110:97-105, 1991.
93. Gueugniaud PY, Gaussorgues P, Garcia-Darennes F et al: Early effects of nimodipine on intracranial and cerebral perfusion pressures in cerebral anoxia after out-of-hospital cardiac arrest, *Resuscitation* 20:203-212, 1990.
94. Orlowski JP, Shiesley D, Vidt DG et al: Labetalol to control blood pressure after cerebrovascular surgery, *Crit Care Med* 16:765, 1988.
95. Van Aken H, Puchstein C, Schweppe M-L et al: Effect of labetalol on intracranial pressure in dogs with and without intracranial hypertension, *Acta Anaesth Scand* 26:615, 1982.
96. Drummond JC, Patel PM, Cole DJ et al: The effect of the reduction of colloid oncotic pressure, with and without reduction of osmolality, on post-traumatic cerebral edema, *Anesthesiology* 88:993-1002, 1998.
97. Olesen J, Hougard K, Hertz M. Isoproterenol and propranolol: ability to cross the blood-brain barrier and effects on cerebral circulation in man, *Stroke* 9:344, 1978.
98. Guell A, Geraud G, Jauzac P et al. Effects of a dopaminergic agonist (pirlbedil) on CBF in man, *J Cereb Blood Flow Metab* 2:255, 1982.
99. Olesen J: The effect of intracarotid epinephrine, norepinephrine, and angiotensin on the regional CBF in man, *Neurology* 22:978-987, 1972.
100. Werner C, Hoffman WE, Thomas C et al: Ganglionic blockade improves neurologic outcome from incomplete ischemia in rats: partial reversal by exogenous catecholamines, *Anesthesiology* 73:923, 1990.
101. Werner C, Hoffman WE, Kochs E et al: Captopril improves neurologic outcome from incomplete cerebral ischemia in rats, *Stroke* 22:910, 1991.
102. Yoshida K, Watanabe H, Nakamura S: Intraarterial injection of amrinone for vasospasm induced by subarachnoid hemorrhage, *AJNR* 18:492-496, 1997.
103. Harris AL, Grant AM, Silver PJ et al: Differential vasorelaxant effects of milrinone and amrinone on contractile responses of canine coronary, cerebral, and renal arteries, *J Cardiovasc Pharmacol* 13:238-244, 1989.
104. Marion DW, Segal R, Thompson ME: Subarachnoid hemorrhage and the heart, *Neurosurgery* 18:101, 1986.

105. DiPasquale G, Pinelli G, Andreoli A et al: Forsade de pointes and ventricular flutter-fibrillation following spontaneous cerebral subarachnoid hemorrhage, *Int J Cardiol* 18:163, 1988.

106. Estanol Vidal B, Badui Dergal E, Cesarman E et al: Cardiac arrhythmias associated with subarachnoid hemorrhage: prospective study, *Neurosurgery* 5:675, 1979.

107. Neil-Dwyer G, Walter P, Shaw HJH et al: Plasma renin activity in patients after a subarachnoid hemorrhage: a possible predictor of outcome, *Neurosurgery* 7:578, 1980.

108. Myers MG, Norris JW, Hachinski VC et al: Plasma norepinephrine in stroke, *Stroke* 12:200, 1981.

109. Smith D, Orkin FK, Gardner SM et al: Prolonged sedation in the elderly after intraoperative atropine administration, *Anesthesiology* 51:348-349, 1979.

110. Sakabe T, Maekawa T, Ishikawa T et al: The effects of lidocaine on canine cerebral metabolism and circulation related to the electroencephalogram, *Anesthesiology* 40:433-441, 1974.

111. Bedford RF, Persing JA, Pobereskin L et al: Lidocaine or thiopental for rapid control of intracranial hypertension? *Anesth Analg* 59:435-437, 1980.

112. Evans DE, Kobrine AI: Reduction of experimental intracranial hypertension by lidocaine, *Neurosurgery* 20:542-547, 1987.

113. Chiang YY, Tseng KF, Lih YW et al: Lidocaine-induced CNS toxicity: a case report, *Acta Anaesthesiol Sin* 34:243-246, 1996.

114. Fujitani T, Adachi N, Miyazaki H et al: Lidocaine protects hippocampal neurons against ischemic damage by preventing increase of extracellular excitatory amino acids: a microdialysis study in Mongolian gerbils, *Neurosci Lett* 179:91-94, 1994.

115. Wolf PA, Cobb JL, D'Agostino RB: Epidemiology of stroke. In Barnett HJM, Mohr JP, Stein BM et al, editors: *Stroke: pathophysiology, diagnosis, and management,* ed 2, New York, 1992, Churchill Livingstone, pp 3-29.

116. Rossen R, Kabat H, Anderson JP: Acute arrest of cerebral circulation in man, *Arch Neurol Psychiatr* 50:510, 1943.

117. Michenfelder JD, Theye RA: The effects of anesthesia and hypothermia on canine cerebral ATP and lactate during anoxia produced by decapitation, *Anesthesiology* 33:430, 1970.

118. Hossmann K-A, Sato K: The effect of ischemia on sensorimotor cortex of the cat. Electrophysiological, biochemical, and electronmicroscopical observations, *J Neurol* 198:33, 1970.

119. Kleihues P, Kobayashi K, Hossmann K-A: Purine nucleotide metabolism in the cat brain after one hour of complete ischemia, *J Neurochem* 23:417, 1974.

120. Kleihues P, Hossmann K-A, Pegg AE: Resuscitation of the monkey brain after 1 hour complete ischemia. III. Indications of metabolic recovery, *Brain Res* 95:61, 1975.

121. Ljunggren B, Ratcheson RA, Siesjo BK: Cerebral metabolic state following complete compression ischemia, *Brain Res* 73:291, 1974.

122. Hinzen DH, Muller U, Sobotka P et al: Metabolism and function of dog's brain recovering from longtime ischemia, *Am J Physiol* 223:1158, 1972.

123. Kogure K, Kato H: Neurochemistry of stroke. In Barnett HJM, Mohr JP, Stein BM et al, editors: *Stroke: pathophysiology, diagnosis, and management,* ed 2, New York, 1992, Churchill Livingstone, pp 69-102.

124. Araki T, Kato H, Kogure K: Selective neuronal vulnerability following transient cerebral ischemia in the gerbil: distribution and time course, *Acta Neurol Scand* 80:548, 1989.

125. Kirino T: Delayed neuronal death in the gerbil hippocampus following ischemia, *Brain Res* 239:57, 1982.

126. Pulsinelli WA, Brierley JB, Plum F: Temporal profile of neuronal damage in a model of transient forebrain ischemia, *Ann Neurol* 11:491, 1982.

127. Kofke WA, Garman RH, Stiller R et al: Striatal extracellular dopamine levels are not increased by hyperglycemic exacerbation of ischemic brain damage in rats, *Brain Res* 633:171, 1994.

128. Garcia JH, HO K-L, Caccamo DV: Pathology of stroke. In Barnett HJM, Mohr JP, Stein BM et al, editors: *Stroke: pathophysiology, diagnosis, and management,* ed 2, New York, 1992, Churchill Livingstone, pp 125-146.

129. Wardlaw JM, Warlow CP: Thrombolysis in acute ischemic stroke: does it work? *Stroke* 23:1826, 1992.

130. Barr JD, Mathis JM, Wildenhain SL et al: Acute stroke intervention with intraarterial urokinase infusion, *J Vasc Interv Radiol* 5:705, 1994.

131. Brott T, Broderick J, Kothari RZ: Thrombolytic therapy for stroke, *Curr Opin Neurol* 7:25, 1994.

132. Jungreis CA, Wechsler LR, Horton JA: Intracranial thrombolysis via a catheter embedded in the clot, *Stroke* 20:1578, 1989.

133. Hacke W, Zeumer H, Ferbert A et al: Intra-arterial thrombolytic therapy improves outcome in patients with acute vertebrobasilar occlusive disease, *Stroke* 19:1216, 1988.

134. The NINDS Stroke Study Group: tissue plasminogen activator for acute ischemic stroke, *N Engl J Med* 333:1581-1587, 1995.

135. Ueda T, Hatakeyama T, Kumon Y et al: Evaluation of risk of hemorrhagic transformation in local intra-arterial thrombolysis in acute ischemic stroke by initial SPECT, *Stroke* 25:298, 1994.

136. Barr JD, Horowitz MB, Mathis JM et al: Intraoperative urokinase infusion for embolic stroke during carotid endarterectomy, *Neurosurgery* 36:606, 1995.

137. Furlan AJ, Busse O, Ringelstein EB: Special aspects in the treatment of severe hemispheric brain infarction. In Hacke W, Hanley DF, Einhaupl KM, editors: *Neurocritical care,* New York, 1994, Springer-Verlag, pp 578-595.

138. Kondziolka D, Fazl M: Functional recovery after decompressive craniectomy for cerebral infarction, *Neurosurgery* 23:143, 1988.

139. Adams HP, Brott TG, Crowell RM et al: Guidelines for the management of patients with acute ischemic stroke. A statement for health care professionals form a special writing group of the stroke council, American Heart Association, *Stroke* 25:1901, 1994.

140. Fisher CM, Ojemann RG: Bilateral decompressive craniectomy for worsening coma in acute subarachnoid hemorrhage. Observations in support of the procedure, *Surg Neurol* 41:65, 1994.

141. Chen H-J, Lee T-C, Wei C-P: Treatment of cerebellar infarction by decompressive suboccipital craniectomy, *Stroke* 23:957, 1992.

142. Forsting M, Reith W, Schabitz WR et al: Decompressive craniectomy for cerebral infarction. An experimental study in rats, *Stroke* 26:259-264, 1995.

143. Kalia KK, Yonas H: An aggressive approach to massive middle cerebral artery infarction, *Arch Neurol* 50:1293, 1993.

144. Powers WJ: Acute hypertension after stroke: the scientific basis for treatment decisions, *Neurology* 43:461, 1993.

145. Myers MG, Norris JW, Hachinski VC et al: Cardiac sequelae of acute stroke, *Stroke* 13:838, 1982.

146. Kolin A, Norris JW: Myocardial damage from acute cerebral lesions, *Stroke* 15:990, 1984.

147. Dimant J, Grob D: Electrocardiographic changes and myocardial damage in patients with acute cerebrovascular accidents, *Stroke* 8:448, 1977.

148. Goldstein D: The electrocardiogram in stroke with relationship to pathophysiological type and comparison with prior tracings, *Stroke* 10:253, 1979.

149. Myers MG, Norris JW, Hachinski VC et al: Cardiac sequelae of acute stroke, *Stroke* 13:838, 1982.

150. Norris JW, Froggart GM, Hachinski VC: Cardiac arrhythmias in acute stroke, *Stroke* 9:394, 1978.

151. Lavy S, Yaar I, Melamed E et al: The effect of acute stroke on cardiac functions as observed in an intensive care unit, *Stroke* 5:775, 1974.

152. Norris JW, Hachinski VC, Myers MG et al: Serum cardiac enzymes in stroke, *Stroke* 10:548, 1979.

153. Cruickshank JM, Neil-Dwyer G, Lane J: The effect of oral pro-pranolol upon the ECG changes occurring in subarachnoid hem-orrhage, *Cardiovasc Res* 9:236, 1975.

154. Myers MG, Norris JW, Hachinski VC et al: Plasma norepineph-rine in stroke, *Stroke* 12:200, 1981.

155. Brewer DB, Fawcett FJ, Horsfield GI: A necropsy series of non-traumatic cerebral hemorrhages and softenings, with partic-ular reference to heart weight, *J Pathol Bact* 96:311, 1968.

156. Kaufman HH, Schochet SS: Pathology, physiology, and model-ing. In Kaufman HH, editor: *Intracerebral hematomas*, New York, 1992, Raven Press, pp 13-22.

157. Mohr JP, Caplan LR, Melski JW et al: The Harvard Cooperative Stroke Registry: a prospective registry, *Neurology* 28:754, 1978.

158. Furlan AJ, Whisnant JP, Elveback LR: The decreasing incidence of primary intracerebral hemorrhage: a population study, *Ann Neu-rol* 5:367, 1979.

159. Mutlu N, Berry RG, Alpers BJ: Massive cerebral hemorrhage: clinical and pathological correlations, *Arch Neurol* 8:74, 1963.

160. Stehbens WE: *Pathology of the cerebral blood vessels*, St Louis, 1972, CV Mosby.

161. Ojemann RG, Mohr JP: Hypertensive brain hemorrhage, *Clin Neurosurg* 23:220, 1976.

162. McCormick WF, Rosenfield DB: Massive brain hemorrhage: a review of 144 cases and an examination of their causes, *Stroke* 4:946, 1973.

163. Brott T, Thalinger K, Hertzberg V: Hypertension as a risk factor for spontaneous intracerebral hemorrhage, *Stroke* 17:1078, 1986.

164. Schutz H, Bodeker R-H, Damian M et al: Age-related spontane-ous intracerebral hematoma in a German community, *Stroke* 21:1412, 1990.

165. Gilles S, Brucher JM, Khoubesserian P et al: Cerebral amyloid angiopathy as a cause of multiple intracerebral hemorrhages, *Neurology* 34:730, 1984.

166. Kase CS, Mohr JP, Caplan LR: Intracerebral hemorrhage. In Barnett HJM, Mohr JP, Stein BM et al, editors: *Stroke: pathophysi-ology, diagnosis, and management*, ed 2, New York, 1992, Chur-chill Livingstone, pp 561-616.

167. Hayashi M, Kobayashi H, Kawano H et al: Treatment of systemic hypertension and intracranial hypertension and intracranial hy-pertension in cases of brain hemorrhage, *Stroke* 19:314, 1988.

168. Mohr JP, Kistler JP, Fink ME: Intracranial aneurysms. In Barnett HJM, Mohr JP, Stein BM et al, editors: *Stroke: pathophysiology, diagnosis, and management*, ed 2, New York, 1992, Churchill Livingstone, pp 617-644.

169. Sahs AL: Preface. In Sahs AL, Nibbelink DW et al, editors: *Aneu-rysmal subarachnoid hemorrhage. Report of the cooperative study*, Baltimore, 1981, Urban and Schwarzenberg.

170. Espinosa F, Weir B, Noseworthy T: Nonoperative treatment of subarachnoid hemorrhage. In Yeomans JR, editor: *Neurological surgery*, ed 3, Philadelphia, 1990, WB Saunders, pp 1661-1689.

171. Fodstad H, Forssell A, Liliequist B et al: Antifibrinolysis with tranexamic acid in aneurysmal subarachnoid hemorrhage: a consecutive controlled clinical trial, *Neurosurgery* 8:158, 1981.

172. Kassell NF, Boarini DJ: Perioperative care of the aneurysm pa-tient, *Contemp Neurosurg* 6:1, 1984.

173. Kassell NF, Torner JC: Epidemiology of intracranial aneurysms, *Int Anesthesiol Clin* 20:13, 1982.

174. Torner JC, Kassell NF, Wallace RB et al: Preoperative prognostic factors for rebleeding and survival in aneurysm patients receiv-ing antifibrinolytic therapy: report of the cooperative aneurysm study, *Neurosurgery* 9:506, 1981.

175. Nishioka H, Torner JC, Goettler LC: Cooperative study of intra-cranial aneurysms and subarachnoid hemorrhage: a long-term prognostic study. II. Ruptured intracranial aneurysms managed conservatively, *Arch Neurol* 41:1142, 1984.

176. Heros RC: Acute hydrocephalus after subarachnoid hemorrhage, *Stroke* 20:715, 1989.

177. vab Gijn J, Hijdra A, Wijdicks EFM: Acute hydrocephalus after aneurysmal subarachnoid hemorrhage, *J Neurosurg* 63:355, 1985.

178. Black P McL: Hydrocephalus and vasospasm after subarachnoid hemorrhage from ruptured intracranial aneurysms, *Neurosurgery* 18:12, 1986.

179. McNealy DE, Plum F: Brainstem dysfunction with supratentorial mass lesions, *Arch Neurol* 7:26, 1962.

180. Mohr G, Ferguson G, Khan M et al: Intraventricular hemorrhage from ruptured aneurysm. Retrospective analysis of 91 cases, *J Neurosurg* 58:482, 1983.

181. Kassell NF: The natural history and treatment outcome of SAH: comments derived from the national cooperative aneurysm study. In Battye R, editor: *Calcium antagonists: possible therapeutic use in neurosurgery*, New York, 1983, Raven Health Care Commu-nications, p 24.

182. Weir BK: Pathophysiology of vasospasm, *Int Anesthesiol Clin* 20:39, 1982.

183. Ropper AH, Zervas NT: Outcome one year after subarachnoid hemorrhage from cerebral aneurysm. Management, morbidity, and functional status in 112 consecutive good-risk patients, *J Neurosurg* 60:909, 1984.

184. Schucart WA, Hussain SK, Cooper PR: epsilon-Aminocaproic acid and recurrent subarachnoid hemorrhage: a clinical trial, *J Neurosurg* 53:28, 1980.

185. Gurus IN, She MT, Richardson AE: The value of computerized tomography in aneurysmal subarachnoid hemorrhage, *J Neuro-surg* 60:763, 1984.

186. Hayward RD: Subarachnoid hemorrhage of unknown aetiology: a clinical and radiological study of 51 cases, *J Neurol Neurosurg Psychiatry* 40:926, 1977.

187. Herdt, Jr, D, Chiro G, Doppman JL: Combined arterial and arteriovenous aneurysms of the spinal cord, *Radiology* 99:589, 1971.

188. Pritz MB, Giannotta SL, Kindt GW et al: Treatment of patients with neurological deficits associated with cerebral vasospasm by intravascular volume expansion, *Neurosurgery* 3:364, 1978.

189. Senguptu RP, So SC, Villarego Ortega FJ: Use of epsilon-aminocaproic acid (EACA) in the preoperative management of ruptured intracranial aneurysms, *J Neurosurg* 44:479, 1976.

190. Allcock JM, Drake CG: Ruptured intracranial aneurysms: the role of arterial spasm, *J Neurosurg* 22:21, 1965.

191. Suzuki J, Yoshimoto T, Onuma T: Early operation for ruptured intracranial aneurysms: study of 31 cases operated on within the first four days of ruptured aneurysm, *Neurol Med Chir (Tokyo)* 18:82, 1978.

192. Mohr JP, Kase CS: Cerebral vasospasm, *Rev Neurol* 139:99, 1983.

193. Tannenbaum H, Nadjmi M, Gruss P: Therapeutic considerations in the treatment of vasospasm in aneurysms, *Acta Neurochir (Wien)* 52:158, 1980.

194. Sundt, Jr, TM: Management of ischemic complications after sub-arachnoid hemorrhage, *J Neurosurg* 43:418, 1974.

195. Winn HE, Richardson AE, Jane JA: The assessment of the natural history of single cerebral aneurysms that have ruptured. In Hopkins LN, Long DM, editors: *Clinical management of intracra-nial aneurysms*, New York, 1982, Raven Press, pp 1-10.

196. Espinosa F, Weir B, Overton T et al: A randomized placebo-controlled double-blind trial of nimodipine after SAH in mon-keys. Part 1. Clinical and radiological findings, *J Neurosurg* 60: 1167, 1984.

197. Espinosa F, Weir B, Schnitka T et al: A randomized placebo-controlled double-blind trial of nimodipine after SAH in mon-keys. Part 2: Pathological findings, *J Neurosurg* 60:1176, 1984.

198. Kistler JP, Crowell RM, Davis KR et al: The relation of cerebral vasospasm to the extent and location of subarachnoid blood visualized by CT scan. A prospective study, *Neurology* 33:424, 1983.

199. Silver AJ, Pederson, Jr, ME, Ganti SR et al: CT of subarachnoid hemorrhage due to ruptured aneurysm, *AJNR* 2:13, 1981.

200. Pasqualin A, Rosta L, DaPian R et al: Role of computed tomography in the management of vasospasm after subarachnoid hemorrhage. *Neurosurgery* 15:344, 1984.

201. Wilkins RH: Cerebral vasospasm, *Crit Rev Neurobiol* 6:51, 1990.

202. Wilkins RH: Intracranial vascular spasm in head injuries. In Vinken PJ, Bruyn GW, editors: *Handbook of clinical neurology*, vol 23, *Injuries of the brain and skull, Part I*, Amsterdam, 1975, North-Holland, p 163.

203. Echlin FA: Spasm of basilar and vertebral arteries caused by experimental subarachnoid hemorrhage, *J Neurosurg* 23:1, 1965.

204. Kanamaru K, Waga S, Kojima T et al: Inhibition of endothelium dependent relaxation by hemoglobin and cerebrospinal fluid from patients with aneurysm subarachnoid hemorrhage: a possible mechanism and relation to cerebral vasospasm. In Wilkins RH, editor: *Cerebral vasospasm: proceedings of the Charlottesville conference held April 29-May 1, 1987*, New York, 1988, Raven Press, pp 163-168.

205. Afshar JK, Pluta RM, Boock RJ et al: Effect of intracarotid nitric oxide on primate cerebral vasospasm after subarachnoid hemorrhage, *J Neurosurg* 83:118-122, 1995.

206. Minegishi A, Ishizaki T, Yoshida Y et al: Plasma monoaminergic metabolites and catecholamines in subarachnoid hemorrhage. Clinical implications, *Arch Neurol* 44:423, 1987.

207. Cruickshank JM, Neil-Dwyer G, Stott AW: Possible role of catecholamines, corticosteroids, and potassium in production of electrocardiographic abnormalities associated with subarachnoid hemorrhage, *Br Heart J* 36:697, 1974.

208. Loach AB, Benedict CR: Plasma catecholamine concentration associated with cerebral vasospasm, *J Neurol Sci* 45:261, 1980.

209. Dilraj A, Botha JH, Rambiritch V et al: Levels of catecholamine in plasma and cerebrospinal fluid in aneurysmal subarachnoid hemorrhage, *Neurosurgery* 31:42, 1992.

210. Wilkins RH: Hypothalamic dysfunction and intracranial arterial spasm, *Surg Neurol* 4:472, 1975.

211. Peerless SJ, Griffiths JC: Plasma catecholamines following subarachnoid hemorrhage. In Smith RR, Robertson JT, editors: *Subarachnoid hemorrhage and cerebrovascular spasm*, Springfield, Ill, 1975, Charles C. Thomas, pp 148-156.

212. Cruickshank JM, Neil-Dwyer G, Brice J: Electrocardiographic changes and their prognostic significance in subarachnoid hemorrhage, *J Neurol Neurosurg Psychiatry* 37:755, 1974.

213. Cruickshank JM, Neil-Dwyer G, Stott AW: Possible role of catecholamines corticosteroids, and potassium in production of electro-cardiographic abnormalities associated with subarachnoid hemorrhage, *Br Heart J* 36:697, 1974.

214. Neil-Dwyer G, Cruickshank J, Stott A et al: The urinary catecholamine and plasma cortisol levels in patients with subarachnoid hemorrhage, *J Neurol Sci* 22:375, 1974.

215. Fraser RAR, Stein BM, Barrett RE et al: Noradrenergic mediation of experimental cerebrovascular spasm, *Stroke* 1:356, 1970.

216. Peerless SJ, Kendall MJ: The innervation of the cerebral blood vessels. In Smith RR, Robertson JT, editors: *Subarachnoid hemorrhage and cerebrovascular spasm*, Springfield, Ill, 1975, Charles C. Thomas, pp 38-54.

217. Neil-Dwyer G, Walter P, Cruickshank JM: Beta-blockade benefits patients following a subarachnoid hemorrhage. *Eur J Clin Pharmacol* 28(suppl):25, 1985.

218. Gascon P, Ley TJ, Toltzis RJ et al: Spontaneous subarachnoid hemorrhage simulating acute transmural myocardial infarction, *Am Heart J* 105:511, 1983.

219. Stober T, Kunze K: Electrocardiographic alterations in subarachnoid hemorrhage: correlation between spasm of the arteries of the left side of the brain and T inversion and QT prolongation, *J Neurol* 227:99, 1982.

220. Brouwers PJAM, Wijdicks EFM, Hasan D: Serial electrocardiographic recordings in aneurysmal subarachnoid hemorrhage, *Stroke* 20:1162, 1989.

221. Cruickshank JM, Neil-Dwyer G, Stott AW: Possible role of catecholamines, corticosteroids, and potassium in production of electrocardiographic abnormalities associated with subarachnoid hemorrhage, *Br Heart J* 36:697, 1974.

222. Davies KR, Gelb AW, Manninen PH : Cardiac function in aneurysmal subarachnoid hemorrhage: a study of electrocardiographic and echocardiographic abnormalities, *Br J Anaesth* 67:58, 1991.

223. Pollick C, Cujec B, Parker S et al: Left ventricular wall motion abnormalities in subarachnoid hemorrhage: an echocardiographic study, *J Am Coll Cardiol* 12:600, 1988.

224. Kono T, Morita H, Kuroiwa T et al: Left ventricular wall motion abnormalities in patients with subarachnoid hemorrhage: neurogenic stunned myocardium, *J Am Coll Cardiol* 24:636, 1994.

225. Fabinyi G, Hunt D, McKinley L: Myocardial creatine kinase isoenzyme in serum after subarachnoid hemorrhage, *J Neurol Neurosurg Psychiatry* 40:818, 1977.

226. Neil-Dwyer G, Cruikshank J, Stratton C: β-Blockers, plasma total creatinine kinase and creatine kinase myocardial enzymes, and the prognosis of subarachnoid hemorrhage, *Surg Neurol* 25:163, 1986.

227. Feibel JH, Campbell RG, Joynt RJ: Myocardial damage and cardiac arrhythmias in cerebral infarction and subarachnoid hemorrhage: correlation with increased systemic catecholamine output, *Trans Am Neurol Assoc* 101:242, 1976.

228. Svengaard NA, Brismar J, Delgado TJ et al: Subarachnoid hemorrhage in the rat: effect on the development of cerebral vasospasm of lesions in the central serotonergic and dopaminergic systems, *Stroke* 17:86, 1986.

229. Svengaard NA, Brismar J, Delgado TJ et al: Subarachnoid haemorrhage in the rat: effect on the development of vasospasm of selective lesions of the catecholamine systems in the lower brain stem, *Stroke* 16:602, 1985.

230. Delgado TJ, Diemer NH, Svendgaard NA: Subarachnoid hemorrhage in the rat: CBF and glucose metabolism after selective lesions of the catecholamine systems in the brainstem, *J Cereb Blood Flow Metab* 6:600, 1986.

231. Svendgaard NA, Delgado TJ, Arbab MAR: Catecholaminergic and peptidergic systems underlying cerebral vasospasm: CBF and CMRgl changes following an experimental subarachnoid hemorrhage in the rat. In Wilkins RH, editor: *Cerebral vasospasm: proceedings of the Charlottesville conference held April 29-May 1, 1987*, New York, 1988, Raven Press, p 175.

232. Kassell NF, Boarini DJ: Perioperative care of the aneurysm patient, *Contemp Neurosurgery* 6:1-6, 1984.

233. Keranen T, Tapaninaho A, Hernesniemi J et al: Late epilepsy after aneurysm operations, *Neurosurgery* 17:897-900, 1985.

234. Adams HP, Love BB: Medical management of aneurysmal subarachnoid hemorrhage. In Barnett HJM, Mohr JP, Stein BM et al, editors: *Stroke: pathophysiology, diagnosis, and management*, ed 2, New York, 1992, Churchill Livingstone, pp 1029-1054.

235. Disney L, Weir B, Grace M et al: Trends in blood pressure, osmolality, and electrolytes after subarachnoid hemorrhage from aneurysms, *Can J Neurol Sci* 16:299, 1989.

236. Koskelo P, Punsar S, Sipila W: Subendocardial hemorrhage and ECG changes in intracranial bleeding, *Br Med J* 1:1479, 1964.

237. Touho H, Karasawa J, Shishido H et al: Neurogenic pulmonary edema in the acute stage of hemorrhagic cerebrovascular disease, *Neurosurgery* 25:762, 1989.

238. Wauchob TD, Brooks RJ, Harrison KM: Neurogenic pulmonary edema, *Anaesthesia* 39:529, 1984.

239. Wijdicks EFM, Vermeulen M, Hijdra A et al: Hyponatremia and cerebral infarction in patients with ruptured intracranial aneurysms: is fluid restriction harmful? *Ann Neurol* 17:137, 1985.

240. Weisman SJ: Edema and congestion of the lungs resulting from intracranial hemorrhage, *Surgery* 6:722, 1939.

241. Crowell RM, Zervas NT: Management of intracranial aneurysm, *Med Clin N Am* 63:695, 1979.

242. Simmons RL, Martin AM, Heisterkamp CA et al: Respiratory insufficiency in combat casualties. II. Pulmonary edema following head injury, *Ann Surg* 170:39, 1969.

243. Peerless SJ: Pre- and postoperative management of cerebral aneurysms, *Clin Neurosurg* 26:209, 1979.

244. Schell AR, Shenoy MM, Friedman SA et al: Pulmonary edema associated with subarachnoid hemorrhage, *Arch Int Med* 147:591-592, 1987.

245. Maroon JC, Nelson PB: Hypovolemia in patients with subarachnoid hemorrhage: therapeutic implications, *Neurosurgery* 4:223, 1979.

246. Theodore J, Robin ED: Pathogenesis of neurogenic pulmonary edema, *Lancet* 2:749, 1975.

247. Solomon RA, Post KD, McMuirtry III, JG: Depression of circulating blood volume in patients after subarachnoid hemorrhage: implications for the management of symptomatic vasospasm, *Neurosurgery* 15:354, 1984.

248. Colice GL: Neurogenic pulmonary edema, *Clin Chest Med* 6:473, 1985.

249. Nelson PB, Seif SM, Maroon JC et al: Hyponatremia in intracranial disease: perhaps not the syndrome of inappropriate secretion of antidiuretic hormone(SIADH), *J Neurosurg* 55:938, 1981.

250. Fein IA, Rackow EC: Neurogenic pulmonary edema, *Chest* 81:318, 1982.

251. Widjicks EFM, Vermeulen M, Ten Haaf et al: Volume depletion and natriuresis in patients with a ruptured intracranial aneurysm, *Ann Neurol* 18:211, 1985.

252. Hund EF, Bohrer H, Martin E et al: Disturbances of water and electrolyte balance. In Hacke W, Hanley DF, Einhaupl KM et al, editors: *Neurocritical care*, Berlin, 1994, Springer-Verlag, Chapter 87, pp 917-927.

253. Diringer M, Ladesnon PW, Stern BJ et al: Plasma atrial natriuretic factor and subarachnoid hemorrhage, *Stroke* 19:1119, 1988.

254. Rosenfeld JV, Barnett GH, Sila CA et al: The effect of subarachnoid hemorrhage on blood and CSF atrial natriuretic factor, *J Neurosurg* 71:32, 1989.

255. Jourdan C, Artru F, Convert J et al: [Hyperthermia in meningeal hemorrhage. Contribution of daily determination of inflammation proteins]. Hyperthermie au cours des hemorragies meningees. Apport du dosage quotidien des proteines de l'inflammation, *Agressologie* 31:380, 1990.

256. Simpson, Jr, RK, Fischer DK, Ehni BL: Neurogenic hyperthermia in subarachnoid hemorrhage, *South Med J* 82:1577, 1989.

257. Rousseaux P, Scherpereel B, Bernard MH et al: Fever and cerebral vasospasm in ruptured intracranial aneurysms, *Surg Neurol* 14:459, 1980.

258. Dietrich WD: The importance of brain temperature in cerebral injury, *J Neurotrauma* 9(suppl 2):S475-485, 1992.

259. Kassell NF, Torner JC: Aneurysmal rebleeding: a preliminary report from the cooperative aneurysm study, *Neurosurgery* 13:479-481, 1983.

260. McKissock W, Richardson A, Walsh L: Middle cerebral aneurysms: further results in the controlled trial of conservative and surgical treatment of ruptured intracranial aneurysms, *Lancet* 2:417-421, 1962.

261. Nibbelink DW, Torner JC, Henderson WG: Intracranial aneurysms and subarachnoid hemorrhage—report of a randomized treatment study: IV. A. Regulated bed rest, *Stroke* 8:202-218, 1977.

262. Jane JA, Kassell NF, Torner JC et al: The natural history of aneurysms and arteriovenous malformations, *J Neurosurg* 62:321-323, 1985.

263. Sundt, Jr, TM, Kobayashi S, Fode NC et al: results and complications of surgical management of 809 intracranial aneurysms in 722 cases, *J Neurosurg* 56:753, 1982.

264. Hunt WE, Miller CA: The results of early operation for aneurysm, *Clin Neurosurg* 24:208, 1976.

265. Kori S, Suzuki J: Early intracranial operation for ruptured aneurysms, *Acta Neurochir (Wien)* 46:93, 1979.

266. Sano K, Saito I: Timing and indication of surgery for ruptured intracranial aneurysms with regard to cerebral vasospasm, *Acta Neurochir (Wien)* 41:49, 1978.

267. Bolander HG, Kourtopoulos H, West KA: Retrospective analysis of 162 consecutive cases of ruptured intracranial aneurysms: total mortality and early surgery, *Acta Neurochir (Wien)* 70:31, 1984.

268. Hugenholtz H, Elgie R: Considerations in early surgery on good-risk patients with ruptured intracranial aneurysms, *J Neurosurg* 56:180, 1982.

269. Kassell NF, Boarini DJ, Adams, Jr, HP et al: Overall management of ruptured aneurysm: comparison of early and late operation, *Neurosurgery* 9:120, 1981.

270. Ljunggren B, Brandt L, Saveland H et al: Early management of aneurysmal subarachnoid hemorrhage, *Neurosurgery* 11:412, 1982.

271. Taneda M: Effect of early operation for ruptured aneurysms on prevention of delayed ischemic symptoms, *J Neurosurg* 57:622, 1982.

272. Weir B, Aronyk K: Management mortality and the timing of surgery for supratentorial aneurysms, *J Neurosurg* 54:146, 1981.

273. Yamamoto I, Hara M, Ogura K et al: Early operation for ruptured intracranial aneurysms: comparative study with computed tomography, *Neurosurgery* 12:169, 1983.

274. Ohman J, Heiskanen O: Timing of operation for ruptured supratentorial aneurysms: a prospective randomized study, *J Neurosurg* 70:55, 1989.

275. Kassell NF, Torner JC, Haley EC et al: The International Cooperative study on the timing of aneurysm surgery. I. Overall management results, *J Neurosurg* 73:18, 1990.

276. Kassell NF, Torner JC, Haley EC et al: The International Cooperative study on the timing of aneurysm surgery. II. Surgical results, *J Neurosurg* 73:34, 1990.

277. Allen GS, Ahn HS, Presiosi TJ et al: Cerebral arterial spasm: a controlled trial of nimodipine in patients with subarachnoid hemorrhage, *N Engl J Med* 308:619, 1983.

278. Mee E, Dorrance D, Lower D et al: Controlled study of nimodipine in aneurysm patients treated early after subarachnoid hemorrhage, *Neurosurgery* 22:484, 1988.

279. Neil-Dwyer G, Mee E, Dorrance D et al: Early intervention with nimodipine in subarachnoid hemorrhage, *Eur Heart J* 8:41, 1988.

280. Petruk KC, West M, Mohr G et al: Nimodipine treatment in poor grade aneurysm patients: results of a multicenter double-blind placebo-controlled trial, *J Neurosurg* 68:505, 1988.

281. Pickard JD, Murray GD, Illingworth R et al: Effect of oral nimodipine on cerebral infarction and outcome after subarachnoid hemorrhage. British Aneurysm Nimodipine Trial, *Br Med J* 298:636, 1989.

282. Terttenborn D, Dycka J: Prevention and treatment of delayed ischemic dysfunction in patients with aneurysmal subarachnoid hemorrhage, *Stroke* 21(suppl):85, 1990.

283. Jan M, Buchheit F, Tremoulet M: Therapeutic trial of intravenous nimodipine in patients with established cerebral vasospasm after rupture of intracranial aneurysm, *Neurosurgery* 23:154, 1988.

284. Flamm ES, Adams, Jr, HP, Beck DW et al: Dose-escalation study of intravenous nicardipine in patients with aneurysmal subarachnoid hemorrhage, *J Neurosurg* 68:393, 1988.

285. Haley EC, Torner JC, Kassell NF and participants: Cooperative randomized study of nicardipine in subarachnoid hemorrhage. Preliminary report. In Sano K, Takakara K, Kassell NF et al, editors: *Cerebral vasospasm. Proceedings of the Fourth International Conference on Cerebral Vasospasm*, Tokyo, 1990, University of Tokyo Press, p 519.

286. Ishii R: Regional CBF in patients with ruptured intracranial aneurysms, *J Neurosurg* 50:587, 1979.

287. Levy ML, Rabb CH, Zelman V et al: Cardiac performance enhancement from dobutamine in patients refractory to hypervolemic therapy for cerebral vasospasm, *J Neurosurg* 19:494, 1993.

288. Levy ML, Giannotta SL: Cardiac performance indices during hypervolemic therapy for cerebral vasospasm, *J Neurosurg* 75:27, 1991.

289. Awad IA, Carter LP, Spetzler RF et al: Clinical vasospasm after subarachnoid hemorrhage: response to hypervolemic hemodilution and arterial hypertension, *Stroke* 18:365, 1987.

290. Brown FD, Hanlon K, Mullan S: Treatment of aneurysmal hemiplegia with dopamine and mannitol, *J Neurosurg* 49:525, 1978.

291. Kassell NF, Peerless SJ, Durward QJ et al: Treatment of ischemic deficits from vasospasm with intravascular volume expansion and induced arterial hypertension, *Neurosurgery* 11:337, 1982.

292. Muizelaar JP, Becker DP: Induced hypertension for the treatment of cerebral ischemia after subarachnoid hemorrhage. Direct effect on CBF, *Surg Neurol* 25:317, 1986.

293. Otsubo H, Takemae T, Inoue T et al: Normovolaemic induced hypertension therapy for cerebral vasospasm after subarachnoid hemorrhage, *Acta Neurochir (Wien)* 103:18, 1990.

294. Solomon RA, Fink ME, Lennihan L: Prophylactic volume expansion therapy for the prevention of delayed cerebral ischemia after early aneurysm surgery. Results of a preliminary trial, *Arch Neurol* 45:325, 1988.

295. Stanek B, Zimpfer M, Fitzal S et al: Plasma catecholamines, plasma renin activity and haemodynamics during sodium nitroprusside-induced hypotension and additional beta-blockage with bunitrolol, *Eur J Clin Pharmacol* 19:317, 1981.

296. Wood JM, Kee DB: Hemorrheology of the cerebral circulation in stroke, *Stroke* 16:765, 1985.

297. Awad IA, Carter LP, Spetzler RF et al: Clinical vasospasm after subarachnoid hemorrhage: response to hypervolemic hemodilution and arterial hypertension, *Stroke* 18:365, 1987.

298. Kassell NF, Peerless SJ, Durward QJ et al: Treatment of ischemic deficits from vasospasm with intravascular volume expansion and induced arterial hypertension, *Neurosurgery* 11:337, 1982.

299. Petrozza PH, Prough DS: Postoperative and intensive care. In Cottrell JE, Smith DS, editors: *Anesthesia and neurosurgery*, ed 3, St Louis, 1994, Mosby, Chapter 30, pp 625-659.

300. Darby JM, Yonas H, Marks EC et al: Acute CBF response to dopamine-induced hypertension after subarachnoid hemorrhage, *J Neurosurg* 80:857, 1994.

301. Nakagomi T, Kassell NF, Johshita H et al: Blood-arterial wall barrier disruption to various sized tracers following subarachnoid haemorrhage, *Acta Neurochir (Wien)* 99:76, 1989.

302. Doczi T, Joo F, Adam G et al: Blood-brain barrier damage during the acute stage of subarachnoid hemorrhage, as exemplified by a new animal model, *Neurosurgery* 18:733, 1986.

303. Doczi T: The pathogenetic and prognostic significance of blood-brain barrier damage at the acute stage of aneurysmal subarachnoid hemorrhage. Clinical and experimental studies, *Acta Neurochir (Wien)* 77:110, 1085.

304. MacKenzie ET, McCulloch J, Harper AM: Influence of endogenous norepinephrine on CBF and metabolism, *Am J Physiol* 231:489-494, 1976.

305. Olesen J: The effect of intracarotid epinephrine, norepinephrine, and angiotensin on the regional CBF in man, *Neurology* 22:978-987, 1972.

306. Ekstrom-Jodal B, Haggendal E, Larsson LE: CBF and oxygen uptake in endotoxic shock. An experimental study in dogs, *Acta Anaesth Scand* 26(3):163-170, 1982.

307. Swift DM, Solomon RA: Unruptured aneurysms and postoperative volume expansion, *J Neurosurg* 77:908, 1992.

308. Buckland MR, Batjer HH, Giesecke AH: Anesthesia for cerebral aneurysm surgery: use of induced hypertension in patients with symptomatic vasospasm, *Anesthesiology* 69:116, 1988.

309. Hasan D, Vermeulen M, Wijdicks EFM et al: Effect of fluid intake and antihypertensive treatment on cerebral ischemia after subarachnoid hemorrhage, *Stroke* 20:1511, 1989.

310. Newell DW, Eskridge JM, Mayberg MR et al: Angioplasty for the treatment of symptomatic vasospasm following subarachnoid hemorrhage, *Neurosurgery* 71:654, 1989.

311. Clouston JE, Numaguchi Y, Zoarski GH : Intraarterial papaverine infusion for cerebral vasospasm after subarachnoid hemorrhage, *AJNR* 16:27, 1995.

312. Barr JD, Mathis JM, Horton JA: Transient severe brain stem depression during intraarterial papaverine infusion for cerebral vasospasm, *AJNR* 15:719, 1994.

313. McAuliffe W, Townsend M, Eskridge JM et al: Intracranial pressure changes induced during papaverine infusion for treatment of vasospasm, *J Neurosurg* 83:430-434, 1995.

314. Mathis JM, DeNardo A, Jensen ME et al: Transient neurologic events associated with intraarterial papaverine infusion for subarachnoid hemorrhage-induced vasospasm, *AJNR* 15:1671, 1994.

315. Hendrix LE, Dion JE, Jensen ME et al: Papaverine-induced mydriasis, *AJNR* 15:716, 1994.

316. Guglielmi G, Vinuela F, Duckwiler G et al: Endovascular treatment of posterior circulation aneurysms by electrothrombosis using electrically detachable coils, *J Neurosurg* 77:515, 1992.

317. Casasco A, Arnaud O, Gobin P et al: [Giant intracranial aneurysm. Elective endovascular treatment using metallic coils]. Anevrysmes geants intracraniens. Traitement endovasculaire electif par des spires metalliques, *Neurochirurgie* 38:18, 1992.

318. Crompton MR: Hypothalamic lesions following the rupture of cerebral berry aneurysms, *Brain* 301, 1963.

319. Busto R, Harik SI, Yoshida S et al: Cerebral norepinephrine depletion enhances recovery after brain ischemia, *Ann Neurol* 18:329, 1985.

320. Nevin C: Neuropathologic changes in the white matter following head injury, *J Neuropathol Exp Neurol* 26:77, 1967.

321. Nilsson B, Ponten U, Voigt G: Experimental head injury in the rat. Part 1: Mechanics, pathophysiology, and morphology in an impact acceleration trauma model, *J Neurosurg* 47:241-251, 1977.

322. Povlishock JT: Experimental studies of head injury. In Becker DP, Gudeman SK, editors: *Textbook of head injury*, Philadelphia, 1989, WB Saunders, pp 437-450.

323. Muttaqin Z, Uozumi T, Kuwabara S et al: Hyperaemia prior to acute cerebral swelling in severe head injuries: the role of transcranial Doppler monitoring, *Acta Neurochir (Wien)* 123:76, 1993.

324. Wald SL, Shackford SR, Fenwick J: The effect of secondary insults on mortality and long-term disability after severe head injury in a rural region without a trauma system, *J Trauma* 34:377, 1993.

325. Wahl M, Schilling L, Unterberg A et al: Mediators of vascular and parenchymal mechanisms in secondary brain damage, *Acta Neurochir Suppl (Wien)* 57:64, 1993.

326. Graham DI, Adams JH, Doyle D et al: Quantification of primary and secondary lesions in severe head injury, *Acta Neurochir Suppl (Wien)* 57:41, 1993.

327. Unterberg A, Kiening K, Schmiedek P et al: Long-term observations of intracranial pressure after severe head injury. The phenomenon of secondary rise of intracranial pressure, *Neurosurgery* 32:17, 1993.

328. Braughler JM, Hall ED: Involvement of lipid peroxidation in CNS injury, *J Neurotrauma* 9(suppl 1):S1, 1992.

329. Kanthan R, Shuaib A: Clinical evaluation of extracellular amino acids in severe head trauma by intracerebral in vivo microdialysis, *J Neurol Neurosurg Psychiatry* 59:326, 1995.

330. Hayes RL, Jenkins LW, Lyeth BG: Neurotransmitter-mediated mechanisms of traumatic brain injury: acetylcholine and excitatory amino acids, *J Neurotrauma* 9(suppl 1):S173, 1992.

331. Kochanek PM: Ischemic and traumatic brain injury: pathobiology and cellular mechanisms, *Crit Care Med* 21(suppl 9): S333-335, 1993.

332. Marmarou A: Intracellular acidosis in human and experimental brain injury, *J Neurotrauma* 9(suppl 2):S551, 1992.

333. Hovda DA, Becker DP, Katayama Y: Secondary injury and acidosis, *J Neurotrauma* 9(suppl 1):S47, 1992.

334. Martin NA, Doberstein C, Zane C et al: Posttraumatic cerebral arterial spasm: transcranial Doppler ultrasound, CBF, and angiographic findings, *J Neurosurg* 77:575, 1992.

335. Jaggi JL, Obrist WD, Gennarelli TA et al: Relationship of early CBF and metabolism to outcome in acute head injury, *J Neurosurg* 72:176, 1990.

336. Bouma GJ, Muizelaar JP: CBF, cerebral blood volume, and cerebrovascular reactivity after severe head injury, *J Neurotrauma* 9(suppl 1):S333, 1992.

337. Sharples PM, Stuart AG, Matthews DS et al: CBF and metabolism in children with severe head injury. Part 1: Relation to age, Glasgow coma score, outcome, intracranial pressure, and time after injury, *J Neurol Neurosurg Psychiatry* 58:145, 1995.

338. Obrist WD, Langfitt TW, Jaggi JL et al: CBF and metabolism in comatose patients with acute head injury. Relationship to intracranial hypertension, *J Neurosurg* 61:241-253, 1984.

339. Muizelaar JP: CBF, cerebral blood volume, and cerebral metabolism after severe head injury. In Becker DP, Gudeman SK, editors: *Textbook of head injury*, Philadelphia, 1989, WB Saunders, pp 221-240.

340. Miller JD, Becker DP, Ward JD et al: Significance of intracranial hypertension in severe head injury, *J Neurosurg* 47:503, 1977.

341. Maxwell WL, Watt C, Graham DI et al: Ultrastructural evidence of axonal shearing as a result of lateral acceleration of the head in non-human primates, *Acta Neuropath* 86:136, 1993.

342. Povlishock JT: Traumatically induced axonal injury: pathogenesis and pathobiological implications, *Brain Pathol* 2:1-12, 1992.

343. Robertson GL: Thirst and vasopressin function in normal and disordered states of water balance, *J Lab Clin Med* 101:351, 1983.

344. Arieff AI: Central nervous system manifestations of disordered sodium metabolism, *Clin Endocrinol Metab* 13:269, 1984.

345. Miller M, Dalakos T, Moses AM et al: Recognition of partial defects in antidiuretic hormone secretion, *Ann Intern Med* 72: 721, 1970.

346. Marshall SB, Marshall LF, Vos HR et al: *Neuroscience critical care*, Philadelphia, 1990, WB Saunders, Chapter 10, pp 285-306.

347. Seckl JR, Dunger DB, Lightman SL: Neurohypophyseal peptide function during early postoperative diabetes insipidus, *Brain* 110:737, 1987.

348. Verbalis JG, Robinson AG, Moses AM: Postoperative and post-traumatic diabetes insipidus. In Czernichow P, Robinson AG, editors: *Diabetes insipidus in man: frontiers of hormone research*, vol 13, Basel, 1984, Karger, pp 247-265.

349. Robinson AG: DDAVP in the treatment of central diabetes insipidus, *N Engl J Med* 294:507, 1976.

350. Chauveau ME: Pathology of posterior pituitary. In Pinsky MR, Dhainaut J-F A, editors: *Pathophysiologic foundations of critical care*, Baltimore, 1993, Williams and Wilkins.

351. Chanson P, Jednyak CP, Czernichow P: Management of early postoperative diabetes insipidus with parenteral desmopressin, *Acta Endocrinol (Copenh)* 117:513, 1988.

352. Seidman PA, Kofke WA, Policare R et al: Anaesthetic complications of acromegaly, *Br J Anaesth* 84:179-182, 2000.

353. Marshall SB, Marshall LF, Vos HR et al: *Neuroscience critical care*, Philadelphia, 1990, WB Saunders, Chapter 8, pp 249-264.

354. Adams RD, Victor M: *Principles of neurology*, ed 5, New York, 1993, McGraw-Hill, Chapter 31, pp 554-559.

355. Taylor WA, Thomas NW, Wellings JA et al: Timing of postoperative intracranial hematoma development and implications for the best use of neurosurgical intensive care, *J Neurosurg* 82:48, 1995.

356. Kalfas IH, Little JR: Postoperative hemorrhage: a survey of 4992 intracranial procedures, *Neurosurgery* 11:337, 1988.

357. Stone JL, Schaffer L, Ramsey RG et al: Epidural hematomas of the posterior fossa, *Surg Neurol* 11:419, 1979.

358. Guidelines for the determination of death: report of the medical consultants on the diagnosis of death to the President's Commission for the Study of Ethical Problems in Medicine and Biomedical and Behavioral Research, *JAMA* 246:2184-2186, 1981.

359. Grenvik A: Brain death and permanently lost consciousness. In Shoemaker WC, Thompson WL, Holbrook PR, editors: *Textbook of critical care*, Philadelphia, 1984, Saunders, pp 968-980.

360. Bleck TP, Smith MC: Diagnosing brain death and persistent vegetative suites, *J Crit Illn* 4:60, 1989.

361. Guidelines for the determination of death: report of the medical consultants on the diagnosis of death to the President's Commission for the Study of Ethical Problems in Medicine and Biomedical and Behavioral Research, *JAMA* 246:2184, 1981.

362. Kofke WA, Darby J: Evaluation and certification of brain death. In Grande M et al, editors: *Textbook of trauma anesthesia and critical care*, Philadelphia, 1993, Mosby Yearbook.

363. Powner DJ: The diagnosis of brain death in the adult patient, *Intensive Care Med* 2:181, 1987.

364. Powner DJ, Darby JM, Stein KL: Organ donor management in the intensive care unit. In Grande M et al, editors: *Textbook of trauma anesthesia and critical care*, Philadelphia, 1993, Mosby-Yearbook.

365. Clifton GL, Ziegler MG, Grossman RG: Circulating catecholamines and sympathetic activity after head injury, *Neurosurgery* 8:10-13, 1981.

366. Hamill RW, Woolf PD, McDonald JV et al: Catecholamines predict outcome in traumatic brain injury, *Ann Neurol* 21: 438-443, 1987.

367. Payen D et al: Head injury: clonidine decreases plasma catecholamines, *Crit Care Med* 18:392-395, 1990.

368. Trento A, Hardesty RL, Griffith BP: Early function of cardiac homografts: relationship to hemodynamics in the donor and length of ischemic period, *Circulation* 74:77-79, 1986.

369. Darracott-Cankovic S et al: Biopsy assessment of myocardial preservation in 160 human donor hearts, *Transplant Proc* 20: 44-48, 1988.

370. Connor RCR: Focal myocytolysis and fuchsinophilic degeneration of the myocardium of patients dying with various brain lesions, *Ann NY Acad Sci* 156:261-270, 1969.

371. Nagareda T et al: Clinicopathological study of livers from brain-dead patients treated with a combination of vasopressin and epinephrine, *Transplantation* 47:792-797, 1989.

372. Novitzky D et al: Electrocardiographic, hemodynamic and endocrine changes occurring during experimental brain death in the Chacma baboon, *J Heart Transplant* 4:63-69, 1984.

373. Adomian GE, Laks MM, Billingham ME: The incidence and significance of contraction bands in endomyocardial biopsies from normal human hearts, *Am Heart J* 95:348-351, 1978.

374. Rose AG, Novitzky D, Copper DKC: Myocardial and pulmonary histopathologic changes, *Transplant Proc* 20:29-32, 1988.

375. Novitzky D et al: Prevention of myocardial injury by pretreatment with verapamil hydrochloride prior to experimental brain death, *Am J Emerg Med* 5:11-18, 1987.

376. Novitzky D et al: Prevention of myocardial injury during brain death by total cardiac sympathectomy in the Chacma baboon, *Ann Thorac Surg* 41:520-524, 1986.

377. Novitzky D et al: Improved cardiac function following hormonal therapy in brain dead pigs: relevance to organ donation, *Cryobiology* 24:1-10, 1987.

378. Finkelstein I, Toledo-Pereyre LH, Castellanos J: Physiologic and hormonal changes in experimentally induced brain dead dogs, *Transplant Proc* 19:4156-4158, 1987.

379. Griepp RB et al: The cardiac donor, *Surg Gynecol Obstet* 133:792-798, 1971.

380. Kinoshita Y et al: Clinical and pathological changes of the heart in brain death maintained with vasopressin and epinephrine, *Pathol Res Pract* 186:173-179, 1990.

381. Jastremski M, Powner DJ, Snyder JV: Problems in brain death determination, *Forensic Sci* 11:201-212, 1978.

382. Nygaard CE, Townsend RN, Diamond DL: Organ donor management and organ outcome: a 6-year review from a Level I trauma center, *J Trauma* 30:728-732, 1990.

383. Emery RW et al: The cardiac donor: a six-year experience, *Ann Thorac Surg* 41:356-362, 1986.

384. Feibel JH: Reduced catecholamine excretion at onset of brain death, *Lancet* 1:890-891, 1981.

385. Toledo-Pereyra LH, Castellanos J, Finkelstein I: Improved donor kidney function and hemodynamics following naloxone administration, *Transplant Proc* 20:733-735, 1988.

386. Wetzel RC et al: Hemodynamic responses in brain-dead organ donor patients, *Anesth Analg* 64:125-128, 1985.

387. Okamoto R et al: Influence of dopamine on the liver assessed by changes in arterial ketone body ratio in brain-dead dogs, *Surgery* 107:36-42, 1990.

388. Gores PF et al: The influence of donor hyperglycemia and other factors on long-term pancreatic allograft survival, *Transplant Proc* 22:437-438, 1990.

389. Wright FH et al: Pancreatic allograft thrombosis: donor and retrieval factors and early postperfusion graft function, *Transplant Proc* 22:439-441, 1990.

390. Whelchel JD et al: The effect of high-dose dopamine in cadaver donor management on delayed graft function and graft survival following renal transplantation, *Transplant Proc* 18:523-527, 1986.

391. Iwai A et al: Effects of vasopressin and catecholamines on the maintenance of circulatory stability in brain-dead patients, *Transplantation* 48:613-617, 1989.

392. Hernandez LA, Granger N: Role of antioxidants in organ preservation and transplantation, *Crit Care Med* 16:543-549, 1988.

393. Zenati M et al: Organ procurement for pulmonary transplantation, *Ann Thorac Surg* 48:882-886, 1989.

394. Novitzky D et al: Electrocardiographic, hemodynamic and endocrine changes occurring during experimental brain death in the Chacma baboon, *J Heart Transplant* 4:63, 1984.

395. Novitzky D, Cooper DKC, Reichart B: Hemodynamic and metabolic responses to hormonal therapy in brain-dead potential organ donors, *Transplantation* 43:852, 1987.

396. Powner DJ et al: Hormonal changes in brain-dead patients, *Crit Care Med* 18:702, 1990.

397. Robertson KM, Hramiak IM, Gelb AW: Endocrine changes and haemodynamic stability after brain death, *Transplant Proc* 21:1197, 1989.

398. Debelak L, Pollak R, Reckard C: Arginine vasopressin versus desmopressin for the treatment of diabetes insipidus in the brain dead organ donor, *Transplant Proc* 22:351, 1990.

CHAPTER 20

Obstetric Procedures

Regina Y. Fragneto, M.D.

OUTLINE

Cardiac disease complicates 0.4% to 4.1% of pregnancies.[1] Depending on the type and severity of the disorder, maternal and fetal outcome may be adversely affected by cardiac disease.[2] Advances in medical and surgical management have changed the composition of cardiac lesions encountered in parturients. Many patients with congenital heart disease are now reaching childbearing age because of improved surgical treatments and constitute an increasing proportion of the pregnant cardiac patients.[3] In contrast, the number of pregnant patients with rheumatic heart disease is declining. Regardless of the cause of the heart disease, the physiologic changes of pregnancy produce added stress on the already compromised cardiovascular system and may result in cardiac decompensation. These patients require close observation and careful management throughout pregnancy, labor, and delivery, and frequently require intensive monitoring and management to optimize outcome. An interdisciplinary approach, involving obstetricians, anesthesiologists, cardiologists, and nurses working closely together, results in optimal patient care.

PHYSIOLOGIC CHANGES OF PREGNANCY

The cardiovascular physiologic changes of pregnancy (summarized in Table 20-1) place added stress on the already compromised cardiovascular system of parturients with cardiac disease. Cardiac output increases 50%[4] and blood volume increases 45% during pregnancy.[5] Parturients develop a "dilutional anemia of pregnancy" because the 30% rise in red cell mass is significantly less than the 50% to 55% rise in plasma volume.[5] Systemic vascular resistance (SVR) is decreased by 20%.[5] These changes may result in cardiac decompensation in parturients with compromised cardiovascular states. The greatest rise in blood volume occurs during the second trimester[6] and the peak rise in cardiac output occurs by the end of the second trimester.[7] The first signs of cardiac decompensation generally occur in the late second or early third trimester.

The cardiovascular system is further stressed during labor, delivery, and the immediate postpartum period. Cardiac output increases an additional 25% during the active phase of labor, and 40% during the second stage of labor.[8] Uterine involution produces

TABLE 20-1
Cardiovascular Physiologic Changes of Pregnancy

Blood volume	Increased 45%
Systemic vascular resistance	Decreased 20%
Heart rate	Increased 15%
Stroke volume	Increased 30%
Cardiac output	Increased 50%
During active labor	Increased additional 25%
During second-stage labor	Increased additional 40%
During immediate postpartum period	Increased additional 80%
Pulmonary capillary wedge pressure	No change
Central venous pressure	No change

significant autotransfusion and increased venous return in the immediate postpartum period, increasing cardiac output 80% above prelabor levels.[9] Patients who tolerated pregnancy may experience cardiac decompensation during labor and delivery. The immediate postpartum period is an especially critical time. These patients should be closely observed in a critical care setting with invasive monitors for at least 24 hours after delivery.

Other physiologic changes of pregnancy also affect the anesthetic management of parturients with cardiac disease. Tidal volume increases 45% and respiratory rate increases slightly or remains unchanged during pregnancy. This results in a 45% increase in minute and alveolar ventilation.[10] Functional residual capacity (FRC) is decreased 20% at term.[10] Oxygen consumption is increased 60% during pregnancy as a result of the increased work of breathing and increased metabolic rate.[11] These changes place the parturient at greater risk for developing hypoxemia, especially during the induction of general anesthesia. Oxygen consumption can increase as much as 75% above prelabor values during labor and delivery, largely because of the hyperventilation associated with painful labor. Epidural analgesia significantly attenuates this additional increase in oxygen consumption.[12]

The gravid uterus displaces the stomach upward and alters the gastroesophageal junction, so that lower esophageal sphincter tone is decreased.[13] Gastrin produced by the placenta raises the acidity of stomach contents.[14] Pregnant patients are therefore at increased risk of pulmonary aspiration. Balancing the benefits of a rapid-sequence induction of general anesthesia to prevent aspiration with the benefits of a slower, heomdy-

namically stable induction is clinically challenging in the parturient with cardiac disease.

CONGENITAL HEART DISEASE

In the past, few patients with complex congenital heart disease survived to child-bearing age and became pregnant. Improvements in the diagnosis and surgical treatment of congenital heart defects have increased the number of pregnant patients with congenital heart disease.[3] Many of these women had successful surgical repair of the defects during childhood and are asymptomatic with normal cardiac function. These patients often require only standard monitoring and anesthetic management during labor and delivery, but should undergo cardiology evaluation early during pregnancy. Echocardiography is beneficial for evaluating patients for asymptomatic residua of the surgical correction that may be exacerbated by the cardiovascular changes of pregnancy. Some of these patients require antibiotic prophylaxis for bacterial endocarditis during labor and vaginal delivery.

Tetralogy of Fallot

Tetralogy of Fallot includes (1) right ventricular outflow tract obstruction, (2) ventricular septal defect (VSD), (3) right ventricular hypertrophy, and (4) an overriding aorta. This is the most common congenital heart defect that produces a right-to-left shunt and cyanosis. It is rare for these patients to reach adulthood without surgical correction. Most pregnant patients who had surgical repair, including closure of the VSD and widening of the pulmonary outflow tract, are asymptomatic. A small VSD may occasionally recur or hypertrophy of the pulmonary outflow tract may develop. Patients with these defects require additional attention during pregnancy, labor, and delivery. Symptoms experienced by these patients depend on the size of the VSD, the magnitude of outflow tract obstruction, and the degree of right ventricular dysfunction. While epidural analgesia is advantageous for preventing the hemodynamic changes associated with labor pain, it is important to maintain SVR to prevent an increase in right-to-left shunting. Phenylephrine should be available. The α-adrenergic effects of phenylephrine have the potential to compromise uteroplacental perfusion. Although ephedrine has generally been the drug of choice for treating hypotension during regional anesthesia in pregnancy, the choice of drug should be based primarily on the pathophysiology of the cardiac defect. Phenylephrine is equally effective as ephedrine in maintaining normal neonatal acid-base status in low-risk pregnancies.[15] Maintenance of venous return is also important for these patients. Patients with severe right ventricular dysfunction benefit from high filling pressures that improve right ventricular output and pulmonary blood flow.

Left-to-Right Shunts

Parturients with a surgically corrected VSD or atrial septal defect (ASD) are usually asymptomatic and require no special anesthetic considerations. Patients with small, asymptomatic VSDs and ASDs generally tolerate pregnancy, labor, and delivery without difficulty and do not require special monitoring. However, it is important to consider that the pain of uterine contractions increases maternal catecholamine levels,[16] resulting in increased SVR. This increased SVR may produce greater left-to-right shunting that ultimately leads to pulmonary hypertension. Epidural analgesia should be used early in labor to prevent these consequences. The mild decrease in SVR associated with epidural analgesia also provides further benefit by reducing left-to-right shunting through the defect. The anesthesiologist must be careful to slowly titrate the onset of epidural anesthesia because a rapid decrease in SVR could produce right-to-left shunting that leads to hypoxemia.

Patients with a VSD or ASD are at risk for systemic embolization. All air should be removed from intravenous tubing before infusion of intravenous fluids. Use of the loss-of-resistance to air technique should not be used when performing an epidural procedure. Supplemental oxygen should be administered during labor and delivery because even mild hypoxemia could lead to increased pulmonary vascular resistance and right-to-left shunting.

Patients with a large VSD or ASD commonly have chronically increased pulmonary blood flow that produces pulmonary hypertension. These patients require special attention during labor and delivery, including radial artery and pulmonary artery pressure monitoring. Increases in heart rate and systemic and pulmonary vascular resistance must be avoided. Marked decreases in systemic and pulmonary vascular resistance are also not well tolerated. Adequate labor analgesia is required to attenuate changes in SVR. While carefully titrated epidural analgesia is acceptable, a combined spinal-epidural (CSE) technique using primarily spinal opioids may be preferable in some patients because decreases in SVR are minimized.[17]

Eisenmenger's Syndrome

Eisenmenger's syndrome results when chronic pulmonary volume overload from an uncorrected left-to-right shunt leads to pulmonary hypertension (Fig. 20-1). Initially the left-to-right shunt becomes bidirectional with acute changes in pulmonary vascular resistance or SVR

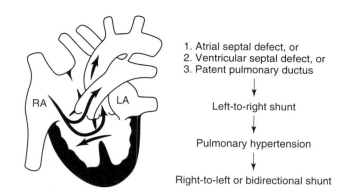

1. Atrial septal defect, or
2. Ventricular septal defect, or
3. Patent pulmonary ductus

↓

Left-to-right shunt

↓

Pulmonary hypertension

↓

Right-to-left or bidirectional shunt

FIG. 20-1   Pathophysiology of Eisenmenger's syndrome. *LA*, Left atrium; *RA*, right atrium.

(From Mangano DT: Anesthesia for the pregnant cardiac patient. In Shnider SM, Levinson G, editors: *Anesthesia for obstetrics*, ed 3, Baltimore, 1993, Williams and Wilkins, p 504.)

determining the direction of flow. Eventually, the pulmonary hypertension becomes irreversible, and shunt flow reverses. Right-to-left shunting occurs when pulmonary artery pressure exceeds systemic pressure.

Patients with Eisenmenger's syndrome do not tolerate pregnancy well. The decreased SVR during pregnancy may increase the shunt fraction. In addition, the decreased FRC and increased oxygen consumption associated with pregnancy exacerbate maternal hypoxemia. Maternal hypoxemia compromises oxygen delivery to the fetus, leading to many pregnancies that are complicated by intrauterine growth restriction and fetal demise.[18,19] Maternal mortality is as high as 36%.[20]

Anesthetic management of the pregnant Eisenmenger's patient is extremely challenging. If the obstetrician chooses to attempt a vaginal delivery, it is essential that adequate labor analgesia be provided. Labor pain causes an increased release of catecholamines that increase pulmonary vascular resistance and right-to-left shunting. Pulse oximetry monitoring is maintained throughout labor and delivery, and supplemental oxygen is administered. Worsening hypoxemia must be treated aggressively to avoid increased pulmonary vascular resistance. Because prevention of hypotension and decreased SVR is also essential in the management of these patients, an intraarterial catheter should be inserted to provide continuous blood pressure monitoring. Left uterine displacement throughout labor is also important to avoid aortocaval compression.

Central venous pressure (CVP) monitoring is very beneficial in the management of these patients,[21] because maintenance of adequate preload is important. Most experts do not recommend the use of a pulmonary artery catheter[22,23] because very little useful information is derived from pulmonary artery pressure monitoring in these patients with fixed pulmonary hypertension and a large intracardiac shunt. Insertion of the catheter into the pulmonary artery in patients with Eisenmenger's syndrome is difficult and the risks associated with catheter insertion are great. The risk of pulmonary artery rupture is high and passing the catheter through the cardiac defect is possible. Finally, common complications associated with placement of the catheter, such as arrhythmias and pneumothorax, could be life threatening for these patients who lack cardiac reserve.

The anesthesiologist faces a significant clinical challenge in providing adequate labor analgesia without deleterious hemodynamic changes. A CSE technique is an excellent choice. Rapid and profound analgesia can be provided during the first stage of labor with an intrathecal opioid without causing a sympathetic block.[17] Fentanyl 15 to 25 μg and sufentanil 5 to 10 μg are the most commonly used opioids for this technique. These opioids reliably produce analgesia for only 1 to 2 hours.[24,25] The addition of 2.5 mg isobaric bupivacaine prolongs the analgesia without causing significant motor block[25] and is unlikely to cause a sympathectomy. Intrathecal morphine provides a longer duration of analgesia,[26] reducing the need for epidural local anesthetic during the first stage of labor. The problem, however, is that the incidence of intrathecal opioid-induced side effects, including pruritus, nausea or vomiting, and respiratory depression, is greater with morphine than with fentanyl or sufentanil.[27]

Small incremental doses of dilute local anesthetic are administered to achieve a T10 to S1 segmental block if the spinal opioid analgesia resolves before completion of the first stage of labor. While 0.25% bupivacaine has been safely used for labor analgesia, 0.25% levobupivacaine or 0.2% ropivacaine might be better choices for cardiac patients because these drugs possess less cardiac toxicity.[28] A continuous infusion of very dilute local anesthetic and opioid (such as 0.125% or 0.0625% levobupivacaine plus 2 μg/ml fentanyl) is administered for the duration of labor. Decreases in SVR associated with the sympathetic block are avoided by slow incremental dosing of the epidural catheter, continuous blood pressure monitoring with an intraarterial catheter, and careful intravenous fluid administration. A phenylephrine infusion is used by careful titration to treat decreases in SVR.

Intrathecal opioid is insufficient for providing anesthesia for the second stage of labor, particularly if an instrumented delivery is planned to minimize maternal expulsive efforts. A higher concentration of local anesthetic in the epidural is required for sacral anesthesia during a forceps-assisted delivery. Ropivacaine, levobupivacaine, or lidocaine are preferred over bupivacaine because of less cardiac toxicity.

A continuous spinal technique or epidural analgesia alone are other options for providing satisfactory analgesia and anesthesia for labor and delivery.[21] Intra-

thecal opioid dosing could be repeated as needed via a continuous spinal catheter during the first stage of labor, and small doses of local anesthetic could be injected to provide anesthesia for the second stage of labor. A high incidence of spinal headache is a disadvantage of this technique because of the intentional dural puncture with a 17- or 18-gauge epidural needle. Dosing with local anesthetics beginning in early labor is the major disadvantage of epidural analgesia. Significant sympathectomy and decreased SVR are more likely to occur compared with the CSE and continuous spinal techniques.

Epidural anesthesia is the preferred anesthetic technique for a cesarean delivery.[29,30] Sudden onset of decreased SVR worsens the right-to-left shunt. This problem is prevented by the slow induction of epidural anesthesia, maintenance of adequate preload with careful monitoring of CVP, and use of a phenylephrine infusion to maintain SVR. Ropivacaine, levobupivacaine, and 2% lidocaine without epinephrine are all reasonable local anesthetic choices. Two-chloroprocaine is not a good choice because of its rapid onset. Anxiolysis may be used to prevent increases in catecholamine release associated with maternal anxiety.

Single-shot spinal anesthesia for cesarean delivery is contraindicated in patients with Eisenmenger's syndrome because of the hypotension and rapid drop in SVR that can occur. A continuous spinal technique may be used because the blockade level is slowly raised to provide adequate anesthesia.

There are several disadvantages to the use of general anesthesia in patients with Eisenmenger's syndrome. Decreased venous return associated with positive pressure ventilation is not tolerated well in these patients. The patient's cardiovascular compromise requires a slow induction of general anesthesia, preferably with a high-dose opioid technique to maintain cardiovascular stability. However, these parturients are also at significant risk for pulmonary aspiration. Measures must be taken to lessen the aspiration risk during a slow, controlled anesthetic induction. A nonparticulate antacid, metoclopramide, and an H_2-receptor antagonist are administered preoperatively. Throughout the induction, cricoid pressure is applied. A neonatologist is present for neonatal resuscitation because the infant is likely to experience respiratory depression associated with a high-dose opioid technique.

The risk of mortality persists into the postpartum period, so that extended hemodynamic monitoring in an intensive care setting is essential. The use of nitric oxide in the peripartum period was recently reported in a patient with Eisenmenger's syndrome.[31,32] This should be considered in patients with severe pulmonary hypertension who decompensate during the peripartum period. Thromboembolic events are a significant cause of maternal death. Prophylactic anticoagulation is considered when the risk of bleeding has subsided in the postpartum period.

VALVULAR HEART DISEASE

Anesthesiologists are caring for fewer patients with rheumatic valvular disease because the incidence of rheumatic fever has markedly decreased in the United States.[33] More parturients may have aortic stenosis and insufficiency associated with a congenital bicuspid valve as more women delay child bearing to the fourth and fifth decade. Parturients with infective endocarditis may be seen with the resurgence of intravenous heroin abuse. Mitral valve prolapse (MVP) remains the most common cardiac abnormality in pregnant women,[34] but is a benign lesion in most patients.[35]

Mitral Valve Prolapse

MVP is the most common cardiac abnormality in women of childbearing age.[34] Most patients are asymptomatic. The diagnosis is made after a midsystolic click is heard during physical examination and echocardiography is performed. The prognosis is usually benign even in patients who experience palpitations and chest pain. The degree of prolapse often improves during pregnancy because of the physiologic changes of pregnancy.[36] Significant mitral regurgitation (MR) occurs in a small percentage of patients who require special care during labor and delivery. Management of these patients is discussed in more detail in the MR section of this chapter. MVP is associated with other serious medical problems, including Marfan syndrome, Ehlers-Danlos syndrome, and Wolff-Parkinson-White syndrome. It is important to evaluate parturients with MVP for these disorders because anesthetic management will differ when one of these disorders is present.

The greatest controversy in the management of parturients with MVP is the need for endocarditis prophylaxis during labor and delivery. Many institutions provide prophylaxis to any woman with a diagnosis of MVP. The most recent recommendations of the American Heart Association (AHA) do not support this practice.[37] Their rationale is that cesarean delivery is not classified as a high-risk procedure requiring antibiotic therapy in patients at risk for endocarditis. Vaginal delivery also does not require prophylaxis, but it should be considered in high-risk patients. Patients with MVP, however, are considered to be at moderate risk. When a procedure does warrant antibiotic prophylaxis, the AHA recommends therapy only in patients with MVP and MR as demonstrated by a murmur of MR or echocardiographic evidence of regurgitation (Fig. 20-2). Patients with MVP and no regurgitation do not require antibiotic therapy.

Mitral Stenosis

Mitral stenosis is the most common cardiac lesion associated with rheumatic heart disease in pregnant women.[38] While the incidence of rheumatic heart disease has declined significantly in the United States, most anesthesiologists who care for high-risk obstetric patients can expect to encounter patients with this valvular disorder. In fact, 25% of women with mitral stenosis experience their first symptoms during pregnancy because of the cardiovascular changes of pregnancy.[39] The necessary increase in cardiac output during pregnancy is impeded by the stenotic lesion. The heart rate increase that occurs during pregnancy decreases the diastolic time for left ventricular filling. This leads to increases in left atrial and pulmonary arterial pressures and ultimately to pulmonary edema. These increased demands placed on the cardiovascular system are especially not well tolerated by parturients with severe mitral stenosis.

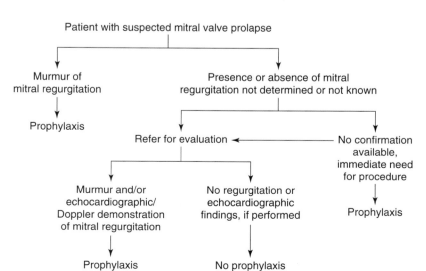

FIG. 20-2 Clinical approach to determination of the need for prophylaxis in patients with suspected mitral valve prolapse.

(From Dajani Ad, Taubert KA, Wilson W et al: *JAMA,* 277:1796, 1997. Copyrighted 1997, American Medical Association.)

These patients must be closely monitored by a cardiologist throughout pregnancy. A multidisciplinary approach is essential during labor and delivery, using obstetricians, anesthesiologists, and cardiologists.

Effective management throughout pregnancy prevents some complications associated with mitral stenosis in parturients. Particular attention should be paid to heart rate and rhythm. β-Adrenergic blockade is used to maintain a slow heart rate. One study demonstrated a decreased incidence of pulmonary edema in parturients receiving β-blockers with no ill effects on the fetus or infant.[40] Maintenance of normal sinus rhythm is also essential for these patients to prevent pulmonary edema and decreased cardiac output. Digoxin and β-adrenergic blockers are used for treating atrial fibrillation and maintaining normal sinus rhythm. If medical therapy is unsuccessful, cardioversion is performed.

Patients with mild to moderate mitral stenosis who remain asymptomatic throughout pregnancy generally tolerate labor and delivery. It is prudent to observe these patients closely during labor and maintain continuous pulse oximetry monitoring. These patients do not usually require invasive monitoring. Patients who are symptomatic during pregnancy or are diagnosed with severe stenosis require invasive monitoring, including a pulmonary artery catheter. Adequate filling pressures must be maintained and fluid overload avoided because these patients are at significant risk for developing pulmonary edema, especially in the immediate postpartum period. Maintenance of adequate SVR is necessary to provide adequate perfusion pressure because the ability to increase cardiac output is limited by the stenotic lesion. These patients may not tolerate a sudden increase in venous return associated with the Valsalva maneuver during maternal expulsive efforts. A passive second stage of labor and instrument-assisted vaginal delivery is often planned. Cesarean delivery is usually reserved for obstetric indications.

Adequate analgesia is needed to prevent undesirable tachycardia associated with labor pain. A dense anesthetic block is required during the second stage of labor to prevent the urge to push and to facilitate a forceps or vacuum-assisted delivery. A CSE anesthesia technique is a good choice for these patients. Intrathecal opioid can provide initial analgesia during the first stage of labor without producing a significant drop in SVR or requiring a large fluid bolus to maintain adequate preload. As further labor analgesia and ultimately anesthesia for delivery is required, slow incremental dosing of the epidural catheter with close observation of the invasive hemodynamic monitors minimizes disastrous decreases in SVR and venous return while also preventing inadvertent volume overload. Phenylephrine is preferred over ephedrine in patients with mitral stenosis if a vasopressor is required to treat hypotension associated with epidural local anesthesia. Phenylephrine maintains SVR and avoids maternal tachycardia. Continuous epidural or spinal anesthesia are also acceptable methods for providing anesthesia and analgesia. Monitoring and hemodynamic management are similar regardless of the technique.

Epidural anesthesia is the preferred technique for cesarean section in most cases.[41] Using invasive monitors to guide fluid management, the slow induction of anesthesia with lidocaine, ropivacaine, or levobupivacaine is generally well tolerated while hemodynamic stability is maintained. A significant sympathectomy is expected with the sensory level of T4 to T6 that is required to provide adequate anesthesia for surgery. Phenylephrine is administered by slow infusion or small, intermittent bolus doses to prevent a hemodynamically significant decrease in SVR. A single-shot spinal technique is not recommended for anesthesia for cesarean delivery in patients with mitral stenosis because of the greater probability of larger and more rapid drops in venous return and SVR.

General anesthesia may be required for cesarean delivery in parturients with a history of atrial fibrillation who are receiving anticoagulant therapy. The patient's ventricular function determines whether she will tolerate a rapid-sequence induction of general anesthesia, or will require a high-dose opioid induction technique. If a high-dose opioid technique is used, all possible modes of aspiration prophylaxis are administered. A β-adrenergic blocker or a small dose of opioid is administered during rapid-sequence induction to blunt tachycardia and hypertension associated with laryngoscopy. Remifentanil is a good choice when a high-dose opioid technique is chosen. Scott et al[42] reported no neonatal respiratory depression when remifentanil was used during cesarean section in a parturient with mitral valve disease.

Patients with mitral stenosis are at high risk for developing pulmonary edema in the immediate postpartum period because of the marked increase in cardiac output and venous return. Patients require close observation and hemodynamic monitoring continued for at least 24 hours postpartum. Epidural anesthesia that is continued for several hours postpartum inhibits the increased preload from resolution of the epidural-induced vasodilatation from coinciding with the increased preload associated with the postpartum period.

Mitral Regurgitation

The majority of parturients with MR have chronic MR caused by rheumatic heart disease or MVP. Slow dilation of the left atrium develops as left atrial pressure increases. The incidence of pulmonary edema and pulmonary hypertension in women of child-bearing age with MR is much less than in women of the same age with mitral stenosis. The physiologic changes of pregnancy, including decreased SVR and mildly increased heart rate, are advantageous in patients with MR. Most of these women tolerate pregnancy well.

Continuous electrocardiogram (ECG) monitoring is warranted during labor and delivery because of the increased risk for atrial fibrillation during pregnancy.[43] Rapid treatment of this arrhythmia is essential. No other special monitoring is required for asymptomatic patients during labor and delivery. Symptomatic patients and patients with a history of pulmonary edema require invasive monitoring with an intraarterial catheter and pulmonary artery catheter.

Increased SVR caused by labor pain or the Valsalva maneuver during expulsive efforts must be avoided. Epidural anesthesia that provides labor analgesia and anesthesia for an instrumented delivery prevents undesirable increases in SVR associated with labor and delivery, and produces a mild decrease in SVR. Decreased SVR improves forward flow, reduces regurgitation, improves cardiac output, and decreases the likelihood of developing pulmonary edema. Careful attention is given to maintaining adequate venous return during epidural anesthesia and to providing adequate left ventricular filling. CSE analgesia is an acceptable technique for these patients; however, epidural local anesthetics are preferred over spinal opioids because of the significant decrease in SVR associated with local anesthetic sympatholysis.

Epidural anesthesia is the anesthetic of choice during cesarean section for patients with MR. A continuous spinal anesthetic also provides cardiovascular effects that are advantageous in these patients. However, the larger-gauge epidural needle and catheter used for this continuous spinal technique increases the risk of postdural puncture headache. Ephedrine is the vasopressor of choice for treating hypotension. Phenylephrine is avoided because the associated increased SVR and decreased heart rate are deleterious to MR. When general anesthesia is required for cesarean delivery, anesthetic agents that produce decreased afterload and a slightly increased heart rate are chosen. Myocardial depressants are avoided.

Aortic Stenosis

Aortic stenosis during pregnancy usually results from rheumatic heart disease or a congenital bicuspid valve. Women with mild stenosis generally tolerate pregnancy well. Many of the physiologic changes of pregnancy are deleterious to patients with moderate to severe stenosis. One study reported a maternal mortality rate of 17% and a perinatal mortality rate of 32% in parturients with aortic stenosis.[44] More recent literature suggests that more aggressive hemodynamic monitoring improves outcome in the mother and fetus.[45] Risk remains significant, however, and aortic valve replace-

ment is recommended before conception in women with moderate to severe stenosis.

The increased cardiac output and oxygen consumption and the decreased SVR that occur during pregnancy are disadvantageous to the patient with severe aortic stenosis. Because stroke volume is relatively fixed with the stenotic lesion, cardiac output increases primarily by an increase in heart rate. Tachycardia decreases time for diastolic coronary perfusion and increases myocardial oxygen demand. The increased left ventricular end-diastolic pressure and left ventricular hypertrophy of aortic stenosis also decrease myocardial perfusion. The decreased SVR of pregnancy reduces coronary filling during diastole and decreases perfusion to the hypertrophied left ventricle. These parturients are therefore at risk for myocardial ischemia. Cardiac output increases even further during labor and delivery, creating a critically dangerous clinical scenario for these patients.

Many obstetricians favor cesarean delivery only for obstetric indications for these patients and prefer a vaginal delivery. An instrumented delivery with minimal maternal expulsive efforts is usually planned to avoid the adverse hemodynamic effects of the Valsalva maneuver. Some obstetricians choose a cesarean delivery to avoid the uncertain duration and course, and the hemodynamic stress of labor for these high-risk patients.[46] There is little consensus in the literature as to the ideal anesthetic management of these patients for labor and vaginal delivery and cesarean delivery.[47,48] The unique characteristics of each patient are used to determine an anesthetic plan.

Regardless of the anesthetic technique, certain hemodynamic conditions are maintained when anesthetizing these patients. A normal heart rate with sinus rhythm is essential. Tachycardia is not well tolerated for the reasons mentioned earlier, and bradycardia provides inadequate cardiac output because of the fixed stroke volume. The atrial "kick" contributes 40% to the ventricular filling and cardiac output. Prompt and effective treatment is necessary when dysrhythmias occur. SVR is maintained to ensure adequate myocardial perfusion. Normal venous return is required for adequate end-diastolic volume to maintain adequate left ventricular stroke volume. Left uterine displacement is used to avoid aortocaval compression, and prevention of myocardial depression is essential. Invasive monitors, including an intraarterial catheter and a CVP or pulmonary artery catheter, are necessary to optimize management of these parturients. A pulmonary artery catheter is preferable for these patients because the measurements are more indicative of left-sided pressures with additional information (cardiac output, SVR) provided that is not available with a CVP catheter. Because the risk of ventricular arrhythmias associated with pulmonary artery catheters in these fragile patients might in some cases be greater than the benefit of additional information, some clinicians prefer a CVP catheter.[49]

Excellent analgesia for labor and vaginal delivery is a challenge to provide, given the hemodynamic goals of aortic stenosis. Some anesthesiologists avoid regional anesthesia in these patients because of the decrease in venous return and SVR associated with the technique. Intravenous opioids for first-stage labor pain and a pudendal nerve block for second-stage labor pain and instrumented delivery is another alternative. Systemic opioids may not provide adequate analgesia and the tachycardia associated with inadequate pain management is deleterious to these patients. With the aid of invasive monitors to assess and quickly treat any decreases in venous return or SVR, slow and careful titration of epidural analgesia provides safe and effective labor analgesia and perineal anesthesia for an instrumented delivery.[46,50] Opioids are added to the local anesthetic to minimize the amount of local anesthetic required. Because of their relatively less cardiac toxicity, ropivacaine or levobupivacaine are preferred over bupivacaine for epidural anesthesia in these high-risk cardiac patients. Intravenous fluids and phenylephrine are used to treat or prevent hypotension; ephedrine is less desirable because of the risk of tachycardia.

Intrathecal opioids are another alternative for labor analgesia for patients with aortic stenosis. A CSE technique provides excellent intrathecal analgesia initially with opioids, and the decreased venous return and SVR associated with epidurally administered local anesthetics are avoided. As the initial intrathecal analgesia resolves, labor analgesia and anesthesia for instrumented delivery are achieved with the epidural catheter. A continuous spinal catheter technique permits intermittent intrathecal opioid injection for analgesia throughout the first stage of labor. Small doses of intrathecal local anesthetic are titrated to provide adequate anesthesia for the second stage of labor and delivery. A significant advantage of this technique is that hemodynamic stability is more easily achieved because the decrease in SVR and venous return associated with a local anesthetic-induced sympathectomy is avoided for the majority of the labor process. A disadvantage of this technique is the increased incidence of spinal headache, but this can be easily treated with an epidural blood patch.

The risks and benefits of regional and general anesthesia are considered for each individual patient with aortic stenosis facing a cesarean delivery. Successful outcomes have been reported with both techniques. A single-shot spinal technique is not an acceptable option because of the rapid hemodynamic changes that occur. Use of invasive monitors to guide management allows slow titration of epidural or spinal anesthesia with a continuous catheter to provide excellent and hemodynamically safe anesthesia in many patients.[51-53] A regional anesthetic technique avoids the risks of aspiration and difficult intubation that are present in all pregnant patients undergoing general anesthesia. The deleterious effects of tachycardia associated with laryngoscopy are also avoided.

The most important risk of a continuous catheter regional technique is hypotension and decreased SVR, which could be catastrophic in a patient with aortic stenosis. It is for this reason that some anesthesiologists prefer using general anesthesia during cesarean section for these patients. Precautions to prevent aspiration during induction are required and anesthetic agents that maintain hemodynamic stability are used. The successful use of etomidate, alfentanil, and succinylcholine for induction has been reported.[54] Others recommend the use of a slow, high-dose opioid induction technique.[55] Regardless of which drugs are chosen for the primary induction, administration of opioids before delivery of the neonate is necessary to prevent tachycardia during laryngoscopy. A neonatologist must be present at delivery to manage any potential neonatal respiratory depression. Volatile agents produce myocardial depression and should either be avoided or used very cautiously in small doses. Anesthesia maintenance is best achieved with a high-dose opioid anesthetic. Remifentanil is a good choice because of its high potency and short duration of action. If remifentanil is used intraoperationly, smaller doses of morphine or fentanyl must also be administered for adequate postoperative after-delivery pain control.

Patients with aortic stenosis must be monitored closely in the postoperative period, regardless of route of delivery. Cardiac decompensation could occur in response to the marked increase in cardiac output after delivery. Invasive monitors are maintained for 24 to 48 hours postpartum. Excellent postoperative analgesia is particularly important in the management of postcesarean patients to prevent tachycardia.

Aortic Regurgitation

Rheumatic heart disease is the most common cause of chronic aortic regurgitation in pregnant women. Acute aortic insufficiency from infective endocarditis has been reported during pregnancy, but is less common than rheumatic disease. Left ventricular volume overload results from regurgitation of blood into the left ventricle from an incompetent aortic valve and ultimately leads to left ventricular failure. Left ventricular hypertrophy and dilation occur. As end-diastolic volume increases, ventricular function declines and forward stroke volume decreases. Progressive deterioration of left ventricular function leads to marked increases of left ventricular end-diastolic volume and pressure, and pulmonary edema develops. These changes occur over many years in patients with chronic regurgitation. Many parturients with aortic regurgitation are asymptomatic.

The physiologic changes of pregnancy are beneficial to the patient with aortic regurgitation. The decreased SVR associated with pregnancy decreases the regurgitant fraction and improves forward stroke volume. The small increase in heart rate that occurs during pregnancy decreases time in diastole, allowing less time for regurgitation and a smaller end-diastolic volume. Patients with mild to moderate aortic regurgitation usually tolerate pregnancy well. However, patients with severe aortic regurgitation in whom significant declines in left ventricular function have occurred before pregnancy require intensive management throughout pregnancy, labor, and delivery. These patients are often unable to compensate for the increased blood volume of pregnancy. Invasive hemodynamic monitors, including an arterial catheter and pulmonary artery catheter, are indicated for these patients during labor and delivery.

Labor analgesia is an important part of the management of patients with aortic regurgitation during labor and delivery. Increased SVR associated with painful labor results in a significant increase in left ventricular volume overload and could lead to pulmonary edema. Epidural analgesia is an ideal technique for providing pain management.[56] The excellent analgesia not only attenuates any increases in SVR, but also the local anesthetic-induced sympathetic blockade decreases SVR, improving forward stroke volume and cardiac output. The pulmonary artery catheter is used in patients with severe disease to guide fluid management during the induction and maintenance of epidural analgesia. It is important to maintain adequate preload and avoid hypotension. The vasopressor of choice for treating hypotension precipitated by the sympathetic block is ephedrine. The small increase in heart rate associated with this drug is beneficial for these patients. Phenylephrine is not preferred because of its potential to produce bradycardia and increase SVR. Bradycardia is harmful to the patient with aortic regurgitation because the time for regurgitant flow across the valve is increased, leading to greater left ventricular volume overload.

CSE analgesia is another acceptable technique for management of labor pain in the parturient with aortic regurgitation. This technique also prevents the undesirable increase in SVR associated with pain. The initial analgesia provided by the spinal opioid does not produce a sympathetic block.[17] Therefore the additional benefit of decreased SVR described earlier is not achieved until later in the labor process when the epidural catheter is dosed with local anesthetic.

For the same reasons mentioned previously for labor, epidural anesthesia is the preferred technique for cesarean delivery. Slow and careful titration of local anesthetic with invasive monitors guiding fluid and vasopressor management is essential. Cardiac arrest

has been reported in a parturient with aortic regurgitation when epidural anesthesia was too quickly achieved.[57] If the clinical situation requires general anesthesia, the severity of the patient's condition determines the type of anesthetic induction. Asymptomatic patients with mild to moderate aortic regurgitation tolerate a rapid-sequence induction with etomidate. A slow induction with high-dose opioids and precautions to prevent aspiration are used for patients with severe regurgitation and severe left ventricular dysfunction. Anesthetic agents that depress myocardial function are avoided or used cautiously for anesthesia maintenance in patients with severe disease.

Infective Endocarditis

Infective endocarditis is a life-threatening infection that may complicate pregnancy. The incidence of endocarditis is rare during pregnancy; however, maternal and fetal mortality are very high when it does occur.[58] One might expect the incidence of this disease in pregnancy to have declined with the significant decrease of rheumatic valvular heart disease in women of child-bearing age. However, intravenous drug abuse is now the major cause of this illness in young adults.[59] Because of the recent resurgence of intravenous drug abuse, anesthesia personnel are more likely to care for patients with infective endocarditis.[60] These patients may be critically ill with acute mitral or aortic regurgitation and may require emergency cardiac surgery even during pregnancy. Management during labor and delivery generally follows that described for valvular lesions. Because of the acute development of valvular lesions, these patients are more likely than patients with chronic valvular lesions to suffer serious cardiac deterioration when confronted with the cardiovascular stresses of pregnancy, labor, and delivery.

The use of regional anesthesia in parturients with infective endocarditis is controversial. Many anesthesiologists avoid regional anesthesia because of legitimate bacteremic concerns and the risk for meningitis or epidural abscess. Regional anesthesia is contraindicated in patients with sepsis. The risk/benefit ratio favors regional anesthesia for labor and delivery in patients receiving antibiotic therapy who are afebrile with no signs of sepsis. Such patients are monitored very closely postpartum for any signs of epidural abscess or meningitis.

A more common issue related to infective endocarditis is antibiotic prophylaxis. Many obstetricians administer prophylaxis during labor and delivery to any parturient with a valvular lesion or history of congenital heart disease. Some studies report the incidence of endocarditis after a normal vaginal delivery to be minimal and do not recommend routine antibiotic prophylaxis in these patients.[58,61] The most recent report of the AHA[37] does not advocate routine endocarditis prophylaxis for vagi-

TABLE 20-2
Cardiac Conditions Associated with Endocarditis

Endocarditis Prophylaxis Recommended
High-risk category
    Prosthetic cardiac valves, including bioprosthetic and homograft valves
    Previous bacterial endocarditis
    Complex cyanotic congenital heart disease (e.g., single ventricle states, transposition of the great arteries, tetralogy of Fallot)
    Surgically constructed systemic pulmonary shunts or conduits
Moderate-risk category
    Most other congenital cardiac malformations (other than above and below)
    Acquired valvular dysfunction (e.g., rheumatic heart disease)
    Hypertrophic cardiomyopathy
    Mitral valve prolapse with valvular regurgitation and/or thickened leaflets

Endocarditis Prophylaxis Not Recommended
Negligible-risk category (no greater risk than the general population)
    Isolated secundum atrial septal defect
    Surgical repair of atrial septal defect, ventricular septal defect, or patent ductus arteriosus (without residua beyond 6 mo)
    Previous coronary artery bypass graft surgery
    Mitral valve prolapse without valvular regurgitation
    Physiologic, functional, or innocent heart murmurs
    Previous Kawasaki disease without valvular dysfunction
    Previous rheumatic fever without valvular dysfunction
    Cardiac pacemakers (intravascular and epicardial) and implanted defibrillators

From Dajani AS, Taubert KA, Wilson W et al: *JAMA* 277:1795, 1997. Copyrighted 1997, American Medical Association.

nal delivery or cesarean section. Prophylaxis is optional for vaginal delivery in high-risk patients. The AHA's risk categories are listed in Table 20-2. Patients with rheumatic heart disease and some congenital heart defects are classified as moderate rather than high risk. Patients with repaired atrial and ventricular septal defects are considered at no greater risk of developing endocarditis than the general population. The recommended drug regimens for endocarditis prophylaxis are described in Table 20-3. Indiscriminate antibiotic usage escalates concerns for the development of antibiotic-resistant organisms. Physicians are urged to follow the guidelines of the AHA and administer prophylaxis during labor and delivery to parturients in whom prophylaxis is truly indicated.

IDIOPATHIC HYPERTROPHIC SUBAORTIC STENOSIS

Idiopathic hypertrophic subaortic stenosis (IHSS), also known as *asymmetric septal hypertrophy* or *hypertrophic obstructive cardiomyopathy,* is an autosomal dominant genetic disorder that usually appears in childhood or young adulthood.[62] This disorder may be encountered in parturients and is characterized by dynamic obstruction of the left ventricular outflow tract resulting from asymmetric hypertrophy of the ventricular septum. The left ventricle is small, nondilated, and relatively noncompliant. Patients present with congestive heart failure, arrhythmias, syncope, or even sudden death.

The cardiovascular changes of pregnancy are variable in their effect on this disorder. Increased blood volume improves left ventricular filling and decreases the severity of outflow tract obstruction.[63] Other cardiovascular changes of pregnancy, including increased heart rate, increased contractility, and decreased SVR, worsen the outflow tract obstruction.[64] The majority of parturients with IHSS tolerate pregnancy fairly well,[65] but significant complications including pulmonary edema and maternal death[65,66] have been reported.

Patients require close observation and monitoring by the obstetrician and anesthesiologist during labor and delivery. While the fetal effects of β-adrenergic receptor blockade are somewhat controversial,[67] most obstetricians continue this mainstay of treatment for IHSS during pregnancy because of the significant maternal benefits. β-Blockade is maintained during labor and delivery. Prevention of aortocaval compression with continual left uterine displacement and aggressive fluid management of any peripartum hemorrhage are very important to avoid a decrease in venous return and worsening of the outflow tract obstruction. Adequate labor analgesia is important to prevent increased catecholamine levels associated with labor pain that result in detrimental increases in heart rate and contractility. Atrial dysrhythmias are treated promptly because the atrial "kick" contributes 40% to ventricular filling.

Adequate intravascular hydration and SVR is essential during labor and delivery to avoid worsening of the outflow tract obstruction. Invasive monitoring, including an intraarterial catheter and a CVP or pulmonary artery catheter, is warranted in these patients to guide hemodynamic management. Nam et al[68] reported the use of transesophageal echocardiography to guide anesthetic management during cesarean section under general anesthesia.

While labor analgesia plays an important role in the effective management of these patients during labor and delivery, the appropriate form of analgesia is con-

TABLE 20-3
Prophylactic Regimens for Genitourinary Procedures

SITUATION	AGENTS*	REGIMEN†
High-risk patients	Ampicillin plus gentamicin	Adults: ampicillin 2.0 g intramuscularly (IM) or intravenously (IV) plus gentamicin 1.5 mg/kg (not to exceed 120 mg) within 30 min of starting the procedure; 6 hr later, ampicillin 1 g IM/IV or amoxicillin 1 g orally Children: ampicillin 50 mg/kg IM or IV (not to exceed 2.0 g) plus gentamicin 1.5 mg/kg within 30 min of starting the procedure, 6 hr later, ampicillin 25 mg/kg IM/IV or amoxicillin 25 mg/kg orally
High-risk patients allergic to ampicillin/amoxicillin	Vancomycin plus gentamicin	Adults: vancomycin 1.0 g IV over 1-2 hr plus gentamicin 1.5 mg/kg IV/IM (not to exceed 120 mg); complete injection/infusion within 30 min of starting the procedure Children: vancomycin 20 mg/kg IV over 1-2 hr plus gentamicin 1.5 mg/kg IV/IM; complete injection/infusion within 30 min of starting the procedure
Moderate-risk patients	Amoxicillin or ampicillin	Adults: amoxicillin 2.0 g orally 1 hr before procedure, or ampicillin 2.0 g IM/IV within 30 min of starting the procedure Children: amoxicillin 50 mg/kg orally 1 hr before procedure, or ampicillin 50 mg/kg IM/IV within 30 min of starting the procedure
Moderate-risk patients allergic to ampicillin/amoxicillin	Vancomycin	Adults: vancomycin 1.0 g IV over 1-2 hr; complete infusion within 30 min of starting the procedure Children: vancomycin 20 mg/kg IV over 1-2 hr; complete infusion within 30 min of starting the procedure

From Dajani AS, Taubert KA, Wilson W et al: *JAMA* 277:1799, 1997. Copyrighted 1997, American Medical Association.
*Total children's dose should not exceed adult dose.
†No second dose of vancomycin or gentamicin is recommended.

troversial. Some clinicians avoid regional anesthesia because of the effects of decreased SVR and preload[65] and advocate systemic opioids and pudendal block. Sympathetically mediated tachycardia secondary to inadequate analgesia is a risk with this technique. The safe administration of epidural[69] and CSE[70] analgesia has been reported in parturients with IHSS, and is preferred by the author for labor pain management. Epidural analgesia is slowly achieved without causing significant decreases in SVR or venous return by using invasive monitors to guide fluid management. Phenylephrine is the vasopressor of choice to treat hypotension. Ephedrine is avoided because the associated increased heart rate and contractility are detrimental. A CSE or continuous spinal catheter technique provides analgesia while minimizing decreases in venous return and afterload associated with local anesthetic-induced sympathetic blockade. Local anesthetic administration is optimally delayed until the second stage of labor, when a decrease in SVR from the sympathetic blockade is offset by an increase in SVR associated with the maternal expulsive efforts.

Obstetricians usually reserve cesarean delivery for obstetric indications in parturients with IHSS. Advantages and disadvantages to both general and regional anesthesia for cesarean section exist and successful use of both have been reported.[71,72] General anesthesia with a halogenated volatile agent causes decreased myocardial contractility that reduces left ventricular outflow obstruction. Tachycardia caused by laryngoscopy must be avoided. Esmolol administered by bolus or continuous infusion helps prevent this response. The use of esmolol does raise concerns about fetal bradycardia and hypoxemia caused by this drug.[73-75] The disadvantages of regional anesthesia for cesarean delivery are the same as those discussed for labor, namely, decreased venous return and SVR resulting in greater outflow obstruction. A recent study showed no difference in outcome between general and regional anesthesia in patients with IHSS undergoing noncardiac surgery.[76] Epidural anesthesia is probably the better choice given the increased risk of general anesthesia in parturients as a result of aspiration and difficult intubation. Single-shot spinal anesthesia is avoided because of the rapid onset of sympathetic blockade and greater acute decreases in afterload and preload.

PRIMARY PULMONARY HYPERTENSION

Primary pulmonary hypertension is a disease of unknown etiology that occurs in the absence of underlying cardiac or pulmonary disease. Pulmonary hypertension and pregnancy is a deadly combination. Maternal mortality was recently reported as 30%.[20] Most obstetricians recommend that these patients not become pregnant. Much of the anesthetic management of patients with primary pulmonary hypertension is similar to that described for patients with Eisenmenger's syndrome. However, the pulmonary vasculature in some patients remains responsive to vasodilator drugs.

Invasive monitoring is required for management of labor and delivery, including an intraarterial catheter and either a CVP or pulmonary artery catheter. Some clinicians argue that the risks associated with pulmonary artery catheter placement in these seriously ill patients are greater than the benefits obtained from the additional information and do not advocate use of a pulmonary artery catheter.[77] However, many patients have pulmonary vasculature that is responsive to the newer, more effective pulmonary artery vasodilators. A pulmonary artery catheter used to titrate these drugs and improve pulmonary hypertension is beneficial and often outweighs the risks of pulmonary artery catheter placement.

Anesthetic management includes supplemental oxygen throughout labor and delivery. Increased oxygenation and decreased hypercarbia improve pulmonary artery pressures in patients with responsive pulmonary vasculature. Adequate venous return is essential for the successful management of pulmonary hypertension. It is important to prevent aortocaval compression, replace significant blood loss, and maintain adequate preload with the sympathectomy induced by epidural blockade. Increases in pulmonary vascular resistance related to labor pain lead to right ventricular failure, which results in decreased left ventricular output, systemic hypotension, and cardiovascular collapse. Adequate labor analgesia is therefore mandatory in patients with primary pulmonary hypertension.

The pulmonary artery catheter is used to guide management, including the administration of pulmonary artery vasodilators to optimize the hemodynamic status of these patients during labor and delivery. Intravenous infusions of nitroglycerin and sodium nitroprusside decrease pulmonary artery pressure in some patients. However, significant decreases in systemic blood pressure can limit their clinical usefulness. Fetal cyanide toxicity is a concern when nitroprusside is administered for a prolonged period. Newer treatments for primary pulmonary hypertension offer greater promise for the parturient with this life-threatening illness. Intravenous prostacyclin is a potent pulmonary vasodilating drug that causes a sustained decrease in pulmonary vascular resistance with long-term therapy.[78] Effective short-term use selectively decreases pulmonary artery pressure during cesarean delivery.[79] Its use is limited by systemic effects, including increased bleeding (because of its inhibition of platelet aggregation) and systemic hypoten-

sion. Aerosolized forms of prostacyclin and iloprost, a more stable analog of prostacyclin, effectively produce selective pulmonary vasodilation.[80] Aerosolized prostacyclin and iloprost were used in the successful management of parturients with primary pulmonary hypertension.[79,81] Inhaled nitric oxide also selectively produces pulmonary artery vasodilation and is being used increasingly for the treatment of pulmonary hypertension. Its successful use during pregnancy has been reported,[82] with expectations that nitric oxide will be used with increasing frequency during labor and delivery for patients with pulmonary hypertension.

Adequate labor analgesia is essential in these patients. As with Eisenmenger's syndrome, anesthesiologists previously avoided epidural analgesia because of the detrimental effects of decreased venous return and SVR caused by the local anesthetic-induced sympathectomy. The alternative of systemic opioids and pudendal block often does not provide adequate analgesia. The risk of pain-induced increases in pulmonary vascular resistance is greater than the risk of decreased SVR and preload if epidural analgesia is titrated slowly and invasive monitors are used to guide fluid management. Epidural labor analgesia has been used successfully in patients with pulmonary hypertension.[21,83,84]

CSE analgesia and continuous spinal analgesia are attractive alternatives for labor pain management in these parturients. Intrathecal opioids provide profound first-stage labor analgesia with minimal cardiovascular changes. As labor progresses or the opioid analgesia resolves, small doses of epidural local anesthetic (in the case of CSE) or spinal local anesthetic and opioid (in the case of continuous spinal analgesia) are slowly and carefully titrated to maintain adequate analgesia. Intrathecal morphine for first-stage labor analgesia and pudendal block for second-stage analgesia have also been used.[85]

The Valsalva maneuver during maternal expulsive efforts in the second stage of labor causes increased pulmonary vascular resistance and must be avoided in these patients. A dense sensory block is necessary during the second stage of labor to prevent the urge to push as the fetal head descends and to provide adequate anesthesia for an instrumented delivery.

Regardless of the anesthetic technique, management of the parturient with primary pulmonary hypertension undergoing cesarean section is extremely challenging. There is no consensus on the ideal technique because successful use of both general[79,86,87] and epidural anesthesia[81,88,89] has been reported. Decreased preload with either technique decreases cardiac output. The decrease in cardiac output during epidural anesthesia for cesarean section is greater than during epidural labor analgesia because a higher, more dense epidural block is required. Meticulous attention to intravenous hydration reduces the degree of hypotension. Vasopressors used to treat hypotension by α agonism are avoided whenever possible because they also increase pulmonary artery pressure. The risk associated with general anesthesia include the hemodynamic responses to laryngoscopy and intubation that may precipitate increases in pulmonary artery pressure. Decreased venous return caused by positive-pressure ventilation during general anesthesia is not well tolerated by these patients. Cardiovascular hemodynamic stability is best maintained during general anesthesia with a high-dose opioid technique for induction and maintenance of anesthesia. Inhalational agents causing myocardial depression are either avoided or used at low concentrations. Most anesthesiologists consider single-shot spinal anesthesia to be relatively contraindicated in these patients.

Most maternal deaths in patients with primary pulmonary hypertension occur in the postpartum period, and frequently occur several days postpartum.[20] Patients should be monitored closely with invasive monitoring until at least 48 hours postpartum in an intensive care setting.

MARFAN SYNDROME

Marfan syndrome is an autosomal dominant disorder affecting connective tissue metabolism. Many organ systems are affected by the disease but cardiovascular involvement is the most serious and potentially life threatening. The parturient with Marfan syndrome often has MVP and possibly MR. These cardiac lesions are managed in the pregnant patient as previously discussed. Cystic medial necrosis of the aorta with resulting aortic root dilation occurs with Marfan syndrome and is especially troublesome for parturients. While the risk of aortic dissection is increased in any Marfan patient with aortic root dilation, the risk is further increased during pregnancy because the increased cardiac output and blood volume associated with pregnancy increases the pulsatile shear stress on the aortic wall. These physiologic changes of pregnancy account for the fact that 50% of all aortic dissections in women younger than 40 years occur during pregnancy.[90] In one review of parturients with Marfan syndrome, nearly two thirds of the patients developed an aortic dissection and 50% of all patients died from aortic dissection.[91] Patients must be followed closely throughout pregnancy, labor, and delivery. Particular attention is given to avoiding increased shear stress on the aorta by minimizing increases in contractility and avoiding sudden changes in blood pressure.[92]

An echocardiogram is performed during pregnancy to determine the presence of aortic root dilation, aortic regurgitation, and MR. β-Blockade is generally recommended in patients with aortic root dilation to minimize shear stress. Labetalol is preferred for use in parturients because of the controversy concerning the effects of pure β-blockade on the fetus. Parturients with Marfan syndrome who lack cardiovascular involvement on the basis of echocardiographic evaluation are at

significantly less risk and usually tolerate pregnancy well. They do not require invasive monitoring during labor and delivery, but are monitored closely to maintain hemodynamic stability. Acute increases in blood pressure are minimized by providing effective labor analgesia.

The increases in cardiac output that occur during labor and delivery place the parturient with known aortic root dilatation at significant risk for aortic dissection. Meticulous blood pressure control with intraarterial catheter monitoring is necessary. CVP monitoring is not necessary unless significant mitral or aortic regurgitation is present. A central line is useful for administration of vasoactive medications for blood pressure control.

β-Blockade medications are continued during labor and delivery. If a parturient with aortic root dilation has not been previously treated with β-blockers, initiation during labor is strongly recommended. Effective labor analgesia is essential for these parturients to avoid increases in endogenous catecholamine levels and associated increases in blood pressure, heart rate, and cardiac output. Epidural analgesia or CSE analgesia are both excellent techniques for the patient with Marfan syndrome. Epinephrine-containing local anesthetics are avoided because an unintentional intravascular injection would cause detrimental tachycardia and hypertension. Intravenous fluids and phenylephrine are used to treat hypotension associated with epidural anesthesia. Ephedrine is avoided because its β-agonist property increases shear stress. A passive second stage of labor with an instrumented vaginal delivery is used to optimize hemodynamic stability. Dense epidural blockade is required during this second stage of labor.

Scoliosis associated with Marfan syndrome may make an epidural or CSE procedure technically challenging. Previous Harrington rod placement for scoliosis decreases the success rate of epidural analgesia further. If epidural or CSE analgesia is unsuccessful, other analgesic options must be considered because effective analgesia is a key component of the management for these parturients. While not as ideal as epidural or CSE analgesia, systemic opioids provide analgesia during the first stage of labor. Intravenous fentanyl or meperidine with a patient-controlled administration pump is more effective than intermittent dosing. A pudendal or subarachnoid block provides effective anesthesia for the second stage of labor and instrumented delivery. Spinal anesthesia is technically easier and more effective than epidural anesthesia in patients with scoliosis or Harrington rods.

Obstetric indications dictate the need for cesarean section. Epidural anesthesia is the preferred anesthetic because an adequate sensory level is obtained slowly while hemodynamic stability is maintained. Single-shot spinal anesthesia is less desirable because of the sudden onset of sympathetic blockade and hypotension. Regional anesthesia (epidural or spinal) is preferable to

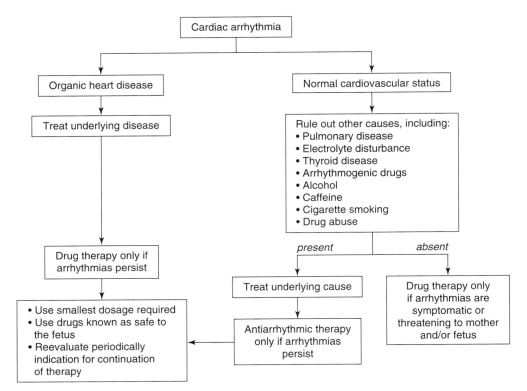

FIG. 20-3 Management of cardiac arrhythmias during pregnancy.
(Reprinted from Rotmensch HH, Rotmensch S, Elkayam U: *Drugs* 33[6]:623-633, 1987. Adis International, Inc.)

general anesthesia because of the potential hemodynamic consequences of laryngoscopy and emergence. If a general anesthetic is required, the response to laryngoscopy and emergence must be attenuated. A rapid-sequence induction is required but labetalol or lidocaine should be used as pretreatment medications. An intraarterial catheter allows for prompt treatment of increased blood pressure with vasoactive agents such as sodium nitroprusside or nitroglycerin.

Some medications commonly used during pregnancy, labor, and delivery are avoided or used with extreme caution in patients with Marfan syndrome. Terbutaline, a β-agonist used for tocolysis of premature labor and for uterine hypertonicity during term labor, increases the force of ventricular contractility and hence the shearing force on the aortic wall. Methergine, used to treat postpartum uterine atony, can cause significant hypertension. Other management options for postpartum hemorrhage secondary to uterine atony should be tried before using Methergine.

CARDIAC ARRHYTHMIAS

Cardiac arrhythmias are more frequently encountered during pregnancy than most cardiac disorders. The incidence of atrial and ventricular ectopy and tachycardia is increased during pregnancy,[93] but in most cases the arrhythmia is benign. Dysrhythmias during pregnancy require evaluation because the arrhythmia may be a sign of underlying organic heart disease or may cause hemodynamic instability that jeopardizes the mother or fetus. An algorithm for diagnosis and treatment of cardiac arrhythmias during pregnancy is outlined in Fig. 20-3.

Special consideration of antiarrhythmic drug therapy during pregnancy include the potential for adverse effects on the fetus and the influence of physiologic changes of pregnancy on the pharmacology of antiarrhythmic drugs. The loading dose of some drugs needs to be increased because of the increased blood volume of pregnancy. Increased renal perfusion of pregnancy increases drug clearance for renally excreted drugs, and decreases in serum protein concentration reduce protein-binding of antiarrhythmic drugs. The unbound fraction of the drugs produces the electrophysiologic effect. The clinical effect is enhanced therefore by the increased unbound fraction for a particular dosage.[93]

Many antiarrhythmic drugs are relatively safe during pregnancy on the basis of absent reported fetal side effects. Table 20-4 reports the FDA use-in-pregnancy ratings and other important safety information for several of these drugs. The absence of controlled studies of antiarrhythmic drugs during pregnancy precludes their

TABLE 20-4
Antiarrhythmic Drugs in Pregnancy

DRUG	CLASS VW	CLASS FDA	PLACENTAL TRANSFER	ADVERSE EFFECTS	TERATOGENIC	BREAST MILK	RISK
Quinidine	1A	C	Yes	Thrombocytopenia, rarely oxytocic	No	Yes*	Minor
Procainamide	1A	C	Yes	None	No	Yes*	Minor
Disopyramide	1A	C	Yes	Uterine contraction	No	Yes*	Minor (L)
Lidocaine	1B	C	Yes	Bradycardia, CNS side effects	No	Yes*	Minor
Mexiletine	IB	C	Yes	Bradycardia, low weight, Apgar, sugar	No	Yes*	Minor (L)
Tocainide	1B	C	Unknown	Unknown	Unknown	Unknown	Minor (L)
Phenytoin	1B	X	Yes	Mental and growth retardation, fetal hydantoin syndrome	Yes	Yes*	Significant
Flecainide	1C	C	Yes	None	No	Yes*	Minor (L)
Propafenone	IC	C	Yes	None (L)	No	Unknown	Minor (L)
Moricizine	1	B	Unknown	Unknown	No	Yes	Minor (L)
Propranolol	2	C	Yes	Growth retardation, bradycardia, apnea, hypoglycemia	No	Yes*	Minor
Sotalol	3	B	Yes	β-Blocker effects	No	Yes*	Minor (L)
Amiodarone	3	D	Yes	Hypothyroidism, growth retardation, premature birth, large fontanelle	Yes?	Yes	Significant
Bretylium	3	C	Unknown	Unknown	Unknown	Unknown	Moderate (L)
Verapamil	4	C	Yes	Bradycardia, heart block, hypotension	No	Yes*	Moderate
Diltiazem	4	C	No	Unknown	Unknown	Yes*	Moderate (L)
Digoxin	NA	C	Yes	Low birth weight	No	Yes*	Minor
Adenosine	NA	C	No (L)	None	No	Unknown	Minor (L)

From Page RL: *Am Heart J* 130:871-876, 1995.

Breast milk, transfer to breast milk; *(L),* very limited experience; *NA,* not applicable; *Risk,* risk of causing injury to fetus; *VW,* Vaughan Williams.
FDA class (use-in-pregnancy rating):
A, Controlled studies show no risk. Adequate, well-controlled studies in pregnant women have failed to demonstrate risk to the fetus.
B, No evidence of risk in human beings. Either animal findings show risk, but human findings do not or, if no adequate human studies have been done, animal findings are negative.
C, Risk cannot be ruled out. Human studies are lacking, and animal studies are either positive for fetal risk, or lacking as well. However, potential benefits may justify the potential risk.
D, Positive evidence of risk. Investigational or postmarketing data show risk to the fetus. Nevertheless, potential benefits may outweigh the potential risk.
X, Contraindicated in pregnancy. Studies in animals or humans, or investigational or postmarketing reports have shown fetal risk that clearly outweighs any possible benefit to the patient.
*American Academy of Pediatrics considers drug to be "usually compatible with breast feeding."

labeling as absolutely safe to the fetus. Obstetricians and cardiologists initially recommend conservative, non-pharmacologic treatment of arrhythmias, including vagal maneuvers and the avoidance of precipitating factors, such as caffeine ingestion, cigarette smoking, and stress. Pharmacologic therapy is instituted if conservative measures fail, the arrhythmia is sustained, and the arrhythmia is causing hemodynamic instability or intolerable symptoms to the mother. Whenever an arrhythmia poses a threat to the mother or fetus, drug therapy is initiated.[94]

Arrhythmias are not uncommon during labor and delivery. The stress and pain of labor and delivery may cause a recurrence of arrhythmias that were previously well controlled. Paroxysmal supraventricular tachycardia (PSVT) is the most common arrhythmia occurring in pregnant patients.[94] β-Blockers have been used successfully to treat PSVT[95] with some authors reporting no ill effects on the fetus.[96] Other reports, however, caution their use in pregnant patients because of associated fetal bradycardia and neonatal hypoglycemia.[67,74] Administration of esmolol, a very short-acting β-blocker, has necessitated emergency cesarean delivery because of fetal bradycardia.[75] Fetal hypoxemia also occurred in pregnant sheep with long-term administration of esmolol.[73] Verapamil is another agent used frequently for conversion of PSVT. Like the β-blockers, successful use during pregnancy has been reported without adverse fetal effects.[97] The disadvantage of verapamil is the high incidence of hypotension that could compromise uteroplacental perfusion. Verapamil also easily crosses the placenta, and may cause fetal bradycardia.[98] Adenosine is considered by many to be the first-line agent for the acute treatment of PSVT in parturients.[93,99] It is very effective with a rapid onset and brief duration of action. Adenosine appears to have a better safety profile than many of the other agents,[100] but because it is a relatively new drug, it does not have a long safety record for use during pregnancy. The safe use of adenosine in several parturients has been reported.[101] One recent report of very brief fetal bradycardia (5 seconds) associated with maternal administration[102] suggests however that it should also be used with caution during pregnancy and certainly encourages its use over other agents, but emphasizes the need for fetal heart rate monitoring, whenever an antiarrhythmic agent is administered.

The goal of therapy for new-onset atrial fibrillation is to decrease the ventricular rate and restore sinus rhythm. Digoxin has a long safety record during pregnancy[93] and is commonly used to slow the ventricular rate. Verapamil, diltiazem, or a β-blocking agent can also be added to control the rate.[95] Quinidine is the drug of choice for pharmacologic conversion to sinus rhythm. It is effective and has the longest safety record for use during pregnancy among drugs commonly used for conversion.[94] Quinidine does have mild oxytocic effects and poses a slight risk of precipitating premature labor.[94]

Ventricular arrhythmias, including ventricular tachycardia, occur more frequently during pregnancy and are more symptomatic. Lidocaine is the first-line drug for pharmacologic treatment of sustained ventricular tachycardia in hemodynamically stable parturients.[94] Procainamide is indicated when lidocaine is unsuccessful at converting the rhythm.[94] Both drugs have long safety records for use during pregnancy and are considered relatively safe.[94] β-Blocking agents are considered the first-line therapy for long-term suppression of ventricular arrhythmias during pregnancy.[94] Procainamide, sotalol, and flecainide are added if the

β-blocking agent is not effective.[94] While sotalol and flecainide do not have a long history of use during pregnancy, the data suggest an equivalent fetal safety profile as the other drugs discussed earlier.[103] Certain antiarrhythmic agents do cause significant fetal or neonatal adverse effects. These drugs are avoided unless safer treatment options have failed and the deteriorating maternal condition dictates further management. Amiodarone has been associated with intrauterine growth restriction (IUGR), neonatal thyroid dysfunction, and neurologic abnormalities.[104,105] Phenytoin is rarely used to manage ventricular arrhythmias, especially those associated with digitalis toxicity. The fetal hydantoin syndrome, which includes microcephaly, mental retardation, and dysmorphic craniofacial features, has been reported in 5% to 10% of fetuses whose mothers received phenytoin.[106]

Atrial and ventricular arrhythmias cause hemodynamic instability in some parturients, compromising both maternal and fetal well-being. Treatment must be prompt and rapid, usually necessitating electrical cardioversion. This procedure is safe during all stages of pregnancy.[107,108] The higher threshold required to provoke arrhythmias in the fetal heart and the small amount of electrical current penetrating the uterus contribute to the safety of electrical cardioversion.[93] Transient fetal arrhythmias can occur during maternal cardioversion.[109] So fetal heart rate monitoring is performed during and after the procedure. The anesthetic technique chosen for electrical cardioversion must account for the increased risk of gastric aspiration during pregnancy and the increased risk of difficult intubation in the pregnant patient. The unique characteristics of each patient are used to determine the best anesthetic approach. Rapid-sequence induction of general anesthesia with tracheal intubation is indicated for electrical cardioversion in some patients, whereas others tolerate the procedure with careful intravenous sedation and maintenance of intact airway reflexes.

Placement of an implantable cardioverter-defibrillator (ICD) is indicated for young women with serious arrhythmias. A recent multicenter study demonstrated that pregnancy, labor, and delivery are well tolerated by parturients with these devices. The number of ICD discharges during pregnancy were equivalent to prepregnancy values. No discharges occurred during labor and delivery. The device should remain activated during labor, allowing prompt intervention if an arrhythmia occurs. The incidence of device-related complications does not increase during pregnancy, even for ICDs implanted in the abdomen, despite the significant increase in abdominal girth.[110]

Placement of an ICD is considered for women who first develop serious arrhythmias during pregnancy. Radiofrequency ablation of accessory pathways causing hemodynamically significant PSVT can also be performed during pregnancy.[111] The major disadvantage to these techniques is the fetal radiation exposure during the procedure. The risks of congenital malformations and mental retardation are increased when the fetus is exposed to radiation during the first or second trimester. Exposure during the second or third trimester is associated with a higher incidence of childhood malignancies.[112]

Bradyarrhythmias and heart block are rare during pregnancy. Asymptomatic patients with complete heart block that become symptomatic with the increased cardiovascular demands of pregnancy should receive a permanent pacemaker. A ventilation-sensing, rate-responsive pacemaker is preferable in pregnant patients because it adapts to the changing cardiac demands of pregnancy, labor, and delivery.[113] Patients who are asymptomatic during pregnancy may become symptomatic (including syncope) during labor and delivery because of the increased cardiovascular demands. Placement of a prophylactic temporary pacemaker before the onset of labor is recommended for these patients. Labor and delivery are generally tolerated well by patients with pacemakers, provided they do not have significant cardiac dysfunction resulting from the underlying heart disease that caused the heart block.[114]

ISCHEMIC HEART DISEASE

Ischemic heart disease is rare in pregnant women. The incidence of myocardial infarction during pregnancy in 1970 was estimated at one per 10,000 pregnancies.[115] It is likely that the incidence of ischemic heart disease in parturients has increased and will continue to increase because of various societal factors. These factors include (1) increased percentage of pregnant women older than 35 years of age and (2) the prevalence of cocaine abuse in parturients (estimated as high as 20% in the United States).[116] It is important for the anesthesiologist to understand the implications of ischemic heart disease in the laboring patient.

Myocardial ischemia occurs when myocardial oxygen demand exceeds oxygen supply. Although myocardial ischemia is generally associated with coronary artery disease, ischemia in the pregnant population is often due to another cause. A review of the medical literature by Aglio and Johnson[117] demonstrated that significant coronary atherosclerosis was present in only 40% of parturients suffering a myocardial infarction when coronary angiography or postmortem examination was performed. Coronary thrombus within normal coronary arteries was found in 40% to 45% of the cases, and normal coronary arteries were found in 10% of the cases. The hypercoagulability of pregnancy and the severe hypertension and coronary artery vasospasm associated with cocaine toxicity are precipitating factors in many pregnant women who experience myocardial ischemia.

The physiologic changes of pregnancy increase the

risk of myocardial ischemia because the increased heart rate and cardiac output produce a significant increase in myocardial oxygen consumption. The balance between myocardial oxygen demand and supply is further jeopardized during labor and delivery with the additional increase of cardiac output and tachycardia that result from the pain and stress of labor. The goal of anesthetic management is to minimize increases in oxygen consumption by providing excellent labor analgesia while maximizing oxygen supply.

The anesthetic plan is dictated by the mode of delivery. There is no consensus within the obstetric community as to the optimal mode of delivery. Elective cesarean delivery prevents the significant and sometimes prolonged hemodynamic stress associated with labor and vaginal delivery. The timing of delivery is also controlled so that maximal resources are available for the care of this high-risk parturient.[118] Conversely, the increased blood loss and increased risk of infection or pulmonary morbidity associated with cesarean delivery are especially harmful to these high-risk patients. Therefore, some obstetricians argue that the risks versus benefits does not warrant routine cesarean delivery,[119] especially because much of the stress response of labor can be avoided with excellent labor analgesia.

If labor and vaginal delivery is planned for the patient with ischemic heart disease, the anesthetic management is affected by the physical status of the patient. Continuous 5-lead ECG monitoring and supplemental oxygen is indicated for all parturients at risk for myocardial ischemia. An intraarterial catheter is also beneficial for management of these patients. A pulmonary artery catheter is indicated only in patients who have sustained a myocardial infarction within the last 6 months or who have significant left ventricular dysfunction. There are many benefits to providing excellent labor analgesia to these parturients. The pain-related increases in heart rate and blood pressure that increase myocardial oxygen demand are minimized. Labor analgesia also prevents increases in maternal catecholamine levels and minimizes hypocapnia secondary to hyperventilation. Attenuation of these responses is especially important for these patients because of their role in coronary artery vasoconstriction.

Epidural analgesia is an excellent method for providing relief of labor pain.[117,120] The drugs and doses discussed previously in this chapter are recommended. It is crucial that adequate intravenous fluid loading occur before instituting the epidural block so that hypotension, which can jeopardize myocardial oxygen supply, is avoided. If pharmacologic treatment of epidural-induced hypotension is required, phenylephrine is preferred over ephedrine. Phenylephrine produces a reflex bradycardia and ephedrine causes an increase in heart rate that is detrimental for these patients. CSE analgesia is another excellent choice for providing analgesia to these patients.[121]

If cesarean delivery is required, epidural anesthesia

is an ideal anesthetic technique.[117] The anesthetic level is slowly raised and hemodynamic stability is maintained. Generous intravenous fluid loading and aggressive treatment of hypotension with phenylephrine is important for the management of these patients. A T4 sensory level is obtained to provide adequate surgical anesthesia. Sympathetic blockade of the cardiac accelerator fibers is an added benefit for obtaining a block in the high thoracic segments. The decrease in heart rate diminishes myocardial oxygen consumption. A continuous spinal technique is another acceptable method for providing anesthesia for cesarean section. The high incidence of spinal headache is one disadvantage of this technique compared with epidural anesthesia.

General anesthesia is avoided for these patients because the tachycardia and hypertension associated with laryngoscopy and intubation lead to a detrimental imbalance between myocardial oxygen demand and supply. If a general anesthetic is required, induction with a potent dose of opioids is used to maintain hemodynamic stability and blunt responses to laryngoscopy and surgery. Precautions are taken to prevent aspiration and the neonatologist is present because the infant is likely to experience respiratory depression.

PARTURIENT WITH CARDIAC TRANSPLANT

The frequency and long-term success of cardiac transplantation has increased significantly over the past several years because of continuing improvements in immunosuppressive therapy. Many women of child-bearing age who have undergone cardiac transplant have subsequently become pregnant. The literature reports successful outcomes for both mother and infant in the vast majority of cases.[122-125] The number of pregnant patients with previous heart transplant is expected to increase.

Parturients with a cardiac transplant usually have excellent ventricular function. The anesthetic and obstetric management of these patients is the same as for normal, healthy parturients. Cesarean delivery is reserved for obstetric indications. Some special considerations for the management of these patients should be noted, however. The transplanted heart is a denervated heart, void of autonomic innervation. Because of the lack of vagal innervation, the patient's heart rate is fast (usually 100-120 beats/min) and does not respond to vagolytic agents, such as atropine. Only direct-acting vasoactive agents produce reliable inotropic or chronotropic effects.[126] The transplanted heart is dependent on the Starling mechanism to provide adequate cardiac output. Maintenance of adequate preload is essential for these patients. Finally, coronary atherosclerosis is accelerated in the transplanted heart,[127] but these patients do not have angina during myocardial ischemia because of denervation.

The results of any recent cardiac catheterization is important to determine the risk for ischemia during labor and delivery. Patients receiving chronic corticosteroids require stress doses during labor and delivery. Invasive monitoring is not required in most cases because left ventricular function is usually normal. The benefit obtained from invasive hemodynamic data is usually outweighed by the risk of infection for these immunosuppressed patients.

Epidural and CSE analgesia are both good choices for labor analgesia.[123,124,128] Generous intravenous fluid loading is essential, given the reliance on adequate preload to maintain cardiac output. Because ephedrine acts by both direct and indirect mechanisms, it is less effective for the treatment of hypotension than phenylephrine. Epidural anesthesia is a good choice for cesarean delivery.[129] Spinal or general anesthesia may be required in certain obstetric situations (such as fetal distress). Both of these techniques have been used successfully in the parturient with a transplanted heart.[124,125]

PERIPARTUM CARDIOMYOPATHY
Epidemiology and Etiology

Peripartum cardiomyopathy is a rare disorder that occurs in 1 of every 3000 to 15,000 pregnancies in the United States.[130,131] This wide variation of incidence is due to differences in the definition of peripartum cardiomyopathy used by various authors. Geography also plays a role in the incidence of the disease. In Africa, an incidence of 1 in every 1000 pregnancies has been reported.[132] Identified risk factors for developing the disease include advanced maternal age, obesity, multiparity, multiple gestation, preeclampsia, chronic hypertension, and black race,[133] but women of all races and ages have developed peripartum cardiomyopathy.

The etiology of peripartum cardiomyopathy remains unknown although much investigation has focused on identifying a cause. One possible cause is some form of myocarditis.[134-136] Both viral and autoimmune processes have been proposed. Endomyocardial biopsies in women with peripartum cardiomyopathy have demonstrated myocarditis in many patients,[134,135] but biopsy results differ markedly among studies. One of the most recent series identified myocarditis by biopsy in only 8.8% of the patients.[136] The etiology remains unclear because of the uncertainty over whether peripartum cardiomyopathy is a distinct disease or a pregnancy-related exacerbation of another form of cardiomyopathy.

Diagnosis and Presentation

Patients with peripartum cardiomyopathy have signs and symptoms of left ventricular failure (Table 20-5). The diagnosis of cardiomyopathy in pregnant women is difficult to make by signs and symptoms alone.

TABLE 20-5
Presenting Features of Peripartum Cardiomyopathy

SYMPTOMS	SIGNS
Dyspnea	Jugular venous distention
Chest pain	Tachycardia
Cough	Gallop rhythm
Tachypnea	Mitral regurgitation murmur
Orthopnea	Loud P2
Paroxysmal nocturnal	Rales
dyspnea	Thromboemboli
Pedal edema	Hepatomegaly
Anorexia	Hepatojugular reflux
Fatigue	Ascites
Mental status changes	Peripheral edema

From Brown CS, Bertolet BD: *Am J Obstet Gynecol* 178:409-414, 1998.

Symptoms such as fatigue, orthopnea, and pedal edema are common among normal parturients during late pregnancy. Further testing is required to establish the diagnosis. Chest x-ray film consistently demonstrates cardiomegaly and pulmonary edema. Echocardiography confirms ventricular failure with increased left ventricular end-diastolic dimensions and decreased fractional shortening.[137]

Once the diagnosis of cardiac failure is established, peripartum cardiomyopathy must be differentiated from other etiologic factors. The cardiovascular stresses of pregnancy frequently unmask previously asymptomatic heart disease, especially during the third trimester. Diagnostic criteria for peripartum cardiomyopathy include (1) development of cardiac failure during the last month of pregnancy or within 5 months of delivery, (2) absence of a known cause for cardiac failure (such as valvular heart disease), and (3) absence of demonstrable heart disease before the last month of pregnancy.[138] Unlike other causes of heart failure associated with pregnancy, the majority of peripartum cardiomyopathy cases occur after the immediate postpartum period.[131]

Prognosis

Maternal mortality from peripartum cardiomyopathy in the United States has been reported to be 25% to 50%.[139,140] Causes of death include progressive left ventricular failure and associated complications, such as thromboembolic events and arrhythmias. Thromboembolism accounts for approximately 30% of these deaths.[141] Approximately half of the maternal deaths occur during the first 3 postpartum months.[138]

Return to a normal heart size and resolution of congestive heart failure within 6 months after delivery is a good prognostic sign.[138] Patients who survive the disease have a significantly higher ejection fraction and smaller left ventricular end-diastolic diameter at the time of diagnosis compared with patients who do not survive.[139] The incidence of resolution is unclear. Early series reported that 50% of patients experienced resolution,[138,139] whereas a more recent study reported only a 7% incidence of disease regression. The majority of patients in the most recent series either died, required cardiac transplant, or experienced continued cardiac impairment.[142]

Patients with peripartum cardiomyopathy require counseling concerning the risks of subsequent pregnancy. Patients without resolution of their cardiomyopathy are at significant risk for death or exacerbation of the disease[138] and should be advised to avoid pregnancy. There is no consensus on recommendations for subsequent pregnancy in women who have resolution of their cardiomyopathy. One of the earliest studies demonstrated that only 25% of these patients experienced a temporary exacerbation during subsequent pregnancy.[138] Sutton et al[143] reported that left ventricular function, based on echocardiography, remained normal during and after pregnancy in patients who had previously recovered from peripartum cardiomyopathy. A more recent study reported a return to normal ventricular function based on echocardiography but reduced contractile reserve during a dobutamine challenge test.[144] Therefore, patients who have recovered from peripartum cardiomyopathy may be unable to tolerate the increased cardiovascular demands of pregnancy.

Medical and Obstetric Management

Medical treatment of peripartum cardiomyopathy is similar to that for other dilated cardiomyopathies. Management goals include preload optimization, afterload reduction, and increased contractility (Table 20-6). Anticoagulation is recommended because of the high incidence of thromboembolism. Some special modifications in treatment are required when the patient develops cardiac failure during pregnancy. Angiotensin-converting enzyme inhibitors are used for afterload reduction in nonparturients with congestive heart failure. These drugs are contraindicated during pregnancy because of fetal effects.[145] Amlodipine or a combination of hydralazine and nitroglycerin are suggested alternatives.[146]

The development of peripartum cardiomyopathy in the antepartum period requires a plan for management of the pregnancy that is dictated by the clinical condition of the mother. If the cardiac status is stabilized with medical therapy, induction of labor at term is recom-

TABLE 20-6
Treatment of Peripartum Cardiomyopathy

Nonpharmaceutical Therapy
Low-sodium diet (<4 g/day)
Fluid restriction (<2 L/day)
Modest daily exercise (i.e., walking)

Oral Pharmaceutical Therapy
Prepartum
  Amlodipine
  Hydralazine/nitrates
  Digoxin
  Diuretics
  α-Blockers
Postpartum
  Angiotensin-converting enzyme inhibitors or angiotensin II
    receptor blockers
  Digoxin
  Diuretics
  β-Blockers (low dose)
  Amlodipine
  Hydralazine/nitrates
  α-Blockers

**Intravenous Pharmaceutical Therapy for Patients
with Severe Symptoms**
Unresponsive to above oral therapy
  Dobutamine
  Dopamine
  Milrinone
  Nitroprusside

From Brown CS, Bertolet BD: *Am J Obstet Gynecol* 178:409-414, 1998.

mended, with cesarean section reserved for obstetric indications. However, if the parturient experiences cardiac decompensation, premature delivery may become necessary. Frequently in this situation fetal distress related to maternal instability or inability of the mother to tolerate the prolonged stress of labor will require cesarean delivery.

Anesthetic Management

Parturients with peripartum cardiomyopathy who present for labor and delivery require special attention from the anesthesiologist. Management of these patients is optimized with invasive monitoring, including a pulmonary artery catheter. The cardiovascular stress of labor and delivery sometimes causes stable patients to experience cardiac decompensation. The anesthesiolo-

gist then needs to infuse intravenous vasoactive agents, such as nitroprusside or nitroglycerin for preload and afterload reduction, and dopamine, dobutamine, or milrinone for inotropic support. Pulmonary artery catheter data help determine the appropriate pharmacologic support for each patient.

Early administration of labor analgesia is essential to minimize further cardiac stress associated with pain. Slow induction of epidural analgesia, by using invasive monitoring data to guide fluid management and titration of vasoactive infusions, is an excellent technique for these parturients. The afterload reduction from the sympathetic block contributes to the improvement of myocardial performance.[147] CSE analgesia is another excellent analgesic option. The initial analgesia is accomplished with spinal opioids, thus avoiding sympathetic blockade for a few hours. Hemodynamic stability is more easily maintained with spinal opioids compared with epidural analgesia. The advantage of afterload reduction is also obtained when local anesthetic is administered into the epidural catheter. Preoperative anticoagulation therapy necessitates confirmation of a normal coagulation status before proceeding with regional anesthesia.

A continuous epidural or spinal anesthetic is usually the best anesthetic option for cesarean section.[147] The patient's hemodynamic status is carefully followed with invasive monitoring while the anesthesia level is slowly raised. As mentioned earlier for labor management, the afterload reduction associated with central neuraxial blockade is especially advantageous for these patients. A single-shot spinal technique is not recommended because the rapid hemodynamic changes associated with this technique are not well tolerated in these fragile patients. General anesthesia is sometimes used when cesarean section is required because of fetal distress or acute maternal decompensation. Myocardial-depressant anesthetic drugs, including pentothal and the volatile agents, are avoided. Cardiac arrest during induction of general anesthesia in a patient with undiagnosed peripartum cardiomyopathy has been reported.[148] Induction and maintenance of anesthesia with a high-dose opioid such as remifentanil is preferred when general anesthesia is required.

CARDIAC SURGERY DURING PREGNANCY

The increased cardiovascular demands of pregnancy often result in cardiac decompensation in parturients with preexisting heart disease, particularly for patients with valvular heart disorders. The prevalence of intravenous drug abuse in our society has increased the number of parturients with severe valvular dysfunction resulting from infective endocarditis. Parturients with Marfan syndrome are at increased risk for aortic dissection during pregnancy. Medical treatment may not be adequate for some of these patients and surgical repair of the defect during pregnancy may be deemed necessary for maternal and fetal well-being. Optimal patient care requires close communication among the obstetrician, cardiologist, cardiac surgeon, and anesthesiologist.

A review of cardiac surgery performed during pregnancy between 1984 and 1996 reported a maternal mortality rate of 5% to 6%.[149] While this is not a particularly high rate, it was higher than the mortality rate in nonpregnant patients of the same age group. Cardiac surgery during pregnancy is reserved for patients whose condition is life threatening, accounting for the higher mortality rate in parturients. Of even greater concern is the fetal-neonatal mortality rate of 30%.[149] Because fetal mortality rates are so high, cesarean delivery before initiation of cardiopulmonary bypass should be considered if the fetus is at least 28 to 30 weeks' gestation. A fetus at 34 weeks' gestation should be delivered before proceeding with maternal cardiac surgery.

The etiology of the high fetal mortality is multifactorial. The poor maternal condition contributes to inadequate uteroplacental perfusion and subsequent fetal hypoxemia. Cardiopulmonary bypass (CPB) is not physiologic and may have deleterious effects on the fetus. There are multiple reports of fetal bradycardia associated with CPB.[150,151] Recommendations to minimize the fetal effects of CPB include (1) higher pump flows (greater than 2 L/min/m^2), (2) a mean perfusion pressure of at least 60 mm Hg because placental perfusion is pressure dependent,[152] and (3) pulsatile flow rather than nonpulsatile flow. Pulsatile flow has been used successfully for CPB during pregnancy.[153] Although some authors suggest that hypothermia is protective for the fetus,[154] most believe that hypothermia is deleterious, and recommend normothermia or moderate hypothermia (32° C or greater). Therefore the ideal management of CPB during pregnancy is likely high-flow, high-pressure, normothermic pulsatile perfusion.[152] Fetal death can still occur despite use of this technique.

Fetal heart rate monitoring by trained professionals is very helpful during cardiac surgery. Fetal bradycardia is common during bypass. However, pharmacologic manipulations and adjustments to pump flow sometimes improve perfusion to the fetoplacental unit. Fetal heart rate monitoring evaluates the effects of these hemodynamic and pharmacologic manipulatives on the fetus. Anecdotal reports in the literature have documented fetal heart rate improvements after increases in pump flow.[155,156] The trained personnel who interpret the fetal monitor must be available throughout surgery. A decision is made before surgery for patients at viable gestation (24 weeks or greater) as to whether an emergency cesarean section is to be performed if severe fetal distress develops during surgery.

There are no data to support recommendations for a

BOX 20-1
Food and Drug Administration Safety-in-Pregnancy Category Ratings

Category A: Controlled studies in humans demonstrate no fetal risk
Category B: Animal studies demonstrate no fetal risk but no controlled human studies have been performed; or animal studies demonstrate adverse fetal effects but well-controlled human studies do not
Category C: No well-controlled animal or human studies exist; or animal studies demonstrate adverse fetal effects but no human studies exist
Category D: Human data demonstrate fetal risk but benefits of drug might outweigh risks
Category X: Contraindicated in pregnancy; studies demonstrate fetal risk that clearly outweighs any benefits of the drug

particular anesthetic technique or agent in terms of better maternal or fetal outcome after cardiac surgery. During early pregnancy, concerns about the teratogenic effects of anesthetic agents exist. Box 20-1 explains the Food and Drug Administration's use in pregnancy category ratings, and Table 20-7 lists the ratings for many commonly used anesthetic drugs. The drugs listed as Category B and C have received that rating because either human studies have not been performed or teratogenesis was found in animals. Controlled drug studies in pregnant patients are virtually nonexistent, and teratogenicity of agents differs markedly among species. All of the anesthetic agents listed as Category B and C have been used in pregnant patients without evidence of teratogenicity. Controversy exists over the safety of benzodiazepines and nitrous oxide during pregnancy. It is reasonable to avoid their use unless the well-being of the mother warrants it. The anesthetic technique and drugs used are based on the patient's condition and the physician's experience.

CARDIOPULMONARY RESUSCITATION IN PREGNANT PATIENTS

Cardiac arrest is a rare event in pregnant women. Survival for both the mother and fetus depends on prompt and appropriate intervention. The management of cardiac arrest in a parturient follows the same algorithms used for nonpregnant patients, but with certain modifications based on the physiologic changes of pregnancy.[157] Prompt intubation of the trachea prevents aspiration and provides adequate oxygenation and ventilation to the mother and fetus. After 20 weeks' gestation, significant aortocaval compression occurs in the supine position, reducing venous return. Effective cardiopulmonary resuscitation (CPR) is not achieved with-

TABLE 20-7
U.S. Food and Drug Administration Category Ratings of Specific Anesthetic Agents

ANESTHETIC AGENT	CLASSIFICATION*	ANESTHETIC AGENT	CLASSIFICATION
Induction agents		Opioids	
Etomidate	C	Alfentanil	C
Ketamine	C	Fentanyl	C
Methohexital	B	Sufentanil	C
Propofol	B	Meperidine	B
Thiopental	C	Morphine	C
Inhaled agents		Neuromuscular blocking drugs	
Desflurane	B	Atracurium	C
Enflurane	B	Cisatracurium	B
Halothane	C	Curare	C
Isoflurane	C	Mivacurium	C
Sevoflurane	B	Pancuronium	C
Local anesthetics		Rocuronium	B
2-Chloroprocaine	C	Succinylcholine	C
Cocaine	C	Vecuronium	C
Bupivacaine	C	Benzodiazepines	
Lidocaine	B	Diazepam	D
Ropivacaine	B	Midazolam	D
Tetracaine	C		

From Beilin Y: *Prog Anesthesiol* 9:219-226, 2000.
For explanation of categories, see Box 20-1.

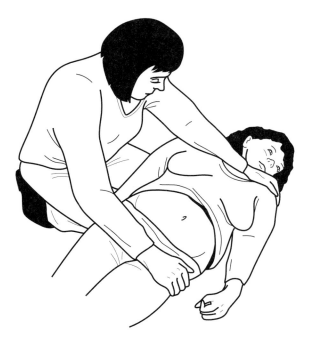

FIG. 20-4 The human wedge position for cardiopulmonary resuscitation of a pregnant woman.

(From Camann WR, Thornhill ML: Cardiovascular disease. In Chestnut DH, editor: *Obstetric anesthesia: principles and practice,* ed 2, St Louis, 1999, Mosby, p 797.)

out maintenance of left uterine displacement throughout the resuscitative efforts. A pillow or wedge device is placed under the right hip, but this may become dislodged during the often chaotic resuscitative efforts. A Cardiff wedge is specifically designed to provide uterine displacement and a hard surface for effective chest compressions.[158] Unfortunately, this equipment is frequently not available during an unexpected cardiac arrest. A "human wedge" provides adequate left uterine displacement during CPR efforts[159] by designating a person to kneel on the floor and sit on their heels. The patient is positioned with her back on the thighs of the kneeling person. The "human wedge" uses one arm to stabilize the patient's shoulders and the other arm to stabilize the pelvis (Fig. 20-4).

Prompt cesarean delivery is performed in the parturient who has reached 24 weeks' gestation if initial resuscitative efforts are unsuccessful. The AHA recommends that cesarean delivery occur within 4 to 5 minutes from the time of the arrest.[160] Neonatal survival occurs in 70% of cases when a prompt delivery is executed.[161] Delivery of the fetus relieves aortocaval compression, improves maternal venous return and cardiac output, and possibly improves the mother's chances for survival. Successful maternal resuscitation has been reported with delivery of the infant.[162,163] The cesarean section is performed at the bedside while CPR continues. Time should not be wasted in moving the patient to an operating room. Emergency cesarean section instruments should be readily available in labor and delivery units, operating room suites, and emergency rooms.

Many of the drugs used during CPR, such as epinephrine and norepinephrine, could theoretically compromise uteroplacental perfusion. However, fetal survival is dependent on maternal survival. Any drug therapy necessary to revive the mother is administered despite its possible adverse effects on uteroplacental perfusion. De-

fibrillation is similarly performed when indicated. A neonatologist is called to resuscitate the neonate if delivery occurs during the resuscitation. The infant will likely be hypoxic, acidotic, and exhibit cardiac arrhythmias related to maternal defibrillation.

Open-chest cardiac massage has been recommended if all other resuscitative efforts (including perimortem cesarean section) have failed, or the resuscitation is expected to be prolonged.[164] This author is not aware of any existing data to support this treatment. Each specific clinical situation is evaluated before deciding if such treatment is warranted.

KEY POINTS

1. Successful management of the parturient with cardiac disease requires an interdisciplinary approach with close communication among the anesthesiologist, obstetrician, and cardiologist.

2. For parturients with a history of congenital heart disease, a sound understanding of the structural anomaly and any previous surgical correction of the anomaly is necessary to devise an appropriate anesthetic plan. Labor and delivery is tolerated well in the majority of patients with corrected congenital heart disease without a need for special management, including invasive monitors.

3. The immediate postpartum period, with its marked increase in cardiac output, is an especially critical time for parturients with cardiac disease. These patients are monitored closely during this period for signs of cardiac decompensation. When invasive monitors are placed to guide management of labor and delivery, they are maintained for at least 24 hours postpartum.

4. Regional anesthesia is usually the technique of choice for labor and cesarean delivery in parturients with cardiac disease. When maintenance of SVR and venous return is critical to the patient's cardiac stability, CSE analgesia using intrathecal opioids is ideal for labor analgesia. Very slow induction of epidural anesthesia for cesarean delivery is usually well tolerated even in seriously ill cardiac

patients when invasive monitors are used to guide management.

5. According to recommendations of the AHA, subacute bacterial endocarditis prophylaxis is optional for vaginal delivery in patients with high-risk heart defects. However, the majority of cardiac defects encountered in parturients are considered moderate or negligible risk. Subacute bacterial endocarditis prophylaxis is not recommended for cesarean delivery.

6. Parturients with Eisenmenger's Syndrome and primary pulmonary hypertension are especially vulnerable to the stresses of labor and delivery. Close monitoring with the use of invasive monitors is essential to optimize maternal and neonatal outcome.

7. The risk of aortic dissection is significant in parturients with Marfan syndrome and aortic root enlargement. Careful blood pressure control throughout labor and delivery is important to minimize the risk.

8. Labor analgesia to avoid tachycardia and the associated increase in myocardial oxygen demand is extremely important in the management of parturients at risk for myocardial ischemia.

9. Maintenance of uterine displacement and early delivery of the fetus are important components of CPR in parturients. All resuscitation drugs indicated in advanced cardiac life support protocols, regardless of their theoretic effects on uteroplacental perfusion, are administered during cardiac arrest.

KEY REFERENCES

Brown CS, Bertolet BD: Peripartum cardiomyopathy: a comprehensive review, *Am J Obstet Gynecol* 178:409-414, 1998.

Dajani AD, Taubert KA, Wilson W et al: Prevention of bacterial endocarditis recommendations by the American Heart Association, *JAMA* 277:1794-1801, 1997.

Dildy GA, Clark SL: Cardiac arrest during pregnancy, *Obstet Gynecol Clin North Am* 22:303-314, 1995.

Gordon CF, Johnson MD: Anesthetic management of the pregnant patient with Marfan syndrome, *J Clin Anesth* 5:248-251, 1993.

Page RL: Treatment of arrhythmias during pregnancy, *Am Heart J* 130:871-876, 1995.

Parry AJ, Westaby S: Cardiopulmonary bypass during pregnancy, *Ann Thorac Surg* 61:1865-1869, 1996.

Pittard A, Vucevic M: Regional anaesthesia with a subarachnoid microcatheter for caesarean section in a parturient with aortic stenosis, *Anaesthesia* 53:169-172, 1998.

Siu SC, Sermer M, Harrison DA et al: Risk and predictors for pregnancy-related complications in women with heart disease, *Circulation* 96:2789-2794, 1997.

Smedstad KG, Cramb R, Morison DH: Pulmonary hypertension and pregnancy: a series of eight cases, *Can J Anaesth* 41:502-512, 1994.

Soderlin MK, Purhonen S, Haring P et al: Myocardial infarction in a parturient, *Anaesthesia* 49:870-872, 1994.

Spinnato JA, Kraynack BJ, Cooper MW: Eisenmenger's syndrome in pregnancy: epidural analgesia for elective cesarean section, *N Engl J Med* 304:1215-1217, 1981.

Weiss BM, Zemp L, Deifert B et al: Outcome of pulmonary vascular disease in pregnancy: a systematic overview from 1978 through 1996, *Journal of the American College of Cardiology* 31:1650-1657, 1998.

References

1. Sullivan JM, and Ramanathan KB: Medical problems in pregnancy—severe cardiac disease, *N Engl J Med* 313:304-309, 1985.
2. Siu SC, Sermer M, Harrison DA et al: Risk and predictors for pregnancy-related complications in women with heart disease, *Circulation* 96:2789-2794, 1997.
3. Pitkin RM, Perloff JK, Koos BJ et al: Pregnancy and congenital heart disease, *Ann Intern Med* 112:445-454, 1990.
4. Robson SC, Hunter S, Boys RJ et al: Serial study of factors influencing changes in cardiac output during human pregnancy, *Am J Physiol* 256:H1060-5, 1989.
5. Conklin KA: Maternal physiological adaptations during gestation, labor, and the puerperium, *Semin Anesth* 10:221-234, 1991.
6. Cheek TG and Gutsche BB: Maternal physiologic alteration during pregnancy. In Shnider SM, Levinson G, editors: *Anesthesia for obstetrics*, ed 3, Baltimore, 1993, Williams and Wilkens, p 7.
7. Elkayam U, Gleicher N: Cardiovascular physiology of pregnancy. In Elkayam U, Gleicher N, editors: *Cardiac problems in pregnancy: diagnosis and management of maternal and fetal disease*, New York, 1982, Alan R Liss, p 5.
8. Robson SC, DunlopW, Boys RJ et al: Cardiac output during labour, *Br Med J* 295:1169-1172, 1987.
9. Hansen JM and Ueland K: The influence of caudal analgesia on cardiovascular dynamics during labour and delivery, *Acta Anaesthesiol Scand* 23(suppl):449-452, 1966.
10. Alaily AB and Carrol KB: Pulmonary ventilation in pregnancy, *Br J Obstet Gynaecol* 85:518-524, 1978.
11. Spatling L, Fallenstein F, Huch A et al: The variability of cardiopulmonary adaptation to pregnancy at rest and during exercise, *Br J Obstet Gynaecol* 99(suppl 8):1-40, 1992.
12. Hagerdal M, Morgan CW, Sumner AE et al: Minute ventilation and oxygen consumption during labor with epidural analgesia, *Anesthesiology* 59:425-427, 1983.
13. Ulmsten U and Sundstrom G: Esophageal namometry in pregnant and nonpregnant women, *Am J Obstet Gynecol* 132:260-264, 1978.
14. Attia RR, Ebeid AM, Fischer JE et al: Maternal-fetal and placental gastrin concentrations, *Anaesthesia* 37:18-21, 1982.
15. LaPorta RF, Arthur GR and Datta S: Phenylephrine in treating maternal hypotension due to spinal anaesthesia for caesarean delivery: effects on neonatal catecholamine concentrations, acid base status and Apgar scores, *Acta Anaesthesiol Scand* 39:901-905, 1995.
16. Abboud TK, Artal R, Henriksen EH et al: Effect of spinal anesthesia on maternal circulating catecholamines, *Am J Obstet Gynecol* 142:252-254, 1982.
17. Riley ET, Walker D, Hamilton CL et al: Intrathecal sufentanil for labor analgesia does not cause a sympathectomy, *Anesthesiology* 87:874-878, 1997.
18. Heytens L and Alexander JP: Maternal and neonatal death associated with Eisenmenger's Syndrome, *Acta Anaesth Belg* 37:45-51, 1986.
19. Yentis SM, Steer PF, Plaat F: Eisenmenger's syndrome in pregnancy: maternal and fetal mortality in the 1990s, *Br J Obstet Gynaecol* 105:921-922, 1998.
20. Weiss BM, Zemp L, Seifert B et al: Outcome of pulmonary vascular disease in pregnancy: a systematic overview from 1978 through 1996, *Journal of the American College of Cardiology* 31:1650-1657, 1998.
21. Smedstad KG, Cramb R, Morison DH: Pulmonary hypertension and pregnancy: a series of eight cases, *Can J Anaesth* 41:502-512, 1994.
22. Robinson S: Pulmonary artery catheters in Eisenmenger's syndrome: many risks, few benefits, *Anesthesiology* 58:588-589, 1983.
23. Schwalbe SS, Deshmukh SM, Marx GF: Use of pulmonary artery catheterization in parturients with Eisenmenger's syndrome, *Anesth Analg* 71:442-443, 1990.
24. Palmer CM, Cork RC, Hays R et al: The dose-response relation of intrathecal fentanyl for labor analgesia, *Anesthesiology* 88:355-361, 1998.
25. Campbell DC, Camann WR, Datta S: The addition of bupivacaine to intrathecal sufentanil for labor analgesia, *Anesth Analg* 81:305-309, 1995.
26. Wu JL, Hsu MS, Hsu TC et al: The efficacy of intrathecal coadministration of morphine and bupivacaine for labor analgesia, *Acta Anaesthesiol Sin* 35:209-216, 1997.
27. Grieco WM, Norris MC, Leighton BL et al: Intrathecal sufentanil labor analgesia: the effects of adding morphine or epinephrine, *Anesth Analg* 77:1149-1154, 1993.
28. Morrison SG, Dominguez JJ, Frascarolo P et al: A comparison of the electrocardiographic cardiotoxic effects of racemic bupivacaine, levobupivacaine, and ropivacaine in anesthetized swine, *Anesth Analg* 90:1308-1314, 2000.
29. Spinnato JA, Kraynack BJ, Cooper MW: Eisenmenger's syndrome in pregnancy: epidural analgesia for elective cesarean section, *N Engl J Med* 304:1215-1217, 1981.
30. Tampakoudis P, Grimbizis G, Chatzinicolaou K et al: Successful pregnancy in a patient with severe pulmonary hypertension, *Gynecol Obstet Invest* 42:63-65, 1996.
31. Goodwin TM, Gherman RB, Hameed A et al: Favorable response of Eisenmenger syndrome to inhaled nitric oxide during pregnancy, *Am J Obstet Gynecol* 180:64-67, 1999.
32. Lust KM, Boots RJ, Dooris M et al: Management of labor in Eisenmenger syndrome with inhaled nitric oxide, *Am J Obstet Gynecol* 181:419-423, 1999.
33. Denny FW: A 45-year perspective on the streptococcus and rheumatic fever, *Clin Infect Dis* 19:1110-1122, 1994.

34. Hanson EW, Neerhut RK, Lynch C: Mitral valve prolapse, *Anesthesiology* 85:178-195, 1995.

35. Shapiro EP, Trimble EL, Robinson JC et al: Safety of labor and delivery in women with mitral valve prolapse, *Am J Cardiol* 56:806-807, 1985.

36. Rayburn WF, LeMire MS, Bird JL et al: Mitral valve prolapse: echocardiographic changes during pregnancy, *J Reprod Med* 32:185-187, 1987.

37. Dajani AD, Taubert KA, Wilson W et al: Prevention of bacterial endocarditis: recommendations by the American Heart Association, *JAMA* 277:1794-1801, 1997.

38. Clark SL, Phelan JP, Greenspoon J et al: Labor and delivery in the presence of mitral stenosis: central hemodynamic observations, *Am J Obstet Gynecol* 152:984-988, 1985.

39. Sullivan JM, Ramanathan KB: Management of medical problems in pregnancy: severe cardiac disease, *N Engl J Med* 313:304-309, 1985.

40. Al Kasab SM, Sabag T, Al Zeibag M: Beta adrenergic blockade in the management of pregnant women with mitral stenosis, *Am J Obstet Gynecol* 165:37-40, 1990.

41. Ziskind Z, Etchin A, Frenkel Y et al: Epidural anesthesia with the trendelenburg position for cesarean section with or without a cardiac surgical procedure in patients with severe mitral stenosis: a hemodynamic study, *J Cardiothorac Anesth* 4:354-359, 1990.

42. Scott H, Bateman C, Price M: The use of remifentanil in general anaesthesia for caesarean section in a patient with mitral valve disease, *Anaesthesia* 53:695-697, 1998.

43. Szekely P, Turner R, Snaith L: Pregnancy and the changing pattern of rheumatic heart disease, *Br Heart J* 35:1293-1303, 1973.

44. Arias F, Pineda J: Aortic stenosis and pregnancy, *J Reprod Med* 4:229-232, 1978.

45. Lao TT, Sermer M, MaGee L et al: Congenital aortic stenosis and pregnancy-a reappraisal, *Am J Obstet Gynecol* 169:540-545, 1993.

46. Suelto MD, Vermillion ST, Vick PG et al: Management of labor and delivery in a parturient with severe aortic stenosis, *Am J Anesthiol* 26:443-445, 1999.

47. Brighouse D: Anaesthesia for caesarean section in patients with aortic stenosis: the case for regional anaesthesia, *Anaesthesia* 53:107-109, 1998.

48. Whitfield A, Holdcroft A: Anaesthesia for caesarean section in patients with aortic stenosis: the case for general anaesthesia, *Anaesthesia* 53:109-112, 1998.

49. Johnson MD, Saltzman DH: Cardiac disease. In Datta S, editor: *Anesthetic and obstetric management of high-risk pregnancy*, ed 2, St Louis, 1996, Mosby-Year Book, Inc., p 237.

50. Easterling TR, Chadwick HS, Otto CM et al: Aortic stenosis in pregnancy, *Obstet Gynecol* 72:113-118, 1988.

51. Colclough G: Epidural anesthesia for cesarean delivery in a parturient with aortic stenosis, *Reg Anesth* 15:273-274, 1990.

52. Brian JE, Seifen AB, Clark RB et al: Aortic stenosis, cesarean delivery, and epidural anesthesia, *J Clin Anesth* 5:154-157, 1993.

53. Pittard A, Vucevic M: Regional anaesthesia with a subarachnoid microcatheter for caesarean section in a parturient with aortic stenosis, *Anaesthesia* 53:169-172, 1998.

54. Redfern N, Bower S, Bullock RE et al: Alfentanil for caesarean section complicated by severe aortic stenosis, *Br J Anaesth* 59:1309-1312, 1987.

55. Johnson MD, Saltzman DH: Cardiac disease. In Datta S, editor: *Anesthetic and obstetric management of high-risk pregnancy*, ed 2, St Louis, 1996, Mosby-Year Book, Inc., p 237.

56. Sheikh F, Rangwala S, DeSimone C et al: Management of the parturient with severe aortic incompetence, *J Cardiothorac Vasc Anesth* 9:575-577, 1995.

57. Alderson JD: Cardiovascular collapse following epidural anaesthesia for caesarean section in a patient with aortic incompetence, *Anaesthesia* 42:643-645, 1987.

58. Seaworth BJ, Durack DT: Infective endocarditis in obstetric and gynecologic practice, *Am J Obstet Gynecol* 154:180-188, 1986.

59. Cox SM, Leveno KJ: Pregnancy complicated by bacterial endocarditis, *Clin Obstet Gynecol* 32:48-53, 1989.

60. Cox SM, Hankins GD, Leveno KJ et al: Bacterial endocarditis: a serious pregnancy complication, *J Reprod Med* 33:671-674, 1988.

61. Sugrue D, Blake S, Troy P et al: Antibiotic prophylaxis against infective endocarditis after normal delivery-is it necessary?, *Br Heart J* 44:499-502, 1980.

62. Fananapazir L, Epstein ND: Prevalence of hypertrophic cardiomyopathy and limitations of screening methods, *Circulation* 92:700-704, 1995.

63. Oakley GG, McGarry K, Limb DG et al: Management of pregnancy in patients with hypertrophic cardiomyopathy, *Br Med J* 1:1749-1750, 1979.

64. Kolibash AJ, Ruiz DE, Lewis RP: Idiopathic hypertrophic subaortic stenosis in pregnancy, *Ann Intern Med* 82:791-794, 1975.

65. Shah DM, Sundjeri SG: Hypertrophic cardiomyopathy and pregnancy: report of a maternal mortality and review of literature, *Obstet Gynecol Surv* 40:444-448, 1985.

66. Tessler MJ, Hudson R, Naugler-Colville MA et al: Pulmonary oedema in two parturients with hypertrophic obstructive cardiomyopathy, *Can J Anaesth* 37:469-473, 1990.

67. Pruyn SC, Phelan JP, Buchanan GC: Long-term propanolol therapy in pregnancy: maternal and fetal outcome, *Am J Obstet Gynecol* 135:485-489, 1979.

68. Nam E, Toque Y, Quintard JM et al: Use of transesophageal echocardiography to guide the anesthetic management of cesarean section in a patient with hypertrophic cardiomyopathy, *J Cardiothor Vasc Anesth* 13:72-74, 1999.

69. Minnich ME, Quirk JG, Clark RB: Epidural anesthesia for vaginal delivery in a patient with idiopathic hypertrophic subaortic stenosis, *Anesthesiology* 67:590-592, 1987.

70. Ho KM, Kee WN, Poon MC: Combined spinal and epidural anesthesia in a parturient with idiopathic hypertrophic subaortic stenosis, *Anesthesiology* 87:168-169, 1997.

71. Boccio RV, Chung JH, Harrison DM: Anesthetic management of cesarean section in a patient with idiopathic hypertrophic subaortic stenosis, *Anesthesiology* 65:663-665, 1986.

72. Autore C, Brauneis S, Apponi F et al: Epidural anesthesia for cesarean section in patients with hypertrophic cardiomyopathy: a report of three cases, *Anesthesiology* 90:12057, 1999.

73. Eisenach JC, Castro MI: Maternally administered esmolol produces fetal beta-adrenergic blockade and hypoxemia in sheep, *Anesthesiology* 71:718-722, 1989.

74. Losasso TJ, Muzzi DA, Cucchiara RF: Response of fetal heart rate to maternal administration of esmolol, *Anesthesiology* 74:782-784, 1991.

75. Ducey JP, Knape KG: Maternal esmolol administration resulting in fetal distress and cesarean section in a term pregnancy, *Anesthesiology* 77:829-832, 1992.

76. Haering JM, Comunale ME, Parker RA et al: Cardiac risk of noncardiac surgery in patients with asymmetric septal hypertrophy, *Anesthesiology* 85:254-259, 1996.

77. Weiss BM, Atanassoff PF: Cyanotic congenital heart disease and pregnancy: natural selection, pulmonary hypertension, and anesthesia, *J Clin Anesth* 5:332-341, 1993.

78. McLaughlin VV, Genthner DE, Panella MM et al: Reduction in pulmonary vascular resistance with long-term epoprostenol (prostacyclin) therapy in primary pulmonary hypertension, *N Engl J Med* 338:273-277, 1998.

79. O'Hare R, McLoughlin C, Milligan K et al: Anaesthesia for caesarean section in the presence of severe primary pulmonary hypertension, *Br J Anaesth* 81:790-792, 1998.

80. Olschewski H, Walmrath D, Schermuly R et al: Aerosolized prostacyclin and iloprost in severe pulmonary hypertension, *Ann Int Med* 124:820-823, 1996.

81. Weiss BM, Maggiorinie M, Jenni R et al: Pregnant patient with primary pulmonary hypertension: inhaled pulmonary vasodilators and epidural anesthesia for cesarean delivery, *Anesthesiology* 92:1191-1194, 2000.

82. Robinson JN, Banerjee R, Landzberg MJ et al: Inhaled nitric oxide therapy in pregnancy complicated by pulmonary hypertension, *Am J Obstet Gynceol* 180:1045-1046, 1999.

83. Robinson DE, Leicht CH: Epidural analgesia with low-dose bupivacaine and fentanyl for labor and delivery in a parturient with severe pulmonary hypertension, *Anesthesiology* 68:285-288, 1988.

84. Slomka F, Salmeron S, Zetlaoui P et al: Primary pulmonary hypertension and pregnancy: anesthetic management for delivery, *Anesthesiology* 69:959-961, 1988.

85. Abboud TK, Raya JA, Noueihed R et al: Intrathecal morphine for the relief of labor pain in a parturient with severe pulmonary hypertension, *Anesthesiology* 59:477-479, 1983.

86. Roberts NV, Keast PJ: Pulmonary hypertension and pregnancy—a lethal combination, *Anaesth Intens Care* 18:366-374, 1989.

87. Cuenco J, Tzeng G, Wittels B: Anesthetic management of the parturient with systemic lupus erythematosus, pulmonary hypertension, and pulmonary edema, *Anesthesiology* 91:568-570, 1999.

88. Breen TW, Janzen JA: Pulmonary hypertension and cardiomyopathy: anaesthetic management for caesarean section, *Can J Anaesth* 38:895-899, 1991.

89. Tampakoudis P, Grimbizis G, Chatzinicolaou et al: Successful pregnancy in a patient with severe pulmonary hypertension, *Gynecol Obstet Invest* 42:63-65, 1996.

90. Husebye KO, Wolff JH, Friedman LL: Aortic dissection in pregnancy: a case of Marfan syndrome, *Am Heart J*, 55:662-676, 1958.

91. Pyeritz RE: Maternal and fetal complications of pregnancy in the Marfan syndrome, *Am J Med*, 71:784-790, 1981.

92. Gordon CF, Johnson MD: Anesthetic management of the pregnant patient with Marfan syndrome, *J Clin Anesth* 5:248-251, 1993.

93. Page RL: Treatment of arrhythmias during pregnancy, *Am Heart J* 130:871-876, 1995.

94. Chow T, Galvin J, McGovern B: Anitarrhythmic drug therapy in pregnancy and lactation, *Am J Cardiol* 82:58I-62I, 1998.

95. Rotmensch HH, Rotmensch S, Elkayam U: Management of cardiac arrhythmias during pregnancy, *Drugs* 33:623-633, 1987.

96. Cox JL, Gardner MJ: Treatment of cardiac arrhythmias during pregnancy, *Prog Cardiovasc Dis* 36:137-178, 1993.

97. Bryerly WG, Hartmann A, Foster DE et al: Verapamil in the treatment of maternal paroxysmal supraventricular tachycardia, *Ann Emerg Med* 20:552-554, 1991.

98. Kleinman CS, Copel JH, Weinstein EM et al: Treatment of fetal supraventricular tachyarrhythmias, *J Clin Ultrasound* 13:265-273, 1985.

99. Joglar JA, Page RL: Treatment of cardiac arrhythmias during pregnancy: safety considerations, *Drug Saf* 20:85-94, 1999.

100. Mason BA, Ricci-Goodman J, Koos BJ: Adenosine in the treatment of maternal paroxysmal supraventricular tachycardia, *Obstet Gynecol* 80:578-580, 1992.

101. Hagle MT, Cole PL: Adenosine use in pregnant women with supraventricular tachycardia, *Ann Pharmacother* 28:1241-1242, 1994.

102. Dunn JS, Brost BC: Fetal bradycardia after IV adenosine for maternal PSVT, *Am J Emerg Med* 18:234-235, 2000.

103. Wagner X, Jouglard J, Moulin M et al: Coadministration of flecainide acetate and sotalol during pregnancy: lack of teratogenic effects, passage across the placenta, and excretion in human breast milk, *Am Heart J* 119:700-702, 1990.

104. DeCatte L, DeWolf D, Smitz J et al: Fetal hypothyroidism as a complication of amiodarone treatment for persistent fetal supraventricular tachycardia, *Prenat Diagn* 14:762-765, 1994.

105. Magee LA, Downar E, Sermer M et al: Pregnancy outcome after gestational exposure to amiodarone in Canada, *Am J Obstet Gynecol* 172:1307-1311, 1995.

106. Hanson JW, Smith DW: The fetal hydantoin syndrome, *J Pediatr* 87:285-290, 1975.

107. Klepper I: Cardioversion in late pregnancy-the anaesthetic management of a case of Wolff-Parkinson-White syndrome, *Anaesthesia* 36:611-616, 1981.

108. Ogburn PL, Schmidt G, Linman J et al: Paroxysmal tachycardia and cardioversion during pregnancy, *J Reprod Med* 27:359-366, 1992.

109. Finlay AY, Edmonds V: D.C. cardioversion in pregnancy, *Br J Clin Pract* 33:88-94, 1979.

110. Natale A, Davidson T, Geiger MJ et al: Implantable cardioverter-defibrillators and pregnancy: a safe combination?, *Circulation* 96:2808-2812, 1997.

111. Dominguez A, Iturralde P, Hermosillo AG et al: Successful radiofrequency ablation of an accessory pathway during pregnancy, *PACE* 22:131-134, 1999.

112. Presbitero P, Prever SB, Brusca A: Interventional cardiology in pregnancy, *Eur Heart J* 17:182-188, 1996.

113. Lau CP, Lee CP, Wong CK et al: Rate responsive pacing with a minute ventilation sensing pacemaker during pregnancy and delivery, *PACE* 13:158-163, 1990.

114. Jaffe R, Gruber A, Fejgin M et al: Pregnancy with an artifical pacemaker, *Obstet Gynecol Surv* 42:137-139, 1987.

115. Ginz B: Myocardial infarction in pregnancy, *J Obstet Gynaecol Br Commonw* 77:610-615, 1970.

116. Schutzman DL, Frankenfield-Chernicoll M, Clatterbaugh HE et al: Incidence of intrauterine cocaine exposure in a suburban setting, *Pediatrics* 88:825-827, 1991.

117. Aglio LS, Johnson MD: Anesthetic management of myocardial infarction in a parturient, *Br J Anaesth* 65:258-261, 1990.

118. Cohen WR, Steinman T, Pastner B: Acute myocardial infarction in a pregnant woman at term, *JAMA* 250:2179-2181, 1983.

119. Frenkel Y, Barkai G, Reisin L et al: Pregnancy after myocardial infarction: are we playing safe? *Obstet Gynecol* 77:822-825, 1991.

120. Soderlin MK, Purhonen S, Haring P et al: Myocardial infarction in a parturient, *Anaesthesia* 49:870-872, 1994.

121. Abramovitz SE, Beilin Y: Anesthetic management of the parturient with protein S deficiency and ischemic heart disease, *Anesth Analg* 89:709-710, 1999.

122. Scott JR, Wagoner LE, Olsen SL et al: Pregnancy in heart transplant recipients: management and outcome, *Obstet Gynecol* 82:324-327, 1993.

123. Kim KM, Sukhani R, Slogoff S et al: Central hemodynamic changes associated with pregnancy in a long-term cardiac transplant recipient, *Am J Obstet Gynecol* 174:1651-1653, 1996.

124. K Troche V, Ville Y, Fernandez H: Pregnancy after heart or heart-lung transplantation: a series of 10 pregnancies, *Br J Obstet Gynecol* 105:454-458, 1998.

125. Morini A, Spina V, Aleandri V et al: Pregnancy after heart transplant: update and case report, *Human Reprod* 13:749-757, 1998.

126. Leachman RD, Colliinas DV, Cabrera R: Response of the transplanted, denervated human heart to cardiovascular drugs, *Am J Cardiol* 27:272-276, 1971.

127. Uretsky BF, Murali S, Reddy PS et al: Development of coronary disease in cardiac transplant patients receiving immunosuppressive therapy with cyclosporine and prednisone, *Circulation* 76:827-834, 1987.

128. Camann WR, Jarcho JA, Mintz KJ et al: Uncomplicated vaginal delivery 14 months after cardiac transplantation, *Am Heart J* 121: 939-941, 1991.

129. Camann WR, Goldman GA, Johnson MD et al: Cesarean delivery in a patient with a transplanted heart, *Anesthesiology* 71:618-620, 1989.

130. Cunningham FG, Pritchard JA, Hankins GD et al: Peripartum heart failure; idiopathic cardiomyopathy or compounding cardiovascular events, *Obstet Gynecol* 67:157-167, 1986.

131. Veille JC: Peripartum cardiomyopathies: a review, *Am J Obstet Gynecol* 148:805-817, 1984.

132. Desai D, Moodley J, Naidoo D: Peripartum cardiomyopathy: experiences at King Edward VIII Hospital, Durban, South Africa and a review of the literature, *Trop Doct* 25:118-123, 1995.

133. Heider AL, Kuller JA, Strauss RA et al: Peripartum cardiomyopathy: a review of the literature, *Obstet Gynecol Surv* 54:526-531, 1999.

134. Melvin KR, Richardson PJ, Olson EJ et al: Peripartum cardiomyopathy due to myocarditis, *N Engl J Med* 307:731-734, 1982.

135. Midei MG, Dement SH, Feldman AM et al: Peripartum myocarditis and cardiomyopathy, *Circulation* 81:922-928, 1990.

136. Nizeq MN, Rickenbocker PR, Fowler MB et al: Incidence of myocarditis in peripartum cardiomyopathy, *Am J Cardiol* 74: 74-77, 1994.

137. Witlin AG, Mabie WC, Sibai BM: Peripartum cardiomyopathy: a longitudinal echocardiographic study, *Am J Obstet Gynecol* 177: 1129-1132, 1997.

138. Demakis JG, Rahimtoola AI, Sutton GC et al: Natural course of peripartum cardiomyopathy, *Circulation* 44:1053-1061, 1971.

139. O'Connell JB, Costanzo-Nordin MR, Subramanian R et al: Peripartum cardiomyopathy: clinical, hemodynamic, histologic, and prognostic characteristics, *J Am Coll Cardiol* 8:52-56, 1986.

140. Lee W: Clinical management of gravid women with peripartum cardiomyopathy, *Obstet Gynecol Clin North Am* 18:257-271, 1991.

141. Homans DC: Current concepts: peripartum cardiomyopathy, *N Engl J Med* 312:1432-1437, 1985.

142. Witlin AG, Mabie WC, Sibai BM: Peripartum cardiomyopathy: an ominous diagnosis, *Am J Obstet Gynecol* 176:182-188, 1997.

143. Sutton MSJ, Cole P, Plappert M et al: Effects of subsequent pregnancy on left ventricular function in peripartum cardiomyopathy, *Am Heart J* 121:1776-1778, 1991.

144. Lampert MB, Weinert L, Hibbard J et al: Contractile reserve in patients with peripartum cardiomyopathy and recovered left ventricular function, *Am J Obstet Gynecol* 176:189-195, 1997.

145. Hanssens M, Keirse MJ, Vankelecom F et al: Fetal and neonatal effects of treatment with angiotensin-converting enzyme inhibitors in pregnancy, *Obstet Gynecol* 78:128-135, 1991.

146. Brown CS, Bertolet BD: Peripartum cardiomyopathy: a comprehensive review, *Am J Obstet Gynecol* 178:409-414, 1998.

147. George LM, Gatt SP, Lowe S: Peripartum cardiomyopathy: four case histories and a commentary on anaesthetic management, *Anaesth Intens Care* 25:292-296, 1997.

148. McIndoe AK, Hammond EJ, Babington R: Peripartum cardiomyopathy presenting as a cardiac arrest at induction of anaesthesia for emergency cesarean section, *Br J Anaesth* 75:97-101, 1995.

149. Weiss BM, von Segesser LK, Alon E et al: Outcome of cardiovascular surgery and pregnancy: a systematic review of the period 1984-1996, *Am J Obstet Gynecol* 179:1643-1650, 1998.

150. Koh KS, Friesen RM, Livingstone RA et al: Fetal monitoring during maternal cardiac surgery with cardiopulmonary bypass, *Can Med Assoc J* 112:110204, 1975.

151. Werch A, Lambert HM: Fetal monitoring and maternal open heart surgery, *South Med J* 70:1024, 1977.

152. Parry AJ, Westaby S: Cardiopulmonary bypass during pregnancy, *Ann Thorac Surg* 61:1865-1869, 1996.

153. Tripp HF, Stiegel RM, Coyle JP: The use of pulsatile perfusion during aortic valve replacement in pregnancy, *Ann Thorac Surg* 67:1169-1171, 1999.

154. Assali NS, Westin B: Effects of hypothermia on uterine circulation and on the fetus, *Proc Soc Exp Biol Med* 109:485-488, 1962.

155. Lamb MP, Ross K, Johnstone AM et al: Fetal heart monitoring during open heart surgery, *Br J Obstet Gynaecol* 88:669-674, 1981.

156. Koh KS, Friesen RM, Livingstone RA et al: Fetal monitoring during maternal cardiac surgery with cardiopulmonary bypass, *Can Med Assoc J* 112:1102-1104, 1975.

157. Dildy GA, Clark SL: Cardiac arrest during pregnancy, *Obstet Gynecol Clin North Am*, 22:303-314, 1995.

158. Rees GD, Willis BA: Resuscitation in late pregnancy, *Anaesthesia*, 43:347-349, 1988.

159. Goodwin AL, Pearce AJ: The human wedge, *Anaesthesia* 47: 433-434, 1992.

160. American Heart Association: Guidelines for cardiopulmonary resuscitation and emergency cardiac care: special resuscitation situations, *JAMA* 268:2242-2250, 1992.

161. Katz VL, Dotters DJ, Droegemueller W: Perimortem cesarean delivery, *Obstet Gynecol* 68:571-576, 1986.

162. Marx GF: Cardiopulmonary resuscitation of late pregnant women, *Anesthesiology* 56:156, 1982.

163. Parker J, Balis N, Chester S et al: Cardiopulmonary arrest in pregnancy: successful resuscitation of mother and infant following immediate caesarean section in labour ward, *Aust NZ J Obstet Gynaecol* 32:207-210, 1996.

164. Camann WR, Thornhill ML: Cardiovascular disease. In Chestnut DH, editor: *Obstetric anesthesia: principles and practice*, ed 2, St Louis, 1999, Mosby, Inc., p 797.

CHAPTER 21
Ambulatory Surgery

Thomas J. Conahan III, M.D.

OUTLINE

PREOPERATIVE EVALUATION

As the population of ambulatory surgery cases has grown, so has the number of patients coming to surgery with significant heart disease. The first major challenge for the clinician is to determine which patients are appropriate to be scheduled as outpatients.

The patient alone does not determine suitability for outpatient surgery. The proposed procedure itself exerts a major influence. In addition to having recovered from anesthesia, the patient must be free of bleeding, able to walk well enough to move into a place of comfort at home, have pain that is controllable with oral medication, and be capable of retaining food and drink. At one time, invasion of a major body cavity was considered grounds for inpatient surgery. The advent of endoscopes has revised that perspective. Outpatient cholecystectomy has been a reality for years. Surgeon skill and patient motivation also play important roles in returning the ambulatory surgery patient home.

The preoperative evaluation of the patient for ambulatory surgery and anesthesia may be the first opportunity for a systematic health evaluation. Careful history taking for lifestyle (stress, inactivity), smoking, history of hypertension, stroke, heart failure, chest pain, palpitations or arrhythmias, and other indications of cardiac disease is imperative. Additional questioning may reveal indications of significant disease in other organ systems.

The history aimed at detection of cardiac problems would obviously include questions about angina or angina equivalents (arm, shoulder, neck or jaw pain, short-

ness of breath). Symptoms of congestive heart failure (shortness of breath, limb swelling, paroxysmal nocturnal dyspnea or orthopnea) and cardiac arrhythmias (palpitations, light-headedness, fainting loss of consciousness, or other signs of transient cerebral ischemia) should also be sought. The preanesthetic physical examination should also be geared to detecting signs of congestive heart failure and arrhythmias.

A primary prerequisite for ambulatory anesthesia and surgery in any patient is stability. While the patient may have ongoing disease, the disease process must be stable. This applies to pulmonary, metabolic, and other disorders as well as to cardiac disorders.

Ischemic Heart Disease

Most studies involving patients with cardiac disease have been done on inpatients who are having operations that are longer, more invasive, and that have longer postoperative courses than the usual outpatient procedure. It is impossible (and probably inappropriate to try) to apply these data to cardiac patients who are having outpatient procedures. Realize that there are no absolutes. We are dealing with patients with significant disease of a vital organ system. Further disease may be manifest at any time. The overall goal is to identify patients who are at high risk of significant intraoperative and postoperative myocardial ischemia and prevent the damage which that ischemia may cause (myocardial infarction, congestive heart failure, arrhythmia). This is best accomplished by placing those patients in a postoperative milieu (inpatient) where detection and immediate therapy of myocardial ischemia are possible.

Many investigators have demonstrated the occurrence of perioperative myocardial ischemia and have documented that most of this ischemia is silent and is not related to changes in heart rate or blood pressure. One of the more interesting studies[1] documented myocardial ischemia by using perioperative Holter monitoring of inpatients with known coronary disease or of those who were at high risk for it. The investigators found that the lowest incidence of myocardial ischemia occurred preoperatively and the highest incidence occurred in the postoperative period. The vast majority of patients who demonstrated ischemia in all of the studies did not proceed to have an adverse cardiac event. Ellis summarized a series of studies that examined the prevalence of postoperative ischemia and the prevalence of cardiac events in those patients.[2] The prevalence of postoperative ischemia ranged from 28% to 62%, and between 3% and 33% of patients had postoperative cardiac events[1,3-6] (Table 21-1). Because of the documented seriousness of myocardial ischemia, the detection of such ischemia is important in the ambulatory patient with cardiac disease. The history, physical examination, and resting 12-lead electrocardiogram (ECG) are the primary modalities available to the anesthesiologist in evaluating the potential ambulatory surgery patient. Assuming that most, if not all, ambulatory surgery is elective, the evaluation of the patient can be more selective than it is for patients undergoing nonelective surgery.

What patients are at risk for postoperative myocardial ischemia? Hollinberg et al[7] identified five factors: (1) left ventricular hypertrophy by ECG, (2) a history of hypertension, (3) diabetes mellitus, (4) definite coronary artery disease, and (5) the use of digoxin. The American College of Cardiology/American Heart Association Task Force on Practice Guidelines for Perioperative Cardiovascular Evaluation for Non-cardiac Surgery identified clinical markers that are predictors of increased perioperative cardiovascular risk[8] (Box 21-1). The adverse perioperative events of most concern were myocardial infarction, congestive heart failure, and death.

Fleisher and Barash[9] proposed a functional approach to preoperative cardiac evaluation (Fig. 21-1). Their algorithm is based primarily on history and exercise tolerance. Patients with documented coronary disease or who were at risk for coronary artery disease but who had good exercise tolerance were to be scheduled for surgery with no further preoperative testing. Patients with poor exercise tolerance were suggested for further evaluation by dipyridamole thallium testing. A study that evaluates outcomes based on this approach has not

TABLE 21-1
Postoperative Ischemia and Cardiac Events

| STUDY (YEAR) | PATIENTS | | PREVALENCE | |
	NUMBER	CHARACTERISTICS	POSTOP ISCHEMIA	CARDIAC EVENTS
Mangano (1990)[1]	474	NCS: Known or suspected CAD	194/474 = 41%	3.2% 2 deaths 8 infarcts 1 UA
Ouyang (1989)[3]	24	Vascular surgery with CAD	15/24 = 62%	33% 2 infarcts 6 UA
McCann (1989)[4]	50	Lower extremity vascular surgery	19/50 = 38% (overall periop ischemia)	8% 2 deaths 2 infarcts
Pasternack (1989)[5]	200	Vascular surgery	57/200 = 28%	6.5% 2 deaths 9 infarcts
Landesberg (1993)[6]	151	Vascular surgery	88/151 = 58% (overall periop ischemia)	5.3% 6 infarcts 2 UA

From Ellis JE: *Myocardial ischemia and postoperative management*, 1997 annual refresher course lectures, Park Ridge, Ill, 1997, American Society of Anesthesiologists.
CAD, Coronary artery disease; *NCS*, noncardiac surgery; *UA*, unstable angina.

BOX 21-1
Clinical Predictors of Increased Perioperative Cardiovascular Risk

Major (Intensive Management Indicated: Probably Precludes Ambulatory Anesthesia)

Unstable coronary syndromes
  Recent myocardial infarction with evidence of important ischemic risk by clinical symptoms or noninvasive study
  Unstable or severe angina
Decompensated congestive heart failure
Significant arrhythmias
  High-grade atrioventricular block
  Symptomatic ventricular arrhythmias in the presence of underlying heart disease
  Supraventricular arrhythmias with uncontrolled ventricular rate
Severe valvular disease

Intermediate (Careful Assessment of Current Status Needed: Further Workup Likely)

Mild angina pectoris
Prior myocardial infarction by history or pathologic Q waves
Compensated or prior congestive heart failure
Diabetes mellitus

Minor (Not Proven to Independently Increase Perioperative Risk)

Advanced age
Abnormal ECG (left ventricular hypertrophy, left bundle-branch block, ST-T abnormalities)
Rhythm other than sinus (e.g., atrial fibrillation)
Low functional capacity (e.g., inability to climb one flight of stairs with bag of groceries)
History of stroke
Uncontrolled systemic hypertension

From Eagle KA, Brundage BH, Chaitman BR et al: *J Am Coll Cardiol* 27:910-948, 1996.
ECG, Electrocardiogram.

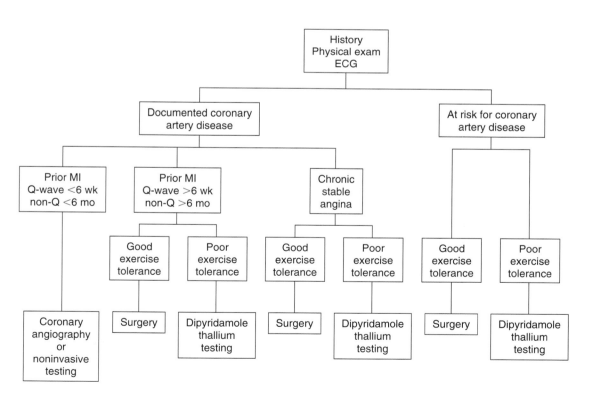

FIG. 21-1   Proposed algorithm for evaluation of patients undergoing surgical procedures associated with low to moderate risk of perioperative ischemia. *ECG,* Electrocardiogram; *MI,* myocardial infarction.

(From Fleisher LA, Barash PG: *Anesth Analg* 74:586-589, 1992.)

been reported. Fleisher and Barash extrapolate their approach from two articles,[10,11] making the distinction that patients who survive a non-Q-wave myocardial infarction are more likely to reinfarct than are those who survive a Q-wave infarction. The Q-wave infarction is usually associated with more extensive myocardial injury, whereas the non-Q-wave myocardial infarction may have a border zone of ischemic tissue along the infarcted tissue that remains at high risk of subsequent ischemia and infarction. Fleisher and Barash postulate abandoning the traditional 6-month interval after a myocardial infarction and basing the assessment of appropriateness of the patient for surgery and anesthesia on the patient's functional status.

The resting 12-lead ECG is of little value if it is normal. Many patients with significant coronary artery disease demonstrate the changes of ischemia only under stress. For this reason, the exercise ECG or the pharmacologically stressed ECG has become an important step in the evaluation of the patient with coronary artery disease.[12] From a practical standpoint, in evaluating the potential outpatient anesthesia candidate with a remote history of coronary artery disease who has a normal ECG, the absence of angina and the presence of a reasonable exercise level become a practical screening test. The patient with a history of prior myocardial infarction who has poor exercise tolerance is at greater risk for a perioperative cardiac event than is the patient with a distant myocardial infarction who has returned to strenuous activity.

There are three categories of patients potentially coming to the ambulatory surgical facility: the patient without symptoms of ischemia or risk factors, the asymptomatic patient at risk for coronary artery disease, and the patient with known coronary artery disease. The patient whose coronary disease is identified by prior myocardial infarction may be stable or unstable. The data relating to incidence of reinfarction with surgery after a myocardial infarction were gathered on inpatients; extrapolation to the outpatient venue is difficult. While Rao et al[13] documented a reduction in the incidence of perioperative myocardial infarction in patients with previous infarctions, they achieved this result with complex invasive monitoring in an inpatient setting.

The patient who comes for evaluation for ambulatory anesthesia with a myocardial infarction in the distant past or other indication of coronary artery disease must be evaluated for stability of the disease process. Chronic stable angina is not a contraindication to ambulatory anesthesia and surgery. But a changing pattern of the occurrence of angina with increasing frequency or severity or with decreasing intensity of stimulus necessary to evoke the angina is a warning sign.

Postoperative ischemia remains a threat for up to 7 days. The greatest threat (the highest frequency of events) occurs 1 to 3 days postoperatively. The ambulatory setting is obviously not appropriate for patients with this sort of a monitoring requirement.

There have been many studies documenting perioperative myocardial ischemia. Few have examined specific interventions and fewer still have followed long-term outcome. Wallace et al[14] reported that prophylactic atenolol reduced myocardial ischemia in the postoperative period and the reduction in myocardial ischemia was associated with a reduced risk for death at 2 years postoperatively.

Influence of Surgical Procedure. Surgery-specific risk was also identified in the American College of Cardiology guidelines.[8] Operations were characterized as high (>5%), intermediate (between 1% and 5%), and low (<1%) risk of cardiac death or nonfatal myocardial infarction (Box 21-2).

Valvular Heart Disease

Patients with valvular heart disease are also subject to a functional evaluation. The ability to walk into the front door of the institution implies the ability to double cardiac output above resting levels. Given a carefully crafted anesthetic of relatively short duration, this level of functioning is usually adequate to see the patient through the operation.

BOX 21-2
Cardiac Risk* for Noncardiac Surgery

High (Reported Cardiac Risk Often >5%)
Emergent major operations
Aortic and other major vascular
Peripheral vascular
Anticipated prolonged surgical procedures associated with large fluid shifts and/or blood loss

Intermediate (Reported Cardiac Risk Generally <5%)
Carotid endarterectomy
Head and neck
Intraperitoneal and intrathoracic
Orthopedic
Prostate

Low (Reported Cardiac Risk Generally <1%)
Endoscopic procedures
Superficial procedures
Cataract
Breast

From Eagle KA, Brundage BH, Chaitman BR et al: *J Am Coll Cardiol* 27:910-948, 1996.
*Cardiac death or nonfatal myocardial infarction.

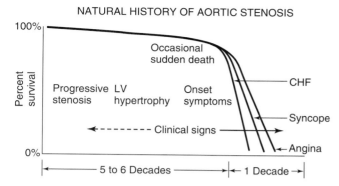

FIG. 21-2 Natural history of aortic valve stenosis. *CHF*, Congestive heart failure; *LV*, left ventricular.

(From Ewy GA, Tempkin LP: Acquired valvular disease—natural history and clinical diagnosis. In Conahan TJ, editor: *Cardiac anesthesia*, Menlo Park, Calif, 1982, Addison Wesley.)

BOX 21-3
Considerations in Congenital Heart Disease

Associated anomalies
Hemoglobin/blood viscosity
Coagulation
SBE prophylaxis
Hydration/NPO status
Upper respiratory infection
Bubbles in IV
Postoperative analgesia

IV, Intravenous; *NPO*, nothing by mouth; *SBE*, subacute bacterial endocarditis.

Aortic Stenosis. The natural history of aortic stenosis is illustrated in Fig. 21-2.[15] This lesion is the only cardiac valvular lesion predictive of death.[16] Patients with symptomatic aortic stenosis are not candidates to be anesthetized as outpatients, and some authors have suggested that either balloon dilation of valve or valve replacement be performed before undergoing anesthesia for other (major) surgery.

Aortic Regurgitation. Chronic aortic regurgitation can be without symptoms until the regurgitant fraction is over 40% of the stroke volume. If a patient's murmur arouses suspicion, the patient should be referred for further evaluation before elective surgery.

Mitral Stenosis. The scarring and fibrosis of the valve typically occur over many years. A patient may be totally asymptomatic with a valve area only 25% of normal. Problems arise when demand for increased cardiac output exceeds the flow capability of the stenotic valve. Exercise tolerance is a useful screening parameter in evaluating such patients for ambulatory surgery.

Mitral Regurgitation. Dysfunction of the mitral valve may be rheumatic or myxomatous in origin, or it may be a manifestation of cardiac dilation or papillary muscle dysfunction secondary to ischemia. Mitral regurgitation may be difficult to quantitate without sophisticated studies.

Congenital Heart Disease

The range of patients with congenital heart disease who may come for an ambulatory procedure is broad: pediatric or adult; corrected, palliated, or uncorrected; cyanotic or not. The first challenge is determining who is an appropriate candidate for anesthesia and surgery in the ambulatory setting.

The patient's history should be reviewed carefully, seeking details of previous surgical procedures (both cardiac and noncardiac) and anesthetics, current medications, activity levels, and symptoms of cardiac failure or cyanotic spells. The child who is growing normally and can run and play and keep up with peers indicates a degree of cardiac reserve. The child with "failure to thrive" invites further evaluation and consultation with a pediatric cardiologist.

Physical examination should seek signs of heart failure (distended jugular veins, rales, enlarged liver). Any unexplained murmur that concerns the anesthesiologist is grounds for requesting evaluation by a pediatric cardiologist. Also, some congenital cardiac lesions are associated with noncardiac abnormalities or airway problems.

Given the complexity of the interactions between the lesion, the operation, and the anesthetic, the decision to perform the procedure in a hospital where consultation and support are immediately available is very attractive. Given a benign course and agreement among the consultants, some patients with more complex problems may be discharged on the day of surgery, assuming that adequate care is available at home. Minor procedures on patients with simple lesions (small atrial septal defect, patent ductus) can often be performed on an outpatient basis.

The anesthesiologist must have a thorough understanding of the congenital defect and any repairs or palliative procedures that have been performed. A major concern is the effect that anesthesia and surgery may have on the cardiac lesion. Systemic vasodilation may change shunt flow, hypercarbia can increase pulmonary vascular resistance, and even brief periods of hypoxia can play havoc with a failing myocardium. Induction and maintenance of anesthesia must be tailored to the individual patient and based on typical pediatric anesthesia techniques. Additional areas of concern are listed in Box 21-3.

Baum and Perloff[17] reviewed the anesthetic implications of congenital heart disease in adults. Anesthetic concerns and perioperative management of congenital heart disease is discussed in more detail in Chapter 10.

Summary

In a practical sense, the patient who has been able to walk into the ambulatory surgery facility has demonstrated an ability to at least double cardiac output above resting level. If this can be done without signs of ischemia or congestive heart failure, an important milestone has been passed. A key concept in evaluating the potential ambulatory surgery patient is determining whether in fact the patient is appropriate to be cared for in an ambulatory procedure unit. Preoperative evaluation should be directed at identifying patients who are either inappropriate for the ambulatory surgical facility or who require further evaluation before the decision can be made.

ANESTHESIA AND SURGERY
Preoperative Medications

Many patients with cardiac disease who come to surgery receive chronic medication. In general, most of these medications should be continued on the day of surgery. They should be taken with as small an amount of water as possible, which allows swallowing. Some practitioners recommend withholding digitalis preparations on the day of the surgery, especially if the indication is a history of congestive heart failure. The blood level will not fluctuate a great deal, and it is preferable to have a waning blood level if any arrhythmias or other signs of digitalis toxicity were to appear. The respiratory alkalosis associated with hyperventilation during induction of general anesthesia may lead to hypokalemia and increase the arrhythmogenic risk during the period of elevated digitalis level.

Most antihypertensive medications should be continued. Diuretics may be withheld on the day of surgery, in part for convenience and patient comfort and in part to maintain intravascular volume before induction of anesthesia. Other antihypertensive medications should be continued. β-Blocking drugs are useful in controlling heart rate and thereby reducing myocardial oxygen demand. Calcium channel blocking drugs also reduce myocardial work and myocardial oxygen demand by peripheral vasodilatation and by direct effects on the myocardium.

Choice of Anesthesia

A major determination to be made is whether the proposed surgical procedure can be performed under local anesthesia with or without sedation, or whether general or regional anesthesia is required. The choice of local anesthesia with little or no sedation and little or no monitoring should be reserved for the healthier patients. This seems in contradiction to the often-heard statement, "he is too sick for any anesthesia, let's do it with local." However, that "too sick" patient is just the one who needs every potential stumbling block removed for a smooth operative course. This includes the provision of adequate sedation, regional or general anesthesia to minimize the stress—both physiologic and psychologic—to which the patient is being subjected.

Sedation can be used to provide anxiolysis, amnesia, and analgesia to supplement locally injected anesthetics and regional or neuraxial blocks. Commonly used anxiolytics are the benzodiazepines, either diazepam or midazolam. Short-acting narcotic analgesics such as fentanyl are often added. A low-dose infusion of propofol has become increasingly popular to provide obtundation of the sensorium in the operating room. Propofol has the added advantage of lowering the incidence of nausea and vomiting in the perioperative period. Characteristics of commonly used sedative and analgesic drugs are given in Table 21-2.

The use of conduction anesthesia (spinal or epidural) in the ambulatory surgical area is a topic of continuing controversy. Many practitioners are reluctant to perform conduction anesthesia because of the potential for delayed recovery and discharge, late complications occurring while the patient is at home, and the potential for rapid changes in peripheral vascular resistance and sympathetic tone. Others argue that awake patients are their own best monitors for angina. Given the fact that a majority of ischemic episodes detected in perioperative Holter monitoring are silent, this argument appears rather weak.

The availability of relatively short-acting anesthetic agents has made general anesthesia in the ambulatory surgery patient more practical. Propofol is used as both an induction agent and as an infusion for maintenance of anesthesia. The short-acting narcotics—fentanyl, alfentanil, and sufentanil—and ultrashort-acting drugs (remifentanil) are popular anesthesia adjuvants. Care must be taken with remifentanil because of its short half-life. Plans for postoperative analgesia must be implemented before the end of the surgery because the drug's effects dissipate rapidly after the discontinuation of the infusion. A smooth transition to postoperative analgesia is a desired pattern for any patient, but it is imperative in the patient with cardiac disease.

The choice of inhalation agent is probably not as important as the skill of the person who delivers it. The age-old warning of "avoid hypoxia and hypotension" has become "avoid hypoxia, hypotension, hypertension, and tachycardia." Inhalation agents such as isoflurane and desflurane, which can cause increased sympathetic stimulation, must be administered carefully to avoid tachycardia. Sevoflurane is less prone to sympa-

TABLE 21-2
Intravenous Sedation

	INITIAL DOSE	ONSET (IV)	PEAK	SIDE EFFECTS
Midazolam	0.5-2 mg	1-2 min	3-5 min	Drowsiness Amnesia
Diazepam	1-3 mg	1-2 min	8 min	Drowsiness Amnesia
Fentanyl	12.5-50 mcg	2 min	4-6 min	Respiratory depression Nausea
Meperidine	12.5-25 mg	2 min	6 min	Respiratory depression Nausea
Morphine	2-5 mg	2 min	20 min	Respiratory depression Nausea
Propofol	Infusion 10-70 µg/kg/min			Respiratory depression Drowsiness

thetic outflow stimulation, but the discussion and controversy over renal cell compromise are not complete. The question of whether or not nitrous oxide is a contributor to perioperative nausea and vomiting will probably never be resolved definitively. The drug is a useful adjuvant to general anesthesia.

Intraoperative Monitoring

Patients whose cardiac disease requires invasive monitoring are rarely candidates for ambulatory surgery. Given the nature and timing of postoperative complications, such patients are best cared for in a hospital setting.

Noninvasive blood pressure, ECG (with appropriate lead placement), pulse oximetry, and carbon dioxide (CO_2) excretion comprise the standard parameters. Temperature monitoring is indicated for longer cases and in situations where significant temperature changes might be expected.

Noninvasive blood-pressure recording may give the first clue that an adverse event is about to occur. Hypertension may indicate pain or anxiety, or may herald the onset of congestive heart failure and pulmonary edema. Among the potential causes of hypotension are myocardial ischemia, arrhythmia, hypovolemia (relative or absolute), and deep anesthesia.

Electrocardiography is useful for detection of both arrhythmias and ischemia. Many ambulatory centers use only a three-lead configuration. In such cases, modification of lead I (placement of the left arm electrode in the V_5 position) provides a view of left-ventricular electrical activity. Lead II is most commonly observed for arrhythmias. Five-lead ECG systems can allow two channels of ECG monitoring, and newer monitors include automated ST analysis.

Pulse oximetry is probably the single most significant safety advance in anesthesia during the past 50 years. Properly applied to a site with an adequately pulsatile arterial bed, the pulse oximeter supplies information about heart rate, rhythm, and oxygen saturation in both visual and audible forms. The pulse oximeter can be rendered ineffective or inaccurate by peripheral vasoconstriction, arteriovenous shunts, intravenous (IV) dyes, excessive ambient light, movement of the probe, and significant concentration of abnormal hemoglobins.

End-tidal CO_2 monitoring has been adopted by the American Society of Anesthesiologists as a standard for basic anesthesia monitoring in all patients receiving general anesthesia. A sudden decrease in end-tidal CO_2 in the anesthetized cardiac patient may indicate cardiac failure or pulmonary embolus.

POSTOPERATIVE COURSE
Recovery and Discharge

The goal of recovery in the ambulatory patient is to have the patient vertical, comfortable (not necessarily pain free), and capable of enough mobility to transfer from the ambulatory procedure area to a vehicle and to home. With the use of relatively short-acting drugs, there are many centers that actually have the patient bypass the traditional recovery area and recover in a step-down unit. This requires, of course, that the determination be made in the operating room that the patient is sufficiently awake and stable. In some institutions as many as 60% of patients undergoing general anesthesia can follow this course. Marshall and Chung[18] recently reviewed discharge and complications after ambulatory surgery. They describe two quantitative scoring systems, one to determine when patients are ready for

TABLE 21-3

TABLE 21-3
Modified Aldrete—Postanesthesia Recovery Score (PARS) for Determining Readiness for Discharge from Acute Postanesthesia Care Unit*

Activity

Able to move 4 extremities voluntarily or on command	2
Able to move 2 extremities voluntarily or on command	1
Unable to move extremities voluntarily or on command	0

Respiration

Able to breathe deeply and cough freely	2
Dyspnea or limited breathing	1
Apneic	0

Circulation

BP ± 20% of preanesthetic level	2
BP ± 20% to 49% of anesthetic level	1
BP ± 50% of preanesthetic level	0

Consciousness

Fully awake	2
Arousable on calling	1
Not responding	0

O_2 Saturation

Able to maintain O_2 saturation >92% on room air	2
Needs O_2 inhalation to maintain O_2 saturation >90%	1
O_2 saturation <90% even with O_2 supplement	1

From Aldrete JA: *J Clin Anesth* 7:89-91, 1995.
BP, Blood pressure; *O_2*, oxygen.
*A score of ≥9 required for discharge from acute postanesthesia care unit.

TABLE 21-4
Modified Postanesthesia Discharge Scoring System (PADSS)*

Vital Signs
Vital signs must be stable and consistent with age and preoperative baseline.

BP and pulse within 20% of preoperative baseline	2
BP and pulse 20%-40% of preoperative baseline	1
BP and pulse >40% of preoperative baseline	0

Activity Level
Patient must be able to ambulate at preoperative level.

Steady gait, no dizziness, or meets preoperative level	2
Requires assistance	1
Unable to ambulate	0

Nausea and Vomiting
The patient should have minimal nausea and vomiting before discharge.

minimal: successfully treated with oral medication	2
moderate: successfully treated with intramuscular medication	1
severe: continues after repeated treatment	0

Pain
The patient should have minimal or no pain before discharge.
The level of pain that the patient has should be acceptable to the patient.
Pain should be controllable by oral analgesics.
The location, type, and intensity of pain should be consistent with anticipated postoperative discomfort.

Acceptability	yes	2
	no	0

Surgical bleeding
Postoperative bleeding should be consistent with expected blood loss for the procedure.

minimal: does not require dressing change	2
moderate: up to two dressing changes required	1
severe: more than three dressing changes required	0

From Marshall SI, Chung F: *Curr Opin Anesthiol* 10:445-450, 1997.
BP, Blood pressure.
*Maximum score is 10; patients scoring 9 or more are fit for discharge.

discharge from the postanesthesia care unit (Table 21-3),[19] and the second as guidelines for safe discharge after ambulatory surgery (Table 21-4).[20] Postoperative nausea is a major factor in delaying discharge and increasing patient distress. Commonly used antiemetics are summarized in Table 21-5.

Postoperative pain is a major complaint in ambulatory surgery patients. The overall anesthetic plan must include provisions for dealing with postoperative pain. Many procedures involving bone and joint surgery, although performed on an outpatient basis, can be very stimulating. Analgesics as potent as morphine may be required to render the patient comfortable in the recovery period. In cases of severe postoperative pain, the transition from parenteral to oral opioid analgesics should be made before the patient is discharged. Less severe pain may be treated with nonsteroidal antiinflammatory drugs either parenterally or orally. The combined use of opioid analgesics and nonsteroidal anti-

inflammatories can be synergistic in some patients, leading to a more comfortable postoperative course and more rapid discharge from the postanesthesia care unit. Other techniques for control of postoperative pain include infiltration of wound sites with long-acting local anesthetics or regional nerve blocks, such as an interscalene nerve block that is used for shoulder surgery.

TABLE 21-5
Commonly Used Antiemetics

	DOSE	DURATION	SIDE EFFECTS
Droperidol (Inapsine)	0.625-1.25 mg (IV)	2-4 hr	Sedation may last 12 hr Hypotension Extrapyramidal signs
Metoclopramide (Reglan)	10 mg (IV)	1-2 hr	Drowsiness
Ondansetron (Zofran)	4 mg (IV)	4-12 hr	Headache Dizziness
Prochlorperazine (Compazine)	5-10 mg (IV)	4-12 hr	Extrapyramidal signs Hypotension Tachycardia
Trimethobenzamide (Tigan)	200-mg rectal suppository	2-3 hr	Drowsiness

Even mild (1°-2° C) postoperative hypothermia can be associated with significant cardiovascular morbidity. The incidence of arrhythmias is increased, coagulation may be impaired, and surgical wound infections are more common.[21] Many ambulatory surgical procedures are too brief to cause significant hypothermia. Both regional and general anesthesia predispose the patient to heat loss; therefore conservation of body heat increases in importance as the surgical procedure increases in duration. Forced warm-air blankets are the best currently available devices to conserve body heat and supply additional warmth.

Many centers do not insist that patients eat or drink before being eligible for discharge. There have been no studies that demonstrate significant complications from not requiring patients to retain fluids or food before discharge.

A major factor in expediting discharge of patients is adequate hydration. While the general trend is to be wary of overloading cardiac patients with IV fluids, the practitioner must remember that the typical patient has not had anything to eat or drink for 6 to 8 hours before surgery. In addition, patients undergo fluid translocation and blood loss during various procedures. A reasonable amount of fluid administration is 20 to 25 ml/kg for most patients deemed healthy enough to be cared for in an ambulatory unit.

Many institutions require patients to void before discharge, regardless of surgical procedure or anesthetic. A recent study demonstrated that most patients can be discharged before voiding and will not suffer any complication.[22]

OVERVIEW

This chapter discussed risks and complications, and it emphasized patient selection for ambulatory surgery. Data from inpatient studies have been discussed and their applicability questioned, and yet conclusions have been drawn. The patient at high risk for cardiac complications should be cared for in the location where those complications can be readily treated. Risk should be reduced whenever possible. Invasive monitoring may be indicated, but is usually inappropriate in the ambulatory setting. The McSPI study of an at-risk inpatient population[14] made a strong argument for the perioperative administration of β-adrenergic blocking drugs. That study followed patients for up to 2 years after discharge, and found a decreased incidence of cardiac events in those patients who received atenolol.

The safety of ambulatory anesthesia must be kept in perspective. The vast majority of patients undergoing surgery and anesthesia on an ambulatory basis have no problems. In a study of more than 45,000 ambulatory procedures, Warner et al[23] found only 33 patients who suffered major morbidity or died in the 30 days following surgery. Two of the four deaths were in automobile accidents, and none of the patients died of medical causes within 1 week of the surgery.

KEY POINTS

1. Not every patient is appropriate for ambulatory surgery.
2. An unstable disease process is a relative contraindication to ambulatory anesthesia.
3. Most stable patients with good exercise tolerance probably do not require extensive cardiac workup before superficial outpatient surgery.
4. Most perioperative myocardial ischemia is silent.

5. Patients who demonstrate perioperative myocardial ischemia are more likely to suffer postoperative myocardial infarctions.

6. Interaction between congenital cardiac lesions, their palliation or repair, and anesthesia can be complex,

and should be fully appreciated before undertaking anesthesia in an ambulatory setting.

7. Local anesthesia, with or without sedation, may be more stressful than a carefully crafted general or regional anesthetic.

KEY REFERENCES

Eagle KA, Brundage BH, Chaitman BR et al: Guidelines for perioperative cardiovascular evaluation for noncardiac surgery. Report of the American College of Cardiology/ American Heart Association task Force on Practice Guidelines (Committee on Perioperative Evaluation for Noncardiac Surgery), *J Am Coll Cardiol* 27:910-948, 1996.

Fleisher LA, Barash PG: Preoperative cardiac evaluation for noncardiac surgery: a functional approach, *Anesth Analg* 74:586-598, 1992.

Palda, VA, Detsky, AS: Perioperative assessment and management of risk from coronary artery disease, *Ann Intern Med* 127:313-328, 1997.

Warner MA, Lunn RJ, O'Leary PW et al: Outcomes of noncardiac surgical procedures in children and adults with congenital heart disease, *Mayo Clin Proc* 73:728-734, 1998.

References

1. Mangano DT, Browner WS, Hollenberg M et al: Association of perioperative ischemia with cardiac morbidity and mortality in men undergoing noncardiac surgery, *N Engl J Med* 323: 1781-1788, 1990.

2. Ellis JE: *Myocardial ischemia and postoperative management*, 1997 annual refresher course lectures, Park Ridge, Ill, 1997, American Society of Anesthesiologists.

3. Ouyang P, Gerstenblith G, Furman WR et al: Frequency and significance of early postoperative silent myocardial ischemia in patients having peripheral vascular surgery, *Am J Cardiol* 64: 1113-1116, 1989.

4. McCann RL, Clements FM: Silent myocardial ischemia in patients undergoing peripheral vascular surgery: incidence and association with perioperative cardiac morbidity and mortality, *J Vasc Surg* 9:583-587, 1989.

5. Pasternack PF, Grossi EA, Baumann FG et al: The value of silent myocardial ischemia monitoring in the prediction of perioperative myocardial infarction in patients undergoing peripheral vascular surgery, *J Vasc Surg* 10:617-625, 1989.

6. Landesberg G, Luria MH, Cotev S et al: Importance of long-duration postoperative ST-segment depression in cardiac morbidity after vascular surgery, *Lancet* 20:715-719, 1993.

7. Hollenberg M, Mangano DT, Browner WS et al: Predictors of postoperative myocardial ischemia in patients undergoing non-cardiac surgery, *JAMA* 286:205-209, 1992.

8. Eagle KA, Brundage BH, Chaitman BR et al: American College of Cardiology/American Heart Association Task Force on Practice Guidelines for Perioperative Cardiovascular Evaluation for Non-cardiac Surgery, *J Am Coll Cardiol* 27:910-948, 1996.

9. Fleisher LA, Barash PG: Preoperative cardiac evaluation for non-cardiac surgery: a functional approach, *Anesth Analg* 74:586-589, 1992.

10. Gibson RS: Non-Q wave myocardial infarction: prognosis, changing incidence, and management. In Gersh BJ, Rahimtoola SH, editors: *Acute myocardial infarction*, New York, 1991, Elsevier.

11. Benhorin J, Moss AJ, Oaks D et al: The prognostic significance of first myocardial infarction type (Q-wave vs. non-Q-wave) and Q- wave location, *J Am Coll Cardiol* 15:1201-1207, 1990.

12. Chaitman BR, Miller DD: Perioperative cardiac evaluation for noncardiac surgery: noninvasive cardiac testing, *Prog Cardiovasc Dis* 40:405-418, 1998.

13. Rao TLK, Jacobs HK: El-Etr AA reinfarction following anesthesia in patients with myocardial infarction, *Anesthesiology* 59:499-505, 1983.

14. Wallace A, Layug B, Tateo I et al: Prophylactic atenolol reduces postoperative myocardial ischemia, *Anesthesiology* 88:7-17, 1998.

15. Ewy GA, Tempkin LP: Acquired valvular disease—natural history and clinical diagnosis. In Conahan TJ, editor: *Cardiac anesthesia*, Menlo Park, Calif, 1982, Addison Wesley.

16. Palda VA, Detsky AS: Perioperative assessment and management of risk from coronary artery disease, *Ann Intern Med* 127:313-328, 1997.

17. Baum VC, Perloff JK: Anesthetic implications of adults with congenital heart disease, *Anesth Analg* 76:1342-1358, 1993.

18. Marshall SI, Chung F: Discharge criteria and complications after ambulatory surgery, *Anesth Analg* 88:508-517, 1999.

19. Aldrete JA: The post anesthesia recovery score revisited, *J Clin Anesth* 7:89-91, 1995.

20. Marshall SI, Chung F: Assessment of home readiness: discharge criteria and postdischarge complications, *Curr Opin Anesthesiol*, 445-450, 1997.

21. Sessler, DI, Current concepts: mild perioperative hypothermia, *N Engl J Med*, 336:1730-1737, 1997.

22. Fritz WT, George L, Krull N et al: Utilization of a home nursing protocol allows ambulatory surgery patients to be discharged prior to voiding, *Anesth Analg* 84:S6, 1997.

23. Warner MA, Shields SE, Chute CG: Major morbidity and mortality within 1 month of ambulatory surgery and anesthesia, *JAMA* 270:1437-1441, 1993.

CHAPTER 22
Thoracic Surgery

E. Andrew Ochroch, M.D. ■ Albert T. Cheung, M.D.

OUTLINE

The demands for providing safe and effective anesthetic and perioperative care for thoracic surgical patients changed during the course of the twentieth century in accordance with the types of procedures performed and the patient characteristics. Thoracic procedures performed in the early part of the century were primarily for the treatment of infections such as empyema and tuberculosis. The early diagnosis of pulmonary diseases after World War II and advances in antibiotic therapy, chest tube drainage, and lung isolation techniques changed the nature of thoracic surgery. Presently, thoracic operations are performed most commonly for the diagnosis or treatment of lung cancer. Cigarette smoking is recognized as an important risk factor for the development of pulmonary disease and lung cancer, but is also an important risk factor for ischemic coronary artery and other cardiovascular diseases. As a consequence, patients requiring thoracic operations for lung cancer are typically older, often have coexisting pulmonary and cardiovascular diseases, and are at increased risk for perioperative cardiac and pulmonary complications.

Thoracic surgery is a significant risk factor for the development of postoperative life-threatening or fatal cardiac complications, and it contributed three points to the cardiac risk index in the classic report by Goldman.[1] In the American College of Cardiology/American Heart Association guidelines for perioperative cardiovascular evaluation of noncardiac surgery, intrathoracic operations were considered an intermediate risk, with perioperative cardiac events occurring in 1% to 5% of cases.[2] Nevertheless, an increasingly complex variety of thoracic operations have since been performed on high-risk patients and operative mortality rates for thoracotomy have actually decreased. Thirty-day mortality rates after lung resections have decreased from a range of 10% to 15% in the 1960s to present rates of less than 2%.[3,4,5] The decrease in mortality rates is attributed to technologic advances in the surgical and anesthetic management of patients in the perioperative period. In addition, better patient evaluation and selection, postoperative pain management, specialized nursing care, and the ability to treat surgical complications in the intensive care unit (ICU) have also developed. Advances in technology have permitted routine thoracic procedures to be performed relatively safely in higher risk patients and permitted the successful conduct of more complex procedures such as lung volume reduction, pulmonary thromboembolectomy, and lung transplantation. Because of the increasingly complex nature of the thoracic surgical procedure and of the patient population, it is anticipated that perioperative complications from known or occult cardiopulmonary disease will continue. Manifestation of these complications is in response to the stress of surgery in patients with limited cardiopulmonary reserve. The importance of suspecting, diagnosing, and treating coexisting cardiac and pulmonary diseases perioperatively may lead to additional reductions in the mortality and morbidity associated with thoracic operations.

The medical and anesthetic management of patients undergoing thoracic surgical procedures is particularly challenging in the patient with cardiac disease. The heart and lungs that form the cardiopulmonary unit for respiration and gas transport are anatomically contiguous and physiologically coupled. This interdependence permits pulmonary disorders to manifest as cardiovascular dysfunction and cardiac disorders to manifest as pulmonary dysfunction, complicating the processes necessary to monitor and identify the source of problems. The treatment of cardiovascular diseases with agents such as β-adrenergic antagonists may exacerbate pulmonary dysfunction in patients with asthma or obstructive airways disease. In contrast, bronchodilator therapy for obstructive pulmonary disease may trigger cardiac arrhythmias or angina in susceptible patients with cardiac disease. In addition, general anesthesia, epidural anesthesia, thoracotomy, one-lung ventilation, and lung resection cause unique physiologic alterations and stresses to the pulmonary and cardiovascular systems that may unmask the presence of disease in otherwise asymptomatic individuals. This chapter describes current approaches for the preoperative assessment and medical optimization of patients undergoing thoracic surgical procedures. The effects of cardiac disease on pulmonary function and pulmonary disease states are reviewed. General considerations for the anesthetic care, medical management, and intraoperative monitoring of patients with cardiac diseases undergoing thoracic operations are discussed. Finally, the impact of specific thoracic operations on cardiac function is addressed.

PREOPERATIVE EVALUATION AND RISK ASSESSMENT

The decision to undergo surgery and its associated risks is made in perspective of the anticipated benefits of the operation.[6] The main benefit of thoracic surgery is the detection and cure of malignancy. Surgical resection offers the only chance for cure in patients with primary non–small cell cancer of the lungs. Survival 5 years after lung resection for non–small cell lung cancer ranges from 15% to 65%. Variability in survival rates reflects the amount of functional lung that is re-

sected, the presence of occult metastasis, and the natural history of patients with coexisting and smoking-related diseases.[7,8]

Although it is important to consider the risk of pulmonary complications in patients undergoing thoracic operations, epidemiologic studies have shown that perioperative cardiac complications remain the leading cause of death after anesthesia and surgery.[9] Most of the existing data regarding perioperative myocardial risk come from studies of noncardiac surgical patients, of whom thoracic surgical patients are only a small proportion. For example, The Coronary Artery Surgery Study (CASS) registry reported 1600 operations over a 3-year period. Of those, only 89 were thoracic operations.[10] Consequently, the published estimates of perioperative cardiac morbidity do not address the risks incurred specifically from the perturbations of thoracic surgery on the typical patient undergoing thoracic surgery. Instead, they address the average risk of a patient with coronary risk factors undergoing either high-risk or low-risk procedures. While few studies have addressed the incidence of perioperative cardiovascular complications in thoracic surgical patients selectively, it is likely that cardiovascular events account for the major cause of perioperative mortality in this subgroup. Cigarette smoking is a significant risk factor for carcinoma of the lung, emphysema, and cardiovascular disease. In addition to its role in the etiology and pathophysiology of atherosclerosis, cigarette smoking decreases coronary blood flow by causing direct constriction of coronary vessels. Hypertension, peripheral vascular disease, and systemic vasoconstriction caused by the acute and chronic effects of tobacco use also increase myocardial oxygen demand by increasing myocardial wall stress.[11]

Traditional scoring systems for estimating the risk of perioperative cardiac complications have been applied to the evaluation of the thoracic surgical patient. In the Goldman risk index, previous myocardial infarction (MI), MI within 6 months of operation, congestive heart failure (CHF), and the presence of ventricular dysrhythmias were significant risk factors for a perioperative cardiac event. In the Goldman score, the risk of a cardiac event was increased when thoracotomy was performed. However, not all clinical studies support the Goldman score as a predictor of outcome after surgery.[12,13] While useful in epidemiologic studies, clinical risk factors such as previous MI, angina, CHF, hypertension, diabetes mellitus, arrhythmias, and peripheral vascular disease are less useful for predicting the risk of perioperative cardiac morbidity in an individual surgical patient.[9] A recent study that compared the cardiac risk index proposed by Goldman to the American Society of Anesthesiologists physical status (ASA-PS) assessment in predicting the risk of mortality after noncardiac thoracic surgery demonstrated that only the information derived from the ASA-PS correlated independently with mortality.[14] Melindez and Carlon[15] investigated the predictive value of a cardiopulmonary risk index to specifically address the risks of thoracic operations. The cardiopulmonary risk index comprised modified Goldman criteria, an estimate of the left ventricular ejection fraction, and the pulmonary risk factors of obesity, cough, elevated resting arterial carbon dioxide tension ($Paco_2$), poor spirometric performance, diffuse wheezing, and recent cigarette smoking. However, this elaborate collection of preoperative history and testing was not useful for predicting the risk of complications after thoracic surgery.[15]

History and Physical Examination

A careful medical history and physical examination are performed to distinguish symptoms attributable to the underlying pulmonary disease processes from those attributable to cardiac disease. Identification of significant cardiac disease in older patients with chronic emphysema or bronchitis is often difficult and subtle (Tables 22-1 and 22-2). Orthopnea is generally considered a symptom of CHF, but patients with chronic obstructive pulmonary disease (COPD), pulmonary hypertension, or pericardial disease may also experience dyspnea in the supine position. Paroxysmal nocturnal dyspnea is a more specific symptom of left ventricular dysfunction. Dependent edema is a physical finding in patients with either CHF or cor pulmonale. Dyspnea caused by pulmonary edema is usually associated with rapid shallow breathing, inspiratory rales, and arterial oxygen hypoxemia. Wheezing as a manifestation of pulmonary edema secondary to heart failure is often referred to as *cardiac asthma*. Although cardiac asthma is believed to be a manifestation of airway narrowing from peribronchiolar cuffing or mucosal edema, the beneficial effect of bronchodilator therapy suggests a component of reactive bronchoconstriction.

The radiologic examination of the chest is useful for detecting the presence of pulmonary edema, pleural effusion, or cardiac chamber enlargement caused by cardiac disease. Increased hilar size; Kerley A, B, and C lines; widened fissures; peribronchial and perivascular cuffs; pleural effusion; and increased alveolar densities are radiographic signs of pulmonary edema. Cephalization or the prominence of vascular markings in the upper lung zones caused by CHF may not be apparent in patients with emphysema and decreased pulmonary vasculature in the apices of the lungs. Pleural effusions are present in approximately 25% of patients with CHF and are more common on the right side. Cardiomegaly is also a nonspecific indicator of cardiac disease.

Although anginal symptoms of coronary artery disease (CAD) are distinguishable from pleuritic pain, the electrocardiogram (ECG) is a useful test for differentiating cardiac from pulmonary processes. The presence of Q waves on the ECG suggests CAD and prior MI. Electrocardiographic evidence of left ventricular hypertrophy or left bundle-branch block also suggests the presence of cardiac disease. Low QRS amplitude, complete or incomplete right bundle-branch block, right-axis deviation of the QRS vector, and increased P-wave amplitude in leads II, III, and aVF (P-pulmonale pattern) are associated with COPD. Right ventricular hypertrophy from cor pulmonale is also associated with a P-pulmonale pattern, right-axis deviation of the QRS axis (to the right of 110 degrees), R/S amplitude ration in V_1 >1, and R/S amplitude ratio in V_6 <1 on the ECG (Figs. 22-1 and 22-2 and Table 22-3). Multifocal atrial tachycardia is a unique cardiac rhythm disturbance associated with chronic bronchitis or emphysema and indicates severe pulmonary disease (Fig. 22-3). Other supraventricular tachyarrhythmias, including atrial fibrillation and flutter, are manifestations of either pulmonary or cardiac disease. In general, radio-

---

TABLE 22-1
Cardiac Diseases that Often Present as Pulmonary Complaints

DISEASE	PULMONARY FINDINGS
Ischemia	Shortness of breath, hypoxemia
CHF	Shortness of breath, hypoxemia, restrictive pattern on PFTs
Right-to-left shunt	Shortness of breath, hypoxemia
Left-to-right shunt	Easy fatigability, restrictive pattern on PFTs
Mitral valve regurgitation	Shortness of breath, restrictive pattern on PFTs
Cardiac asthma	Shortness of breath, peribronchial cuffing on CXR

CHF, Congestive heart failure; *CXR*, chest X-ray; *PFTs*, pulmonary function tests.

TABLE 22-2
Pulmonary Diseases that Often Present as Cardiac in Origin

DISEASE	CARDIAC COMPLAINT
COPD/emphysema	Fatigability, shortness of breath
Pneumothorax	Chest pain
Pulmonary hypertension	Peripheral edema, fatigability

COPD, Chronic obstructive pulmonary disease.

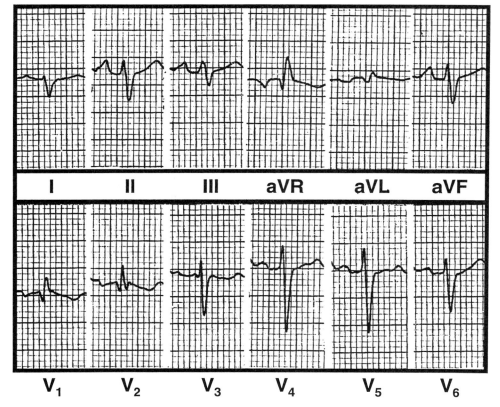

FIG. 22-1 A 12-lead electrocardiogram from a patient with chronic bronchitis and emphysema, showing electrocardiographic signs of cor pulmonale in the presence of chronic obstructive pulmonary disease. The wide deep S waves in leads I, II, III are consistent with an $S_1S_2S_3$ pattern caused by an anomalous wave from rightward and superiorly oriented and opposed to the electrical forces of the ventricular free wall. The peak P waves in leads II, III, and aVF are consistent with the P-pulmonale pattern. The P-wave axis of greater than 90° indicates right atrial overland, and a dominant R wave in V_1 and V_2 with an rS pattern in V_5 to V_6 indicates right ventricular hypertrophy.

(From Holford FD: The electrocardiogram in pulmonary disease. In Fishman A, editor: *Pulmonary diseases and disorders,* ed 2, New York, 1988, McGraw-Hill.)

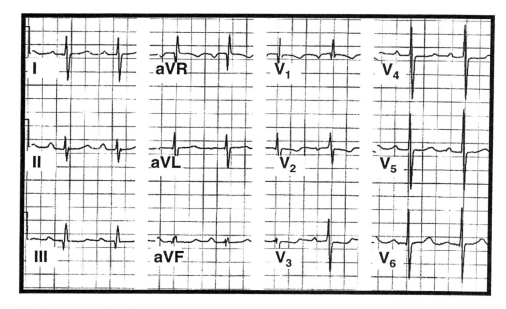

FIG. 22-2 A 12-lead electrocardiogram in a patient with primary pulmonary hypertension and cor pulmonale without lung hyperinflation. There is right-axis deviation with a QRS axis of 149° and clockwise rotation of the electrical axis in the precordial leads with RS complex in V_5 and V_6. The dominant R wave in V_1 and V_2 and the P-pulmonale pattern with peaked P waves in leads II, III, and aVF are also consistent with right ventricular hypertrophy.

nuclide imaging, stress testing, or coronary angiography are necessary to determine the presence and clinical significance of CAD.

Tests of Pulmonary Function

Clinical spirometry is widely available, is easy to perform, and provides a means to detect and quantify the severity of mechanical ventilatory and chest wall dysfunction in an objective and reproducible manner. In 1954, Gaensler et al[16] demonstrated a relationship between tests of preoperative pulmonary function and outcome after operation. Although their retrospective study was based on surgery for tuberculosis, the rationale for preoperative pulmonary function testing was demonstrated and prompted the clinical use of pulmonary function testing and additional studies to refine the use of these tests to predict morbidity and mortality after thoracic surgery.

In 1990, a position paper was endorsed by the American College of Physicians that recommended preoperative spirometry for all patients undergoing lung

---

TABLE 22-3
Electrocardiographic Signs of Cor Pulmonale

With COPD
P-wave axis $\geq 90°$ (P-wave amplitude in lead I < P-wave amplitude in lead III)
$S_1S_2S_3$ pattern (deep, wide S waves in leads I, II, and III)
S_1Q_3 (S wave in lead I; Q wave in lead III)
Right bundle-branch block
Right ventricular hypertrophy defined by one of the following patterns:
    Type A: Dominant R wave in V_1-V_2 and rS pattern in V_5-V_6
    Type B: rS pattern in V_1 and R-wave amplitude maintained V_1-V_6

Type C: Small R waves and deep S waves in V_1-V_6
Low-voltage QRS

Without COPD
Right-axis deviation (mean QRS axis $>110°$)
R-wave amplitude > S-wave amplitude in V_1
R-wave amplitude < S-wave amplitude in V_6
Clockwise rotation of the electrical axis in precordial leads (equiphasic QRS, RS complex V_{5-6})
P-pulmonale pattern (peaked P waves in leads II, III, and aVF)

COPD, Chronic obstructive pulmonary disease.

Multifocal Atrial Tachycardia (MAT)

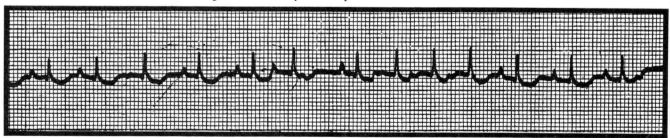

Atrial Fibrillation

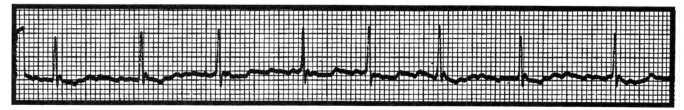

FIG. 22-3 Comparison of multifocal atrial tachycardia (MAT), associated with obstructive airways disease, with atrial fibrillation, which can be associated with either lung disease or primary cardiac disease. In MAT, discrete P waves can be identified preceding each QRS complex.

resection.[17] This recommendation was based on studies that demonstrated that patients undergoing surgery with values for forced expiratory volume in the first second of exhalation (FEV_1) or forced vital capacity (FVC) less than 70% of the predicted value or an FEV_1/FVC ratio of less than 65% were at increased risk of pulmonary complications.[18] However, a review of clinical studies investigating the use of pulmonary function testing for preoperative risk assessment found that the predictive value of the test was highly variable and did not offer an advantage for risk assessment over bedside clinical assessments.[19]

Peters et al[20] performed a retrospective analysis of 49 "sicker" patients undergoing thoracotomy and found no relation between FEV_1, vital capacity (VC), and outcome. In another retrospective study, Keagy et al[21] reviewed the cases of 90 patients who underwent pneumonectomy. They found no correlation between preoperative VC, FEV_1, and FEV_1/VC and postoperative events such as arrhythmia, pneumonia, atelectasis, dyspnea, and 30-day mortality rate. The findings of an early retrospective study that indicated a 50% incidence of pulmonary death in patients with a maximal breathing capacity of less than 50% predicted have not been reproduced.[16] The findings from other early studies such as the prospective demonstration of a relationship between low FEV and pulmonary complications by Miller et al[22] were limited by the small number of subjects and the exclusion of sicker patients. Nevertheless, clinical spirometry continues to be used selectively to assess the severity of pulmonary dysfunction and to predict the expected impact of lung resection on high-risk patients undergoing thoracic procedures.

As with preoperative spirometry, the use of arterial blood gas analysis for predicting operative risk is of limited value. The level of arterial oxygen saturation is not predictive of postoperative outcome.[23] Carbon dioxide retention manifested by increased resting arterial carbon dioxide tension, chronic respiratory acidosis, or increased serum bicarbonate concentration suggests the presence of end-stage lung disease and minimal respiratory reserve. A $Paco_2$ tension greater than 45 mm Hg is considered a major risk factor for postoperative pulmonary complications. Patients with hypercarbia typically exhibit clinical signs and symptoms of respiratory insufficiency and marked airflow restriction with spirometry.[24] In contrast, a recent study by Kearney et al[25] demonstrated that patients with $Paco_2$ above 45 mm Hg tolerated lung resection and that the elevation in $Paco_2$ was not an important risk factor for postoperative complications.

Diffusion capacity of the lung for carbon monoxide (DLco) has also been investigated as a predictor of morbidity and mortality after thoracic surgery. Although no definitive studies exist, one study demonstrated that a predicted postoperative DLco of less than 40% was a marker of increased mortality.[26] Others have shown that

a preoperative DLco of less than 60%, corrected for lung volume and hemoglobin concentration, indicates an increased risk of operative mortality.[27] These authors suggested that the DLco value correlates with the amount of functional pulmonary vasculature and therefore predicts the likelihood of developing pulmonary hypertension or right ventricular failure leading to increased mortality. However, an abnormal DLco is nonspecific and is observed in various pulmonary, vascular, and cardiac disease states.

When interpreting the results of clinical spirometry, it is important to recognize the effect of cardiac diseases on these standard tests of pulmonary function. Pulmonary edema secondary to CHF alters the result of pulmonary function testing. Left ventricular failure typically produces a restrictive ventilatory defect, but a degree of obstruction can also be detected. Congestion and increased pulmonary blood volume decrease pulmonary compliance. VC and other subdivisions of the total lung capacity (TLC) are decreased in the presence of interstitial edema with relative sparing of the residual volume (RV), resulting in an increased RV/TLC ratio. Peribronchiolar cuffing and mucosal edema cause compression of the terminal airways, resulting in a higher closing volume and increased small airway resistance. Hypocarbia and respiratory alkalosis from hyperventilation usually accompany the acute phase of pulmonary edema, and hypercarbia in the chronic phase indicates respiratory fatigue. The diffusing capacity of the lungs is reduced by alveolar or interstitial edema. Successful treatment of decompensated heart failure is demonstrated by a marked improvement in pulmonary function testing. Serial measurements of VC reflect the clinical course and severity of pulmonary edema in patients with heart failure.[25-27]

There have been many studies that use preoperative pulmonary function to stratify the risk of thoracotomy in terms of the overall risk of surgery in patients with pulmonary disease, and of mortality associated with the removal of functional lung tissue. Unfortunately, the role of basic pulmonary function measurements, including VC, FVC, RV, TLC, FEV, FEV_1, maximum breathing capacity, and maximum voluntary ventilation, remains unclear.

Studies of basic spirometry measurements from the late 1970s and early 1980s cast significant doubt on the use of these measurements as primary predictors of morbidity and mortality. The often-quoted number of an FEV_1 greater than 800 ml as providing reasonable respiratory reserve comes from a study by Segall and Butterworth.[28] Their study did not examine surgical patients, but delineated ventilatory failure based on FEV_1 in patients with chronic bronchitis. Furthermore, there was no normalization of FEV_1 to body size. An FEV_1 of 800 ml represents 48% predicted FEV_1 for an elderly woman but only 21% for a young man.[29] Boysen et al[30] used a postoperative predicted FEV_1 of 800 ml as inclusion criteria for pneumonectomy. The 30-day mortality rate of 15% was acceptable to these investigators, who noted that the use of this inclusion criterion allowed them to offer surgery to patients whom they would otherwise have assumed to be too sick. Recently, Markos et al[26] demonstrated that a postoperative predicted FEV_1 of less than 40% was associated with a 50% mortality rate.

Other studies have focused on whether a patient would tolerate the removal of lung tissue for a curative operation. Currently, ventilation and perfusion scanning is the most widely used method for predicting postoperative pulmonary function. When this is performed in conjunction with spirometry, accurate predictions of postoperative spirometric values are obtained.[6] The residual lung function is calculated preoperatively by subtracting the proportion of ventilation provided by the lung to be removed. Because of the close linking of ventilation and perfusion, this calculation is made from either a ventilation scan or a perfusion scan. If the extent of the surgery is unclear preoperatively, residual lung function is calculated by subtracting 4% of lung function for each segment. Unfortunately, no good data exist that determine the exact cutoff of postoperative lung function that provides a good quality of life.

The predictive strength of combining postoperative predicted DL_{CO} and room air alveolar-arterial oxygen gradient into a predictive respiratory quotient (PRQ) was tested by Melindez and Barrera.[31] They used logistic regression to assign the relative contribution of each factor. Ten of 12 patients who had a PRQ of less than 2200 suffered serious pulmonary complications with a relative risk of complications of 54:1. All 49 patients with a PRQ of greater than 2200 did not suffer any pulmonary complications. No prospective evaluation of the PRQ has been published.

Currently, there is no clear practice guideline aiding in pulmonary risk assessment. Virtually every patient coming to the operating room for pulmonary resection has a set of pulmonary function tests. Even in patients with severe pulmonary compromise or those undergoing large resections (bilobectomy or pneumonectomy), V/Q scans or split lung function studies may not add to the assessment of relative risk, because no absolute or relative minimum residual lung function has been established that clearly indicates excessive risk. The often-quoted value of 800 ml FEV_1 residual function has little support in the literature. Until further research produces a better risk assessment tool, the anesthesiologist, surgeon, intensivist, and patient must weigh the benefit of increased survival with the risk of developing pulmonary or cardiac disabilities.

Cardiac Stress Testing

The limited value of clinical predictors of perioperative cardiac risk has led to the development and common

use of specific diagnostic tests of cardiac function and reserve to quantify the severity of CAD and predict the risk of perioperative MI or heart failure. An abnormal test result prompts a reevaluation of the anticipated risks of the operation versus the need for intervention to decrease the risk of cardiovascular complications. Potential preoperative interventions consist of changes in medical therapy, coronary revascularization, or valvuloplasty. The utility of preoperative cardiovascular diagnostic testing aimed specifically at the thoracic surgical patient has not been addressed directly but must be inferred from the information gained from large studies done on patients undergoing vascular and other major operative procedures.

Exercise stress testing is used to assess the risk of perioperative cardiac complications resulting from coronary insufficiency. Several studies demonstrated that ischemic responses to exercise were associated with poor outcome after surgery. Ischemic responses consisted of the onset of angina, at least 1 mm horizontal or down-sloping ST-segment depression or elevation, or a subnormal increase in blood pressure that occurs in the early stages of the exercise regimen. Unfortunately, not all studies are consistent with these findings.[9] A metaanalysis of published reports comparing exercise testing to coronary angiography found exercise testing to have a mean sensitivity of 68% and a mean specificity of 77% for detecting significant disease.[32] Some studies showed that the ability to complete the exercise regimen alone, regardless of ECG changes, was associated with favorable outcomes. Increasing the number of monitoring leads during exercise electrocardiography improves the detection of CAD. Michaelides et al[33] showed that monitoring right precordial ECG leads increased the sensitivity for exercise stress testing for the detection of CAD from 52% to 89%. This level of sensitivity is comparable to thallium-201 scintigraphy. Tests that provide information regarding perfusion of the right ventricle are of particular value for the thoracic surgical patient. Patients with lung disease are predisposed to pulmonary hypertension and right ventricular hypertrophy. Increased pulmonary vascular resistance (PVR) during one-lung ventilation and surgical manipulation increases the afterload stress on the right ventricle and increases the risk of right ventricular ischemia and infarction in patients with CAD. Unfortunately, exercise stress testing is difficult to perform in patients with advanced lung disease because of their inability to exercise within 85% of their predicted maximum heart rate (HR).

Pharmacologic stress imaging is used for patients who cannot exercise to the necessary level or who have a left bundle-branch block, left ventricular hypertrophy, or other electrocardiographic changes that make it difficult to interpret the ECG for ischemia. Pharmacologic stress testing is performed by using dipyridamole, adenosine, or dobutamine (Table 22-4). Radionuclide imag-

TABLE 22-4
Comparison of Thallium Stress Testing with Echocardiography Stress Testing

THALLIUM	ECHO
Determine percentage of myocardium at risk	Determine percentage of myocardium at risk
Determine regions of myocardium at risk	Determine regions of myocardium at risk
Rate-related ischemia found on ECG analysis	Rate-related ischemia found directly
Cardiopulmonary reserve tested when an exercise test is performed	Echo data available: EF, valvular function, pulmonary pressures estimated

ECG, Electrocardiogram; EF, ejection fraction.

ing with pharmacologic stress testing has a reported sensitivity of 80% to 90% in detecting significant CAD and is generally more sensitive than standard 12-lead ECG exercise testing.[34] While pharmacologic stress testing has an excellent record of safety, dipyridamole and adenosine can provoke severe bronchospasm in patients with asthma or COPD. The increase in coronary blood flow by dobutamine is less than that achieved with dipyridamole, but is sufficient for demonstrating heterogeneous perfusion by radionuclide imaging. Dobutamine stress echocardiography alone or in combination with radionuclide imaging is also used to detect significant CAD. Dobutamine increases myocardial contractility and enhances left ventricular wall motion in patients with normal coronary blood flow. Areas of limited coronary perfusion are detected by using echocardiography to locate decreased myocardial wall thickening and excursion in comparison to normal segments. The sensitivity of dobutamine stress echocardiography for detecting coronary artery stenosis is generally considered to be similar to dipyridamole stress imaging, but a satisfactory transthoracic echocardiographic examination is sometimes technically difficult in patients with COPD because of hyperinflated lungs.

Eagle et al[35] suggested that combining information from thallium imaging and clinical information improved the preoperative assessment of cardiac risk in vascular surgery patients. Dipyridamole-thallium stress imaging had a positive predictive value of 17% to 50% and a nearly 100% negative predictive value, making it useful for identifying patients without significant coronary artery stenosis.[35] While not all studies have validated the accuracy of dipyridamole-thallium imaging for predicting the cardiac risk of operation, pharmacologic stress imaging or stress echocardiography is rou-

tinely performed preoperatively in patients considered at risk for CAD.

Hemodynamic Assessment

Determination of right ventricular function, pulmonary artery pressure, and PVR is useful for predicting perioperative outcome after thoracic surgery. Significant right ventricular dysfunction after pulmonary resection was demonstrated by Reed et al[36] and Okada et al,[37] who made serial measurements of right heart performance by using right ventricular ejection fraction (RVEF) pulmonary artery catheters. Okada et al showed a decrease in RVEF from 43% to 37%, an increase in right ventricular end-diastolic volume, and a decrease in stroke volume. Other investigators, however, found that measuring RVEF, PVR, and right ventricular filling pressures in patients scheduled for pneumonectomy was not useful for predicting early postoperative cardiopulmonary morbidity.[38] Dynamic measurements of right ventricular performance before the operation and 3 weeks after surgery reveal that patients with preoperative exercise-induced decreases in RVEF are at significantly greater risk for developing postoperative cardiopulmonary complications than are patients with exercise-induced increases in RVEF. Decreases in RVEF in response to exercise indicate a limited cardiopulmonary reserve. Reduction of the pulmonary vascular bed with pulmonary resection stresses the limited reserve and leads to an increased risk of cardiopulmonary decompensation and complications.[39] A significant decrease in arterial oxygen tension (Pao_2) during exercise also increases the surgical risk.[40] Because of conflicting reports and the risk of invasive monitoring, the role of preoperative right heart catheterization combined with exercise testing for the assessment of surgical risk in thoracic surgical patients is unclear.

Echocardiographic Assessment

Transthoracic echocardiography is a noninvasive tool for evaluating cardiac function and anatomy and is useful for determining whether respiratory symptoms are attributable to cardiac disease. Recent improvements in instrumentation and techniques have improved the accuracy and sensitivity of the echocardiographic examination for detecting cardiac disease. Excessive lung volume from hyperexpansion because of COPD may limit the acoustic windows available for a satisfactory transthoracic echocardiographic examination, but does not effect the transesophageal examination. Left ventricular segmental hypokinesis, akinesis, or dyskinesis suggest the presence of ischemic heart disease.[41] Fixed left ventricular wall-motion abnormalities indicate a previous MI. Reversible left ventricular wall-motion abnormalities with exercise testing indicate myocardial ischemia.

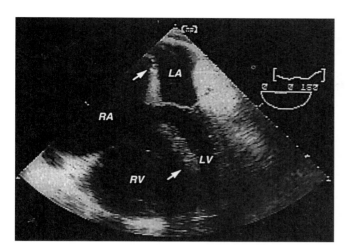

FIG. 22-4 Transesophageal midesophageal four-chamber view in a patient with severe pulmonary hypertension. Marked dilation of the right atrium (*RA*) and right ventricle (*RV*) with leftward deviation of the interatrial septum (*arrow*) and interventricular septum (*arrow*) indicate right ventricular hypertrophy from chronic pressure overload. The small left atrium (*LA*) and left ventricle (*LV*) indicate decreased left ventricular preload from impaired pulmonary blood flow.

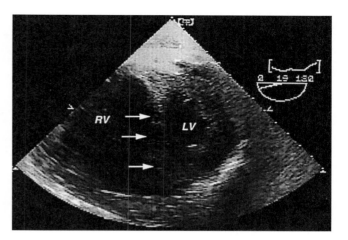

FIG. 22-5 Transesophageal transgastric midventricular short-axis view of the right ventricle (*RV*) and left ventricle (*LV*) in a patient with severe pulmonary hypertension. The normally crescent-shaped right ventricular cavity has become dilated and circular in shape as a consequence of pressure overload. The interventricular septum (*arrow*) that normally bulges toward the right has become flattened because right ventricular systolic pressure is nearly equal to the left ventricular systolic pressure. The left ventricular cavity is small, indicating underfilling from impaired pulmonary blood flow.

Echocardiography provides a reasonably accurate estimation of the left ventricular ejection fraction.[42] Left ventricular dilation or global systolic dysfunction with an ejection fraction less than 35% indicates a limited cardiac reserve, the potential for CHF, and increased risk of cardiovascular mortality independent of surgical risks.[43] Right ventricular hypertrophy and right ventricular chamber enlargement are associated with pulmonary hypertension and cor pulmonale (Fig. 22-4). Flattening or leftward deviation of the interventricular septum, leftward deviation of the interatrial septum, right atrial chamber enlargement, and tricuspid regurgitation are echocardiographic signs of pulmonary hypertension (Fig. 22-5).

Doppler-derived pressure gradients provide a noninvasive estimate pulmonary artery pressure by measuring the velocity of tricuspid or pulmonic regurgitant jets.[44,45] Doppler echocardiographic measurements demonstrate a 20% increase in right ventricular systolic pressure after pneumonectomy, but no significant change after lobectomy.[46] Although postoperative right ventricular enlargement is associated with postoperative respiratory failure, routine preoperative echocardiographic examination is not useful for predicting the risk of postoperative pulmonary complications in patients undergoing lung resection.[46] The presence of cardiac valvular disease such as mitral stenosis, mitral regurgitation, aortic stenosis, or aortic regurgitation is reliably detected and accurately quantified by using two-dimensional imaging and Doppler velocity measurements. Patients with an atrial septal defect or patent foramen ovale may suffer hypoxemia or paradoxical

cerebral embolization from right-to-left intracardiac shunting as a consequence of mechanical ventilation, one-lung anesthesia, or other interventions that increase pulmonary artery and right atrial pressures. Transesophageal echocardiography (TEE) with saline-contrast injection and provocative testing by the release of positive airway pressure is more sensitive than the transthoracic echocardiographic examination for detecting the presence of a patent foramen ovale[47] (Fig. 22-6).

Combined Cardiopulmonary Exercise Testing

Exercise tolerance and maximum oxygen consumption evaluate the performance and endurance of the cardiopulmonary system as a unit. Limitation in the ability to increase cardiac output or increase the capacity for gas exchange in response to increased metabolic demands limit the amount of exercise that can be performed and the rate of oxygen consumption. Though nonspecific, exercise testing provides a measure of cardiopulmonary reserve or endurance to predict the risk of postoperative cardiopulmonary complications. In addition, exercise testing reveals unrecognized cardiac or pulmonary disease in the patient who is asymptomatic at rest. The ability to climb two flights of stairs is a useful means of stratifying patients undergoing pneumonectomy into a high- or low-risk category for postoperative complications.[48] The inability to climb three flights of stairs is predictive for prolonged postoperative mechanical ventilation, longer hospital stay, and a greater frequency of complications, but not mortality.[49] Gerson et al[50] showed that an inability to perform 2 minutes of supine bicycle exercise was the most important predictor of cardiac and pulmonary complications in 277 surgical patients, 29 of whom underwent thoracic operations. In patients undergoing lung resection, inability to perform a symptom-limited bicycle exercise test correlated with an increased risk of perioperative morbidity and mortality.[51]

Changes in arterial oxygen content in response to exercise provide a more specific predictor of pulmonary complications after lung resection.[52] In a retrospective study of 46 patients, Ninan et al[52] found that arterial desaturation of more than 4% below baseline values during exercise predicted serious pulmonary morbidity defined as an ICU stay of 4 or more days, pneumonia, adult respiratory distress syndrome (ARDS), prolonged ventilation, and reintubation. Unfortunately, their study was too small to determine the predictive value of desaturation for short- or long-term morbidity.

Quantification of oxygen uptake ($\dot{V}_{O_2}$), maximum oxygen uptake ($\dot{V}_{O_{2max}}$), minute ventilation ($\dot{V}_E$), HR, and respiratory exchange ratio ($\dot{V}_{CO_2}/\dot{V}_{O_2}$) during exercise provides more precise clinical information on exercise tolerance. Most normal patients can achieve 85% of their predicted $\dot{V}_{O_{2max}}$. The anaerobic threshold is determined by measuring $\dot{V}_{CO_2}/\dot{V}_{O_2}$. $\dot{V}_{CO_2}/\dot{V}_{O_2}$ increases when metabolic demands exceed oxygen delivery and normally occurs at 60% of the $\dot{V}_{O_{2max}}$. In a series of 25 patients undergoing thoracotomy considered to be at increased risk for postoperative complications on the basis of an FEV_1 less than 2 L, a DL_{CO} less than 50%, or a New York Heart Association dyspnea score less than or equal to 2, those with postoperative complications achieved a $\dot{V}_{O_{2max}}$ of less than or equal to 62.8% ± 7.5% of that predicted on preoperative symptom limited-cycle ergometry. In contrast, patients without postoperative complications achieved a $\dot{V}_{O_{2max}}$ equal to or greater than 84.6% ± 19.7% on preoperative ergometric testing. Mortality was associated with an absolute value of $\dot{V}_{O_{2max}}$ of less than 10 ml/kg/min.[53] In a separate study, the ability to achieve a $\dot{V}_{O_{2max}}$ less than or equal to 14.5 ml/kg/min on preoperative exercise testing separated patients undergoing lung resection into high- versus low-risk groups. Based on these findings, a $\dot{V}_{O_{2max}}$ of less than 20 ml/kg/min is a reasonable threshold for discriminating patients who are at high risk for postoperative complications after lung resection.[54]

Occult cardiac disease is also detected with cardiopulmonary exercise testing. The onset of cardiac arrhythmias or electrocardiographic evidence of ischemia indicate the presence of CAD. A disproportionate increase in HR in relation to the increase in oxygen uptake, referred to as the "O_2 pulse" ($\dot{V}_{O_2}/HR$) reflects a limited ability to increase the cardiac stroke volume and is an indication of cardiac dysfunction. An early anaerobic threshold or increase in V_{CO_2} relative to $\dot{V}_{O_2}$ may also indicate a limited ability to increase cardiac output as a result of cardiac disease.

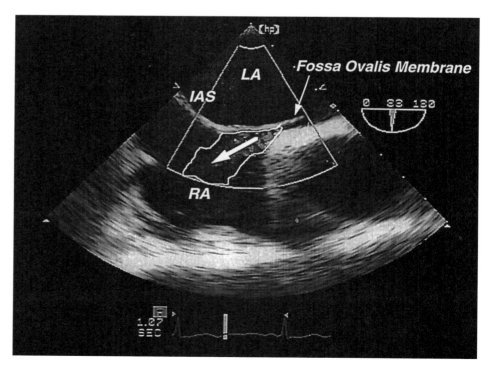

FIG. 22-6   Transesophageal midesophageal right ventricular inflow-outflow view with Doppler flow imaging, showing left-to-right intracardiac shunting (*arrow*) through a patent foramen ovale. If the right atrial pressure exceeds the left atrial pressure, the fossa ovalis membrane can be lifted off the interatrial septum (*IAS*), providing a communication for right-to-left intracardiac shunting and paradoxical embolism. *LA*, Left atrium; *RA*, right atrium.

PREOPERATIVE PREPARATION

Morbidity and mortality from pulmonary complications of surgery often arise from the immediate postoperative reduction in pulmonary function. Functioning lung is removed by the surgical procedure and pulmonary function is impaired by surgical trauma and anesthesia. Thoracotomy in the absence of lung resection causes a decrease in VC and predisposes the patient to hypoventilation, atelectasis, hypoxemia, hypercarbia, and retention of pulmonary secretions. Patients are at risk for wound infections, tracheobronchitis, and pneumonia. These consequences of thoracic surgery may persist for months after the operation. The dynamic perioperative changes in pulmonary function necessitate an aggressive approach to minimize this source of morbidity and mortality. Common steps include ordering incentive spirometry, chest physiotherapy, early mobilization, nutritional support, antibiotic prophylaxis, and continuing treatment of preoperative lung disease throughout the perioperative period (Table 22-5).

Despite lack of evidence that improving pulmonary function and respiratory reserve before surgery decreases the risk of thoracic surgery, the concept of pulmonary rehabilitation remains an integral part of the preoperative preparation. For many patients, preoperative preparation begins with smoking cessation and pulmonary toilet. Cessation of smoking for 24 hours before surgery has the theoretical benefit of increasing oxygen delivery by decreasing carboxyhemoglobin levels. Discontinuing smoking 10 weeks before surgery is required to restore ciliary function and decrease sputum production.[55] Abstinence from cigarette smoking for 4 or more weeks before surgery is associated with a decreased incidence of postoperative respiratory complications in general surgical patients.[56] Weight loss also serves to improve pulmonary reserve despite fixed lung disease. Optimizing bronchodilator therapy to minimize the severity of obstructive airway disease and delaying surgery for treatment of pulmonary infection also increases pulmonary reserve and decreases the risk of postoperative respiratory complications.[57]

Compared with other noncardiac procedures, thoracic and thoracoabdominal operations are associated with greater risk for adverse cardiac events.[1,58,59] There is a paucity of information on strategies that decrease the risk of cardiac complications specifically for thoracic surgical patients. It is likely that preoperative β-blocker therapy, which decreases the risk of perioperative MI and cardiac death in vascular surgical patients, would also benefit thoracic surgical patients at risk for CAD.[60,61] Medical management that optimizes the cardiac function of patients with decompensated cardiac conditions is also recommended. Such medical therapy includes diuretic therapy for the treatment of pulmonary edema or CHF. Angiotensin-converting enzyme inhibitors and β-adrenergic agonists have been shown to extend survival in patients with heart failure.[62] Percutaneous coronary angioplasty with stenting in patients with life-threatening CAD and suitable anatomy,[63] and antiarrhythmic therapy for patients with hemodynamically destabilizing cardiac arrhythmias should also be considered.[63] Medically optimizing the condition of a patient before surgery provides improved pulmonary and cardiovascular reserve to handle the physiologic stresses associated with thoracic surgery (Table 22-6). Preoperative medical preparation of the thoracic surgical patient requires urgent intervention because elective operations for cancer cannot be delayed because of the perceived risk of tumor extension or metastasis.

INTRAOPERATIVE MONITORING

Routine intraoperative monitoring for patients undergoing thoracic surgical procedures under anesthesia includes electrocardiography, blood pressure, pulse oximetry, capnography, and spirometry. Invasive or specialized hemodynamic monitoring is reserved for patients at high risk for cardiopulmonary complications.

TABLE 22-5
Preoperative Checklists

PULMONARY	CARDIAC
Smoking cessation	Smoking cessation
Bronchodilator therapy	β-Blockade/antianginals
Treatment of infection	Weight loss
Physical rehabilitation	Physical rehabilitation
Breathing training	Tests for ischemia
Training in incentive spirometry	Consider revascularization
Pulmonary consult	Cardiology consult

TABLE 22-6
Postoperative Changes in Pulmonary Function

Inhibition of ciliary clearance mechanism
Reduction in FVC by 20% to 35%
Reduction in FEV_1 by 15% to 35%
Inhibition of cough by pain
Blood or retained secretions in bronchial stump

FEV_1, Forced expiratory volume in the first second of exhalation; FVC, forced vital capacity.

Physiologic monitoring allows detection of problems associated with general anesthesia, regional anesthetic techniques, lateral decubitus positioning, one-lung ventilation, and surgical manipulation of the lung and mediastinal structures. The specific monitoring requirements of a specific patient are individualized and based on preexisting cardiac or pulmonary disease, type of anesthetic technique used, and planned operative procedure.

Pulse oximetry and capnography are normally used to assess the adequacy of ventilation and gas exchange during thoracic operations. Measurement of the expired CO_2 concentration and observation of the CO_2 wave form identifies the integrity of the breathing circuit used for ventilation. Normally, the end-tidal CO_2 concentration is 5 to 8 mm Hg less than the $Paco_2$ concentration. It is not uncommon for the discrepancy to be greater during thoracic surgery because of increased dead space ventilation. The end-tidal CO_2 concentration is lower in patients with cardiogenic shock, despite an increased $Paco_2$ concentration, because of reduced pulmonary blood flow. Monitoring the arterial oxygen saturation with pulse oximetry ensures safe levels of arterial oxygenation during one-lung ventilation. Arterial hypoxemia is observed because of transpulmonary shunting through nonventilated lung regions. Intracardiac right-to-left shunting through an atrial septal defect or patent foramen ovale should also be considered in the differential. Primary cardiac dysfunction with pulmonary edema also produces a decrease in arterial oxygen saturation. Cardiac dysfunction with peripheral vasoconstriction impairs the ability to use pulse oximetry because of the decreased amplitude of the plethysmographic pulse. Arterial blood gas analysis is used to distinguish between acidosis caused by respiratory insufficiency and acidosis from hypoperfusion or metabolic disturbances. Placement of an indwelling radial arterial catheter is a low-risk intervention and provides a rapid means to obtain blood samples for arterial blood gas analysis in addition to continuous monitoring of arterial pressure. For this reason, most centers routinely use arterial catheters for patients undergoing thoracotomy.

Auscultation of the chest with a precordial or esophageal stethoscope detects wheezing from bronchospasm, rales from CHF, cardiac murmurs from valvular heart disease, the absence of breath sounds as a consequence of malpositioning of the endotracheal or endobronchial tube, and disconnections in the ventilator circuit. Monitoring the airway pressure, tidal volume, and minute ventilation is used to detect changes in lung or airway compliance. Increased airway pressure or decreased tidal volume during positive-pressure ventilation are associated with bronchospasm, airway obstruction, airway secretions, malpositioning of the endotracheal or endobronchial tube, kinking of the endotracheal tube, or pulmonary edema as a consequence of intravascular fluid overload.

The ECG is used to detect cardiac arrhythmias and myocardial ischemia during surgery. Electrocardiographic monitoring for ischemia is less sensitive than the reported incidence of 50% to 75% achieved during exercise testing under optimal conditions in patients with CAD. There is less sensitivity for detecting myocardial ischemia by using ECG monitoring in the operative setting, particularly in patients undergoing thoracic surgical procedures. Electrocautery interference, the lack of uniform criteria for diagnosing myocardial ischemia, the inconsistent use of automated algorithms for the detection and quantification of ST-segment changes, episodic assessment of the ECG waveform, failure to calibrate the ECG monitor, electronic filtering of the ECG signal, and variable ECG lead placement all add to the difficulties inherent in ECG monitoring for ischemia in the setting of surgery. Lateral decubitus positioning for thoracotomy rotates the heart relative to the chest wall and causes unpredictable changes in the ECG pattern. Thoracotomy and one-lung ventilation further changes the position of the heart relative to the chest wall. In the right lateral decubitus position for left thoracotomy, it is not possible to routinely monitor precordial leads V_2 to V_6 because lead placement is within the surgical field. As a consequence, ECG monitoring for patients undergoing left thoracotomy is limited to the limb leads and the V_1 precordial lead for ischemia monitoring of the anterior-septal wall of the left ventricle.

Body temperature monitoring is important to ensure that normothermia is maintained. Hypothermia during general anesthesia for thoracotomy is common because of prolonged exposure of the lung, heart, great vessels, and other structures. Intraoperative hypothermia increases metabolic requirements and increases the risk of myocardial ischemia in patients with CAD. A randomized trial conducted in 300 patients at risk for CAD undergoing major vascular, abdominal, or thoracic surgical procedures demonstrated that maintenance of normothermia decreases risk of perioperative cardiac morbid events by 55%.[64] Cardiac morbid events were defined as cardiac arrest, MI, or unstable angina. The incidence of postoperative ventricular tachycardia was also less in the normothermic patient group. For these reasons, forced-air warming and other interventions to prevent hypothermia are routinely used for all major thoracic operations to decrease the risks associated with inadvertent hypothermia and reduce the potential for cardiovascular morbidity.

Invasive hemodynamic monitoring with a pulmonary artery thermodilution cardiac output catheter permits measurement of central venous pressure (CVP), pulmonary artery pressure, estimation of the left atrial pressure, cardiac output, and mixed venous oxygen saturation. Although the effectiveness of pulmonary artery

TABLE 22-7
Indications for Pulmonary Artery Catheter Monitoring in Thoracic Surgery

Severe left ventricular dysfunction (LVEF <30%)
History of pulmonary edema, CHF, or right heart failure
Renal insufficiency (creatinine >1.7 mg/dl)
Anticipated major blood loss
Pulmonary hypertension
Severe valvular heart disease
Lung transplantation
Pulmonary thromboarterectomy

CHF, Congestive heart failure; *LVEF,* left ventricular ejection fraction.

catheters for preventing morbidity has been debated because information from clinical outcome studies are limited,[65,66,67] the hemodynamic information provided by the pulmonary artery catheter is more accurate than routine clinical assessment in complicated cases.[68] For this reason, the pulmonary artery catheter is often used for the intraoperative and postoperative management of patients with combined cardiac, pulmonary, or renal disease subjected to operations associated with blood loss or intravascular fluid shifts (Table 22-7). The pulmonary artery catheter is rarely used for the routine care of thoracic surgical patients without heart disease. Measurement of cardiac output, CVP, and pulmonary artery pressure enables precise perioperative fluid and circulatory management of patients with pulmonary hypertension or heart failure. The routine use of perioperative epidural analgesia and anesthesia in combination with general anesthesia further complicates the clinical assessment of hemodynamic status because it is often difficult to distinguish hypotension caused by heart failure from the hypotension caused by sympatholysis without the aid of a pulmonary artery catheter. The cardiovascular condition of patients with pulmonary hypertension or cor pulmonale is very sensitive to changes in PVR, right ventricular contractility, and intravascular fluid status. Hemodynamic data derived from the pulmonary catheter are useful for identifying mechanisms contributing to right ventricular failure or pulmonary hypertension and for directing appropriate management. In addition, the hemodynamic information provided by the pulmonary catheter is useful for assessing the efficacy of therapeutic interventions used to treat hypotension, heart failure, or pulmonary hypertension.

When using information derived from the pulmonary artery catheter in thoracic surgical patients it is important to distinguish the changes in hemodynamic parameters caused by patient positioning in the lateral

decubitus position, one-lung ventilation, and an open thoracic cavity from the final intravascular pressures at the conclusion of the operation. Interpretation is further complicated in patients requiring right lung collapse for pulmonary resection, pneumonectomy, or lung transplantation. Pulmonary artery catheters inserted via the internal jugular veins pass into the right main pulmonary artery 90% of the time. Data derived from a pulmonary artery catheter positioned in a collapsed lung are unreliable. During pneumonectomy, there is a small risk that the catheter is located in the lung to be removed. The tip of the pulmonary artery catheter should be positioned safely within the main pulmonary artery by withdrawing the catheter into the right ventricular outflow tract and then advancing it only a few centimeters past the pulmonic valve. In this position, the pulmonary artery pressure is continuously monitored and cardiac output by thermodilution remains accurate. Alternatively, the pulmonary artery catheter can be positioned by using fluoroscopy or TEE guidance, but maintaining it in a fixed position cannot be guaranteed during the entire course of the operation. The decision to use a pulmonary artery catheter is not without risk. Although reports of serious complications from pulmonary artery catheterization are rare,[69] patients undergoing thoracic operations are at increased risk of pulmonary infarction, pulmonary artery rupture, and misleading hemodynamic information obtained from the catheter.

An oximetric pulmonary artery catheter provides continuous mixed venous oxygen saturation monitoring. In the absence of intracardiac shunting, this provides a constant assessment of global oxygen delivery. This monitoring is useful for surgery requiring extensive dissection near the hilum or manipulation of cardiac structures. Pulmonary artery desaturation is a sign of hemodynamic decompensation and signals a cessation of the maneuver leading to desaturation. In the absence of surgical manipulation, mixed venous desaturation may require fluid, inotropic therapy, or transfusion therapy.

CVP monitoring is useful for assessing intravascular volume status and right ventricular function. Changes in the CVP correlates with changes in pulmonary artery diastolic pressure, pulmonary capillary wedge pressure, and left ventricular cavity size during graded hypovolemia, but is not as sensitive as the other parameters for detecting small decreases in intravascular volume.[70] Acute increases in the CVP or the appearance of central venous v waves suggest right ventricular failure, right ventricular dilation, or tricuspid regurgitation, and these signs are useful for detecting cardiovascular decompensation in patients with pulmonary hypertension or cor pulmonale (Table 22-8, Figs. 22-7 and 22-8). Evaluation of CVP is complicated by the changes in patient position from supine to lateral, which necessitates an adjustment of the "zero" position of the transducer. The

TABLE 22-8
Hemodynamic Differentiation of the Causes of Right Ventricular Failure

CAUSE	BLOOD PRESSURE	CVP	PAP	PCWP	CARDIAC OUTPUT	LV SIZE*
Volume overload	Normal	↑	↑	↑	Normal	↑
LV failure	↓	↑	↑	↑	↓	↑
Mitral regurgitation	↓	↑	↑	↑†	↓	↑
Tricuspid regurgitation	↓ or normal	↑†	↑ or normal	Normal	↓ or normal	↓ or normal
Primary pulmonary HTN	↓	↑	↑	↓	↓	↓
RV ischemia/infarction	↓	↑	↓ or normal	↓	↓	↓
Diastolic dysfunction	↓	↑	↑	↑	↓	↓

↑, Increased; ↓, decreased; *CVP*, central venous pressure; *HTN*, hypertension; *LV*, left ventricular; *PAP*, pulmonary artery pressure; *PCWP*, pulmonary capillary wedge pressure; *RV*, right ventricular.
* Measured by echocardiography.
† V wave from regurgitant flow increases measurement.

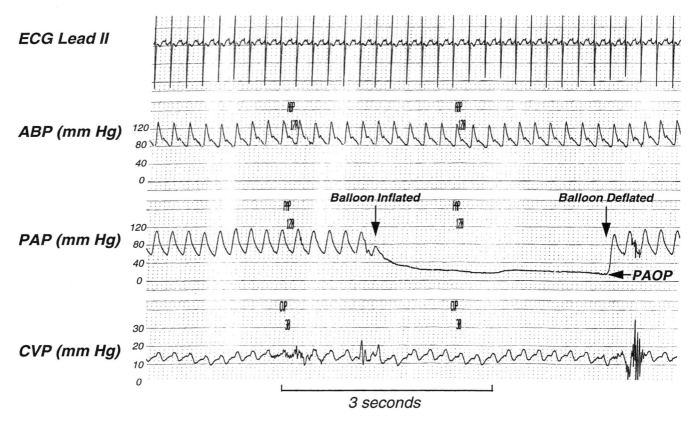

FIG. 22-7 Strip-chart recording showing the electrocardiogram (*ECG*), radial artery pressure (*ABP*), pulmonary artery pressure (*PAP*), and central venous pressure (*CVP*) in a patient with severe primary pulmonary hypertension. The pulmonary artery systolic pressure is nearly equal to the systolic arterial pressure. The central venous pressure is elevated because of right ventricular pressure overload. The pulmonary artery occlusion pressure (*PAOP*) is much less than the pulmonary artery diastolic pressure, indicating high pulmonary vascular resistance in the presence of a relatively low left atrial pressure. The pulmonary artery occlusion pressure would be elevated if left ventricular failure, mitral regurgitation, or mitral stenosis caused pulmonary hypertension.

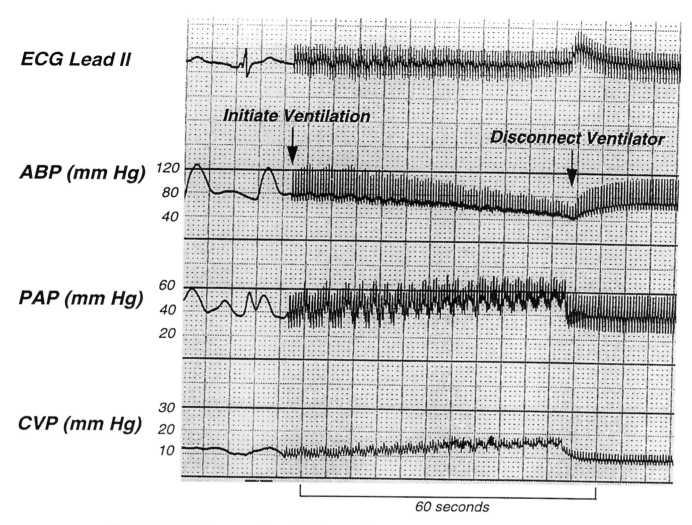

ECG Lead II

ABP (mm Hg)

Initiate Ventilation

Disconnect Ventilator

PAP (mm Hg)

CVP (mm Hg)

60 seconds

FIG. 22-8   Strip-chart recording of the electrocardiogram (*ECG*), radial artery pressure (*ABP*), pulmonary artery pressure (*PAP*), and central venous pressure (*CVP*) in a patient with severe bullous emphysema showing hemodynamic effects of lung hyperinflation or "autopositive end-expiratory pressure (PEEP)." The onset of positive pressure mechanical ventilatory support (*initiate ventilation*) after the induction of general anesthesia caused pulmonary air trapping that progressively increased intrathoracic pressure. The increase in intrathoracic pressure was associated with an increase in CVP, increase in PAP, and decrease in ABP as a consequence of decreased venous return. The condition resolved on discontinuation of positive pressure ventilation (*disconnect ventilator*). Dynamic lung hyperinflation during positive pressure ventilation in patients with severe obstructive airways diseases can be avoided by using lower tidal volumes, avoiding PEEP, and allowing for complete exhalation by increasing the exhalation time.

CVP wave form can also change with the opening of the thorax and a change from two-lung to one-lung ventilation. A central venous catheter also provides reliable vascular access for the administration of vasoactive and inotropic medications.

Intraoperative TEE accurately assesses intravascular volume by determining left ventricular cavity size,[70] assesses myocardial ischemia by determining left ventricular regional wall motion,[71] and detects the presence and severity of valvular heart disease.[72] It is not routinely used during thoracic surgery, even in patients with known cardiac disease, because of equipment expense and the need for constant attention by certified personnel. Clinical evidence suggests that TEE is best reserved for the intraoperative evaluation and diagnosis of life-threatening acute or persistent hemodynamic instability in the setting of thoracic surgery.[73] TEE would be specifically useful for the evaluation of intracardiac shunting through an atrial septal defect or patent foramen ovale, particularly if intraoperative hypoxemia was precipitated by pulmonary hypertension or right ventricular failure (see Fig. 22-6).

TEE is used to estimate pulmonary artery systolic pressure by measuring the velocity of the tricuspid regurgitant jet.[72] TEE data are used to determine the cause of pulmonary hypertension. If pulmonary hypertension is caused by intrinsic lung disease, the left ventricular and left atrial cavities are small. When pulmonary hypertension is caused by left ventricular systolic dysfunction, the left ventricular cavity is dilated and the estimated left ventricular ejection fraction is decreased. When pulmonary hypertension is caused by left ventricular diastolic dysfunction resulting from restrictive cardiomyopathy, the left ventricular size is small, but the left atrium is enlarged. Pulmonary hypertension caused by pulmonary venous congestion from mitral stenosis or mitral regurgitation is also identified by using TEE. Each of these causes of pulmonary hypertension requires different treatments. The effectiveness of the interventions are judged by serial TEE measurements.

In summary, pulmonary artery catheters are rarely used during routine thoracotomy for lung resections. The intraoperative physiologic changes associated with the anesthesia and surgery can usually be anticipated and blood loss is usually minimal. Routine management during thoracic surgery does not necessitate the added hemodynamic information. A pulmonary artery catheter or TEE can be used during acute intraoperative or postoperative hemodynamic decompensation to determine the cause of the problem and monitor the course of treatment.

ANESTHETIC MANAGEMENT

Although limited thoracic procedures have been accomplished using regional anesthesia alone, lung isolation during general anesthesia has permitted more extensive and varied surgery. General anesthesia is often combined with placement of a thoracic epidural. Use of the epidural intraoperatively is controversial. The advantages of using the epidural are to decrease the anesthetic requirement and improve postoperative convalescence by improving postoperative pulmonary function,[74] decreasing major postoperative infections,[75] shortening ICU stay,[76,77] and decreasing hospital cost.[78] The role of epidural anesthesia in preemptive analgesia to improve short-term comfort and long-term outcome is another advantage. The major potential disadvantage to the use of epidural analgesia is the associated decrease in vascular tone necessitating additional fluid administration or use of exogenous catecholamines.

A major consideration in the choice of anesthetic agents is to provide short-term hemodynamic control while minimizing postoperative respiratory depression. This is commonly achieved during induction by the use of short-acting induction agents and carefully titrated doses of narcotics. Lidocaine, esmolol, nitrous oxide, and potent inhalational agents are useful adjuncts during induction of anesthesia. A potent inhalational agent and neuromuscular blocking drugs are used for anesthesia maintenance. Intraoperative analgesia is often achieved by epidural administration of local anesthetics and opiates. Narcotics need to be titrated carefully. These patients do not tolerate respiratory depression superimposed on preexisting pulmonary problems and the postoperative alterations in pulmonary function that are discussed in the following paragraphs.

Potent inhalational agents allow high inspired concentrations of oxygen, blunting of airway irritability, and rapid elimination. However, use of high concentrations of inhaled agents that are sufficient to inhibit hypoxic pulmonary vasoconstriction (HPV)[79-81] potentially decrease Pao_2 by increasing shunt flow to the nondependent, nonventilated lung.

The lateral decubitus position, commonly used during thoracic surgery, is associated with serious hazards. Attention to proper alignment of the cervical spine minimizes stretch of nerve plexuses and vascular compromise. A roll or edge of the soft contour bag ("bean bag") positioned under the chest at the axilla prevents compression of the neurovascular bundle by the humoral head. The nondependent arm is secured and stabilized in a position that elevates the scapula away from the surgical field but does not stretch the brachial plexus. Slight flexion of the dependent hip balances the patient and decreases stretch of the sciatic nerve. A bed strap secures the patient across the hip. All pressure points are checked and well padded, particularly the dependent eye and ear.

The lateral decubitus position affects pulmonary and cardiovascular physiology. The dependent lung has decreased functional residual capacity (FRC), increased atelectasis, and airway closure. The effects of these factors on worsening V/Q mismatch are exacerbated during one-lung mechanical ventilation. These changes are not completely reversed after surgery and may persist postoperatively. The effect of V/Q mismatching is reduced by the homeostatic mechanism of HPV. On initiation of isolated dependent lung ventilation, the nonventilated lung collapses by passive exhalation and absorption atelectasis. Hypoxia in the nonventilated lung activates pulmonary vasoconstriction, decreasing blood flow in this lung from 50% to 20%. The onset of HPV occurs in about 10 to 20 minutes and achieves peak effect over the next hour.

The lateral decubitus position and one-lung ventilation predisposes the patient to hypoxia and hypercapnia. Appropriate management strategies include increasing inspired concentration of oxygen, adjusting the ventilatory parameters, and checking the integrity of the oxygen delivery system. Proper positioning of the double-lumen endotracheal tube and patency of the airway is determined with a pediatric bronchoscope.

Hypoxia is addressed by inspecting equipment and manipulating ventilators in an attempt to improve oxygenation. The inspired concentration of oxygen is increased to 100% and the tidal volume (10 ml/kg) and rate (8-14 breaths/min) are adjusted. The addition of positive-end expiratory pressure (PEEP) to the dependent lung eliminates atelectasis and decreases V/Q mismatch. However, the use of PEEP will raise the peak inspiratory pressure and shift blood flow to the nonventilated lung, worsening V/Q matching. Application of continuous positive airway pressure (CPAP) to the nonventilated lung may increase oxygen saturation. CPAP is increased until adequate oxygenation is achieved, but its use is limited because partial inflation of the lung by CPAP interferes with surgical exposure. If the patient is critically hypoxemic, two-lung ventilation is reestablished. In certain clinical circumstances, the surgeon can clamp the pulmonary artery of the nonventilated lung. Clamping the pulmonary artery eliminates shunt flow through the nonventilated lung.[82] The disadvantage to this maneuver is the potential for increasing pulmonary artery pressure to the point of right ventricular failure.

General anesthesia greatly increases the risk of postoperative hypoxemia. Hypoxemia is caused by an increase in shunting, atelectasis, or worsening of ventilation and perfusion matching. There is conflicting evidence on the mechanism of hypoxemia after general anesthesia. In a study of upper abdominal surgery, patients were noted to be hypoxemic 24 hours after surgery. Their shunt had increased nearly 5%; however, their venous admixture had increased by 17% of total cardiac output, so that the predominant effect was worsening of V/Q matching.[83] A second study conflicted with these findings. On the first, third, and fifth postoperative days, the alveolar-arterial gradient was significantly increased because of shunting and not from V/Q mismatch.[84]

There is no clear mechanism for postoperative changes in oxygenation. There are mechanisms suggested by the changes in lung volumes (Table 22-9). FRC is reduced after general anesthesia for upper abdominal surgery. FRC is reduced by 20% after surgery and slowly recovers to baseline after 12 days.[85] This effect diminishes as the surgical site is located farther from the thorax or upper abdomen.[86] VC is reduced by 50% after upper abdominal surgery; FEV and FEV_1 are also greatly decreased. Tidal volume decreases to 80% of preoperative values. Furthermore, sigh breaths (defined as twice the volume of preoperative tidal volume breaths) do not spontaneously occur after upper abdominal surgery.[87] It has been proposed that the combination of decreased lung volumes, smaller tidal breaths, and elimination of sigh breaths combine to promote atelectasis, leading to hypoxemia and postoperative pneumonia.

TABLE 22-9
Effects of General Anesthesia

ON PULMONARY FUNCTION	ON CARDIAC FUNCTION
Decrease in FVC	Arterial vasodilation decreases myocardial oxygen demand
Decrease in FEV_1	Hypotension $\Rightarrow$ ischemia, especially in hypertrophic myocardium
Inhibition of ciliary transport	Venous vasodilation $\Rightarrow$ $\downarrow$RV filling, $\downarrow$PAP, $\downarrow$PCWP $\Rightarrow$ $\downarrow$CO
Increase in V/Q mismatch	

$\downarrow$, Decrease; $\Rightarrow$, leads to; *CO*, cardiac output; FEV_1, forced expiratory volume in the first second of exhalation; *FVC*, forced vital capacity; *PAP*, pulmonary artery pressure; *PCWP*, pulmonary capillary wedge pressure; *RV*, right ventricular; *V/Q*, ventilation/perfusion.

Regional Anesthetics and Analgesics

Despite controversy over the best location for an epidural catheter (lumbar versus thoracic) for perioperative analgesia for thoracotomy, there is agreement that this method of pain control is superior to any of the other available forms. Epidural infusions of opiates or opiates combined with local anesthetic provide pain relief to the affected dermatomes while minimizing respiratory depression. Pain relief is superior,[88] and pulmonary function is improved.[89]

The authors recommend the preoperative placement of a T5 to T7 epidural. After a test dose is given, an infusion of local anesthetic and opiate are started while the patient is being positioned. The typical combination of drugs is ropivacaine or bupivacaine 2.5 mg/ml to 5 mg/ml with 3 mcg/cc fentanyl. The epidural is bolused with 6 to 8 ml and infused at a rate of 5 to 8 ml/hr. With this regimen, the patient requires minimal amounts of isoflurane (0.3% to 0.6% end-tidal concentration) to remain hemodynamically stable throughout the procedure. There is often mild to moderate hypotension that is treated with fluid administration (limited to 5 ml/kg bolus) and vasopressors.

The specific physiologic effects of high epidural blockade with local anesthetics are myriad for the cardiac and pulmonary systems (Table 22-10). For the cardiovascular system, the initial effect of blockade is usually a decrease in sympathetic nervous system tone. Blockade of the sympathetic chain leads to a decrease in mean arterial pressure, an increase in venous capacitance, a decrease in CVP and pulmonary artery pressures and a fall in cardiac output. The decrease in sympathetic tone to the myocardium does not greatly effect cardiac output. Decreasing inotropy and Starling force stretch that decreases cardiac force generation is balanced by the decreased afterload that increases LVEF.[90,91] Similar effects are observed for right heart function where high local anesthetic blockade decreases both pulmonary artery pressure and right ventricular preload.[92]

It has been postulated that the physiology of high epidural blockade outlined in the previous paragraph could decrease the risk of myocardial ischemia through several mechanisms. Decreasing myocardial work by decreasing afterload, wall stress, and inotropy shifts the balance of myocardial oxygen supply and demand toward a surplus of oxygen supply. Thoracic epidural blockade with local anesthetic in the distribution of T1 through T7 increases coronary blood flow to the endocardium, which is at greatest risk of ischemia. This may be another protective effect of epidural blockade.[93] Finally, epidural blockade restores contractility to stunned myocardium in a canine model.[94] Epidural sympathetic blockade may decrease the risk of myocardial ischemia by decreasing coronary artery vasoconstriction. Blomberg et al[95] demonstrated an increase of the luminal diameter of stenotic coronaries in 64% of patients with CAD. They noted no change in the diameter of nonstenotic vessels.[95] The decrease in platelet aggregation and thrombus formation seen in experimental applications of thoracic epidural blockade may also play a role in decreasing the risk of myocardial ischemia.[96]

The pulmonary effects of thoracic epidural analgesia, like the cardiac effects, are protean. Unlike general anesthesia, arterial oxygenation is not altered by epidural blockade as long as normal hemodynamics are maintained. FRC, VC, airway closure, and intrapulmonary gas distribution are unchanged by local anesthetic blockade.[97] V/Q relationships are maintained during thoracic

epidural blockade.[98] Studies from the late 1960s and early 1970s demonstrated no difference in postoperative hypoxemia when intravenous opiates were compared with thoracic epidural blockade. These studies, however, were flawed, because intravenous opiate analgesia was inadequate and aggressive pulmonary toilet was not promoted in patients with epidural analgesia.

As discussed previously, invasive monitors are used on the basis of the patient's operation and disease. The authors routinely use arterial catheters during open thoracotomies. Continuous arterial pressure monitoring is particularly useful when the surgeon is dissecting near the heart or great vessels. CVP monitoring is occasionally used when the patient is undergoing a decortication or extrapleural pneumonectomy, particularly if the patient previously received external beam radiation therapy. Radiation disrupts tissue plains and leads to greater blood loss. Pulmonary artery catheters are almost never used because of the unpredictable position of the catheter tip and the difficulty of interpreting pressure changes within the context of the dramatic alterations in intrathoracic pressures. The authors prefer to use TEE if there is a question of cardiac performance.

POSTOPERATIVE CARE

Postthoracotomy patients are monitored in an ICU setting, or overnight in the postanesthesia care unit, where nursing-to-patient ratios are 1 to 2. Patients receive aggressive pulmonary toilet including incentive spirometry, breathing coaching, nebulized bronchodilators, and chest percussion. Analgesia is optimized with epidural infusions. The authors use an epidural infusion of bupivacaine 0.5 mg/ml with 5 mcg/ml fentanyl, given via patient-controlled epidural analgesia with a constant infusion of 4 to 6 ml/hr and a patient-controlled demand bolus of 3 ml every 10 minutes. An anesthesiologist is continuously available to titrate the infusions. Patients commonly receive ketorolac 15 to 30 mg every 6 hours for the first 24 hours. Nonsteroidal antiinflammatory drugs (NSAIDs) are very effective in treating the ipsilateral shoulder pain that patients often experience after thoracotomy. While there is no clearly defined etiologic factors for this pain, ketorolac is 80% effective in eliminating or significantly reducing this pain within an hour of its administration. Bolusing the epidural in an attempt to relieve the shoulder pain is minimally effective.

Patients are transferred to a general postsurgical floor, and are mobilized to a chair on the first postoperative day. Pulmonary toilet continues and the patients begin walking on the second postoperative day. Epidural infusions are maintained until the thoracostomy tubes are removed, usually on postoperative day 4 or 5. Patients are then prescribed oral opiates and NSAIDs. No continuous monitoring is used on the general floors. Pa-

TABLE 22-10 Effects of Thoracic Epidural Blockade	
PULMONARY	**CARDIAC**
No change in spirometric values: FVC, FEV$_1$, TLC, FRC	T1-T7 sympathectomy Coronary vasodilation Bradycardia
Sympathectomy causes a minor decrease in DL$_{CO}$	Possible increase in lusitropy
V/Q mismatch may worsen if hypotension develops	Hypotension may cause ischemia

DL$_{CO}$, Diffusing capacity for carbon monoxide; FEV$_1$, forced expiratory volume in the first second of exhalation; FRC, functional residual capacity; FVC, forced vital capacity; TLC, total lung capacity; V/Q, ventilation/perfusion.

tients with a significant cardiac history will go to a telemetry-monitored bed on the first preoperative day, with pulse oximetry checks performed along with vital signs three times a day. Patients are discharged 12 to 24 hours after removal of their thoracostomy tubes if a follow-up chest x-ray film shows no residual pneumothorax.

SPECIFIC ASPECTS OF DRUG THERAPY
Treatment of Perioperative Pulmonary Hypertension and Cor Pulmonale

One of the most challenging medical conditions encountered in thoracic anesthesia and surgery is the management of patients with cor pulmonale or right ventricular failure caused by pulmonary hypertension. Acute or chronic increases in PVR precipitate right ventricular pressure overload and CHF. Tricuspid regurgitation, right atrial pressure increase, hepatic congestion, and impaired venous return are consequences of right ventricular failure. Low cardiac output resulting from the under-filled left ventricle produces hypotension and cardiogenic shock. Intravascular volume expansion in an attempt to treat hypotension and low cardiac output may further increase right ventricular size, worsening tricuspid regurgitation, increasing the CVP, and further compromising splanchnic perfusion. Intracardiac right-to-left shunting through a preexisting patent foramen ovale occurs when the mean right atrial pressure exceeds the mean left atrial pressure, resulting in hypoxemia and further pulmonary vasoconstriction (see Fig. 22-6). Acute perioperative cor pulmonale is caused by a partial loss of the pulmonary vascular bed as a direct consequence of lung resection, right ventricular failure caused by the negative inotropic actions of general anesthetics or myocardial ischemia, or acute increases in PVR

caused by the release of inflammatory mediators, hypoxia, hypercarbia, hypothermia, or metabolic acidosis. Prompt treatment of cor pulmonale is important to prevent rapid decompensation and cardiopulmonary arrest.

Nitric oxide (NO) is one of the most effective treatments for pulmonary hypertension and cor pulmonale (Table 22-11). NO was identified as the endothelium-derived relaxing factor in 1987, and in 1991 Frostell and Zapol[99] reported that inhaled NO selectively caused pulmonary vasodilation and reversed the pulmonary vasoconstriction caused by hypoxia. Subsequent studies of inhaled NO demonstrated increased Pao_2 in patients with lung disease by improving perfusion to ventilation and decreasing PVR in patients with pulmonary hypertension.[100,101] Inhaled NO during thoracic surgery, administered in concentrations ranging from 4 ppm to 40 ppm, almost instantaneously increases Pao_2, decreases pulmonary artery pressure, and consequently decreases right ventricular afterload. Although inhaled NO is effective in acutely improving oxygenation and circulatory function in patients with perioperative cor pulmonale, outcome studies have not demonstrated a long-term benefit of the treatment. Nevertheless, inhaled NO is widely used in the setting of postoperative cor pulmonale or refractory hypoxemia. Side effects are rare, allowing temporary cardiorespiratory support until the underlying problem is corrected. Administration of inhaled NO is not effective or practical for the treatment of hypoxemia during one-lung ventilation[102] (Fig. 22-9).

Milrinone and its predecessor amrinone are selective phosphodiesterase type III inhibitors that have both positive inotropic, positive lusitropic, and vasodilatory properties. These agents increase both right and left ventricular contractility and decrease left ventricular after-

TABLE 22-11
Effects of Common Perioperative Drugs on Right Ventricular Parameters

	RV PRELOAD	DIASTOLIC RELAXATION	PULMONARY VASCULATURE TONE	INOTROPY
Dobutamine	↓ or normal	↑ or normal	↓	↑
Epinephrine	↑ or normal	↓ or normal	↑ or normal	↑
Milrinone	↓	↑	↓	↑
NO	↓ or normal	↑ or normal	↓	No change
Nitroglycerin	↓	No change	↓	No change
Nitroprusside	↓	No change	↓	No change
Prostaglandin	↓	No change	↓	No change
Diltiazem	↓ or normal	↑ or normal	↓ or normal	↓ or normal
β-Blockers	No change	↑ or normal	↑ or normal	↓ or normal

↑, Increased; ↓, decreased; *NO*, nitric oxide; *RV*, right ventribular.

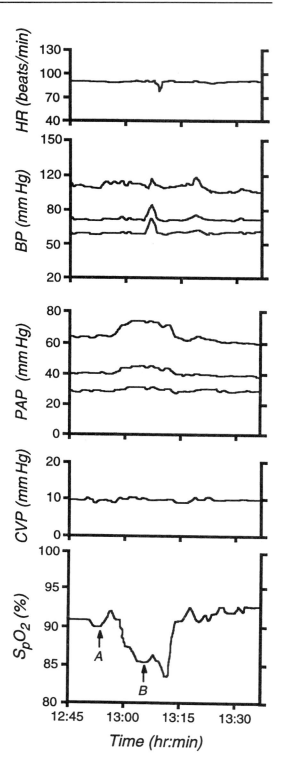

FIG. 22-9 Hemodynamic and arterial oxygen saturation tracings displaying the temporal effects of inhaled nitric oxide (NO) administration in a patient with pulmonary hypertension and respiratory failure after pulmonary thromboembolectomy. Inhaled NO was temporarily discontinued (*A*) and readministered (*B*) at an inhaled concentration of 40 ppm during mechanical ventilation with a percent inspired oxygen (Fio$_2$) of 45%. Discontinuation of inhaled NO was associated with an acute increase in pulmonary artery pressures (*PAP*), a decrease in arterial oxygen saturation measured by pulse oximetry (*Spo$_2$*), and only minor changes in arterial pressures (*BP*), heart rate (*HR*), and central venous pressure (*CVP*). The temporal lag between monitored parameters and the deliberate changes in NO concentration can be explained by the time required for NO to be washed out of and into the lungs and ventilator circuit.

load.[103,104] The direct effects of milrinone and amrinone on PVR are difficult to elucidate. These drugs decrease PVR by nearly 50% in patients with pulmonary hypertension associated with heart failure. These pulmonary vascular actions could be attributed to decreased pulmonary venous pressure as a consequence of increased left ventricular contractility or improved left ventricular diastolic relaxation.[105] Amrinone has only a relatively modest pulmonary vasodilating effect.[106] Both clinical experience and experimental models indicate that milrinone is effective for the treatment of right ventricular dysfunction associated with pulmonary hypertension, promoting increases in cardiac output, decreases in PVR, and decreases in CVP.[107,108] The increase in right ventricular contractility produced by milrinone can increase pulmonary artery pressure if the PVR remains fixed.

Isoproterenol, epinephrine, dobutamine, and dopamine are also used to support the circulation in patients with right ventricular failure in the setting of acute or chronic pulmonary hypertension. The α_1-adrenergic vasopressor action of epinephrine and dopamine is necessary for treatment of systemic hypotension to preserve myocardial and central nervous system perfusion. Patients have severely underfilled left ventricles because of decreased pulmonary blood flow. In the absence of vasopressor support, acute administration of vasodilatory inotropes such as milrinone, dobutamine, or isoproterenol may precipitate life-threatening systemic hypotension (Table 22-11).

Calcium channel antagonists, prostaglandin E_1 (PGE$_1$; Alprostadil), and prostacyclin I_2 (PGI$_2$; Epoprostenol) are also used for the treatment of pulmonary hypertension. The calcium channel antagonists, nifedipine or diltiazem, produce immediate but nonselective pulmonary vasodilation in some patients, decreasing symptoms and improving survival, but may also cause myocardial depression.[109,110] PGE$_1$ is a stable prostaglandin analogue that is a potent vasodilator and undergoes most first-pass elimination in the lung.[111] Intravenous PGE$_1$ is effective for treating pulmonary hypertension associated with ARDS or following mitral valve replacement.[112] At dosages ranging from 20 ng/kg/min to 100 ng/kg/min, PGE$_1$ decreases PVR, systemic vascular resistance, and arterial blood pressure. Despite nonselective vasodilation, PGE$_1$ does not increase intrapulmonary shunt fraction and does not impair oxygenation.[113] Prostacyclin has both vasodilator and antithrombotic actions.[114] PGI$_2$ lowers PVR and increases cardiac output in patients with primary pulmonary hypertension.[115,116] Although short-term actions of prostacycline for the treatment of acute decompensation caused by pulmonary hypertension have not been studied, the routine use of prostacyclin prevents postoperative pulmonary hypertension after pulmonary thromboembolectomy.[117]

Few studies have compared the effects of PGI$_2$ and PGE$_1$. One study noted that PGE$_1$ caused less alteration in blood pressure as a result of faster clearance and a mild vasoconstriction of the veins.[118] Another study of isolated rat lung showed that, while both drugs caused pulmonary vasodilation, PGI$_2$ led to edema formation.[119]

β-Blockers and Obstructive Airways Diseases

Treatment of hypertension, ischemic heart disease, heart failure, and cardiac arrhythmias with β-adrenergic antagonists is becoming more common as clinical studies demonstrate their efficacy and consensus statements endorse their use.[62,120] An increasing number of patients with preexisting heart disease undergoing thoracic operations receive either β-blocker therapy or are candidates for β-blocker therapy. The only absolute contraindications to β-blockade in thoracic surgical patients is asthma or CHF with concurrent verapamil or diltiazem. Although many thoracic surgical patients are labeled with COPD, they tolerate β-blocker therapy if pulmonary function testing does not demonstrate improvement with β-agonists.

Because many thoracic surgery patients are prone to bronchospasm, β-receptor antagonism is not widely used. One rational approach is a perioperative trial by using an esmolol infusion. Esmolol has a very short half-life, and if it is tolerated, patients are converted to a β-blocker with a longer half-life. Atenolol (100 mg/day for 1 week) and celiprolol (200 mg/day for 1 week) have minimal impact on FEV$_1$ in patients with COPD who respond to inhaled β-agonist therapy. Propranolol (80 mg/day for 1 week), however, significantly reduces FEV$_1$ in these patients.[121] Selective β$_1$-adrenergic antagonists such as metoprolol or atenolol can be administered, but bronchoconstriction may occur with higher dosages. It may be necessary to increase the dosage of the bronchodilating β-agonist if a patient develops bronchospasm with β-blocker therapy.[122] Calcium channel blockade does not alter airway reactivity and is an alternative to β-blockade for the treatment of hypertension, angina, or heart failure. Concurrent administration of β-blockade to patients with heart failure who are also receiving calcium channel blockade may exacerbate or precipitate CHF. Calcium channel blockade should be discontinued before instituting β-blockade.

Several studies suggest a possible link between β-blockade and obstructive sleep apnea.[123] One large study of patients with CHF found 29% of patients had evidence of central sleep apnea and 32% of patients had evidence of obstructive sleep apnea.[124] The anesthetic implications of this finding in thoracic surgical patients with heart disease have not been studied, but it is important to consider this as a potential postoperative complication.

Vasodilators, Angiotensin-Converting Enzyme Inhibitors, and Hypoxic Pulmonary Vasoconstriction

HPV is an important physiologic adaptation that reduces hypoxemia during one-lung ventilation. Inhaled anesthetics and vasodilatory drugs such as nitroglycerin and nitroprusside attenuate HPV and potentially increase the risk of hypoxemia during one-lung ventilation.[125] Angiotensin-converting enzyme inhibitors and angiotensin-II receptor antagonists used to treat hypertension and heart failure produce vasodilation and can potentially attenuate HPV. This effect appears to be clinically insignificant.[126-128]

Angiotension-converting enzyme inhibitors are widely used for the treatment of heart failure, hypertension, and diabetic nephropathy.[129] Approximately 10% of patients who receive angiotensin-converting enzyme inhibitors develop cough.[130] The cough mechanism caused by this class of drugs is incompletely understood, but drug-induced increases in bradykinin, increases in substance P, or stimulation of vagal C fibers may play a role. Patients who do experience cough while receiving angiotensin-converting enzyme inhibitors exhibit increased airway reactivity.[131] Angioedema with swelling of the lips, tongue, mouth, throat, and nose is an uncommon but recognized side effect of angiotensin-converting enzyme inhibitors and may occur idiosyncratically even in asymptomatic patients who have been on chronic long-term therapy.[132]

Amiodarone and Pulmonary Toxicity

The use of intravenous amiodarone in patients with heart disease is increasing.[133] Clinical studies demonstrate that intravenous amiodarone is more effective than other antiarrhythmic agents for the acute treatment of patients with hemodynamically destabilizing ventricular tachycardia and ventricular fibrillation.[134,135] Intravenous amiodarone increases early survival when administered during the resuscitation of patients with ventricular tachycardia or fibrillation.[136] Oral and intravenous amiodarone is effective and well tolerated for the treatment of both acute and chronic atrial fibrillation[137] and reduces the incidence of postoperative atrial fibrillation in cardiac surgical patients.[138,139] Amiodarone therapy reduces the incidence of sudden death in high-risk patients with MI or CHF.[140]

Despite widespread use of amiodarone in patients with cardiac disease, the use of amiodarone in patients undergoing thoracic surgery remains controversial. Long-term amiodarone therapy is associated with drug-induced pneumonitis and pulmonary fibrosis in 1% to 17% of patients.[141] Although this condition is sometimes fatal, reversal of the pulmonary symptoms is observed after discontinuation of the drug. A distinct syndrome of acute pulmonary toxicity has been described in patients receiving amiodarone therapy who undergo surgery.[141] In the acute syndrome, ARDS, characterized by diffuse pulmonary infiltrates with a normal pulmonary capillary wedge pressure, occurs between 1 and 5 days after surgery and is associated with a high mortality rate. The risk of amiodarone-induced perioperative lung injury became apparent during a clinical trial that tested the efficacy of intravenous amiodarone for the prevention of postoperative supraventricular tachycardia in patients undergoing pneumonectomy.

The trial was discontinued when 3 of 11 patients receiving amiodarone developed postoperative ARDS.[142] Recent clinical studies in large patient populations have not demonstrated an increased risk of pulmonary complications in patients who received perioperative amiodarone for arrhythmia prophylaxis. This suggests that the pulmonary risks associated with amiodarone in thoracic surgical patients may have been exaggerated.[138,139] Nevertheless, based on the present understanding of the drug and its associated risks, amiodarone should not be used indiscriminately in thoracic surgical patients. It is reserved for the treatment of hemodynamically destabilizing cardiac rhythm disturbances that are refractory to conservative therapy in the perioperative period. Because of the long half-life of amiodarone, discontinuation of the drug before thoracic procedures does not affect the incidence of perioperative pulmonary complications.

The Risk of Bleeding with Aspirin, Antiplatelet Drugs, and Heparin

Aspirin tops the list of recommended pharmacotherapy in a consensus statement by the American Heart Association for treatment of patients with CAD.[143] It is likely that patients with suspected cardiovascular disease undergoing thoracic surgery receive aspirin therapy. The efficacy of aspirin is attributed to its antithrombotic action by inhibiting cycloxygenase and the generation of platelet thromboxane A_2. Aspirin prevents MI and decreases the incidence of adverse cardiovascular events in asymptomatic patients, patients with chronic stable angina, and patients with suspected acute MI.[144] There is no evidence to suggest that preoperative aspirin therapy increases the amount of blood lost during thoracic surgery. The use of preoperative aspirin therapy raises a concern for intraspinal hematoma with placement of a thoracic epidural catheter. Several large clinical series evaluating low-dose aspirin therapy, NSAID therapy, and low-dose heparin therapy did not demonstrate an increased risk of bleeding complications with epidural anesthesia and analgesia, despite clinically significant increased bleeding times.[145-147] Based on the available clinical evidence, and in the absence of additional risk factors for bleeding, aspirin in the dosage range of 60 to 325 mg per day can be continued during the perioperative thoracic surgical period. Aspirin therapy alone does not constitute a contraindication for the use of epidural anesthesia or analgesia.

The risk of spinal hematoma after epidural anesthesia or increased bleeding after thoracotomy with the use of the newer antiplatelet medications such as ticlopidine, clopidogrel, tirofiban, and abciximab has not been established. Limited experience has suggested that these potent antiplatelet drugs are associated with excessive bleeding during cardiac surgery and may have been attributed to the development of a spontaneous hemothorax after trauma.[148,149] Low-molecular-weight heparin use has been associated with an increased risk of spinal hematoma in patients undergoing neuraxial blockade, especially on removal of an indwelling epidural catheter.[150] Neuraxial anesthesia or analgesia in patients receiving low-molecular-weight heparin or potent antiplatelet therapy is not recommended.

Bronchodilator Therapy in Patients with Heart Disease

Bronchodilator therapy is the most important class of medication used for the treatment of dyspnea in patients with asthma or COPD.[151] The sympathomimetic action of bronchodilator therapy may have adverse effects in patients with cardiac arrhythmias or ischemic heart disease. Bronchodilator therapy is associated with cardiac arrhythmias, tachycardia, and sudden cardiac death in patients with heart disease.[152-155] The risk of sudden cardiac death in patients with heart disease taking bronchodilator therapy appears to be dose dependent. The risk is greater with theophylline, oral, or nebulized β_2-agonists as compared with β_2-agonists administered by metered-dose inhalers. Hypoxemia increases the cardiovascular actions of bronchodilator therapy.[156] β_2-Adrenergic stimulation decreases serum potassium concentration, further contributing to the arrhythmic potential in vulnerable patients.[152,157] Recently developed bronchoselective β_2-agonists, such as levabuterol, have improved potency. Cardiovascular side effects are present but with slightly less tachycardia.[158]

Epinephrine and isoproterenol, used as inotropic agents to treat acute heart failure, also cause bronchodilation. Epinephrine is a useful vasopressor agent for patients with reactive airways disease who require perioperative cardiovascular support. Isoproterenol is a potent inotropic agent that produces bronchodilation combined with pulmonary and systemic vasodilation. The small decrease in Pao_2, caused by medically inhibiting HPV, is negligible compared with the cardiovascular and bronchodilatory effects. Isoproterenol is useful for treating isolated right ventricular failure in patients with pulmonary hypertension when tachycardia is not a major concern.

Standard therapy for cardiac disease may not always be compatible with standard therapy for pulmonary disease. This dilemma creates challenges for the perioperative management of patients with heart disease undergoing thoracic surgical procedures. Understanding potential drug interactions and adverse effects is important for improving the margin of safety for treatments used in patients with combined pulmonary and cardiac diseases undergoing general or regional anesthetic procedures.

LONG-TERM CARDIOPULMONARY EFFECTS OF LUNG RESECTION

Recent investigation has focused on the long-term effects of pulmonary resection on cardiac and pulmonary function. Improved survival has increased the likelihood of patients with previous thoracotomy undergoing surgery. The timing and risk of those operations are better understood as the impact of the initial operation becomes further elucidated.

Pelletier et al[159] prospectively studied 56 patients, 24 of whom had previous pneumonectomy and 32 who had lobectomy. Spirometry, exercise tolerance, and minute ventilation were measured during standardized cycle ergometry before and shortly after surgery. The investigators demonstrated a decrease in mean FEV_1 from 79% to 53% after pneumonectomy and from 89% to 74% after lobectomy. Maximum workload decreased from 78% to 58% after pneumonectomy and from 77% to 67% after lobectomy. There was a positive relationship between the intensity of dyspnea and maximal ventilation after pneumonectomy, but not after lobectomy. Leg discomfort occurred sooner during exercise after both pneumonectomy and lobectomy. The investigators concluded that there was a significant decrease in maximal work, but their study could not discriminate between whether the decrease was attributed to cardiac or pulmonary deconditioning.

Additional studies also demonstrated exercise limitation after pulmonary resection.[160] Nishimura et al[161] studied nine patients (five lobectomies and four bilobectomies). The patients underwent pulmonary function tests and pulmonary artery catheterization with supine bicycle ergometry before and 6 months after their operations. All of the pulmonary function data collected showed a significant decrease in pulmonary function. FEV_1 decreased from 2.23 L to 1.72 L. This corresponded to a decrease from 63.3% to 50% of predicted FEV_1. DLco decreased from 87.8% predicted to 77.3% predicted postoperatively. These findings are consistent with previous reports by Berend et al.[162]

The hemodynamic data from Nishimura's study suggest that pulmonary flow limitation plays a role in decreased exercise tolerance. Cardiac index at 50 watts cycling load decreased from 8.96 L/min/m² to 7.74 L/min/m² (p <0.05). Mean pulmonary artery pressure increased from 33.6 mm Hg to 38.9 mm Hg (p <0.5). PVR index increased from 1.92 mm Hg/L/min/m² to 3.30 mm Hg/L/min/m² (p <0.5). Pao_2 and Vo_2 decreased, but did not reach significance. This indicates that the reduction in the pulmonary vascular bed plays a central role in cardiopulmonary changes after lung resection.

Meighem and Demedts performed a similar, but much larger, study of the effects of lobectomy and pneumonectomy on pulmonary and cardiac performance.[163] Patients were studied before and 6 months after their surgery with pulmonary artery catheterization and cycle ergometry. Fourteen patients had lobectomy and 14 had pneumonectomy. FEV_1, VC, and RV decreased significantly after both lobectomy and pneumonectomy. DL_{CO} decreased only after pneumonectomy. In contrast to the findings of Nishimura et al, none of the cardiac, workload, or oxygen delivery indices at maximal workload changed significantly in the lobectomy group. At maximal workload, the pneumonectomy group had a significant reduction in cardiac output (CO), stroke volume (SV), HR, Pao_2, Vo_2, and V_E, and an increase in arterial-venous O_2 difference. At identical workloads, CO fell significantly in both the lobectomy and the pneumonectomy groups. The authors concluded that the loss of recruitable pulmonary vascular bed is the causative factor for postoperative decrease in cardiopulmonary performance at maximal workloads.

The implications of the alterations in pulmonary and cardiac performance measurements during exercise following thoracic surgery has not been fully elucidated. The potential impact on morbidity and mortality in patients with underlying cardiac disease is important. Additional studies are necessary to better address the clinical significance of alterations in exercise capacity after pulmonary resection on meaningful outcome issues such as quality of life, daily activity levels, or survival.

PNEUMONECTOMY

Pneumonectomy was first described in 1933 and, until the introduction of antibiotics and chest tube drainage, had an in-hospital mortality rate of 56.5%.[164] The recent mortality figures for pneumonectomy are less than 3%.[165,166] These improved figures are the result of advances in perioperative management and include patient selection, surgical technique, pain management, ICU use, and preoperative optimization.

The relative proportion of pulmonary resections that are pneumonectomies has decreased. The American Lung Cancer Study Group report in 1983 showed a rate of 25.6%.[167] A study of all thoracic surgeries in Japan reported a pneumonectomy rate of 8.3% in 1998.[165] The decreasing rate could be attributed to improved screening programs that allow lung cancer to be detected earlier, the increased use of sleeve resection to preserve lung tissue, and the absolute increase in the number of thoracic procedures performed.

The risk factors associated with increased mortality vary depending on the study. Patient factors that are consistently associated with increased mortality after pneumonectomy include age greater than 70 years, right-sided pneumonectomy, advanced lung disease, extrapleural pneumonectomy, concomitant CAD, CHF, and hypertension.[168,169] Atrial fibrillation, completion pneumonectomy, and diabetes were inconsistent risk

TABLE 22-12
Risks of Right Pneumonectomy
Increased mortality
3× risk of postoperative pulmonary edema
Increased risk of cardiac herniation
Increased postoperative arrhythmias
Increased risk of empyema
Increased risk of bronchial stump breakdown

factors for mortality after pneumonectomy. Mortality within 30 days of pneumonectomy is predominately pulmonary and cardiac related. Pneumonia or respiratory failure accounts for more than half of the early mortality. Cardiac death (cause undefined) accounts for nearly 20%. Pulmonary embolus and empyema account for fewer than 5% of deaths after pneumonectomy.

Right-sided pneumonectomies carry a greater risk of morbidity and mortality (Table 22-12). The rate of postoperative pulmonary edema after right pneumonectomy is three times higher than after left pneumonectomy and this edema is associated with a greater than 50% mortality rate. Bronchopleural fistulae (BPF) are more common because the right main bronchus stump resides in the pleural space. Empyema is also more common. Right heart strain and pulmonary failure occurs more frequently because the right lung accounts for 55% to 58% of lung mass and right-sided cardiac output. Rare but life-threatening events such as cardiac herniation are more common after right pneumonectomy. Morbidity after pneumonectomy remains very high with reported rates between 40% and 60% in recent series.[24,170] Cardiac arrythmias are more common after pneumonectomy than they are after lobectomy or wedge resection, with reported rates as high as 34%.[171] Atrial fibrillation accounts for nearly two thirds of the arrhythmias, and ventricular arrhythmias account for only 6%. Perioperative arrythmias are associated with a decreased 18-month survival rate.[172] Prophylactic use of digoxin was traditionally advocated in the past in an effort to decrease the incidence of postoperative arrhythmia and to improve myocardial contractility against the increased right heart afterload. Digoxin use may have contributed to arrhythmogenesis. Reassessment of this practice by Ritchie et al[174] brings this routine practice into question. These investigators found that digoxin was not effective in preventing postoperative arrhythmias, and that patients suffered the side effects of digoxin therapy.[173]

A recent study by Amar et al[174] prospectively compared digoxin, diltiazem, and placebo for the prevention of perioperative arrhythmias after pneumonectomy. The incidence of arrhythmia was not different between the digoxin group and the placebo group. Only diltiazem was found to be effective in preventing arrhythmias. A 20-mg load followed by 10 mg intravenously every 4 hours (changed to 180-240 mg PO qd postoperatively) decreased the incidence of atrial fibrillation from 8/21 to 0/21 in the pneumonectomy group. When extrapleural (intrapericardial dissection) pneumonectomies were included, the incidence of atrial fibrillation decreased from 11/35 to 5/35. Unfortunately, none of the findings reached statistical significance.[174]

Verapamil has also been considered as a prophylactic treatment for atrial fibrillation after lung surgery. The treatment regimen used by Van Mieghem et al[175] consisted of a continuous infusion of verapamil, which resulted in a slight decrease in the incidence of atrial fibrillation. The treatment was accompanied by a high incidence of hypotension that often required discontinuation of the verapamil infusion. Consequently, diltiazem has been favored over verapamil for perioperative arrhythmia treatment.[175]

Other researchers have examined the efficacy of β-receptor antagonism for preventing or terminating perioperative arrhythmias. The theoretical basis for the use of β-blockers is that increased plasma catecholamine levels have an important role in provoking the postoperative arrhythmia. Patients given metoprolol, 100 mg PO, have a 6.7% incidence of atrial fibrillation compared with 40% of patients who receive placebo.[176] Patients who receive metoprolol have a slight increase in blood pressure and decrease in cardiac index. Postoperative bronchospasm is not problematic.[176]

The etiology of postoperative atrial arrhythmias after pneumonectomy has not been elucidated. Right atrial stretch or enlargement resulting from increased right ventricular afterload from the reduction in pulmonary vasculature following resection is not consistently observed with transthoracic echocardiography. An increase in tricuspid regurgitant jet velocity, a reliable measure of systolic pulmonary artery pressure does correlate with the incidence of arrhythmia.[177] Existing studies do not show a correlation between postoperative atrial fibrillation and postoperative hypoxia, preoperative pulmonary dysfunction, pericardial disease, electrolyte imbalance, or theophylline use.[171,178]

Postpneumonectomy pulmonary edema (PPE) is a dreaded complication of pneumonectomy. It occurs in approximately 4% of all pneumonectomies, with a fourfold greater incidence after right-sided pneumonectomy. Symptoms of dyspnea with desaturation usually begin 48 to 72 hours after surgery, but radiologic evidence of pulmonary edema may present earlier. Treatment is usually supportive. Diuretic therapy in the absence of intravascular volume overload does not alleviate the condition. The edema fluid is usually exudative with high protein content. Pulmonary artery pressures in PPE do not have a consistent pattern. Pulmonary

capillary wedge pressures are usually normal. Mortality after the onset of symptoms is greater than 50%.[179] Because the outcome is so grave, attention is focused on developing a schema of perioperative care that minimizes the risk of postoperative pulmonary edema. Zeldin et al[180] published a retrospective review of 10 patients that reported three significant risk factors: right-sided pneumonectomy, increased perioperative fluid administration, and increased postoperative urine output. The authors attempted to corroborate these findings in an experimental model where postoperative pulmonary edema was caused by excessive fluid administration, but their results were not conclusive.

The findings of Zeldin et al have been supported and refuted by many reports in the literature. Subsequently, the two largest studies that included 402 lung resections from Leeds, England,[180] and 806 pneumonectomies from the Mayo Clinic[181] showed no association between the volume of perioperative fluid administration and the development of PPE. Both studies supported the increased risk of developing postoperative pulmonary edema after right-sided pneumonectomy.

The data from the Mayo Clinic[181] indicated a possible overlap of ARDS with PPE. Of 21 patients who died from postoperative pulmonary edema, 17 showed pulmonary changes consistent with ARDS. Endothelial damage appears to play a role and could account for the high protein content of the edema fluid despite normal pulmonary artery occlusion pressures. Pulmonary injury from active and passive hyperinflation of the residual lung may play a role, especially because of the increased risk of dynamic hyperinflation resulting from the high incidence of obstructive pulmonary disease in this patient population.[182]

Beyond PPE, there are several short- and long-term risks that are unique to pneumonectomy. Thromboembolism, always a threat after any operation, can originate from the pulmonary artery stump.[183] Cardiac herniation through a defect in the pericardium is rare but often fatal. Most cases occur within the first 24 hours of surgery and patients undergo acute cardiovascular collapse. Cardiac herniation occurs with equal frequency after right-sided or left-sided pneumonectomy.[168] Treatment initially consists of positioning the patient with the operative side into the nondependent position. Emergency cardiopulmonary bypass may be necessary if conservative methods of resuscitation fail. By the third postoperative day adhesions form and the risk of herniation is greatly diminished.

A rare long-term complication of pneumonectomy is the postpneumonectomy syndrome. The syndrome consists of proximal airway obstruction with distal air trapping because of an extreme shift and rotation of the mediastinum. Patients have dyspnea and shortness of breath. It has been reported to occur from 6 months to 9 years after thoracotomy. Treatment requires reoperation to reposition and anchor the mediastinum. Induction of general anesthesia and control of the airway is challenging in patients with this condition because of the angulation of the airway and the limited cardiopulmonary reserve of the patient.[184]

Completion pneumonectomy is more complex than a primary pneumonectomy because of dense adhesions from the prior thoracotomy and tissue injury caused by radiation therapy. The reasons for performing a completion pneumonectomy vary widely from progression or spread of the primary disorder to emergency surgery for bleeding.[185] The number of completion pneumonectomies that are being performed has been increasing. The incidence ranges from 8% to 15% of all pneumonectomies performed, as more centers perform sleeve resections to spare pulmonary tissue. Reported operative mortality rates for completion pneumonectomy range from 0% to 15.2%. Five-year actuarial survival rates range from 18% to 44.5% for patients with lung cancer.[186] The anesthesia for completion pneumonectomy depends on the reason for surgery, but is generally similar to that of a primary pneumonectomy. Increased blood loss from dissection of adhesions should be expected. If the patient had radiation therapy, the likelihood of intrapericardial dissection to gain access to the hilum increases. Intrapericardial dissection creates an increased risk of arrythmia and herniation of the heart.

ANTERIOR MEDIASTINAL MASS

Preoperative workup for a patient with an anterior mediastinal mass includes seeking signs and symptoms suggesting pulmonary, cardiac, and vascular impingement. Severity of the patient's preoperative respiratory and cardiac symptoms does not always predict the degree of compromise or collapse occurring during the induction of general anesthesia. It is often useful to determine if a specific body position improves or worsens cardiopulmonary performance while awake or asleep, because that position may be important for the treatment of cardiopulmonary disturbances under anesthesia, and may be the induction position of choice.

Computed tomography (CT) and magnetic resonance imaging scans are often useful for determining the static anatomy of the mediastinum, airway, and vascular structures. Upright and supine flow-volume loops are sensitive, noninvasive studies that indicate obstruction to major airways. The inspiratory limb provides information about extrathoracic obstruction, and the expiratory limb provides information about intrathoracic obstruction. Similarly, upright and supine echocardiography can detect potential positional cardiac compromise. Awake fiberoptic bronchoscopy is considered if there is evidence suggesting dynamic airway collapse.

Masses adjacent to the carina may cause simultaneous obstruction of the left mainstem bronchus and the right pulmonary artery. This situation results in severe hypoxemia resulting from transpulmonary shunting of blood from the right lung into the poorly ventilated left lung.

A clear plan for emergency airway and hemodynamic management needs to be worked out in advance of the induction of anesthesia. While the use of a rigid bronchoscope or emergent tracheostomy can often be life saving for other causes of airway obstruction, an obstruction below the level of the carina requires cardiopulmonary bypass or extracorporeal membrane oxygenation for effective resuscitation.

LUNG-VOLUME-REDUCTION SURGERY

The surgical resection of emphysematous lung (LVRS) as a treatment for COPD has undergone a renaissance since Cooper et al[187] reported a series of 20 successful operations in 1995. LVRS surgery has become popular again because improvements in care have decreased perioperative morbidity and mortality. The operation offers the potential for improvements in FEV_1 and functional status in patients awaiting lung transplants who have a 30% 1-year mortality rate associated with an FEV_1 of less than 0.75 L.[188]

There is much debate in the literature concerning the effect of LVRS. Cooper et al did not provide any long-term follow-up data. The proliferation of treatment sites caused the Health Care Financing Administration to end reimbursement for LVRS in 1998. The current surgical status of LVRS has been recently reviewed, raising concerns that the benefits attributed to LVRS may be overly optimistic.[189] There is no clear indication of benefit, or lack of benefit, from LVRS. Most studies provide follow-up data for 3 to 6 months. FEV_1 is followed, but functional status or exercise ability is not. The effect of pulmonary rehabilitation is often not considered.

Because of increased patient demand for the procedure and the lack of definitive outcome data, the National Emphysema Treatment Trial (NETT) was begun in 1998. Its screening process requires a history and physical examination that meet established clinical criteria for emphysema. The patient must have abstained from tobacco use for 4 months. Furthermore, the following criteria must be met:

- Postbronchodilator TLC greater than or equal to 100% of predicted
- Postbronchodilator RV greater than or equal to 220% of predicted
- Postbronchodilator FEV_1 equal to or less than 45% and if the patient is older than 70 years, a postbronchodilator FEV_1 greater than or equal to 15% of predicted
- FEV_1 postbronchodilator therapy increase equal to or less than 30% or equal to or less than 300 ml

- DLco equal to or less than 70% of predicted
- High-resolution CT scan of moderate to severe bilateral emphysema
- Approval for surgery by cardiologist if the following criteria are met:
  Ejection fraction less than 45%
  Unstable angina
  Dobutamine stress test reveals CAD or ventricular dysfunction
  Greater than five premature beats/min
  S_3 gallop on examination

The NETT patients are enrolled in rigorous pulmonary rehabilitation for 9 weeks. At the end of that period the patients are randomized to medical therapy (one third) or surgical therapy (two thirds). Of the patients randomized to surgery, 50% undergo LVRS by a video-assisted thoracoscopic procedure and 50% undergo LVRS via a median sternotomy. Follow-up includes pulmonary testing, exercise status, and quality-of-life measurements.

The perioperative management of patients undergoing LVRS is complex and often challenging. There is little standardization of care between different centers for patients not enrolled in the NETT study. Presumably, all patients undergo a rigorous cardiac and pulmonary examination. Preoperative pulmonary function is improved with variable amounts of rehabilitation, bronchodilator therapy, and treatment of infections. Intraoperative management generally includes the placement of a thoracic epidural, the avoidance of long-acting respiratory depressant medications, and close attention to pulmonary mechanics and oxygenation. Intraoperative hypoxemia can be critical for these patients because they have severely limited pulmonary function. Patients are subjected to general anesthesia and a bilateral procedure, which further compromises lung function.

Treatment of intraoperative hypoxemia is challenging. CPAP with 100% oxygen to the nondependent (nonventilated) lung is used with caution and only with direct communication with the surgeons. During the resection, surgeons attempt to remove nonfunctional emphysematous lung. They judge those areas on the basis of ventilation/perfusion scans and appearance on CT scan, and then directly in the surgical field. They remove areas of lung that are bullous and remain inflated in the absence of ventilation. CPAP can make normal lung appear bullous and nondeflated. Consequently, the use of CPAP is very confusing to the surgeon and increases the likelihood that normal lung tissue may be removed.

During median sternotomy, the surgeon can temporarily occlude the ipsilateral pulmonary artery to decrease shunt. While this maneuver will nearly always increase the oxygenation during one-lung ventilation, it is undertaken with the understanding that it may lead to right heart failure in a patient with preexisting right heart compromise. The surgeon does not have access to the pulmonary artery during thoracoscopic volume reduction. Consequently, other measures to improve oxygenation during one-lung ventilation are used if hypoxemia occurs during one-lung ventilation. Adequate oxygenation, saturation of arterial hemoglobin with oxygen (Sao_2) greater than 95%, can usually be achieved during one-lung ventilation, but care must be taken to avoid hyperinflation. While avoiding hyperinflation, minute ventilation may not be adequate, and arterial CO_2 will exceed preoperative values. This permissive hypercapnia usually causes minor changes in arterial pH, and resumption of two-lung ventilation returns the patient to preoperative CO_2 level.

Extubation of patients after LVRS continues to be a challenge. Before surgery most patients have marginal pulmonary function and no pulmonary reserve. All means to improve postoperative pulmonary function are used, and respiratory depressants are avoided. The use of narcotic analgesics to prevent inadequate respiration due to pain is weighed against drug-induced respiratory depression. Bronchodilators are administered before extubation. The endotracheal tube and airway are well suctioned. The lungs are gently reexpanded to eliminate areas of atelectasis but not to the point of disrupting the staple line and developing an air leak. Epidural analgesia is used for optimal pain control and ketorolac is used as an adjunct in all patients without contraindications to NSAIDs. The trachea is extubated and the patient is placed in a sitting position with administration of supplemental oxygen. The patients are transferred when stable to a unit where the nurses are skilled in recovering these patients and providing optimal pulmonary care.

As with all thoracic surgery patients, most morbidity and mortality arises from the cardiac and pulmonary systems. Prolonged air leak and BPF are constant hazards for these patients. Limited cardiopulmonary reserve increases the risk of postoperative respiratory failure, pneumonia, and wound infection.

COMBINED CARDIAC AND PULMONARY OPERATIONS

Because cardiac and pulmonary disease share smoking as a common risk factor, patients are occasionally examined for coronary artery bypass graft (CABG) with subsequent discovery of a lung mass. Alternatively, during workup for a lung mass, they are found to have significant CAD. More recently, patients who are candidates for LVRS often have underlying CAD amenable to CABG. The issue becomes a choice between attempting to decrease perioperative cardiac morbidity by improving coronary vascular perfusion before a definitive lung cancer operation, or remove the lung cancer first to minimize the time for the cancer to metastasize. Similarly, the choice between the timing of LVRS and CABG must be weighed between the risk of MI after LVRS or respiratory failure after CABG. Combining the operations may reduce the morbidity from an additional operation and reduce the time of treatment for CAD or cancer. In centers where combined operations occur, approximately 1% of patients with CABG undergo simultaneous procedures.

Arguments against combining CABG and major thoracic surgery come from technical aspects of median sternotomy and potential immunologic effects of bypass. Median sternotomy, the incision of choice for CABG surgery, provides limited access to the left lower lobe and the posterior mediastinum for lymph node sampling. Furthermore, the risk of pulmonary parenchymal bleeding with anticoagulation is an important source of perioperative mortality.[190] Finally, the immunologic effects of bypass may diminish long-term survival.

Several case series reviews of combined cardiac revascularization and lung resection have been reported in the literature.[191-194] The findings suggest that combined CABG and pulmonary resection can be performed simultaneously. The in-hospital and 30-day mortality figures do not vary from either operation alone. Although surgeons may choose to perform the pulmonary resection before, during, or after bypass, most of the resections are performed before or after bypass to avoid pulmonary resection while the patient is heparinized. In some cases, coronary revascularization can be performed without cardiopulmonary bypass, but full anticoagulation is still required for the procedure.

The most interesting data on concomitant cardiac and pulmonary surgery come from two reviews from the Mayo Clinic. In 1985, Piehler et al[195] reported on 43 combined procedures performed between 1965 and 1983. There were two deaths that occurred within 30 days of the operation. There were six postoperative complications, two of which were attributed to the pulmonary surgery. The authors concluded that the combined procedure was safe and effective. The second review from the Mayo Clinic that was published in 1995, reported cases performed from 1965 to 1992, in which 30 patients with primary lung cancer underwent combined cardiac and pulmonary operations. (Piehler et al included all pulmonary resections, both benign and malignant.) During the same period 15 patients underwent cardiac procedures followed by pulmonary resection. The 5-year survival rate of patients having concomitant CABG and pulmonary resection was 36.5%. The 5-year survival rate of the patient having separate procedures was 53%. The authors concluded that the short-term benefits of a combined operation were clearly outweighed by the increased long-term survival conferred by staging the procedures. The authors did not speculate whether the observed difference in survival rates was due to immunologic factors, technical differences in the quality of the operation, or the increased risk of complications when the procedures were combined.[196]

The 5-year survival advantage conferred by staged cardiac and pulmonary operations for lung cancer was more recently questioned by Rao et al.[196] They reviewed 30 patients who underwent combined cardiac and pulmonary resection between 1982 and 1995 and demonstrated a 5-year survival rate of 64%. The majority of the late deaths were due to cardiac events.[196] The long-term benefits of improved adjuvant therapy for cancer or control of comorbid diseases could explain the more favorable outcome observed in the more recent study by Rao et al. Unfortunately, the overall limited experience with combined pulmonary and cardiac surgery does not favor a general approach to either staging or combining the procedures. The decision to stage or combine the operations must be made on an individual basis.

KEY POINTS

1. Patients undergoing thoracic surgical procedures often have concomitant heart and lung disease. One goal of preoperative preparation is to identify the extent of cardiac and pulmonary disease, improve the patient's status with medication and rehabilitation, and reduce the risk of surgery.

2. Thoracic surgery is performed on patients with more severe pulmonary disease than in previous years. Previous exclusion criteria are no longer applicable. Combinations of pulmonary, cardiac, and exercise testing are used to determine and reduce perioperative risk.

3. There is no universally accepted system to predict perioperative morbidity and mortality. The risks and benefits of thoracic surgery are individualized to each patient by the surgeon, anesthesiologist, and internist.

4. Altered right ventricular performance is an important risk factor for perioperative morbidity and mortality. Many of the common maneuvers and therapies used during thoracic surgery profoundly impact right ventricular function.

5. Newer therapies such as NO, prostaglandins, and milrinone are beneficial in supporting failing contractility and reversing pulmonary hypertension.

6. HPV is a homeostatic mechanism that limits perfusion to nonoxygenated alveolae. Many anes-

thetics and common perioperative medications inhibit HPV.

7. More complex thoracic surgeries such as sleeve resections and lung volume reduction surgeries require specialized care. CPAP and hyperinflation can interfere with the surgery and compromise the patient's cardiopulmonary status.

8. Thoracic epidural analgesia has a significantly positive impact on the balance of myocardial oxygen delivery and demand.

KEY REFERENCES

Chen EP, Craig DM, Bittner HP et al: Pharmacologic strategies for improving diastolic dysfunction in the setting of chronic pulmonary hypertension, *Circulation* 97:1606-1612, 1998.

Eagle KA, Brundage BH, Chaitman BR et al: ACC/AHA Guidelines for perioperative cardiovascular evaluation for noncardiac surgery, *Circulation* 93:1280-1317, 1996.

Mangano DT: Perioperative cardiac morbidity, *Anesthesiology* 72:153-184, 1990.

Mangano DT, Layug EL, Wallace A et al: Effect of atenolol on mortality and cardiovascular morbidity after noncardiac surgery. Multicenter Study of Perioperative Ischemia Research Group, *N Engl J Med* 335:1713-1720, 1996.

Nezu K, Kushibe K, Tojo T et al: Recovery and limitation of exercise capacity after lung resection for lung cancer, *Chest* 113:1511-1516, 1998.

Rao V, Todd TRJ, Weisel RD et al: Results of combined pulmonary resection and cardiac operation, *Ann Thorac Surg* 62:324-327, 1996.

Ribas J, Diaz O, Barbera JA et al: Invasive exercise testing in the evaluation of patients at high risk for lung resection, *Eur Respir J* 12:1429-1435,1998.

Slinger PD: Perioperative fluid management for thoracic surgery: the puzzle of postpneumonectomy pulmonary edema, *J Cardiothorac Vasc Anesth* 9:442-451, 1995.

Smetana GW: Preoperative pulmonary evaluation, *N Engl J Med* 340:937-944, 1999.

Utz JP, Hubmayr RD, Deschamps C: Lung volume reduction surgery for emphysema: out on a limb without a NETT, *Mayo Clin Proc* 73:552-566, 1998.

References

1. Goldman L, Caldera DL, Nussbaum SR et al: Multifactorial index of cardiac risk in noncardiac surgical procedures, *N Engl J Med* 297:845-850, 1977.

2. Eagle KA, Brundage BH, Chaitman BR et al: ACC/AHA Guidelines for perioperative cardiovascular evaluation for noncardiac surgery, *Circulation*93:1280-1317, 1996.

3. Deslauriers J, Ginsberg RJ, Dubois P: Current operative morbidity associated with elective surgical resection for lung cancer, *Can J Surg* 32:335-339, 1989.

4. Ishida T, Yokoyama H, Kaneko S: Long-term results of operation for non-small cell lung cancer in the elderly, *Ann Thorac Surg* 50:919-922, 1990.

5. Weiss W: Operative mortality and five-year survival rates in men with bronchogenic carcinoma, *Chest* 66:483-487, 1974.

6. Cottrell JJ, Ferson, PF: Preoperative assessment of the thoracic surgical patient, *Clin Chest Med* 13:47-53, 1992.

7. Read RC, Yoder G, Schaeffer RC: Survival after conservative resection for t1 n0 m0 non-small cell lung cancer, *Ann Thorac Surg* 49:391-400,1990.

8. Putnam JB, Lammermeier DE, Colon R et al: Predicted pulmonary function and survival after peumonectomy for primary lung carcinoma, *Ann Thorac Surg* 49:909-915, 1990.

9. Mangano DT: Perioperative cardiac morbidity, *Anesthesiology* 72: 153-184, 1990.

10. Foster ED, Davis KB, Carpenter JA et al: Risk of noncardiac operation in patients with defined coronary disease: The Coronary Artery Surgery Study (CASS) Registry experience, *Ann Thorac Surg* 41:42-50, 1986.

11. Nicod P, Rher R, Winniford MD et al: Acute systemic and coronary hemodynamic and serologic responses to cigarette smoking in long-term smokers with atherosclerotic coronary artery disease, *J Am Coll Cardiol* 4:964-971,1984.

12. Detsky AS, Abrams HB, McLaughlin JR et al: Predicting cardiac complications in patients undergoing non-cardiac surgery, *J Gen Intern Med* 1:211-219, 1986.

13. Zeldin RA, Math B: Assessing cardiac risk in patients who undergo non-cardiac surgical proceedures, *Can J Surg* 27:402-404, 1984.

14. Prause G, Offner A, Ratzenhofer-Komenda B et al: Comparison of two preoperative indices to predict preioperative mortality in non-cardiac thoracic surgery, *Eur J Cardiothorac Surg* 11: 670-675, 1997.

15. Melendez JA, Carlon VA: Cardiopulmonary risk index does not predict complications after thoracic surgery, *Chest* 144:69-75, 1998.

16. Gaensler EA, Cugell DW, Lindgern I et al: The role of pulmonary insufficiency in mortality and invalidism following surgery for pulmonary tuberculosis, *J Thoracic Surg* 24:163, 1954.

17. Anonymous: Preoperative pulmonary function testing. American College of Physicians, *Ann Intern Med* 112:793-794, 1990.

18. Gass GD, Olsen GN: Preoperative pulmonary function testing to predict postoperative morbidity and mortality, *Chest* 89: 127-135, 1986.

19. Smetana GW: Preoperative pulmonary evaluation, *N Engl J Med* 340:937-944, 1999.

20. Peters RM, Clausen JL, Tisis GM: Extending resectability of the lung in patients with impaired pulmonary function, *Ann Thorac Surg* 26:250-259, 1978.

21. Keagy BA, Schorlemmer GR, Murray GF et al: Correlation of preoperative pulmonary function testing with clinical course in patients after pneumonectomy, *Ann Thorac Surg* 36:253-257, 1983.

22. Miller WF, Wu N, Johnson RL: Convenient method of evaluating pulmonary function with a single breath test, *Anesthesiology* 17:480-493, 1956.

23. Melendez JA, Fischer ME: Preoperative pulmonary evaluation of the thoracic surgical patient, *Chest Surg Clin N Am* 7:641-654, 1997.

24. Stein M, Koota GM, Simon M et al: Pulmonary evaluation of surgical patients, *JAMA* 181:765-770, 1962.

25. Kearney DJ, Lee TH, Reilly JL et al: Assessment of operative risk in patients undergoing lung resection: importance of predicted pulmonary function, *Chest* 105:753-759, 1994.

26. Markos J, Mullan BP, Hillman CR: Preoperative assessment as a predictor of mortality and morbidity after lung resection, *Am Rev Respir Dis* 139:902-910, 1989.

27. Ferguson MK, Little L, Rizzo L et al: Diffusing capacity predicts morbidity and mortality after pulmonary resection, *J Thorac Cardiovasc Surg* 96:894-900, 1988.

28. Segall JJ, Butterworth BA: Ventilatory capacity in chronic bronchitis in relation to carbon dioxide retention, *Scand J Resp Dis* 47:215-219, 1966.

29. Gass GD, Olsen GN: Preoperative pulmonary function testing to predict postoperative morbidity and mortality, *Chest* 89: 127-135, 1986.

30. Boysen PG, Block J, Olsen GN et al: Prospective evaluation for pneumonectomy using ^{99m}technecium quantitative perfusion lung scan, *Chest* 72:422-425, 1977.

31. Melindez J, Barrera R: Predictive respiratory complication quotient (PRQ) predicts pulmonary complications in thoracic surgical patients, *Ann Thorac Surg* 66:220-224, 1998.

32. Gibbons et al: ACC/AHA Guidelines for exercise testing, *Circulation* 96:345-354, 1997.

33. Michaelides AP, Psomadaki ZD, Dilaveris PE et al: Improved detection of coronary artery disease by exercise electrocardiography with the use of right precordial leads, *N Engl J Med* 340: 340-345, 1999.

34. Cahalan MK, Litt L, Botvinick EH et al: Advances in noninvasive cardiovascular imaging: implications for the anesthesiologist, *Anesthesiology* 66:356-372, 1987.

35. Eagle KA, Coley CM, Newell JB et al: Combining clinical and thallium data optimizes preoperative assessment of cardiac risk before major vascular surgery, *Ann Intern Med* 110:859-866, 1989.

36. Reed CE, Spinale FG, Crawford FA: Effect of pulmonary resection on right ventricular function, *Ann Thorac Surg* 53:578-582, 1992.

37. Okada M, Ota T, Okada M et al: Right ventricular dysfunction after major pulmonary resection, *J Thorac Cardiovasc Surg* 108: 503-511, 1994.

38. Lewis, Jr, JW, Bastanfar M, Gabriel F et al: Right heart function and prediction of respiratory morbidity in patients undergoing pneumonectomy with moderately severe cardiopulmonary dysfunction, *J Thorac Cardiovasc Surg* 108:169-175, 1994.

39. Okada M, Okada M, Ishii N et al: Right ventricular ejection fraction in the preoperative risk evaluation of candidates for pulmonary resection, *J Thorac Cardiovasc Surg* 112:364-370, 1996.

40. Ribas J, Diaz O, Barbera JA et al: Invasive exercise testing in the evaluation of patients at high risk for lung resection, *Euro Respir J* 12:1429-1435, 1998.

41. Schiller NB, Shah PM, Crawford M et al: Recommendations for quantitation of the left ventricle by two-dimensional echocardiography. American Society of Echocardiography Committee on Standards, Subcommittee on Quantitation of Two-Dimensional Echocardiograms, *J Am Soc Echocardiogr* 2:358-367, 1989.

42. Niebauer J, Clark AL, Anker SD et al: Three year mortality in heart failure patients with very low left ventricular ejection, *Int J Cardiol* 70:245-247, 1999.

43. CIBIS-II Investigators and Committees: The cardiac insufficiency bisoprolol study II (CIBIS-II): a randomized trial, *Lancet* 353:9-13, 1999.

44. Tramarin R, Torbicki A, Marchandise B et al: Doppler echocardiographic evaluation of pulmonary artery pressure in chronic obstructive pulmonary disease. A European muticentre study. *Eur Heart J* 12:103, 1991.

45. Berger M, Haimowitz A, VanTosh A et al: Quantitative assessment of pulmonary hypertension in patients with tricuspid regurgitation using continuous wave Doppler ultrasound, *J Am Coll Cardiol* 6:359, 1985.

46. Amar D, Burt ME, Roistacher N et al: Value of perioperative Doppler echocardiography in patients undergoing major lung resection, *Ann Thorac Surg* 61:516-520, 1996.

47. Rafferty TD: Intraoperative transesophageal saline-contrast imaging of flow-patent foramen ovale, *Anesth Analg* 75:475-480, 1992.

48. Van Nostrand D, Kyelsberg MO, Humphrey EW: Preresectional evaluation of risk from pneumonectomy, *Surg Gynecol Obstet* 127:306-312, 1968.

49. Olsen GN, Bolton JW, Weiman DS et al: Stair climbing as an exercise test to predict the postoperative complications of lung resection. Two years' experience, *Chest* 99:587-590, 1991.

50. Gerson MC, Hurst JM, Hertzberg VS et al: Prediction of cardiac and pulmonary complications related to elective abdominal and noncardiac thoracic surgery in geriatric patients, *Am J Med* 88:101-107, 1990.

51. Epstein SK, Faling J, Daly BDT et al: Inability to perform bicycle ergometry predicts increased morbidity and mortality after lung resection, *Chest* 107:311-316, 1995.

52. Ninan M, Sommers E, Landreneau RJ et al: Standardized exercise oximetry predicts postneumonectomy outcome, *Ann Thorac Surg* 64:328-333, 1997.

53. Bollinger C, Wyser C, Roser H et al: Lung scanning and exercise testing for the prediction of postoperative performance in lung resection candidates at increased risk for complications, *Chest* 108:341-348, 1995.

54. Torchio R, Gulotta C, Parvis M et al: Gas exchange threshold as a predictor of severe postoperative complications after lung resection in mild-to-moderate obstructive pulmonary disease, *Monaldi Arch Chest Dis* 53:127-133, 1998.

55. Warner MA, Offord KP, Lennon RL et al: Role of preoperative cessation of smoking and other factors in postoperative pulmonary complications: blind prospective study of coronary artery bypass patients, *Mayo Clin Proc* 64:609-616, 1989.

56. Pearce AC, Jones RM: Smoking and anesthesia: preoperative abstinence and perioperative morbidity, *Anesthesiology* 61:576, 1984.

57. Stein M, Cassara EL: Preoperative pulmonary evaluation and therapy for surgical patients, *JAMA* 211:787-790, 1970.

58. Tiret L, Hatton F, Desmonts JM et al: Prediction of outcome of anaesthesia in patients over 40 years: a multifactorial risk index, *Stat Med* 7:947-954, 1988.

59. Cohen MM, Ducan PG, Tate RB: Does anesthesia contribute to operative mortality? *JAMA* 260:2859-2863, 1988.

60. Poldermans D, Boerma E, Bax JJ et al: The effect of bisoprolol on perioperative mortality and myocardial infarction in high risk patients undergoing vascular surgery. Dutch echocardiographic cardiac risk evaluation applying stress echocardiography study group, *N Engl J Med* 341:1789-1794, 1999.

61. Mangano DT, Layug EL, Wallace A et al: Effect of atenolol on mortality and cardiovascular morbidity after noncardiac surgery. Multicenter Study of Perioperative Ischemia Research Group. *N Engl J Med* 335:1713-1720, 1996.

62. Williams JF, Bristow MR, Fowler MB et al: Guidelines for the evaluation and management of heart failure. Report of the American College of Cardiology/American Heart Association Task Force on Practice Guidelines (Committee on Evaluation and Management of Heart Failure), *Circulation* 92:2764-2784, 1995.

63. Scanlon PJ, Faxon DP, Audet AM et al: ACC/AHA guidelines for coronary angiography. A report of the American College of Cardiology/American Heart Association Task Force on Practice Guidelines (Committee on Coronary Angiography), *Circulation* 99:2345-2357, 1999.

64. Frank SM, Fleisher LA, Breslow MS et al: Perioperative maintenance of normothermia reduces the incidence of morbid cardiac events: a randomized clinical trial, *JAMA* 277:1127-1134, 1997.

65. Practice guidelines for pulmonary artery catheterization. A report by the American Society of Anesthesiologists Task Force on Pulmonary Artery Catheterization, *Anesthesiology* 78:380-394, 1993.

66. Dalen JE, Bone RC: Is it time to pull the pulmonary artery catheter? *JAMA* 276:916-918, 1996.

67. Connors AF, Speroff T, Dawson NV et al: The effectiveness of right heart catheterization in the initial care of critically ill patients, *JAMA* 276:889-897, 1996.

68. Eisenberg PR, Jaffe AS, Schuster DP: Clinical evaluation compared to pulmonary artery catheterization in the hemodynamic assessment of critically ill patients, *Crit Care Med* 12:549-553, 1984.

69. Shah KB, Rao TLK, Laughlin S et al: A review of pulmonary artery catheterization in 6,245 patients, *Anesthesiology* 61:271-275, 1984.

70. Cheung AT, Savino JS, Weiss SJ et al: Echocardiographic and hemodynamic indexes of left ventricular preload in patients with normal and abnormal ventricular function, *Anesthesiology* 81:376-387, 1984.

71. Smith JS, Cahalan MK, Benefiel DJ et al: Intraoperative detection of myocardial ischemia in high risk patients: electrocardiography versus two-dimensional transesophageal echocardiography, *Circulation* 72:1015-1021, 1985.

72. Lee RT, Satinder JS, St John Sutton MG: Assessment of valvular heart disease with doppler echocardiography, *JAMA* 262:2131-2135, 1989.

73. Practice guidelines for perioperative transesophageal echocardiography. A report by the American Society of Anesthesiologists and the Society of Cardiovascular Anesthesiologists Task Force on Transesophageal Echocardiography, *Anesthesiology* 84:986-1006, 1996.

74. Bromage PR: Spirometry in assessment of analgesia after abdominal surgery, *BMJ* 2:589, 1955.

75. Sackner MA, Hirsch J, and Epstein S: Effect of cuffed endotracheal tubes on tracheal mucous velocity, *Chest* 68:774, 1975.

76. Applefeld JJ, Caruthers TE, Reno DJ et al: Assessment of the sterility of long-term cardiac catheterization using a thermodilution Swan-Ganz catheter, *Chest* 74:337, 1978.

77. Neustein SM, Eisenkraft JB: Anesthetic considerations during thoracic procedures using the laser. In *Cardiothoracic and vascular anesthesia update*, vol 1, Philadelphia, 1990, WB Saunders.

78. Yeager MP, Glass DD, Neff RK et al: Epidural anesthesia and analgesia in high-risk surgical patients, *Anesthesiology* 66:729, 1987.

79. Benumof JL, Augustine SD, and Gibbons JA: Halothane and isoflurane only slightly impair arterial oxygenation during one-lung ventilation in patients undergoing thoracotomy, *Anesthesiology* 67:910, 1987.

80. Bjertnaes LJ: Hypoxia-induced vasoconstriction in isolated perfused lungs exposed to injectable or inhalation anesthetics, *Acta Anaesthesiol Scand* 21:133, 1977.

81. Rees DI, Gaines GY: One-lung anesthesia—a comparison of pulmonary gas exchange during anesthesia with ketamine or enflurane, *Anesth Analg* 63:521, 1984.

82. Anderson HW, Benumof JL: Intrapulmonary shunting during one-lung ventilation and surgical manipulation, *Anesthesiology* 55:A377, 1981.

83. Georg J, Hornum I, Mellemgaard K: The mechanism of hypoxemia after laparotomy *Thorax* 22:382, 1967.

84. Siler JN, Rosenberg H, Mull TD et al: Hypoxemia after upper abdominal surgery: comparisons of venous admixture and ventilation/perfusion inequality components, using a digital computer, *Ann Surg* 179:149, 1974.

85. Beecher HK: The effect of laparotomy on lung volume. Demonstration of a new type of pulmonary collapse, *J Clin Invest* 12:651, 1933.

86. Alexander JI, Spence AA, Parikh RK et al: The role of airway closure in postoperative hypoxeamia, *Br J Anaesth* 35:34, 1973.

87. Zikria BA, Spencer JL, Kinney JM et al: Alterations in ventilatory function and breathing pattern following surgical trauma, *Ann Surg* 179:1, 1974.

88. Cousins JM, Mather LE: Intrathecal and epidural administration of opiods, *Anesthesiology* 61:276-310, 1984.

89. Rawal N, Sjostrand U, Christoffersson E et al: Comparison of intramuscular and epidural morphine for postoperative analgesia in the grossly obese: influence on postoperative ambulation and pulmonary function, *Anesth Analg* 63:583-592, 1984.

90. Ottesen S, Renck H, Jynge P: Thoracic epidural analgesia, *Acta Anaesthesiol Scand Suppl* 69:1-16, 1978.

91. Kock M, Blomberg S, Emanuelsson H et al: Thoracic epidural anesthesia improves global and regional left ventricular function during stress-induced myocardial ischemia in patients with coronary artery disease, *Anesth Analg* 71:625-630, 1990.

92. Lynn RB, Sancetta SM, Simone FA, Scott RW: Observation on the circulation in high spinal anesthesia, *Surgery* 32:195-199, 1952.

93. Klassen GA, Bramwell RS, Bromage PR et al: Effect of acute sympathectomy by epidural anesthesia on canine coronary circulation, *Anesthesiology* 52:8-15, 1980.

94. Rolf N, Van de Velde M, Wouters PF et al: Thoracic epidural anesthesia improves functional recovery from myocardial stunning in dogs, *Anesth Analg* 83:935-940, 1996.

95. Blomberg S, Emanuelsson H, Kvist H et al: Effects of thoracic epidural anesthesia on coronary arteries and arterioles in patient with coronary artery disease, *Anesthesiology* 73:840-847, 1990.

96. Rosenfeld BA, Beattie C, Christopherson R et al: The effects of different anesthetic regimens on fibrinolysis and the development of postoperative arterial thrombosis. Perioperative Ischemia Randomized Anesthesia Trial Group, *Anesthesiology* 79:435-443, 1993.

97. Mc Carthy GS: The effect of thoracic extradural analgesia on pulmonary gas distribution, functional residual capacity and airway closure, *Br J Anaesth* 48:243-248, 1976.

98. Lundh R, Hedenstierna G, Johansson H: Ventilation-perfusion relationships during epidural analgesia, *Acta Anaesthesiol Scand* 27:410-416, 1983.

99. Frostell C, Fratacci MD, Wain JC et al: Inhaled nitric oxide: a selective pulmonary vasodilator reversing hypoxic pulmonary vasoconstriction, *Circulation* 83:2038-2047, 1991.

100. Rossaint R, Falke KJ, Lopez F et al: Inhaled nitric oxide for the adult respiratory distress syndrome, *N Engl J Med* 328:399-405, 1993.

101. Pepke-Zaba J, Higinbottam TW, Dinh Xuan AT et al: Inhaled nitric oxide as a cause of selective pulmonary vasodilation in pulmonary hypertension, *Lancet* 338:1173-1174, 1991.

102. Fullerton DA, McIntyre RC: Inhaled nitric oxide: therapeutic applications in cardiothoracic surgery, *Ann Thorac Surg* 61:1856-1864, 1996.

103. Bottorff MB, Rutledge DR, Peiper JA: Evaluation of intravenous amrinone: the first of a new class of positive inotropic agents with vasodilator properties, *Pharmacotherapy* 5:227-237, 1985.

104. Konstam MA, Cohen SR, Salem DN et al: Effect of amrinone on the right ventricle: predominance of afterload reduction, *Circulation* 74:359-366, 1986.

105. Deeb GM, Bolling SF, Guynn TP et al: Amrinone versus conventional therapy in pulmonary hypertension patients awaiting cardiac transplantation, *Ann Thorac Surg* 48:665-669, 1989.

106. Nyhan DP, Pribble CG, Peterson WP et al: Amrinone and the pulmonary vascular pressure-flow relationship in conscious control dogs and following left lung autotransplantation, *Anesthesiology* 78(6):1166-1174, 1993.

107. Chen EP, Bittner HP, Davis RD et al: Milrinone improves pulmonary hemodynamics and right ventricular function in chronic pulmonary hypertension, *Ann Thorac Surg* 63:814-821, 1997.

108. Chen EP, Craig DM, Bittner HP et al: Pharmacologic strategies for improving diastolic dysfunction in the setting of chronic pulmonary hypertension, *Circulation* 97:1606-1612, 1998.

109. Rich S, Kaufman E, Levy PS: The effect of high doses of calcium-channel blockers on survival in primary pulmonary hypertension, *N Engl J Med* 327:76-81, 1992.

110. Rich S, Brundage BH: High-dose calcium-channel blocking therapy for primary pulmonary hypertension: evidence for long-term reduction in pulmonary artery pressure and regression of right ventricular hypertrophy, *Circulation* 76:135-141, 1987.

111. Ferreira SH, Vane JR: Prostaglandins: their disappearance from and release into the circulation, *Nature* 216:868-873, 1967.

112. Kunimoto F, Arai K, Isa Y et al: A comparative study of the vasodilator effects of prostaglandin E_1 in patients with pulmonary hypertension after mitral valve replacement and with adults respiratory distress syndrome, *Anesth Analg* 85:507-513, 1997.

113. Heerdt PM: Intrapulmonary shunt fraction and prostaglndin E_1, *Anesth Analg* 87:233, 1998.

114. Kadowitz P, Chapnick BM, Feigen LP et al: Pulmonary and systemic vasodilator effects of the newly discovered prostaglandin PGI_2, *J Appl Physiol* 45:408-413, 1978.

115. McLaughlin VV, Genthner DE, Panella MM et al: Reduction in pulmonary vascular resistance with long-term epoprostenol (prostacyclin) therapy in primary pulmonary hypertension, *N Engl J Med* 338:273-277, 1998.

116. Rich S, McLaughlin CC: the effects of chronic prostacyclin therapy on cardiac output and symptoms in primary pulmonary hypertension, *J Am Coll Cardiol* 34:1184-1187, 1999.

117. Jamieson SW, Auger WR, Fedullo PF et al: Experience and results with 150 pulmonary thromboendarterectomy operations over a 29-month period, *J Thorac Cardiovasc Surg* 106:116-127, 1993.

118. Sinzinger H, Silberbauer K: Contractile response of veins to prostaglandin E_1 in humans, *Vasa* 8:268, 1979.

119. Misselwitz B, Brautigam M: A comparative study of the effects of iloprost and PGE_1 on pulmonary artery pressure and edema formation in the isolated perfused rat lung, *Prostaglandins* 51(3): 179-190, 1996.

120. Cleland JGF, McGowan J, Cowburn PJ: β-Blockers for chronic heart failure: from prejudice to enlightenment, *J Cardiovasc Pharmacol* 32(suppl 1):S52-S60, 1998.

121. Fogari R, Zoppi A, Tettamanti F et al: Comparative effects of celiprolol, propranolol, oxprenolol, and atenolol on respiratory function in hypertensive patients with chronic obstructive lung disease, *Cardiovasc Drugs Ther* 4:1145-1150, 1990.

122. Lofdahl C: Antihypertensive drugs and airway function, with special reference to calcium channel blockade, *J Cardiovasc Pharmacol* 14(suppl 10):S40-S51, 1989.

123. Longstaff M: Do β-blockers pose an unacceptable risk to patients with obstructive sleep apnea (OSA)? *Sleep* 20:920, 1997.

124. Sin DD, Fitzgerald F, Parker JD et al: Risk factors for central and obstructive sleep apnea in 450 men and women with congestive heart failure, *Am J Respir Crit Care Med* 160:1101-1106, 1999.

125. Hill AB, Sykes MK, Reyes A: A hypoxic pulmonary vasoconstrictor response in dogs during and after infusion of sodium nitroprusside, *Anesthesiology* 50:484-488, 1979.

126. Krebs MO, Boemke W, Simon S et al: Acute hypoxic vasoconstriction in conscious dogs decreases renin and is unaffected by losartan, *J Appl Physiol* 86:1914-1919, 1999.

127. Kiely DG, Cargill RI, Lipworth BJ: Angiotensin II receptor blockade and effects on pulmonary hemodynamics and hypoxic pulmonary vasoconstriction in humans, *Chest* 110: 698-703, 1996.

128. Cargill RI, Lipworth BJ: Lisinopril attenuates acute hypoxic pulmonary vasoconstriction in humans, *Chest* 109:424-429, 1996.

129. McKelvie RS, Benedict CR, Yusuf S: Evidence-based cardiology: prevention of congestive heart failure and management of asymptomatic left ventricular dysfunction, *BMJ* 318:1400-1402, 1999.

130. Brown NJ, Vaughan DG: Angiotensin converting enzyme inhibitors, *Circulation* 97:1411-1420, 1998.

131. Bucknall CE, Neilly JB, Carter R et al: Bronchial hyperreactivity in patients who cough after receiving angiotensin converting enzyme inhibitors, *BMJ* 296:86-88, 1988.

132. Brown NJ, Ray WA, Griffin MR et al: Black Americans have an increased rate of angiotensin converting enzyme inhibitor-associated angioedema, *Clin Pharmacol Ther* 60:8-13, 1996.

133. Podrid PJ: Amiodarone: reevaluation of an old drug, *Ann Intern Med* 122:689-700, 1995.

134. Kowey PR, Levine JH, Herre JM et al: Randomized, double-blind comparison of intravenous amiodarone and bretylium in the treatment of patients with recurrent hemodynamically destabilizing ventricular tachycardia or fibrillation, *Circulation* 92:3255-3263, 1995.

135. Levine JH, Massumi A, Scheinman MM et al: Intravenous amiodarone for sustained hypotensive ventricular tachyarrhythmias, *J Am Coll Cardiol* 27:67-75, 1996.

136. Kudenchuk PJ, Cobb LA, Copass MK et al: Amiodarone for resuscitation after out-of-hospital cardiac arrest due to ventricular fibrillation, *N Engl J Med* 341:871-878, 1999.

137. Disch DL, Greenberg ML, Holzberger PT et al: Managing chronic atrial fibrillation: a Markov decision analysis comparing warfarin, quinidine, and low-dose amiodarone, *Ann Intern Med* 120:449-457, 1994.

138. Guarnieri T, Nolan S, Gottlieb SO et al: Intravenous amiodarone for the prevention of atrial fibrillation after open heart surgery: the amiodarone reduction in coronary heart (ARCH) trial, *J Am Coll Cardiol* 34:343-347, 1999.

139. Daoud EG, Strickberger SA, Man KC et al: Preoperative amiodarone as prophylaxis against atrial fibrillation after heart surgery, *N Engl J Med* 337:1785-1791, 1997.

140. Amiodarone Trials Meta Analysis Investigators: Effect of prophylactic amiodarone on mortality after acute myocardial infarction and in congestive heart failure: meta-analysis of individual data from 6500 patients in randomised trials, *Lancet* 350:1417-1424, 1997.

141. Balser JR: The rational use of intravenous amiodarone in the perioperative period, *Anesthesiology* 86:974-987, 1997.

142. Van Mieghem W, Coolen L, Malyssse I et al: Amiodarone and the development of ARDS after lung surgery, *Chest* 105: 1642-1645, 1994.

143. Gibbons RJ, Chatterjee K, Daley J et al: ACC/AHA/ACP-ASIM Guidelines for the management of patients with chronic stable angina: Executive summary and recommendations. A report of the American College of Cardiology/American Heart Association Task Force on Practice Guidelines (Committee on Management of Patients with Chronic Stable Angina, *Circulation* 99: 2829-2848, 1999.

144. Collins R, Peto R, Baigent C et al: Aspirin, heparin, and fibrinolytic therapy in suspected acute myocardial infarction, *N Engl J Med* 336:847-860, 1997.

145. Sibai BM, Caritis SN, Thom E et al: Low-dose aspirin in nulliparous women: safety of continuous epidural block and correlation between bleeding time and maternal-neonatal bleeding complications, *Am J Obstet Gynecol* 172:1553-1557, 1995.

146. Horlocker TT, Wedel DJ, Schroeder DR et al: Preoperative antiplatelet therapy does not increase the risk of spinal hematoma associated with regional anesthesia, *Anesth Analg* 80:303-309, 1995.

147. Wulf H: Epidural anaesthesia and spinal hematoma, *Can J Anaesth* 43:1260-1271, 1996.

148. Gammie JS, Zenati M, Kormos RL et al: Abciximab and excessive bleeding in patients undergoing emergency cardiac operations, *Ann Thorac Surg* 65:465-469, 1998.

149. Quinn MW, Dillard TA: Delayed traumatic hemothorax on ticlopidine and aspirin for coronary stent, *Chest* 116:257-260, 1998.

150. Horlocker TT, Heit JA: Low molecular weight heparin: biochemistry, pharmacology, perioperative prophylaxis regimens, and guidelines for regional anesthetic management, *Anesth Analg* 85:874-885, 1997.

151. British Thoracic Society guidelines for the management of chronic obstructive pulmonary disease, *Thorax* 52(suppl 5), 1997.

152. Crane J, Burgess C, Beasley R: Cardiovascular and hypokalaemic effects of inhaled salbutamol, fenoterol, and isoprenaline, *Thorax* 44:136-140, 1989.

153. Suissa S, Hemmelgarn B, Blais L, et al: Bronchodilators and acute cardiac death, *Am J Resp Crit Care Med* 154:1598-1602, 1996.

154. Seider N, Abinader EG, Oliven A: Cardiac arrhythmias after inhaled bronchodilators in patients with COPD and ischemia heart disease, *Chest* 104:1070-1074, 1993.

155. Conradson TB, Eklundh G, Olofsson B et al: Cardiac arrhythmias in patients with mild-moderate obstructive lung disease: comparison of β-agonist therapy alone and in combination with a xanthine oxidase derivative, enprofylline or theophylline, *Chest* 88:537-542, 1985.

156. Bremmer P, Burgess CD, Crane J et al: Cardiovascular effects of fenterol under conditions of hypoxemia, *Thorax* 47:814-817, 1992.

157. Libretto SE: A review of the toxicology of salbutamol (alberterol), *Arch Toxicol* 68:213-216, 1994.

158. Anonymous: Levalbuterol for asthma, *Med Lett Drugs Ther* 41:51-53, 1999.

159. Pelletier C, Lapointe L, LeBlanc P: Effects of lung resection on pulmonary function and exercise capacity, *Thorax* 45:497-502, 1990.

160. Nezu K, Kushibe K, Tojo T et al: Recovery and limitation of exercise capacity after lung resection for lung cancer, *Chest* 113:1511-1516, 1998.

161. Nishimura H, Haniuda M, Morimoto M et al: Cardiopulmonary function after pulmonary lobectomy in patients with lung cancer, *Ann Thorac Surg* 55:1477-1484, 1993.

162. Berend N, Woolcock AJ, Marlin GE: Effects of lobectomy on lung function, *Thorax* 35:145-150, 1990.

163. Van Mieghem W, Demedts M: Cardiopulmonary function after lobectomy or pneumonectomy for pulmonary neoplasm, *Respir Med* 83:199-206, 1989.

164. Wilikins EW, Scannell JG, Craver JG: Four decades of experience with resections for bronchogenic carcinoma at the Massachusetts General Hospital, *J Thorac Cardiovasc Surg* 76:364-368, 1978.

165. Wada H, Nakamura T, Nakamoto K et al: Thirty-day operative mortality for thoracotomy in lung cancer, *J Thorac Cardiovasc Surg* 115:70-73, 1998.

166. Patel RL, Townsend ER, Fountain SW: Elective pneumonectomy: factors associated with morbidity and operative mortality, *Ann Thorac Surg* 54:84-88, 1992.

167. Ginsberg RJ, Hill LD, Eagan RT et al: Modern thirty-day operative mortality for surgical resections in lung cancer, *J Thorac Cardiovasc Surg* 86:654-658, 1983.

168. Kopec SE, Irwin RS, Umali-Torres CB et al: The postpneumonectomy state, *Chest* 114:1158-1184, 1998.

169. Romano PS, Mark DH: Patient and hospital characteristics related to in-hospital mortality after lung cancer resection, *Chest* 101:1332-1337, 1992.

170. Mitsudomi T, Mizoue T Yoshimatsu T et al: Postoperative complications after pneumonectomy for treatment of lung cancer: multivariate analysis, *J Surg Oncol* 61:218-222, 1996.

171. Von Knorring J, Lepantalo M, Lindgren L et al: Cardiac arrhythmias and myocardial ischemia after thoracotomy for lung cancer, *Ann Thorac Surg* 53:642-647, 1992.

172. Amar D, Burt M, Reinsel RA et al: Relationship of early postoperative dysrhythmias and long term outcome after resection of non-small cell lung cancer, *Chest* 110:437-439, 1996.

173. Ritchie AJ, Bowe P, Gibbons JRP: Prophylactic digitalization for thoracotomy: a reassessment, *Ann Thorac Surg* 50:86-88, 1990.

174. Amar D, Roistacher N, Burt ME et al: Effects of diltiazem versus digoxin on dysrhythmias and cardiac function after pneumonectomy, *Ann Thorac Surg* 63:1374-1382, 1997.

175. Van Mieghem W, Tits G, Demuynck K et al: Verapamil as prophylactic treatment for atrial fibrillation after lung operations, *Ann Thorac Surg* 61:1083-1086, 1996.

176. Jakobsen CJ, Bille S, Ahlburg P et al: Perioperative metoprolol reduces the frequency of atrial fibrillation after thoracotomy for lung resection, *J Cardiothorac Vasc Anesth* 111:746-751, 1997.

177. Amar D, Roistacher N, Burt M et al: Clinical and echocardiographic correlates of symptomatic tachydysrhythmias after onocardiac thoracic surgery, *Chest* 108:349-354, 1995.

178. Krowka MJ, Pairolero PC, Trastek VF et al: Cardiac dysrhythmias following pneumonectomy: clinical correlates and prognostic significance, *Chest* 91:490-495, 1987.

179. Waller DA, Gebitekin C, Saunders NR et al: Noncardiogenic pulmonary edema complicating lung resection, *Ann Thorac Surg* 55:140-143, 1993.

180. Zeldin RA, Normadin D, Landtwing BE et al: Post pneumonectomy pulmonary edema, *J Thorac Cardiovasc Surg* 87:359-365, 1984.

181. Turnage WS, Lunn JL: Postpneumonectomy pulmonary edema. A retrospective analysis of associated variables, *Chest* 103:1646-1650, 1993.

182. Slinger PD: Perioperative fluid management for thoracic surgery: the puzzle of postpneumonectomy pulmonary edema, *J Cardothorac Vasc Anesth* 9:442-451, 1995.

183. Chaung TH, Dooling JA, Connolly JM et al: Pulmonary embolization from vascular stump thrombosis following pneumonectomy, *Ann Thorac Surg* 2:290-298, 1966.

184. Valji AM, Maziak DE, Shamji FM et al: Postpneumonectomy syndrome, *Chest* 114:1766-1769, 1998.

185. Verhagen AFTM, Lacquet LKMH: Completion pneumonectomy: a retrospective analysis of indications and results, *Eur J Cardiothorac Surg* 10:238-241, 1996.

186. Muysoms FE, De la Riviere AB, Defauw JJ et al: Completion pneumonectomy: analysis of operative mortality and survival, *Ann Thorac Surg* 66:1165-1169, 1998.

187. Cooper JD, Trulock EP, Triantafillou et al: Bilateral pneumectomy (volume reduction) for chronic obstructive pulmonary disease, *J Thorac Cardiovasc Surg* 109:106-116, 1995.

188. Hodgkin J: Prognosis in chronic obstructive pulmonary diseases, *Clin Chest Med* 11:555-569, 1990.

189. Utz JP, Hubmayr RD, Deschamps C: Lung volume reduction surgery for emphysema: out on a limb without a NETT, *Mayo Clin Proc* 73:552-566, 1998.

190. Miller DL, Orszulak TA, Pairolero PC et al: Combined operation for lung cancer and cardiac disease, *Ann Thorac Surg* 58: 989-994, 1994.

191. Rosalion A, Woodford NW, Clarke CP et al: Concomitant coronary revascularization and resection of lung cancer, *Aust N Z J Surg* 63:336-340, 1993.

192. Danton MHD, Anikin VA, McManus KG et al: Simultaneous cardiac surgery with pulmonary resection: presentation of series and review of literature, *Eur J Cardiothorac Surg* 13:667-672, 1998.

193. La Francesesca S, Frazier OH, Radovanevic B et al: Concomitant cardiac and pulmonary operations for lung cancer, *Tex Heart Inst J* 22:296-300, 1995.

194. De la Riviere AB, Knaepen P, Van Swietan H et al: Concomitant open heart surgery and pulmonary resection for lung cancer, *Eur J Cardiothorac Surg* 9:310-314, 1995.

195. Piehler JM, Trastek VF, Pairolero PC et al: Concomitant cardiac and pulmonary operations, *J Thorac Cardiovasc Surg* 90: 662-667, 1985.

196. Rao V, Todd TRJ, Weisel RD et al: Results of combined pulmonary resection and cardiac operation, *Ann Thorac Surg* 62: 324-327, 1996.

Index

Page references followed by "f" indicate figures, "t" indicate tables, and "b" indicate boxes.